Total Rehabilitation

Total Rehabilitation

George Nelson Wright, Ph.D.
University of Wisconsin–Madison

Boston
Little, Brown and Company

To my wife,
Patricia Adele Gilmer Wright,
and to our children,
John, Elizabeth, Robert, and James

Contents

Preface

Total Rehabilitation covers the complex process of overcoming a handicap through comprehensive vocational and life adjustment services to disabled or disadvantaged individuals. This book was written to help remove several obstacles to the full utilization of rehabilitation technology. The major difficulty was that the voluminous literature had never been compiled and organized for a definitive coverage of the subject. Previous material was fragmented and generally scattered and inaccessible. Because an inclusive publication on rehabilitation techniques did not exist, a clear perception of the gestalt of the process was not possible, and its utilization as a unique, interrelated body of knowledge within the helping professions was restricted. Another problem has been the lack of standardization of the nomenclature, impeding conceptualization and communication.

The fields of knowledge encompassed by rehabilitation are integrated in this volume. Forty chapters are bound together in five major parts:

Foundations—overview and orientation;
Resources—facilities and services;
Assessment—client evaluation and planning;
Counseling—adjustment areas and methods;
Placement—employment techniques and alternatives.

Essential information for rehabilitation practice is provided in the first two parts, while the last three parts describe professional techniques. However, this order of presentation—knowledge then skills—is not followed rigidly because these five parts (and the chapters in them) also follow the steps of the rehabilitation process from case-finding to closure.

Rehabilitation technology, presented here for practical application, has developed greatly since 1954 from federal grant support for rehabilitation research, development, demonstration, innovation, and training programs. Unfortunately, much of the substantial body of knowledge accumulated through these and other projects and experience is not generally available. As a consequence, much of what is known about rehabilitation technique has not been communicated effectively to practitioners; the growth of knowledge has proceeded more rapidly than its application in improving the lives of handicapped persons.

The present volume resulted from a monumental literature search spanning 15 years and representing an estimated 20,000 reviewed documents reduced to a working bibliography of nearly 5,000 screened titles, of which the most important and useful (including ideas or quotations) are referred to in the text. These references provide a perspective of the field of rehabilitation and document its advanced development.

Glossaries defining hundreds of relevant terms are built into the chapters to clarify technical concepts. The conceptualizations expressed by these terms are the building blocks of rehabilitation practice. Moreover, professionals within this field communicate with one another through their common language. Professional jargon in rehabilitation has been confusing because it lacked a standardized nomenclature. Selection of glossary terms and the composition of their definitions followed an extensive investigation of their usage to reconcile differences and thus to permit the writing of uniform definitions. Terms of specific interest can be located in the index. Subjects that are discussed in another context elsewhere in the book are cross-referenced in the text by chapter, section, and subsection numbers.

Words that label people prejudicially, another problem in the rehabilitation of disabled and disadvantaged people, presented an editorial issue. Sexist language has been eliminated in the text—except in direct quotations, which sometimes imply sex roles such as the "physician, he . . ." and the "nurse, she . . ." Another type of verbal stereotyping that can have negative consequences derives from labels such as "the crippled," and "the trainable class of MRs." Stigmatizing labels were avoided in the writing, although reference is made to "disabled people" rather than using the more acceptable but cumbersome expression, "the population of people who have a disability." Words of positive regard are always important in human relationships.

G. N. W.

Acknowledgments

While I am solely responsible for everything written in this publication, many people assisted in its preparation. Appreciation is expressed to everyone who helped by reviewing the literature, typing successive drafts, editing copy, reading the manuscript, and preparing and printing this work. I would like to express my gratitude to all, but space limits me to the following listing.

Literature searches used in this volume were conducted over a 15-year period beginning in 1965. This work was published by the University of Wisconsin–Madison Rehabilitation Research Institute (U.W.-RRI) as research monographs on rehabilitation counselor functions, a digest of rehabilitation research, an annotated bibliography of rehabilitation literature, and abstracts entitled "Rehabilitation Information Series," and "Vocational Counseling of the Severely Disabled: Transcript of a Literature Search."

The last-mentioned abstract was part of a project sponsored by the federal Region Five Developmental Disabilities Office and the Wisconsin Division of Vocational Rehabilitation. The earlier documentary publications were primarily supported by grants to the U.W.-RRI from the federal rehabilitation agency, although funding was also obtained from the university and other sources. My co-authors in the earlier volumes that presented literature searches included Alfred Butler, Kenneth Reagles, and Ann Beck (Trotter) Meyer. They also collaborated with me in some of the 24 monographs in the three-volume U.W.-RRI *Wisconsin Studies in Vocational Rehabilitation.*

Other important U.W.-RRI research collaborators and co-authors of publications relevant to rehabilitation counselor functions include the following University of Wisconsin–Madison Rehabilitation Counselor Education Program faculty members and/or doctoral graduates: M. Jane Ayer, Norman Berven, Thomas Blaskovics, David Bogost, Brian Bolton, Donn Brolin, Winfield Bronson, Philip Browning, Suzanne Bruyere, Veronica Butler, Keith Byrd, Robert Chope, Ralph Crystal, Donald Dellario, Neil Dumas, William English, Robert Fraser, Keith Gardner, Mary Garfield, Dennis Gay, Michael Goldman, Michael Greenwald, Bruce Growick, Andrew Halpern, Clarence Hammond, Robert Harbach, William Hauck, Richard Holman, James Jacks, Hollis Jellinek, Schlomo Katz, Yoko Kojima, Schlomo Kravetz, Jerome Lorenz, John Mathews, Brian McMahon, Ann Meissner, James Organist, Jerry Parham, Jackson Pease, John Rasch, Carolyn Rayford, Gerald Rose, William Sather, James Scorzelli, Ami Sha'ked, Woodrow Smith, Jr., Stanley Smits, LeRoy Spaniol, Kenneth Thomas, Richard Thoreson, and Josh Walling. All of these joint endeavors contributed information included in the present work, and many are explicitly cited.

For the Developmental Disabilities project, mentioned earlier, as well as subsequent literature searches, a number of graduate assistants contributed magnificently: Patricia Fenner, Virginia Fraser, Rochelle Habeck, Leslie Halverson Hall, James Hill, Marie Iwanski, Linda Lingen, Richard Klun, Dennis Maki, Brian McMahon, Deborah Pape, Robert Pullo, Michael Scofield, and Joe Thompson. Scofield, Maki, Pape, and Thompson, who have subsequently completed doctoral studies, did most of the documentation for Parts I through IV, Foundations, Assessment, Counseling, and Placement (respectively), while Hill's work was mostly on Part V, Resources.

Materials reviewed included not only my own collection gathered over 30 years but also those found in the libraries of the University of Wisconsin; the Library of Congress and its depository in Madison, Wisconsin; the library of the National Society of Crippled Children and Adults, and other university and agency libraries. The National Clearing House of Rehabilitation Training Materials, housed at Oklahoma State University and directed by Paul Gains, provided hundreds of otherwise unobtainable documents. John Muthard of the University of Florida at Gainesville loaned his personal collection. The National Rehabilitation Association and the federal rehabilitation agency made one-of-a-kind documents available. A search of the world literature was made through the libraries of the United Nations and the International Labor Organization and in university and agency collections in several European countries. These literature searches were organized and combined with the previous literature reviews and research reports as well as my unpublished notions about rehabilitation.

Early suggestions for contents and organization were derived from a conference with Thomas Porter, Leonard Miller, and Roger Decker. John Muthard was a continuing consultant. Chapter outlines, however, were developed over time, being continually revised to accommodate usable information. Most of the relevant literature was reviewed and systematically screened for what the rehabilitationist needs to know. A 50-page manual was written to provide consistent guidelines in the selection and processing of material.

Typists of the many thousands of pages of manuscript drafts deserve special thanks. They are my wife, Patricia; my secretary, Elizabeth Rentschler; and typists Ruth Severson and Susan Schaaf. The librarian throughout the literature search and writing was Nancy Wynn, whose dedication was invaluable. The list of references was painstakingly verified by Christopher Pape. Joyce Sexton edited every word as written and again after each revision. Dr. Sexton, a teacher of English and technical writing, provided indispensable expertise.

Every chapter was read critically by an authority on the subject and some were read by several. These readers (listed below) were asked to flag inaccuracies or omissions of coverage, suggest additional references, and check the definitions of terms. Their contributions reinforce the authoritative nature of the text.

Adrian Towne, nationally respected rehabilitation authority and long-time Director of the Wisconsin Division of Vocational Rehabilitation, with a lifetime of first-hand knowledge, corrected all of the chapters (except selected chapters on counseling, which were reviewed by other people). His work is especially noteworthy and appreciated. Edward Pfeifer, a psychologist, university lecturer, and former rehabilitation (state and private agency) administrator, read Chapters 1, 2, and 3.

Chapters 4, Impact of Disability, and 5, Functional Limitations, were reviewed by Friedrich Klutzow, M.D., of the Veterans Administration Hospital, Brockton, Massachusetts.

Esco Obermann and E. B. Whitten both read and contributed to Chapter 6, History of Rehabilitation. Dr. Obermann wrote the definitive book on that subject and gave permission for use of that material as "digested" in the present chapter; Whitten has helped make history over more than a quarter-century as the Executive Director of the National Rehabilitation Association.

Chapter 8, Rehabilitation Facilities, was read by Richard Harvey, M.D., Chairman of the University of Wisconsin–Madison Rehabilitation Medicine Department and also by several professional staff members of his program, including the head of rehabilitation counseling, Robert Haskin.

Irene Cooperman of the U.S. Veterans Administration contributed material on her agency and reviewed the history and description of it given in Chapters 6 and 12.

Paul Lustig of the University of Wisconsin–Madison Rehabilitation Counselor Education Program constructively criticized Chapters 13 and 14, Adjustment Training and Educational Services.

Protection and Advocacy, Chapter 16, was reviewed by Jenny Armstrong, who has doctoral degrees in both special education and law and makes protection and advocacy of disabled people her specialty.

Donn Brolin, University of Missouri Professor of Rehabilitation Counselor Education and well-known author read most of the chapters in Part III, Assessment—Chapters 17, 18, 21, 22, 23, and 24. Chapters 21, 22, and 23 were also read by Tennyson Wright of the Singer Education Division. Chapter 19, Occupational Information, was reviewed by Kenneth Thomas of the University of Wisconsin–Madison Rehabilitation Counseling Education Program. Chapter 20, Psychological Testing, was read by William LeBold of Purdue University.

Counseling chapters in Part IV were reviewed by the following individuals: Alfred Butler of the University of Wisconsin–Madison Rehabilitation Counseling Education Program, Chapter 25; Robert Harback of the University of Nevada–Las Vegas Rehabilitation Counseling Education Program, Chapter 26; David Hershenson of Boston University, Brian McMahon of the Illinois Institute of Technology Rehabilitation Counseling Education Program, and John Muthard of the University of Florida Rehabilitation Counseling Education Program, Chapter 27, Vocational Counseling; Leonard Stein of the University of Wisconsin–Madison Department of Psychiatry, Chapter 28, Personal

Adjustment; Ray Hosford of the University of California–Santa Barbara and William Gardner of the University of Wisconsin–Madison, Chapter 29, Behavior Techniques; Norman Berven of the University of Wisconsin–Madison Rehabilitation Counselor Education Program, Chapter 30, Group Counseling; Ami Sha'ked, formerly of the Indiana-Purdue University Rehabilitation Counseling Education Program and the late Bruce Thomason, Professor Emeritus of the University of Florida, Chapter 31, Family Counseling.

Chapters 33 to 39 in Part V, Placement, were read not only by Adrian Towne but also by a number of rehabilitation counselors and placement specialists. Chapter 40, Independent Living, was read by Jean Kiernat, Professor of the University of Wisconsin–Madison Department of Occupational Therapy and teacher of a course on independent living, and also by Melanie Pullo, who practices as a rehabilitation counselor in Madison, Wisconsin. The final section, Rehabilitation Recreation, was constructively criticized by H. Clifton Hutchins, Professor Emeritus of the University of Wisconsin–Madison.

The publisher, Little, Brown and Company, has my appreciation for its assistance. There were many noteworthy contributions from the highly competent staff of this publisher—editors, designers, printers, and others who produce attractive books.

Full acknowledgment is given to all those who have written before about their research and experience in rehabilitation and whose material I have used. So far as possible, all original thoughts have been credited, although only direct quotes are signified by page reference. (Many statements published by others are paraphrased or rewritten for consistency of style and usage.) Credits to authors and publishers are acknowledged in the text.

Last, but most important, I thank my many rehabilitation counseling clients for teaching me about disability and rehabilitation. Much of what I have learned since 1947 about this helping process came from direct work with individuals who have overcome their handicaps. My appreciation for rehabilitation and those it serves has grown with the experience of supervising the clinical practice of students in the Rehabilitation Counselor Education Program of the University of Wisconsin–Madison.

G. N. W.

Part I
Foundations

Chapter 1

Introduction

Rehabilitation is a facilitative process enabling a person with a handicap to attain usefulness and satisfaction in life. The individual's handicap may result from any type of disablement (i.e., physical, mental, or emotional) and from various causes (e.g., birth defects, sickness and disease, industrial and road accidents, or the stresses of war, work, and daily life). People are likewise handicapped by cultural disadvantage (i.e., social, financial, or educational). Whenever any of these conditions cause difficulties in life adjustment, the person is handicapped. Rehabilitation then equalizes opportunity for life attainments as a human right and societal obligation.

Any kind of rewarding activity considered useful or satisfying—not merely paid employment—is the goal of rehabilitation. To overcome the handicap, rehabilitation provides individualized services including assessment, counseling, and planning; through community resources it arranges help in the form of medical care, adjustment or occupational training, financial assistance, employment opportunities, and whatever else is needed. These services are available to eligible people through a system of public and private agencies, many of which date back to the World War I period.

A substantial portion of the world population is disabled and their number grows each year. While these data vary geographically, even the most advanced nations have their underdeveloped population of handicapped people, a wasted resource. Most of these people will need rehabilitation services to achieve their potential for productivity and independence. But since any disability limits only selected functions, almost everyone can be made suitable for rewarding work. Often the greatest barrier is ignorance, stigma, and prejudice toward disablement on the part of the public—one's would-be employers, friends, family—and even one's self.

Program success depends upon the availability of public and private funds and facilities, technological development and dissemination, the supply and qualifications of professional rehabilitation workers, and the nature of the environment (e.g., the social climate, work incentives, physical accommodations, and the labor market). Success also depends upon the recipient of service, who is not just the target but the one ultimately responsible for the rehabilitation process and its positive (or sometimes negative) outcome.

More than anything else, rehabilitation is intended to help handicapped individuals to help themselves—to know and to use their assets. This is the role of the rehabilitation professional. It is not always easy, not even always successful, but it is invariably a human obligation worthy of the effort. And the process is remarkably effective in the hands of the well-prepared rehabilitation counselor working with a team of specialists. Fortunately there exists a very substantial body of practical knowledge to help the helper in rehabilitation. This broad and advanced technology explicit to modern rehabilitation and applicable for professional practice is documented throughout this volume.

Rehabilitation for vocational objectives has been expanded conceptually so that by 1980 "total" rehabilitation, meant: (1) a complete scope of program goals for medical, social, and occupational as well as independent-living rehabilitation; (2) a comprehensive array of available rehabilitation services in a multidimensional program; and (3) an extended rehabilitation program to serve the entire disabled population, including the most severely handicapped of all ages. Under this concept no one should be turned down because of being "too handicapped" or "not feasible." Total rehabilitation programming may never be fully implemented, but it gained greatly in the United States with federal rehabilitation legislation in the 1970s covering severe disablement and independent living. Consequently, rehabilitation is no longer exclusive but has broadened its client population, service program, and goal alternatives.

The public rehabilitation program was expanded operationally by a redefinition of the term *vocational* to make it inclusive of broader goals. Originally the vocational objective was restricted to competitive employment for regular pay; over the years the objective has been extended to include any remunerative employment or gainful work. Programming for independent living continued the expanding goal of public rehabilitation: self-care and self-determination are viewed as proper objectives for severely handicapped persons who cannot otherwise work. This latest expansion was justified because increased independence is socially or economically rewarding in that this relieves dependence upon the efforts or dictates of other people. James Garrett, in the foreword to a 1979 book by James Bitter, said, "What is important to keep in mind is that the rehabilitation process is applicable regardless of the goal—employability or not" [p. viii]. The objective for an individual may start with independent living and then, with reappraisal, shift to paid employment—or vice versa. This flexibility of services and goals is inherent in the individualized nature of the process that is rehabilitation.

1.1. The Meaning

Rehabilitation as just described simply means helping a handicapped individual live rewardingly. The clients of rehabilitation are disabled or otherwise handicapped, the help is individualized from a broad selection of services, and the goal is maximal adjustment. The process of total rehabilitation includes both independent living as well as vocational services referred to collectively as "rehabilitation." In vocational rehabilitation (VR) the contraction *voc. rehab.* and initials *VR* are commonly heard in conversation among rehabilitation professionals.

1.1.1. CONCEPTUALIZATIONS
Multiple affixes cause *re-ha-bil-i-ta-tion* to be a difficult and rather unglamorous word. But it has a highly positive quality due to the constructive work represented. Despite the favorable connotations of the term, however, some people would replace it with a more euphonious or apt label. As they point out, the prefix *re* implies "putting back to a former state of unimpairment"; consequently, strictly speaking, the term is inappropriate for congenital conditions (e.g., mental retardation). Thus, the substitute *habilitation* is often favored by persons associated with early childhood development as opposed to the public rehabilitation program for the adult disabled. While these critics do have a linguistic argument, the tradition associated with the word *rehabilitation* is of overriding value. This volume, adhering to well-accepted American ter-

[Handwritten annotation across top margin: Total Rehab includes Physical, Mental, economic, Familial, social, Environmental, Personal, Vocational]

minology, uses *rehabilitation* as synonymous with *habilitation*. The term *resettlement*, which is used in England and some other countries for complete rehabilitation, will not be used in this book. However, the term *rehabilitation* should always imply thorough service for sustained adjustment.

Over the years rehabilitation has been defined in a number of ways. The classical definition of rehabilitation, adopted internationally, came from a May 25, 1942 symposium in New York of the National Council on Rehabilitation [1944]: "restoration of the handicapped to the fullest physical, mental, social, vocational, and economic usefulness of which they are capable." John McGowan [1960] used essentially the same definition in his first orientation manual for state rehabilitation employees. While this objective of "total rehabilitation" [Wright, Gibbs, & Linde, 1962] is idealistic and never fully realized, it serves as a goal to be sought for every person who is handicapped in life.

There are three fundamental courses of action available when a disability imposes limitations that handicap the individual: one can (1) remedy the cause of the person's handicap by restoring ability, (2) compensate for the handicap by enhancing other characteristics of the person, or (3) change the environmental circumstances so that the impact of the disability is avoided or negated. The best foundation for rehabilitation incorporates all of these approaches, utilizing and developing all needed resources of the community and embracing all professions that can contribute to the process.

Various authors on the subject stress particular dimensions of rehabilitation according to their conception of the problem, process, or philosophy: Thus we have descriptions of medical or other phases of rehabilitation that are only partial answers. Total rehabilitation includes physical, mental, economic, familial, social, environmental, personal, and vocational goals in life as part of the comprehensive process of rehabilitation. In practice, however, it is found that improvement in the ability to work and to live independently bring about a concurrent adjustment in other areas of an individual's life.

Total rehabilitation can be regarded as the culmination, the payoff, of all other services to the person who has a disability. "Special education is only a preparatory stage of occupational adjustment and medical rehabilitation is sense-

less without helping the patient use restored function," observed a physician with an appreciation for comprehensive rehabilitation. Despite a theoretical continuum, total rehabilitation does have discrete phases, each with its distinct identity, methods, and purposes. Professionals are apt to regard their contribution as paramount, and the nature of rehabilitation as a common effort is rarely appreciated by disabled persons as patients and clients of the process. It is clear, however, that without the restoration of independence and/or productivity the term *rehabilitation* is a misnomer for the unfinished effort. Thus it is misleading to call rehabilitation the "third phase of medicine." Medicine is rather the first phase of rehabilitation.

Rehabilitation as it is described in this volume is applicable to a broad clientele. It is not restricted to the medically disabled (i.e., those with physical, mental, or emotional impairments). The process can be applied to the even larger population of culturally disadvantaged people, to help them realize their vocational and personal potential and help them change their underprivileged social and financial status to one of self-sufficiency [Wright & Reagles, 1973a].

Despite the type of handicap or service provided, the goal of rehabilitation should be to help each person achieve whatever life adjustment that person is capable of attaining. The U.S. White House Conference on Handicapped Individuals [n.d.] expressed this: "At one end, the maximum attainable goal may be progress from bed to wheelchair or an increased capacity for self-care. At the other extreme it may be aimed at restoration to paid employment" [p. 25]. The former is designated as rehabilitation for "independent living" while the latter is referred to as "vocational rehabilitation." These two categories of rehabilitation and their life adjustment goals are on a continuum from self-determination and self-care to self-support. It is noted that all definitions of the term *adjustment* offered by psychologists include the concepts of independence and productivity.

Belief in the right of independency and productivity is deeply ingrained in rehabilitation. An extension of this concept of self-sufficiency is the right of people to be themselves, to work out their own problems, and to make personal decisions. Rehabilitation, then, can be viewed as a method through which handicapped people are enabled to mobilize their own resources, decide what they wish and are able to be, and achieve goals through their own efforts and in their own way. This "reflects the ultimate goal of rehabilitation philosophy," an observation of Marceline Jaques [1970, p. 4].

"The object of all help is to make help superfluous," according to the philosopher Paulson [1899, p. 429]. With this quotation Henry Kessler, M.D., introduced his first book on rehabilitation, *The Crippled and Disabled,* in 1935. It was his published thesis for his second doctorate, a PhD. degree from Columbia University in Political Science. Already noted as a pioneer in rehabilitation medicine, Kessler studied legislation to develop an "adequate and comprehensive program which will facilitate the vocational adjustment of the disabled person." He had found that the help offered through medical and vocational rehabilitation workers could not serve its purpose fully with the legal and social restrictions faced by disabled people. Thus, Kessler not only identified the goal of rehabilitation, but also the difficulties and he charted broad action programs.

1.1.2. PUBLIC SERVICE IMPACT

Persons given to social and human service considerations agree that rehabilitation is a human right of disabled people, one that should be provided by governments to citizens who need the service. Rehabilitation for those who need it is not offered as charity but rather as a public service to be accepted without humiliation or stigma by the recipient of services. Thus, rehabilitation is comparable to public schooling as a responsibility of government. Even though clients may be required to pay what they can afford for most services provided, comprehensive rehabilitation is too costly for most of those who need it. Consequently, rehabilitation is an obligation that must be supported by taxation because the cost is beyond family resources or voluntary contributions to private agencies.

Objectives of public rehabilitation are both societal and individual. Explicit objectives include increasing productivity of an expanded work force, and facilitating a life of independence for otherwise dependent people. Moreover, a developed society demonstrates its humanitarianism through rehabilitation programs. Objectives for the disabled individual involve tangible benefits—economic well-being, health and physical capabilities, and satisfying social

relations—and intangibles, such as wholesome self concepts.

A persuasive argument is the proof that rehabilitation is a good investment of tax funds [Conley, 1965]. The government benefits from the more productive citizenry that rehabilitation provides. One study of the economic impact of vocational rehabilitation as measured by benefit-cost analysis revealed that for every dollar of public funds spent to rehabilitate the medically disabled, more than $25.00 is returned in increased, taxable, lifetime earnings [Wright & Reagles, 1971]. When rehabilitation services were extended to culturally disadvantaged people the yield was a benefit-cost ratio of 70 to 1 [Reagles & Wright, 1972]. Other research shows that living independently, even with ongoing attendant care, is less costly than institutionalization. But there is a far greater value in rehabilitation: governmental services to the disabled and disadvantaged population express the humanitarian values of a people.

Before the meaning of rehabilitation can be fully appreciated, it is necessary to know about its objectives and methods, its service organization and workers, and its philosophy and theoretical perspectives, but most of all one needs to know about its clients with their handicaps and their resources for overcoming problems.

1.1.3. PERSONAL IMPACT

While sophisticated analyses of the financial effectiveness of rehabilitation provide impressive documentation, the story of real people is more moving. Dollar ratio data do not describe the humanitarian values of the program. Roger Barker, Beatrice Wright, and Mollie Gonick [1946], in their historic survey of disability research, extensively reviewed studies on the effectiveness of rehabilitation and concluded: "Actually the case examples which accompany some reports are the most convincing evidence" [p. 294].

Courage Facing Handicaps, a collection of case histories from state rehabilitation agencies, was the first major publication of the National Rehabilitation Association [1933]. "A book intended to give a picture of the new hope that vocational rehabilitation brings to the physically handicapped, and to provide a storehouse of inspiration for the thousands who yearly undertake the difficult but wholly worthwhile struggle to come back,'' was an explanatory note on the title page. Innumerable personal accounts of "living with a handicap"—or with "special people"—have been published. There is, for example, Shirley Cohen's [1977] helpful story. Most moving, however, is Henry Kessler's [1968] autobiography, the fascinating story of a physician astounded by the resilience of the catastrophically disabled. His portraits of patients graphically illustrate the great resources available in a human personality. Recognizing the "tremendous potential in the individual," Kessler advised that it is the job of the rehabilitationist "to dredge that reservoir of dormant abilities and translate them into effective economic and social terms" [p. 134]. "Fundamentally and finally, the lifeline for the disabled is rehabilitation," said Kessler.

Rehabilitation is the unfinished business of the medical profession and the community. It is more than the rebuilding of shattered lives. It is a fierce belief in our individual responsibilities for what happens to our fellow man.

I am reminded of Lewis Mumford, who wrote in *The Culture of Cities:* "We can live three weeks without food, three days without water, yes, we can even live for three minutes without air, but we cannot live without hope."

Rehabilitation is, finally, the precious gift of hope—hope translated into action [p. 286].

With these words Dr. Kessler ended his autobiography, *The Knife is not Enough.*

The greatness of the rehabilitation model, of preferring self-sufficiency to dependency, came about through the vision and work of many devoted leaders. Many of these strategists in the war against disability and handicaps will be cited in reference to their contributions. To appreciate fully the effort of these great pioneers one should read the autobiography of Howard Rusk, M.D. [1977] *A World to Care For*. Dr. Rusk, who established the Institute of Rehabilitation Medicine in the New York University Medical Center and the World Rehabilitation Fund, exemplifies rehabilitation's tradition of great leadership.

Henry Viscardi, Jr. personifies rehabilitation leadership from the ranks of those who are severely disabled. Born with unformed legs, he was three feet eight inches tall when fully grown. After Viscardi became a successful businessman he founded [in 1952] Abilities, Inc., a company that hires only severely disabled workers at pre-

vailing wages. His insightful personal account of overcoming disability, *A Man's Stature*, was published in 1952. Abilities, Inc. has expanded to other innovative and model programs and Viscardi, as its president, continues as an exceptionally devoted and valuable spokesperson for disabled individuals.

1.1.4. EARLY NOTIONS

There has been much improvement in society's view of the disabled and their rehabilitation. In 1883 Samuel Fallows, University of Wisconsin Professor of Rhetoric and Logic, published a book of synonyms and antonyms including *rehabilitation* and *disability*. *Disability* was seen as synonymous with *impotency, unfitness, incompetency,* and *disqualification,* all the opposite of *deserving* and *merit* in the language of that time. Even then, however, the word *rehabilitate* represented completely positive ideas: "reinstate, reempower, recapacitate, requalify." Rev. Fallows saw rehabilitation as "wiping out the effects of disablement" and said that the antonym of rehabilitation was "deprive."

The concept and methods of vocational rehabilitation for the handicapped were first proposed by a Scottish minister, Thomas Chalmers (1780–1847), according to Friedlander and Apte [1974]. Rev. Chalmers observed that poverty was often caused by personal and health problems and that public and private financial assistance was demoralizing, destroying the pauper's will to be independent. He developed the principle of individually investigating each case of destitution and attempting a solution to the cause of distress. It was his theory that poor-relief was ineffective and that the client needed "rehabilitation" in order to support self and family. Chalmers' early proposals for vocational rehabilitation were carried out by the London Charity Organization Society; they investigated applications individually, established a personal relationship with each case and gave advice, financially sponsored vocational training, furnished occupational tools and equipment, provided rent for setting up a workshop or small business, and funded personal and family maintenance for the purpose of vocational rehabilitation until the process was completed. Gordon Hamilton [1940, 1951] in her classic text, *Theory and Practice of Social Casework,* charted the rehabilitation ancestry and consequent orientation of social and human service.

Robert Lassiter [1970] has written a scholarly history of the social trends and forces in America from 1890 leading up to vocational rehabilitation legislation. With increasing industrialization, all social problems became more complex. Labor unions were organized as a revolt against the long hours, low pay, and poor working conditions that prevailed then. Striking progress was being made in medicine and public health. Worker compensation provisions were being legislated for industrial illness and accidents. The mental health movement of Dorothea Dix, and later Clifford Beers, got under way. Psychology as a practical field was developing assessment, therapeutic, and vocational guidance methods. Social work pioneers such as Jane Addams at the Hull House in Chicago were active in social reforms. The American free public education system developed during the period so that by 1920 all states had compulsory attendance laws. Religion too provided a stimulant for the awakening American social conscience. These are the forces described by Lassiter from which the vocational rehabilitation concept evolved.

The history of disability and rehabilitation will be discussed later in Chapter 6. It suffices to say here that rehabilitation was started as a government service to war-injured veterans and disabled citizens during the World War I era in Europe, the United States and Canada. These many years of an uninterrupted and growing program provide a rich heritage for philosophy, operational principles, and applicable techniques.

1.1.5. DEFINITIONS

The nomenclature of a field provides the basis for precise labeling of concepts. Throughout this volume, terms are defined for better understanding of the subject. It is important for those contemplating entering a profession to learn the precise meanings of terms since professionals within a field communicate with one another through their common language. (Casual readers will find the text understandable without reading these glossaries, however.)

Unfortunately, the rehabilitation nomenclature is unstandardized because many of its words are derived from other disciplines and are contaminated by varied uses. Feingold [1969] referred to it as "a babel of tongues" [p. 39]. Lay dictionaries and popular thesauruses fail to give clear descriptions of rehabilitation problems and populations. A universal, scientific vocabulary designating explicit names for rehabilitation concepts has not yet been authoritatively expounded.

The evolution of a language progresses through the acceptance of users, consequently, the conceptions, definitions, and terms presented in this volume are based not only upon a search of the relevant literature, but also the denotations of words used by rehabilitation workers. Several basic terms are defined below.

REHABILITATION. The International Labor (Labour) Office (ILO) [1973] and others have adopted a broad definition of rehabilitation: "The restoration of handicapped persons to the fullest physical, mental, social, vocational and economic usefulness of which they are capable" [p. 1]. This all-inclusive statement suggests an ideal goal seldom, if ever, achieved in practice. Operationally defined, rehabilitation is the provision of any kind of service provided individuals to correct, avoid, or compensate for their handicapping problems. This latter, more practical definition is framed for the purposes of this book. It does not restrict the term to the medically disabled but embraces all who need rehabilitation, including culturally disadvantaged people. Moreover, total rehabilitation incorporates the full range of rehabilitation services for the broad objectives of social usefulness and personal satisfaction in restored productivity and independence.

VOCATIONAL REHABILITATION. The ILO [1973] has presented this definition for vocational rehabilitation: "The continuous and coordinated process of rehabilitation which involves the provision of those vocational services, e.g., vocational guidance, vocational training and selective placement, designed to enable a disabled person to secure and retain suitable employment" [p. 4]. Operationally defined, vocational rehabilitation is the provision of any rehabilitative services (including medical, educational, social, etc.) to a vocationally handicapped person for the purpose of occupational (re)adjustment in work that may or may not be financially remunerative.

INDEPENDENT LIVING REHABILITATION. 1978 federal rehabilitation legislation authorized public funds for independent living rehabilitation services to severely handicapped individuals who may not have a vocational objective. Independent living rehabilitation services are "aimed at assisting a severely handicapped individual to gain maximum control over the management of his or her life activities and to minimize reliance on others in providing for one's self-maintenance" according to regulations of the federal rehabilitation agency. Chapter 40, Independent Living, describes purposes and processes of rehabilitation for self-care and self-determination.

REHABILITANT. The recipient of rehabilitation is a rehabilitant (viz., a handicapped person who is receiving services). Because it may also refer to a person who has already experienced a rehabilitation program, *rehabilitant* can mean either a person who is an "active" (current) case, or a "closed" case who has received and completed rehabilitation previously. The impersonal term *case* is sometimes used interchangeably with *client* but strictly speaking, the latter implies a helping relationship, such as counseling, with a professional worker.

REHABILITATIONIST OR REHABILITATOR. Both terms are used to refer to the professionals who provide rehabilitative services. In this book the term *rehabilitationist* generally refers to the rehabilitation counselor, but the title implies a broader function than counseling and includes other professional or technical specialists on the rehabilitation team.

PREVENTIVE REHABILITATION. In preventive rehabilitation measures are taken to avoid the need for rehabilitative services or the need for more extensive rehabilitative services at some point in the future. The position of some physicians that rehabilitation is the third phase of medicine (with preventive and curative care respectively, the first and second phases) would seem to disassociate them from the preventive area. In truth, however, all of the professions involved in rehabilitation are concerned with preventive measures. Prevention is seen not only as a public health measure to avoid disabling accidents and illnesses, but also as the rehabilitation objective of early intervention following a disablement to avoid or reduce its negative effects. Preventive rehabilitation calls for interventions

at different levels: first-level prevention is action taken to reduce the occurrence of disability; second-level prevention is intervention directed toward prevention of the development of functional limitations resulting from disablements; and third-level prevention is intervention taken to prevent the transition of irreversible functional limitations into handicaps. According to the World Health Organization [1977], with the technology of the last quarter of the twentieth century, over half of all disability could be prevented or postponed.

REHABILITATION DELIVERY SYSTEM. The rehabilitation delivery system covers the whole organization for the provision (delivery) of rehabilitation services to handicapped people, including all the various agencies involved. Agency programs should be coordinated (if not unified) to meet the complex needs of the whole person. Often, however, a proliferation of agencies divide recipients according to cause and type of disability, age, specific service, rehabilitation objective, method of payment, and administrative control and financing (e.g., public or private).

REHABILITATION PROCESS. The rehabilitation process generally follows acute medical or special education services, although both may be a part of the program for a handicapped person. Provision is made for any and all unmet needs of the rehabilitant as planned by the rehabilitationist and client to achieve the latter's life-adjustment objectives.

DISABILITY. This term in the nomenclature of American rehabilitation counselors means a medically defined condition (i.e., impairment) and use here follows that tradition. This word and the related words, *functional limitation* and *handicap,* will be defined in detail later. It suffices now to explain that a disability is any physical, mental, or emotional condition that is chronic or long-lasting (not acute or temporary), which is severe enough to limit the individual's functioning, and which results in, or threatens to be, a handicap to productive activity (see 4.1.1).

All the above terms are understood by rehabilitationists, although this nomenclature is not universally accepted. The choice of terms and the definitions in this book derive from an extensive search of the relevant literature, including a number of published glossaries on rehabilitation and associated fields [Goodwill Industries of America, 1975; International Labour Office, n.d.; Kelly, L. J. & Vergason, 1978; Northwest Association of Rehabilitation Industries, 1975; Vocational Evaluation and Work Adjustment Association, 1975]. Also consulted were several glossaries from related fields and standard dictionaries: American Psychiatric Association [1975]; Drever [1968]; Heber [1959]; Hopke [1968]; Oxford English Dictionary [1971];

Webster's New Collegiate Dictionary [1976]. Concepts used are labeled according to the apparently best accepted yet professionally precise nomenclature. Likewise, the definitions and descriptions given are composites derived from the several different sources and arbitrarily rephrased for clarity, precision and widest acceptance. Since the various glossaries in this book are unique to it, the above agencies and authors are not responsible for the terminology and definitions.

1.2. Human Philosophy

Social adjustments and improvement were seen as the pragmatic goals of life by philosopher-psychologist William James [1842–1910]. Mankind's concern for self has continued to be the basis of many philosophic works in the twentieth century. Modern philosophers are concerned with humanity's situation on earth, and rehabilitation psychology shares this philosophical focus on how people can survive in and adjust to a changing world. In fact, the concern of rehabilitationists extends to the survival of handicapped persons and how they can adjust to the demands of the world; the adjustment processes of disabled people are all the more precarious because of the adaptations required in a changing environment.

Philosophy leads to clear thinking by providing both a unified view of the whole subject of rehabilitation and precise thought about its components. Reasoned thought on the meaning of rehabilitation can give the worker an articulated foundation for a set of beliefs. With this rational framework, professionals can fully appreciate the work and the goals of rehabilitation and, more importantly, the way in which they themselves relate emotionally and behaviorally to its principles. From one's philosophy emerge behavioral guidelines for professional practice. This is essential for consistency in rehabilitation techniques, in linking "means" with "purpose" [Strickland, 1969]. So both philosophic content and strategy of thought, as exemplified by the concepts listed below, have direct relevance to rehabilitation.

1.2.1. HOLISTIC NATURE
Holistic is a Gestaltist term meaning "whole," "entire," or "complete." In her discussion of the philosophic assumptions of rehabilitation, Marceline Jaques [1970] also listed first the "whole person" approach in rehabilitation. As she pointed out, it is not possible in life to divide people into individual parts—physical, mental, psychological, social, economic. In science and professional practice, however, there are arbitrary divisions of the unitary being of the person for the convenience of collecting, classifying, and utilizing knowledge about human behavior. Thus, there are many organized professions based upon bodies of knowledge about artificially defined aspects of humanity. In rehabilitation it becomes clear that these divisions are not only simplistic interpretations but also quite inadequate in practice; but, because the professions are so organized and their bodies of knowledge so large, and because the problems of the disabled person are so multi-faceted, a team approach has been developed to enable each of the specialists on human nature to contribute pieces of knowledge toward understanding the whole person.

The human development process is also dynamic, each of its continuing stages affecting the next, as Jaques said. This is a tenet of human behavior and it has a practical message for the practitioner: it says that in order to know the client, one must investigate the case history and in particular, search for the constructive patterns of the past and build upon a favorable foundation. Finally, as Jaques pointed out, human problems tend to cluster together; that is, disability does not ordinarily appear as a single entity. The highest incidence of disability occurs among the financially disadvantaged who are, as a group, also undereducated and underemployed. Social pathology epitomizes the interacting influences of associated poverty, family deterioration, unhealthy environments, mental illness, substance abuse, and crime. A holistic approach for helping intervention systems is needed because of this so-called clustering phenomenon.

Rehabilitation can deal with the clustering of problems and the human being's holistic nature, since it is comprehensive in scope. The rehabilitation process is an orderly sequence of activities planned to meet the individual's total needs (see 10.2.1). To provide services related to one aspect of a person's functioning without considering other aspects and their interdependency could result in failure of the rehabilitation effort [Sohoni, 1977].

1.2.2. SELF-DETERMINATION

All people have a right to self-determination insofar as they are capable of responsible judgments; people should make their own decisions, set their own goals, and also decide how they achieve those goals. This does not mean that the rehabilitationist must assume a passive role or be totally nondirective. Active intervention by the rehabilitation counselor helps the client make decisions by providing needed information, by fostering the development of self-confidence, and by facilitating problem-solving.

The client is the primary person in rehabilitation with ultimate decision-making authority—and responsibility. Essential conditions for successful rehabilitation are the clients' knowledge that self-determination is a right and full acceptance of their responsibility for their decisions. This has practical implications because the clients are often overcoming a dependency upon others. In fact, independent action is a fundamental client purpose of total rehabilitation. Sincere appreciation of the final authority of clients also relieves the rehabilitation counselor of unwarranted feelings of personal responsibility for the client who fails. Andrew Adams [1977], a former administrator of the federal rehabilitation agency and a severely disabled person himself, stressed as a premise to any re-

habilitation concept that the "disabled must have a voice in their own destiny: in the rehabilitation care and services they receive, in their employment, and in where and how they live" [p. 25].

Rehabilitation is an individualized process, if for no other reason than the uniqueness of each client. All efforts are adapted to meet the particular needs and choices of the individual concerned. As such, it is a democratic process and a permissive relationship, in which the handicapped person shares fully. By present federal law there must be a unique and personalized rehabilitation plan for each disabled individual, a plan developed and carried out with full involvement of the disabled person in the decision-making process. Clients' rights have not always been so respected. In the rehabilitation literature since the beginning of the public program, a gradual progression in the use of the term *advisement* to *guidance* to *counseling* can be noted. This development, which seems to suggest a movement toward less authoritarianism on the part of the rehabilitationist, coincides with the increasing awareness of client rights for self-determination.

1.2.3. SOCIETAL CONTRIBUTION

Each individual is a social organism motivated to work and contribute as a member of society, beginning with self-support and progressing outward to a commitment to family, community, and the nation. This urge to participate in the achieving of communal objectives is deeply ingrained in the human culture and may be more or less instinctive due to eons of tribal existence. A variation of what might be termed mutual dependency is still an economic necessity in today's complex materialistic age. All sorts of reward systems have been developed to assure individual productivity, and punishment is meted out for anything perceived as less than a full contribution. Thus, disability was reacted to as a socioeconomic handicap until productivity is restored. The accomplishment of vocational rehabilitation still results in high positive regard by the social community and the handicapped person alike.

E. B. Whitten [1971a], long-term Director of the National Rehabilitation Association, defined vocational rehabilitation as "the organized effort to help physically and mentally handicapped people attain and maintain the ability to work."

Services, Whitten thought, are justified on the basis that "work is profoundly important to all adults, and disability may prevent meaningful participation in the world of work and in the satisfactions that come from work; and society needs the productive effort of every person" [p. 236].

Joseph Fenton [1972] echoed these ideas about disability and rehabilitation for social contribution: "The emphasis on the employment concept in the vocational rehabilitation program reflects a striving to secure for the disabled the same opportunities as are available for other persons, and the conviction that the economic, social, scientific, and cultural life of the nation are adversely affected if serious disability is neglected" [p. 7].

Fenton also suggested services for independent living as another philosophical dimension. Rehabilitation, he said, should prepare disabled persons to move toward "integration" into normal life situations, rather than segregation according to housing, working, medical care, family life, social life, or other phases of living.

1.2.4. RIGHT TO BE EQUAL

Equalization of ability is a fit description of total rehabilitation. The right of equality among people is recognized in various societies as "God-given," meaning inherent in all humans. For over 200 years in America the right has had constitutional sanctions. The evolving implementation of this concept has led to the granting of opportunity to all citizens without regard to heritage, race, sex, creed, national origin, disability, or other personal characteristics. For those who are handicapped, rehabilitation is provided because every member of a democratic society has a right to contribute to society. Thus, society has the obligation to equalize, through rehabilitation services, the handicapped population's opportunity for independence and productivity.

McGowan and Porter [1967] explained society's obligation to make the disabled person's opportunity equal to that possessed by nondisabled members. They went on to point out that these assumptions are particularly important in American society: "The status of independence is self-sufficiency, hard work, industriousness, contribution to society, and upward social mobility of the individual. To the extent that the handicapped individual is unable to reach these

goals, he suffers a loss of personal dignity, prestige, and self-esteem, both as a member of society and as a member of a family" [p. 5].

1.2.5. HUMAN SPIRIT

Belief in the spirit of human beings comes from witnessing miraculous recoveries accomplished by case after case in rehabilitation. The rehabilitation literature written by the disabled themselves and by professional workers has amazing accounts documenting this indefatigable will to recover and to do so in the face of utter hopelessness. Recommended for reading for more sensitivity to this ill-defined human spirit as exhibited by disabled persons are two outstanding books: the beautiful story of his life and his patients by Dr. Henry Kessler [1968], which was mentioned before, and also *Tongue Tied*, the fantastic personal account of life in a subnormality hospital by Joseph John Deacon [1974]. It is the great pleasure of the career rehabilitationist to witness firsthand how some persons forestall death and then go on to overcome great barriers to enjoy useful lives despite—some say because of—catastrophic limitations.

The concept of rehabilitation as a therapeutic philosophy has been advanced by Whitehouse [1961]: "Rehabilitation is primarily and fundamentally a therapeutic philosophy that is generic to the whole treatment field. Each profession utilizes this common philosophy through the operations characteristic of its training and knowledge. . . . All professions owe allegiance to the general principles, but each apply them through its own . . . special practice skills" [p. 20]. This therapeutic goal is based upon the hope and spirit of the person as much as the skill and collaboration of the professionals.

1.2.6. FOCUS ON ASSETS

A tenet in rehabilitation is that the focus must be on the assets a person has left following disablement. This is not only philosophically wise but also operationally sound in practice. All physical tasks, activities, and jobs demand abilities; consequently, rehabilitation requires the development and utilization of abilities—not disability. "Hire the handicapped: it is ability that counts," a slogan of the President's Committee on Employment of the Handicapped, is not controverted by experienced employers. Scientifically based procedures for the selective placement of handicapped workers involves a process of matching the demands of a specified job with the abilities of a specific applicant. The professional then accentuates the positive while not ignoring the limitations resulting from disability. Within this frame of reference residual assets come into better focus through a greater appreciation for strengths and weaknesses, both of which are objectively accepted.

A healthy mind-set for both counselor and client is implied by positivism of this kind. The "can-do" attitude expresses the spirit of prophecy that facilitates positive outcomes. Beatrice Wright [1968] said, "Man not only submits to reality; he also shapes it. Being unrealistic can be a source of hope, achievement and redefinition of the boundaries of new realities" [p. 296]. While the rehabilitation professional must be realistic about the deficits of clients, there is one universally characteristic attitude for successful rehabilitation workers—optimism.

The goal of rehabilitation is to identify and utilize residual capacities for functional independence. This broad goal subsumes economic self-sufficiency as well as personal, social, and community living skills [Morris, 1973]. Functional independence must be defined for each individual on the basis of residual capacities so that rehabilitation success is meaningful to each client.

1.2.7. MOTIVATION FOR GOOD

People are motivated for good. In psychological terms this means that individuals are capable of changing: of changing for the better, in the instance of rehabilitation. A person can be rehabilitated no matter how ingrained the negative attitudes and behavior patterns have become because of the deprivations and insult of disablement. From a practical standpoint many potential candidates for rehabilitation are judged "infeasible" because their attitudes and resources and those of society do not support the extraordinary effort required. But the potential strength of people is limitless.

Coping behavior by disabled persons (and conversely succumbing behavior) has been studied by rehabilitation psychologists. According to Jaques [1970], coping represents the attainment of "positive adaptive reaction to deviance" [p. 7]. She warned, however, that it must be properly reinforced to be effective.

1.2.8. INFLUENCE OF ENVIRONMENT

The positive and negative influences of the past and present social and physical environment help to shape what one becomes. Despite initially strong motivation, barriers can overwhelm and eventually defeat the inner spirit. Thus it is a tenet of rehabilitation not only to improve individuals and make them able, but also to improve their environments for enabling social and physical circumstances. Not only is the client who has an amputated leg taught how to drive, but also the car is fitted with hand controls. The emotionally troubled trainee, while being taught a trade, is counseled on interpersonal problems. People must be understood and treated within the context of their environment—both of which are subject to improvement for purposes of rehabilitation.

Kenneth Hamilton, in his fundamental 1950 book, provided many insights into the destructive power of disablement and nonacceptance:

The writer is convinced of one thing perhaps more strongly than any other with reference to the desires of disabled persons. They desire full-fledged acceptance as active participating members of the community. Despite the abundance of folklore to the contrary, few disabled persons develop compensating gifts or talents. Most of us, if overtaken by handicap, can expect to be pushed to the side-lines of life, to become at least partially dependent, financially and otherwise. Unless some coordinated group effort is made toward rehabilitation, that is the usual end result of a handicap. . . . The need which we all have for some type of success experience, for self-respect, self-support, self-determination, and full group acceptance can best be achieved by the handicapped through regaining their highest degree of employability. This is one of the more subtle significances of vocational adjustment [p. 9].

1.2.9. INTRINSIC VALUE

There is intrinsic value in the human being. This principle is fundamental in rehabilitation. People have an inherent dignity and value simply because they are human beings. Hamilton said: "The philosophical premises of rehabilitation are such that they will not be questioned in a democratic society. Regardless of the race, creed, or color of a handicapped person or the nature of the handicap he presents, we accept him as a human being, having intrinsic dignity as such. He has basic political, social, and human rights, among the last being the right to function at his maximum level of personal satisfaction and social usefulness" [p. 9]. The human dignity of the disabled individual is a thing apart from any consideration of enfeeblement, repulsiveness, or dependency. There is no insinuation of privilege in this, because acceptance of the value of every person is a universal human right.

Governments sometimes drastically limit the number of disabled people who shall be served, selecting only the most "worthy" or best potential wage earners. Compliance with the stated principle that all people are inherently valuable would dictate that every disabled person is worthy, without regard to monetary considerations. Rehabilitation practitioners do not make the laws and budgets that invariably screen out people for rehabilitation benefits. They can only follow the criteria set forth for eligibility and case selection. Basic respect for all people for their intrinsic value is still the prime consideration of the professional; it is expressed by positive regard for all clients.

1.2.10. CONCERN FOR INDIVIDUALS

The ultimate premise of the rehabilitation philosophy is an all-encompassing concern for the handicapped individual. Twelve principles formulated by B. Wright [1959] that outline the centrality of individualization in rehabilitation were summarized by DiMichael [1969] as follows:

1. Every human being has an inalienable value and is worthy of respect for his own sake.
2. Every person has membership in society, and rehabilitation should cultivate his full acceptance.
3. The assets of the person should be emphasized, supported, and developed.
4. Reality factors should be stressed in helping the person to cope with his environment.
5. Comprehensive treatment involves the "whole person," because life-areas are interdependent.
6. Treatment should vary and be flexible to deal with the special characteristics of each person.
7. Each person should assume as much initiative and participation as possible in the rehabilitation plan and its execution.
8. Society should be responsible, through all possible public and private agencies, for the providing of services and opportunities to the disabled.
9. Rehabilitation programs must be conducted with interdisciplinary and interagency integration.
10. Rehabilitation is a continuous process that applies as long as help is needed.
11. Psychological and personal reactions of the individual are everpresent and often crucial.
12. The rehabilitation process is complex and must be subject to constant reexamination—for each individual and for the program as a whole [pp. 12–13].

While these points may seem abstract, they have great value for practice.

A basic characteristic of the rehabilitation process is that it is always individualized. Each person is unique in skills, limitations, resources, and desires; and the manifestations of disabilities, different in each individual, have varying meanings and implications. Successful rehabilitation must identify the unmet needs of a particular client and plan a treatment program that satisfies the unique pattern of that individual's needs and desires.

1.3. Process Overview

The rehabilitation process consists of a planned and orderly sequence of individualized services tailored to meet the needs of a handicapped person. Through coordination by a rehabilitation counselor, an appropriate set of services is planned and provided to help the client solve those problems that interfere with life adjustment.

Rehabilitation services are an established right of disabled Americans. Public rehabilitation is provided by state agencies under federal guidelines and with matching (80%) federal funds. The state rehabilitation agency is respon-

sible for providing all services to its disabled clients but many of its client services are purchased or obtained from other community resources.

The public rehabilitation program was recently expanded to include independent living as well as vocational objectives. Vocational rehabilitation is intended for physically, mentally, or emotionally disabled persons who need service in order to secure employment. Independent living rehabilitation is provided to disabled individuals of all ages to enable those without a job objective to "function more independently in their family or community." All of the services of the public program for vocational rehabilitation clients are available to independent living rehabilitation clients plus additional services needed by the latter because of the severity of their handicaps.

Initiated with casefinding or referral, the process closes with the successful completion of services and resulting adjustment of the handicapped individual. Services are obtained from virtually the full span of community resources, depending on individual needs. Private physicians, public and private hospitals, specialized clinics, rehabilitation centers, workshops, public and private schools, and employers are but some of the resources utilized for effective rehabilitation. In the public rehabilitation program such services are often purchased for the client. Practically any service needed to complete the eligible client's rehabilitation plan can be provided through the state rehabilitation agency. Available services include medical and other evaluation, physical or mental restoration, therapeutic treatment, health maintenance, artificial appliances and technological devices, vocational or personal adjustment training, maintenance and transportation, family services, housing accommodations, attendant care, interpreter (deaf) or reader (blind) services, rehabilitation teacher and mobility instruction, recreation, assistance for starting a small business, placement in suitable employment, postemployment services, and other needed goods and services. Professional counseling is provided to the client throughout the process from referral to case closure and subsequently as indicated.

The program marshals all needed resources in a coordinated way. In the public agency and many other rehabilitation programs, the rehabilitation counselor is the key staff member in the adjustment process. The counselor makes the determination as to whether applicants are eligible and "feasible," plans with clients the objectives and strategy of their rehabilitation, manages the arrangements for the necessary services, makes client referrals to other agencies, provides ongoing counseling, keeps in contact during the entire process, and conducts or participates in placement.

Descriptions of the processes of rehabilitation have been published by the authors or editors of numerous books on the subject. Many of these works are credited in context—for example, a federal manual for the orientation of state rehabilitation counselors by John McGowan and Thomas Porter [1967]. Other notable texts and reference books on rehabilitation are cited frequently in the present volume. A number of other books were reviewed for material and are referenced here for their bibliographic value: Harris [1919]; Kessler [1947]; Rusk and Taylor [1949]; Soden [1949]; Pattison [1957]; Lofquist [1957]; Jacobs, Jordan, and DiMichael [1961]; Sussman [1965]; Malikin and Rusalem [1969]; Cull and Hardy [1972]; Malikin [1973]; Browning [1974]; Hardy and Cull [1974a]; Mallik, Yuspeh, and Mueller [1975]; Jenkins, Anderson, and Dietrich [1976]; Rusalem and Malikin [1976]; Chigier [1978]; Goldenson [1978]; and Bitter [1979]. Still other important rehabilitation text and reference books and works of historical interest are referred to elsewhere and listed in the References. Additional rehabilitation documents are listed and abstracted in books by Graham and Mullen [1956], Riviere [1949], and Wright and Butler [1968].

1.3.1. PROCESS VARIABLES

The rehabilitation process as applied from case to case is never the same. There can be no "production line" due to the varying configurations of client objectives, problems, and resources. What goes into the process depends upon the disabled person as well as outside considerations, and in relation to both there are many influencing elements.

Many separate but interacting components of the rehabilitation process influence the outcome of each case. Statisticians refer to causal components as independent variables in a process, the outcome of which is called the dependent variable. Sometimes an independent variable can be manipulated to produce change in its influence. But even when a component of the process (an independent variable) cannot be changed, it may be helpful to know what its influence (relationship) is on the outcome (dependent variable). So it is with understanding the variables of the rehabilitation process and their ability to cause successful client outcomes.

The relationship of rehabilitation process variables and outcomes has been extensively studied. The first issue is the definition of rehabilitation success. Many reasonable outcome criteria have been suggested: increased income from application to case closure, decreased dependency (financial or otherwise), improved psycho-social adjustment, reduced needs or problems, and enhanced satisfaction or style of life. Sophisticated measurement techniques have been developed for a weighted combination of outcome variables such as cost-effectiveness analyses or service-need-reduction scales.

Studies that reveal the relationship of process variable to outcome are useful in two ways. Such results help in the task of determining feasibility for rehabilitation and for setting alternative goals. The other value of such knowledge is that it allows for the identification of significant variables that require attention for successful life adjustment. Most of the independent variables in the rehabilitation process can be manipulated. This means that negative influences can be either changed or neutralized: they can be neutralized by being made irrelevant (e.g., the client's functional limitations can be made irrelevant through the wise choice of a job); they can also be changed at times (e.g., the client's lack of job skills can be overcome by vocational training).

Variables associated with rehabilitation difficulty are by no means limited to client *problems* such as severity of disability or lack of motivation. In fact, it is found that even the most catastrophically disabled persons can successfully adjust because of counterbalancing attributes. Moreover, the old excuse for rejecting cases with the reason "unmotivated" is now challenged. In the first place, the problem is likely to be a barrier to motivation, which can be removed by counseling or other assistance. Even "disincentives," caused by fear of losing financial or other assistance, can often be overcome through counseling. Few people really prefer the status of dependency, and it is incumbent upon the rehabilitationist to try to cope with the basic problems.

Difficulties in rehabilitation may also be attributed to external variables. Examples include poor labor market conditions, housing and transportation barriers, and negative family attitudes and practices (e.g., over-protection). Changing some of these negative conditions may seem to be beyond the power of the rehabilitationist; for example, placement workers may not be able to create appropriate new jobs in local business. However, experience shows that even in periods of substantial unemploy-

ment, with extra effort they do find appropriate openings for rehabilitants. Traditionally, rehabilitation counselors go out into the community and become involved in advocating changes for their clients such as arrangements for special housing or transportation. Likewise, rehabilitationists reach out to the homes of clients and attempt to help families develop informed attitudes and facilitative relationships.

Who are the tough rehabilitation cases? What personal variables represent high-risk cases? Which characteristics indicate greater effort to achieve program effectiveness? These issues have been studied in depth (e.g., Wright, 1976; Wright & Reagles, 1973a; Wright & Butler, 1968a). There are several approaches to identifying case difficulty before the process even begins. Assessment can be based on two types of applicant information. The first is measurements from formal instruments, including results of tests taken by the person and questionnaires answered by others (e.g., the counselor, the parents). The second is demographic data on the client.

The following indicators of vocational rehabilitation case difficulty, based upon client variables, seem valid:

1. Having many self-perceived problems of a social, psychological, familial, and/or vocational nature.
2. Performing poorly on intelligence and achievement tests.
3. Being a member of a particularly "vulnerable" client group such as the elderly or the multiply and severely disabled.
4. Being single and having no dependents and few (if any) property acquisitions.
5. Having a negative employment history, such as being unemployed for long periods of time, earning low weekly wages, having depended on some type of welfare support.
6. Having no vocational training and possessing few job skills.
7. Having indefinite or unrealistic plans for the future.
8. Being disabled later in life and having other medical problems (e.g., alcoholism) in addition to the disability.
9. Having had fewer years of formal education or being mentally retarded.
10. Having a "poor" family relationship and little financial support from the family.
11. Having few friends, leisure-time activities, and social skills.
12. Having weak ego-strength and a negative self-concept.

13. Having severe or long-standing psychiatric problems.

Negative variables in combination may be far more destructive. Conversely, there are personal characteristics that may be either positive or negative, depending upon other circumstances; minority racial membership (black, oriental), for example, differs in its influence on the unskilled person as compared to the professionally educated person.

The essential human elements in the process are: recognition of the multiple impact of disability, consideration of the need for overall rehabilitation rather than concentration on a particular aspect of the rehabilitation process, and awareness of the role that the prejudice of society plays in causing a disablement to be a handicap. But it is wrong to focus on negative considerations. It is because disability can have a pervasive impact that the proper approach in rehabilitation is to mobilize the abilities of the individual and the facilities of the environment. With so many variables, both positive and negative, always present in a unique configuration, it is essential that rehabilitation be a coordinated process.

The significant variables change according to the phase and objectives of the rehabilitation process. Rehabilitation services, broadly defined, may be employed at various points in time to attain a number of different objectives. According to Rusalem and Baxt [1970] these may include: prevention (e.g., ensuring proper prenatal care and providing dietary supplements and immunizations); correction (e.g., medical treatment for cure or remission of symptoms); adaptation (i.e., adapting the handicapped to the environment or vice versa); protection (e.g., providing family casework, housekeeping services, guardianship, institutionalization); and integration (i.e., obtaining the acceptance of society).

Jaques [1970], referring to the temporal and objective variables, listed four stages: curative or ameliorative, convalescent, transitional and developmental, and the therapeutic community stage. These focus upon medical and independent living objectives. Later stages of the total rehabilitation process are more directly associated with vocational objectives.

Perhaps the most important set of variables influencing the rehabilitation outcome is the process itself. It is here that the rehabilitation coun-

selor's knowledge of these principles is crucial:

1. The active involvement of the client is necessary and must be secured before adequate rehabilitation can be accomplished.
2. Action must be based upon adequate evaluations and accurate and realistic interpretation of the information that is secured.
3. Each rehabilitation client must be served on the basis of a sound plan developed with the rehabilitant.
4. Each service must be carefully selected and properly and thoroughly rendered.
5. Counseling of clients and close monitoring of all services are essential at each step of the process.
6. Every aspect of the client rehabilitation plan is individualized (for a unique pattern of needs and resources) and dynamic (in order to make strategic changes in objectives or services on the basis of ongoing evaluation).

1.3.2. SERVICE PROVISION

The American rehabilitation system is based on a goal that is "vocational" in the broadest sense of the term: to assist a rehabilitant to perform adequately in a productive role [Gellman, 1973]. It involves developing the desire and capacity to function productively in competitive employment, sheltered work, unpaid work, or independence from other people. The steps are self-determination, self-care, work competence (the ability to function in a job), employability (the ability to secure employment), and occupational security (the capacity for continued adaptation to a work environment). If the rehabilitant cannot be placed in competitive employment, the rehabilitation objective becomes employment in a nonprofit facility or in productive activity in the home. Freedom from dependence upon other people is also a productive role.

Structurally, the American service system is a network of rehabilitation agencies (public and voluntary, national and local) and major service systems (health, welfare, manpower, and education) that relate to the special needs of disabled people through a reciprocal referral process in the provision or use of service (see 9.2). The node of the rehabilitation system is the state-federal civilian rehabilitation program (see Chapter 7, Public Rehabilitation). The public agency influences the operating policies and programs of collaborating agencies at the local level though government grants and the purchase of service contracts. The administration of services to disabled individuals is conducted by the state rehabilitation agencies in the fifty states, the Commonwealth of Puerto Rico, the District of Columbia, and other jurisdictions.

Government funds are dispersed through the state rehabilitation agencies, which provide direct services for clients and purchase or procure from other public or private agencies such services as are not directly provided by the state rehabilitation agency. State agency rehabilitation counselors are responsible for locating candidates for service, determining applicant eligibility and rehabilitation potential (with the aid of evaluative reports from other professionals), providing ongoing counseling to clients, planning with clients a program of services required for a rehabilitation objective, arranging for and supervising needed services, and arranging either directly or indirectly for client placement. State agencies refer rehabilitants to, and purchase (other) client services from other public or private sources of needed services.

Resource agencies and facilities in the rehabilitation system include centers, workshops, hospitals, and clinics. Comprehensive rehabilitation centers offer a diversified array of services—integrating the medical, phychological, social, independent living, and vocational spheres. The several thousand rehabilitation workshops in the United States use work activity methodologically to provide work evaluation, work adjustment, and sheltered employment services. Several hundred speech and hearing clinics make up another large group of facilities providing rehabilitation service.

In many instances the provision of services to an individual involves a number of agencies and professionals in a multidisciplinary team approach. The team can include people in any of the disciplines, such as physicians, physical therapists, occupational therapists, social workers, speech and hearing therapists, psychologists, job placement specialists, special educators, and vocational educators, as well as rehabilitation counselors.

The focal points of the rehabilitation system then are: active casefinding; an individualized plan of service developed with the client; a coordinated and goal-oriented service approach; the use of a multidisciplinary team; and follow-through for optimal and sustained life adjustment.

1.3.3. ADMINISTRATION

The administration and financing of rehabilita-
tion services vary from country to country. A detailed examination of the administrative structure of American rehabilitation agencies will be offered later. Alternative system approaches operate well elsewhere.

The variations among countries are on several dimensions. (1) Operation may be centralized or decentralized. In the United States there is a rather effective partnership of state and federal government in the public program. (2) Control may be in a single agency or it may be fragmented [Reagles, Katz, & Wright, 1974]. In some countries, rehabilitation services are provided by several different ministries of government (e.g., Welfare, Education, Labor, Defense, Health, Insurance). (3) Funding can come from either voluntary contributions or from taxes. (In most countries the increase of human service expenditures has forced a greater financial participation by governments.) (4) Responsibility for all categories of disability (e.g., blindness) and all categories of services (e.g., medical) are not always under the same administration. (5) National social security insurance programming is often closely allied with rehabilitation service delivery, particularly independent living rehabilitation.

The increased size and complexity of the processes and organizations of rehabilitation have made critical the issue of administration. The whole problem is further complicated by the explosion of knowledge which forces ever greater specialization among the human service professionals. Coordination at the professional or local service delivery level is the immediate solution. Still there is need for better program planning and staff preparation at all levels to assure the handicapped individual of complete and high quality service, promptly rendered.

Coordinating bodies on rehabilitation of the disabled are recognized as an important mechanism of the rehabilitation delivery system. Such bodies have usually been set up on the national level, but in some countries they have been established on the regional and local levels as well. Sometimes the coordinating and advisory functions are delegated to a specific agency, for example the U.S. National Council on the Handicapped. These issues will be discussed in later chapters on rehabilitation resources. (Chapter 11, Resource Coordination, describes the mechanics of agency collaboration and cooperation.)

Chapter 2

The Profession

The term *rehabilitation* may refer to a process, a service system, or a discipline. The process of rehabilitation is structured by the needs of handicapped people and by the relevant resources available in the community. The service delivery system of rehabilitation is composed of government and private agencies, the organizational configuration of which varies from one nation to another. As a disciplinary area it includes rehabilitation specialists with knowledge of numerous professions and skills that can be taught and practiced anywhere for the benefit of all people who are handicapped. The process, agency, and professional components of rehabilitation are interdependent but distinguishable. While the professional components in the various phases are multidisciplinary, the focus here is on the rehabilitation counselor.

In its present stage of technological advancement the profession of rehabilitation counseling has the capacity for extending effective services far beyond the level of present programming.

This professional capacity, based upon applicable research and accumulated experience, is quite substantial and continues to expand rapidly. Inadequacies in practice are due not so much to lack of known techniques as to inadequate community resources, inadequate funding levels, inadequate organization, and insufficient numbers or preparation of professional personnel.

The depth and breadth of knowledge and techniques in rehabilitation counseling as reported in this book document the substantive foundation of rehabilitation counselor practice. This is the profession that encompasses the full scope of rehabilitation—client identification, assessment, counseling, planning, advocacy, resource utilization, placement, and continuing services indicated for the adjustment of the handicapped individual. It is necessary to have this central professional person for the total rehabilitation process because it represents a Gestalt, with the phases so intertwined that the process cannot be fragmented. The rehabilitation counselor keeps a continuous focus on a single client for whom the goal is life adjustment. This requires knowledge of the whole set of rehabilitation techniques. While the expertise of various other rehabilitationists may be called upon, the service system for vocational and independent living rehabilitation has an explicit identity personified by a unique professional entity, the rehabilitation counselor.

It matters not what this profession of rehabilitation counseling is called. What is important is that this body of knowledge—developed over the years to help handicapped persons to adjust—be recognized for its value and disseminated and utilized in effective professional practice. A new rehabilitation counseling technology has been developed that, although unique in its approaches and purposes, is enriched by several other disciplines. The fact is that in developing their technology, rehabilitation counselors borrowed from many professional fields. Until recent years there was no explicit research effort to discover effective techniques for rehabilitation counseling practice. Nor were there professional programs in colleges for rehabilitation counselor preparation.

Initially rehabilitation counselors were recruited from related occupations. They brought with them a variety of orientations, information, and skills to apply to the life adjustment problems of disabled and handicapped people. Medicine, social work, vocational education, special education, educational guidance, academic psychology, personnel management, labor economics, occupational and physical therapy, nursing education, and sociology—all contributed to the emerging rehabilitation counseling profession, which freely borrowed and adapted that which others could contribute. Yet the profession that has emerged is not solely descended from any one of its relative disciplines.

Professionally, rehabilitation counseling is identified with psychology as the science of human behavior. In practice it relies heavily upon several fields of psychology, namely, counseling, clinical, industrial and personnel, measurement, and rehabilitation psychology (the new subdiscipline for the study of reaction to disability). In the United States most rehabilitation counselor-educators are psychologists, although few university rehabilitation counseling education (RCE) programs are located in academic psychology departments. University RCE programs are usually autonomous; ideally they will form separate departments, although they are now often organizationally associated with school guidance, special education, educational psychology, or other graduate programs (such as those for health related services). In most countries around the world, social work generally has been accepted as the parent profession encompassing rehabilitation. Curricula of schools of social work provide instruction in generic human services. The professional preparation of American RCE programs, however, is specific to the understanding of the problems of handicapped persons, their life adjustment, and explicit rehabilitation techniques.

Whether rehabilitation counseling is a separate and independent discipline, a subprofession of psychology, or an integral part of social service still seems an unresolved issue in some quarters. Despite this, in the United States the central professional person in the total rehabilitation process is indisputably the rehabilitation counselor. But roles and functions—and even the titles—of those doing rehabilitation counseling vary according to their preparation and other qualifications, and are dictated by the difference in clientele and by the employing agency's goals, structure, and regulations.

Another complication in the definition of work roles is inherent in the phases of rehabilitation counseling. It is being questioned whether the counselor's functions should include all of the professional tasks of the counseling process or whether separate professions should be established for the various functions. Specifically, work evaluation and job placement are seen by some as distinct from counseling, and separate professional associations have been organized. The idea of a fragmented rehabilitation professional responsibility was argued a number of years ago by a few early rehabilitation counselor-educators who did not appreciate the differences between counseling and psychotherapy and would have confined the setting, techniques, and goals of the rehabilitation counselor. Their published idea was that to be "professional" rehabilitation counselors must do only counseling, do it only for personal adjustment, and only at the office. A broader view of rehabilitation counseling has evolved that includes community involvement, client assessment, and job placement as a part of the continuum of professional service. This broader position is shaped by total client needs rather than the dictates of either an agency or the profession. This newer model for preparation in and implementation of the rehabilitation technology is reflected in the organization of the present volume which describes the techniques needed for the continuum of professional functions in the whole counseling process. Today's rehabilitation counselors can be and are appropriately employed in widely different settings to perform a variety of functions serving handicapped clients.

2.1. *Characteristics*

Rehabilitation counseling has the unique distinction of being the only profession established by an Act of the United States Congress. Actually, a series of federal actions, both legislative and administrative, shaped the structure and status of rehabilitation practice. However, Public Law 565 of the 83rd Congress in 1954, which provided for research foundations and university education programs, elevated rehabilitation counseling to the level of a profession. It now has its own identity, extending beyond the public rehabilitation agency realm—for services to all types of handicapped individuals throughout the human services system. The profession is now adapting to other cultures around the world for the adjustment of their handicapped people [Wright, 1969, 1978].

2.1.1. HELPING PROFESSION

A profession is an occupation based upon a specialized knowledge that requires long and extensive academic preparation. This level and type of vocation is sometimes further delimited as one providing a direct human service. The even more circumscribed and newer term *helping profession* implies humanitarian service to individuals in need of specialized knowledge and skill.

Definition of Profession

The term *profession* can be viewed from the following perspectives, according to Whitehouse [1969]. A profession is an organized and structured body of knowledge within a certain philosophical framework, a certain part of the universe of knowledge. It is a vocation in which the practitioner devotes energy to some noble cause by engaging in certain circumscribed activities. A profession is distinguished as an occupation that requires certain credentials that are regulated by an official body. It is a group of prac-

titioners who establish their own qualification standards and offer protection and enhancement, as a body, to all those who meet those qualifications. Finally, a profession is a group that adheres to certain demands and expectations of the public and therefore receives its approval to provide certain services.

Usually thought of as a rather homogeneous group of individuals, a profession actually consists of a variety of different but related work groups. All members share a common, general role and typically have similar levels of training and education, but they engage in different functions. While they all have the same role, certain groups within a profession represent certain specialties requiring unique knowledge, skills, and interests. Some of the segments within a profession may be better established, wield more influence and power, and enjoy more status than others. At any point in the history of a profession, some segments are just emerging, others are attempting to become firmly established, and others are striving to maintain their viability. Along with the organization of a profession according to various specialties, there is a social organization that consists of relationships among the various segments that are determined by the practice and tactics of these groups [S. J. Miller, 1971].

Every profession, Miller said, exercises a certain degree of exclusivity in order to maintain its integrity as a specialized group providing unique services. It is assumed that the nature of the work is too difficult or complex for anyone but the specially trained members of the profession to engage in, and thus the profession's claim to the exclusive privilege of providing such services is protected. Certain mechanisms therefore are developed through which the profession exerts control over entrance into the profession and the criteria for admittance.

Given that a profession serves a special need that must be met, the profession has certain "correlative characteristics," which were viewed by Richardson [1968] as the following. First, the members of a profession have mastered their discipline through rigorous training. Second, these skills are used to render a needed social service. Third, there is some official sanction or some system of credentials through which an individual is granted permission to enter a profession and engage in its practices. Fourth, the profession maintains a high degree of autonomy, which includes a responsibility to set up standards of practice, educational requirements, selection procedures, a code of ethics, guarantees for the continuing professional development of practitioners, and a system of disciplining members who violate professional ethics or standards.

Another critical aspect of a profession, as Obermann [1962] emphasized, is that the body of knowledge special to each profession has a sound research base so that the knowledge is not only specialized but also systematized. It is through this research base that the profession develops its own scientific technique. It is the responsibility of professional people to extend this scientific base by engaging in research endeavors or by verifying research findings in their own practice. However, the professional member is more than just a skilled craftsman applying systematized techniques since a distinguishing feature of a profession is that its members must exert discretion and judgment while performing their duties.

Professionalization involves more than objective characteristics such as obtaining training and credentials, meeting social needs, providing unique services, and establishing a research base. There are intangible attributes that distinguish professionals. By claiming the title "professional" one is stating that one's primary values lie in providing a needed service to society, rather than in income, power, and prestige. At least this is an ideal toward which one strives. In this commitment to service, the practitioner must be mature and responsible, dedicated to personal growth, and willing to take risks while exercising discretion.

Nature of the Counseling Professions

Rehabilitation counseling education has its academic roots in counseling psychology. Counseling psychology emerged to prominence following World War II, initially to meet the educational and vocational needs of veterans. At that time there was an integration of vocational guidance, psychometrics, and personality psychology to help individuals who needed assistance in vocational and educational planning. Unlike clinical psychology, which deals with clients with overriding difficulties and in need of intense psychotherapeutic intervention, counseling psychology attends to the needs of the otherwise adjusted person who is seeking optimal fulfillment and positive growth. All counseling specialties, including educational, vocational, and rehabilitation counseling, rely on psychological principles and techniques for assessment, intervention, and personal growth [Muthard, 1963]. Rehabilitation counseling, however, has developed additional assessment methods and intervention strategies for the unique needs of handicapped individuals [Cottingham & Swanson, 1976].

In this day of mass delivery of human services, it is important to remember that the key to effective helping is the individualization of services. In regard particularly to the focus on individuals, Feingold [1977] provided a set of tenets (condensed below) basic to any counseling philosophy.

1. Each person is important, possessing human dignity and the right to equal opportunity.
2. Counselors are concerned individuals who have a real interest in the welfare of all people.
3. All clients must be afforded complete freedom of choice, which includes the risks involved in allowing them to make a wrong choice.
4. Every person has the potential to make a contribution to self, family, and society.
5. The counselor does not impose a personal philosophy on clients but rather serves to assist people in making their own decisions.
6. As a result of freedom of choice and individual dignity, each person has a right to be unique and different.
7. In assisting a client, counselors must remember their responsibility not only to their clients but also to the public, to their institutions, and to their work settings.
8. As society and technology change, it be-

comes increasingly important for counseling philosophies to recognize the need for inter-disciplinary functioning.

9. The results of research are professionally helpful, and therefore it is incumbent upon the counselor to keep abreast of current re-search, incorporate it into practice, and participate in it when possible.

10. The counselor's knowledge, skills, and abil-ities are not static but must be constantly developed through participation in continu-ing educational experiences.

*Counseling and Rehabilitation
Counseling Compared*

All counseling professions appreciate that fa-cilitating client growth requires understanding of the cognitive (knowing) and affective (emo-tional or feeling) aspects of behavior. This is the psychological basis of these fields. Rehabilita-tion counseling, then, uses this knowledge to aid in the adjustment of persons who have hand-icaps to employment and independence. This differentiates the rehabilitationist from other types of counselors, because the rehabilitation client population consists of people who are handicapped. Here the practitioner must rely heavily on the specialized body of knowledge and techniques in rehabilitation that have been shown to be effective with this special needs group.

The rehabilitation counselor, Williamson [1965] maintained, blends three streams of thought in understanding and helping the person with a disability. First, the medical model ex-plains the disability and the restorative services that are necessary. Second, the vocational guid-ance model provides direction for vocational choice and decision-making. Third, the mental health model addresses personal and social ad-justment.

Owing to the "clustering effect" of human problems the rehabilitationist must often help the client deal with a variety of barriers rather than merely overcoming the adjustment difficul-ties imposed by society. As Jaques [1970] wrote, the work of the rehabilitation counselor there-fore extends much beyond the interpersonal exchange methods traditionally associated with most counseling fields.

The modern concept of total rehabilitation developed out of years of experience with

handicapped persons and repeated demon-strations of the need for treating the whole per-son. The efficacy of medical and nonmedical treatment within the person's total life sphere in a comprehensive rehabilitation program has been dramatically demonstrated in the restora-tion of severely handicapped persons to inde-pendent and useful lives. It is this recognition that underlay the emergence of rehabilitation counseling as an accepted profession; it is now known that large medical expenditures may be of little ultimate value unless implemented by a plan for working and living that is congruent with the handicapped person's physical and mental condition. In such a process, the re-habilitation counselor is called upon to perform the crucial task of helping people make the best use of their positive attributes for life adjust-ment. The role of rehabilitation counseling in al-lied health professions has been described by Robert Boudreaux and associates at the Texas School of Allied Health Sciences in Dallas [Boudreaux, Pool, Henke, & McCollum, 1978].

The concept of the "rehabilitation team" conveys the idea of a cooperative effort by people in a number of professional disciplines working toward a common goal (i.e., maximum rehabilitation of a handicapped person). The re-habilitation counselor is on the team as a full-fledged member, not just at the end stage but from the acute medical care stage on. Ac-ceptance as a member of the rehabilitation team in hospitals and clinics has made the counselor's effort more effective in preventing adjustment problems before they develop.

2.1.2. THE UNIQUENESS

Rehabilitation counseling is now an established profession with a history of more than 60 years of development. With an extensive research lit-erature, developed primarily through an invest-ment of several hundred million dollars from the federal government, the profession rests upon a deep foundation of specialized knowledge. Broad recognition of the importance and unique contribution of this profession is demonstrated by the fact that nearly 100 American universities offer graduate degree (masters) programs in re-habilitation counseling. Graduates are eligible for membership in professional associations with high standards of excellence.

Knowledge Base

An examination of the relevant literature shows the depth and breadth of knowledge underlying the profession of rehabilitation counseling. For example, in 1968 Wright and Butler identified 1,413 documents, published within a 10-year period, specifically related to the roles and functions of rehabilitation counselors. Also in 1968, Wright, Butler, and Aldridge in their *Rehabilitation Information Series* (*RIS*) compiled 2,000 references pertinent to rehabilitation counseling and service delivery. The working bibliography for the present volume consisted of over 5,000 documents selected for relevant and practical information. A number of journals are devoted exclusively to rehabilitation literature, and many other periodicals publish articles related to this field.

Rehabilitation as a process is made meaningful and effective for the handicapped person by the extensive knowledge of the counselor. In order to help people whose physical, mental, and social limitations are so serious as to have resulted in a handicap to employment or to daily living activities, one must be skilled in helping them use their personal and environmental resources. It is important to attend to the individual's adjustment in all aspects of life.

The rehabilitation counselor, as Jaques [1970] summed it up, operates from a psychological base and functions as part of a psychosocial and health-related professional team providing a broad range of services for disabled persons. Primarily community-based, the rehabilitation counselor works within and through a number of different agencies, services, and facilities and effectively coordinates all the available resources. Moreover, an effective relationship with the client is essential for the proper operation of the counseling process.

The Impact of Service

From the beginning of the public program the services of the rehabilitationist had a profound effect on the lives of disabled individuals, and organized professionalism in rehabilitation counseling has made for far better service. For example, through accreditation and certification, incompetent persons are excluded from this profession in order to protect clients; through its associations and agencies the profession influences legislators for the improvement of rehabilitation client services and the initiation of new services; and because of its prestige, rehabilitation counseling has an impact on the attitudes and behaviors of other professionals who work with clients. Most importantly, the professionalization of rehabilitation counseling has resulted in increased counselor effectiveness and efficiency.

A systematic attempt to assess the impact of rehabilitation counseling was reported by Tinsley and Gaughan [1975]. Data obtained from nearly 4,000 closed cases were analyzed to determine the relationship of rehabilitation counseling to client adjustment. Their conclusion was that rehabilitation counseling has a lasting effect on the vocational adjustment of the client. This finding agrees with the results of other research indicating that professional rehabilitation service helps handicapped people achieve their goals in life.

One result of rehabilitation counseling is a substantial increase in the employment rate and a shift toward appropriate occupations for the disabled clientele. Gains from the service are largely maintained, according to follow-up studies. Although the employment rate drops some after cases are closed, it is still markedly higher than the employment rate before rehabilitation. The sustention of this gain for most rehabilitants has been well established. In addition, the tendency for former clients to be employed in proper occupations is maintained. Qualitatively, research subjects generally report that working at their jobs does not aggravate their handicaps, that their handicaps usually do not interfere with doing a good job, and that they are satisfied with the rehabilitation service and with their jobs.

While there are those in rehabilitation who are uncomfortable with its vocational emphasis, Samler [1966] noted that it is a critical, though complex function. He said:

The disenchantment with vocational guidance arose out of its concern with only part of the person. This is not to say that specified abilities—for example, scholastic aptitude or eye-hand coordination—are not important to identify, but they do not constitute all of a person's life or even its most important aspects . . . . It passes understanding that the person who everywhere else—as a family member, in social settings, as a citizen, lover, worker—is regarded as having various needs and as being quite complex somehow becomes something less than these at the point of exploring himself relative to work [p. 40].

But this complexity should not be used as an argument for neglecting the vocational needs of adults. In fact, vocational adjustment often satisfies emotional and other needs when psychotherapists have failed.

The potential impact of vocational counseling services is increasingly being recognized in many human service agencies. Trained vocational counselors for the handicapped are hired by private rehabilitation facilities, hospitals, nursing homes, psychiatric facilities, schools, worker compensation carriers, industrial personnel offices, labor organizations, and various other rehabilitation, employment, and human service agencies. Some are in private practice as disability consultants, halfway house operators, work evaluators, and work adjustment counselors. Others maintain private practices for traditional rehabilitation counseling as well as for avocational counseling, leisure counseling, and career change counseling [Wilkinson, 1977].

2.1.3. THE NEED

Hamilton's remarks in 1950 concerning the need for the rehabilitation counselor demonstrate that the problems of the disabled and the services offered by the rehabilitationist are enduring over time, rather than being peculiar to a particular span of years.

When one refers to the "field" of work with crippled children or with the disabled, one hardly in fact refers to a field at all. Rather, the community presents its handicapped persons with a vertical segment of many fields piled one atop the other, like the cross section of an anthill. The pyramided segments of services which comprise the rehabilitation services of the community cut through the specialized fields of medicine, . . . , family casework, vocational guidance, and employment. The handicapped individual seeking assistance is also confronted with the services of medical social work, occupational therapy, and industrial medicine [p. 201].

Personnel Shortage

The problem in 1950 involved the need for a central professional person to understand the whole person and to stay with that handicapped individual through the maze of treatment. Getting diverse specialties to effectively coordinate their work presupposes a sustained individualized contact all the way through to the point of readjustment. The person who maintains this

contact is the rehabilitation counselor. But there are not enough qualified rehabilitation counselors to fill the potential demand for their services—this is an ongoing problem.

Future Personnel Needs

The U.S. Department of Labor, Bureau of Labor Statistics [1976a, 1978, 1980], studies manpower needs throughout the country in all notable occupations. The following analysis for rehabilitation counseling is selected from recent editions of their *Occupational Outlook Handbook*:

About 19,000 persons, one-third of them women, worked as rehabilitation counselors in 1976. About 70 percent worked in State and local rehabilitation agencies financed cooperatively with Federal and State funds. Some rehabilitation counselors and counseling psychologists worked for the Veterans Administration. Rehabilitation centers, sheltered workshops, hospitals, labor unions, insurance companies, special schools, and other public and private agencies with rehabilitation programs and job placement services for the disabled employ the rest.

Employment opportunities for rehabilitation counselors are expected to be favorable through the mid-1980's. Persons who have graduate work in rehabilitation counseling or in related fields are expected to have the best employment prospects.

Contributing to the long-run demand for rehabilitation counselors will be population growth and the extension of service to a greater number of the severely disabled, together with increased public awareness that the vocational rehabilitation approach helps the disabled to become self-supporting. The extent of growth in employment of counselors, however, will depend largely on levels of government funding for vocational rehabilitation. In addition to growth needs, many counselors will be required annually to replace those who die, retire, or leave the field for other reasons.

The supply of rehabilitation counselors has leveled off as has the pressing demand in many state rehabilitation agencies. But there are many new areas of vocational services for handicapped persons that are being staffed with untrained personnel, for example, the mammoth manpower programs for the culturally handicapped population. Also, currently many areas of counseling the medically disabled person are understaffed. And the anticipated expansion of independent living rehabilitation will create a shortage of qualified counselors.

The Nature of the Work

The next chapter will address the functions and specific tasks performed by rehabilitationists. However, a general overview of the rehabilitation counselor's work and of the vocational counseling aspects of the rehabilitationist's work would be helpful here for an understanding of the professional nature of the role. Statements from recent editions of the *Occupational Outlook Handbook*, as paraphrased below, describe the work of the rehabilitation counselor.

Rehabilitation counselors help people with physical, mental, or social disabilities to adjust their vocational plans and personal lives. Counselors learn about client's interests, abilities, and limitations. They then use this information, along with available medical and psychological data, to help disabled persons evaluate themselves for the purpose of pairing their physical and mental capacity and interests with suitable work.

Together, the counselor and client develop a plan of rehabilitation, with the aid of other specialists responsible for the medical care and occupational training of the handicapped person. As the plan is put into effect, the counselor meets regularly with the disabled person to discuss his progress in the rehabilitation program and help resolve any problems that have been encountered. When the client is ready to begin work, the counselor helps him find a suitable job, and usually makes follow-up checks to insure that the placement has been successful.

Rehabilitation counselors must maintain close contact with the families of their handicapped clients, other professionals who work with handicapped people, agencies and civic groups, and private employers who hire the disabled. Counselors in this field often perform related activities, such as informing employers of the abilities of the handicapped and arranging for publicizing the rehabilitation program in the community.

An increasing number of counselors specialize in a particular area of rehabilitation; some may work almost exclusively with blind people, alcoholics or drug addicts, the mentally ill, or retarded persons. Others may work almost entirely with persons living in poverty areas.

The amount of time spent in counseling each client varies with the severity of the disabled, person's problems as well as with the size of the counselor's caseload. Some rehabilitation counselors are responsible for many persons in various stages of rehabilitation; on the other hand, less experienced counselors or those working with the severely disabled may work with relatively few cases at a time.

Lamb and Mackota [1975] developed the thesis that rehabilitation counseling should be considered a "high status profession requiring sophisticated skills." They described how rehabilitation counseling demands a high degree of sensitivity and perception about people: "In order to be of help to clients in the crucial area of career selection, it is essential that the counselor be skillful in judging those elements of a client's temperament which would have an effect on his succeeding in certain occupations. Conversely, the counselor must also be fully informed about the personality traits demanded by occupations so that he can effectively counsel in career choice" [p. 23]. As they pointed out, the rehabilitation counselor's help in the client's selection of an occupation can have profound and far-reaching effects. The trained counselor can identify problems and avoid further failures that might be emotionally devastating to clients.

2.2. Qualifications

The concept of qualifications as applied to a profession is a vague one, but it takes on meaning by a process of professionalization. Tangible aspects of professionalization include the development of membership associations, ethical standards, and credentials. Each are described in this section.

2.2.1. PROFESSIONAL ASSOCIATIONS

A professional association, as defined by Sussman, Haug, and Krupnik [1965], is "an organization of individuals engaged in the same work whose objectives include setting standards for practice and entrance into the field through control of the educational process, self-regulation of members' behavior, and political activity to establish a position within the body of professions and to create a public image of professionalism. The image contains notions of an orientation of service to others, based upon a scientific body of knowledge" [p. 1].

Purposes and Professionalization

Professionalization of an occupation involves setting up a professional association to regularize the interactions between practitioners, practitioners and clients, and practitioners and society. Regulation becomes a professional endeavor, the profession seeking a mandate to control itself rather than submitting to the governance of society. In demonstrating its right to this mandate, the association may need to lobby on a large scale for certification, licensure, and legal definition of relationships with other occupations. If the occupation is not well known, public relations efforts are usually necessary.

Members join professional organizations on a voluntary basis. Those who do not join may or may not have difficulty advancing within the field. However, since the purpose of the association is essentially to foster the profession, those who do not belong to the association still benefit from its work, especially in improved status, higher salaries or larger fees, and greater acceptance by the public.

The association provides the incentives needed to encourage excellence as well as social and moral support to individual members. These functions are essential, especially in salaried professions such as rehabilitation counseling in which employees do not determine the work situation, especially their relationships with clients, and therefore depend on group action for protection of professional interests.

The association is always attempting to improve standards, an effort that may be resisted by workers who feel threatened by changes in practice. In order to deal with this, association by-laws usually have a "grandfather" clause allowing membership for all those who were practicing prior to the certification or licensure period. Research, demonstration, and dissemination are aimed at upgrading practice, self-regulation, and the public image of the emergent profession. Research is encouraged and supported, and journals for dissemination of new knowledge as well as newsletters for information about the profession are published by the typical association. Most professional associations sponsor annual conventions for the entire membership to participate in organizational affairs and to exchange new knowledge through scientific papers.

The professional association may assume responsibility for standards of training and education in its field. It does this by establishing criteria for entrance requirements into the field and implements its demand by "certifying" qualified practitioners or by making arrange-

ments for licensure through state legislation, or both. A close link between training institutions and the professional association evolves. The association is instrumental in the establishment and operation of academic accreditation—a mechanism for the regulation of preprofessional preparation programs. Education is not limited to new students: Programs of continuing education, most notably in annual conferences, are conducted to upgrade qualifications, disseminate new knowledge concerning practice, and raise motivation.

Professional associations frequently originate by a process of differentiation from older groups. In this way the American Rehabilitation Counseling Association became a division of the Americal Personnel and Guidance Association (APGA).

Through the association the members gain a sense of identity and community that sets the profession apart from others. This and the association's systems of education, professional development, and awards, encourage the member to make a lifelong commitment to the field. The social and moral support of colleagues sustains motivation for excellence and defines success or satisfaction with the job.

Associations of Rehabilitation Counselors

Two independent associations represent the profession of rehabilitation counseling: American Rehabilitation Counseling Association (ARCA) and National Rehabilitation Counseling Association (NRCA). ARCA and NRCA were both organized in the late 1950s and they share similar goals as to the advancement of professional standards and the status of professionals. They hold separate annual meetings, and each publishes its own journal. Jointly they help to sponsor the same organizations for accreditation and certification.

Although the existence of two rehabilitation counseling associations is regarded as inefficient and confusing, substantial advantages derive from their separate though cooperative efforts. They do represent different constituencies (overlapping membership is relatively small); more importantly, however, they solicit support from different power bases: ARCA draws the support of the American counseling community and NRCA has the influential support of all rehabilitation organizations. This broad support is crucial for the advancement of the profession (e.g., favorable congressional action). Recognizing their mutual goals, ARCA and NRCA work closely and amicably on all issues beneficial to the profession. They conduct joint board meetings regularly and cosponsor important projects. Membership in both ARCA and NRCA is beneficial to rehabilitation students and practitioners and also benefits the profession.

A number of professional and other organizations, to be described in Chapter 12, are of interest to rehabilitationists. The American Psychology Association (APA) and its divisions for counseling and rehabilitation psychology have been mentioned. Several NRA divisions in addition to NRCA are important because they represent important professional concerns to all rehabilitation personnel. A listing of other NRA divisions and their purposes follows: National Rehabilitation Administration Association (NRAA)—the purpose of the NRAA is to advance the field of practice in rehabilitation supervision and administration; Job Placement Division (JPD)—has as its purpose the advancement of the employment of handicapped persons; National Association of Rehabilitation Instructors (NARI)—the purpose of this association is to help disabled persons by improving their functional abilities (e.g., mobility) through special instruction; Vocational Evaluation and Work Adjustment Association (VEWAA)—this association works to improve and advance the field of vocational evaluation and work adjustment training of handicapped persons by the use of simulated or real work, or both, to enhance their rehabilitation; National Association of Rehabilitation Secretaries—purposes of this association of clerical and secretarial workers in rehabilitation include the promotion of ethical conduct and needed practices; National Congress on the Rehabilitation of Homebound and Institutionalized Persons—NRA members employed in the rehabilitation of institutionalized or homebound people belong to this organization. In addition to these divisions, NRA has state chapters throughout the country, as do ARGA and APA. The national offices of NRA, APGA, and APA are in the Washington, D.C. area.

Of all the associations, the National Rehabilitation Association most comprehensively represents the interests of all those concerned about the needs of the disabled. According to an NRA (n.d.) membership promotion flyer, "If you are a rehabilitation professional, consumer, volunteer, student, or concerned citizen, you can unite in a common effort to advance rehabilitation and achieve opportunity for all handicapped people` by joining the National Rehabilitation Association." With a membership of over 30,000 persons, the Association, which was founded in 1925, is an effective advocate for handicapped people, articulating their rights and needs, and pursuing means to meet those needs.

2.2.2. ETHICAL ISSUES

Incorporated within the principles of all helping professions is a code of ethics that controls the practitioner's behavior for the protection of the client's welfare. And as Scorzelli [1977] said, the professional code of ethics helps the counselor through a specific set of guidelines for making ethical decisions.

Code of Ethics

The necessity for a code of ethical standards becomes even more important, as Scorzelli pointed out, in view of the recent concern over professional liability and the increased emphasis on the rights of handicapped people. Rehabilitationists identify for themselves a set of values through the development of their career and are given opportunity to validate and crosscheck them as different situations arise. However, because their encounters with ethical situations have been limited, the inexperienced must depend upon the experience of others.

The rights and responsibilities of a profession are explained to the student by a code of ethics. It provides guidelines for practice and sets forth criteria for eliminating those who are unqualified. "The promulgation of a code of ethics by an occupation is an advanced stage of professionalization, and usually occurs simultaneously with efforts to obtain legislation that sanctions a profession by having its claims officially recognized and protected by the law" [Milller, 1971, p. 985].

A number of codes of ethics contain principles relevant to the rehabilitationist. The National Rehabilitation Counseling Association (NRCA) code of ethics is organized according to the counselor's relationships—with clients, family, employers, other professions, agencies, and the community. The American Personnel and Guidance Association code is organized according to counselor functions—general, counseling, assessment, research, publication, consulting, and administration. The American Psychological Association code of ethics addresses broader questions such as responsibility, competency, and confidentiality.

The Commission on Rehabilitation Counselor Certification [n.d.] has published an abridgement of the NRCA code of ethics to which the certification applicant is required to ascribe. A product of the major organizations concerned with the rehabilitationist's practice, it is perhaps the most succinct statement of ethical standards for the rehabilitationist. It reads as follows:

A rehabilitation counselor has a commitment to the effective functioning of all human beings: his emphasis is on facilitating the functioning or refunctioning of those persons who are at some disadvantage in the struggle to achieve viable goals. While fulfilling this commitment he interacts with many people, programs, institutions, demands, and concepts, and in many different types of relationships. In his endeavors he seeks to enhance the welfare of his clients and of all others whose welfare his professional roles and activities will affect. He recognizes that both action and inaction can be facilitating or debilitating and he accepts the responsibility for his action and inaction.

The primary obligation of the rehabilitation counselor is to his client. In all relationships he will protect the client's welfare and will diligently seek to assist the client towards his goals.

The rehabilitation counselor recognizes that the client's family is typically a very important factor in the client's rehabilitation. He will strive to enlist the understanding and involvement of the family as a positive resource in promoting the client's rehabilitation plan and in enhancing his continued effective functioning.

The rehabilitation counselor is obligated to protect the client-employer relationship by adequately apprising the latter of the client's capabilities and limitations. He will not participate in placing a client in a position that will result in damaging the interests and welfare of either or both the employer and the client.

The rehabilitation counselor will relate to his colleagues in the profession so as to facilitate their ongoing technical effectiveness as professional persons.

Typically, the implementation of a rehabilitation plan for a client is a multi-disciplinary effort. The rehabilitation counselor will conduct himself in his interdisciplinary relationship in such a way as to facilitate the contribution of all the specialists involved for maximum benefit of the client and to bring credit to his own profession.

The rehabilitation counselor will be loyal to the agency that employs him and to the administrators and supervisors who supervise him. He will refrain from speaking, writing, or acting in such a way as to bring discredit on his agency.

The rehabilitation counselor will regard his professional status as imposing on him the obligation to relate to the community (the public) at levels of responsibility and morality that are higher than are required for persons not classified as "professional." He will use his specialized knowledge, his special abilities, and his leadership position to promote understanding and the general welfare of handicapped persons in the community, and to promote acceptance of the viable concepts of rehabilitation and of rehabilitation counseling.

In his relationships with other programs, agencies and institutions that will participate in the rehabilitation plan of the client, the rehabilitation counselor will follow procedures and insist on arrangements that will foster maximum mutual facilitation and effectiveness of services for the benefit of the client.

The rehabilitation counselor is obligated to keep his technical competency at such a level that his clients receive the benefit of the highest quality of services the profession is capable of offering.

The rehabilitation counselor is obligated to assist in the efforts to expand the knowledge needed to serve handicapped persons with increasing effectiveness.

Keith Wright [1977] at the Virginia Commonwealth University has provided insightful thoughts on professional values and behavior in rehabilitation. Wright's monograph, *Ethics in Rehabilitation*, followed his many previous publications on this important subject.

Legal Aspects of Ethical Conduct

Rehabilitation counselors become involved with legal issues in at least three ways. One may be called upon to testify in court as an "expert witness." Material revealed during counseling may be relevant to a trial or hearing. And involvement in a civil lawsuit is possible when it is alleged that, by either omission or commission in the professional relationship, the counselor must be held liable for the acts of a client.

Every counselor wonders what to do if subpoenaed to testify in court about confidential information revealed by a client. Questions center around the counselor's legal rights, the risk of being held in contempt of court, societal obligations to tell the truth, and the ethical obligation to the client regarding confidential information. As Berven [1968] advised, counselors should be prepared for the time when they will have to answer these questions for themselves. Generally rehabilitation counselors are not legally immune from being compelled to testify in court about clients. Still they should have some knowledge of the notion of "privileged communication" so that they can respond knowledgeably if the situation arises.

An Institute on Rehabilitation Issues [U.S. IRI, 1976] discussed confidential information, "privileged communication," and the possible consequences of a breach of confidence. The concept of confidentiality is based on the individual's right to privacy, expressed or implied, and has both legal and ethical implications. Confidentiality means that disclosures of the client to the professional will not be revealed to others except under certain circumstances. A breach of confidence may make the professional liable for damages in a tort action for invasion of privacy or for defamation.

Privileged communication is granted by statute to protect a client's confidential communication with a professional (one who is included under the state's statutes) from being disclosed against the client's will in a legal proceeding. Unless the client has waived these rights, he or she has the privilege of preventing the professional from answering questions about their communication when the professional is called as a witness in court. It is important, therefore, that professionals know the relevant law, if any, in their jurisdiction.

Since privileged communication is a right, the client is free to waive it. When the privilege is waived, all relevant information that the professional has must be disclosed in court—neither the client not the professional may withhold any particular items that could be detrimental to the case. There is usually no liability for invasion of the right to privacy or for defamation when a person does what the law compels.

When a professional believes that a client may inflict self-injury, there is an obligation to take the action necessary to protect the person, including commitment to a mental institution, even though the counselor may have to reveal information given in confidence. Although primary consideration must be given to the client, it is also necessary to consider the welfare and safety of others. If a client informs a counselor of the intention to kill someone and the counselor believes this possible, the counselor has a duty to disclose this information to the police if the client cannot otherwise be prevented from carrying out the threat.

Issues of confidentiality are also encountered in determinations regarding an individual's right of access to personal case record information collected by public and private agencies. Recent federal legislation has been designed to expand and further protect the constitutional right of privacy of individuals concerning whom identifiable information is recorded and to make such records available to them so that they may exert control over the content and accuracy of the information.

The rehabilitation counseling profession has not, as yet, received the statutory recognition that would protect a client's confidential communication as intrinsically privileged. Support for refusal to disclose information regarded as confidential can be found, however, in the various federal and state laws and regulations that dictate the administration of the public vocational rehabilitation program. The mere fact that a communication was made in confidence to a professionally competent person is not enough for the relationship to be granted a privilege, however. The courts have generally held in fact that no privilege does exist for the particular relationship.

When counselors are subpoenaed to testify in court as to a client's confidential disclosures, they face a severe dilemma. If they reveal confidential information, they may be inflicting irreparable damage upon untold numbers of counseling relationships, as well as violating a personal and professional trust. If they refuse to testify, they may be held in contempt of court and be subjected to court-imposed penalties. If they attempt to shade the truth, they may face perjury charges. Under the circumstances they must carefully weigh many factors in making a decision whether to testify or not to testify. Fortunately this is a relatively unusual problem for rehabilitation counselors.

In public agencies and most private agencies, professional employees are provided legal services for problems encountered in connection with their appointed and properly executed duties. This may include legal representation if the counselor is sued by a client or guardian for alleged malpractice. While civil action against counselors is uncommon, the American Personnel and Guidance Association does sponsor a low-cost malpractice insurance coverage for members (including ARCA members) through a commercial insurance carrier. This insurance may cover lawyer fees as well as possible damages if a counselor is sued.

2.2.3. CREDENTIALS

The evidence that provides assurance of the competency of the professional to practice and use the title is provided through several devices that are collectively referred to as credentials.

Certification

A rehabilitation counselor can now be recognized as a professional by qualifying for the title "Certified Rehabilitation Counselor," indicated by the letters "CRC" after the worker's name. As Hansen [1977] said, certification is intended mainly to establish standards by which disabled people, other professionals, administrators, and the general public can assess the competence of persons practicing rehabilitation counseling. The major objective is to provide assurances that professionals engaged in rehabilitation counseling will meet acceptable standards of quality in their practice.

The certification program for rehabilitation counselors was an outgrowth of the concern of NRCA and ARCA. They hoped to set standards that would consequently stabilize the field of rehabilitation counseling and thus lay the foundation for future professional growth. They established a joint committee on certification that became an independent incorporation now known as the Commission on Rehabilitation Counselor Certification (CRCC). It consists of five appointees from NRCA; five from ARCA; one each from the National Council on Rehabilitation Education (NCRE), the Council on Rehabilitation Education (CORE), the Council of State Administrators of Vocational Rehabilitation (CSAVR), the (International) Association of Rehabilitation Facilities (ARF), and the National Association of Non-White Rehabilitation Workers; and three consumer representatives from the American Coalition of Citizens With Disabilities.

Certification is a salient issue for rehabilitation counselors and their employers. The program for rehabilitation counselor certification was begun July 1, 1974 by CRCC. It provides professional recognition of minimum standards of counselor competency as reflected by education, experience, peer and supervisor evaluation, and a standardized national examination. At a 1976 meeting of the Rehabilitation Services Administration (RSA) Advisory Council on Rehabilitation Counseling, the Advisory Council advised that the RSA advocate legislation and other measures to require state-federal and private rehabilitation agencies to employ only certified rehabilitation counselors [Feinberg, 1977].

Licensure

The requirement of a license to practice a trade or profession is provided by state legislation, which regulates the practice and the title of the occupation. Because of its legal basis, licensure subjects violators to greater legal sanctions than does certification. For this reason and because it is broader in coverage, licensure is generally regarded as desirable when a considerable percentage of people in a profession are in private practice. Licensure boards usually have quasi-legislative power to make rules and examine applicants for licenses [Forster, 1977].

Licensing protects an unwary public from charlatans or from well-intentioned but inadequately trained practitioners. Rehabilitation counseling is clearly an occupation in which practice may result in harm or exploitation by the uninformed or the unscrupulous practitioner. Still the attempts to obtain licensure for rehabilitation counselors are only beginning. Closely allied professions (e.g., counseling psychology) are subject to licensing requirement in most states, however.

Registration

It is through licensing or certification that one becomes "registered." A person becomes registered by paying a fee after being licensed or certified in the profession. An annual fee maintains the registration. [Gianforte, 1976].

Education Program Accreditation

In this process an independent accrediting agency certifies that an educational institution meets certain established standards as determined through evaluations. In some professions, graduates of accredited preparation programs are considered to have all of the required credentials of the profession.

The accreditation of rehabilitation counselor education (RCE) programs followed the development at the University of Wisconsin Rehabilitation Research Institute (UW-RRI) of a new method of program evaluation, published in 1970 as *A Device for Systematic Planning and Evaluation of Rehabilitation Counselor Education* by Wright, Reagles, and Lewin. Recognizing that this research approach could be the basis for RCE accreditation, the principle author, as director of the Institute, organized the founding meetings of the accreditation mechanism subsequently incorporated as the Council on Rehabilitation Education (CORE). Selected leaders from several associations were invited to review the UW-RRI program evaluation strategies as the basis for an accrediting mechanism. The resulting organization, CORE, was mainly composed of representatives from this initial group. Consequently the Council has had two representatives from each of the following five associations: ARCA, NRCA, NCRE, CSAVR, and ARF.

The basic purpose of all accreditation efforts is to ensure quality education. The CORE accreditation procedure promotes program self-improvement as a regular system. These efforts assist in placing rehabilitation counseling on a par with other professional disciplines. Finally, and most importantly, such procedures ensure a level of excellence in professional training, with the ultimate goal of improving service delivery to rehabilitation clients. CORE, with the research assistance of the UW-RRI and federal-grant funds developed an evaluation and consulting procedure that provides for information input from students, graduates, and employers as well as faculty in the RCE evaluation for ac-

creditation [Wright & Reagles, 1973; Berven & Wright, 1978].

Daniel McAlees and Brocman Schumacher have been recognized for their administrative leadership in the successful program outcome of rehabilitation counselor certification (CRCC) and RCE accreditation (CORE), respectively.

2.2.4. PROFESSIONAL COMMITMENT

"When a person enters a profession," as Whitehouse [1969] said, "he engages in a way of life. The nature of this passage and the personal dedication it requires is tied to the substance and purposes of the profession. Rehabilitation counseling penetrates deeply into the stream of humanity. Consequently, it carries a responsibility that should not be entered upon unless the person entering recognizes the kind of commitment it requires and accepts its demands" [p. 246].

Qualification does mean responsibility. Whitehouse wrote of "the hours freely given; the discomfort and frustration borne with good grace; the anxiety of honest, but uncertain decisions; the promotion of courage when a great deal is required; the devotion to continued learning; the dedication to ideals; the empathetic strain on emotions; the lack of capricious freedom that others enjoy but that costs us too much in time." But as he pointed out, it is more difficult for the rehabilitationist to be patient with a society that treats disabled people harshly than to be patient with the clients themselves.

2.3. Preparation

A very good summary of the importance of professional preparation for rehabilitation counseling is the following material, from the testimony of Carl Hansen [1973], as president of the National Rehabilitation Counseling Association, to a Select Subcommittee of the Congress that was considering the continuation of federal support (grants) for rehabilitation education.

The rehabilitation counseling profession represents the best system yet designed to coordinate all community services to meet all the rehabilitation needs of the handicapped individual. The rehabilitation counselor is the synthesizer for understanding the handicapped person's problems globally, and through his

training, experience and understanding, attempts to meet the disabled individual's needs [p. 210].

Extensive research strongly indicates a need for rehabilitation counselors trained at the masters degree level. It has been found that graduates of Rehabilitation Counselor Education (RCE) masters degree programs are more willing to accept the "high risk" cases (the severely handicapped who require greater time and skill) and that they are more sensitive to and concerned with improving service delivery systems [Ayer, Wright, & Butler, 1968]. Furthermore, clients served by these professionally prepared rehabilitation counselors are more satisfied with the services they receive [Reagles, Wright, & Butler, 1970]. And well-served clients maintain a suitable level of vocational adjustment at follow-up [Gay, Reagles, & Wright, 1971]. Moreover, as Hansen testified, the state-federal rehabilitation system "supports the belief that masters level rehabilitation counselors serve clients better by showing a preference to hire people with a masters degree. These and other studies support the need for graduate level trained rehabilitation counselors" [p. 213].

A convincing argument for the support of RCE grants is that graduates make use of their professional preparation. A high percentage of RCE graduates go into the field of rehabilitation, as reported in research by Wright, Reagles, and Scorzelli [1973]. Of 534 randomly selected graduates who had received federal rehabilitation stipends while in graduate school, 83 percent were employed full-time, and 87.6 percent of those were employed in a rehabilitation setting with 43.7 percent working for state rehabilitation agencies. The RCE programs are clearly meeting the manpower needs of rehabilitation agencies and so the Congress has approved educational grant support since 1954.

Rehabilitation counselor education programs are obliged to continue this excellent record. This can best be assured by their own evaluation efforts as described by Geist, Hershenson, and Hafer [1975].

2.3.1. REHABILITATION EDUCATION

While the emphasis here is on rehabilitation counselor education, there are a number of higher education degree programs interfluent with rehabilitation work. Specialization in rehabilitation is offered in schools of medicine, social work, and other instructional programs. The level of instruction ranges from undergraduate to postdoctoral. With the encouragement of federal-grant support for training (discussed elsewhere), American colleges and universities have responded to the need for special preparation to work with rehabilitation clients [Wright & Katz, 1969].

Prior to the establishment of rehabilitation education programs it was necessary for the state rehabilitation agencies and other employers to try to train new staff members who had little previous experience or relevant education. Critics of rehabilitation counselor educa-

tion thought that the only needed attribute of a rehabilitationist was a desire to help. They were unaware of the complexity of the problems of handicapped people and the solutions available in the developing technology. Good performance actually requires both academic instruction (including knowledge and skills) and the development of certain personality attributes such as emotional adjustment, projected warmth, and interest in other individuals. The dilemma is solved by a student selection policy in rehabilitation education of screening applicants not only for academic potential but also for nonintellectual requirements [Pepper, 1976]. Evaluative criteria include not only previous grade-point average and aptitude test scores but also personal data from letters of reference, personal interview, and experience record.

Preparation for a profession is more complex than training for a skilled trade. For many years, though, it was thought that rehabilitation counselors, after a general education, could be trained on the job. Perceptive individuals, through self-study in counseling, human behavior, and other critical studies did indeed master the prerequisite education. And in time, they developed their skills through on-the-job practice with disabled people who sought their counsel. Many of these rehabilitation agency employees eventually became qualified in their work because of the remarkable opportunity to learn from experience as clients were followed through the rehabilitation process from beginning to end.

Preprofessional education and continuing or on-the-job instruction should not be seen as separate alternatives for rehabilitation counselor preparation. Both education and training have a role. The locus for formal preparation, however, is the university, which in preservice education provides the fundamental, generalized, and systematic knowledge essential to performance. Education prepares professionals who "infuse the real with the ideal," as Sinick [1973] said, "who are proactive rather than merely reactive" [p. 170]. Education provides the background for ongoing development in a dynamic field of study. It is a career-long endeavor.

Education, on the other hand, should not be cluttered with agency rules and specific procedures. Some tasks are best learned on the job, but these are activities that the rehabilitationist engages in that require supervised experiential learning. In rehabilitation counselor education, clinical practice that builds professional skills is integrated with the acquisition of theory and principles through classroom instruction.

A sound professional education program must prepare students to deal with the future—not only for the time immediately following their graduation but also for their entire professional careers. In other words, one of the bases of a professional education is to teach students to continue learning throughout their lives. Programs preparing students for professions that serve the needs of others must, especially, take into account these changing needs to determine what kinds of professional knowledge and skills are required both for the present and for the future [Anthony, Slowkowski, & Bendix, 1978].

The number of rehabilitation education programs has grown steadily since the 1954 Amendments to the Vocational Rehabilitation Act (PL 565), which authorized federal subsidy. By 1965 about 40 colleges and universities offered graduate degrees in rehabilitation counseling with nearly 100 programs by 1980. Federally sponsored traineeships for students and financial support for the institutions providing professional education were instrumental in encouraging universities and prospective students to go into RCE programs, thus meeting the need for qualified rehabilitationists.

Word of the success of American RCE programs has spread over the world. A number of other nations are starting training projects based on adaptations of the American model and utilizing the new technology of vocational rehabilitation.

2.3.2. STANDARDS AND STRUCTURE

The rapid development of rehabilitation technology makes it necessary for RCE programs to demand higher standards. The content of such programs has developed to the point that what one learns is not merely important, but necessary for the provision of adequate services. This goal is reflected in the "Statement of Policy on the Professional Preparation of Rehabilitation Counselors" by the American Rehabilitation Counseling Association [1974], drafted by Richard Thoreson at the request of the ARCA president and approved by its board and membership:

A statement of Professional Preparation and Standards from a professional organization must necessarily serve the broad interests of the professional community. Such a statement should not constrain or discourage the application of research and demonstration findings and should possess inherent durability to survive the daily successes, failures, and conflicts associated with dynamic professional growth.

I. Statement Objectives—A Statement on Professional Preparation and Standards in Rehabilitation Counselor Education Should:
  A. Promote concern for quality in the establishment and review of professional education programs in rehabilitation counseling that in turn will lead to better services for people with handicaps.
  B. Encourage self-study and improvement of rehabilitation counseling programs to insure the maintenance of competencies relevant to the professional field.
  C. Help to meet manpower needs of agencies providing rehabilitation services by insuring that graduates have been instructed in the skills and knowledge necessary for delivering vocational rehabilitation services to disabled and disadvantaged people.
  D. Protect the needs and rights of students who wish to acquire the knowledge and skills requisite for obtaining adequate employment as counselors in the vocational rehabilitation field and who wish to continue their professional development as the field evolves.
  E. Offer an articulated standard of professional education in vocational rehabilitation counseling through which mutual respect and cooperation with programs in other helping professions can be fostered.

II. Objectives of Professional Education in the Field—The Objective of Graduate Education is to Prepare the Individual for Entering Upon a Lifelong Profession, not for a Specific Job or Position. Therefore, a Rehabilitation Counselor Education Program Should:
  A. Provide students with basic education in rehabilitation counseling and promote the knowledge and skills necessary to provide adequate vocational rehabilitation services to handicapped people.
  B. Foster in the learner the development of habits of scholarship and professionalism, a commitment to respecting individual human values, support of high ethical standards and personal integrity, and maintenance of an objective and inquiring attitude.
  C. Foster the development of practitioners, educators, and researchers, through a program of academic study, clinical training, continuing education, and consultation that will lead to effective practice in the field.
  D. Promote the advancement of knowledge and skill in the field of rehabilitation counseling by conducting research and demonstration ac-

tivities and facilitating the incorporation of new and improved practices in the educational process and, where possible, in the field through continuing education consultation [pp. 3–4].

In addition to these objectives, the ARCA Policy Statement also outlines the following:

III. Standards for the academic program, including both generic and specialized knowledge and skill components.
IV. Standards for supervised experience in both practicum and internship forms of clinical practice.
V. Standards for faculty in relation to profession, academic, and community service activities.
VI. Standards for student recruitment and retention.
VII. Standards for student rights and responsibilities.

The discerning student can become more familiar with the specific standards by referring to the original work.

Undergraduate Education

The originator of undergraduate rehabilitation education was Kenneth Hylbert [1963], a professor who pioneered his program at Pennsylvania State University despite early opposition from officials of the federal rehabilitation agency and some rehabilitation counselor educators. Finally the federal rehabilitation agency decided in 1972 to support the development of bachelor's degree level rehabilitation programs. Consequently, a large number of graduate RCE programs began to develop new undergraduate components, and many other colleges began offering undergraduate majors in rehabilitation. Incentives in the form of federal support aside, these institutions of higher education were responding to both students who sought new opportunities to major in the human service areas and to rehabilitation agencies that needed generically trained bachelor's degree level rehabilitation personnel. By the end of the decade about 50 new undergraduate rehabilitation programs were well established or underway. Curricula were usually set up in accordance with the federal training guidelines, which called for generic programs in rehabilitation [Feinberg, Sunblad, & Glick, 1974].

Although it is widely believed in America that professional training in counseling is for graduate students only, vital needs are served by the various (noncounseling) undergraduate "rehabilitation education" programs. Pennsylvania State University, when it broke new ground on the undergraduate level, provided a sound foundation upon which later programs could be based. Hylbert [1963] discussed certain aspects of the curriculum:

Originally the curriculum was considered to exist primarily to prepare students for employment immediately upon graduation. However, . . . it now provides undergraduate preparation appropriate for students who desire graduate study in a variety of helping relationships.

It continues to serve as a terminal program for students wishing to take entry positions with public and private agencies and institutions concerned with rehabilitation, job placement, health and welfare, and related services, such as rehabilitation caseworker, industrial therapist, and employment interviewers [p. 23].

More recently, Steger [1974] has discussed undergraduate rehabilitation education not only from the perspective of paraprofessional training and preliminary study for the potential graduate student, but also as a basis for multidisciplinary training for the various professions involved in the broad field of rehabilitation. He suggested a common core for undergraduate rehabilitation education with eight categories of skill and knowledge.

1. Multidisciplinary collaboration: Basic group skills and productive experience in working with people from other disciplines.
2. Communication skills: The ability to communicate with clients and colleagues clearly and to understand the professional vocabulary.
3. Problem-solving: The ability to secure the information needed to identify goals and alternatives and to implement them for a client in the most appropriate manner.
4. Use of resources: The skill required to identify community resources and see that the client is put in touch with them.
5. Knowledge of the individual: The basic physical, psychological, and social elements of human development.
6. Knowledge of social variables: Along with the general implications of social variables, rehabilitation workers need to understand the social aspects of stigma.
7. Knowledge of the effects of disability: An understanding of the complexity of the consequences of disability.

8. Knowledge of rehabilitation: The history, philosophy, legal basis, and organizational structure of rehabilitation.

Graduate Education

Among American rehabilitation organizations there is consensus that the professional entry level for a rehabilitation counselor should be the masters degree. This requires two years of explicit education and skills training beyond an appropriate bachelors degree (i.e., four years of undergraduate study in psychology and rehabilitation-related subjects).

As long recognized, successful rehabilitation counselors need competence in a number of areas concerned with the adjustment of people disabled [Lee, 1955]. An early conference report in 1956 by Hall and Warren identified the competencies required. (That one-week workshop, sponsored by the National Rehabilitation Association and the National Vocational Guidance Association, provided the initial guidelines for curriculum planning by the new, federally funded, RCE programs.) The knowledge and skills needed by rehabilitation counselors in the performance of their functions were listed (not necessarily in order of importance) as follows:

1. An understanding of human growth and development; the effect of childhood and adolescent experiences upon adult behavior.
2. An understanding of human anatomy and physiology; the effects of disease or injury on body structure, functions, behavior, and personality.
3. An understanding of mental and emotional conditions affecting social and vocational adjustment, their nature, course, and probable cause.
4. The ability to detect and identify the manifestations of disability, mental or physical, and to understand their relationships to vocational and social adjustment.
5. Familiarity with medical information, therapies, prosthesis, services, and equipment designed to remove or minimize the effects of disability.
6. The ability to use accepted methods and techniques of individual case study, recording, evaluation, and reporting, and to adapt procedures to the practices of employing agencies.
7. The ability to establish and maintain a satisfactory counseling relationship.

8. The ability to use methods and techniques of vocational and personal counseling to assist clients in achieving an understanding of their problems and potentialities and in planning constructively for their rehabilitation.
9. The ability to analyze occupations in terms of skills, physical demands, training requirements, and working conditions.
10. An understanding of relationships of aptitudes, skills, interests, and educational background of the handicapped person to occupational requirements.
11. An understanding of community organizations and of the facilities and procedures, policies, and limitations under which their services are made available to applicants.
12. The ability to make use of available community services and resources in meeting problems of disabled persons and to maintain effective relationships with such sources.
13. The ability to analyze the rehabilitation needs of a community and to organize resources to meet these needs.
14. An understanding of the relationship of administrative policies and procedures to the counselor's work.
15. The ability to organize work to make the most economical use of one's time.
16. The ability to analyze reports furnishing medical, psychological, or social data and to interpret the relationship of such data to the needs of the client.
17. The ability to carry on basic study and research growing out of rehabilitation work and to interpret and apply the findings.
18. The ability to use consultative services both within and outside the rehabilitation agency.
19. The ability to utilize national, regional, and state reports concerning industrial, occupational, and labor market trends, and to analyze specific community job information and opportunities.
20. The ability to collect occupational information and use it effectively in counseling.
21. The ability to orient employers to the employment of disabled persons.
22. An understanding of federal, state, and local laws pertaining to rehabilitation and an understanding of related social legislation.
23. An understanding of agency policies, practices, and standards as they apply to the counselor's work.

24. The ability to interpret agency policy, laws, and regulations to clients and others.

The rehabilitation leaders and counselor educators who, in July, 1955, compiled this competency list at the University of Virginia in Charlottesville, had remarkable foresight. A quarter of a century later rehabilitation graduate programs are still following these guidelines. There is different emphasis today, however, due to changing responsibilities of rehabilitation counselors. The state rehabilitation agency was once the only large employer of graduates, but applicants now have a broad selection of opportunities. Thus the role is a broader one and educators have responded with a broader curriculum. New courses include vocational assessment, job placement, group counseling, independent living, and behavioral modification. The original list of 24 competencies has been expanded because of the greater awareness of the problem-solving approach to successful rehabilitation that has grown out of a sound research base. In addition there are variations in university rehabilitation counseling curricula due to specializations, unique models, and program goals.

The clinical practice component of professional training is essential in the development of counselor abilities. For accreditation, CORE requires that a graduate program for rehabilitation counseling students include at least 600 hours of supervised clinical practice. Relevance to rehabilitation and client needs should dictate the choice of what types of agencies and facilities are used for field experiences.

Supervision of clinical practice is primarily the responsibility of an RCE faculty member (perhaps with the assistance of a doctoral student working under the direction of the doctoral level faculty member). Also sharing the supervisory responsibility is a professional employee of the agency in which the clinical practice student is placed. There is general agreement that agency supervisors should have the RCE masters degree and be certified rehabilitation counselors. Some agencies pay the advanced clinical practice students (Interns) because their contribution to the agency outweighs the supervisory time they require [Geist, 1977].

The preferred method of practicum supervision at the university level is the individual conference. This is supplemented by audio and/or video tapes or vision screens [Taylor, Sales, & Lavender, 1971].

2.3.3. CONTINUING DEVELOPMENT

Any profession should encourage the continuing development of its members. Part of this responsibility falls upon the individual practitioner, who must seek out experiences that will facilitate professional growth. However, this responsibility is shared by agencies employing the rehabilitation counselors, by universities, and by professional associations, all of which organize vehicles for continuing education, professional development, research utilization, and knowledge dissemination. A primary means of providing this experience is through in-service training offered by and within agencies.

In-service education for rehabilitation counselors and for persons with assigned supervisory duties became increasingly important in the 1950s and 1960s because of a rapid growth in personnel and a broadening of their responsibilities. With the expansion of rehabilitation programs and appropriations, many more clients came to state-federal rehabilitation agencies. The need for staff competency was again stressed as cases became more difficult after the Congress in 1973 mandated priority acceptance of the severely handicapped and in 1978 authorized services for independent living.

Regional Rehabilitation Continuing Education Programs (RRCEP), authorized in 1974 and funded by the federal rehabilitation agency, offer a program of staff training to improve and renew professionally relevant rehabilitation knowledge and skills. While they appear to be serving an important need for most state rehabilitation agencies, the emphasis of the RRCEP projects is on staff training as contrasted with professional development and advanced education.

The following purposes for RRCEP grantees are from federal rehabilitation agency guidelines:

1. To train newly employed and inexperienced rehabilitation counseling personnel of state rehabilitation agencies in the basic knowledge and skills of rehabilitation counseling practice in the public rehabilitation program.
2. To train newly employed state agency staff at the administrative, supervisory, professional, subprofessional, or clerical levels in order to develop needed skills for effective agency performance.
3. To provide training opportunities for experienced state agency personnel at all levels of practice to upgrade their skills and to develop

mastery of new program developments dealing with significant issues, priorities, and legislative thrusts of the public rehabilitation program.

4. To develop and conduct training programs for staff of private rehabilitation agencies and facilities that participate closely with state rehabilitation agencies in the delivery of services.

It is apparent that continuing improvement and effort are justified for in-service and out-service training since quality varies greatly. Perhaps the most successful staff instruction was the work-study approach as described by Porter and Settles [1968]. The work-study programs, now largely replaced by the RRCEP centers, were conducted by local universities for the state rehabilitation agencies. The participants were usually caseload-carrying counselors who were given study time to obtain the masters degree in rehabilitation counseling. A large number of state rehabilitation counselors obtained their masters degree in RCE through these programs. Unfortunately, these arrangements with local universities generally have not been continued for state agency staff wishing postmasters instruction for further advancement.

2.3.4. STAFF DEVELOPMENT MATERIALS

The federal rehabilitation agency throughout its long history has sponsored programs and materials for state agency staff development. Even when the federal agency was seriously understaffed, they managed to stimulate and participate in practitioner training sessions.

In September, 1920, the rehabilitation staff of the U.S. Federal Board for Vocational Education issued a bulletin titled *Industrial Rehabilitation—A Statement of Policies to be Observed in the Administration of the Industrial Rehabilitation Act*. This was the first of the Industrial Rehabilitation Series of booklets published for state staff instruction. Others included: *General Administration and Case Procedures* [March, 1921] covering topics such as "cooperation with social agencies," "records," "the case method," "making the contact," "interviewing the disabled person," "determination of eligibility," "determination of job objective," "types of training," "realization of job objective," and "follow-up"; and *Services of*

Advisement and Cooperation [October, 1921b], which covered "stimulation of courage and interest," "maintenance," "physical restoration," "prosthetic appliances," "knowledge of occupations," "training," "placement," and "work conditions." Also in 1921, the Federal Board [1921a] published *Bibliography on Vocational Guidance*.

Training materials continued to be printed for state rehabilitation professionals. The need to improve standards was pointed out by Blauch, who wrote a 1938 U.S. Government Printing Office book [Staff Study Number 9] titled *Vocational Rehabilitation of the Physically Disabled*. He proposed that the state rehabilitation field agents, then numbering 330 (including supervisors and administrators), should have a "minimum of two years of training at the college level" [p. 53]. He further noted the need for in-service training since "institutions do not offer special courses of study as preparation for the work" [p. 54].

Over the years, with changes in staff qualifications, professional standards, agency practices, and available resources, the federal agency has shifted its training policies. For example, as mentioned above, in the 1970s the concept of regional training centers for state agency staff preparation replaced state university out-service work-study plans. The greatest impact on training directions came with the advent of federal training grants in 1954.

2.3.5. WORKSHOPS AND INSTITUTES

The most effective method for the production of rehabilitation staff development materials has been in use since 1947 [Massie, 1974]. After advance planning and with staff leadership, the federal agency sponsored a workshop in Washington for state rehabilitation agency "guidance, training, and placement supervisors." The proceedings of this first "Workshop for Guidance, Training, and Placement" (GTP) were published in 1947 by the Office of Vocational Rehabilitation of the Federal Security Agency. The second GTP workshop was held two years later and the same procedure—with refinements, expansions, and name changes—has continued annually thereafter.

In 1962, following review of the GTP workshop experience, it was decided to involve universities as sponsors of study groups to broaden the scope of ideas from participant. That year the name was changed to the Institute on Rehabilitation Services (IRS), but the proceedings were still published by the federal rehabilitation agency, then the U.S. Department of Health, Education, and Welfare, Vocational Rehabilitation Administration (U.S. HEW, VRA). Additional changes occurred in 1973 with new funding arrangements for an annual Institute on Rehabilitation Issues (IRI). The proceedings of the Institutes were thereafter published by several federally sponsored university Rehabilitation Research and Training (R & T) Centers (namely, the universities of Arkansas, Wisconsin-Stout, and West Virginia). The annual Insti-

tutes were still sponsored, however, by the federal rehabilitation agency, the Rehabilitation Service Administration (RSA).

Cumulatively the product of this uninterrupted series of annual workshops (or institutes) contains most of what is known about rehabilitation counselor techniques. (Every one of these reports to date has been researched and utilized in the preparation of this book.) In the References section at the end of this book there is a complete listing of all U.S. GTP, IRS, and IRI references, arranged chronologically under the special heading, "U.S. [Rehabilitation Institute Publications]."

2.4. Related Areas

A number of occupations are so closely associated with rehabilitation counseling that they could be regarded as specializations. This occupational cluster encompasses the professional functions traditionally performed by the generalist rehabilitation counselor—disability determination, work evaluation, vocational assessment, rehabilitation planning, personal and vocational adjustment counseling and instruction, and job placement. The public rehabilitation agency generally recognizes "rehabilitation counseling"—with various qualification grades and specializations—as the legitimate title of the profession. Private rehabilitation facilities, however, are likely to have separate job titles, even though the differences are nominal as to qualifications. The following occupational descriptions are from various sources.

2.4.1. WORK EVALUATOR

The primary responsibility of the work evaluator (cf. vocational evaluator), regardless of setting, is to help determine the rehabilitation client's vocational potential and rehabilitation strategy. Work evaluators must first identify the vocational problems and gain an understanding of the rehabilitation needs of each individual client. Their primary method of evaluation is to present clients with real or simulated work activities in order to observe, analyze, and predict the client's future work performance. Moreover, they must consider if an inadequate performance by a client is due to physical or mental limitations, inappropriate work habits, or lack of

work skills or experiences, and what rehabilitative services could minimize these problems [U.S. IRS, 1972a].

According to the Vocational Evaluation and Work Adjustment Association [1975], the primary difference between the vocational evaluator and the rehabilitation counselor is that the evaluator usually has a much better opportunity to observe a client over a protracted period of time (e.g., half a day to a year or more). The evaluator thus becomes an expert in conducting and recording behavioral observations, concretely and factually, so that they are understandable to subsequent readers. The work evaluator then helps the counselor with the difficult task of synthesizing these data with other types of client evaluations into meaningful interpretations.

The evaluator utilizes psychometric tests, standardized work samples, and temporary placement in actual job settings, either within a rehabilitation facility or in competitive employment, to produce a work evaluation report. Job analysis is an important ancillary technique that provides information for matching a person with a job and creating work samples [Hoffman, 1972].

Work evaluators are employed in rehabilitation facilities; in institutions for the mentally ill, the retarded, and the public offender; in schools with special education students; and in vocational and technical schools. The evaluator can also be employed as an expert consultant to perform vocational appraisals for compensation insurance companies, to report disability determination evaluations to social security examiners, and to advise industrial firms on the selection of workers.

Individuals employed as work evaluators come from varied backgrounds, including industry, the skilled trades, business, and education. The fact that these evaluators are employed in a variety of facilities with different goals and objectives complicates the formation of personnel qualifications. Until recently, most facilities established their own employment standards with regard to education and work experience. However, the trend is now toward employing evaluators with graduate training and toward increasing the professional status of this discipline.

The status of work evaluation has been furthered by the formation of the Vocational Evaluation and Work Adjustment Association (VEWAA) as a Division of the National Rehabilitation Association, by the publication of a journal, by in-service training, and by various projects [Ross, 1971].

2.4.2. WORK ADJUSTMENT SPECIALIST

A good way to define a work adjustment specialist is to start with a definition of work adjustment. *Work adjustment* is a rather vague term, more often than not defined operationally to fit whatever service is being offered. Those facilities that try to define work adjustment services precisely often describe it as work-habit training, work hardening, work readiness training, personal (or social) adjustment training, or work-skill training. Many facilities assume that all work is therapeutic and that therefore work adjustment training means offering the client some type of work activity. Others have specific procedures and curricula to conduct the work adjustment program. These sophisticated programs often use behavior modification techniques [Pruitt, 1973]. An all-encompassing definition of work adjustment, however, has been developed by participants in the Tenth Institute on Rehabilitation Services [U.S. IRS, 1972a]:

Work adjustment is a treatment/training process utilizing individual and group work, or work related activities, to assist individuals in understanding the meaning, value, and demands of work; to modify or develop attitudes, personal characteristics, and work behavior; and to develop functional capacities, as required, in order to assist individuals toward their optimum level of vocational development [pp. 3–4].

The responsibilities of the work adjustment specialist might include: educating clients as to the proper conduct of a worker (e.g., when to take breaks, why it is important to be on time, how a work situation is different from school); adjusting schedules and work assignments to help clients build physical stamina and work tolerance; using behavior modification techniques to improve work performance (e.g., use of production charts to show improvement); counseling clients on interpersonal problems affecting their work performance; dealing with day-to-day client problems (e.g., handling money and arranging transportation to work); report writing; and meeting with other members of the rehabilitation team.

There are no certificates or degree programs for a work adjustment specialist, perhaps because of the similarity to the education required for a rehabilitation counselor. There are short-term training programs for workshop personnel in this field, and several universities offer courses in work adjustment.

2.4.3. EMPLOYMENT COUNSELOR

The employment counselor (sometimes called a "vocational counselor") performs many of the same functions as a rehabilitation counselor although the title differs according to setting. The employment counselor is typically associated with the state employment service agency and works with handicapped job seekers. Job seekers may include youth with little work experience, older workers, the disabled, veterans, and individuals unhappy with their present jobs or displaced because of automation. This clientele, which includes former prison inmates, welfare recipients, and the educationally or socially disadvantaged, may have underdeveloped skills or various other difficulties in getting jobs. Like the rehabilitation counselor, the employment counselor interviews the job seeker, arranges testing, and gathers information from other sources when necessary to develop a vocational plan with the individual. The plan may specify further education, job training, work experience, or other activities needed to enhance employability. Employment counselors can help people learn appropriate job-seeking skills and contact employers, although the client is usually encouraged to appear for placement interviews following counseling.

While employment counselors work mainly in state employment service offices, some are employed by the Veterans' Administration, Bureau of Indian Affairs, prisons, training schools for delinquent youths, and mental institutions. First-level employment counselors in the state employment services must meet the national qualification standard of 30 graduate semester hours beyond a bachelors degree, or one year of counseling experience in lieu of 15 graduate semester hours. All states require counselors in their employment service offices to pass state civil service or merit system requirements. Private and community agencies often do not have standardized entrance requirements for employment counselors, but many prefer masters level training in vocational counseling or a related field.

2.4.4. JOB PLACEMENT SPECIALIST

The title *job placement specialist* is used often in facilities, although individual agency labels include *placement counselor, manpower specialist, rehabilitation specialist (job placement), placement representative, manpower coordinator, placement consultant*, and *program specialist for employment development* [Hutchison & Cogan, 1974].

As with other specializations listed in this section, job placement is trying to establish itself as a professional entity in the field of rehabilitation. However, as a group, placement specialists have not had either the graduate education or the professional recognition that rehabilitation counselors have obtained. The importance and uniqueness of placement activities have been promoted by William Usdane [1976] who said there is "far more spillover and reinforcement of job functions within a rehabilitation facility among the psychologist, social worker and rehabilitation counselor than there would be between any of these professions and that of the placement worker" [p. 165].

According to the participants in the 1971 Institute on Rehabilitation Services [U.S. IRS, 1971], the following surveyed opinions reflect how rehabilitation placement workers have been regarded in state rehabilitation agencies.

Placement Consultant: Serves as an advisor to the rehabilitation staff in all phases of the placement process. May assist with staff development training to provide higher level of competence in the field of placement. Assists counselors to evaluate client readiness for employment. Provides occupational information relative to specific job objectives. May accompany placement personnel on job development visits to prospective employers. Works with counselor on job adjustment problems which need to be taken into consideration in bringing a case to successful closure. Is usually a rehabilitation supervisor with orientation to the business world and with a thorough knowledge of rehabilitation.

Job Development Specialist: Acts as liaison between the rehabilitation agency and the business and industrial community. Seeks placement opportunities for rehabilitation clients and promotes a favorable attitude with employers toward consideration of hiring the handicapped. Provides rehabilitation staff with occupational information and listings of job opportunities. May engineer special job opportunities for the severely handicapped. Is business, industry, and job analysis oriented. May, on request, get involved in the actual placement action on behalf of some clients.

Placement Counselor: A counselor with skills and orientation to the business and industrial field. Generally works as a teammate with a caseload-carrying counselor. At a given period in the rehabilitation process, assumes the major role of the counseling relationship with the client, providing services during the placement process.

Placement Specialist: The placement specialist for the blind, as originally conceived, was a special combination of the placement counselor and the job development specialist. One of the major tasks was to demonstrate to prospective employers that a blind client could perform certain jobs. The placement specialist did some job re-engineering in order to set up job requirements specifically suited to given situations, and also provided specific job performance instruction to newly-employed clients as well as job adjustment counseling. This same type of service might well be provided to clients from other disability groups needing specific services during the placement process beyond those normally provided [pp. 36–37].

It was recognized in a survey of state rehabilitation directors by Hutchison and Cogan [1974] that job placement specialists should have at least a bachelors degree and experience in job placement or vocational counseling, employment relations, occupational analysis, personnel, and/or technical or managerial experience in business and public relations. Job placement specialists are typically employed by rehabilitation facilities and, to a lesser extent, by state rehabilitation agencies.

2.4.5. WORKSHOP SUPERVISOR

Workshop floor supervisors work with handicapped individuals in a supervisory role. Tasks include inspecting work for quality and adherence to production requirements, assigning workers to production activities, ordering supplies, instructing workers in how to perform their job assignments, keeping attendance and production records, and supervising the work of volunteers and assistants, depending on the size of the workshop.

Floor supervisors have perhaps the most direct and most continuous involvement with the handicapped worker during the course of the day. Because of this, they serve as important role models for clients and are often in the most advantageous position to reinforce good work behaviors, to handle problems as they arise, and to carry out the rehabilitation plans laid out by the work adjustment specialist, rehabilitation counselor, psychologist, and others. They are crucial members of the rehabilitation team. They may be involved with a variety of industrial subcontract jobs or may supervise a specialized training area such as maintenance, food service, upholstering, or radio-television repair. It is often the floor supervisor who finds ways to help clients perform job tasks without letting their handicaps interfere with performance. The recording of work behaviors and other daily observations is another important function. In some rehabilitation facilities, the work adjustment specialist is also the floor supervisor.

Requirements for this position are highly variable. Frequently industrial arts instructors, skilled craftsmen, or industrial supervisors are selected for workshop supervision.

2.4.6. DISABILITY EXAMINER

The disability examiner or adjudicator generally works in a state rehabilitation agency and determines whether or not applicants for social security disability payments are eligible. The state rehabilitation program usually acts as an agent for the federal Social Security Administration in performing this function.

Rosse, Marra, and Novis [1962] conducted a study in which questionnaires were sent to adjudicators throughout the country and found the following rank order of disability adjudicator duties:

1. Determines through facts, standards, and guides whether the claimant is under a disability.
2. Evaluates evidence to determine if an immediate finding can be made or if additional evidence is required.
3. Secures additional medical evidence to confirm or refute existing evidence.
4. Explains disability insurance benefits requirements to other agencies, employers, medical and psychological professions, and others expressing interest.
5. Reviews and analyzes vocational rehabilitation case records using medical, vocational, social, educational, and other information as they relate to determining disability.
6. Analyzes part-time work or lowered earnings in terms of established criteria to determine substantiality of employment or "made" work.
7. Reviews wage record and other earnings data for coincidence of work stoppage with alleged date of onset of disability.
8. Secures clarification or additional pertinent evidence from claimant or other sources, as required.
9. Evaluates all case data to determine vocational rehabilitation potential of each claimant for possible referral.
10. Makes necessary recommendations when gaps exist in services.
11. Redevelops, reviews, and reevaluates evidence in cases at the appellate level.
12. Recognizes manifestations of physical and mental disabilities and their relationship to vocational adjustment.
13. Utilizes occupational information to assess work potential.
14. Secures information about the claimant's personality traits, attitudes, educational background, work experience, special interests, and social and economic circumstances.
15. Interviews claimant to help prepare requests to sources of medical information.
16. Establishes and maintains close working relationships with other agencies and professionals.
17. Provides for administration and interpretation of psychological tests when indicated.

Appropriate preprofessional preparation for this professional group is through the existing rehabilitation education programs, although relatively few disability examiners (adjudicators) are so prepared.

2.4.7. REHABILITATION TEACHER

The rehabilitation teacher or instructor (formerly called "home teacher") is a recently expanded professional role. Traditionally, rehabilitation programs for blind people have employed a staff to instruct clients for various activities of living in an environment designed for a sighted population. These instructors were often blind themselves and were not necessarily credentialed (e.g., teacher college degree or special education preparation).

Skills that are taught to blind clients by the rehabilitation teacher include: personal management (e.g., table etiquette, hygiene, and grooming); communication (e.g., reading and writing braille, techniques for listening to recorded materials, dialing a telephone); home management (e.g., cooking, laundering, caring for a child, budgeting); and leisure time activities (e.g., handicrafts, games). The rehabilitation teacher helps clients to obtain, adapt, and use special aids and devices such as braille watches, and household appliances. The instruction may be with individuals or small groups.

Extension of public rehabilitation to include severely handicapped individuals with nonvocational objectives will create a demand for qualified instructors attending to other disability (sighted) categories. Some Centers for Independent Living may follow an "educational model"

emphasizing instruction in self-care and coping with environmental and personal-social barriers to life adjustment.

2.4.8. ORIENTATION-MOBILITY TEACHER

This specialization (peripatology) in the rehabilitation of the blind or low-vision clients includes instruction in both orientation and mobility. Orientation involves an understanding of the layout of the environment and how to get from one location to another; mobility is considered to be the process of moving safely and efficiently from place to place in a socially acceptable manner.

The orientation and mobility teacher or specialist is responsible for assisting visually handicapped individuals to learn to travel independently. They must learn techniques such as the use of other senses and residual vision and the use of the long cane or other devices. Through individualized instruction, the visually impaired person can develop mobility skills and improve the self-confidence and problem-solving ability necessary for independent travel in familiar (or unfamiliar) environments. Mobility instructors for blind clients must have functional vision (no less than 20/40 visual acuity in the better eye with correction). Limitation in mobility may be caused by disabilities other than impaired vision (e.g., retardation, paraplegia); therefore mobility instruction is an important component of any comprehensive center for independent living serving a clientele with the full range of mental, emotional, and physical disabilities.

Chapter 3

Role and Functions

While the terms *role* and *function* are related, a conceptual distinction between them underlies the understanding of any occupation—including rehabilitation counseling. The separation of role from function is acknowledged in the 1968 American Rehabilitation Counseling Association policy statement on the preparation of rehabilitation counselors. ARCA proclaimed:

The functions of a counselor . . . vary according to the mandates under which the agency operates and the characteristics of the clientele. Although these functions may vary in nature, their ultimate objective is the same—to mobilize both client and environmental resources to meet client objectives. The role of the counselor, however, is the same from agency to agency. The role of the professional rehabilitation counselor is, primarily, to utilize face-to-face communication between counselor and client to bring about improved personal, educational, vocational, and social adjustment.

The role and function of rehabilitation counselors have been extensively studied. John Muthard at the State University of Iowa and later Florida State University has devoted much of his career to the topic. A notable study on the subject was published by the American Rehabilitation Association [Muthard & Salomone, 1969]. Over a 10-year period, the University of Wisconsin-Madison, Rehabilitation Research Institute (UW-RRI) conducted programmatic research on rehabilitation counselor functions. Much of the thought in this chapter in fact was stimulated by 16 of the UW-RRI monographs—the first two volumes of the *Wisconsin Studies in Vocational Rehabilitation* (Wright & Butler, 1968a; Wright & Reagles, 1973a).

3.1. Professional Role

Role is a composite of service functions dictated by the needs of a specified clientele as perceived by an organized profession. These service functions are facilitated by the competencies derived from a body of knowledge and skills. The helping competencies can be operationally described by the content of preprofessional preparation. To understand the contemporary role of rehabilitation counselors, it will be helpful to review first the history of their role development.

3.1.1. HISTORICAL PERSPECTIVE

Use of the term *vocational counseling* in rehabilitation and a description of the counseling function in rehabilitation appeared, probably for the first time, in January, 1920, in an article in *The Vocational Summary,* a monthly journal published by the U.S. Federal Board for Vocational Education (1920a), entitled "Problems of the Vocational Adjustment and Counseling of the Disabled Soldier and Sailor under the Vocational Rehabilitation Act"; its authorship was anonymous. The administrators of the Federal Board, however, did not appreciate the proper role of counselors. The rehabilitation program for the war-disabled adhered to authoritarian model: (1) the Bureau of War-Risk Insurance was given the power and duty to order disabled veterans to "follow suitable courses of vocational rehabilitation to be prescribed and provided by the Federal Board for Vocational Education;" and (2) benefits from War-Risk Insurance could be withheld from persons who "willfully failed to follow the prescribed course of vocational rehabilitation."

Over the years there has been a gradual shift of authority in determining what services will be provided, reflecting recognition of the need for handicapped people to make their own decisions rather than being told what to do, even by a vocational expert. Initially in the civilian vocational rehabilitation program as well as in the World War I veterans' rehabilitation program, the "vocational advisor" decided what types of services were to be provided. In the veterans' program, a client's federal pension for disability could be withdrawn if the veteran did not agree to the plan for his vocational rehabilitation. In the civilian rehabilitation program, a client who did not accept the advice and plan of services

could be closed as "uncooperative." This authoritarian role of the rehabilitation worker gradually changed toward freedom of informed choice by the client. In agency literature the term *advising* was gradually replaced by the word *guidance,* and still later by *counseling.* Since the 1973 Rehabilitation Act, it has been mandatory for the rehabilitation counselor to include the client in planning. In fact, the client (or parent or guardian in appropriate cases) must formally agree to the plan of rehabilitation services—the individualized written rehabilitation program or IWRP—which then serves as a kind of contract for joint responsibility in achieving the service objectives.

Marceline Jaques [1970] provided a developmental history of the rehabilitation counselor's role from the early 1920s through the late 1960s. She suggested that the history of rehabilitation counseling reflected developmental phases, and because these phases followed each other chronologically, they tended to be additive rather than discrete. Each phase presented a gross description of the evolving view as to the "proper" thrust of the rehabilitation worker's roles and functions. Inherent in each description is a conception of what constitutes "help" for disabled clients. In the earliest phase the narrow, paternalistic, and authoritarian view of the role of rehabilitationists dominated.

In the beginning it was believed that rehabilitation workers should be vocationally competent in various occupations so that they could advise their clients about specific training and work; for this reason in some states people representing job skill areas were chosen as rehabilitation workers. However, because of the great number of jobs and occupations the impracticality of this became obvious. This link between vocational rehabilitation and occupational information, however, was to some extent responsible for the idea that professional employees should be men. Women were thought naive in this domain and were presumed to be unable to advise men about the work world.

Although some early rehabilitationists thought social work, with its dual emphasis on the individual and the community social setting, should be the role model, the dominant view favored following the methods of vocational guidance.

From its inception the leadership of rehabilitation saw the complexity of vocational readjustment and the need for competent workers.

Gradually there developed general recognition of the importance of the individual and of the idea that a person's greater knowledge of self should be the basis for vocational choice. Thus relationship and evaluation counseling became accepted practice. Tests, interviews, and job analysis techniques from psychology also contributed to vocational rehabilitation technological development [Williamson, 1965].

It also came to be acknowledged that because goals for total rehabilitation were multidimensional they could be best attained when a group of professionals pooled their skills and knowledge to help the client. Team members came from medicine, social work, education, nursing, psychology, and the therapies (physical, occupational, and speech). It was realized, too, that these professionals had to coordinate their efforts with one another and with the community at large. Because they were legally central in the process, the public rehabilitation agencies took over the coordinating function. The main goal, however, continued to be employment for each client, and the role of the rehabilitationist as a professional who specialized in vocational counseling became fairly well established.

It was recognized that individualized goals should be set by each client—goals that represented each person's highest level of personal adjustment. The goal of psychosocial development was given as much importance as working. That phase was influenced by the then current counseling theory: The client-centered approach caused professionals to reevaluate former methods and objectives and consequently to examine the client's role along with the counselor's [Rogers, 1942, 1951].

Rehabilitation counselors learned more about both personality and vocational development. The public rehabilitation agency concept of disability became progressively broader so that emotional and social problems like mental illness, retardation, and alcoholism were included. Counselors became more aware that the physical, vocational, and other facets of a person's life could not be treated in isolation, that disability caused multiple problems for each client and this required a comprehensive treatment approach.

The Community Centered Team Counselor Model was the fourth—future—phase of rehabilitation counseling, according to Jaques [1970]. This model, Jaques thought, would help disabled clients to participate in services without the actual or perceived stigma that she believed had been associated with rehabilitation in the past. She anticipated broad but highly educated counseling psychologists for rehabilitation. The decade of the 1970s with its deceleration of public social programs, however, did not bring such a development of the profession and program of rehabilitation. The practice of using "generalists" as broadly based rehabilitation workers did emerge in some states during the 1970 decade, but it was done to reduce government personnel cost rather than to improve the delivery of professional services. So, as the community-center model actually evolved it represented a step backward in the use of untrained or improperly prepared workers for rehabilitation and social services.

Human services have become so complex that the expertise of specialists is essential. Client needs and technological advancements should influence future changes in the role of rehabilitation counselors. The final section (3.4) in this chapter presents a proposed rehabilitation counselor specialization model.

3.1.2. ROLE DEFINITION

A lag in the development of a role model for rehabilitation counseling arose from an erroneous and narrow view of counseling that focused on the therapeutic relationship; this psychotherapeutic model of counseling ignored its foundation in a psychology that encompasses socioenvironmental considerations. The profession of rehabilitation counseling must consider both internal and external barriers to the adjustment of handicapped persons. This broader professional responsibility is facilitated by the vast resources at the command of the rehabilitation counselor, who has more "situational" power than any other practitioner in the country [McCauley, 1967].

Progress has been made in articulating a clear description of the proper role and functions of the rehabilitation counselor. Many knowledgeable people have contributed to the definition of the domain of this profession. This literature, reviewed in part below, attempts to provide a distinct role structure.

At the University of Minnesota, the vocational counselor has been described as an expert in the measurement of abilities and needs and the location and interpretation of job ability requirements leading to vocational diagnosis and prognosis; the counselor was also seen as an expert in influencing client decisions regarding vocational selection through some form of communication or effective manipulation of client experiences [Dawis, England, & Lofquist, 1964].

The concept of a counselor-rehabilitationist was described by Cubelli [1967] in the context of longitudinal rehabilitation. The rehabilitation specialists or "enablers" devote all of their time to moving clients in and out of needed rehabilitation services. In addition to facilitating such movement through the use of the counseling relationship, these personnel also need community organization skills.

Obermann [1965] subscribed to the position that all professional rehabilitation workers should serve as "rehabilitationists" without regard to professional identification. Switzer [1967] pleaded for a new perspective in rehabilitation to clarify the complex problem of putting together the vast array of services that may be needed by an individual—keeping that individual in mind at all times.

One concept is that the particular activities engaged in by the rehabilitation counselor vary according to the employment setting, which Hall and Warren [1956] noted in their discussion of the rehabilitation counselor's role. A counselor's role of course depends on the agency's program and clientele requirements and also on the social and resources (e.g., financial) environment. This is especially important in counseling, which is affected by all of these variables.

Though these early role statements recognized the multiplicity of tasks performed by the rehabilitation counselor, such completely flexible definitions of role militate against a clear understanding of the unique nature of the profession.

Stone [1978] differentiated between rehabilitation counseling and other forms of counseling, favoring the view that rehabilitation is a distinct professional entity. The objective (i.e., vocational adjustment), the client (i.e., a disabled person), and the treatment (i.e., not only the service of the counselor but full utilization of all the appropriate community resources)—all are unique in rehabilitation counseling.

In Smits' [1976] discussion of the counselor's role and function in rehabilitation he suggested increasing specificity: first, "counseling," then "rehabilitation counseling," and finally "vocational rehabilitation counseling." Though the position in this volume is that "rehabilitation counseling" implies a broad concern with a client's total adjustment, the point to be made is that the role of this rehabilitationist falls within certain boundaries.

Perhaps the clearest way to view role is as the general structure that describes the purpose of the rehabilitation counselor's activities [Maki, McCracken, Pape, & Scofield, 1978]. It is important for any role definition to relate directly to the needs of the client. The effective role of the rehabilitationist is one of problem-solver. A counselor helps the client to identify problems that are barriers to life adjustment, to explore with the client a variety of possible solutions, to decide on an appropriate course of action, and to evaluate the results of that action. The main characteristic of the rehabilitation counselor in this role is the ability to perceive the handicapping problems of each client and to then plan the appropriate intervention strategies.

Sinick [1977] described the professional role as a composite of responsibilities and functions. Once the client's problem is identified and a strategy selected, it is up to the rehabilitation counselor to assume responsibility for the coordination of the integrated pattern of services that address the client's needs. Additional responsibilities are to serve as a client advocate and a resource for the community.

Functions are performed by the rehabilitation counselor to fulfill the role and responsibilities of the profession. Functions are determined by the needs of a particular client, the nature and demands of the particular work setting, and the requirements of the community. Within the generic role of the problem-solver the counselor performs many and varied functions.

3.1.3. ADVOCACY

Modern definitions of the rehabilitation counselor's role incorporate "advocacy" as a primary responsibility. Although certain activities involved in advocacy are more correctly labeled as functions, this core responsibility permeates not only professional activities, but also the worker's attitudes, values, and ethics.

An advocate is a person who represents an individual and his or her interests or any person who pleads the causes of another. Rehabilitation also can be defined as the process of representing and pleading for disabled people, for their dignity and rights as full participants in society. Rehabilitation counselors have always been advocates for their clients in arranging for needed services [De Simone, 1979].

Certainly one of the goals of advocacy is to change the attitudes of the nondisabled toward disabled people in a positive direction. Rehabilitation counselors have been engaging in this process of attitudinal change since the beginning of rehabilitation counseling. By interpreting the capacities of the person with a disability for an employer, the counselor tries to influence or change the attitudes of that employer. Also, by giving talks to civic groups and interested citizens, the rehabilitation counselor is creating a more positive attitudinal climate for clients. Recognizing the complexities of attitudes and attitude change, the rehabilitation counselor helps to educate the citizenry about the facts and myths of disability. In a general sense this is advocacy for a clientele but it does affect the individual client.

The implementation of advocacy necessitates that a most important variable prized by the disabled and the nondisabled alike, be recognized: power. The rehabilitation counselor can be influential within the community through professional knowledge and the respect of others. The counselor who is action-oriented can and does bring about changes in a community.

Sponsors of the advocate system have the impression that there is an inherent conflict between being an employee of an organization and being a representative (counselor) of a client of that organization. This issue has been discussed and dismissed in Chapter 16, Protection and Advocacy. The position taken is that advocacy is an inherent function of any profession—the law, the ministry, or rehabilitation counseling.

3.1.4. PUBLIC SERVANT ROLE

Most rehabilitation counselors are public servants and their employment in this role raises issues regarding possible conflict of loyalties. While there are a variety of private rehabilitation organizations in every community staffed by rehabilitationists, the majority of American rehabilitation counselors are employed by government. This employment pattern is due to the fact that rehabilitation is generally recognized as the human right of all disabled people who qualify to be provided for from tax-collected funds, just as with public schooling. Relatively few rehabilitation counselors are in private practice, in which they are paid by the client.

Government Career Advantages

Many professional people prefer a career in government service because of singular advantages. Self-employment or work in private organizations (either competitive business or private agencies) does not afford the structure or protections of public employment. For example, government civil service regulations are designed to select, place, promote, pay, and otherwise reward employees through objective assessment of the individual's job qualifications.

Career ladders constructed in government agencies tend to be clear and stable. For example, a state agency Rehabilitation Counselor-I (Trainee) can move from that classification to Rehabilitation Counselor-II upon completion of the masters degree in rehabilitation counselor education or other requirements, then on up the qualifications hierarchy to Counselor-III and -IV with experience and demonstrated qualification—and with graduated pay raises at each step of the ladder. Moreover, promotions to counselor supervisor, which also has several levels, and on up in agency administration are charted. A promotional procedure such as this is found in most state (and federal) civil service career fields and is generally based on merit.

Other rewards of government employment include a comfortable income level with considerable assurance against layoff or termination. Discharge from employment is generally subject only to proved charges of either misfeasance (wrongdoing) or nonfeasance (not performing) in office. Career government employees usually work until retirement and receive good fringe benefits (e.g., vacation and sick leave, insurance coverage) throughout. Many people are attracted by the prestige of government office and by the privilege of helping people and country. State rehabilitation agencies traditionally have had less bureaucratic regulation of professional decisions and fewer procedures that would restrict counselor authority for client programming.

Conflicts of Profession and Government

With so many rehabilitation counselors working for the government, there is a possible conflict of interest between profession and government. Rehabilitation counselors, just as other employees, need to voice their demands to the employing agency for salary adjustments and personal benefits. Yet over and above natural self-interests as an employee, the professional person has an inherent obligation to represent the clientele through governmental negotiations for social change. These altruistic goals of rehabilitation are personified by its members who both individually and collectively further the cause of the handicapped.

The interests of the rehabilitationist are appropriately both personal and professional. These are not necessarily incompatible. One's personal interests may be achieved by bargaining, perhaps through union organizations. Altruistic goals are traditionally represented by group action, supported through professional association membership. Achievement of both personal and professional goals ultimately depends upon the effectiveness of the workers' rehabilitation effort in helping handicapped people.

Professionalism and Goals

To avoid conflicts of interest and short-sighted goals, it is essential to focus upon the needs of the client population. In the early years of rehabilitation counselor education (RCE) programs so much emphasis was put upon counseling instruction that other aspects of student preparation such as job placement techniques were neglected. State rehabilitation agency administrators complained that RCE graduates were inappropriately prepared for the agencies' work. RCE educators countered by accusing the state agencies of failure to make proper use of the counseling expertise of professional rehabilitation graduates. One educator used the medical model as an example for state rehabilitation agency employers, pointing out that hospitals adapt to facilitate the professional practice of practitioners (doctors). Such educators and administrators overlooked the overriding consideration that hospitals and physicians both

exist to serve sick patients; so also must the government agencies and professional workers in rehabilitation alike accommodate the needs of handicapped clients. This dialogue has led to a growing awareness that while the profession does not exist for the agency, the agency does not exist for the profession; both exist to serve the rehabilitation needs of handicapped individuals. This focus upon the client as a consumer of service has led to substantial curricular improvements in RCE programs as well as better agency utilization of RCE graduates.

The Broad Professional Role in State Rehabilitation

In the United States the administration by government of a comprehensive rehabilitation process under a single public agency has accommodated a full range of expertise in its professional workers. Their central function is counseling, broadly defined to include client assessment, adjustment, and arrangement for outside rehabilitative services and placement. While this broad professional involvement from client acceptance through case closure is quite desirable, other countries and many rehabilitation facilities in the United States restrict the rehabilitation counselor's role. In fact, there is no absolute assurance that the future functions of the state rehabilitation counselor will not be fragmented or even deprofessionalized. If for no other reason, then, the professional concerns of the rehabilitationist must be viably expressed when necessary to promote high standards.

Undue Influence of Government upon Professions

Professor Yoko Kojima of Japan Women's University has published an account of governmental influence on professionalization in Japan. The development of the profession of social work (which provides rehabilitation to the disabled in Japan) was curtailed during the period of the suppression of democratic institutions by the Japanese government from 1930 to 1945. The totalitarian government felt threatened by the democratic ideas rooted in social work. It placed colleges under close surveillance. According to Kojima [1977a]: ''The word 'social' was seen as synonymous with 'anti-governmental' so the term 'social work' (shakaijigyo) was replaced with 'welfare work' (koseijigyo), and the word 'social' was eliminated from course names in the universities. The existence of social work education as a philosophy as well as a name was discouraged in the 1930's and early 1940's" [p. 25]. This is a vivid example of government interference with professional education.

Kojima went on to provide a recent example of conflict in the governmental role of employer of professionals. With Western influence there was a reawakening of professionalism, and new social work training programs were established in the late 1940s to staff the new social and rehabilitation agencies started by the democratic government in Japan. Still, government selection policy for social workers involved an administratively oriented test that screened in graduates of law and business schools. Some social work graduates left the field in the face of continuing resistance to the profession by a government that placed higher value on academic science than the human service profession. Recognition from the Japanese government has been obtained now by the social work professional and educational associations. This accomplishment by the associations depended upon the demonstration of the effectiveness of professional practitioners as compared with that of unprofessional employees. This account by Kojima, who has an American doctorate degree in rehabilitation counseling, shows that while professionals and their practice can be thwarted by the government as the employer, the concerted effort of the profession through good work and organized pressure can change government policy for the benefit of clientele.

3.2. *Professional Functions*

The functions engaged in by professional human service workers are determined by their role as practitioners, as well as by their education and training, the demands of the employer, and most importantly, the needs of the client. Specifically, functions are those tasks performed by the individual that allow fulfillment of one's role. For rehabilitation counselors, then, these functions are any and all of those activities that these practitioners are prepared for through training and that enable them to solve problems relevant to clients' life adjustment needs.

3.2.1. EXPLANATION

The goal of rehabilitation counseling, McCauley [1967] said, "is to put the client into the mainstream of living as soon as possible. The most therapeutic modality for its practice is life itself. To participate in, to partake of and to give to life itself are the highest forms of therapy" [p. 55].

The rehabilitation counselor is a "totalist." In sheer power-status function in their field of practice, rehabilitation counselors have a larger field of action and greater autonomy of direction than other counseling practitioners. It follows that they can affect people more deeply than other counselors.

The rehabilitation counselor has many modalities for service available over and above the practice of counseling, and more rights and attributes for using a greater variety of methods with which to approach client problems. With regard to goals and potential outcomes in their client's lives, they have greater freedom in planning services. They have greater coordinating powers and deal with more professional and nonprofessional people about client needs and problems.

The number of economic, social, and human resources that rehabilitation counselors can use to help clients is tremendous. These counselors selectively apply the complete array of professional and institutional resources for rehabilitation in the community. And, they are likely to have the most information about any one client, receiving client evaluations on the basis of their own practice and that of other professionals.

Rehabilitation counselors create links between the often isolated world of handicapped people and their community, between their capabilities and their opportunities. They do so by working on both sides. They help clients to accept and minimize their disabilities, to acknowledge their assets and limitations, and to prepare for the fullest lives they can lead. Rehabilitation counselors also work in the environment to find or make opportunities so that handicapped people can join in society's activities and, frequently, earn their livelihood, and the counselor encourages community agencies and employers to accept them.

Rehabilitation uses all of the relevant resources both within the disabled individual and within the community. Disabled individuals usually cannot utilize these resources themselves and sometimes do not even know that they exist. It is the rehabilitation counselor who helps clients to identify, select, and obtain needed services; more importantly the counselor helps clients understand the relationship of rehabilitation services to their personal values and goals. To do this the rehabilitation counselor must know clients as they are and must be sensitive to their hopes and fears, self-perceptions, and views [Ogg, 1966].

3.2.2. COMPETENCIES

In order to be successful, rehabilitation counselors must possess a certain core of competencies that relate directly to the performance of their functions. McGowan and Porter [1967] characterized the skills, knowledge, and duties of the rehabilitation counselor. Their principal descriptions are summarized here, with updating where indicated.

Necessary Skills

The rehabilitation counselor must have various types of ability for:

1. Establishing and maintaining a wholesome counseling relationship.
2. Relating various professional competencies, including one's own, to the needs of the client as a person.
3. Understanding and accepting human behavior as it relates to a particular client.
4. Realizing the broad, pervasive effects of the environment in shaping human motivation.
5. Evaluating the personality dynamics, skills, aptitudes, interests, and capacities of the client throughout the rehabilitation processes.
6. Assessing the potential of the client in choosing a suitable objective and making plans for achieving that objective.
7. Applying human relations skills to not only clients but other key people in the agency

and community for a more effective professional (and personal) life.

8. Understanding community organization, including job structure, job requirements, and training facilities.
9. Understanding employment procedures in all fields and relating them to the needs of the client.
10. Developing and utilizing community resources.
11. Working collaboratively with a rehabilitation team of professionals representing other disciplines and other agencies.
12. Functioning effectively in a public relations role in order to improve community understanding of rehabilitation.

Necessary Knowledge

The rehabilitation counselor must acquire professional knowledge of many variables:

1. Human behavior as it relates to personal, social, and vocational adjustment.
2. Significance of client aptitudes, skills, interests, and educational backgrounds.
3. The effects of handicaps on personality as they relate to emotional and community adjustment.
4. Federal, state, and local laws pertinent to rehabilitation.
5. Employment policies regarding persons with physical and mental handicaps.

Necessary Duties

The rehabilitation counselor also has many job responsibilities:

1. Collecting, analyzing, and evaluating pertinent information about the client.
2. Arranging for medical diagnosis.
3. Determining client eligibility for agency services.
4. Collecting further information about a client, including making provision for psychological, social, and work evaluations.
5. Integrating information into a comprehensive program of rehabilitation services.
6. Assisting the client in learning new techniques for coping with life adjustment problems.
7. Arranging for purchased services (e.g., physical or psychological restoration, personal adjustment and vocational training, transportation and maintenance).

8. Developing job opportunities suitable for agency clientele.
9. Assisting clients in securing employment consistent with their personality, capacities, and preparation.
10. Following up the client after employment in order to evaluate vocational adjustment.

Cohen, Cole, Galloway, Hedgeman, and Schmones [1971] view the rehabilitation counselors as having some responsibilities that are administrative and others related to the counseling function. As adapted from their descriptive categories, the functions of the rehabilitation "counselor-administrator" are record keeper, administrative supervisor, correspondent, budget analyst, program evaluator, consultant, job developer, and public relations expert. These administrative functions may be time-consuming, tedious, and even boring sometimes, but they are necessary in rehabilitation client counseling. The functions of the rehabilitation "counselor-practitioner" are all client-oriented. As practitioners, they serve as intake interviewer, coordinator, evaluator, psychometrist, adjustment counselor, vocational guidance worker, case worker, service supervisor, training advisor, and job placement officer. These are functions in which the counselors can utilize those professional characteristics for which they were trained.

Wherever a counselor is employed—in a rehabilitation or other setting—there is a mix of administrative and counseling activities. In fact it is most unlikely that any counselor would do nothing but counsel clients. The proper balance will depend upon the needs of the agency, the client, and the staff. Too much time spent in either client contact or administration is at the expense of the other obligation.

3.2.3. PLACES OF EMPLOYMENT

Rehabilitation counselors are mainly employed in the areas of education, labor, health, and welfare. Although government agencies are still the predominant employer, with broader recognition of the counselors' unique qualifications, many other opportunities have developed. The largest single employer continues, as in the past, to be the public rehabilitation program. Other important employers among government agencies are the Veterans Administration, the state Employment Services, manpower training proj-

ects, departments of health, hospitals, and mental health clinics, and prisons, as well as agencies dealing with manpower, education and training, public assistance, social security, workers' compensation, corrections, and special disability groups.

Voluntary, nonprofit agencies constitute a very significant employer of rehabilitation counselors and related personnel. Rehabilitation counselors are employed by rehabilitation facilities (workshops, independent living centers, etc.), vocational advisory services, disabled veterans' organizations, and special disability organizations. The latter includes the organizations working in behalf of their blind, deaf, mentally retarded, cerebral palsied, or other disability groups.

General and special hospitals in every community have great need for the services of rehabilitation counselors and represent a prospect for future counselor utilization. An increasing number of rehabilitation counselors work in special schools for handicapped students, including schools for those who are blind, deaf, emotionally disturbed, or mentally retarded.

Colleges and universities also employ rehabilitation counselors. They are located in student counseling programs for handicapped students and also the university personnel office for the employment of handicapped workers. The needs of handicapped students and workers alike must be met to satisfy the affirmative action provisions of federal rehabilitation law.

Many rehabilitation counselors are now in private practice, either on their own or with corporations. These private practitioners provide evaluation, counseling, and other rehabilitation services to handicapped individuals for a fee, or, under contract, for workers' compensation insurance carriers and other companies. They also serve attorneys in a capacity known as "expert witness" in legal action having to do with personal injury claims (e.g., workers' compensation hearings) and also for the Social Security Administration in appealed disability cases.

Earnings and peripheral benefits for state agency rehabilitation counselors are comparable to those of other public employees such as social workers and school teachers who have a masters degree. Although counselors employed in private agencies may have different functions, qualifications, and salary ranges, there is general awareness of the need for practitioners with professional level (graduate) training. This results in competitive pay and benefits for rehabilitation counselors in their various work settings.

3.2.4. ENUMERATION OF FUNCTIONS

As discussed earlier, the functions performed by the rehabilitation counselor depend upon the particular needs of the client, the administrative and programmatic goals of the agency, and the practitioner's particular responsibilities within that setting. The University of Wisconsin Rehabilitation Research Institute analyzed counselor functions and contextual variables [Wright, Smits, Butler, & Thoreson, 1968]. The research model was based on the premise that the client rehabilitation process is influenced by counselor functions in interaction with the context of those functions. In this model, key counselor functions were conceptualized: case finding; eligibility determination; vocational assessment; counseling and vocational planning; provision of client training; restoration and supportive services, job development and employment placement; and administrative functions such as consultation and public relations. Contextual covariables include attributes of the client, the counselor, the agency, and the community. The counselor performs these functions with the client, with others related to the client's welfare, and within agency structure.

With the disabled client the rehabilitation counselor: (1) helps the client through discussion to work toward the fullest possible self-realization; (2) gives information about resources that can be used in moving in this direction; (3) assists the client to identify strengths and limitations; and (4) makes plans for use of services and resources and helps put these plans into operation.

With others in the community the counselor: (1) works in conjunction with other professionals to help the client adjust fully; (2) establishes a community climate that will support the client in striving toward self-actualization goals; and (3) organizes others' services into a planned whole.

Within agency structure, the counselor: (1) implements policy and applies criteria for service to the client; (2) evaluates policy and standards as they support service goals; and (3) stimulates and promotes better practice and standards through communication to administrative personnel.

Decision-making

A central theme runs through every function performed by the rehabilitation counselor: decision-making, the common denominator in the many aspects of rehabilitation services. Rehabilitation counseling results in a great many decisions by the client, from the choice of a career or other objective to every step in the rehabilitation plan. The decision-making process, therefore, determines the kinds of services provided and their outcomes [Page, Apostal, & Lipp, 1977].

Case Management

The function of case management requires knowledge of where clients are in the rehabilitation process in order to keep them moving through their program of services. A counselor needs to follow a management system whereby rehabilitants are given case work load priority according to needs. In the state rehabilitation program a listing of every counselor's case load by client name and status serves this purpose. The system informs the counselor which specific cases are ready for further attention.

"In case management skills, the counselor takes a case and evaluates the next step to be taken, considers the decision which needs to be made, and then makes the decision" according to Henke, Connolly, and Cox [1975, p. 224]. But every decision must be dictated by client needs and client wishes. Even "case management" need not be authoritarian.

In describing a theoretical model of vocational redevelopment for the adventitiously disabled, McMahon [1977] discussed functions relating to case managing activity. On the basis of management theory he described four operations that together constitute the functions of management: planning, organizing, directing, and controlling.

Guidelines for this important counselor function are provided in a section entitled "Case Management" in Chapter 7, Public Rehabilitation.

Pervasiveness of the Counseling Function

No matter what other functions and responsibilities are engaged in by the rehabilitation counselor, counseling is the central function that is provided continuously throughout the rehabilitation process.

It should be repeated that counseling is inherent in rehabilitation: this is a nontransferable obligation of the rehabilitation counselor. Consultant and rehabilitative services of other kinds may or should be purchased, but the ultimate professional responsibility for the function of counseling cannot be delegated. Professional counseling is indispensable to the proper selection, provision, and ultilization of the other rehabilitation services. Handicapped people tend to see this when they look back and attempt to analyze the reasons for the success they have experienced.

In a study directed by John Muthard, Jaques [1959] evaluated "critical incidents" in client-counselor interactions to identify the components of counseling in a rehabilitation setting. Her findings break down this function into a number of essential parts, the key requirements of which are as follows:

1. The creation of a climate in which the client feels understood and safe to explore problems and plans.
2. The interaction between counselor and client, their working together to arrive at some solution to the problem at hand.
3. The evaluation of the client's problems by means of eliciting the client's ideas and observing the conditions relevant to the vocational potential of the client.
4. The communication of information, explanations, and professional knowledge, while permitting the client to decide.
5. The definition of the limits within which counseling takes place in terms of time, the nature of counseling, and the responsibilities of both counselor and client.
6. The gathering of information about the client for a comprehensive understanding of the individual and the present situation.
7. The administrative arrangements made for the client such as appointments, referrals, and future contacts.

It can be seen that counseling is a kind of catalyst that permits clients to benefit from other services. As such it typically provides the crucial impetus for successful rehabilitation.

Functions as a Team Member

The rehabilitationist rarely works alone. The complex needs of people with disabilities and the nature of rehabilitation settings make this almost impossible. No amount of individual skill in one's own particular profession can circumvent the necessity for group skills when there is need for understanding and treating the whole individual with multiple and interrelated problems. It is therefore a function of every rehabilitationist to participate actively as a member of a "team." The team may consist of those individuals from the various disciplines in a rehabilitation facility who are working with a client. It may be made up of representatives of the various community agencies that are contributing services to the client. The team may include staff members within an organization and outside professionals. The most important purpose of any rehabilitation team, however, is to combine efforts toward alleviation of the client's varied problems. Team success depends upon staff implementation of the following principles: freedom of communication, sharing of responsibility for decision-making and leadership, respect for individuals, encouragement of independent functioning, development of congenial interpersonal feelings, and continuous evaluation of clinical functioning.

A number of elements can contribute to effective teamwork, especially with regard to interagency cooperation. Some of the most important were suggested by Roessler and Mack [1977]:

1. Involvement to build staff cooperation.
2. Leadership to minimize service duplication and maximize service coordination.
3. Program design to define concepts such as coordination, case management, progress monitoring, shared intake, and so on.
4. Communication to inform personnel of all project activities.
5. Community relationships to provide valuable resources.

When the team functions as a unit to decide the most effective and efficient means of delivering services to an individual, the client is the most important team member. "If the rehabilitation process is to be effective, the person to be helped must be a very important contributor to the helping process," said Jaques [1970]; she went on to say, "clients need to feel that their lives are in their own hands and that they are in control of themselves and their own world" [p. 9]. Rehabilitationists opposed to authoritarian methods accept the client's right of decision-making.

3.2.5. PARAPROFESSIONALS

Beginning in the mid-1960s, concern for minority groups and their underemployment led to various schemes to develop career opportunities for them in human service agencies. Under the leadership of the U.S. Department of Labor, a number of programs were financed, the objective being to prepare these "new careerists" and to induce employers to accommodate them. An example is the "career ladder" model in which recruits start at unskilled work, then by experience and study work up to technical or even professional levels. Priority of employment was given to the culturally disadvantaged to begin at the first "rung" as "nonprofessionals" (variously known as paraprofessionals, support personnel, aides, subprofessionals, or assistants). The use of paraprofessionals in rehabilitation has been described by Mitra, Fitzgerald, Hilliad, and Baker [1974] and by McMahon and Fraser [1978].

State rehabilitation agencies have attempted to employ a larger number of disadvantaged minority workers. One strategy was the creation of entry level, professional-track jobs. Theoretically, the aide could develop through work-study to a counseling position. Wright and Fraser [1975, 1976], in fact, demonstrated a hierarchical categorization of tasks in rehabilitation counselor-track jobs.

Unfortunately, the various schemes for a rehabilitation career ladder have been disappointing. Fully prepared masters degree rehabilitation counselors are generally available at not much greater total cost to the agency than untrained workers. Generally speaking it seems better to prepare professionals for competent practice before employment. (An exception, perhaps, is the indigenous worker whose location and personal similarities with a clientele group may justify extensive on-the-job preparation.) Rehabilitation education programs give priority to qualified minority members and handicapped people for admission to and financial support for full-time professional training.

3.3. *Personal Characteristics*

It is important to realize that one needs characteristics other than the skills, knowledge, and abilities required to perform the rehabilitation counselor's functions. There are other attributes that, though difficult to measure, are as necessary for the counselor to possess as any technical skill.

3.3.1. ESSENTIALS

Essentials, according to Feingold [1977], are those characteristics that the best counselors seem to have: a belief that life is worthwhile, a belief in the counseling profession, a sense of concern and involvement, and belief in the value of self-knowledge. The sense that life is worth living is expressed in the phrase "reverence for life." It is doubtful that a counselor whose life philosophy is cynical and negative can be very helpful; people with positive attitudes toward life can probably identify and handle frustration better.

It is important for a counselor to feel convinced that people can learn, with help, to live more creatively and constructively. Faith in the process benefits the professional person as well as the individuals being served. It is essential to believe that human behavior can be altered and improved. Equally important are concern and involvement with people, expressed in the counselor's behavior and embodied in a working philosophy. Without this the counselor cannot help people change. Finally, self-knowledge is a major vehicle for self-improvement, although it is difficult in many cases to obtain.

A number of authors have discussed the personal characteristics necessary for the rehabilitationist (e.g., Hilliard [1972]). A listing of these traits demonstrates the "well-roundedness" required of the practitioner. The characteristics needed are suggested by the fact that the rehabilitation counselor is usually a counselor, an administrator, a coordinator of services, and a public relations person. Many of the qualities named are valuable for any counselor but especially significant in the context of rehabilitation [Hall & Warren, 1956].

There is no single ideal rehabilitation counselor; many different types of people can fulfill the role successfully. Beyond the requirements of stamina, intelligence, and appropriate academic credentials, however, the following characteristics suggested by Ogg [1966] are desirable:

1. A strong desire to help.
2. A strong commitment to life.
3. A realistic view of everyday life.
4. Faith in people.
5. Enthusiasm and vitality.
6. The ability to communicate effectively.
7. The ability to get along successfully with different types of people.
8. Sensitivity, perceptiveness, and the ability to empathize.
9. Ability to accept clients and their values as they are.
10. The ability to derive pleasure from others' successes.
11. The ability to put others' needs before one's own.
12. Objectivity and optimism.
13. Patience and perseverance.
14. Open-mindedness toward innovative attitudes about the handicapped, and the ability to see new possibilities.
15. Imagination, creativity, initiative.

Obermann [1962] listed several essential characteristics for a rehabilitation counselor: competence, effectiveness, the ability to facilitate others' efforts, integrity, and the ability to communicate. Competence is not the result of good intentions alone but of much hard work through which knowledge and skills are acquired. Counselors should continually read and study the literature related to their work; should participate in conventions, conferences, and conversation with colleagues; should engage in research, evaluation, and criticism. They should make the effort to become exceptionally competent in their special fields and should gain the respect of their peers when discussing these areas of expertise. They should achieve a degree of self-assurance without becoming arrogant and work toward chosen ideals with pride.

To be successful the rehabilitation counselor must be a person of action: initiating, making decisions, teaching, and guiding. Sometimes there is no one else who can do what is necessary, and the responsibility that then falls on the counselor cannot be abdicated because of a sense of personal inadequacy. To make the necessary decisions one must be competent and knowledgeable, and these qualities stem from commitment to the profession.

The client must be the focal point of concern, and the satisfaction that the counselor derives from the helping relationship must be considered secondary or the client will in a sense be exploited.

Finally, the rehabilitation counselor must have the integrity that comes from fundamental self-esteem. Adherence to accepted rules out of a fear of being criticized does not constitute integrity; instead the person with true integrity behaves according to the rules out of a sense of self-esteem.

3.3.2. SELF-UNDERSTANDING

The rehabilitation counselor is constantly confronted with the heavy burdens that can be thrust upon an individual's life. Facing the multitude of problems wrought by disability in the life of a client demands that the professional human service worker have a keen sense of reality and a firm grip on personal values. Such a strong constitution is not necessarily an inherent trait. Counselors must work hard at personal growth and develop a complete openness for understanding all dimensions of the human experience.

As a rehabilitation counselor, one's ultimate goal is to help clients solve problems that are inhibiting life adjustment. One must keep in mind that the individual is much more than simply a potential resource for the nation's manpower needs. Oftentimes, an individual's worth is measured by the status of a job or the amount of money earned, but this viewpoint denies the essential characteristics of the individual's uniqueness. Frequently, clients who are unable to work competitively have absorbed society's view that paid employment is a requisite to personal worth. They must be helped to discover values that are more meaningful and realistic and learn to appreciate other contributions that they are able to make [Leung, 1972].

3.3.3. PROFESSIONAL STRESSES

Rehabilitation counselors will always be faced with the frustrations and stresses of the profession. Their responsibility is to work with the client as a total human being, to be sensitive to a wide variety of needs (psychological, medical, social, economic, and vocational), and to be considerate and responsive in every way. Eventually one realizes that it is impossible to fulfill this responsibility completely. Although the client's problems become the counselor's concerns and the stress is shared, the counselor must remain objective and not become emotionally frustrated by the failures that inevitably occur.

There was much discussion in the counseling literature of the 1970s about "burn out" of practitioners after a few years. Many counselors do experience this to a degree, but there are techniques that help prevent such deterioration. The problem has been recognized and avoided for many years by other professionals who have intensive client involvement. It *is* possible to remain dedicated, with continued effectiveness, to individuals dependent upon the service. One approach uses what can be called "critical empathy": the helper understands the client's problems and feelings but remains outside as to personal, emotional involvement. This objectivity allows for a critical stance in empathetic understanding, increasing the counselor's immediate usefulness to the client while avoiding the emotional burden that can be cumulative and eventually crippling to any human service worker.

3.3.4. CULTURAL BARRIERS

Most rehabilitation counselors come from the predominant culture of our society. However, a large number of clients are not members of this cultural mainstream. This fact is yet another variable of which the practitioner must be aware as it exerts an influence on relationships with clients. Counselors, like other people, adopt the values of their cultural surroundings and are bound by what D. L. Morrow [1972] called "cultural addiction."

Counselor attitudes, according to Wicas and Carluccio [1971], can be affected by biases, stereotypes, and habitual reactions. Of special concern to American rehabilitationists are the negative effects of stereotyping and culture-bound attitudes toward blacks, the ethnic minority group most represented in the disabled population. Rehabilitation personnel should take measures to obtain information and experience that

will enable them to increase their understanding of blacks, a disproportionate number of whom are vocationally handicapped. These measures, according to Ayers [1969], are to:

1. Develop a desire to help black clients and make a commitment to do so.
2. Gather, within the agency, a collection of literature about black history and culture.
3. Become familiar with the linguistic patterns of black people.
4. Work against the dehumanizing procedures within the rehabilitation system.
5. Talk to many black people and visit black neighborhoods.
6. Create and take part in sensitivity training programs aimed at working on attitudes toward black people.
7. Create and take part in training programs geared toward helping rehabilitation workers understand the black experience.
8. Listen to the statements made by black clients about rehabilitation.
9. Participate in community projects involving black neighborhoods.

Effective rehabilitation of disabled black people, and other minority members, can contribute to the solution of racial problems.

The following considerations suggested by William English [1972] pertain, not only to black clients, but to any client group from a cultural minority. The disadvantaged disabled could be helped more effectively under the following circumstances:

1. Such individuals must have increased opportunities to bring their cultures into rehabilitation facilities. Motivation and the chance for success are decreased when people cannot relate what they are doing to their cultural backgrounds.
2. Rehabilitation facilities should be made more accessible to the poor: getting there should be made easy, hours should correspond to their schedules, information about the service should be disseminated, and referral procedures perfected in order to reach those in need.
3. Counseling methods need to be creative, even unconventional, for this group. Traditional counseling and psychotherapy techniques have not been effective with poor people; they were evolved, of course, to help other groups with well-developed communi-

cation skills and considerable education. Recently, more attention has been given to approaches that do not necessitate verbal and intellectual skills in the client. Counseling poor people should be active and practical in nature; it should teach problem-solving. Finally, counseling should concentrate on "critical behaviors," those behaviors that spell success or failure.

Rehabilitation counseling with minority group members involves a number of unique issues. While it would be unreasonable to assign only black counselors to serve black clients, agencies should recognize the need for special considerations for culturally different rehabilitants. Charles Vander Kolk [1977] has studied counselor stress when dealing with minority clients and found it greater than with disabled clients.

3.4. Specialization

Rehabilitation counseling as a profession possesses an extensive body of knowledge and technology. It is a rich heritage of experience derived from the operation of a single public rehabilitation system since 1921, as well as from the explicit contributions of federally sponsored research and university graduate education since 1954. However, this great and expanding accumulation of information and skill applicable to the readjustment of handicapped people has grown beyond the grasp of the practicing generalist. Consequently it is necessary for rehabilitation counseling organizations and agencies to accommodate and utilize this professional knowledge through a systematic plan of specialization for practitioners. This section reviews the history of rehabilitation counselor specialization and proposes an organizational and professional plan for a new method of specialization.

3.4.1. TRADITIONAL GENERALIST
Rehabilitation counselors were obliged to be generalists in years past when there was only one rehabilitation "agent" charged with a territory having a population of several hundred thousand people. Even now it is expedient to assign a single state counselor in sparsely populated areas; this requires extensive driving for home calls and community contacts. When there were only several rehabilitation workers to serve an entire state it was reasonable to simply assign each staff person to a geographic district. As the public program and staff expanded, the geographic assignments were smaller but the generalist tradition for state counselors continued.

The rehabilitation generalist role makes the counselor responsible for everything and every-

one in a specified area. All generalists do essentially the same thing without regard to their level or type of qualifications or the unique needs of the particular clientele. Rehabilitation counselors are often still assigned to general practice in a given geographic area by state rehabilitation agencies. Graduate rehabilitation counselor preparation covers all basic professional competencies required of the generalist; consequently RCE graduates are qualified for this general role.

Why should the state agencies continue to follow the traditional staffing pattern in the face of clear evidence—from personnel practice and rehabilitation research—of a better way? The customary method is archaic in that it denies the fact of individual differences. While an increasing number of rehabilitation counseling positions are created to handle special situations and client groups, many counselors remain generalists with inherently broader role responsibilities and indiscriminate case assignments.

It is for some very sound reasons that state rehabilitation administrators cling to the idea of generalists who handle a variety of services and clients throughout their entire rehabilitation from case finding to placement and follow-up. This general responsibility for a district has proven values: it provides for more intimate knowledge of the individual client and of what community resources are available to help. Such continuity and personal knowledge is lacking if professional services are fragmented in such a way as to make more than one staff person responsible. Moreover, state rehabilitation counselors have found it satisfying and challenging to have the entire responsibility for the whole rehabilitation process for a given client. Successful client outcomes are directly rewarding to the responsible counselor. Also, in each closure the longitudinal experience becomes a "continuing education" as selected case services and successful outcomes are assessed and linked.

3.4.2. SPECIALISTS BY DISABILITY

In about half of the states, rehabilitation services for the blind are independent of the general rehabilitation agency for all other disabilities. Before public rehabilitation began, many states already had a Commission for the Blind, which sponsored industrial workshops and other vocational and welfare services, and this separation has been maintained by the U.S. Congress in subsequent rehabilitation legislation. In this traditional specialization, many workers for the blind are themselves visually disabled.

Not only administrative specialization, but also the appointment of disabled people to state rehabilitation agency positions was proposed for years by people who had organized to foster this personal interest. The usual argument was that the rehabilitation counselor had to be disabled to understand the problems of disability; that workers for the blind should be blind themselves, deaf workers deaf, and so on. The nonhandicapped professionals then facetiously asked, "But who is to serve the mentally retarded and emotionally disturbed?" The suggestion that one had to experience a particular handicap to understand it was often taken as an affront to rehabilitation counseling; after all, physicians treated all kinds of illnesses, and attorneys represented all kinds of felons. These arguments—heard often during the 1950s—were unsettling to the new profession of rehabilitation counseling. Attempts were oftentimes made to obtain the appointment of disabled people to rehabilitation jobs, perhaps just to get them work. These arguments and pressures subsided as masters level graduates in rehabilitation counseling demonstrated the value of their preparation and as public agencies developed more informed personnel hiring practices.

It is well for rehabilitation agencies to demonstrate leadership in affirmative action for the employment of handicapped applicants for all staff positions, but it is as unreasonable to claim that disability makes one a more competent professional rehabilitation counselor as it would be to accept the opposite bias. Such stereotyping leads to vocational segregation. Nevertheless, there are sound reasons for choosing counselors matched to the needs of their clients and to the unique tasks of special case loads. For example, a deaf clientele requires a counselor who "signs" for communication; blind clients seeking industrial jobs benefit from having a blind placement counselor demonstrate to employers how people without sight can perform job tasks; older counselors may find it easier than younger ones to develop relationships with middle-aged clients.

This obligation to train and hire disabled people for rehabilitation agency jobs is more than public relations to demonstrate the general qualifications of a segment of the population. A legion of outstanding workers for and of the disabled attests to the effect of their extraordinary dedication and talents. The fact remains, however, that being disabled is neither a necessary nor a sufficient condition for the successful performance of rehabilitation counseling.

3.4.3. CHANGING ROLE MODEL

The roles and functions of rehabilitation counselors have undergone continuing modification from the earliest days. Important trends may be identified from an analysis of various rehabilitation counselor roles.

The first of these is the "jack of all trades" role, which was initiated in 1920 with the advent of public rehabilitation and which dominated for well over a quarter of a century. In this role the counselor—actually, the more accurate title of "agent" was often used—was all things to all clients. These practitioners were ordinarily untrained or, at best, self-taught in counseling and other professional knowledge and skills. Theoretical-speculative papers throughout this period proposed interdisciplinary training for the rehabilitation counselor (Levine & Pence, 1953; Lee, 1955).

The mid-1950s brought a second role to the fore, the "counseling" counselor role. Its development relates directly to the institution of federally supported training programs in rehabilitation counselor education (RCE). Generally speaking, recognition of the essential nature of rehabilitation counseling as a complex process necessitating RCE graduate course work gave potent impetus to the field of rehabilitation. However, the singular training focus on the counseling process had the effect of perpetuating an illusory distinction between counseling and other rehabilitative activities.

The third and current role picture for graduate rehabilitation counselors became apparent in the mid-1960s. Counseling was put in proper focus as only one of the facilitating functions in the vocational adjustment of disabled individuals. Counselor education for vocational rehabilitation shifted from a therapeutic to a vocational adjustment emphasis. Moreover, the other, traditional rehabilitation functions were given greater curriculum emphasis in preprofessional education. The maturing RCE programs began preparing graduates to work for state and other rehabilitation agencies as generalists in their various capacities, including client assessment, case planning and management, utilization of community resources, and job placement—as well as counseling.

The fourth role model, as proposed here, would go beyond the generalist concepts and provide for rehabilitation counselor specialization in a realistic personnel configuration of client needs and counselor functions. It includes specialization in counseling for independent living rehabilitation.

3.4.4. HISTORIC PROPOSAL

Oscar M. Sullivan, the state rehabilitation agency director of Minnesota and a national leader during the years 1920–1935, the fifteen formative years of public rehabilitation, developed and articulated the specialization concepts that reappeared in the rehabilitation counseling literature many years later. In the innovative 1926 book by Sullivan and Snortum on the rehabilitation of disabled persons, both generalist and specialist staff models were described. Staff activities in public rehabilitation were characterized as falling under one or the other of two different systems of administration: either (1) generalists were assigned a territorial district, or (2) specialists were assigned to work in a "functional" organization. In some states the two systems may be combined, however. The choice of agency administration was explained as follows:

One consists in a territorial division of the state. Each member of the staff is assigned to a district and works exclusively in that district. Sometimes there are district offices and the administration is so decentralized that even the records are kept in branch offices. . . .

The other plan of organization is a functional one. Under this each staff member is a specialist along

some particular line, even though he is expected to be prepared to take care of any phase of the work or to take complete charge of any case. Some of the specialists that are frequently so represented are placement, rehabilitation of women, agriculture, industrial training, expert in mining, and the like. This system is more practicable in a state where the administration can be fairly centralized and all of the staff can work out of the same office. It makes possible a better type of service in many special cases by bringing to bear expert knowledge. Minnesota and California have made considerable use of the functional plan. Of course the two systems that have been described are not mutually exclusive. A combination of the two is frequently possible and may be found to be best adapted to the needs of some states [pp. 170–171].

3.4.5. COUNSELOR NOT COORDINATOR

C. H. Patterson [1957] is credited with raising the issue of the "Counselor or Coordinator?", the title of his much-quoted 1957 article in the *Journal of Rehabilitation* in which he denounced rehabilitation functions other than counseling as "nonprofessional." Patterson argued against including "coordinator" tasks such as case work and job placement in the preparation of rehabilitation counselors or in their work with clients. The newly established rehabilitation education programs were generally administered by school guidance departments, and few of the rehabilitation counselor educators at that time were experienced in the civilian rehabilitation program. As a consequence many of the early rehabilitation counselor education programs did not prepare their graduates for general competency in vocational rehabilitation of the handicapped. While the notion of a division of staff labor according to level of skills is noteworthy, Patterson's "*coordinator*" suggestion for a subprofessional was not original.

Sullivan and Snortum [1926] had also observed that "much of the rehabilitation agent's work falls within the scope of the term "*coordinator*," for example, supervising clients in training." They thought the addition of a coordinator who would assume this "function" for the agent would have "many points of superiority" over the "unmodified case plan of work under which a staff member keeps charge of a case from the first contact until the closure" [p. 235].

Patterson, in 1965, while continuing to subscribe to his counselor versus coordinator model, acknowledged at a conference on specialization in vocational rehabilitation a serious difficulty in splitting professional functions.

The major disadvantage associated with specialization is the breaking of the individual into parts. The client may be seen and dealt with as a problem, as a disease, or as a disability rather than as a total person. Now it is true that specialization requires concentration upon a part or aspect of the whole person. This is necessary, and specialization would not be possible without it. To an extent, this is a price we must pay for specialization [p. 14].

Specializing in just the counseling function indeed would fragment the client and the total rehabilitation process. However, as Patterson [1967] pointed out, preparation for broad functioning as a specialized counselor was a difficult problem: "Specialized training must be in addition to the present two years of graduate preparation for rehabilitation counselors" [p. 153]. With the subsequent advent of baccalaureate programs in rehabilitation education, this is no longer such a serious barrier; a two-year masters degree in rehabilitation counseling (on top of two years of undergraduate rehabilitation foundation courses) can accommodate some specialized knowledge and skills in the counseling area as well as in other rehabilitation instruction. Moreover, Patterson apparently did not consider the use of continuing professional education for helping mature rehabilitation counselors to develop further (specialized) expertise.

3.4.6. HORIZONTAL AND VERTICAL

A thought-provoking two-way classification of rehabilitation counselor specialization was described by Salvatore DiMichael in 1967: "Horizontal specialists" are restricted to work with a particular type of disability (e.g., mental retardation), while "vertical specialists" attend to only one function in the rehabilitation process (e.g., job placement). In a variation of such specialization rehabilitation counselors are assigned to a facility (e.g., a mental hospital, halfway house, rehabilitation workshop). In vertical and facility specialization clients change counselors as they move along in the rehabilitation process or from one setting to the next.

Many rehabilitation counselors in the public rehabilitation program have been employed in horizontal specialization, for example, in programs for the blind. Perhaps most rehabilitation counselors in other agencies and facilities work

as vertical specialists in that they have circumscribed functions or clientele, or both. The problem for either horizontal or vertical specialization is that of whole person or whole process continuity. DiMichael saw this need for coordination:

In today's and tomorrow's rehabilitation program, the principle of continuity of service will be emphasized very much. With so much specialization today, the need for coordination is almost desperate. I am convinced that the counselor will have to be a coordinator, not a quarterback, nor the coach. I am not speaking of administrative coordination, but of the individual client. The counselor will have to coordinate in a more subtle fashion, keeping an eye on the person's plan and its execution, not looking to be conspicuous, aware of the many community facilities and many specialized professional resources. He must learn to bring these resources together through the consent and actions of the client. As I see it, this form of counselor-coordination through the client's consent and action is an essential ingredient for the job ahead [p. 39].

In other words, DiMichael proposed a role that encompassed both counseling and coordinating. Empirical research later established the soundness of this role orientation [Sather, Wright, & Butler, 1968; Ayer, Wright, & Butler, 1968].

3.4.7. SPECIALIST AND GENERALIST

The older position papers on rehabilitation counselor specialization posed a dilemma: how could coordination be preserved and the benefits that derive from specialization of function still be obtained? The solution arises from a new model in which the specialist treats the whole person through the entire rehabilitation process—and also shoulders territorial community resources responsibilities—just as the "old-fashioned" generalist did. Concentrated efforts of specialization need not fragment the process and delivery system or isolate its clientele.

The term *generalist* may be defined in either of two dimensions: (1) a rehabilitation counselor who is charged with the entire responsibility of a client from intake through closure, or (2) one who has a geographic territory and whose caseload is not selectively assigned. Continuity of responsibility as in the first interpretation is clearly desirable, and the heterogeneous case load implied by the second may be both undesirable and unnecessary. With some operational conversion of role and assignments it is possible to combine the positive characteristics of case continuity of the generalist with the expertise of specialists working with a homogeneous case load.

Specialization in rehabilitation is needed more than ever due to:

1. The challenge of an everexpanding fund of technical knowledge and the difficulty busy practitioners find in keeping up to date on the full range of literature relevant to rehabilitation.

2. The congressionally mandated program for independent living services for the severely handicapped population, which taxes modern technology, existing resources, and professional knowledge and skill.

3. The accountability pressure currently upon rehabilitation—as a process, as an agency, and as a profession—which is vulnerably small in the encompassing human services system.

4. The challenge to maintain an enviable reputation for innovation and flexibility to accommodate expanding needs, services, and client populations.

5. The need for recognition of newly developed groups of rehabilitation specialists performing professional client services not primarily of a counseling nature.

Preparation for the role of specialist should be over and above the usual rehabilitation counseling masters degree program, although this curriculum already allows considerable opportunity to begin a specialization through choice of the clinical practice placement, thesis topic, and electives. However, in rehabilitation facilities especially, several specializations have developed outside of the counseling profession and are not identified as subprofessions. So the dilemma of rehabilitation counselor specialization has assumed still other dimensions.

Most specialists operate within the confines of an established discipline or institution to which they owe allegiance. Moreover, "these specialists are employed to perform functions that are unique to, and consistent with a given discipline or institution and do not overlap with other fields of endeavor," according to a discussion of rehabilitation professionalization by Nadolsky [1975, p. 2]. He went on to discuss the profession of "independent specialist," which emerges

"to perform functions that lie within the province of (and consequently overlap with) an already established discipline, institution or field of endeavor" [p. 2]. Concerned with limited functions of the parent discipline, these new specialists fashion a new role and adopt an independent identity. Nadolsky stated, "The development of specialized fields of endeavor within an overall discipline is accomplished through the elevation of one or more related functions to the status of role" [p. 5]. He believed that vocational evaluation has become a specialized discipline through the elevation to the status of "role," selected functions of the vocational rehabilitation counselor (e.g., use of assessment techniques, provision of occupational information, interviewing, and vocational counseling).

Another case dimension indicative of "special" personnel relates to minority populations—Hispanic, black, native American, and Oriental clients. Reasons given for this kind of specialty include understanding of language, appreciation of culture (ways and values), and ability to establish rapport in the counseling relationship. A number of years ago, a survey of Southern states showed that black people were not served in proportion to population by a predominantly white rehabilitation staff. Apparently no attempt was made to find further inequalities by comparing amounts of time or case funds spent, number of clients in higher education, or the occupational and earning level at case closure. A direct way for agencies to avoid even subtle racial prejudice by counselors against minority groups is to employ minority member counselors for case loads in communities where a substantial number of potential applicants are nonwhite. More effective counseling relationships can result from an initial matching of counselor with client according to similarity of perceptions, personality, age, or other personal variables. Thus, matching has been suggested to avoid disparities in frame of reference. The most readily discernible fit is that of counselor expertise fulfilling the client need or engaging the presenting problem.

3.4.8. SELECTIVE ASSIGNMENT MODEL

The rehabilitation personnel model proposed here can be descriptively referred to as "selective case assignment" or "longitudinal specialization." It is called "longitudinal" because a single rehabilitation counselor has responsibility for the rehabilitation client—the case work is not fragmented by a proliferation of experts throughout phases or agencies of the rehabilitation process. "Selective case assignment" is also descriptive because professional workers are matched with applicants systematically on the basis of the most predominant needs of the case and the appropriate expertise of the counselor assigned.

The selective, longitudinal assignment of the rehabilitation counselor to cases adheres to modern principles of personnel management as well as tenets of professional practice. It is a flexible and practical yet comprehensive procedure, applicable to both public and private rehabilitation agencies. This model derives from both rehabilitation research and experience. Moreover, the strategy is fully operational with instruments available for implementation in public rehabilitation agencies and field offices. Finally, it overcomes the limitations of specialization as proposed in earlier models.

As described, this modified model for rehabilitation counselors provides a needed combination of generalist and specialist roles, but takes full advantage of the positive aspects of both personnel administration strategies. And this new role model accommodates the existing preparation of trained rehabilitation counselors. It does not fragment the established rehabilitation counselor functions, nor does it encourage proliferation of separate subprofessions. It does not necessitate additional training programs for areas of work splintered from rehabilitation counseling.

This longitudinal case responsibility builds upon the general education and functions of the present yet it allows for selective specialization of the rehabilitation counselor. The general masters degree level rehabilitation counselor preparation areas remain viable: counseling theory, techniques, and clinical practice; service resources; client assessment; occupational, medical, and psychosocial impact of disability; case management; job placement; and supporting courses. Both neophytes and specialists should be generically trained, though the specialist must have extra qualifications.

Wright and Fraser [1976] developed a method for a differential assessment of counselor qualifications on the "Rehabilitation Task Performance Evaluation Scale" [Wright & Fraser, 1975]. The 294 items on this Scale, which were obtained largely by agency task analysis, vary greatly as to the type and level of required qualifications. It was concluded from this research for the Council on Rehabilitation Education that state agency supervisors with profiles of staff competency could assign clients selectively (e.g., difficult cases would be given to master counselors).

The method of rehabilitation counselor specialization outlined here can be implemented by allowing supervisors to assign cases in order to achieve a match between the dominant needs of the applicant and the special competencies of the counselor. Every office with a staff of counselors should have different kinds of specializations, chosen according to individual interests and competencies as well as agency program priorities. A variety of staff specializations, both vertical (specialization by function) and horizontal (specialization in a specific disability) are envisioned for larger, urban offices. An applicant with mental retardation as the predominant problem might well be assigned to the specialist in developmental disabilities. Other cases—including some retarded clients—could be selectively assigned to counselor-specialists in vocational assessment, personal adjustment counseling, or job placement according to the presenting problem.

Clients would not be shifted routinely to different specialists as the process progresses but would ordinarily remain with the assigned counselor throughout. The value of total case responsibility and relationship continuity is destroyed in previous specialist models such as the classic experiment by W. R. Ooley reported in Wright and Trotter [1968]. In this 1957–1961 Arkansas study by Ooley, work by a rehabilitation team of specialists was compared with the traditional counselor approach in state rehabilitation offices. All of these other specialization plans, including Ooley's, split the client-rehabilitation responsibility by having someone other than the generalist counselor handle other professional or subprofessional activities. In the new model— the principles of which are being outlined here—the entire counseling staff, except for new members, would be encouraged to prepare for specialization but, like generalists, would still be responsible for the full process.

An obvious side benefit of having local staff specialists is the immediate consultation they can give fellow counselors. For example, the specialist in vocational assessment would get ready advice from the specialist on job placement in that phase of a client's rehabilitation plan, and vice versa. Another professional development advantage is the opportunity for staff members to shift areas of specialization during their careers as program emphases and their own interests and competencies change.

Organizational improvements are needed and are derived from this plan of local office specialists. The basic administrative change is that counselors would be assigned cases selectively. This implies special staff expertise that must be developed and maintained, necessitating an on-going professional development program. Yet it is cheaper to train a single counselor in each office on selective topics than it is to train everyone. In fact, the explosion of knowledge mandates such targeting of subject and student. The need for specialists in each local office exposes the need for state-level programming and state staff expertise for direct consultation between local and state-level program specialists. Local office supervisors should be somewhat relieved of day-to-day professional consultation and training of counselor staff and could spend greater time in administrative and evaluative duties. A state consulting staff of program specialists would provide professional help to field counselors.

In addition to the special client service expertise of the rehabilitation counselor specialist there are other practical values to this model. As "generalists" in rehabilitation agencies have done in the past these new specialists would serve in the full role of the rehabilitationist by building professional contacts for needed community resources—encourage prompt referral; provide professional consultation, collaborative client services, training and placement assistance; engage in public relations. These specialists, however, could sharpen their focus through selected community contact. If the agency had a full complement of qualified specialists, all of the key community resources would be more professionally and more intensively covered by the assigned staff of specialists.

A number of specializations are identifiable and along with each one there are examples of pertinent community resources with which the designated specialist can relate. Actual type and number of specializations would vary according to the size, character, and charge of the local agency staff. (In sparsely populated areas, there is a constriction due to travel expenses and

time.) One staff member may have more than one specialization; conversely, more than one staff member may be required for certain specializations (for example, the agency may work to develop several personal adjustment counseling specialists who are specifically trained to work with the psychosocial problems).

Specializations may be categorized by function as well as by disability or client characteristics. The following list is for purposes of illustrating areas of specialization suitable in rehabilitation counselor preparation and case assignment. (For each specialist area the appropriate community contacts for services and referrals are given parenthetically.) Specialties (and contacts) are as follows:

1. Client assessment specialist (employment service testing staff, psychometrists, work evaluation units, trial work projects).
2. Personal adjustment counseling specialist (clinical and counseling psychologists, psychiatrists, psychiatric social workers).
3. Job development and placement specialist (employers, personnel departments, state employment service offices, government civil service agencies).
4. Developmental disabilities specialist (neurologists; developmental disabilities councils; residential facilities for the mentally retarded; special education teachers; private associations for mental retardation, cerebral palsy, epilepsy, autism).
5. Emotional disturbance specialist (psychiatrists and treatment staff in mental hospitals and clinics, mental health associations, crisis centers).
6. Vision impairment specialist (ophthalmologists, special education classes and state schools for the blind, mobility centers, special services such as sources for talking books and readers, associations of and for the blind).
7. Hard of hearing specialist (otologist, special education classes and state schools for the deaf, hearing aid distributors, private associations).
8. Alcohol and drug abuse specialist (professional staff in treatment centers, Alcoholics Anonymous, private agencies such as the Salvation Army).
9. Severe orthopedic disabilities specialist (orthopedists and physiatrists, rehabilitation hospitals, appliance shops).

10. Disabled-minority specialist (fair employment practice officials, Urban League, National Association for the Advancement of Colored People, other formal and informal groups such as Hispanic, Native American, or Oriental groups).
11. Disabled–public offenders specialist (probation and parole officers, court social workers, corrections institutions).
12. Rehabilitation facilities specialist (community workshops, rehabilitation hospitals).
13. Financial support sources specialist (state workers' compensation board and insurance carriers, student aid officers, Social Security offices and disability determination units, public welfare and social service workers).
14. Small business enterprise specialist (banks, loan agencies, accountants).
15. Independent living rehabilitation specialist (rehabilitation residences and centers, special transportation and housing services, recreational and activities facilities, health maintenance services, self-care and activities-of-daily-living instructors).

This list of specializations (and companion resources) is not complete and does not include rehabilitation agency liaison assignments in universities, hospitals, and other institutions.

Supervision of an administrative nature may be thought of as another area of specialization. It is a form of professional development requiring preparation over and above that offered in the masters degree program of rehabilitation counselor education. Administrative activities also can be distinguished from professional affairs of the counselor, indicating the possibility of a division of task assignment. Selected rehabilitation counselors could be identified for training and special assignment to administrative duties. In fact, there is an implication in this whole specialization model that personnel assignment in state rehabilitation agencies could be organized according to administrative and professional tracks at both practitioner and supervisory levels.

3.4.9. VALUE OF SPECIALIZATION

The continuing controversy over the trend toward an integrated human service delivery system is an ideological conflict between non-categorical versus specialized service with rehabilitation represented by the latter. The strongest argument against absorption by an omnibus social system is the superiority of rehabilitation personnel attributable to their professional expertise (i.e., rehabilitation counselors are more effective in their work for the life adjustment of handicapped individuals). The efficiency claim for merger of human service personnel loses its persuasion in the light of the more effective contribution of expert rehabilitation professional service.

Specialization allows the professional to exercise his or her particular pattern of interests, aptitudes, and abilities. It also makes each counselor unique in the agency or office as its consulting authority on problems within an area of expertise. This has potential for greater job satisfaction than would probably be found in an office of "general practitioners." Moreover, the advent of specialization affords opportunity for a continuing, lifelong challenge of professional enrichment by expanding or even shifting one's specialty.

Higher level civil service status with correspondingly higher pay ranges would be provided for rehabilitation "counseling specialists"—more advanced categories than the present "master counselor" rating in state civil service. The extra preparation and corresponding value to clients and to society of rehabilitation counseling specialists justifies such advancement in recognition and rewards by civil service and agency administrators. Formal implementation by rehabilitation agencies of this modern specialist model would call for continuing education programs by rehabilitation counselor educators, new initiatives for staff development through the federal rehabilitation training grants program, and refinements in the rehabilitation counseling certification and accreditation mechanisms. (In the obsolete "generalist" personnel classification system, masters degree graduates soon reach the top master counselor status and maximum salary, thereby losing financial incentive for further professional development.) Finally, this proposed specialist system could very well help the whole profession of rehabilitation counseling toward a recommitment of professionalism and excellence in client service.

Chapter 4

Impact of Disability

The effects of physical and mental disabilities vary from minor annoyances—or even quite positive influences on the individual such as greater motivation to achieve or more sensitive appreciation of the real meaning of life—to catastrophic destruction. Disability may be temporary, may be overcome by time and medical intervention, or may worsen despite all efforts. Disablement from birth defects, illness, and accidents can take many forms, touching any or all facets of normal living. This chapter covers the postmedical problems of disability.

4.1. Principles

Total rehabilitation as a problem-solving process addresses the limitations and handicaps that remain after a medical condition is treated. The rehabilitation counselor is not concerned with the medical aspects, but rather with the *impact* of the physical, mental, or emotional condition. Differential conceptualizations as discussed in this section provide understanding of the borders of responsibility for the rehabilitationist.

4.1.1. CONCEPTS
Disability, limitation, and *handicap* are important words in rehabilitation because they stand for phenomena impacting upon clients. They refer to key concepts. Yet no other area of the rehabilitation nomenclature produces such semantic confusion as these three words. There are countless words in use for the vague notions implied: *defect, inability, deficit, incapacity, disadvantage, impairment, disablement, invalidity, chronically ill, crippled, unfit,* and more. Worse yet, such words, with their negative connotations, elicit highly emotional reactions and are often misconstrued as being demeaning or interpreted as destructive (even malicious) labeling by the target (disabled) population. Part of the problem is a lack of defined difference in the terms. The definitions given below for these words are arbitrary but

they do reflect traditional connotations and thinking among rehabilitation workers.

DISABILITY. In American rehabilitation nomenclature *disability* means a long-term or chronic condition medically defined as a physiological, anatomical, mental, or emotional impairment resulting from disease or illness, inherited or congenital defect, trauma, or other insult (including environmental) to mind or body. Examples are: (1) epilepsy, (2) mental retardation, (3) poliomyelitis, (4) psychosis, and (5) emphysema.

FUNCTIONAL LIMITATION. The hindrance or negative effect in the performance of tasks or activities, and other adverse and overt manifestations of a mental, emotional, or physical disability is here referred to as a "functional limitation." Examples (cf. above, disabilities) are: (1) activity restrictions due to the danger of unexpected unconsciousness, (2) inability to follow rapid or frequent changes in instructions due to slow learning, (3) restrictions in mobility due to neuromuscular impairment, (4) difficulty in interpersonal relationships associated with peculiar behavior, and (5) necessity of avoiding respiratory infection or dusty conditions due to hypersensitivity reactions.

HANDICAP. A handicap is a disadvantage, interference, or barrier to performance, opportunity, or fulfillment in any desired role in life (e.g., vocational, social, educational, familial), imposed upon the individual by limitation in function or by other problems associated with disability and/or personal characteristics in the context of the individual's environment or role. For example, people in the following occupations would probably be handicapped if the disabilities and functional limitations above were present: (1) arc welder, (2) rehabilitation psychologist, (3) garbage collector, (4) cleric, and (5) hospital janitor.

The above definitions refer to essential concepts in rehabilitation. Specific meanings of the terms referring to the separate phenomena called "disability," "limitation," and "handicap" conceptually accommodate several principles:

1. The definitions distinguish between medical disability, functional limitation, and vocational (or other) handicap so that these phenomena may be understood and treated separately (e.g., the disabled person is not assumed to be handicapped). Each of the three identified phenomena is described by a specific aspect or characteristic and consequently any negative implication of the terms referring to the phenomena does not spread demeaningly to the whole person.

2. The dynamic hierarchy—handicap from functional limitation from medical disability—clarifies possible cause-effect relations, therefore suggesting the point and method of rehabilitation intervention. Yet multiple causation and varying effects of the phenomena are also accommodated. For example, a handicap for an occupation may be attributed to a physical limitation in function, as well as various other reasons, such as lack of knowledge or of job skills. Moreover, descriptions for the various types of handicaps (e.g., legal, social) constitute alternative dimensions for examination of the rehabilitation client or environmental problems.

3. A valid assessment of the severity of a handicap requires nonmedical measures. The disability of epilepsy is an example: when seizures are completely controlled, there are no functional limitations and no occupational handicap, yet the person with the disability label *epilepsy* may still be under an "employment handicap" due to social stigma or even legal restrictions; another case, for example, a writer of fiction, illustrates that severe functional limitations such as uncontrolled grand mal seizures may not constitute a handicap in one's occupation.

4. Three "stages" of rehabilitation are implied in the three types of phenomena, each of which presents different problems and requires different professional expertise. The first phase of rehabilitation addresses the disability as a medical problem requiring physicians and the paramedical team; the next stage begins when the medical treatment has been partially successful and the patient has survived but with some functional limitations requiring a rehabilitation team who can provide physical or technical aid and adjustive services; the final phase—vocational or independent living rehabilitation—occurs when residual limitations causing a handicap call for nonmedical strategies and staff in which the counselor is the central professional person. Thus, total rehabilitation is portrayed as a course of action for preserving a person's life,

functions, and productivity in three identifiable stages.

5. This classification is suitable for rehabilitationists because it conforms to their professional interests and their traditional terminology. Handicapping mostly derives from the client's residual limitations rather than the basic disability. The focus then is upon limitations that are compounded (or alleviated) by other personal characteristics and circumstances. For example, when the functional limitation is immobility or inability to walk, it is less important that this limitation results from paraplegia or from double hip disarticulation than whether or not the client may be trained or placed in a job that does not require functioning lower limbs.

4.1.2. DEFINITIONAL ISSUES

The definition of *disability* as a medical problem distinct from the resulting handicap was stated by Hamilton [1950] in *Counseling the Handicapped in the Rehabilitation Process*. Confusion has prevailed, however, about the meaning of *handicap*, which Hamilton (and others) failed to differentiate from an intervening physical or behavioral variable described here as "functional limitation." Thus, the word *handicap* has been used imprecisely and has meant anything from a limp to unemployability. However, when the word *disability* refers to a medical condition that causes a handicap, it is clearly understood by rehabilitation professionals.

Unfortunately, traditional rehabilitation terminology differs from that of the American medical profession, in which the term *impairment* for the medical condition is preferred to *disability*. Moreover, physicians call the result of the medical impairment a "disability," referring to a narrower range of phenomena than that referred to by *handicap* as defined here for rehabilitation use.

The lack of a uniform nomenclature is troublesome in interprofessional communication and in the interpretation of legislation and agency regulations. It is particularly confusing that the words *disability* and *handicap* in rehabilitation are comparable to *impairment* and *disability*, respectively, in American medicine. Still, the crucial issue is clarity of conceptualization rather than nominal uniformity and, from a practical standpoint, changing this familiar language of rehabilitation is an academic notion that would gain little support among practitioners.

Actually the rehabilitation terms *disability* and *handicap* are broadly used and understood. In its *Glossary—Vocational Rehabilitation and Employment of the Disabled*, the International Labor Office [n.d.] stated:

Handicap occurs as a result of disability; but disability does not always constitute a handicap. A handicap may be said to exist when a disability causes a substantial and continuing reduction in a person's capacity to function socially and vocationally. Handicap may also result from community prejudice and resistance thereby reducing opportunities to the disabled person's functioning [p. 18].

Handicap as defined in the unabridged *Oxford English Dictionary* [1971] means, ". . . to place anyone at a disadvantage by the imposition of any embarrassment, impediment, or disability. . . ." Moreover, *disability* in American glossaries of rehabilitation terms is consistently defined as a medical term; for example, the publication *Words: Work-Oriented Rehabilitation Dictionary and Synonyms* [Northwest Association of Rehabilitation Industries, 1975] gives this definition of *disability*: "A physical or mental defect or impairment that a person is born with, or that is acquired by accident, injury, or disease. (Syn.: impairment)."

Not everyone is satisfied with the nomenclature of the rehabilitation field. Nagi, a professor of sociology, in an address to the 1977 American Rehabilitation Counseling Association conference in Dallas, Texas, objected to the term *handicap* as it ". . . has been widely used in the field of rehabilitation . . ." and expressed his preference for the term *permanent disability* as defined in 1960 by an American Medical Association committee. Nagi assumed erroneously that the use of the term *handicap* emerged in rehabilitation during the development of the rehabilitation counseling profession in an attempt to distinguish its "non-medical" entities from the domain of physicians. The fact is that the rehabilitation words and concepts in question were in common use long before the profession of rehabilitation counseling developed.

Differential meanings of the terms *physical disability* and *occupational handicap* were used in the context of selective placement techniques for World War I disabled veterans—before the civilian Rehabilitation Act was passed by Congress. In 1919 Elizabeth Upham articulated these notions through a major aricle in *The Vocational Summary*, the official publication of the U.S. Federal Board of Vocational Education:

If all men who have physical defects may be considered handicapped, the vast part of the working population is in some degree handicapped. In the popular sense a man is considered handicapped only when his physical defect is such that he is unfitted for certain occupations. The handicap is therefore not dependent on the physical condition of the man, but on its relation to his employment. Thus one man may find himself handicapped in one occupation but not in another. A method of reducing handicaps is therefore the careful selection of the occupation in relation to the disability. . . .

Selective placement aims to place men in those positions which they are by nature, training, and experience best qualified to fill. . . . This involves a knowledge of the physical limitations and assets of every applicant for every position. . . . Vocational education [sic] reduces the effect of handicap; in fact, it eliminates the handicap altogether, since the man is not handicapped by his physical condition, but only by the limitation which his physical condition imposes upon his employment. . . . As a matter of fact, a "handicap" cannot be strictly defined in any but a relative way. . . . Disease produces a variety of conditions which are handicaps in certain employments. Heredity defects, and disease of childhood, environment, and employment produce a number of individual symptoms which must be considered in the placing of the applicant. The problem of finding a job which will eliminate a man's handicap is solved by the scientific analysis of his physical condition in relation to occupation. . . . [pp. 35–36].

In 1924 this distinction between a "disability" and a "vocational handicap," was made by the U.S. Veterans Bureau through their manual of procedures for the vocational rehabilitation of veterans of World War I.

4.1.3. LEGISLATIVE DEFINITIONS

The first federal legislation for civilian vocational rehabilitation, in 1920, provided this definition of *disablement* in Section 2:

. . . for the purpose of this Act the term "persons disabled" shall be construed to mean any person who, by reason of a physical defect or infirmity, whether congenital or acquired by accident, injury, or disease, is, or may be expected to be, totally or partially incapacitated for remunerative occupation . . .

This legal definition of *disablement* has been refined and made more operational over the years.

In 1943 Public Law 113 defined vocational rehabilitation services as ". . . any services necessary to render a disabled individual fit to engage in a remunerative occupation." With the dele-

tion of the word *physical* rehabilitation services were extended by definition to people disabled by mental retardation or emotional disturbance.

The 1973 Rehabilitation Act defined a severely handicapped person as having ". . . a severe physical or mental disability which seriously limits his functional capacities (mobility, communication, self-care, self-direction, work therapy, or work skills) in terms of employability." This phraseology is consistent with the traditional vocational rehabilitation model.

The 1978 Amendments to the 1973 Act, which authorized rehabilitation services for independent living, continued the traditional language. Eligibility for services was extended to any individual "whose ability to function independently" is "limited" by the "severity of his disability." Services were thus authorized to "enhance the ability of a handicapped individual" to live independently.

4.1.4. CONCEPTUAL CLARITY

The terminology of rehabilitation appears to be of greater concern to other professionals than to rehabilitationists. A report on comprehensive rehabilitation service needs by the Urban Institute [1975a] reflected displeasure with the traditional rehabilitation nomenclature. Consequently, J. S. Turem, Director of that project, surveyed about 1,000 rehabilitation workers and asked them if the language of the 1973 Rehabilitation Act, as interpreted in the federal regulations, provided "an adequate operational definition of a severely handicapped individual for vocational rehabilitation purposes." Despite Turem's concerns, an overwhelming 86 percent answered affirmatively and many of the dissenters seemed only to be quarreling with the criteria rather than the clarity of the concepts. It is apparent that despite differences in definition of terms such as *disability* and *handicap* by other agencies and other professions, rehabilitation workers as a group have little difficulty with their traditional terminology.

For state rehabilitation agency purposes of case selection priority and eligibility determination, it is essential to have a clear conception of how vocational handicapping is manifested. While Nagi in 1977 said that ". . . the term handicap has never been operationally defined," state rehabilitation agencies have done so for years. In 1926 Sullivan and Snortum listed the following principles adopted for state vocational rehabilitation services in Minnesota:

A vocational handicap will be considered to exist when there is evidence to support any of the following conditions:

A. Inability to pursue former occupation, or any occupation without special training.
B. Inability to pursue former occupation except at a decrease in efficiency and consequent material reduction in remuneration as compared with that previously received, or inability to pursue another occupation except at a materially lower remuneration.
C. Probability of more frequent periods of unemployment in former occupations, through decreased efficiency resulting in earlier layoffs at slack times, discrimination in re-employment and the like.
D. Existence of unusual hazard of incurring further or total permanent disability if former occupation is continued, e.g., a man who has lost one eye continuing in an occupation where there is a high degree of danger of eye accident [pp. 186–187].

McGowan [1960] explained, ''The rehabilitation process is concerned primarily with the handicapping problems resulting from disability rather than with disability per se'' [p. 16]. And yet textbooks on medical information that are written for courses in rehabilitation counseling education still follow the medical emphasis on disability and are typically organized around body systems (e.g., neurology), as in medical education. The professional concerns of rehabilitation counselors, however, are directed toward the causal factors of handicapping. Thus, the rehabilitation counseling orientation for training and practice needs to be focused on the functional limitations and abilities of clients.

4.2. Medical Implications

It is beyond the scope of this volume to cover the medical aspects of disability comprehensively. The application of medical information, however, is essential in rehabilitation client assessment and planning. This issue in an adjustment context is discussed below in Chapter 5, Functional Limitations.

4.2.1. BOOKS ON THE SUBJECT
There are many notable medical information books appropriate for rehabilitation workers. Those listed here are used as text or reference works in rehabilitation education courses on medical information.

Handbook of Severe Disability, by W. C. Stolov and M. R. Clowers [1980].
Medical Information for Human Service Workers (2nd. rev. ed.), by Kenneth Hylbert [1979].
Rehabilitation Medicine, by Howard Rusk [1977a].
The Merck Manual of Diagnosis and Therapy, by D. N. Holvey [1977].
The Rehabilitation Medicine Services, by Lawrence Ince [1974].
Medical and Psychological Aspects of Disability, by A. Beatrix Cobb [1973].
Handbook of Physical Medicine and Rehabilitation, by F. H. Krusen, F. J. Kottke, and P. M. Ellwood [1971].
An Orientation to Chronic Disease and Disability, by Julian Myers [1965].

Chapter 15, Medical Services, provides information on the relationship of medicine to total rehabilitation.

4.2.2. MEASUREMENT OF SEVERITY
Severity of disablement as a medical term refers to the extent of the disorder of the body or the mind. For example, a convenient measure of the severity of leg amputation is the above knee (A/K) or below knee (B/K) distinction. Similarly the amount of hearing loss is measured in decibels. Mental retardation (MR) is commonly measured by IQ tests: no retardation, 83–100 IQ range; borderline MR, 70–84 IQ; mild (educable), 55–69 IQ; moderate (trainable), 35–54 IQ; severe, 20–34 IQ; profound, 0–19 IQ.

The handicaps resulting from the disability are of various kinds. A medical disability may handicap or limit an individual at school, work, home, or in any of life's situations or pursuits. The types and extent of the handicaps associated with disability are modified or compounded, as the case may be, by many other positive or negative personal characteristics (e.g., motivation and compensating attributes). Moreover, the nature and severity of the handicaps of disability depend upon one's environmental circumstances.

An example is mildly retarded children whose

limitation in learning is based on their mental age subnormality. These children are usually classified as educable and rarely need institutionalization because of their intelligence level. In general, then, for the 90 percent of the mentally retarded population whose IQ is between 55 and 70 (approximately), there are indications regarding the type and severity of their limitation: as a group such people can be educated and can live outside of institutions. Similar predictions about the functional limitation level can be made for the moderately retarded who are considered trainable. In actuality, however, the educational potential of the retarded person is realized only when other personal and environmental circumstances are favorable. Moreover, there is a wide range of individual differences among retarded people with the same IQ level. In fact, intelligence alone may not be a good predictor of employment potential. The severity of disabilities in general has low correlation with the type and degree of handicap.

4.2.3. DISABILITY EVALUATION

The first book of note on disability evaluation, written by Henry Kessler [1935], facilitated the measurement by physicians of the medical factors of functional limitation (e.g., physical units or deviation scores for range of motion, muscle strength, or coordination). More important for this discussion was Kessler's [1970] continuing leadership in isolating the medical component of evaluation of the handicap:

Although the physician is able to estimate the nature and degree of a medical impairment, nothing in his training and little in his experience have prepared him for the task of evaluating the psychological, social, and economic consequences. With little or no knowledge of the ability of handicapped persons to engage in gainful employment and with no means of estimating adaptability to employment, the physician's judgments about disability are likely to be arbitrary and inaccurate. He is trained to observe defects and to measure the variations from the normal, but no system of pathological evaluation includes estimation of the capacity to work and other associated nonmedical factors [p. 25].

Wan [1974], who analyzed the effects of chronic diseases, concluded: "The ability to engage in gainful work despite a disabling condition is determined by a complex relationship between pathological condition and a variety of social, demographic, and environmental attributes" [p. 234]. Thus, the effects of disability may be compounded by other negative attributes or situations.

An example of the complex nature of disability is provided by the problem of unattractiveness. Physical or behavioral unattractiveness may lead to social rejection, which nurtures in the person an expectation of rejection with resulting defensive reactions. A cyclical reaction is thus perpetuated and this leads in turn to a social limitation as well. The self-concept deteriorates as the interaction with others becomes worse. Thus people can become "unacceptable," not merely because of their appearance, but because of their own self-image and untoward social defenses. Such reactions are exemplified by defensive or nonconforming behavior, argumentativeness, and so on. They may become severely handicapping, depending on situational factors. This aspect is discussed in the section that follows.

4.3. Psychosocial Impact

Personal and social resources of the disabled individual are often more important in rehabilitation than residual physical resources. Disabled people are far more than assemblages of mechanical parts—they are spiritual beings influenced by psychological and environmental conditions. The interactions of mind and body and their environs are not easily predicted, but their complex relationships in the human being are at no time more striking than when sudden physical incapacity occurs. Neither the type nor degree of physical disablement foretells the pattern or extent of the psychosocial impact, as it varies with the individual and life circumstances.

While there is no systematic and universal correlation of type or severity of disablement with type or severity of maladjustment, disability can affect personality. Still, it should not be assumed that disability has only disturbing psychological consequences. Along with frustration and grief, disability can generate opportunity and gratification [B. Wright, 1960]. Hope exerts a strong counterforce against despair. Small achievements can be most rewarding when the individual has overcome a large obstacle.

It is the personal meaning of the disability to the individual that is crucial in rehabilitation counseling practice. Somatopsychology is the study of those variations in physique that affect the psychological situation of a person by influencing the effectiveness of the body as a tool for actions or by serving as a stimulus to the self or others [Barker, Wright, Myerson, & Gonick, 1953]. But because psychological processes are not constant from one client to another, psychological treatment must be tailored to meet individual situations and reactions.

Fink [1967] divided the "crisis of disability" into these stages: shock, defensive retreat, acknowledgement, and adaptation. He tied this to motivational theory by pointing out that the early stages of reaction primarily involve security needs while the last stage is directed toward growth.

The psychosocial impact of disability can be measured. An inventory to measure the self-perceived problems caused by disability is published by the Purdue University Research Foundation. The *Handicap Problems Inventory* by Wright and Remmers [1960] is used to understand the impact of any disability upon the individual. Four aspects of life are covered: personal, social, familial, and vocational. Donald Linkowski [1971] has developed a scale (the AD scale) to measure a person's acceptance of disability. A report by Linkowski and Dunn [1974] showed that AD scores were related to the broader perspective of self-conception by the disabled person. Nondisabled people's attitudes toward disability have also been studied and a scale has been developed [Yuker, Block, & Campbell, 1960]. Negative attitudes of society have an effect upon the disabled—not only because of unkind treatment accorded them but also because of how they feel about themselves. This was expressed by Siller, Chipman, Ferguson, and Vann [1967].

Self-depreciation by a handicapped person may be explained as a reflection of prevalent social attitudes. In the newly disabled, negative attitudes that were previously focused on members of a devalued out-group may refocus on the self with devastating results.

4.3.1. EXPLANATIONS FROM THEORY

A number of theoretical ideas on reaction and adjustment to disability have been proposed. Unfortunately there has been a lack of experimental research in the literature on personality and disability. Most of the relevant studies are descriptive in nature and not sufficiently comprehensive. But while the theoretical notions may remain inadequately tested, they still have value to the rehabilitationist as a conceptual framework within which to understand the impact of disability.

Early theorists traced the person's self-concept and values back to interpersonal relations and the way the person is seen by others [Barker, 1947; 1948]. Roger Barker and his colleagues proposed this interpersonal theory. They developed a number of useful concepts: comparative and asset values, containment of disability effects, expectation of discrepancy, spread, and new and overlapping situations.

Body-image theory uses psychoanalytic principles to explain the development in each individual of a conception of self as a bodily unity. Murphy [1957] wrote that it is by way of the "body image" that castration anxiety influences personality in cases of physical disabilities.

Maslow's [1954] theory of motivation has provided a basis for understanding the "prepotency" of human needs: lower level needs such as hunger and safety must be satisfied before one can attend to higher level needs such as interpersonal gratifications and self-esteem. Barry and Malinovsky [1965] have applied Maslow's organization to the literature on rehabilitation client motivation. Studies on society's devaluing attitudes toward disability provide important information for both rehabilitation research and practice [Kojima, 1976; 1977]. However, they do not explain the disabled person's reaction to disablement.

Personality theories generally have had little relevance to disability impact. The exception is Adlerian theory, which postulates compensation for organ inferiority. While Adler's proposal of an inferiority complex has been controverted, there are suggestions of inherent value to rehabilitation workers, and the rehabilitationist should understand the complex dynamics of inferiority. Feelings of inferiority lead to maladaptive behaviors, sometimes with vividly different manifestations. One person succumbs to the impairment as totally crippling and protects self-perceived vulnerability by seeming helplessness, while other people may overcompensate in a desperate effort to overcome what they perceive as personal inferiority.

This section is intended as an introduction to the psychosocial impact of disability, knowledge of which is extremely important to the rehabilitationist. These psychosocial aspects are discussed further in Chapter 28, Personal Adjustment, and in numerous books on the subject, many of which are listed below.

4.3.2. NOTABLE BOOKS

Study of the psychosocial impact of disability is facilitated by a number of outstanding works on the subject. The following are recommended to the student for further reading.

Psychosocial Adjustment to Disability, by Richard Roessler and Brian Bolton [1978].
The Psychological and Social Impact of Physical Disability, by Robert Marinelli and Arthur Dell Orto [1977].
Social and Psychological Aspects of Disability, by Joseph Stubbins [1977].
Physical Disability and Human Behavior, by James McDaniel [1976].
The Psychological Aspects of Physical Illness and Disability, by Franklin Shontz [1975].
Rehabilitation Practices with the Physically Disabled, by James Garrett and Edna Levine [1973].
Medical and Psychological Aspects of Disability, by A. Beatrix Cobb [1973].
The Sociology and Social Psychology of Disability and Rehabilitation, by Constantina Safilios-Rothschild [1970].
Body Image and Personality, by Seymour Fisher and Sidney Cleveland [1968].
Psychological Practices with the Physically Disabled, by James Garrett and Edna Levine [1962].
Physical Disability—A Psychological Approach, by Beatrice A. Wright [1960].
Psychology and Rehabilitation, by Beatrice A. Wright [1959].

In addition there are a number of books on psychosocial aspects of disability that are of value for in-depth study or historical review of the subject:

The Sociology of Physical Disability and Rehabilitation, by Gary Albrecht [1976].
Behavior Modification in Rehabilitation Medicine, by Lawrence Ince [1976].
Dependency and its Implications for Rehabilitation, by George Goldin, Sally Perry, Reuben Margolin, and Bernard Stotsky [1972].
Rehabilitation Psychology, by Walter Neff [1971].
The Measurement of Attitudes Toward Disabled Persons, by Harold Yuker, J. R. Block, and Janet Younng [1970].
Studies in Reaction to Disability. Attitudes of the Nondisabled Toward the Physically Disabled, by Jerome Siller, Abram Chipman, Linda Ferguson, and Donald Vann [1967].
Stigma: Notes on the Management of Spoiled Identity, by Erving Goffman [1963].
Psychological Research and Rehabilitation, by Lloyd Lofquist [1960].
The Denial of Illness, by E. Weinstein and R. L. Kahn [1955].
Psychology of Exceptional Children and Youth, by William M. Cruickshank [1955].
Adjustment to Physical Handicap and Illness: A Survey of the Social Psychology of Physique and Disability, by Roger Barker, Beatrice A. Wright, Lee Myerson, and Mollie Gonick [1953].
Psychological Aspects of Disability, by James Garrett [1952].
Adjustment to Physical Handicap and Illness: A Survey of the Social Psychology of Physique and Disability, by Roger Barker, Beatrice A. Wright, and Mollie Gonick [1946].
The Psychology of the Physically Handicapped, by Rudolf Pintner, Jon Eisenson, and Mildred Stanton [1941].

In addition to the books on the psychological impact of disabilities in general (listed above) there are a number of books that focus on the psychosocial aspects of a specific disability. An outstanding example is *Adjustment to Blindness—Reviewed* by Mary K. Bauman and Norman M. Yoder (1966).

4.4. *Vocational Impact*

Disability reduces the degree of freedom in vocational choice and forces the handicapped person to stay within a more restricted range of occupations. Functional limitations resulting from disability, however, at the worst simply reduce one's employment options. The vocational impact of disability consequently is only selectively handicapping because a limitation is relevant only to a requirement of a particular job.

Functional limitations will be classified and

described in considerable detail in the next chapter. It suffices here to put these restrictions into proper perspective: they must be neither ignored nor overestimated as a factor in rehabilitation planning. For example, deafness is a limitation in the function of communication; some jobs (e.g., telephone operator) require interpersonal communication that a deaf person could not engage in, while a great many other jobs can be performed quite well without hearing (e.g., linotype operator). Still other job requirements ·can be adapted to dispense with the need to hear (e.g., a signal light flasher can be exchanged for a bell sound). Moreover, through rehabilitative devices such as hearing aids or training such as lip reading, deaf and hard of hearing people can overcome the functional limitation and expand the variety of suitable jobs [Myklebust, 1960]. Another approach in vocational rehabilitation is to help the client become so well qualified through, for example, the provision of professional education, that the difficulty in hearing is compensated for by other expertise. (See Chapter 14, Educational Services).

4.4.1. VOCATIONAL HANDICAP

Employment handicap and *occupational handicap* are another pair of terms helpful for understanding the problems of disability and vocational handicapping.

When a disability results in limitations in the functions required to perform the tasks of an otherwise suitable occupation, it is causing an *occupational handicap;* vocational adjustment requires either correcting the functional limitation(s) or changing the occupation. The extent of occupational handicap with even catastrophic medical disablement can be offset by positive job attributes such as general education. Conversely, the disabled person's occupational handicap is compounded by lack of experience or training for work.

Employment handicap denotes difficulty in getting (or retaining) a suitable job because of employer ignorance or prejudice pertaining to physical or other characteristics of an applicant who is able to perform the required work tasks. In addition to mental and physical disablement, many personal characteristics are misunderstood or scorned by employers and others in the community because of individual differences: being of minority race, being poor, speaking a foreign language. Overcoming these

barriers is a frequent challenge in vocational placement. Employment handicapping, also, can be either compounded or compensated for by other characteristics of an individual.

Vocational rehabilitation by definition means helping a person cope with either an occupational or employment handicap. Often it means making the person more competitive. Whether accurately or not, disabled people are sometimes thought to be restricted in these job considerations:

1. Job time schedule: Variations are required in the number or schedule of hours, and time-out periods or absences are needed.
2. Job tenure: Premature retirement due to deterioration of physical or mental condition is probable.
3. Job performance: Quality or speed of production is below normal.
4. Job assistance: Extra help from fellow employees and supervisors is needed.
5. Job flexibility: Shift or transfer to jobs with other tasks requiring another set of abilities is not possible.
6. Job progression: Performance in entry job required of new employees would be inadequate.
7. Job modification: Job or station needs to be changed to eliminate barriers.

None of the above are considerations in the placement of most disabled workers with most employers. *Severity of handicap* is a comparative term indicating the degree of inability to meet the demands of roles or tasks. Severity of handicap must be assessed in relation to all of the important personal and environmental factors that impinge on the individual. Personal variables include age, sex, and physical, mental, social, economic, skill, educational, and cultural factors. Environmental variables include available services, economic conditions, climate, transportation, and the type of employment opportunities existing. Severity of handicap consequently must be analyzed from a comprehensive and individualized perspective.

It is a great mistake to assume that the degree of handicapping can automatically be predicted from the medically diagnosed disability. Highly incapacitating physical conditions do not necessarily result in severe handicapping. The total impact of a disability is either mitigated or compounded by a complex configuration of strengths and weaknesses in the afflicted person and the environment. Still, it is common in our language and legislation to associate specified severe disabilities with severe handicapping.

The vocational handicap from disability and other causes is manifested in various ways. This picture is further complicated when disabilities negatively influence other life areas: thus, along with vocational handicapping there may be a social handicap, family handicap, psychological handicap, and so on. All of these may interact, and any such handicap may itself become a causal factor to other adjustment problems. Extensive research on the correlates of disability or handicaps has been conducted for the U.S. Social Security Administration by Lawrence D. Haber [1971, 1973].

Everyone is occupationally handicapped in one way or another for most jobs. There are in the world an uncounted number of different kinds of jobs—different in that each places a unique set of demands on the worker to perform all component tasks properly. No one individual has ever had the full range of abilities to meet all of the critical requirements of all occupations (e.g., aviator, chaplain, artist, judge, boxer, cabinetmaker).

Stated in a positive way, almost everyone has all of the abilities required for some occupation. Residual functional abilities, whatever they may be, are relevant to the requirements of some kind of employment. In fact, abilities are the only relevant consideration in the determination of what a worker can do.

Only gradually has society recognized that the severely disabled can become active, producing members of society. Lack of appreciation for this was demonstrated over a 100-year period by the erection of institutions for the custodial care of these people. Recently the huge state mental hospitals, colonies for the retarded or epileptic, and residential schools for the blind or the deaf are being replaced by community-based facilities for their social integration and entrance into the community and the world of work. The movement is dubbed "deinstitutionalization." Rehabilitation processes are being employed effectively even with very severely disabled persons whose handicap has worsened through the experience of institutionalization.

Underemployment and unemployment of culturally disadvantaged people has also become a public issue. The techniques of VR are again found effective in bringing the underprivileged masses into the regular labor force. Thus, U.S. Department of Labor programs are improving the employability of socioeconomically deprived people in much the same way as the state rehabilitation agencies have helped medically disabled people overcome vocational handicapping.

4.4.2. CAUSAL VARIABLES

The vocational impact of disability goes far beyond that of physical and mental inability to perform job activities (listed below as 1.). There are many other vocational problems and some are often far more handicapping; many are beyond the power of the person to correct. All of these negative variables, however, may have an impact upon the rehabilitant:

1. Inability (physical or mental) to tolerate job environment or to perform required tasks—explicitly termed an "occupational handicap."
2. Inexperience due to lack of opportunity to develop work personality and adjustment to the world of work.
3. Deficiencies in education or training due to lack of learning opportunities or abilities.
4. Negative self-concepts (e.g., feelings of inferiority, lack of motivation, unrealistic goals).
5. Disincentives such as loss of social security benefits and secondary gains of dependent status, things that may be withdrawn if paid employment is accepted.
6. Lack of positive societal attitudes along with actions that restrict, demoralize, and dehumanize the individual.
7. Employer ignorance and bias about personal characteristics (e.g., disability, race, sex), known as an "employment" or "placement" handicap.
8. Environmental barriers such as unsuitable housing and transportation or unavailable personal and professional services.
9. Unfavorable labor market conditions or decreasing number of jobs in the geographic area, occupation, or industry.
10. No provision to reengineer or restructure jobs to accommodate applicant's positive and negative attributes.

11. Inadequate identification of jobs suitable for the selective placement of disabled people through public employment services.
12. Deficiencies in organization of service to the vocationally handicapped (e.g., lack of referral and collaboration, inefficient and bureaucratic administration, inadequate planning and accountability).
13. Deficiencies in the staffs of rehabilitation agencies (e.g., lack of professional preparation, motivation, or supervision).
14. Lack of public subsidy for substandard production as an incentive to employers to hire handicapped workers in competitive industry.
15. Lack of tax-subsidized jobs in industry, protected factories, or sheltered workshops to employ disabled workers.
16. Inadequate financial support for comprehensive public rehabilitation agencies and facilities to provide service to all who need and would benefit from services.
17. Inadequate number of qualified agency personnel and insufficient resources for preparing rehabilitation professionals.
18. Insufficient public appropriation for research and demonstrations to further technological advancement in vocational counseling, client assessment, independent living, and job placement as well as in rehabilitation medicine and engineering.
19. Constrictions in public rehabilitation regulations (e.g., restricted eligibility, which denies service until the handicap becomes severe).
20. Narrow conceptualization of the potential clientele for "vocational rehabilitation," which fails to include people handicapped by cultural limitations (e.g., chronic poverty, racial or language prejudices, educational or training disadvantages).

4.4.3. VOCATIONAL READJUSTMENT

Disability, even when severe and lasting, does not always impinge upon earning power or even necessitate a change in job duties. But when it does, the vocational handicap can be serious, not only in terms of livelihood but also in other areas of adjustment. In a society strongly oriented toward work, productive employment is seen by most people as indispensable for independence and respect. Work is the mark of adulthood, a sign that the child has come of age.

Return to work is the traditional goal of American rehabilitation. Even the 1978 Rehabilitation Act Amendments authorizing "Independent Living" programs held out the hope of possible remunerative employment. Increased earning power of recipients in fact has been the predominant criterion of rehabilitation success—so much so that the number of "employed closures" has been the basis for program evaluation of the public agency. State rehabilitation counselors in the past received little case work credit for client progress other than gainful employment. As a consequence, improvement in other life areas tended to be neglected even when essential to occupational readjustment. And when improvement of another kind did occur, there was no mechanism for assessing it to justify the rehabilitation effort.

A comprehensive rehabilitation model could relegate vocational adjustment goals to the final stages of effort following personal adjustment and other preparatory services. This would be naive. Despite criticism of its narrow focus, experience with vocational rehabilitation indicates that other problem areas (e.g., family) may not require outside intervention if the disabled person can be returned to work. The impact of working—even the work of self-care—often dramatically and pervasively improves the rehabilitant's life situation, thereby overcoming the need for psychotherapy.

The narrow vocational emphasis in rehabilitation eligibility requirements, however, screened out applicants who were not clearly feasible for remunerative employment. The federal-state rehabilitation program gradually modified criteria for eligibility so that "employment" was defined more liberally, and the rehabilitation objective no longer had to be remunerative. The 1978 Rehabilitation Act Amendments provide rehabilitation for other social gains—"independent living," which means self-care chores. With people who are very severely disabled, any kind of remunerative work may be only a remote possibility. For these people the objective may be to carry on "activities of daily living" (the acronym ADL is used for such services).

Competence in ADL (see 40.2) without ability to work for pay is still seen as only a partial rehabilitation success. Certainly the extra effort required for reemployment in a productive occupation is economically attractive as a public expense. Moreover, rehabilitants place a high value on the opportunity to work at the highest possible level: follow-up studies show that employment status is the key to clients' satisfaction with their rehabilitation (Reagles, Wright, & Butler, 1970a).

The procedure for vocational readjustment of the disabled population in earlier years was limited to job training and placement after medical evaluation. This notion of service was an oversimplification, particularly for severely handicapped cases with multiple problems that impinge upon vocational adjustment. Many clients were not feasible in the simple vocational reeducation model of vocational rehabilitation that existed before World War II. A common excuse for the inadequacy of the process—and the incompetency of the unprofessional rehabilitation worker—was that the applicant was "unmotivated." Speaking of that period, Walter Neff [1971] pointed out that "the tacit assumption prevailed that the rehabilitation expert could really function effectively only with clients who already manifested adequate motivation for employment" [p. 124]. As Neff reported, this limited rehabilitation to a fraction of the target population, since many applicants were uncertain about their ability to perform any kind of useful work.

For the rehabilitation counselor to label a person as "unmotivated" is so meaningless that it is almost an admission of professional failure. There are barriers to client motivation—the so-called disincentives to rehabilitation—that the professional must identify. Examples are the person's prospects of losing insurance benefits or financial security with reemployment, threats by the family if one becomes independent, fear of failure. But there are also various kinds of incentives, and the rehabilitation counselor must find out what motivates this particular client—examples are social status, material possessions, independence from family, personal usefulness. To help the so-called unmotivated client the counselor eliminates that person's barriers to motivation and installs the proper incentives. This kind of counseling service requires a high level of professional preparation.

There are still rehabilitation agencies that do not provide competent counseling to cope with the multiple causes of vocational maladjustment.

To deal with problems of the severely disabled especially, the profession of rehabilitation counseling has changed agency methods from passive facilitation to active helping (see 13.4.5). It addresses the coping behaviors of the person whose disability is detrimental not only vocationally but also in other, interrelated facets of life.

4.4.4. VOCATIONAL OUTCOMES

Work success is the ultimate programmatic criterion of rehabilitation. Yet this does not mean that all disabled people should have self-supporting jobs. Remuneration is a desirable goal of work for most people, but the humanistic purpose of rehabilitation does not exclude those whose work effort will never have a significant monetary value. For the latter there are other values in work activity that make it constructive and personally rewarding.

This broad definition of rehabilitation success as gainful work or simply rewarding activity, however, should not be used to compromise the desirability of an occupational objective. The goal still should be the highest level of occupational success that is reasonable. Altogether too many cases are closed as rehabilitated before their vocational potentials have been maximized. The real meaning of rehabilitation is to restore maximal opportunity for disabled people, not merely to find jobs. Handicapped people as a group suffer far more than others from underemployment, inadequate pay, and insecurity of tenure, which are more frequent problems for this population as a whole than permanent unemployment. When disabled individuals find paid work it is too often submarginal, temporary, and unlikely to lead to career growth. Insufficient service often results in cases closed in marginal employment; and these must often be reopened, with further disappointment and expense.

Ideally, rehabilitation should provide compensatory skills to make the handicapped worker really equal to others in vocational attractiveness by counterbalancing the disability through extra expertise. Case service expenditures are indicated for extended education and extensive training to ensure the rehabilitant's adaptability and ability to compete throughout a career life. Studies [e.g., Gay, Reagles, & Wright, 1971] have shown that this vocational adjustment effort helps to ensure rehabilitation sustention.

A significant negative impact of disabilities on earnings was confirmed in a study by McManus [U.S. HEW, Social Security Administration, 1978]. It was concluded that, "Only vocational training as a form of human capital investment seems to favor the disabled decidedly; it is about four times as important for disabled workers" [p. 24]. Vocational training was found to be particularly valuable for those who had not finished high school as it greatly enhances their potential earnings. (See Chapter 14, Educational Services).

4.5. Impact on People

Who are these people with disabilities? How does this population differ from the nondisabled? These questions may seem out of place here because rehabilitation always addresses the characteristics and needs of persons, not a faceless population vaguely referred to as "the disabled." This focus on individuals is correct because no two persons are alike and disability impinges on lives in unique ways. Yet the general overview of the collective problem of disablement provides rehabilitationists the perspective they require for their role in social planning.

The word *disability* as used here refers to a medical condition that handicaps a person vocationally. The word *prevalence* refers to the total number of cases in the general population at any point in time, while *incidence* refers to the number of new cases per year or during any time span. Epidemiological studies (epidemiology is the science of determining the amount and distribution of a condition or disease in a given population), census data, and other research indicate how many people are disabled. But information is almost nonexistent on the magnitude of the problem of handicapping.

Information on the problems of people who have disabilities is insufficient for social planning and programming. It is necessary to estimate how many members of the disabled population are vocationally handicapped, what percentage are feasible for rehabilitation services, and also, what services (by type and extent) are indicated. To be meaningful in program planning the data obtained about disabled people must be categorized by the functional limitation and treatment indicated. The planning problem is compounded by the interaction of many community and clientele variables.

4.5.1. PREVALENCE OF DISABILITY

The full magnitude of the disability problem is incalculable. Only rough estimates exist on the prevalence of certain disabilities such as epilepsy (some experts estimate that less than one-half of 1 percent of the population has some form of epilepsy while others place the number at over 3 percent). Survey research—the commonly employed method for estimating the extent of a problem—often fails to identify cases of unapparent or undiagnosed conditions. Thus the U.S. census data and various health survey findings underestimate the impact of disability. Ambiguous terms and unstandardized categories further complicate the interpretation of comparative studies.

Estimating Prevalence

A continuing National Health Survey was inaugurated by the U.S. HEW Public Health Service starting in 1957. It is supposed to provide current data, on a regular basis, concerning the health status of the general population. Estimates made over a 30-year period have indicated that nearly half of the men, women, and children in the United States have some degree of chronic illness or impairment. Survey results further show that these problems are far more common among the poor and the aged.

Chronicity

The National Center for Health Statistics of the U.S. Public Health Service uses the "International Classification of Diseases," adapted for use in the United States. They consider a condition chronic if it is described by the respondent in their survey research as having been noticed for more than three months, or if it is one of the following conditions (these are always considered chronic regardless of the date of onset): allergy (any), arthritis or rheumatism, asthma, cancer, cleft palate, club foot, condition present since birth, deafness or serious trouble with hearing, diabetes, epilepsy, hardening of the arteries, hay fever, heart trouble, hemorrhoids or piles, hernia or rupture, high blood pressure, kidney stones, mental illness, missing extremity (fingers, hand, or arm; toes, foot, or leg), palsy, paralysis of any kind, permanent stiffness or deformity of a limb (the foot, leg, fingers, arm, or back), prostate trouble, repeated trouble with back or spine, rheumatic fever, serious trouble with seeing (even when wearing glasses), sinus trouble (repeated attacks of), speech defect (any), stomach ulcer, stroke, thyroid trouble or goiter, tuberculosis, growths (including tumor or cyst), or trouble with varicose veins.

Estimate of Prevalence

Chronic disabilities that cause some degree of vocational handicapping can best be estimated from the various sources referenced in this section. No actual enumeration (head count) has been made of the Americans of work age who need and would benefit from rehabilitation services. Various studies have been made, however, of the number of people having a disability. The following percentages refer to the total population of adults having the category of disability:

9%: Musculoskeletal (arthritis, rheumatism, or trouble with spine or extremities).

8%: Cardiovascular (any heart trouble, stroke, or arterial vascular problem).

4%: Respiratory (tuberculosis, bronchitis, emphysema, asthma, etc.).

3%: Emotional (psychosis, neurosis, drug abuse, etc.).

3%: Retardation (mild, moderate, severe, and profound mental retardation).

3%: Communication (defective vision, hearing, or speech).

2%: Digestive (stomach ulcer, gall bladder or liver trouble, hernia, etc.).

2%: Neurological (epilepsy, multiple sclerosis, cerebral palsy, etc.).

1%: Endocrine (diabetes, thyroid trouble, etc.).

1%: Urogenital (kidney stones and other trouble).

1%: Neoplasm (cancer, tumor, cyst, and other growths).

3%: Other (allergies, abnormal size or appearance, and other).

All of these are rough approximations. Also, due to the phenomena of multiple disablement (one person can have several disabilities) the above percentages are not additive. The total number

of persons having one or more disabilities (as defined) is assumed by some to be over 20 percent of the American adult population; others estimate the grand total of work-age disabled Americans at as low as 10 percent.

The Urban Institute estimated in 1975 that there were 8,280,000 noninstitutionalized persons in the United States with "severe" disabilities (i.e., severely handicapped); over half of these people are in the work-age range (18 to 64 years). Another 1,787,000 severely disabled persons were in institutions, making up a total of over 10 million people. The Urban Institute, in their feasibility study of vocational rehabilitation program expansion to include people previously considered not feasible for service, stated that a comprehensive rehabilitation program for the severely disabled will cost billions of dollars; at that time rehabilitation accounted for only 2 percent of the total federal expenditure for the severely disabled. While the technical knowledge exists to allow all disabled people to realize their rehabilitation potential, the design of the program expansion (authorized in the 1978 Amendments to the Rehabilitation Act) will require a substantial financial commitment. "This commitment must be undertaken," the Urban Institute concluded, "if the promise of providing comprehensive service is to be fulfilled" [p. 41].

None of the above studies report the number of people who are culturally disadvantaged (i.e., minority members, financially dependent, educationally deficient, language-alienated). These individuals are also handicapped and need rehabilitation services.

4.5.2. WORLD PREVALENCE

The World Health Organization (WHO) studies the scope of disability on a worldwide basis. WHO [1977] estimated the following number of disabled people (the percentage of the world population of 4,000,000,000): congenital disturbances—mental retardation (7.7%), hereditary somatic (body) defects (7.7%), nongenetic (but congenital) disorders (3.9%); communicable diseases—trachoma (1.9%), leprosy (0.7%), poliomyelitis (0.3%), onchocerciasis (0.2%), other communicable diseases (7.7%); noncommunicable somatic disease (19.3%); functional psychiatric disturbance (7.7%); chronic alcoholism and drug abuse (7.7%); trauma or injury—traffic accidents (5.8%), occupational accidents (2.9%), home accidents (5.8%), other

(0.6%); malnutrition (19.3%); other (0.4%). A correction (reduction) for possible double accounting of the above data is suggested (i.e., −25%) for a calculation of the total number of disabled people.

4.5.3. CHARACTERISTICS

Counting the number of disabled people is not nearly as difficult as determining how disability affects the lives of the people. But the latter is far more important for planning social programs.

In the United States, the largest series of surveys and multifaceted reports on the impact of disablement—the functional limitations and vocational handicaps—have been published by the staff of the U.S. Department of Health, Education, and Welfare, Social Security Administration, Office of Research and Statistics. Some of their findings are reported in the *Social Security Bulletin,* a U.S. HEW, SSA journal (monthly) publication; others are issued (irregularly) as separate "staff papers" or "reports" through the U.S. Government Printing Office. The data reported below are entirely from that survey research. These publications are far too numerous to reference specifically but many are available from the federal agency.

Social Security Administration surveys of disabled Americans have covered their functional limitations and vocational handicaps, their living arrangements and social relations, their medical problems and financial losses, and many other results of disablement. In the 1966 survey, data were collected on over 8,000 noninstitutionalized adults (ages 18 to 64) with a follow-up of 4,000 of these in 1969; this longitudinal information showed changes in disability impact and SSA insurance entitlement. Institutionalized adults (6,000 patients) were surveyed in 1967. Then in 1971 data were collected in 1,400 personal interviews with recently disabled (noninstitutionalized) adults on the economic and social consequences and the adjustment of the disabled and their families. Finally, in 1972 the SSA conducted the largest survey of all with a follow-up in 1974; results have furnished data for the comprehensive analyses, published over the subsequent years by SSA, that are used here. The 1972 survey included interviews with 18,000 persons. Data from this study focuses on the extent to which disability affects the labor-force activity of working-age adults and examines the effects on income and other variables.

Impact of disability in terms of its dimensions does not change much from one year to the next, just as the total number affected remains fairly constant over time. The data reported below from the 1972 SSA survey are assumed to reflect a representative sample (as to time and subjects) of all people who are vocationally handicapped because of disability, out of the over 100 million noninstitutionalized Americans in the 20 to 64 age range. Three levels of handicapping are used:

1. Work-prevented: people so categorized cannot work at all or cannot work with regularity.
2. Work-revised: these people can work regularly but cannot work at the same occupation they had before they became disabled or they cannot work full-time.
3. Work-restricted: these people can work full-time, regularly, and at the same occupation as before but they have restrictions on the amount or kind of work they can do (this includes keeping house).

For consistency of terms and ease in reporting, the first category (work-prevented) will be referred to as a "total vocational handicap" and the second and third categories (work-revised or work-restricted) will be combined and referred to below as a "partial vocational handicap."

Prevalence

Of all Americans in the group described above, nearly 15 percent are affected in their ability to work because of chronic health conditions and impairments. Half of these people are totally handicapped vocationally while the remainder are only partially handicapped. While similar proportions of men and women are handicapped, one and one-half times as many women are in the totally handicapped category (9 percent of women, 6 percent of men).

Disabilities Causing Handicaps

The SSA survey asked handicapped people to name their main disability. These disabilities were listed (and are given here along with the percentage of the total number) by those who were prevented from working: musculoskeletal (30%), cardiovascular (25%), respiratory (8%), digestive (4%), mental (11%), and other or not reported (22%). The analyses for this report ignored other conditions existing at the time.

Role of Accidents

Accidents or injuries cause a significant percentage of the disabilities. Furthermore, the proportion is much higher among people who are handicapped than among those who are not. Almost one-seventh of the adult population reporting a disability indicated that it was accidental in origin.

Multiple Conditions

The presence of multiple conditions as well as their number increases the likelihood of the person being handicapped. Three-fourths of all handicapped people report two or more disabilities. The presence of severe handicapping increases even more sharply with the number of disabilities.

Age

The median average age for the disabled is much higher than for the nondisabled. The median age for people who cannot work (totally handicapped) is 53 years; of those, 47 percent are in the 55 to 64 bracket.

Most disabilities take years to develop, the result of slow disease processes. It is not surprising that the prevalence of chronic diseases increases substantially with age: from less than 10 percent in the 20 to 44 age range to nearly 30 percent in the 55 to 64 range.

In general, whatever the degree of disability the chance of occupational handicap increases with age: work is prevented in only 2 percent of those aged 20 to 34 while in disabled people aged 55 to 64 the number classified as totally handicapped vocationally is nearly 20 percent. The percentage of disabled people whose work is revised or restricted is also somewhat greater with age.

Race

Just as age compounds the vocational handicap of disability, race is found to be a significant variable. Black people not only have the highest prevalence of disability, they also suffer the greatest degree of vocational handicapping. Over 20 percent of blacks are disabled compared to 14 percent of whites. And twice as many blacks as whites are totally handicapped vocationally.

Geographic Distribution

Proportionately more handicapped people live in the South than any other region. The South also has the largest number of disabled for whom work is prevented: 9 percent as compared to 7 percent for the Northeast and 6 percent each in the North Central states and the West; the lowest rate is in the Northwest. These patterns probably reflect the larger minority population of the South.

Marital Status Impact

The majority of the disabled in this age range (20 to 64), like the nondisabled, are married, but a higher percentage of the disabled are divorced, separated, and widowed (and not remarried) than the nondisabled.

Educational Level

Lower levels of educational attainment are correlated with the level of vocational handicap from disability. About 70 percent of the nondisabled had at least a high school education as compared to only a third of those with total vocational handicaps. Of the latter group, 44 percent had only an elementary education or less. Lack of education clearly compounds the handicapping effect of disablement.

Income

Income (all money received) of those people reporting total vocational handicap is 25 to 50 percent less than that of the nondisabled. Disabled people are more likely than the nondisabled to be in or near poverty. Less than 10 percent of the income of the nondisabled is from public income maintenance programs as compared to as much as 60 percent of the total income of the nonmarried disabled persons whose work is prevented. The nonmarried disabled are much more likely to be poor. The average income (from all sources) for the totally handicapped group is about half that of the nondisabled.

Medical Costs

The cost of medical care for the people classified as totally handicapped vocationally is twice as high as for the nondisabled. Disabled men are much more likely than the nondisabled during a one-year period to be hospitalized (34% vs. 8%) and to visit a physician (86% vs. 67%). These differences are not so great for women but are in the same direction.

Chapter 5

Functional Limitations

Functional limitations that result from physical, mental, and emotional disabilities are many and varied. This chapter represents an attempt to identify and describe the outstanding categories of limitations associated with loss of function. It represents a reconceptualization of the disabled person's problem as it should be viewed by the rehabilitation counselor. For rehabilitation the issue is not a medical condition but the resulting limitation in functioning, in a life adjustment context.

The listing of 14 functional limitations in this chapter most certainly should be expanded and refined. At present it is not exhaustive and the categories, as stated, are not discrete. More-over, the description here of each limitation is necessarily brief. Nevertheless, this presentation of the nonmedical aspects of disability should provide the orientation toward client problems that rehabilitation professionals require.

This classification of limitations and their descriptions has not been previously published but has been successfully utilized for several years in an academic course on medical information. (The help and constructive suggestions of these rehabilitation education students at the University of Wisconsin-Madison is gratefully acknowledged.)

For an overview preceding more thorough descriptions, the functional limitations are defined as follows:

MOBILITY LIMITATION. The function of getting from one location to another is limited. This can result from various medical disabilities (e.g., blindness, paralysis, retardation, emotional disturbance) or from environmental restrictions (e.g., architectural barriers, overprotective family). Immobility is closely associated with social isolation.

COMMUNICATION LIMITATION. There is a breakdown in the process by which information is exchanged between individuals through common symbols, signs, or behavior. Communicating persons engage in and exchange two roles that form the communication process: the expressive role (e.g., speech) and the receptive role (e.g., hearing).

SENSORY LIMITATION. A sensory limitation is the result of defect(s) in the transmission of information from the environment to the mind. It usually occurs as a result of damage in the nervous system which includes the brain and the sense organs. Only the external senses (e.g., vision, hearing, feeling) are included in this category of limitation.

DYSFUNCTIONAL BEHAVIOR. Emotional disorders are associated with deviance from behavior defined by the culture as appropriate. Abnormalities are manifested in many ways and to various degrees. They may stem from physical disabilities or cultural disadvantages, but emotional or dysfunctional behaviors impact upon the total individual.

ATYPICAL APPEARANCE. Atypical appearance refers to the characteristics of an individual's physique and carriage that are inconsistent with what is considered acceptable by a culture. Deformity is an aspect of physical appearance that is outside of society's expectations. The problem is social—not mechanical—and there is a tendency for others to assume atypical behavior in those who appear different.

INVISIBLE LIMITATION. These conditions that are concealed or unapparent but nonetheless limit functions create special problems. People who appear normal are expected to perform work without special considerations. Thus,

someone with a cardiac disability may be unable to lift, but others who have to do extra work because of this person's limitation may be resentful.

RESTRICTED ENVIRONMENT. This is a barrier resulting from a disability that inhibits the choice of where a person can be comfortable and safe. The afflicted person is bound to a place or status, or limited in activity, atmosphere, or progress. This limitation includes situations in which the disabled person would risk injury, health, or well-being because of personal inadequacy in tolerance, agility, perception, or other expression of compatibility with the environment.

MENTAL LIMITATION. Retardation and learning disabilities are grouped as a functional limitation, although again the causal circumstances are quite different. Both refer to a hindrance or negative effect in the learning and performance of activities and to other overt manifestations of inadequate mental function.

SUBSTANCE DEPENDENCY. The term *substance dependency* was developed to encompass psychological dependency (mental or emotional need to take a drug for relief of tensions or discomfort or for pleasure) and/or physical dependency (occurrence of biochemical reaction or physical symptoms when the drug is discontinued.)

PAIN LIMITATION. *Pain* refers to an unpleasant sensation characterized by throbbing, aching, shooting or other unpleasant feelings associated with bodily injury or disorder. While pain serves as a useful warning, when it is continuing, unremitting, uncontrollable, and severe, it may constitute a severe functional limitation to normal living. Much depends upon the individual's tolerance to pain as well as secondary rewards for the suffering of pain.

CONSCIOUSNESS LIMITATION. Unconsciousness and other defects in consciousness constitute a serious functional limitation. Epilepsy is the most dramatic cause, but there are many other disability conditions that contribute to problems of attention, reality orientation, and perception or awareness.

UNCERTAIN PROGNOSIS. This limitation involves the stress and ambiguity of those medical conditions that have an unpredictable course or termination. Some are cyclical; some hold out hope for cure; some appear more or less serious than they actually are. All leave the person with anxiety over the uncertainty of future plans.

DEBILITATION OR EXERTIONAL LIMITATION. Debilitation is a condition in which the individual is in a weakened state for an extended time period. This weakness results in diminished capacity to engage in various physical tasks. It may derive from various physical and mental impairments.

MOTIVITY LIMITATION. As a functional limitation this is the inability properly to produce, direct, and/or control bodily movements as required by specific activities and situations. While related to mobility, it is a different concept. *Motivity* refers to the ability or power to move an object or to do another task normally performed by using the musculoskeletal system, rather than denoting the movement of one's body from one place to another.

Limitations of human functioning as categorized above represent a bridge between medical disabilities (impairments) and handicapping. This categorization is designed for use by the rehabilitation counselor and therefore combines subgroups of physical functions as defined by physical or occupational therapists (e.g., strength of hand grip, ability to move self to and from wheelchair and other seat). A review of these other views and measures of functional limitation was published under a federal grant by Indices, Incorporated in 1979. They described a number of instruments including the following:

1. Barthel Index: An indicator of client independence in mobility and activities of daily living. A summary score of ten items covers self-feeding, moving from wheelchair to bed and returning, doing personal toilet, getting off and on toilet, self-bathing, walking on level surface, propelling wheelchair, ascending and descend-

ing stairs, dressing and undressing, continence of bowels, and controlling bladder.

2. Pulses Profile: A scale designed for medical practitioners, it is intended as a "performance" test of the individual's requirements for assistance in several areas: P—physical condition, including viscera; U—upper extremities; L—lower extremities; S—sensory components; E—excretory function; and S—mental and emotional status.

3. Long-Range Evaluation Summary: A method for estimating the progress of a client in a rehabilitation hospital or facility, it identifies general areas of unmet service needs.

4. Level of Rehabilitation Scale: Forms that are filled in by professional staff after client interviews reflect client progress in medical rehabilitation centers.

5. Functional Capacity Areas: This approach is designed for use with developmentally disabled individuals in work activity centers.

6. Longitudinal Functional Assessment System: This is an attempt to judge client health status, progress, planning, and program impact.

7. Functional Assessment Inventory: A 30-item scale developed by the University of Minnesota to help rehabilitation professionals, it covers in 10 to 15 minutes sensory, motor, psychological and intellectual, social and biographical, and environmental factors.

8. Rehabilitation Indicators: This system is the development of the New York Institute for Rehabilitation Medicine to describe client behaviors and environment including: (1) status (e.g., living arrangement, employment status); (2) activity pattern (i.e., recreational, self-care, educational, and other activities of daily living); (3) skill (e.g., walking up and down stairs, reading newspaper); and (4) environment (physical, social, and personal).

The 14 functional limitations described below differ from previous conceptualizations in that these categories group internally consistent components into a meaningful behavior orientation in assessment for independent living or vocational rehabilitation.

5.1. *Mobility Limitation*

Mobility, moving one's self (or being moved) from one place to another, is a fundamental need in humans. To be mobile the individual must be aware of the physical and the cultural environment and have the mental and mechanical capabilities to manage within it. Limitations on mobility can have broad psychological, social, and occupational repercussions. Immobility restricts the individual's environment and sets the boundaries of a person's very existence.

Mobility limitations may be temporary, for instance, after surgery, but the concentration here is on permanent conditions. There is a range of mobility restrictions from insignificant to severely limiting; this list is not definitive, but only illustrates the broad types of disabling conditions that can result in the functional limitation of an individual's mobility.

There are obvious and subtle causes of limitations in mobility. The more obvious causes are physical disabilities—those that result in a sensory disorder, loss or restriction of motor abilities, or amputation. The subtle causes may be classified as psychosocial and are more indirect in their connection to mobility restrictions. Emotional disorders may reduce mobility—for example, severe depression causing disinterest in the environment, or anxiety creating a fear of people and things. It should be noted that there is a great deal of interaction of the physical and psychosocial causes.

The causes of mobility problems as discussed below are related to other functional limitations.

5.1.1. SENSORY DEFICIENCY

A sensory deficiency is the inability to process stimuli adequately through the affected sense organ. An individual with a hearing loss will have difficulty both in the reception of verbal instructions and in their interpretation. Also, hearing conveys environmental warnings (e.g., the sound of automobile horns, obviously related to transportation).

A vision loss eliminates in varying degrees a vast array of cues and a very important way of learning about the environment. An individual's ability to place the self in space in relation to other objects may be poor. Many cues for transporting the self are visual: for example, numbers on a bus, street signs, architectural and geographic landmarks by which individuals get their bearings.

5.1.2. MUSCULOSKELETAL DEFECTS

Another broad category of disabling conditions that can affect mobility encompasses defects in body movement described under Motivity Limitation. These defects can be a result of either impairment of motion or amputation of an extremity. Loss of motion results from partial or total paralysis: paraplegia, quadriplegia, and hemiplegia. The degree of mobility restriction for the paraplegic client depends on the level of the spinal cord injury. A great deal of energy, including oxygen consumption, is required for proper motor action, and in case of reduced respiratory capacity mobility can be a significant challenge.

Restrictions in motion and range of motion can result from a variety of conditions. Among the major causes are the various forms of arthritis and the neuromuscular disorders. Mobility is interfered with due to stiffening and deformity of the joints and loss of muscle power. Pain such as that associated with chronic back conditions can also interfere with mobility. Since the treatment often requires rest, it could limit mobility. Arthritis can also be the result of the aging process. Debilitation due to aging and to atrophy of the muscles results in a decreased ability to move about freely. Cerebral palsy can result in spasticity, disequilibrium in walking, or a variety of involuntary and uncoordinated movements directly affecting locomotion. A weakness or lack of muscle tone can affect the range of motion. Respiratory diseases can result in shortness of breath, fatigue, and lack of stamina for any activity. An example of this is emphysema, which so curtails oxygen exchange that the amount of tolerable exertion can be drastically restricted.

Amputation, particularly of a lower extremity, creates another locomotor defect that will interfere with mobility. The amputee who cannot be fitted with an artificial leg has to depend on crutches or a wheelchair. Even if the individual has a prosthesis, there may be difficulty in tolerating long periods of walking or standing due to the pressure put on the stump. With either prosthesis or crutches, there may be poor balance due to the loss of the feeling of the foot on the ground. Uneven or slippery surfaces may be dangerous. An individual with a prosthesis may become easily fatigued since more energy has to be expended to move. Chronic skin irritation can result in sustained pain and discomfort that hinder mobility. Another problem with wearing a prosthesis is that even if the individual becomes skilled in its use, occasional failure is possible and the person is likely to fall or be stranded. It should be noted, however, that a properly fitted artificial leg attached to a good stump (particularly in a below-knee amputation) is not considered a serious limitation.

5.1.3. COGNITIVE DEFICITS

Another class of disabling conditions has to do with cognitive deficits. Such deficiencies may be the result of brain injury. Sometimes after brain injury there is difficulty in communication, in speaking and understanding (e.g., in getting directions). Even if the individual's expressive abilities are intact, there may be problems with the receptive process. Mobility problems can result from poor judgment, disorganization, and difficulty adjusting to new situations. Also there may be difficulty in generalizing and shifting from one aspect of a situation to another. Spatial judgment may be impaired. These all can contribute to problems in purposeful maneuvering. Hemiplegics may become lost in new surroundings or ignore or distort objects that confront them on their paralyzed side.

Another cause of cognitive deficit is mental retardation. Retarded individuals lack knowledge about the environment and its general layout. Learning about the environment takes a longer period of time and requires more effort. Limited intelligence may result in inability to deal with new situations and result in problems such as getting lost and needing to ask for directions. There may be an inability to read street signs and bus numbers, hampering mobility further.

5.1.4. PSYCHOSOCIAL PROBLEMS

There are other conditions that result in a functional limitation of mobility; these will be referred to as "psychosocial." Perhaps the most common condition that can be considered as psychosocial in origin is an emotional disorder. People with emotional disorders have difficulty relating to other people and to the environment due to internal processes that disrupt daily interactions. Anxiety, an underlying factor in most emotional disorders, can immobilize an individual. The range of restriction can be illustrated by the individual who is mildly neurotic and exhibits a fear of flying, a fear of high places, or a fear of big cities with all their traffic. At the other extreme are the individuals who are paranoid and dare not go out because they feel everyone is staring at them and talking about them.

Mobility can be limited by almost any kind of severe emotional disturbance. Ability to learn is affected by difficulty in generalizing from one situation to another. Another individual may in effect be limiting potential for mobility because of feelings of depression that result in inactivity. Still others may not be assertive enough to ask for directions or may ask for information in such an aggressive manner that interaction is difficult and thus avoided. In extreme cases, the psychotic individual is placed in a hospital for its protective environment.

5.1.5. SOCIAL BARRIERS

Another subtle reason for limitation of mobility that is strictly environmental lies in the attitudes of the community toward individuals who because of atypical appearance or inappropriate behavior are stigmatized and devalued. In a society that is very much involved with appearance and "normalcy," any individual who deviates makes others uncomfortable and may prompt a wish for their disappearance. In some neighborhoods there may be resistance to having obviously disabled individuals live or work there. A person's mobility is restricted by community resistance to deinstitutionalization and to the setting up of group homes and alternate living situations.

Overprotectiveness and fears on the part of significant others can lead to the incarceration of a handicapped person. The family members may be reluctant to let the person travel around alone because they underestimate the person's abilities to handle situations and because they are afraid to "let go." In this case, the individual may have the ability to travel independently but the social situation or self-devaluation does not allow execution of the function.

Dependency is a problem common among people who live in restricted environments. Moreover, dependency and mobility can be interrelated because overprotection by family members can be the major cause of immobility. On the other hand, restrictions in mobility serve to increase dependency on others. This has intrapersonal and interpersonal impact. Intrapersonally, the disabled person may not be able to reach levels of independent functioning and may have difficulty in feeling fully worthwhile. As a result of this dependency, interpersonal isolation can cause the immobile individual to become socially introverted.

Interpersonally there are many repercussions. In regard to family, limitations in mobility can mean the added burden of continually having to transport the disabled person, cutting into everyone's free time. This can put a strain on family relationships as frustration and resentment build. Because of the dependency on others, normal interactions with peers are disrupted. This can add to feelings of isolation since social interaction is limited and often at the convenience of others.

5.1.6. ARCHITECTURAL BARRIERS

Another situational cause of mobility difficulties lies in architectural barriers, which often pose insurmountable obstacles for aged individuals, people in wheelchairs, and amputees. (See 8.5 and 40.5 for a description of rehabilitation residences.)

Mobility limitations can cause vocational handicapping in two ways. The first is difficulty in getting to and from a job site outside the home; the second one, at the job site, is difficulty in maneuvering around the area. To the person with motor impairment of the lower limbs or the person in a wheelchair, the "normal" public transportation system is difficult to use. Bus steps may be too high, and doors on subways close too quickly to allow individuals moving slowly to get in and out. Large, busy streets are threatening because of the time it takes to get across them. Many environmental barriers figure in transportation to and from the job site—ranging from sign numbers that must be read to the multiplicity of choices that present themselves. Problems with balance and the propensity to fall, poor spatial judgment, and the accompanying inability to place the self into relation to other parts of the environment may also be present.

If transportation to and from the job site is mastered, mobility may still constitute a problem when the individual is maneuvering around the place of employment. First and foremost from a purely physical point of view, the job placement counselor has to be aware of how ac-

cessible places within the building are. If the building has narrow doorways, many staircases without elevators, and no ramps, it will be inaccessible for people in wheelchairs, individuals with hemiplegia, or those with arthritis, musculoskeletal disorders, or cerebral palsy.

With respect to the job, the first difficulty may be to convince the employer that the individual can function independently. Jobs can be modified so that the problem of mobility is minimized. Tools and equipment can be lowered or put within the reach of the individual in a wheelchair or the one who has trouble with ambulation. These measures need not be expensive or complicated.

5.1.7. MOBILITY TRAINING

Mobility and orientation training is a method for developing the skills an individual needs to maneuver about in the environment and to overcome hazardous obstacles encountered in travel. Mobility specialists train blind and other handicapped people to get around independently (see 2.4.8, Orientation-Mobility Teacher). They take into consideration the obvious and subtle factors that can diminish the capacity of disabled people to transport themselves, and then provide appropriate learning situations for each individual according to personal needs.

For people with mobility problems, there are a number of strategies. In addition to using sensory or mechanical devices, deaf or blind people can learn various techniques (e.g., sensitivity to clues from unimpaired senses). Auditory maps can substitute for visual landmarks. Prosthetic and orthotic devices are available from various manufacturers and can be specially built for those who have lower extremity amputations and impairments. Physical therapy helps restore maximum functioning of muscles, and occupational therapy helps people learn to ambulate. For those with gross paralysis, electric wheelchairs are available that can be operated by the mouth or slight movements of the upper extremities. For people with emotional disorders, anxiety can be lessened through psychotherapy, drugs, and the development of social skills.

5.1.8. COMMUNITY CHANGES

The problems of mobility limitations are alleviated through public information and community action programs. Unfavorable attitudes need to be changed so that people and communities are more accommodating and accepting of various disabling conditions. In this way, mobility restrictions such as resistance to deinstitutionalization, the stigma attached to those who are disabled, and the resulting fear and embarrassment connected with moving about the community, are lessened. Unlike a one-time intervention such as installing a special phone for an individual with quadriplegia, changing community attitudes is a continuing effort on the part of many. An individual's ability to navigate from one place to another should be limited only by the progress of science and technology and never by fellow human beings.

5.2. Communication Limitation

Communication as a broad term includes all of the interactions by which one organism affects another. All behavior—oral, written, verbal, tonal, postural, and so on—is communicative. Essential characteristics of the communication process are the transmission of information or feeling and the reception of messages and feedback. The range of disabilities includes those affecting the expressive and receptive mechanisms (auditory, visual, and oral) as well as other disorders. People who do not speak the dominant language are occupationally limited, but the focus here is on physical impairment.

5.2.1. TRANSMISSION PHASE
Communication impairments limit many of the major areas of life activity such as psychosocial adjustment and educational and vocational achievement. The transmission or expressive phase in the communication process is the act of sending or conveying an idea, concept, emotion, or feeling to another person. An individual who is affected by a physical, mental, or emotional disorder may be hindered in the performance of certain tasks or activities related to this phase.

The primary transmitters of encoded information are the articulatory organs of speech, the hands and arms, and the facial muscles. Other body parts may transmit emotion and information signals; for example, the shoulders may be shrugged, the head may be nodded affirmatively or shaken negatively, or the foot stomped angrily. The different functions of transmission can include the expression of ideas and emotions, the inducement of emotions in the listener, the persuasion of the listener to act, and the elicitation of information from the listener (see 26.9).

For the spoken word, the transmitter is the vocal mechanism. The transmission phase is accomplished in four steps: respiration, phonation, resonation, and articulation. Respiration is the process of inhaling and exhaling that occurs by breathing. Phonation occurs as a column of air from the lungs through the windpipe that passes between the vocal folds within the larynx, causing them to vibrate and produce sound. Resonation occurs when the sound is amplified and modulated in the nasal and pharyngeal cavities. Articulation is an interruption in the flow of voiced air by the tongue, teeth, lips, and palate, which shape it so as to produce identifiable speech sounds.

5.2.2. CAUSES
The inability to produce intelligible speech can be a very frustrating limitation. Speech disorders can occur as a result of physical impairment of the mechanisms for respiration, phonation, resonation, or articulation. Intelligible speech can also be limited by central nervous system disorders. Speech inadequacy may result from impairment of the brain because it is responsible for the storage of communication symbols essential for providing meaning for the sounds articulated by the vocal mechanisms of the mouth and face. Organic impairment that affects language functions also can be attributed to neurological damage by strokes, tumors, or traumatic injury to the brain. Rehabilitation approaches toward people with the various aphasias stress the importance of general physical recovery as well as total support and acceptance of the individual person. The most successful outcome occurs when the client is psychologically secure and there is no unrealistic pressure about word by word expression in conversations.

Defective speech is a common complication of mental retardation. Mental deficiency restricts the individual's ability to abstract and highly abstract symbols make up language. The relationship between organic brain damage, speech defect, and mental retardation is evident and is a major limiting factor for life functioning.

Stuttering is differentiated from other types of speech impairment on the basis of a lack of an organic cause. Stuttering is defined as a disturbance in rhythm. The fluency or flow of speech is disrupted by repeated sounds or words, prolonged sounds, pauses, or blockages. Stuttering is usually viewed as a functional disorder that is either a conditioned response pattern with emotional overtones or indicative of an emotional state with a high degree of tension and anxiety. The individual who stutters often exhibits muscle tension, facial tics and grimaces, or spastic movements of other body parts. It is much more common in males and is not associated with level of intelligence. To increase the stutterer's confidence, conversations with the individual should be conducted in a relaxed, accepting atmosphere.

5.2.3. TREATMENT

The treatment program that aims at reducing the limitations imposed by defective speech begins with possible alteration of the anatomical and physiological structure if impaired. A consultation with a physician who specializes in ear, nose, and throat problems or with a neurologist may be necessary. Psychotherapeutic intervention may be the initial step in dealing with problems of a psychological nature. The second step would be to provide speech therapy and training to further reduce the imposed limitations. A qualified speech pathologist and possibly an audiologist would be employed for these services. The third stage would be the development of an occupational plan, which is the rehabilitation counselor's specific responsibility. Since these stages are often overlapping, the rehabilitation counselor serves as a coordinator of the treatment program.

Counseling for the speech-handicapped should take into consideration four areas of client adjustment: psychological, social, educational, and vocational. The psychological problems resulting from speech disorders may be a negative self-concept, low frustration tolerance, high anxiety level, or personality trait disturbances. These psychological problems may diminish with improvement in speech ability, although they may be severe enough to require

intensive psychotherapy and counseling as part of the training process.

5.2.4. PSYCHOSOCIAL ASPECTS

The social problems of the speech-handicapped individual are based upon the reactions of others who respond to the speech rather than to the person as an individual. The social response most commonly associated with speech defects are exclusion from desired social relationships, peer group rejection, and social isolation, as well as public pity and sympathy.

These psychological and social factors magnify the limitations imposed by the speech defects. They have important implications for educational and vocational adjustment as well. Much of the process of educational development depends on the ability to express oneself verbally in the classroom, and social, psychological, and educational factors combine in influencing vocational aspirations. Certain vocations do not have a requirement of quality oral communication. Other vocations, however, such as sales, acting, and teaching may be contraindicated for those with speech difficulties.

Other aspects of expressive communication do not involve the mechanisms of speech but can nevertheless limit vocational and interpersonal functioning. Cultural differences evidenced in various dialects can pose difficulties at times in certain occupational settings. Meanings and intentions can be easily misinterpreted. An even more obvious communication difficulty faces immigrant populations who have not yet assimilated the language of their new culture (e.g., the Mexican-American immigrants and the Vietnamese refugees). This factor has limited the types of employment such people can find, even if they had professional, skilled positions in their home country. Tutoring programs and continuing education courses are helpful, especially for the able-bodied immigrant.

Another aspect of expressive communication not related to defective speech mechanisms but one which has implications for adjustment is the unassertive expression of thoughts and feelings. Feelings of insecurity, low self-concept, defensiveness, and anxiety in social and interpersonal relationships can affect the way individuals present themselves to employers in interviews and the way they communicate with co-workers and supervisors on a job.

The inability to express oneself through written

language is a communication limitation in certain situations. Blind individuals cannot see written language or use it to express themselves. People with motor dysfunctions due to muscle weakness or central nervous system involvement lack hand-motor coordination for writing or typing.

Individuals with upper extremity amputations are also restricted, although amazing adaptations are possible with various devices, for example, hand braces, mouthsticks, and other prosthetic devices. *Receptive* aspects of communication are described below.

5.3. Sensory Limitation

All of the sensory organs are connected to their respective centers in the brain. The person makes use of these sensors to obtain information about the external environment. Sensory impairment usually occurs by damage to the nervous system. This impairment can then lead to functional limitations associated with loss of an external sense (i.e., sight, hearing, smell, taste, or touch).

Internal senses are those that send messages to the brain about changes that take place within the body. They respond to chemical or physical stimuli in the circulatory, digestive, respiratory, excretory, endocrine, or nervous systems as well as to body positions and movements. Hunger, fatigue, pain, and thirst are such sensations. These so-called internal senses are not covered here, although the vestibular sense is described.

5.3.1. VISUAL IMPAIRMENTS

Visual disabilities include both legal blindness and severe visual loss. It is estimated that there are approximately one and one-half times as many severely visually impaired persons (defined as those in whom both eyes are involved who cannot read newsprint even with the best correction) as blind people. Severely visually disabled persons often need extensive rehabilitation services in order to carry on reasonably normal lives.

The most common and least limiting of possible impairments are defects in refraction (the deflection of a light ray when passing obliquely from one medium to another of different density). Specific errors in refraction are hyperopia (far-sightedness), myopia (near-sightedness), astigmatism (distortion in vision), and presbyopia (reduced accommodation). Fortunately corrective lenses are usually all that is necessary to correct these defects.

A second area of disability results from disorders of the cornea, which is highly susceptible

to injury or disease. Some causes for corneal disorders are infections, chemicals, burns, trauma, or degenerative lesions. Corneal disease is the cause of 10 percent of all legal blindness.

Glaucoma is a highly common condition characterized by an increase in intraocular pressure. About 2 percent of the over 40 population have it, and it results in about 12 percent of all legal blindness.

Cataracts can be defined as an opacity of the lens or its capsule. This condition can manifest itself in a variety of ways, and there is no method of preventing or impeding its progress. Surgical removal of either the entire lens or part of it is done. A contact lens is often used as a replacement, the reasoning being that while the removal does not restore any visual acuity, at least nonclouded vision is an improvement.

Disorders of the retina can result from injury, inflammation, diabetes mellitus, tumors, detachment, or circulatory and degenerative disturbances. When the involvement is in only one eye monocular vision results. A client with monocular vision will have problems with depth perception.

Another minor visual impairment is color blindness. As with defects in refraction, color blindness would only be dealt with in work with a client having other disabilities.

5.3.2. BLINDNESS

Finally there is the category of blindness. Legal blindness is defined as visual acuity of 20/200 or less in the better eye with the use of correcting lenses. There are nearly 300,000 legally blind people in the United States.

Blindness can be attributed to any of a number of causes: trauma, degenerative diseases such as glaucoma or cataracts, infections, birth injuries, disorders of the retina, disorders of the cornea, chemical burns, and disease of metabolism. Important considerations are whether the loss of sight was congenital or acquired and whether it is either acute or progressive.

A standard examination of the eye should include a check of the visual fields, testing of the functioning of the muscles of the eye, tests for color discrimination, depth perception, and stereopsis (3-D perception). Not only an accurate diagnosis but also as accurate a prognosis as possible is necessary to enable the counselor and client to develop a rehabilitation plan.

For the blind or visually handicapped individual medical information on any auditory problem (the type and amount of hearing loss, monaural or binaural, and otological treatment) is essential, because hearing is the major sensory substitute for a blind person. Hearing is critical for communication, for orientation by sound-location, and for determining the extent to which a blind person can become a proficient traveler. This is not to say that blind people develop better innate hearing ability. They simply learn to utilize more effectively the hearing ability they do have.

The application of rehabilitation services to the visually disabled population usually does not mean increasing sight. Rather, it means the improvement of visual perception for the person who has residual vision and the provision of sight substitutes for those who are totally blind or who have only light perception. Mobility instruction, discussed earlier, is a sight substitute technique. Another area in which sight substitutes will be necessary is that of communication (i.e., reading and writing), braille being the most common alternative used.

5.3.3. HEARING IMPAIRMENTS

Technically the only people who are actually deaf are those who are born without any practical hearing or who lose their hearing before they develop language or speech. All other kinds of hearing deficits put the person in the hard of hearing category.

A hearing loss, whether it is deafness or not, can be one of three medically defined types. A deficit that is the result of blockage of sounds from the auditory nerves is a conductive hearing loss. A sensory-neural hearing loss occurs when sounds reach the nerves but the nerves are unable to respond and transfer them to the brain. The third (or mixed) type is the result of a combination of problems.

Any of the types of hearing loss can happen at any age and result from a variety of causes. The accumulation of wax, infections, formation of tumors or scar tissue in the middle ear or ear canal because of various diseases, can all cause conduction problems. Diseases and infections can cause inner ear sensorineural loss, which can also be the result of congenital malformations. Finally, excessive noise or vibration in the environment can result in a hearing deficit.

There are a number of factors that affect deaf and hearing loss clients' communicative functioning. The degree and time of onset of the hearing loss and the amount and kind of education and experience the client has had are the major factors involved. Deaf clients usually are unable to develop speech and have somewhat less ability to use language than do people with normal hearing. The later the onset of a hearing loss the greater the ability to use language, since the client will have had more time to acquire normal language skills. Thus, a hard of hearing client, especially one whose hearing loss occurred in adolescence or adulthood, will generally be able to function normally or more nearly normally in the use of language.

Lip reading is a rare skill, one difficult to acquire, and the majority of hearing people have no knowledge of "signing." The person with the hearing deficit who does not learn signing communication is normally limited to writing and pantomime. In the instruction of the deaf, communication is by the "simultaneous method,"—with finger spelling, the language of signs, and speech (for lip reading) all used at the same time.

5.3.4. TACTILE IMPAIRMENT

Skin, the organ associated with the sense of touch, covers almost the entire body. The seriousness of tactile impairment depends on where exactly the loss occurs. On the skin there is a distribution of distinct areas sensitive to different kinds of stimuli. The human body has a total of perhaps 640,000 such tactile areas, but they are not equally thick. On the hands and on the face they are clustered densely together, whereas on the back they are more widely spaced.

The four basic modalities of the tactile sense include touch, pain, pressure, and temperature. Among causes of a loss in the sensitivity of touch are degeneration of nerves, spinal cord lesions, certain medications, congenital defects, burns, and cerebrovascular accidents. All of these cause damage directly to the nerve or nerve pathway. Loss of sensation can also result from paralysis due to spinal cord lesions. In these instances there is an increased probability of developing pressure sores as well as atrophy of areas involved.

The modalities of touch need to be considered. Pain is a warning, a sensation for self-protection, since the perception of pain offers an important biological advantage for the survival of the organism. Someone who has lost touch sensation has lost this warning signal.

Another very important factor for any individual who has lost cutaneous sensation is the necessity to develop an increased awareness or consciousness of body positioning. In particular, one must become aware of one's position in relation to other physical objects in the environment, especially potentially harmful objects. In addition, one must learn to become keenly aware of the temperature of the environment. If a person cannot detect extremes in temperature, there can be serious consequences, such as burning or frostbite.

These limitations produce obvious occupational handicaps. A client who has lost tactile sensation might be injured on machinery without realizing it. Various nonvocational handicaps are also associated with a loss of the cutaneous stimulation. Emotional security is derived from physical touching and handling. The touch sensation is also very important in displays of affection, and skin and touch gratification play a very important role in the sexual realm.

5.3.5. IMPAIRMENT OF OTHER SENSES

Impairment of the senses of taste and smell and inner ear dysfunction can cause serious functional limitations. The impairment may be subtle but it can have a considerable effect on the client's vocational placement, progress, and safety. Generally the loss of taste or smell must accompany another disability before a person is eligible for public rehabilitation services. The other disability will often seem to overshadow the loss of these senses but in dealing with the client the entire problem must be considered.

The functional limitation caused by impairment of the senses of taste and smell can range from a slight annoyance to a total lack of ability to detect any odors or flavors. When the sense of smell is obliterated or impaired, the gustatory sense will reflect this impairment. This phenomenon is commonly experienced during an upper respiratory infection. The loss of ability to detect noxious fumes can be a serious problem in daily living as well as an occupational handicap.

Another important consideration is hygiene. Inability to detect body odor could, with some clients, lead to poor hygiene with resultant health and social problems. On the other hand, people sometimes overcompensate for a deteriorating sense of smell by overusing aftershave lotions or perfume.

Inability to taste is functionally limiting, not just in terms of the pleasure of eating but in relation to the possibility of food poisoning because of the inability to tell when food is tainted. Another problem that can be created is loss of appetite. When everything tastes like cream of wheat, appetite is lost. When there is a partial loss of taste, heavy spicing (e.g., with salt) can lead to health problems.

The seriousness of the loss of the sense of taste or smell, or both, depends on the other residual capacities of the disabled person. For instance, for blind individuals the loss of smell and taste compounds the orientation problem. Loss of taste and smell are also serious limitations for a blind client in food preparation.

A wide range of disabilities can cause the loss or impairment of the olfactory or gustatory senses. One of the most common is trauma, damaging nerve endings in the sinus or blocking the neural pathways to the brain. Facial disfigurement might be the primary problem, accompanied with the sensory loss. Surgical operations for oral or nasal cancer, tumors, or sinus abnormalities may result in the loss of taste or smell.

Trauma by smoke, fumes, or pollution can cause permanent damage to nasal passages and nerves. Specifically, fumes from lead, manganese, phosphorus, mercury, benzene, nitrogen, and chrome, and heavy dust have been identified as causes of damage to the olfactory sense as well as the rest of the respiratory system. Nasal sprays, when used or abused over many years, may cause impairment of the olfactory nerves. Severe or prolonged respiratory infections also lead to permanent damage.

Very small, "mini" strokes are sometimes detectable by the ensuing impairment of taste or smell. Old age alone sometimes causes a breakdown in the ability to taste and smell things.

There are occupational conditions that a person with an impaired olfactory or gustatory sense should avoid: fumes, odors, toxic conditions, dust and poor ventilation. Contraindicated job placements are in chemical plants, grain elevators, steel mills, lumberyards, foundaries, and welding shops.

The vestibular apparatus of the ear is not often taken into account in discussions of the senses. It is unique among the sensory organs in that stimulation of it is not consciously perceived. Stimuli are received through the body's relationship to its surroundings. The mechanism for this sense is located in the labyrinth of the inner ear and when it is impaired, dizziness, loss of balance, nausea, tinnitus, and many other problems occur. These problems are often referred to as "vertigo."

The manifestations of vertigo vary widely. It may occur as a sudden, unpredictable attack or it may be a continuous sensation of light-headedness. It may be the result of certain head movements or changes in position. Consciousness may or may not be maintained during an attack. To some people with vertigo, it appears that the objects around them are floating; others feel as though they themselves are floating. An attack can last for a few moments or for several days or weeks. Some cases can be controlled with medication. When there is a warning or "aura" before an attack of vertigo, the functional limitation is reduced as long as it gives the client time to prepare. Sometimes it takes several years for a person to learn to recognize a forewarning sensation. It is more common for women to experience vertigo than men.

Gait impairment and inability to regain balance after tripping or getting jostled are two problems that people with vertigo sometimes have to deal with. They may stagger to the point of looking drunk. Areas of difficult footing must always be avoided, as well as areas where a temporary loss of balance would be dangerous to the person or others. Physical therapy and gait training may help.

Labyrinth impairment can often result in nausea and vomiting. In normal individuals this "motion sickness" is the typical response when travel by boat, airplane, or car causes fluctuations in the labyrinth (or inner ear). Disturbances in vision can be an associated problem.

The mechanism of the labyrinth is based on the movement of minute hair cells, called "cilia," in a fluid. The cilia move in response to various body motions such as head rotation, bending, turning, or walking. A message is then sent through the neurons of the labyrinth to the brain. The disabilities that cause vertigo or tinnitus result from a breakdown of one or more parts of the system. Tinnitus, an ear condition involving a continuous roaring, ringing, hissing, or other noises within the ear, can be an annoyance to the point of distraction.

Pressure on the inner ear caused by a brain tumor or brain injury can have a negative effect on the labyrinth. Streptomycin treatment, as well as viral infections, can lead to vertigo and deafness. Among the diseases related to this problem are allergies and migraine. The disease most commonly linked with vertigo is Meniere's syndrome, which is characterized by vertigo, tinnitus, and even deafness. All external sensory impairments are associated with environmental *communication limitation*.

5.4. Dysfunctional Behavior

Dysfunctional (emotional) behaviors are manifest in many of the clients seen by rehabilitation counselors. Problems of adaptive behavior may be secondary to the physical problems experienced by a client or they may be the primary factor necessitating help. In either case the rehabilitation process is essentially the same as with other types of handicapping.

As in physical disease, the label assigned—in this case the psychiatric diagnostic classification—does not assist the rehabilitation counselor to recognize the functional limitations asso-

ciated with emotional behavior difficulty. A logical way of approaching limitations is to discuss the areas of an individual's life that are affected. Thus, it is better to discuss cognitive, emotional, and physical, as well as social and interpersonal categories of life.

A nonmedical approach, centering on a functional analysis of behavioral ineffectiveness, is presented here. Classification is according to the area of the client's life that is affected. Chapter 28, Personal Adjustment, provides a more elaborate description of psychological adjustment problems and processes following, in part, the 1980 American Psychiatric Association classification system (see 28.7).

5.4.1. COGNITIVE DISORDERS

Cognition is the ability to think, understand, learn about, and be aware of the environment through the senses. Dysfunction may occur when there is any difficulty with these processes. The first significant area affected is that of learning. If the individual has difficulty organizing and processing information due to distorted thought processes, it is not easy to learn new skills. Distorted thought processes may also make it difficult to maintain logical thought sequences and may cause confusion as to the meaning of words and instructions. Memory loss is a detriment to learning and maintaining skills. This can result from deviations in the cognitive processes or from the medication used to regulate the emotional disorder. An individual's attention may be erratic and concentration may be minimal if the person is attending to internal processes (e.g., is listening to "voices" or "sounds," or has difficulty in deciding which of many environmental stimuli to attend to). Also, an individual may not have the ability to generalize, that is, may deal with learning situations in a very concrete way, in the here and now, and have difficulty with abstractions. (See 5.8.2.)

Another area affected is that of independence. A person may be disorganized and confused as to time and place. If thought processes are in confusion, peculiarities in conversation may be exhibited. There may be an impairment in judgment or in the ability to plan. In some cases, people make impulsive, irrational decisions or completely lack the ability to make decisions at all. Anxiety can be overwhelming. Due to poor self-concept and feelings of inadequacy, the individual may be very reliant upon others.

Finally, reality interpretation may be impaired and the individual may consistently misinterpret and overgeneralize the objective happenings that occur. Such people may substitute their delusional system for an unpleasant reality.

5.4.2. AFFECTIVE DISORDERS

The affective range of human functioning includes subjective feeling and emotional tone. For the person experiencing emotional behavior difficulty, the problems here revolve around inappropriate emotional expression, lack of emotional expression, and consuming feeling states. Since thought processes are sometimes cut off from emotional expression, affect may be inappropriate. An individual may laugh or cry in a situation that does not evoke these as appropriate responses. Due to feelings of paranoia and suspicion of others, one may express hostility although no objective stimulus for this emotion is present in the environment. Instead of expressing inappropriate emotions, a person may have very shallow affect, to the point of expressing little or no emotion at all. An apathy may surround all of the person's activity so that little is communicated on the subjective level.

Finally, the individual may be involved in an all-consuming feeling state: one that can influence the individual strongly is depression: sadness, loneliness, and boredom are experienced. There may be a loss of emotional involvement with other people and feelings of worthlessness. The experiencing of this emotion ranges from mild sadness, which can be relieved, to severe feelings of hopelessness and worry.

Mania, another all-consuming feeling, is a mood state that seems opposite to depression. In effect, the individual exhibits a reaction formation against feelings of worthlessness, and the range can go from mild euphoria and elation to extreme agitation when the individual is confused and disorganized. Though the person may exude overconfidence, there can be a high sensitivity to criticism and a tendency to become easily angered or frustrated.

Anxiety is thought to be the basis of a great deal of emotional behavior difficulty. It is an unpleasant feeling state of generalized fear and apprehension. It increases during periods of stress and potentially threatening situations for the person. It can range from heightened nervousness in particular situations to a total involvement so that the individual is immobilized in all aspects of functioning.

5.4.3. PHYSICAL BEHAVIOR

The effects of emotional difficulty can have expression in abnormal appearance and behavior. With regard to general motor response, the individual may exhibit less than normal activity. This ranges from a reduced rate of activity, when every action is slow and deliberate, to the extreme of total immobility. Reaction time may be extremely slow, and there may be difficulty in the preparation of responses. Hyperactivity in which a great deal of agitation and restlessness is exhibited, occurs. The individual may exhibit fidgeting, handwringing, pacing, and moaning.

Sleeping and eating patterns can be greatly affected by emotional difficulties. The person may have insomnia and resulting fatigue or may sleep in excess, with little desire to do anything else. Deficiency in appetite and gastrointestinal irregularity usually occur.

An individual who feels hostile to or suspicious of others or who is very depressed may engage in antisocial physical behaviors, including physical aggression toward others, self-destructive behaviors (such as mutilation or suicide), and destruction of property. Persons experiencing emotional difficulty may involve themselves in stereotyped behaviors, all excessive in expression and usually seen as repetitive and rapid movements of the extremities or torso. Common examples are ''body-rocking'' and ''hand-flapping.''

Verbal behavior represents another component of human interaction and expression that is subject to dysfunction. Mutism represents a deficiency in verbalization. An example is the individual who refuses to speak in social situations. Excessive manifestations include irrelevant or ''crazy talk'' and nonlinguistic noises (e.g., grunts, moans, and screams).

5.4.4. SOCIAL AND INTERPERSONAL

The person with an emotional disorder may exhibit behavioral idiosyncrasies that in themselves interfere with effective functioning in contacts with other people. Perhaps more than any physical disability, emotional behavior involves the total person; difficulty with interpersonal functioning is a direct result. A common response, and an indication of emotional difficulty, is the tendency to withdraw from the social environment to some degree. This may be the result of suspicion, fear, anxiety, or involvement in an inner world.

Another manifestation of behavioral dysfunction is marked dependence and passive behavior. Often an individual may not show much initiative or motivation to accomplish any activity. The emotional expressions of people with interpersonal difficulties are often inappropriate or flat.

Communication skills are impaired for a variety of reasons. Conversation may be impeded by a slow response time, difficulty in concentration, unique word meanings, and distorted perceptions. These people may have trouble communicating openly and frankly, and may be unable to assert themselves, assertion including the capacity to express feelings, make requests, and make refusals. They may have problems discussing criticisms, asking questions, and expressing ignorance or confusion.

5.4.5. REHABILITATION METHODS

A rehabilitation counselor must be mainly concerned with the manifestations of an emotional disorder rather than with treatment of the abnormality itself. Behavioral limitations in the cognitive, emotional, and physical areas may result in social and vocational handicapping requiring extensive intervention. The treatment of emotional disorders is not like treatment of physical disabilities. Some methods attempt to increase the competence or emotional strength of the individual, while others attack the difficulty through the relief of symptoms. The basic type of treatment is somatic; drug and other medical therapies are the most prevalent. The importance of medical treatment is that it makes certain patients open to other forms of treatment.

Psychotherapy has as its goal a revamping of personality arising out of insight into those parts of the personality that are self-defeating for the person. As a result of this process the individual can see the self in a more positive light and can handle people and problems more effectively. When it is effective, psychotherapy increases ego strength, reduces anxiety, and increases tolerance levels for frustration and pressure.

Behavior therapy, which uses conditioning and learning, focuses on specific aspects of behavior functioning so that effective interaction with the environment can take place.

A rehabilitation counselor can provide a relationship of trust and support, and this relationship can facilitate communication between the counselor and the client. The client can begin to develop the interpersonal social skills that work requires as a social situation. People frequently lose jobs because of interpersonal difficulties rather than the inability to perform specific work tasks. Rehabilitation counselors, however, can help their clients to achieve adaptive behavior. The rehabilitation process introduces to the client a variety of coping devices including self-discipline, the comfort of other people who care, freedom to express one's feelings (e.g., crying, laughing, assertion), and other ways of averting tension, maintaining stability and behaving ef-fectively. Behavior modification techniques used by rehabilitation counselors are described in Chapter 29.

5.5. Atypical Appearance

A functional limitation results from the negative interpersonal impact of atypical appearance. Unusual appearance is associated with a wide variety of human disabilities and conditions apparent to others, such as dwarfism, facial disfigurement, and social or racial difference. Included are disabilities for which atypical appearance would not be considered the primary limitation, that is, amputation, mental retardation, or cerebral palsy. This limitation is most logically considered in the context of a sociopsychological process having three phases: the disabled person's own self-image and reaction to a changed physique; other people's reactions and attitudes toward the disabled individual; and the interaction of the two and the handicapping aspects of this process.

5.5.1. BODY IMAGE

The concept of body image is pertinent. Body image, an element of self-concept, includes one's conception of one's own appearance to others. When a person has a congenital disability, the physical condition is incorporated into the formation of the body image. If the disability occurs later on in life, however, changes must be made in the body image. People resist altering their body image, especially when the change is negatively perceived. A person has an ideal body image and an actual body image. It has been proposed that the greater the discrepancy between the two, the poorer the adjustment to disability. Another factor relating to adjustment is a person's view of the body's purpose. This may be understood in terms of points on a continuum: at one end is the view of the body as a productive tool, and at the other end is the view of the body as an aesthetic stimulus to be enjoyed and to provide pleasure for others. These views can have great impact on adjustment to disability. Thus the person's reaction to becoming disabled is not necessarily correlated with the severity of the condition. One could compare the reactions of a laborer and a model to a facial scar; the psychological consequences

of this disability would probably be much more devastating to the model than to the laborer. Since, too, reactions to disability are highly individualized, relatively superficial disabilities may have serious psychological effects.

Facial disfigurement is especially important to consider because of its social and psychological meaning. Studies of the severely facially disfigured indicate a high incidence of disturbance and difficulty in dealing with life. People with this disability often have poor self-acceptance and do not expect others to accept them. Those who have adequately incorporated their disability into their self-concept have been found to be satisfied with improvement achieved through plastic surgery, while those who had not were dissatisfied with the results.

5.5.2. PSYCHODYNAMICS

During adolescence especially, physique, general appearance, and physical ability are significant determinants of a person's acceptance by peers. The physically disabled adolescent is particularly subject to social rejection. This seems to be more true of the congenitally disabled than of those who become disabled after having had the opportunity to gain peer acceptance. Personality and social development can be more adversely affected when the onset is before maturity.

Acceptance of one's own disability depends, in part, upon one's predisability attitude. In other words, a person who had a positive attitude toward people with a disability prior to becoming disabled is more likely to accept the condition. In adjusting to disability, people need to enlarge their scope of values, replacing values relating to appearance and physical ability with nonphysical values.

5.5.3. SOCIAL ATTITUDES

Prejudice toward disabled people is a negative prejudgment. It reflects the degree of intolerance, expressed in the amount of social distance that viewers place between themselves and the disabled person. These reactions might range from the wish that disabled persons would stay out of sight, to the overt unwillingness of an employer to hire such a person for a job. A visible disability tends to generate a greater amount of prejudgment, both positive and negative, than other characteristics. A person whose face is disfigured, obviously appearing different from others, does not necessarily have a physical restriction. However, hostility and discrimination may follow the belief that the face mirrors the personality. Particularly if one places a high value on physical perfection, disfigured people are considered inferior.

The attitude one forms toward the disabled person is based on four factors. The first has to do with moral accountability, or how the disability was obtained: whether it is congenital; results from natural illness, disease, or injury suffered with honor (war); or from personal fault (self-destructive act); or deviance (criminal act). Second, one decides on the probability that the person will recover from the disability, for instance, from obesity in contrast to severe burn scars. Third, negative reactions are related to a variety of emotional attitudes toward the particular disability. Last, attitudes are influenced by the viewer's feelings of personal involvement ranging from a felt obligation to assist (e.g., assume extra job tasks for a co-worker who has a heart problem) to a deep fear for one's own well-being (e.g., a fear that the condition is contagious or can be transmitted).

Because of all these factors, there is no stereotype of physically disabled persons; the negative attitudes people have tend to be more related to the type of disability. Atypical physique or physical appearance is very influential in producing personal impressions and feelings. In fact, a physical deviation is often seen as the primary key to a person's behavior and personality. This concept, known as "spread," applies both to people with a disability and the persons viewing them. Essentially it involves perception of the physical disability as spreading to other nonimpaired characteristics of the person. For example, a person who is blind is sometimes assumed to be hard of hearing as well, even though there is no connection between the two.

Several personal characteristics influence the viewer's attitudes toward those who appear different. Women, for example, tend to show a more positive attitude toward physically disabled individuals than men do. Also, one's personality plays a significant role in the formation of social attitudes and acceptance of a person who is disabled. To generalize, the most accepting are less aggressive persons, with lower levels of anxiety, higher needs for social approval, and greater ability to tolerate ambiguity. Most people react more negatively to the more visibly handicapped. The unfamiliar disrupts the established rules of social interaction. Especially when a visible impairment is involved, attention is focused on this single physical feature. Generally people tend to like and accept those things and persons they perceive to be most like themselves.

Societal reactions to the disabled are illustrated by the role of appearance across cultures. A facial or overall physical condition that one society views as a defect may be regarded as a positive status symbol by another people. The cultural values one holds determine what is perceived as atypical or as beautiful and may influence subsequent reactions of hostility and avoidance or acceptance and approval.

Individual reactions to those with atypical appearances are explained by various theories. The "body-concept" approach hypothesizes that one's self-perception conditions attitudes toward disabled persons. Individuals who experience minimal discrepancy between their body as it actually is and the body ideal will express more positive attitudes toward the visibly disabled than those who experience extreme discomfort in relation to their own body.

Prejudgments concerning the attributes one assigns to the person with an atypical appearance are not always negative. Sometimes people exaggerate positive qualities in the same way that they do negative ones. In the work situation co-workers are more willing to assist a visibly impaired person (e.g., a person in a wheelchair) than they are a person with a nonvisible handicap.

5.5.4. EMPLOYMENT

The functional limitation of an atypical appearance is not mechanical in nature but rests strictly on the attitudes of others whose behavior may place the disabled person at a disadvantage. The attitudes of the employer toward disabled workers, like those of the general public, are sometimes positive, sometimes negative, but usually more or less indifferent. Employers as a group are basically motivated by pressures of economic competition rather than concern for social welfare. When hiring, employers tend to choose disabled persons primarily in terms of productivity or functional ability as opposed to physical appearance and style in social situations. Too, persons with physical appearance deviations are usually preferred over workers with sensory impairments and brain-related disabilities.

Employers' hiring practices in this regard, of course, depend somewhat on the job for which a person is being hired. Many employers believe that in occupations with extensive public contact the disfigured employee will not be tolerated by customers. This belief rests not only on personal attitudes but those of the general public. A co-worker may also be intolerant of those with apparent disabilities and initially may be distracted by the new employee who is disabled. Grand mal epileptic seizures by an assembly line worker are disrupting—particularly to women —but the sense of disturbance quickly subsides after the initial episode.

Social stigma is a major handicap to disabled persons in job placement. The prejudice and limited expectations others may have for severely disabled persons drastically limit their lives. Especially with congenital deformities, self-images are at least partially a result of the reactions of others during the developmental ages. Over the years there is a continual process of integration in which new feelings and attitudes about oneself are absorbed within old ones, thereby altering one's self-concept for good or bad.

5.5.5. COPING

Self-concept plays an important role in the interpretation of social relationships. Self-assessment affects the way in which people

think others view them. And this affects their public image. The public displays interest in and curiosity about apparent disabilities, and this can be quite hurtful. A disabled person may cope with these reactions in several ways. Disabled persons, however, have the power to set the social climate of an initial encounter; once they are able to accept and be at ease with disability they can begin to establish social techniques that allow other people to be at ease with them. Most people hold both positive and negative feelings toward those who are disabled; it is therefore possible to suppress negative feelings and build on positive ones. One of the major turning points for disabled persons is their insight that other people have interest in or admiration for them as opposed to curiosity or mere pity. Although many disabled people report an initial feeling of pity or embarrassment on the part of another person, they are able to develop positive attitudes as they continue to build the relationships.

Persons who have obvious visible disabilities or physical deformities are constantly vulnerable to public reaction. Even strangers seem to feel free to stare at the person, to ask questions, and to communicate feelings about the disability. Blatant, impudent questioning may be responded to assertively: "Why do you ask?" The situational context is important, however. In some instances it is all right to talk about the disability but at other times it is rude. The personal context is also important; people are most likely to feel comfortable discussing the disability constructively with those they trust.

Interaction can often be as much a problem for the nondisabled as it is for disabled individuals. Many people just do not know how to act around individuals they consider different from themselves. Their initial reactions toward a disabled person may result primarily from their own nervousness and insecurity.

5.6. *Invisible Limitation*

Unapparent conditions—restrictions in behavior resulting from medical impairments that are not visible—create a unique functional limitation. People with such conditions are unable to perform various tasks yet they are expected to act normally because they seem normal to others.

Because outsiders do not understand their impairment and consequently give no special considerations, the person is under social pressure to act as if the disability did not exist, even if this means violating medical orders. Also, when the disablement is not apparent there is ambiguity about what the individual can and should do, and there is less tolerance for substandard performance.

A wide range of medical impairments are unapparent but nonetheless disabling. Some are poorly understood by the general public with the consequence that even when people are aware that an individual has the disability, they cannot assess its effect. Even in the case of heart disease, few lay people understand the impairment and the wide range of functional impact. Some cardiac cases complain that they are treated as invalids and are overprotected, despite typical medical advice to return to normal activity. On the other hand, the worker who has sustained a back injury that curtails lifting may find that people are unable to distinguish between legitimate avoidance of tasks and lazy or faking behavior. Unapparent limitations, which may occur intermittently or be present continuously, can provoke fear in both the individual with the hidden condition and others around that individual.

5.6.1. AMBIGUITY

The ambiguity, the lack of tangible or external evidence of unapparent conditions, affects the disabled person as well as others. There may be a tendency to deny the existence of the impairment and to act as if it were not present. With some hidden impairments the person feels normal until the condition is ignored or is not attended to (e.g., person fails to rest or to take controlling medication). In other cases one is constantly reminded by discomfort or pain of a condition that others do not directly see, for example, emphysema or asthma.

5.6.2. CHARACTERISTICS

There are four basic characteristics of unapparent limitations. First, unapparent limitations are invisible to other members of society. Second, self-management by individuals with these disabilities is indicated because other people do not extend needed help. Third, there is a tendency to fail to accept the disability psychologically (this is not exclusive to unapparent limitations, but it is very important). The fourth characteristic of unapparent limitations is that other members of society expect the individual with the limitation to be "normal."

There are three ways in which the invisibility of these limitations can be a factor. One problem is that a person may not ungrudgingly accept the special considerations given to individuals with more "apparent" disabilities (e.g., wheelchair clients). Another problem involves the issue of disclosure: whether or not the disabled person should inform the prospective employer of the disability. If the job applicant tells an employer of the serious impairment, there is a chance of rejection. However, if the person gets the job after falsifying an application and the employer later learns about it, termination may result. A third factor is safety. Workers with unapparent limitations may be a hazard to themselves or other workers because proper work precautions or assignments were not made by the employer, who did not know of the existence of the disability. Lack of selective placement is common with small firms that do not require a preemployment medical examination.

The second characteristic of unapparent limitations, the need for self-management of the disability, is perhaps the most important. The individual with an unapparent limitation is particularly responsible for maintaining good health since others do now know about the limitation. The person with asthma must make sure to take the medication. The person with diabetes must maintain insulin dosage. Also, someone with a cardiovascular disability must keep track of diet, stress, and exercise levels. The question of self-management is an important matter for the rehabilitation counselor.

The third characteristic of unapparent limitations is the special problem of psychological acceptance. Three types of reactions that occur are fear, depression, and denial. Fear follows the realization that the disability is life-threatening. Depression arises from contemplation of the profound life changes the disability brings. An individual may also deny the disability since it is so frightening; for example, the cancer case may be afraid to face the reality of the situation because of the strong association of cancer with death. These psychological reactions may affect the person's work situation and interpersonal relationships.

A fourth characteristic of unapparent limitations is the expectation of normalcy. Other people will expect someone who appears to be normal to be normal. A person who complains about the disabling condition faces the possibility of being labeled a hypochondriac. On the other hand, when the person does not divulge medical facts and simply avoids work that is harmful, the lack of understanding results in criticism. Reluctance to reveal the disability is common with cancer and epilepsy cases, since these conditions provoke fear in others.

5.6.3. CATEGORIES

The different disabilities associated with invisible or unapparent limitations fall into five main categories: neurological disorders, malignancies, organ and gland dysfunctions, mental and emotional disorders, and other human problems.

Neurological conditions that may be unappar-ent include epilepsy and strokes. Epilepsy, even if only partially controlled, is not observable 99 percent of the time. Malignancy, of course, includes the various internal forms. Inner organ dysfunctions from various diseases include conditions of the heart, lungs, and kidneys. Diabetes involves a dysfunctioning in the endocrine glands. Mental and emotional disorders include both neuroses and psychoses, not all of which are always apparent. Retardation or lack of mental development does not necessarily make one look atypical. The "other" category would include alcoholism and socially deviant predispositions.

5.7. Restricted Environment

A "restricted environment" can be described as a barrier resulting from a disability that inhibits the overall alternatives of a human being. This barrier is reflected in the inability of a person to move freely within a normal life space; its manifestations are infinite. Specific environmental requirements or contraindications, architectural and engineering barriers, homeboundness, overprotection, social rejection, as well as institutional living, provide examples of some of the broad categories involved.

These barriers range from very subtle to blatantly overt. They may affect only a certain specific circumstance or the totality of a person's life-style. Variables include the impact of current legislation, societal attitudes, and public awareness, as well as existing scientific and medical knowledge.

5.7.1. INSTITUTIONALIZATION

The functional limitation associated with environmental restriction is most dramatic for people confined to institutions such as jails and hospitals. Institutional living, which is highly restricted in terms of space, cuts people off from the rest of society, and their human needs are administered by a bureaucratic organization. The setting establishes the functional limitation. Its boundaries strongly limit tasks, activities, and interpersonal relationships normally engaged in "outside."

Institutions include sanitariums, correctional facilities, hospitals, training schools for people with subnormal intelligence, inpatient mental health centers, nursing homes, and residential facilities for the aged or chronically ill. (See 40.1.2).

The handicap results from overt hindrances in the institutional setting. The most obvious restriction is the lack of freedom of movement: locked doors, privilege systems, and the necessity for offgrounds passes severely limit the access of institutional residents to the community and jobs. Loss of driving privileges may result from being institutionalized, and transportation problems may compound the difficulties. In addition, rural and semirural settings are traditional for institutions. Lack of community and employer acceptance of the person living in an institution, when combined with a long lapse in employment or a highly limited, if existent, work history, rounds out the list of vocational problems. Deinstitutionalization is discussed in Chapter 40, Independent Living.

5.7.2. DEHUMANIZATION

A less obvious characteristic—but perhaps the most important—is the loss of responsibility along with all the inherent subtleties characteristic of institutional living. In a society in which independence and self-respect go hand in hand, institutional living reinforces ideas of dependence and loss of identity. Everyday choices like what to eat and when to sleep are all predetermined. This continual process of redefinition of roles and self-concepts by the situation and the institution's staff is called "dehumanization." One step further, the assimilation of and the succumbing to the role by the individual is called "institutionalization." Occupationally, dependency and a limited self-concept are viewed as counterproductive traits. Employers want employees who can exercise initiative and assume responsibility and can deal interpersonally with others as equals. People lacking these fundamentals of self-concept have difficulty entering the working world.

Dehumanization and institutionalization affect the totality of the person's life. Family relationships, sexuality, social functioning, and recreational life are all influenced. Healthy family relationships perhaps contribute more to personal adjustment and growth than any other factor, but due to the restricted environment itself, families are physically divided. Just the lack of physical togetherness can have devastating effects; and specific visiting hours, common lounge areas, and dormitories provide little privacy.

Sexuality within institutions is evaluated with a double standard. While professionals agree upon its importance, sexual behavior is discouraged. Sexual relations, if any, remain secretive. Masturbation, while not condoned, is the type of sexual involvement most tolerated.

5.7.3. CONSTRUCTIVE PROGRAMS

Social functioning and one of its components, recreational life, can provide structure, relaxation, and meaningfulness to an individual's life. While institutional programming may expose participants to these realms in a positive way, two negative themes recur. First, although decisions regarding these activities may involve client input, institution regulations and staff decision-making play a limiting role. Second, activities are designed for groups of people. One-to-one or individually planned activities are rare. Generally, outings and other activities group sizable numbers of clients, thus reinforcing the institutional identity.

Generally two types of programs will meet individual needs. First, it is estimated that less than 10 percent of the institutional population can be rehabilitated to competitive employment. For these people, vocational education, training,

vocational experiences, and transitional employment combined with supportive interpersonal skill-building experiences have proved effective in preparing clients. Second, it has been estimated that half of all institutional cases could participate in sheltered employment if it were available. In-house work activity centers and sheltered workshops within institutions are expanding and developing to meet these needs.

5.7.4. OCCUPATIONAL ASPECTS

In an occupationally restricted environment a person may be bound to a place or status, restricted posturally, assigned to an intolerable setting, or limited in activity or progress. A common example of "postural limitation" occurs when the worker is restricted at the work site to sitting all of the time without standing (or vice versa). The surrounding conditions negatively influence self-determination with respect to where or what the disabled individual will be.

Some occupational environments are regarded as potentially dangerous for even non-handicapped people. Operating dangerous machinery, however, poses a special problem with certain disablements (e.g., epilepsy), and jobs that necessitate exposure to potentially toxic chemical agents are restrictive for some types of disabilities (e.g., skin impairment, respiratory disorders). Toxic agents can include dust, gases, fumes, and mists. Other disabilities can be particularly influenced by intense noise, extremely high and/or low temperatures, or unsanitary surroundings.

American business and government are concerned about health and safety for all workers. Focus is on improvement in various aspects of the environment: industrial ventilation, noise control, and industrial toxicology are being emphasized, as are such problems as exposure to ultraviolet rays, exposure to crystalline silica, exposure to hot environments, air and water pollution, chemical additives in food, pesticides, and exposure to sulphur oxides and particulate matter in the air. Many physical features of work settings can be particularly restrictive to people who have a disability. Efforts to remove architectural barriers and to remove environmental restrictions are discussed elsewhere.

5.8. Mental Limitation

Intellectual and learning deficiencies result in adverse social and vocational status. The mentally deficient individual is hindered in the performance of many tasks, activities, and roles of life, or in the opportunities to perform them. This functional limitation is best characterized as an inability to generalize, but it is referred to as a deficit of the mind or a deficit in learning. Differentiation is made, however, from the diagnostic group called "learning disabled."

5.8.1. CONDITIONS

There are a number of causal conditions of limitations in mental function: (1) Mental retardation is a restriction in cognitive functioning manifested in a slowness to make transitions in assigned tasks. There is also the inability to follow rapid or frequent changes in instruction. With reference to motivation, this means a slowness in identifying the incentive conditions of task performance. (2) Autism resulting from birth trauma is predominantly a limitation of affect (feeling). Typical behavior may be poor interpersonal relationships, regression, lack of self-care, and also self-stimulation. (3) Environmental conditions can cause the person to deteriorate mentally. An example is retirement from an active work life that was the major source of self-esteem or rewarding interpersonal relationships. The onset of physical disability can also result in functional intellectual loss due to a breakdown in personal identity, incentives, and life-style. Cultural deprivation is negatively associated with the acquisition of behaviors appropriate to the work environment.

5.8.2. COGNITIVE PROCESSES

Cognition as a general term refers to all of the processes involved in knowing. As a faculty of the mind it has been associated with common sense and all forms of reasoning and understanding.

Stages of the cognitive process include motivation, apprehension, acquisition, retention, recall, generalization, performance, and feedback. Motivation is defined as the expectation of a desired reward or an incentive condition. It results in the person's ability to accept a task assignment and to follow through to completion without other guidance. The expectation of a reward assists the learner to approach the task, stay with it, and maintain the behaviors required for acquiring a skill or knowledge.

Apprehension, the next stage, is the selective attending of the person to relevant parts or features of the learning situation.

Acquisition is the core of the learning process. In this stage material presented to the learner must enter the person's cognitive storage system as memory so that it may later be recalled and used. The events in this phase are internal and, consequently, only inferences can be drawn about them from subsequent observable events. It is inferred that people have some form of coding facility for information storage. It is difficult to differentiate problems at the acquisition level from problems in retention and recall.

Decision-making is relatively difficult for retarded people as is the mastery of technical skills. Even the ability to follow directions—a requirement of all jobs—may be affected by difficulty in acquisition or retention, or both. Incentives are affected rather directly by one's ability to generalize.

Performance of the retarded person is complicated by nonintellectual factors. Certainly the negative attitudes of society create a vicious circle of low expectation, overprotection, lack of self-confidence, and so on. Personality factors are usually the greatest deterrent to successful employment. Undependability and immaturity cause a high turnover rate in the unskilled jobs for which so many of these people are forced to compete, despite the fact that most of them can be successful in jobs that are well-defined, routinized, and constantly paced. (See 5.4.1.)

5.8.3. DESCRIPTION

Mental retardation can be described in many ways and from many points of view (i.e., educational, medical, cultural, psychosocial). There is a wide range of mental retardation, from profound to mild—a range from total dependency and the need for complete supervision to minimal dependency in which almost no supervision is needed. The IQ scores fall below 70 on the Wechsler child or adult intelligence scale or on instruments that have been modified to test more accurately the cognitive and vocational skills of minority groups. But this disability should be defined in terms of functional limitations as well as IQ scores.

The mildly retarded groups will be the vocational rehabilitation focus for the most part. Having an IQ range of roughly 55 to 70 as measured by standardized intelligence tests, they constitute about 90 percent of all cases of mental retardation. These individuals are usually not distinguishable until they reach school age and are identified by their inability to learn school subjects.

The retarded person learns new information and concepts more slowly than the general population. Consistent slowness in sitting, standing, walking, talking, or toilet training may suggest mild retardation to the parent or the professional person. Some clues may indicate mild retardation at an early age, such as the child's lag in communication, inability to learn colors, hyperactivity, and peculiar social habits.

5.8.4. CAUSES

The causes of mental retardation are organic, sociocultural, and psychological. One or any combination of these factors may result in the inability to function normally.

Among organic factors that cause mental retardation are genetic disorders that result in mongolism and metabolic disorders. The factors that most contribute to mild retardation are prenatal, perinatal, and postnatal events that affect the central nervous system.

Lack of stimulation, which is the most frequent sociocultural cause of mild retardation, occurs because the family situation is impoverished both physically and mentally. Culturally disadvantaged families sometimes cannot provide a stimulating environment for their children because they lack the means and ability to do so, thus creating a cycle of underdevelopment.

The psychological factors involved in the lag in intellectual and adaptive functioning of the child usually relate to the mother and child relationship. When the relationship is severed at a critical time (the first 30 months are the most important) due to the mother's absence, death, or mental illness, the child's mental development can be negatively affected.

5.8.5. ADAPTIVE BEHAVIOR

The concern of the rehabilitationist in working with people who have mental limitations is to help them to develop needed coping skills. Heber [1959] introduced the term *adaptive behavior* as applied to retardation and defined it in the original edition of the *Manual on Terminology and Classification in Mental Retardation,* published by the American Association on Mental Deficiency (AAMD) as referring "primarily to the effectiveness of the individual in adapting to the natural and social demands of his environment. Impaired adaptive behavior may be reflected in: (1) maturation, (2) learning, and/or (3) social adjustment."

Adaptive behavior can be measured by an instrument published by AAMD [Nihara, Foster, Shellhass, & Leland, 1974]. In general the life-coping skills signifying adaptive behavior (as operationally defined in *The AAMD Adaptive Behavior Scale*) include mastery over activities of daily living, being mobile, staying out of trouble, getting along at work and at home with people and obligations, enjoying life and living in a satisfying, satisfactory way.

5.9. Substance Dependency

There are two types of substance dependency: (1) "habituation," which is a psychological need to take a drug for the relief of tension, pain, discomfort, or for pleasure; and (2) "addiction," which is a physical dependence, a biochemical reaction causing unpleasant physical symptoms when the drug is withdrawn. The addict also develops a tolerance for the drug so that ever larger doses are required for satisfaction and to prevent withdrawal. Habituation and addiction are not mutually exclusive classifications.

5.9.1. SUBSTANCES

Drug abuse can damage either mind or body or both and can harm relationships with other people. The drug can become an all-consuming interest, destroying other values. Commonly abused drugs are as follows: (1) alcohol; (2) hallucinogenic (vision-producing) drugs (e.g., lysergic acid diethylamide (LSD), mescaline); (3) marijuana (cannabis); (4) nicotine (as found in tobacco); (5) opiates (e.g., heroin, morphine); (6) sedatives (e.g., barbiturates and other kinds of sleeping pills); (7) stimulants (e.g., cocaine, amphetamines); and (8) inhalants—fumes inhaled (e.g., glue, cleaning fluid). To this list of drugs could be added many more substances that are commonly abused.

5.9.2. HABITUATION

Psychological dependence on drugs or habituation may be mild or severe. In mild dependence people are accustomed to taking a drug that gives a sense of well-being, for example, the caffeine in coffee or nicotine in cigarettes. Such people are said to be habituated and will not readily give up the drug; they tend to feel uneasy when deprived of it. Yet, if they wish, habituated people can usually, of their own accord, give up the drug without resorting to professional help.

Severe psychological dependence on drugs is a neurotic reaction that occurs in people who, once having experienced a feeling from a drug that is particularly satisfying, will continue to compulsively seek out the drug (e.g., heroin). Still it can be seen that habituation is a very human trait that is often socially accepted. Examples, in addition to substance abuse, are seen in various entertainments that can become obsessive, e.g., gambling, sports, collecting. One type of psychological dependence is a habituation to food. The resulting overeating and obesity are serious physical, social, and vocational problems. Excessive fat in the body may elevate the blood pressure and this can lead to stroke, heart attack, or kidney disease. Fat can also disrupt breathing patterns and cause respiratory diseases. Mobility may be a functional limitation. Work is often restricted to sedentary jobs.

5.9.3. ADDICTION

Physical dependence or addiction results in an alteration in the body because of continued ingestion of narcotics or depressants so that the drug is required for the individual to function "normally." The withdrawal from narcotics results in increased autonomic nervous system activity and increased central nervous system excitability. Withdrawal from depressants

(barbiturates, sedative-hypnotics, antianxiety agents) also results in increased excitability of certain regions of the central nervous system, notably those controlling motor and mental functions. The person becomes tremulous and may suffer ·confusion, disorientation, and psychotic reactions.

In physical dependence, which is true addiction, there are two elements: habituation and tolerance (chemical dependence). The addicting drugs provide relief from anguish and pain swiftly and efficiently. They induce a physiological tolerance that requires an increase in dosage on repeated use if it is to be effective. These two features foster the continued need for the drug and lead to its becoming a functional component in the biochemistry of the brain. Sudden removal of the drug provokes a withdrawal syndrome that includes mental and physical pain. This is the hallmark of addiction and the way in which it differs from habituation.

Alcohol is probably the most lethal (i.e., in number of deaths) drug in this category, yet it is the easiest to obtain. *Alcoholism* is the proper term for addiction to alcohol, yet the disease progression would fit any of the addicting drugs. Continued use of alcohol may result in cirrhosis of the liver, heart disease, ulcers, cancer of the esophogus or intestines, and central nervous system damage. Delirium tremens (hallucinations), blackouts, seizures, and tremors are withdrawal symptoms. Withdrawal from alcohol can be life-threatening.

Barbiturates are another type of central nervous system depressant. Large doses can result in unconsciousness and death. Withdrawal is similar to that experienced with alcohol except that it is much more life-threatening.

Another form of addicting drug are those in the opiate family. Opiates leave the bloodstream and are absorbed into the body quickly where they tend to concentrate in the liver and spleen. They have a long half-life and thus easily build up to toxic proportions. Withdrawal from this family, although extremely painful, is not life-threatening. Excessive overdoses can result in death, usually from respiratory failure.

Amphetamines are the last category of the addicting drugs frequently used. Amphetamines are called "uppers"; that is, they speed up the body system. Regular usage of these drugs can cause weight loss, skin reactions, and ulcers. Long-term limitations result because extended use can cause vascular damage or heart failure. Death usually occurs from mental and physical deterioration.

Functional dependency vastly differs from the two types of dependency described above. Physicians prescribe so-called ethical drugs to relieve annoying or disturbing conditions and the particular function involved becomes dependent on the action of a drug. Such drugs are prescribed primarily for relief of symptoms.

5.9.4. REHABILITATION ISSUES

Dependence on drugs may not preclude rehabilitation and subsequent employment as many people engage in gainful employment after addiction. The choice of life-style and the meeting of substance needs are related to the amount of drugs required, length of time on drugs, and most importantly, the basic personality, temperament, predisposition, and skills of the addict in question. Opportunity, resources, and contacts also play a major role in the choice of a drug-oriented life-style.

During the addiction period, substance-dependent people are mainly concerned with "feeding" the habit. Everything in their lives is centered on the need for drugs. Money is used purely to meet this need. Other aspects of life, pleasures, and obligations hardly exist, so all-absorbing is the use of and search for drugs.

The usual, traditional approaches to job training have serious limitations when applied to the substance-dependent population. In addition to a lack of skills, there is frequently a lack of motivation and general education as well. This is further complicated by the attitude of many employers, who screen such people because of their addiction or arrest record. There is also the special situation of the addicted individuals who may have additional limitations. First, their addiction may have been precipitated by another or prior deviance, for example, inability to conform to socially acceptable standards of behavior. The rewards of work, other than money, may be of little interest to them, and they may not want to be restricted to a regular job. It is extremely difficult for most addicts to remain gainfully employed on a continuous basis for an acceptable length of time.

Business and industry are developing programs as they are becoming increasingly concerned about substance dependence within the ranks of the employed. Community clinics and special facilities are generally available where alcoholics and drug abusers can receive treatment for their drug problems. Rehabilitation and preventive rehabilitation must be social as well as medical. Finding socially acceptable jobs that substance-dependent people can perform is a primary part of the process.

5.10. Pain Limitation

The subjectivity of pain gives it a deceptive quality, so, despite the fact that everyone experiences pain, it is hard to communicate its personal meaning. The other's pain sensation itself is not directly observable. Clinically, then, there is no completely adequate way to describe the intensity of pain objectively. However, two methods of evaluation have been devised: the pain estimate and the tourniquet pain ratio. In the pain estimate, the patient is asked to rate pain on a scale of 0 to 100 on which 0 represents no pain and 100 represents pain so severe that the individual would commit suicide if it were necessary to endure it for more than one or two minutes. In the tourniquet pain ratio, on the other hand, a painful stimulus is introduced against which patients can match their clinical pain; this information can be translated into a

score that falls on the same scale as is used for the pain estimate. While both methods have been validated, discrepancies between the two measures frequently occur.

5.10.1. CLASSIFICATIONS OF PAIN

There is no single clearly defined syndrome, no single disability group encompassing this population of people who are limited by pain. A myriad of conditions cause pain: to name a few, arthritis, low back problems, the neuralgias, migraine, and angina. To manage this variety, it is helpful to classify the pain sensation in terms of: (1) duration (acute or chronic); (2) origin (physical or mental); (3) nature of the disease (malignant or benign, static or progressive); (4) the precipitating causes and nature of onset of pain attack; (5) resulting limitations in ordinary life functions and behavior patterns. The use of these classifications will help the rehabilitationist formulate a picture of the extent of the problem and the factors that will be critical in assessing the client's rehabilitation potential and needs.

5.10.2. INTERVENING VARIABLES

A number of factors influence both the perception of the pain sensation and the individual's reaction to it. Awareness of these factors makes possible planned manipulation of the variables so as to alleviate the pain experience. The more obvious factors include the components of the physical environment as they affect the pain sensation; for instance, temperature, noise, light, humidity, and the individual's posture may directly affect the intensity of the sensation. Knowledge of how these factors affect pain will be critical for successful job placement of the client in pain.

More subtle are the factors influencing the subjective experience of the sensation, and, in turn, the reaction to it. These factors are thought to include both stable personality traits and cognitive-motivational influences. The influence of personality traits is still being researched and the evidence is at times conflicting. There is, however, a wide range of cognitive-emotional factors that have more predictable effects on the pain experience. Among these are fatigue, fear, conditioning, cultural norms, attention, anxiety, expectancies, and past experiences.

The factors influencing the pain experience can be broadly categorized into: the sensory attributes of the pain, the nature of the disease, the individual's psychological situation, and cultural norms. These factors account for the variability among individuals in their response to the pain experience, another area that needs to be addressed.

5.10.3. THE PAIN RESPONSE

The individual's response to pain can be divided into three components: the biological reaction to pain, the behavioral response, and the nonbehavioral response. The biological reaction has both voluntary and involuntary aspects. Involuntary reflexes include changes in respiration, perspiration, heart rate, and muscle contraction. Voluntary reactions enable individuals to manipulate both their own posture and the physical environment so as to alleviate the pain.

The behavioral response is a variable composite of several components: motor (e.g., clenching of teeth), vocal (moaning or crying), verbal (complaining or cursing), and social (bad manners or withdrawal). Nonbehavioral responses include the cognitive, emotional, and personal elements of the response. There may be a fear of pain and anxieties about the family and employment. Loneliness develops when the "pain" patient is unable to sleep at night and is unable to participate in activities. Dependency, depression, and guilt are frequent problems.

5.10.4. TREATMENT FOR PAIN

The therapeutic conceptualization of pain can be divided into two fundamental frameworks: the disease model and the learning model. According to the disease model, pain is defined as a combination of observable symptoms and an underlying responsible pathological stimulus; by identifying and treating the pathology, the pain in turn will be alleviated. The phenomenon of pain is defined according to the specificity theory that pain is a specific sensation straight from pain receptors (damaged tissue) to a pain center in the brain. Treatment is directed to the underlying pathology.

Drug therapy is one of the most common methods of treatment. Analgesics treat the symptoms of pain rather than its cause. Nonnarcotic analgesics (e.g., aspirin) are preferred when they are effective. Narcotics such as morphine, heroin, and methadone may produce a tolerance effect as well as result in mental clouding, dizziness, vomiting, and constipation. Surgical procedures are also utilized for relief of pain, although the relief may be only temporary.

In contrast to the disease model for pain control, the learning model deemphasizes the importance of the underlying pathology and focuses on the behavioral manifestations of pain and their consequences. Based on the behavioral approach to learning, this model depicts chronic pain as a series of observable "illness behaviors" or symptoms with associated, identifiable, environmental consequences that serve as reinforcers of the illness behavior. Treatment is concerned with identifying and modifying the behavioral responses to pain, rather than seeking out and trying to eliminate the underlying pathology.

In pain (or contingency) management clinics, treatment is based on the learning model. The basic premise is that the individual's response (behavior) to pain occurs because it is being directly and positively reinforced or because it constitutes an avoidance of some aversive event, such as some other noxious stimulus. This approach is sensitive to the client's "pain game" (i.e., pain behavior to elicit sympathy, attention, or other psychological payoffs from others).

5.10.5. IMPLICATIONS

A serious vocational handicap often results from distraction and disturbance of function as a result of severe, uncontrollable pain. In fact, low back pain following spinal injury—accompanied by perceived restrictions in lifting, alleged distractions of pain, and claimed requirements for frequent changes in posture (from sitting, standing, or reclining)—is the most frequent reason given for long-term disability benefits by industrial workers. Even though there are many sedentary jobs that a person in pain can perform without further injury, many employers are unwilling to risk legal action for further injury.

The client should initially be given physical and neurological examinations and a psychological evaluation. The counselor must then consider possible methods of pain treatment and pain adjustment through purchased services from the staff of a pain clinic or other specialists. Rehabilitation counseling for personal and vocational adjustment is also necessary for successful resolution.

5.11. Consciousness Limitation

Consciousness can be functionally defined through a delineation of its elements: attention, reality orientation, and perception or awareness. Reality orientation is mental contact with actually existing internal and external phenomena; perception is interpreting information received through the senses. Memory, the ability both to encode and decode stimuli, and the emotional state are contributing factors to the functional effectiveness of conscious processes.

5.11.1. DESCRIPTION

Functional limitations of the individual suffering a disorder in consciousness encompass the entirety of life, depending on the length of time involved and the degree of impairment, the range is from a permanent stupor or, more commonly, a continuous inadequate level of consciousness or periodic unconsciousness to the unimportant fleeting distractions everyone experiences. Causes are physical, mental, emotional, and situational. Altered consciousness can be deliberately induced as with alcohol ingestion; this is a kind of "unliving." Sleep is a healthy state—in the proper place and with proper preparation—but sudden loss of consciousness can be disastrous, and even the threat of its occurring is a functional limitation.

5.11.2. CAUSES

A variety of disabilities comprise the category of defects in consciousness. Epilepsy in all of its forms is the principal disability; others are mental illness, cerebral atherosclerosis, drug abuses, extreme fatigue, and metabolic disorders (e.g., diabetes). The function can even be interfered with by preoccupation (absentmindedness) due to other interests.

Because loss of consciousness is most readily identified with epilepsy, epilepsy will be used as the basis for discussion of this functional limitation. Material is from several previous books and journal articles on the rehabilitation of persons with epilepsy [Wright, 1976, 1975, 1961, and Wright, Gibbs, & Linde, 1962]. It is more accurate to speak of "epilepsies" because there are so many different manifestations: petit mal, a brief absence of consciousness; grand mal, a generalized convulsion; psychomotor, an amnesia with irrelevant behavior; and a number of others. Most fits of epilepsy are accompanied by a loss of consciousness, and this is its greatest limitation, other than its social stigma.

5.11.3. PLACEMENT CONSIDERATIONS

A worker is handicapped for a specific job if the consciousness impairment constitutes a func-

tional limitation for any of the critical requirements of that job. Selective placement procedures consequently are especially useful in the
evaluation and placement of persons with disorders of consciousness such as epilepsy.

Occupationally pertinent questions are as follows: Which type or types of seizures are experienced now or have been experienced in the
past? How severe and how long are they? How
frequent and regular? Are there precipitating
factors? When do the seizures occur? Is there an
aura or warning and is it reliable? Is the seizure
behavior (e.g., violent screams) disconcerting to
others? What is the postseizure behavior and
how long does it take for the person to return to
normal? What medication is taken and what is
the apparent effect? How does the person feel
about the disability? Is there mental or emotional impairment?

Persons subject to loss of consciousness
should not be placed in positions in which their
safety or the safety of others may be endangered
by the loss of consciousness or by uncontrollable actions. Environmental conditions to avoid
are exposure to dangerous moving objects or
mechanical and electrical hazards, situations in
which there is danger of falling from one elevation to another or of exposure to burns, and
work in cramped or otherwise hazardous quarters. Examples of unsafe jobs include the operation of a crane; welding, in which the torch may
be dropped or thrown; handling molten metal;
piloting an airliner; performing surgery.

Of all the environmental characteristics and
demands of jobs used by the United States
Employment Service in job analyses, only a
relatively small number would disqualify an applicant because of epilepsy. Many job requirements disqualify disabled persons other than
epileptics: lifting and carrying heavy loads,
crawling, running, jumping, hand-and-finger dexterity, gripping, reaching, back strength, agility, exertion, vision, perception, hearing, talking, and repetitive motion. Work conditions that
would disqualify other disabled persons but not
those with epilepsy are: temperature excesses or
fluctuations, humidity or wet conditions, dusts
and respiratory irritants, and exposure to communicable diseases. Epileptic seizures, including convulsions, do not prevent assignment to

any of these tasks or environments, and these
are merely examples of the many job demands
that are suitable.

Work activity, both mental and physical, is
beneficial for the person with epilepsy. In fact,
seizures may be more likely to occur when
epileptics are idle than when they are occupied.
Excessive emotional stress, however, should be
avoided. The important consideration here is
employment that is consistent with the applicant's physical and mental abilities.

A consciousness disorder does not preclude
most tasks required with most jobs. Admittedly
epilepsy, if not fully controlled, can be a serious
job handicap, preventing placements in dangerous positions. But there is overgeneralization of
the handicap, and epileptic applicants are not
hired although they can meet all of the physical
demands of the job, there is no safety problem,
and the work does not aggravate the disability.

The employment handicap associated with
epilepsy creates a problem for industry as well
as for the epileptic worker. Applicants with epilepsy refuse to reveal it because experience has
taught them that they are rejected for suitable
employment. Consequently because they do not
tell about their seizure history they are often
placed in dangerous situations. The natural anxiety over a new job plus the fear of disclosure
may bring on a seizure. Dismissal typically follows, without understanding or an attempt at
selective placement, and the worker moves on
to another company.

5.11.4. TREATMENT

The most important task in epilepsy rehabilitation is to achieve maximal control of seizures.
Diagnosis and treatment by a neurologist specializing in epilepsy is essential for total rehabilitation. It is necessary to determine the
cause of the impairment of consciousness (e.g.,
possible brain tumor), and also to establish the
best medical control. There are many anticon-
vulsants on the market and the prescription
choice requires an "epileptologist." Physical
restoration—correcting or controlling the medical condition and the resulting episodes of
unconsciousness—has priority over efforts for
vocational adjustment.

5.12. *Uncertain Prognosis*

The functional limitation associated with an uncertain prognosis occurs with any medical condition characterized by uncertainty about the future. This includes the uncertain outlook for decreased mobility and strength in the arthritic, loss of consciousness in the epileptic, and so on. The emotional reaction to future uncertainties is not limited to clearly deteriorating physical conditions.

An individual's reaction to the stress and ambiguity of an uncertain prognosis can cause the person to withdraw socially, which limits interpersonal, vocational, and even intellectual development. Individuals overcome by anger, anxiety, fear, and the like can develop psychological disorders that can pose a real barrier to rehabilitation.

5.12.1. PSYCHOLOGICAL IMPLICATIONS

The fear of becoming a useless, nonproductive, dependent person is very real in many physically disabled individuals. But when a person is faced with a disease process that has an uncertain prognosis, the problem is complicated by destructive uncertainty and ambiguity. This individual has little knowledge of how the disease will progress. Arthritics may not know how long they will be able to walk, bend over, grasp a small object, and so on. The epileptic case wonders when and where a seizure will occur; the diabetic case wonders how long it will be before vision begins to deteriorate, and cancer cases may not know if they will be alive three months hence.

An individual with an uncertain prognosis can manifest any number of psychological reactions: panic, nightmares, fear of losing intellectual abilities as the disease progresses, fear of death and dying, and feelings of rejection and shame, along with thoughts of suicide, denial, isolation, and so on. Such people may react by withdrawing from emotional involvement in close relationships; they may become hostile toward those with physically sound bodies; they may become apathetic, passive, and dependent. The individual and the family may panic and try one "miracle cure" after another, running from specialists to faith healers in a desperate desire to hang on to some hope, no matter how slim. It seems that an uncertain prognosis almost always fosters a good deal of false hope during those periods when the person is practically symptom-free. In a number of cases these remissions, periods of being "normal," are followed by exacerbations, periods of increased disease symptoms; this is much harder to handle than continuous disease. An example is the person with a cardiovascular disease who might experience periods of angina only after engaging in some sort of physical activity and then feel discomfort at other times for seemingly no reason at all. The arthritic may function quite well one day and the next not be able to move without severe pain and stiffness. The individual with multiple sclerosis has episodes of disability that may last several months and recur at intervals of months or years and yet at other times be symptom-free. Even the seizure-free epileptic cannot be sure the medication will continue to control. Those who have seizures do not know where or when they will occur.

The rehabilitation counselor needs to be aware of the client's changing situation and how it is affecting the individual so that realistic vocational planning can evolve. It must be acknowledged that there will be times when the client simply will not be physically able to engage in certain activities and that it is not possible to know when these times will come. This does make for a complicated employment problem because most jobs have to be conducted with regularity.

5.12.2. TERMINAL ILLNESS

Special counseling and understanding are needed for the dying person. Individuals faced with the knowledge that they have a terminal illness obviously go through a variety of psychological reactions. The first reaction is, generally, "It can't be true, not me!" This is characteristic of the first stage in death and dying, that of "denial and isolation." The individual anxiously searches for some other explanation, may shop around for a number of different doctors and ask for reexamination, anything to prolong or avoid the reality of the diagnosis. This temporary state of shock gradually decreases, depending upon how the individual is told, how much time there is to acknowledge the impending death, and how the person has coped with stressful situations in the past. Some denial is used by almost everyone during the course of a terminal illness. The second stage, that of anger, is manifest through feelings of rage, envy, and resentment toward those who are healthy and living. This stage is very difficult for family, friends, doctors, and counselors to deal with. The anger is displaced in all directions, at times almost at random: the doctors are no good, the test cannot tell anything, a concerned relative may be accused of not caring. What the individual really needs at this stage is to be understood, respected, and given time and attention. If the person is made to feel like someone valuable and allowed to function on the highest possible level, including continued gainful employment, the anger soon dissipates. The third stage, that of bargaining, may last for only a short time. It is really an attempt to postpone the inevitable. As his condition begins to degenerate, the individual realizes that life cannot be bargained for and begins to feel a great sense of loss. At this

point the person usually becomes depressed. This fourth stage—terminally ill individuals going through the process of grieving over their own death—is very necessary for letting go of life possessions. In order to progress to a state of acceptance, the person must let go of significant things and people and eventually gain permission from those people to die (through open, honest communication and their acceptance of the death). The final stage of acceptance is the point at which the individual has mourned the impending loss of meaningful people and places and is able to contemplate death with quiet anticipation.

In general, these stages cover fairly well the range of emotions usually experienced, although not all people go through every stage in this particular order. These stages can also be applied to some degree to individuals faced with life-threatening diseases and to those whose capacities may progressively deteriorate.

5.13. Debilitation Limitation

Debilitation (or exertional limitation) is associated with a variety of medical and psychiatric disabilities that weaken the operation of the body or prevent the exercise of its strength (i.e., exertion). Examples are rheumatoid arthritis, malnutrition, emphysema, aging, and infectious mononucleosis, among others. Weakness results partly from endocrine disorders involving the thyroid, adrenal, and pituitary glands. Fatigue accompanies chronic infections such as brucellosis. Debilitating conditions can involve the heart, back, spinal cord, brain, muscles, glands, and sensory organs. Certain medical therapies are debilitating, such as radiation therapy in the form of cancer treatment.

Examples of this condition in the psychiatric area are depression, which has lethargy as a symptom, and neurasthenia (anergy); the latter is characterized by muscular weakness and easy fatigability to a state of exhaustion. Emotionally disturbed people are often apathetic and listless.

5.13.1. CAUSES

During convalescence after illness or surgery muscles often become flabby from lack of use.

Chronic invalids require exercise and activity programs to maintain or regain use of muscles and joints. Orthotic devices can aid function by providing mechanical assistance for inadequate musculature, and other devices such as walkers may be used. Occupational and physical therapists work together to increase strength. Therapy includes exercise, massage, mechanical apparatus, and the applications of electric stimulation, moving water, light, hot or cold temperature, and oil.

Physical lethargy may seem to be a personality trait; conversely, the will to overcome somatic debilitation is highly individualized.

5.13.2. RESTRICTIONS

As with other disabilities, vital restrictions may be required of the person with a debilitating impairment, but unique to this condition is, perhaps, the permanence of these restrictions or their progressive nature. It may seem as though all of the person's energy is now to be directed toward preservation of the body itself and not the gratification of other important needs and drives. Quantity of life becomes the priority, at the sacrifice of quality. A conflict may develop between the individuals' ideal image of themselves (strong, energetic, potent, robust, sturdy, tough) and the empirical situation.

Dependency is also increased. Again this occurs with many disabilities, but it can be especially distressing in a debilitating situation. The individual may sometimes enjoy the dependency but more likely will feel guilty about it. The family may also become quite resentful of their added responsibility.

Even without normal limits there are vast differences in the level of mental and physical energy people exhibit. It is a mistake to assume that the two always go together (as often seen in mental retardation), although the dynamic person with obvious body vigor appears more animated and gives the impression of being intellectually energetic. When physical illness has enervated someone by lessening physical vitality or reducing strength, there is a danger that prospective employers will falsely assume the person is less active mentally.

5.13.3. VOCATIONAL IMPLICATIONS

Physical strength is but one of a number of considerations in job placement of the handicapped. However, occupational exertion requirements are important and must be carefully appraised. The U.S. Employment Service has analyzed and published information about the physical demands of jobs (discussed in Chapter 19, Occupational Information). The strength variables involve four factors: (1) lifting, carrying, pushing and/or pulling; (2) climbing and/or balancing; (3) stooping, kneeling, crouching, and/or crawling; and (4) reaching, handling, fingering, and/or feeling. There are five classifications of work, from sedentary to very heavy work, depending upon these factors, particularly the amount (weight) and frequency of lifting.

Another precaution to consider is that jobs vary in time and place. Even a so-called sedentary or light job may be or may become too strenuous for the exertion (amount) and endurance (time) capacity of the clients who are limited in this respect.

5.14. Motivity Limitation

A functional limitation in motivity is the inability to produce, direct, and/or control bodily movements as required in a specific situation. Motivity and mobility limitation are related but different concepts. Motivity refers to the bodily ability required to move objects and do tasks performed normally by using the musculoskeletal system, whereas mobility means moving the body from one location to another. The term *motive* means "moving or causing motion" while *mobile* means "movable or capable of being moved." The primary physical restrictions in motivity are in reaching forward or performing movements of the hand and fingers, which may be called a "manipulative limitation."

Three types of motivity problems are described here: (1) those involving broad, or gross, movements, such as bending over; (2) those involving precise, or fine, movements, such as writing with a pen; and (3) the complete absence of movement, as in the case of paralysis or amputation. A fourth variation, which could be termed "motivity insufficiency," was discussed under Debilitation Limitation.

Motivity defects vary greatly in their degree of functional limitation, depending on the type and complexity of the task required, the part of the body involved, and the degree of the impairment. This limitation is manifested in most of the physical disabilities, as well as in some mental and psychological disabilities.

The following is a list of the components involved in functional limitation of motivity as defined here: (1) strength, (2) speed, (3) endurance, (4) balance, (5) agility, (6) dexterity, (7) perception, (8) coordination, (9) size, (10) physical demand for movement, and (11) spontaneous uncontrolled movement. Such limitations as are not exertional limitations could be collectively referred to as "manipulative limitations."

5.14.1. STRENGTH

The intensity, power, and scope of movement denote strength. Again, the overall physical condition of people can greatly influence the amount of strength asserted in their movements; for example, when alcoholism has reached the point of damaging the major body organs, the entire body state is weakened. A physiological condition that directly reduces strength in movement is muscular dystrophy, in which the muscles degenerate progressively. Since strength is required more in manual types of work, the client with strength limitations should be encouraged to select skilled or semiskilled jobs that may reduce the need to lift, carry, push, or pull heavy objects.

5.14.2. SPEED

The act of moving swiftly or rapidly is a component of motion. Generally, the more familiar a task is the more quickly an individual can perform it. However, for those persons with motion disorders the rate of speed may not increase even with practice, that is, not to a competitive or normal level. Examples of medical conditions that affect speed include various orthopedic disabilities: cerebral palsy, arthritis, or injuries to the extremities. Such disabilities may preclude employment on an assembly line or other jobs in which efficiency is a criterion of performance.

5.14.3. ENDURANCE

This is the capacity or power to withstand pain, distress, or any very prolonged stress without untoward effect. In terms of motivity this would mean sustaining movement. Examples of medical conditions that might limit endurance include cardiovascular disease so severe that the client cannot continue in stressful or active exertion for very long periods because of chest pains or shortness of breath. Respiratory disorders such as emphysema or asthma would also affect an individual's endurance because of a lack of oxygen.

5.14.4. BALANCE

Balance refers to the ability to keep the body in a state of equilibrium, thus proportioning the weight equally on both sides. The body has a group of reflexes, called the antigravity or stretch reflexes, that (normally) straighten the body upright automatically when balance is disrupted. Disorders involving these muscles may be so severe that the muscles cannot counteract the imbalance as they should.

A number of medical conditions relate to balance. A newly blinded person may have difficulty in walking straight and have a tendency to veer in one direction. Injury or disease involving the labyrinth (inner ear) mechanism may affect balance. Others with this problem include brain-damaged individuals (hemiplegics) and amputees. Counselors working with clients with balance problems should find out whether the difficulty occurs only in motion and the circumstances under which it occurs. Obvious vocational considerations include avoiding high places and dangerous environments.

5.14.5. AGILITY

The ability to move and change direction and position quickly and easily is a natural part of an intact and healthy body. Reduced agility, however, occurs with various physical, mental, and emotional disabilities. For example, the movements of an amputee with an artificial limb will not be as agile as those of a person with unimpaired arms and legs.

5.14.6. DEXTERITY

Dexterity refers to skill and rapidity in physical activity, especially expertise in using the hands and fingers. It also refers to mental skill and quickness. Both of these definitions apply in terms of the limitations of motivity. An example of a medical condition relating to physical dexterity is arthritis in the upper extremities. Arthritic clients whose disability affects the use of hands and fingers would be unable to make the fine movements necessary to do detailed work. Mentally retarded or psychiatric cases may be unable to respond quickly to their environment because judgment and reaction time may be slowed down. Certain types of medications such as tranquilizers or barbiturates may also inhibit mental dexterity. Tests of motor dexterity and eye-hand coordination are discussed in Chapter 20, Psychological Testing and Chapter 23, Work Evaluation Techniques.

5.14.7. PERCEPTION

Perception can be simply described as an awareness of the environment through sensation. In terms of movement, perception involves both tactile (touch) sensation as well as kinesthesis (the effect of moving a body member). Perception allows an individual to know where the body is positioned at any given moment, as well as its relation to the environment. The abilities of seeing, hearing, touching, and feeling greatly affect the way people respond with movement to events. Someone with monocular (one-eyed) vision would have difficulty estimating both distance and depth, in addition to having a smaller field of vision. The person's movements would reflect the visual impairment. Also, those who have lost their sense of touch are adversely affected in their movements.

5.14.8. COORDINATION

The harmonious and integrated action of the various complex movements of the body is referred to as coordination. Ataxia, which may be due to multiple sclerosis, refers to the failure of muscle coordination for voluntary movements. This disability especially affects the more complex movements that involve integration of groups of muscles, such as the arm-leg coordination involved in walking. Because of the irregularity of the action of their muscles, ataxic persons resemble alcoholics in the way they stagger when walking. Eye-hand coordination is generally the most important type of coordination needed for semiskilled job tasks; this would limit the job placement of persons with perceptual disorders or motor problems involving eye-hand coordination.

5.14.9. SIZE

Abnormal size of an individual can also be a limiting factor of motion. Clients whose physical dimensions are unusual may have difficulty with aspects of movement such as speed, coordination, and mobility and may also have difficulty negotiating in an environment of housing and machines designed for average-sized people. Examples are obesity, giantism, and dwarfism. The physical dimensions of a person's hands might limit dexterity in certain job tasks also.

Anthropometry, the study of human body measurements, influences the design of manufactured products. Things are made with only the typical person considered. People who are outside of the average range in their physical proportions consequently may have trouble operating a standard machine.

5.14.10. PHYSICAL MOVEMENT DEMAND

Physical movement demand refers to conditions in which the person feels it is necessary to move in order to relieve the pain or discomfort of a medical condition. Clients with arthritis of the upper extremities or chronic back pain may be unable to sit for extended periods of time without getting up occasionally to move around.

Movement ameliorates the stiffness or tension, or both, that mounts when the person stays in a stationary position. The work station must allow someone to sit or stand, or even recline or walk, at will. (This was mentioned previously as a "postural" limitation.) Clients who are hyperactive, or who have a high degree of anxiety, may also feel the need to move in order to dissipate "excess energy." A vocational consideration would be a job that does not require continuous attention and in which short breaks are permitted.

5.14.11. SPONTANEOUS MOVEMENT

This refers to actions or motions that occur without the individual's intentional effort. Epilepsy is characterized by spontaneous seizures that often involve movement. The spasticity of cerebral palsy is another form of neurological damage. Most striking are the involuntary movements of persons with Huntington's chorea. Another example is the muscular contractions of facial tics, which may be of a psychological origin.

5.14.12. TREATMENT METHODS

Medical rehabilitation—using physical exercise and physical training methods—can serve to restore an individual's functional abilities insofar as possible when the motor defect is due to injury or disease.

Two means of improving motivity involve the use of prosthetic and orthotic devices. Prosthetic devices are made to compensate for the loss of an appendage. A common example is the artificial appliance fitted after an arm amputation. Orthotic devices, on the other hand, straighten or strengthen an existing part of the body and prevent deformity. An upper-extremity orthotic device is the "handy hand" splint used for realigning and giving movement back to the nonfunctional hand (caused by injury, infection, or paralysis) when the digits no longer touch the thumb. Hooks may be used in both orthotic and prosthetic hands. Used in conjunction with cables, levers, and rubber bands, they are employed for prehension (holding) purposes.

Whenever possible in the case of a partial hand amputee, an orthotic device is used to allow what is left of the hand to be as useful as possible. Prosthetic devices to replace lost fingers or the thumb are used also. Sometimes with surgery existing bones are used to create replacements (osteotomy) or the surgeon will even recreate a usable joint (arthroplasty).

Upper-extremity appliances can also be powered by a power pack; this process is called "myoelectric power." Even if the arm is paralyzed or amputated, a measurable electric potential will occur on the skin of the remaining appendage when the person thinks about moving the limb. An oscilloscope probes to find the greatest spot or spots of potential and these are tattooed. Electrodes, attached to the tattooed areas, act as switches to activate the power in the power pack, which then is converted into mechanical energy by way of the splints or hooks in conjunction with the cables.

Lower prosthetic devices are identified by the location of use—above-knee (AK) or below-knee (BK)—and by the way in which they are attached. There are generally three types: the first, which is rarely used, is the shoulder-suspension type; the second, the pelvic-band type, is considered the conventional limb; and the third type is the suction-socket artificial leg. This artificial leg has no attachment to the pelvis or trunk so there is better control and greater freedom of motion. It seems lighter and because the pelvic belt is eliminated, it can be worn by pregnant women or obese patients. The suction-socket leg works on the principle of negative pressure. The stump fits down to within two inches of the chamber floor (unlike the first two types in which the stump fits flush to the floor of the prosthesis). In this space an expulsion valve lets air out as the stump is pushed down. As the stump pulls upward the valve closes, creating negative pressure, which then holds the limb secure.

5.14.13. APPLIANCES DIFFICULTY

Important problems are associated with the loss of a limb and the use of prosthetic devices. The sweating and irritation of a stump confined in a socket requires good sanitation and proper fitting. Lower-extremity amputees should avoid jobs requiring much walking, constant standing, climbing, crawling, kneeling, and the lifting of heavy objects.

Upper-extremity amputees may have difficulties in tasks involving carrying, fingering, grasping, handling, lifting, and throwing. A prosthetic hand is useless in the dark because the wearer directs its operation by vision as opposed to normal feeling. For those who still have one good arm and hand—particularly if on the dominant side—normal motivity is largely a matter of learning to do things differently.

Motivity limitations are pertinent to the fields of biotechnology (the study and application of the integration of biological and engineering techniques) and ergonomics (the study of human relationships with machines and environments). The concerns here are directed toward the anatomical, physiological, and psychological restrictions and capacities of the human operator as well as the application of knowledge of these to engineering or architectural design in order to facilitate or maximize human function. Anthropometry is also relevant. Scientists and engineers as well as practitioners on the rehabilitation team need to examine the motivity variables as well as other functional limitations that influence bodily performance (see 8.4.3).

Chapter 6

History of Rehabilitation

Historians and social planners appreciate that the past has much to teach about the present and that knowledge about the past helps as people try to predict the future. Projections have little validity if they cannot be measured by the events, causes, and effects that have been experienced before.

It is important that work in rehabilitation too be considered in historical perspective. Most of those involved in rehabilitation want to make a constructive contribution to society. Since the quality of their work and of its contribution to the world is shaped by what has gone before, it is important that they be aware of the past. Thus a knowledge of the development of rehabilitation is necessary for an understanding of present programs and issues.

A History of Vocational Rehabilitation in America, a scholarly and comprehensive book, was written by C. Esco Obermann in 1965. Commissioned by a Memorial Fund for William F. Faulkes, founder of the National Rehabilitation Association, with the financial support of the federal rehabilitation agency, the Obermann study of vocational rehabilitation history is the definitive work on the subject. The reader is directed to it for a more extensive account of the history of rehabilitation.

In this chapter the presentation of the history up to 1965 is essentially a digest of Obermann's book, with occasional departures from the original text. These changes include observations and interpretations from several individuals and from other documents. Because of the additions, deletions, and deviations in the present version of the history from that presented by Dr. Obermann, he should not be held accountable for what is presented here. His work should be fully credited, however, since a great bulk of the research and writing was his and much of what is included here has been selected directly from his 1965 book. The history has been updated from various other sources and consulting authorities. Historical references up to 1965 in this account of the history may be found in Obermann's bibliography and for the most part are not listed in the Reference section of this book. A special note of appreciation is due for the permission from Dr. Obermann, the author, T. S. Denison and Company, the publisher, and the National Rehabilitation Association, the sponsor of his writing, to make extensive use of his materials.

Several other accounts of the history of rehabilitation are noteworthy. Russell Dean's [1972] book focused on six pioneers in American rehabilitation: Henry Kessler, Howard Rusk, Frank Krusen, Jeremiah Milbank, and Mary Switzer. E. B. Whitten wrote an account of the National Rehabilitation Association (NRA), which he directed for over a quarter of a century, although his manuscript has not been published. It has provided perspective to events reported in this chapter.

Historical information on events from 1965 to 1980 was gathered from various sources. Two serial publications were so heavily used that general rather than specific references are cited: the *NRA Newsletter*, which is published bimonthly by the NRA in Washington, D.C.; and a periodical publication of the U.S. Department of Health, Education, and Welfare entitled *A Summary of Selected Legislation Related to the Handicapped,* available through the U.S. Government Printing Office in Washington, D.C.

It is necessary as a final note to point out that the history recounted here is oriented toward American and Western European culture. The perspective therefore reflects an unfortunate bias and does represent a limited view of the development and role of rehabilitation in human history.

6.1. Attitudes Toward Disability

A culture inherits all that has gone before. No civilization has come and gone without leaving some legacy. Rehabilitation, a small element of our culture, is what it is and is becoming as a result of all the variations in human interrelationships to date. Judged by contemporary standards in the Western world, the life of the disabled person through the centuries has not been easy. But in a primitive society there were some logical reasons for the treatment of disabled people and the roles they were assigned. This cannot always be said about modern attitudes and practices (see 4.3).

6.1.1. PRIMITIVE PRACTICES

It has been suggested that the common practice of rejecting the atypical specimen among men comes from evolutionary periods much older than those that anthropologists study. Some animals attack the physically inferior or inadequate members of their group, but this is not universal. Some, but not all, ants kill the aged and infirm; some birds will drive off an individual bird with unusual coloring, but black sheep are not ostracized by other sheep.

Some apparent "rejection" by animals of the disabled in their group is probably a manifestation of the pecking order commonly found among animals. When in an animal society there is desperate competition for food, weak or disabled members will frequently be pushed aside and eliminated.

In primitive tribes the disabled or inadequate members are often eliminated. In a society that subsists on hunting and primitive agriculture and that needs its warriors for defense, physical ability is highly prized and the society will only support the healthy young who will later contribute to the welfare of the group. It cannot support members who represent a burden.

6.1.2. RELIGION AND MEDICINE

The Bible has perhaps had a greater impact on Western culture than any other source of information, inspiration, or dogma. From it millions of people draw blueprints for attitudes and behavior. Even people who belong to "liberal" or "reformed" denominations or even to none, are influenced by what their forebears believed. There are many allusions to disability in the Bible. Some of the books reflect an aversion to anyone who has a blemish or other physical disfiguration. Elsewhere it is emphasized that people must have compassion for those who are crippled, deaf, and blind.

The Mohammedans looked at disability more objectively. In the ninth century they established a hospital in Baghdad that provided treatment as dictated by the best scientific knowledge of the day. It is reported that there was a hospital in Cairo where people with all kinds of disorders received free treatment. When discharged, they were given money to meet their needs until they could go back to work again.

In another ancient society, Sparta, deformed and disabled children were systematically eliminated, not because of religious beliefs but as a way of improving the society.

It was usually believed that the gods were on the side of the strong. Without any methods of finding germs or other causes, ancient doctors analyzed disease and physiological disorders in terms of evil spirits; they thought of cures in terms of exorcism and magic. If the gods favored the healthy and the strong, the sick and the disabled must be under the sway of demons. Thus, in addition to experiencing frustration and inadequacy, disadvantaged people were ostracized by their fellows.

In primitive societies even today doctors are trained in the secrets and mysteries of magic and demonology. They reinforce their technical skills by outwitting the evil spirits warring against man.

At particular points in history, courageous and imaginative persons have challenged the established beliefs and those who profited from them. Hippocrates (460–370 B.C.) had the genius and bravery to develop theories and practices that were in conflict with those of the priest-physicians in charge of the temples (hospitals) of Aesculapius, the god of healing. Hippocrates maintained that disease should be treated in a rational and scientific way. While far ahead of his time, he of course did not have the explanations for many diseases and disabilities that are known today. But he did set such a course for medicine that it could become a science and profession. He established a rationale for disability so that hope could be achieved through relief and rehabilitation. Going beyond Aristotle, the anatomist, Hippocrates proposed that joy, despondency, madness, and delirium were products of the operation of the brain and should not be attributed to the influence of demons and evil spirits.

6.1.3. THROUGH THE MIDDLE AGES

Little is known about the status of disabled people during the Middle Ages. Written accounts do not contain much detail about the daily lives of those who could not function normally or effectively. Because physical competence was part of the foundation of feudalism, people with physical impairments must have been held in low regard. It is reasonable to assume that there were few disabled people, that ill and deformed children in weakened physical condition and supposedly in a lowered state of grace were the principal victims of the pestilence, famine, and destruction that resulted in part from poor hygiene, low food production, and continual warfare. More than 70 percent of children born in London through the eighteenth century died before the age of five; the mortality rate among infants with physical disabilities must have been much higher than this.

There were many explanations for disability besides the malevolence of Satan and the harsh judgments of God. Whatever the explanation, among the most common remedies for these misfortunes were purging, scourging, exorcism, and prayer. In 1488 Pope Innocent VIII, intending to rescue the Church from Satan— "Thou shalt not suffer a witch to live" (Exodus 22:18)—issued an order that led to the witch mania that swept across Europe and thrived during the next two centuries. Inquisitors were to discover, try, convict, and punish people who might be in consort with devils. The inquisitors used torture, forced confessions, and destroyed supposed witches, establishing their own reputations on a numerical basis. People skeptical about the charges and procedures were wise to keep silent.

Belief in witchcraft pervaded the intellectual and ethical atmosphere even through the Renaissance and the Reformation. While great accomplishments in learning were taking place in the sixteenth and seventeenth centuries, belief in witchcraft was at its height. At that time a great deal of insight was needed in order to discover other explanations and remedies for physical and mental disabilities, but there were men who possessed this kind of insight.

As credited by Obermann [1965], Reginald Scot, in his 1584 *Discoverie of Witchcraft*, ridiculed notions of witchcraft and suggested that "witches" were really ill persons who needed medical help. King James I of England later became so infuriated by Scot's book that he ordered it burned and wrote a rebuttal. Evidently Scot's ideas had little impact; more than 20,000 "witches" were burned in Scotland alone during the century after his book was written. In 1736 the laws against witches in the United Kingdom were at last repealed, but even this did not put an end to the persecution.

During the Renaissance the notion of the dignity of all human beings began to develop. In Queen Elizabeth the First's reign the first of the Poor Laws was enacted, which provided for asylum care of crippled individuals who could not work. But the disabled people were not meant to be the primary beneficiaries of this legislation, which was intended instead to promote the stability of the master-servant relationship and of the community at large.

Nevertheless, from this time onward the humanitarian spirit grew. It was not engendered either by religious or political forces but rather by people who were liberated and courageous enough to view life rationally and empirically. Robert Burns in the eighteenth century wrote poems about the individual's right to live with dignity; Paine and Jefferson stated the idea as a philosophical proposition. By the end of the eighteenth century enlightened attitudes toward disability could be discerned along with the older beliefs. The latter are illustrated by an English ordinance from this period that placed all people into one of three categories, the lowest of which included "those whose defects make them an abomination." These people, the ordinance stated, had to work. If they refused, the punishment would be "a few stripes and the withdrawal of food and drink." At the same time another force that would oppress disadvantaged persons was gathering momentum: the Industrial Revolution. The oppressor was no longer theology, but technology. The suffering of persons with handicaps was intensified in a system that could not accommodate them.

The first Factory Act became law in England in 1802. Its purpose was to improve working conditions for women and children. This type of legislation was needed because within the existing industrial system children were exploited and literally crippled as they worked. They were recruited for work in the mines and factories under horrendous conditions. In the English cottages of Buckinghamshire they were a major source of labor to make the lace for which this locale became famous. Working in the cottages, which were unclean and overcrowded, the entire family suffered, became crippled and often blind; the children almost inevitably developed distorted spines, premature blindness, and chronic poor health. Children worked in the English country cottages because it was economically necessary in order for families to survive; everyone in the family was a slave to the economic system. In education and other life experiences they were likely to be almost totally deficient.

The move of the world's disabled people forward from primitive times was due to improved social attitudes as well as improved technology and the economy of nations. They moved first to the right to survival, then to the right to dependency, and finally to the right to independency. But the transitional stages have been terribly slow and are still not complete in even the wealthiest and most advanced nations. Social attitudes revert at times to even primitive levels as expressed in the treatment accorded disabled individuals.

6.2. Resources for Disabled Persons

Throughout history people have understood that training is an effective way of bringing youth from a state of inadequacy to a state of adequacy to meet the demands of the culture. Training among primitive peoples was and is essentially on-the-job instruction. Formal training in schools has been known since early medieval times, but the first schools were only for intelligent boys of upper-class families. Modern universal education is of recent origin, as are schools and training for disabled people. (The historical background of rehabilitation facilities is related in 8.1.3.)

6.2.1. TEACHING DEAF CHILDREN

The earliest reports of attempts to educate handicapped children involved those who were deaf or blind. John Wallis (1616–1703) and William Holder (1616–1698) both maintained that they were the first English teachers of deaf pupils. They argued with each other, as have their successors, about whether only "manual" communication, that is, sign language, is appropriate for deaf people or whether they should be taught to speak and "read lips." This controversy impeded then and still impedes the teaching of deaf persons. However, it did draw attention to the needs and possibilities of deaf people in their time.

While the British teachers quarreled among themselves, better progress was being made on the mainland of Europe. In 1760 the first "public" school for deaf children was established in Paris by Charles Michel, Abbé de l'Epée. The Institution Nationale des Sourds-Muets was intended to serve poor children and no one was refused. Samuel Heinicke (1727–1790) taught deaf children to speak in his school at Eppendorf near Hamburg. In 1778, he established at Leipzig the first state school for handicapped children. The "oral" method of teaching deaf children to speak at the Leipzig school came to be called the "German method." The "manual" method taught at the Institution Nationale des Sourds-Muets came to be called the "French method." Heinicke and Michel conducted their debate over the relative merits of the two methods in letters over a long period. A decision by the Zurich Academy, to which the issue was referred, was equivocal and did not settle the argument between the "oralists" and the "manualists," nor has it yet been settled.

The Academy for the Deaf and Dumb, which was established at Edinburgh in 1780 by Thomas Braidwood, taught oral methods of communication. Subsequently the Braidwood family had control of all the schools for the deaf in England.

6.2.2. TEACHING BLIND PERSONS

Special hospices were among the first formal institutions to care for and help rehabilitate blind people. St. Basil is said to have founded a hospice for the blind in the Roman capital of Palestine in the fourth century. The Hospice Nationale des Quinze-Vingts was started in Paris in the mid-thirteenth century by Louis IX as a refuge for soldiers blinded in the Crusades, and it still serves blind people. It is doubtful that any teaching or training was conducted in these hospices. Some encouraged inmates to beg in order to help raise the money that was needed by the facility.

Blind persons were first taught to read by means of an alphabet made up of block letters. This was devised by Didymus, a blind philosopher and theologian at Alexandria during the late years of the Roman Empire. Unfortunately these letters were not practical to use in making books.

The search for an appropriate reading and writing method went on for centuries. In 1651 Harsdorffer in Germany devised wax tablets that allowed blind people to write. Jacob Bernouilli of Switzerland invented a mechanism for guiding a pencil on paper. Still, people who were blind desperately needed to learn to read.

Valentin Hauy, a public servant in pre-Revolutionary France, wanted to help the indigent blind beggars whom he saw on the streets of Paris. With the help of Maria van Paradis, a blind harpsichordist, and the Societé Philanthropique, he established the Institution Nationale in 1784. Five years later 50 people were learning to read by means of embossed type.

Louis Braille (1809–1852), the blind son of a harnessmaker, went to the Institution Nationale at age 10. There he did so well that in seven years he was asked to become an instructor. At about this time he learned of a technique of writing military messages by which the messages could be recorded and read in the dark. It involved combining 12 embossed dots so that they represented various symbols; they were read by touch. In 1829 Braille decreased the number of dots to six; these dots could then be combined in 63 different ways. This was the Braille method.

6.2.3. WORKSHOPS FOR BLIND PEOPLE

The early English institutions for blind trainees placed more stress on vocational rehabilitation than did those on the continent. In 1791 Henry Dannett collected money from charitable people and opened The School of Instruction for the Indigent Blind in Liverpool. Blind children and adults were to learn "music and mechanical arts, and so be rendered comfortable in themselves, and useful to their country." A variety of mechanical arts was taught and the training in music also had a vocational purpose. Most of the trainees learned trades and went back home to look for work. It was from these methods developed in England that methods of rehabilitating blind and deaf children in America were adapted.

6.2.4. EDUCATING CRIPPLED CHILDREN

General education for handicapped children evolved less rapidly. Industrial training and workshop production retained their preeminence, and general education was not offered in many institutions for handicapped children. The British House of Commons did not allocate funds for this purpose until 1833. Begging and the exploitation of begging children were common. The Society for the Suppression of Public Begging was founded in 1812, but the Society for Prevention of Cruelty to Children was not established until 1884.

Improvements began to take place in the second half of the nineteenth century. The care and training of mentally retarded, epileptic, and crippled individuals also improved in quality. The first school exclusively for crippled children was founded in Bavaria in 1832 by John Nepinak. This was followed by the opening of such schools in Germany, France, England, Switzerland, and Italy.

The separation of deaf, blind, or crippled children from those in regular schools has continued to be a problem. The word *asylum*, commonly used to refer to the early institutions for handicapped children and adults, was slowly eliminated but the segregation was not. Although the many disadvantages of segregation were evident, early provisions for helping disabled persons, when attempted at all, were made outside the social, cultural, and economic mainstream.

6.2.5. TRAINING RETARDED CHILDREN

Attempts to help mentally retarded children in social and economic adaptation came later than for most other groups. St. Vincent de Paul (1576–1660) had offered care to mentally retarded adults in the facility in Paris that was to become the Bicêtré. Jean Jacques Rousseau (1712–1778) discussed principles that could be applied to the learning experiences of mentally retarded children; Jean Itard (1775–1838) and Edouard Seguin (1812–1880), his student, applied these ideas to the teaching of such children. In 1848 Seguin came to the United States when he was appointed superintendent of the new Massachusetts School for Idiots and Feeble-Minded Youths.

Institutions to help handicapped children in Europe were established at a relatively late date, but the stress almost from the start was on vocational rehabilitation. Facilities, however, were usually segregated and the isolation imposed on the pupils was often extreme. The general education was of low quality.

6.3. Disability in Early America

It was from Europe, especially England, that the colonies and newly formed American states adapted many ideas and practices relative to disabled people. The American colonists were European for the most part, with European backgrounds in superstition, sorcery, alchemy, astrology, materia medica, and general social and cultural attitudes. Witchcraft and demonology thrived in early America. In New England (notably in Salem, Massachusetts) the witchcraft fanaticism reached its most extreme. Any physical or behavioral variation from the norm was viewed with suspicion. In 1691–1692 about 250 persons were arrested and tried in Salem for witchcraft.

Although there were Poor Laws for the indigent (usually including disabled persons), modeled on the Poor Laws of England, their content did not encourage the restoration of disadvantaged persons to productive lives. Communities tried to decrease dependency by using length-of-residence requirements to prevent people who might wander into their villages from becoming public charges. Traditionally, disabled persons had earned a living by begging, but the colonists tried to ensure that begging would remain a local activity and that beggars would not come in from other places.

Destitute people were "warned out of town," and if they came back, they might receive punishment, such as whipping—"36 lashes on the bare back if a man, and 25 if a woman." In some colonies it was customary to whip poor strangers or vagabonds when they were caught. Almshouses were not widespread in the colonies until the late eighteenth century; dependent individuals who could not be cared for by their families stayed in private homes at public expense. Mentally ill and retarded people were often put in tiny cell-like, unheated structures and kept like dogs in a kennel. Some communities "auctioned off" dependent people, who were then required to serve the buyer in return for their support. People too disabled to attract any bidder were sometimes supported by special appropriations or were maintained in jails or workhouses.

6.3.1. THE FIRST HOSPITALS

The first almshouse was founded in Boston in 1662 for all people who were public charges, including petty criminals, "worthy" poor, vagrants, the sick, the mentally ill, and the disabled. Between 1716 and 1766 the question of segregating some of the inmates was raised many times. In 1746 there was an effort to raise, by general subscription, the money needed for a separate building for those who were disabled. But it failed then and again in 1766, despite a bequest of 600 pounds in 1764 by Thomas Hancock, who thought there should be a separate building for the mentally ill inmates.

The first hospital for mentally ill patients was established in Virginia in 1773. There was medical supervision, but evidently not many of the patients were returned to productivity. Fifty years would pass before the next separate state institution for mentally ill people would be founded in America; in 1824 the Eastern Lunatic Asylum was established in Lexington, Kentucky.

In 1752 the Quakers, with the help of Benjamin Franklin working through the Pennsylvania Provincial Assembly, were responsible for setting up the Pennsylvania Hospital near Philadelphia. This was the first general hospital in the colonies. People with all kinds of illnesses, including mental illness, were accepted and treated. The Pennsylvania Hospital, directed by Dr. Benjamin Rush, used work for treatment and rehabilitation. Rush stressed the significance of work and decent treatment for the patients. The second general hospital founded in America was the New York Hospital, which began operating in 1791.

Hospitals were important in the evolution of concepts of rehabilitation. Medication and surgery were emphasized, but the other needs of patients became apparent to physicians, social reformers, philanthropists, legislators, and educators who could see that the needs of patients extended beyond medical treatment. Hospitals afforded the opportunity for representatives of various disciplines to meet and focus on patient problems and to exchange insights as to how those problems could be solved. The products of such exchanges resulted in much of what later would be called "rehabilitation."

6.3.2. EARLY SPECIAL SCHOOLS

In Baltimore in 1812 the first educational institution for disabled children in America was founded. This was a private school for deaf children. The families of some deaf children went to Scotland for training under Thomas Braidwood and subsequently were instrumental in the movement to set up American schools in which Braidwood's methods could be applied.

Thomas Hopkins Gallaudet went to Britain in 1815 for training in the Braidwood method of teaching deaf persons to speak and develop other communication skills. But, unable to reach agreement with the Braidwood family for instruction in the secret techniques, he continued on to Paris and learned the manual methods of Michel under Abbé Sicard. Upon returning to America he brought with him Laurent Clere, a deaf teacher from the Paris school. With Clere's help and funds from Congress the first public school for deaf people was established in Hartford, Connecticut, in 1817.

The first American school for crippled children, The Industrial School for Crippled and Deformed Children, opened in Boston in 1893. Its purpose was to train disabled children so that they would be able to earn a living.

Mentally retarded people were customarily sent to lunatic asylums, poorhouses, almshouses, or local jails. This was typical through most of the nineteenth century, although there were some attempts to make special provisions for mentally retarded persons by the middle of the century. During this period, Dr. Samuel Gridley Howe, as head of a special Massachusetts legislative committee, wrote an excellent report on the situation of mentally retarded citizens in Massachusetts. The legislature responded, in 1848 making an annual appropriation of $2500 for an experimental school to train 10 pauper idiots for three years. The school opened in October, 1848, as part of the Perkins Institution for the Blind, under the supervision of Dr. Howe, who was Superintendent of the Perkins Institution. Dr. Edouard Seguin, who had been an instructor of mentally retarded children at the Bicêtre in Paris, assisted. The school was very successful and was incorporated in 1851 as The Massachusetts School for Idiotic

and Feeble-Minded Youths. The project was later moved to Waverly, Massachusetts, and renamed the Walter E. Fernald State School.

The Pennsylvania Training School for Feeble-minded Children was started in 1853, supported partially by the state and partially by private subscription. The Ohio State Asylum for the Education of Idiotic and Imbecile Youth and the Connecticut School for Imbeciles were founded in 1857. Kentucky established the Kentucky Institution for the Education of Feeble-Minded Children and Idiots in 1860.

During this time concepts important for rehabilitation and special education were being established. It became apparent that mentally retarded people were teachable, and some of them could learn to function in the community. However, failure to understand that some more severely retarded people or people with asocial tendencies would have to be permanently institutionalized, resulted in disappointment on the part of many who had been enthusiastic about new methods in education and rehabilitation. The new institutions originally were not thought of as custodial in nature but the problem of what to do with people who could not respond to treatment and training was a pressing one. Many institutions consequently became custodial, and the spirit of optimism associated with the founding of the first schools slowly decreased.

At the turn of the twentieth century a reaction of pessimism and even alarm about "feeble-mindedness" set in. Many sweeping generalizations were made from the reports on such families as the Jukes, the Kallikaks, and the Pineys. Information from these studies gave rise to popular beliefs that mental retardation was a genetic trait and that every mentally retarded person could become a social liability. The validity of the tests that were used to measure intelligence was apparently not questioned. The idea of helping the individual through management, training, and rehabilitation became less appealing. The high correlation of mental retardation, crime, and delinquency was given a genetic explanation, and little attention was paid to the social conditions that contributed to such problems.

While around the turn of the century optimism about educating and rehabilitating mentally disabled persons was abating, there was fresh interest in training children with orthopedic problems. In 1897 Minnesota passed the first legislation providing for the treatment, care, and education of crippled children. This was followed by the establishment in Wisconsin, Indiana, Iowa, New York, North Carolina, Nebraska, and Massachusetts of central state institutions. The founding of the federal Children's Bureau attracted new attention to the plight of handicapped young people. Through the health, education, and welfare agencies at the state level, the Bureau stimulated fresh interest in the treatment and prevention of disabilities. This preventive rehabilitation effort has had important program implications because a difficulty with many rehabilitation clients arises when the handicap has been neglected too long. Young people who live with a disability often acquire dependent attitudes that are difficult to surmount when they become adults. Early educational and medical intervention help to prevent or to reduce the handicapping effects of childhood problems.

6.4. Voluntary Organizations

Human beings have always felt a need to help one another; as Donne wrote, "No man is an island." A person's safety and survival can be assured only when the other people in the environment are safe.

Possibly most medieval almsgivers merely hoped to strengthen their claims to a place in heaven. Perhaps many of those who helped the consumptive child in the city slums get medical treatment hoped only to keep the disease from spreading to their own families; perhaps most crusaders against child labor acted out of guilt. If they fought for more sanitary working conditions in slaughterhouses, it might have been because they could not tolerate the stench that reached their own neighborhoods. "Do-gooders" may have been and still may be in search of social status and the satisfactions that come from patronizing less fortunate people. But it is also possible that those who have given time, talent, and tithes to help better the lot of others have acted out of compassion, altruism, and love.

6.4.1. CHARITABLE ORGANIZATIONS

A large number of family-service societies were established between 1840 and 1890, but they were criticized as "pauperizing" the people they helped. These years were difficult ones for economic development in the United States. The concept of "rugged individualism" received strong support and social policy was consciously based on it.

By the beginning of the twentieth century a greater sense of responsibility and guilt was discernible. Rockefeller established his famous Foundation, and the Carnegie Corporation was founded. In 1913 Woodrow Wilson talked about "the human cost" of the great industrial accomplishments of the country and recommended that industry help to assuage the suffering caused by its own evolution. Charity was taking on a new meaning. Social workers and philanthropists were developing what might be called a "rehabilitation attitude." The family-service agencies that had originated in the previous century were emphasizing the need for a "social-work" approach toward indigency and disability. Thus by the beginning of the century a number of the contemporary health and welfare societies had originated, and some started with a rehabilitation emphasis (see 12.1).

6.4.2. THE RED CROSS

The American Red Cross was formed in 1881, although its history goes back to the Civil War when the United States Sanitary Commission and Clara Barton rendered volunteer services to the wounded and sick on both sides of the conflict. Learning about the actions taken in 1864 at Geneva where the International Red Cross movement began, for almost 20 years Barton attempted to persuade the United States government to join in the Geneva Convention. President Chester Arthur signed the treaty in 1882. As the first president of the American Red Cross, she successfully argued for the notion of disaster relief, and the organization acquired a major peacetime purpose.

The Red Cross project most relevant to vocational rehabilitation was its support of the Institute for Crippled and Disabled Men in New York, an experimental school for the vocational rehabilitation of veterans that had been opened

by the federal government in a building donated
for the purpose by Jeremiah Milbank in 1917.
The Red Cross also set up retraining programs
for disabled veterans in Walter Reed and other
Army hospitals. But it was realized very early
that the vocational rehabilitation of disabled veterans would be too expensive for private agencies, and this task was assumed by the federal
government.

The Red Cross took on Braille transcription as
a volunteer service in 1921, after a pioneer effort
in Chicago. While some chapters continue this
work, the national service was transferred to the
Library of Congress in 1942.

6.4.3. TUBERCULOSIS ASSOCIATION

A California laborer named Lawrence Flick
contracted tuberculosis in the year the tubercle
bacillus was identified. Ten years later, in 1892,
he had recovered, earned a medical degree, and
campaigned among his peers for strong action
against the killer disease. The medical profession did not respond as he had hoped, so he did
something unusual. Going to the public for help,
he organized the Pennsylvania Society for the
Prevention of Tuberculosis, the first voluntary
organization in America uniting the efforts and
resources of both medical and lay people to fight
a disease. At the time it was formed, more than
200 fatalities in each 100,000 of population in the
United States resulted from tuberculosis, thus
making it a leading cause of death.

By the turn of the century several organizations were dedicated to the study and treatment
of tuberculosis, some wishing to become the national organization for this purpose. There was a
great deal of arguing among them and much ac-
rimony was generated. At a meeting of some 100
leaders in Philadelphia in 1904, Dr. Flick obtained agreement about a national organization.
It was named the National Association for the
Study and Prevention of Tuberculosis. Its first
president was Edward Trudeau, who identified
public education as its primary task and legislation for the prevention and control of tuberculosis as the next priority. Others, including
Dr. Flick, thought that more attention should
be given to providing care for needy people with
tuberculosis.

Hundreds of thousands of people joined the
"TB" Association. Hundreds of hospitals,
sanitoriums, and treatment centers were established through legislation. The Christmas Seal
campaign originated in 1907. Vocational rehabilitation of tuberculous patients was a primary concern of the Association almost from its
beginning.

6.4.4. GOODWILL INDUSTRIES

Charity and welfare were integral features of the
work of Christian churches from the days of
their origins. Goodwill Industries was taken over
as a charitable enterprise by the Methodist
Church in 1918. Goodwill had been founded in
1902 by Dr. Edgar James Helms (1863–1942), a
Methodist minister at the Morgan Memorial Institutional Church of South Boston. A salient feature of work in this church was the gathering of
used clothing and other items and their distribution to people in need. Sometimes repair or ren-
ovation was required, and sometimes people
preferred to pay for things instead of receiving
them as charity. This led to the idea of hiring unemployed individuals to do the necessary work.
The workers were remunerated from the money
the products brought.

Because it was a time of serious economic depression, many unemployed people who came
to work at the Morgan Church establishment
were skilled workers only temporarily unemployed. When the economy improved they left
Goodwill Industries to go back to their jobs. Dr.
Helms then looked toward disabled persons and
others who were less employable to carry out
the work of collecting, renovating, and distributing donated materials. In this way Goodwill
Industries became more involved in rehabilitation than in welfare. As the enterprise has continued, the objective has been more and more to
"graduate" workers out of Goodwill workshops
to regular jobs.

6.4.5. EASTER SEAL SOCIETY

The National Easter Seal Society for Crippled
Children and Adults, which originated in 1921, is
a federation of state organizations. It has always
focused on crippled children but has been increasingly concerned with rehabilitation of
adults. Its Easter Seal approach to raising funds
was begun in 1934.

Many rehabilitation facilities, workshops,
diagnostic centers, homebound programs, and
other such endeavors have been initiated by the
Society. Through the nearly autonomous state
organizations, the Society raises money to be

used to supply or to buy rehabilitation services needed by handicapped individuals. At its headquarters in Chicago the Society maintains a professional library, a research program, and a group of specialists to whom state society per-

sonnel and others involved in rehabilitation can go for consultation.

Many other voluntary agencies associated with the rehabilitation service delivery system are described in Chapter 12, Agency Structures.

6.5. Rehabilitation of War Veterans

The vocational rehabilitation of disabled veterans in the United States is a topic in itself because of the special legislation and organization that underlie it. There have been advantages and disadvantages in separating veterans' programs from others. Because legislators and their constituents have generously underwritten rehabilitation services for veterans, it has been possible to create programs that could not be attempted otherwise. Probably the keeping of rehabilitation for veterans separate from slower-moving programs made it possible to handle quickly the emergencies created by developments associated with demobilization following armed conflict. But, inadequate communication between those involved in veterans' rehabilitation and the administrators of other rehabilitation activities has been a continuing problem.

War veterans have usually been thought of as a special population within a country; because they have shouldered the burden and braved the dangers of war they have been considered heroes—the American Vietnam War veteran excepted. The soldier's profession has been honored within the ethical framework of western culture: he has defended his people against the invader; he has made the population safe at home. Traditionally they have been generously rewarded—the early kings granted them special privileges and prizes; in modern states, veterans' benefits range from employment preferences to medical care to vocational education.

Legislation for veterans has changed with each American war. The following legislative history is organized by these war periods.

6.5.1. THE REVOLUTIONARY WAR

Veterans' benefits in America originated in the time of the Revolutionary War. On August 26, 1776, the first national pension law, providing

compensation for service-connected disability, was enacted. Any officer, soldier, or sailor losing a limb or being so disabled in service that the ability to earn a living was lost was to receive half pay for life or as long as the disability lasted. Provision was also made for partial disability. Various colonies had made similar provisions for military men, but this was the first national pension plan.

6.5.2. THE CIVIL WAR

Because the consequences of the Civil War were so far-reaching, it was necessary to go about solving national problems in new ways. The veterans of the Union Armies, organized as the Grand Army of the Republic, were an important political force for almost half a century. In 1862, Congress passed the so-called General Law (12 Stat. L., 566) intended to apply to servicemen of the Regular Army and Navy of the Civil War and all subsequent wars. It remained substantially unchanged during the war with Spain and was still in effect when the United States entered World War I. It resembled previous veterans compensation laws in that it stipulated that to receive compensation an individual must have become ill or wounded as a direct result of being in military service. It added some new benefits such as more liberal compensation for widows, children, and dependent relatives of deceased servicemen. For the first time it allowed for a veteran's preference in the federal Civil Service. Medical provisions were especially important with respect to the rehabilitation of war-injured veterans.

A form of self-rehabilitation following the Civil War had particular significance. In the West there was still a great deal of public land, and veterans of the Union forces received special preference in applying for it through homesteading. Time in the service was counted toward the residency requirement for asserting a claim. Taking advantage of this, veterans moved westward with others who settled there. They became part of the established communities and typically needed no more help in readapting to civilian life.

Congressional legislation for veterans of the Spanish-American War and the Boxer Rebellion was similar to that enacted after the Civil War.

6.5.3 WORLD WAR I

The United States entered World War I on April 6, 1917. Before that (though not in anticipation of entering the war) three laws had been passed that would directly affect World War I veterans. The War Risk Insurance Act, passed on September 2, 1914, authorized the government to insure United States ships and cargoes on the high seas. Later amendments of this Act provided for vocational rehabilitation training for certain specified categories of persons disabled in the federal service.

The Smith-Hughes Act (Public Law 347 of the 64th Congress) was passed on February 23, 1917. It was:

An act to provide for the promotion of vocational education; to provide for cooperation with the states in the promotion of such education in agriculture and the trades and industries; to provide for cooperation with the states in the preparation of teachers of vocational subjects; and to appropriate money and regulate its expenditure.

One section of the Act established a Federal Board for Vocational Education, composed of the Secretary of Agriculture, Secretary of Labor, Secretary of Commerce, the U.S. Commissioner of Education, and three citizens to be appointed by the President and approved by the Senate. The Board was formed on July 21, 1917. The United States was already at war the first time the Board met.

The National Defense Act of 1916 reflected the attitude of Congress toward helping men in the armed services in their vocational adjustment. Section 37 of the Act stated:

In addition to military training, soldiers while in active service shall hereafter be given the opportunity to study and receive instruction upon educational lines of such character as to increase their military efficiency and enable them to return to civil life better equipped for industrial, commercial, and general business occupations.

These three pieces of legislation suggested that the nation was willing to set a new course and that it was beginning to recognize the value of vocational education and rehabilitation.

On October 6, 1917 the War Risk Insurance Act of 1914 was amended in significant ways. Section 304 of these amendments stated:

In cases of dismemberment, of injuries to sight or hearing, and of other injuries commonly causing permanent disability, the injured person shall follow such course or courses of rehabilitation, and vocational training as the United States may provide or procure to be provided.

1918 Soldier Rehabilitation (Smith-Sears) Act: Public Law 65-178

Bills introduced in both houses of the 65th U.S. Congress in April of 1918 provided for the vocational rehabilitation of disabled servicemen. The fact that the Federal Board for Vocational Education was charged with the responsibility did not arouse opposition, but the fact that there were no provisions for disabled civilians did. However, this omission of provisions for civilian rehabilitation was defended on three grounds: (1) providing for services to disabled civilians might hold up or even stop the legislation for military men and veterans; (2) the proposal was a war measure; and (3) it would be difficult enough to find teachers who could deal with the soldiers and sailors who needed rehabilitation. The rehabilitation of disabled civilians represented too big a task to take on without preparation.

The bills that came out of the joint hearings and were finally presented in Congress had no provision for rehabilitating civilians. The Soldier Rehabilitation Act, Public Law 178 of the 65th Congress, was passed unanimously by both houses June 27, 1918. Referred to as The Smith-Sears Act, it provided the Federal Board for Vocational Education with the authority to set up and offer programs of vocational rehabilitation to disabled veterans. To organize, recruit, train, coordinate, and set up communications constituted a great challenge for the members of this Board and there was little experience to guide them. Work in vocational education under the Vocational Education Act of 1917 was their greatest advantage.

The eligibility requirements for vocational rehabilitation under the Act were fairly simple.

The veteran had to have a disability resulting from military service for which compensation could be received under the War Risk Insurance Act. The disability had to be vocationally handicapping, and preparation for a realistic occupation had to be feasible. During the rehabilitation process the veteran client was to receive pay equal to that received during the last month spent in service or an amount equal to that awarded under the War Risk Act.

It was the function of the U.S. Department of Labor to locate jobs for the veterans. The Federal Board and the Labor Department worked together to place the individuals who were being rehabilitated.

Administrative Problems Develop

Veterans could not begin a rehabilitation program until after eligibility under the War Risk Insurance Act had been established by the Bureau of War Risk Insurance, an agency independent of the Federal Board. The Bureau could not handle the enormous number of claims that came in immediately after the close of the war, and thousands of disabled veterans who needed and wanted vocational rehabilitation were kept waiting. Not only the veterans but their representatives in Congress voiced angry protests about this situation.

The 66th Congress in 1919 therefore placed the responsibility for establishing eligibility for vocational rehabilitation directly on the Federal Board so that it did not have to await the decisions of the Bureau of War Risk Insurance. This legislation also gave the Board authority and money to pay maintenance and support allowances to those veterans placed in vocational rehabilitation programs.

New laws only partially resolved the difficulties of the Board. It still had trouble recruiting and training competent personnel, structuring and running the organization, working with other agencies, and communicating with veterans and other people whose involvement was necessary. The Board did achieve a tremendous amount, however, as it struggled in unknown territory and made generally sound and productive decisions.

Administrative Structures Provided by the Federal Board

An office in Washington was the administrative center of the rehabilitation program for veterans and 14 district offices were set up. By June 30, 1921, there were 146 local offices. Field contact squads went into outlying areas. They were composed of a medical officer who gave physical examinations to assess the severity of disability; a worker who established eligibility from a legal standpoint; and a counselor who helped veterans prepare their cases, make career decisions, and work toward the various adjustments necessary for rehabilitation. These counselors kept in contact with the veteran until the individual's rehabilitation training was completed.

Various difficulties—social, economic, family, and personal—that were common among the veterans appeared to require special settings in order to be resolved. The Board kept to the practice of using existing facilities such as schools and colleges. However, different types of facilities, and sometimes special communities, had to be set up to meet the needs of thousands of the disabled men. Known as "Community Training Centers," they were sometimes housed in abandoned war plants or other such places. Provisions for family living, vocational training, medical care, recreation, social service, and instruction for wives were made. The Board approached its responsibilities in a bold and innovative manner. In spite of its accomplishments, however, the Board was the object of continual criticism.

Establishment of the Veterans Bureau

Public Law 47 of the 67th Congress, signed by the President on August 9, 1921, provided for the creation of the Veterans Bureau, an independent agency whose Director was to answer directly to the President. This agency was to assume the functions of the Bureau of War Risk Insurance, the Veterans Rehabilitation Division of the Federal Board for Vocational Education, the Pension Bureau, the functions of the Public Health Service related to veterans, and the National Home for Volunteer Soldiers. At the beginning its major responsibility was the rehabilitation of disabled veterans.

In order to solve the numerous problems that grew apparent after it began operating, the Veterans Bureau hired more personnel, including additional employees to supervise trainees and training establishments more closely. It specified rehabilitation objectives and plans more clearly, characterizing training programs explicitly in writing. Better "vocational advisement" was stressed, and improved schools, offices, and industrial plants were sought for academic and on-the-job training. The task of finding jobs for rehabilitated clients received more attention. The vocational rehabilitation staff was increased to 3,000 persons, and several thousand other employees of the Bureau worked on tasks related to rehabilitation.

Eventually the Veterans Bureau (1924) could publish a manual of procedure for the vocational rehabilitation of veterans of World War I, a document that presented the knowledge gained from 1918 to 1924. What the Federal Board and the Veterans Bureau could only look on as theory in earlier years had now become a verified principle. Workable degrees of decentralization and delegation of authority were identified; employee specialties that had been discovered necessary were authorized; effective methods of management, supervision, and review of all operations were outlined or recommended. The manual also specified optimum work loads for employees, defined "disability" and "vocational handicap," defined "need for vocational rehabilitation training," set forth criteria for training programs, and defined "feasibility for training" more precisely.

The manual was useful and valuable. If it could have been prepared in 1918, many problems might have been avoided and the disappointments of the earlier years of the program would have been unnecessary. But it did serve an important purpose. When the task of rehabilitating World War II veterans was encountered twenty years later, this manual helped prevent the making of the same mistakes again.

The War Veterans Act, which became law on June 7, 1924, served as a well-planned legal basis for closing the veterans' vocational rehabilitation program. From the beginning of the program in 1918 to its close ten years later, about 675,000 veterans had applied for training, about 330,000 had been judged eligible, nearly 180,000 entered training, and almost 130,000 finished the program successfully. About 98% of these 130,000 had jobs when their training ended. A total of $645 million was spent in the program.

6.5.4. WORLD WAR II

The fact that the nation supported the World War I program made it a certainty that disabled veterans in later years would find vocational re-

habilitation available. Immediately after the United States entered World War II, Congressmen and people from many official, professional, and voluntary organizations started to plan for the vocational rehabilitation of the disabled servicemen who would return.

1943 Disabled Veterans Rehabilitation (Welsh-Clark) Act: Public Law 78-16

The vocational rehabilitation legislation for veterans of World War II was passed by the Congress and was signed by President Roosevelt on March 24, 1943. It was identified as Public Law 16, 78th Congress. It authorized the Veterans Administration to carry out the rehabilitation programs, giving this agency all the authority necessary to begin immediately with the rehabilitation of disabled and eligible individuals, injured in the service, who needed help in readjusting to the world of work.

Several hundred thousand disabled veterans would take advantage of the provisions of Public Law 16 while it was in effect. Because educational programs would also be authorized for nondisabled veterans, the task facing the Veterans Administration would be staggering. It would necessitate coordinating a work force of many thousands of highly trained people and close cooperation with thousands of job-training establishments, schools, colleges, and universities. The vocational rehabilitation and readjustment of the millions of World War II veterans would become nearly as huge and significant an endeavor as the war mobilization itself.

There was considerable bitterness because this program and state-federal rehabilitation and education programs were not merged, as some strongly advocated, but this was probably fortunate. The Veterans Administration had powers that state-directed agencies did not. The old Veterans Bureau had been reorganized and designated as the Veterans Administration in 1933 by Public Law 2 of the 73rd Congress.

1944 Servicemen's Readjustment Act: Public Law 78-346

A year and three months after Public Law 16 was passed, the 78th Congress enacted the Servicemen's Readjustment Act of 1944 (Public Law 346). Popularly called the "GI Bill of Rights," its implications for rehabilitation and readjustment were extensive and important. It became obvious that many men and women whose educational and vocational pursuits had been interrupted by military service would have serious difficulties upon returning home. These could be as handicapping as physical problems and could be approached in some of the same ways. Public Law 346 provided tuition and subsistence for up to 48 months for veterans who underwent and completed training. Vocational assessment and counseling were offered and training was supervised.

Other federal laws authorized many types of rehabilitation and readjustment benefits for veterans: hospitalization, domiciliary care, guardianship service, disability compensation, mustering-out pay, preferential employment referral, and Civil Service advantages for federal employment and retention in employment. Many states enacted laws that provided supplemental benefits.

In ten years, ending in December, 1953, more than 600,000 World War II veterans received rehabilitation training. Almost 8 million had entered training under Public Law 346. Over $1.2 billion had been spent under Public Law 16, and about $14 billion under Public Law 346. By 1947 more than 28,000 workers—specialists in counseling, training, contract negotiations, and placement—had been oriented. Thousands of educational training facilities had been evaluated and had entered into agreements with the Veterans Administration to work with veterans.

Colleges and universities markedly enlarged their operations so that they could serve the veterans, and in some cases the veterans more than doubled enrollments at these institutions. Many institutions made contracts with the Veterans Administration to provide special counseling services to veterans; this supplemented service resources and made counseling more accessible to veterans.

One of the most important facets of the Veterans Administration's program was the counseling. Early in the vocational rehabilitation program for World War I veterans it had been recognized that vocational counseling and guidance was critically important. Legislators kept this in mind in providing for World War II veterans. Public Law 16 trainees received formal vocational evaluation and counseling before selecting vocational goals. Those training under Public Law 346 received counseling if they wished.

Rehabilitation of Hospitalized Veterans

Many disabled veterans went directly to Veterans Administration hospitals, while others required hospitalization later. The rehabilitation of these long-term patients was an especially sensitive task. Their condition did not always follow a predictable pattern, but the Veterans Administration was responsible not only for their medical treatment but also for motivating them and restoring them to employability. Well-staffed sections on physical medicine were set up in most of the Veterans Administration's general medicine and surgical hospitals. The medical work of these sections was supplemented by vocational counseling and rehabilitation.

6.5.5. SUBSEQUENT CONFLICTS

American participation in the Korean Conflict brought a new need for rehabilitation services for veterans. On December 28, 1950, Public Law 81-894 extended benefits under Public Law 78-16 to veterans disabled as a result of military service after June 27, 1950, and prior to the end of the Korean Conflict period (a date later set at January 31, 1955). The law specified nine years as the duration of the program.

A major development occurred in 1962, when veterans rehabilitation was established as an ongoing program, available to veterans of peacetime as well as war periods. Enacted on October 15, 1962, Public Law 87-815 authorized rehabilitation benefits for veterans who served during the period between WW II and the Korean Conflict or after the Korean Conflict. However, the law did impose one new proviso in the case of veterans of these service periods who were rated less than 30% disabled: they could be provided rehabilitation only if it were shown that the service-connected disability caused a pronounced employment handicap; this requirement was subsequently eliminated by Public Law 93-508, enacted December 3, 1974. However, by that time many veterans of the Vietnam war (the Vietnam era began August 15, 1964) had been denied rehabilitation services on the basis of criteria much more stringent than those that had been applied to similarly disabled WW II and Korean Conflict veterans.

In the program since its inception, veterans have had a specified period of eligibility in which they could use their benefits. As the years passed, however, it became apparent that some veterans, because of medical reasons or other circumstances outside their control, would be unable to pursue training within their basic eligibility period. To remedy this situation, extension of eligibility under certain circumstances has been authorized by law; in October, 1976, Public Law 94-502 completely eliminated eligibility termination dates for seriously disabled veterans. In a report to the Congress in 1978, the Administrator of Veterans Affairs recommended that termination dates on eligibility similarly be removed for all disabled veterans, but eligibility continues to be time-limited. The period generally is nine years after date of discharge, with a four-year extension permissible in cases of medical infeasibility, upgraded discharge, or late determination that compensable disability exists.

Except for increases in rates of subsistence allowance, authorization of pursuit of training on a part-time basis (PL 90-431), provisions for eligibility extension and for nonpay training for work study in federal agencies, the pattern of the veterans vocational rehabilitation program has remained essentially unchanged over the years. Benefits include the full cost of tuition, books, and fees and a monthly subsistence allowance for up to 48 months of training (more if necessary in the individual case); special assistance such as tutorial, reader, and interpreter services; interest-free emergency loans; and whatever medical, prosthetic, and restorative services are required to enable the veteran to enter and remain in training. Counseling and continuing assistance by the Veterans Administration rehabilitation staff throughout training are an integral part of each veteran's program.

By May, 1978, 621,300 WW II veterans, 77,000 Korean Conflict veterans, 23,600 veterans of peacetime periods, and 95,600 veterans of the Vietnam era—a total of 817,500 veterans—had been provided rehabilitation training. Training has covered the entire range of professional, technical, business, and skilled trade occupations, but over the years the frequency of college training has increased steadily. Among WW II trainees, only 25 percent attended college, compared with 65 percent of Vietnam era veterans. On-the-job training, on the other hand, decreased from 38 percent during the WW II program to less than 5 percent for Vietnam veterans.

Just as rehabilitation benefits were extended to veterans of periods subsequent to WW II, so,

too, was the GI Bill educational assistance. The Korean Conflict legislation (PL 82-550) became effective August 20, 1952, and covered service from June 27, 1950, through January 31, 1955. The law specified that the education or training pursued must lead to an identified educational, professional, or vocational objective, thus continuing the prohibition against payment of benefits for pursuit of recreational or avocational courses that was imposed in 1948 (PL 80-862). Instead of tuition and subsistence, benefits in the new program consisted of a monthly educational assistance allowance paid to the veteran for a period equalling one and a half times the duration of his or her active military service up to a total of 36 months.

Effective June 1, 1966, the Veterans Readjustment Benefits Act (PL 89-358) provided a similar program of educational assistance for veterans who served after January 31, 1955 (i.e., after the Korean Conflict). Training entitlement was based on the same rate, but the maximum of 36 months was granted for 18 months of service. Later laws significantly increased the "GI Bill" benefits: "free entitlement" for high school education or for the pursuit of required refresher, remedial, or deficiency courses; tutorial assistance allowance in addition to regular educational allowance; the Predischarge Education Program (PREP), allowing pursuit of education while still in the armed forces; extension of maximum entitlement from 36 to 45 months; education loans; work study allowances; increase in eligibility from 8 to 10 years following discharge, with provision for extension if the veteran is unable to pursue education within the basic eligibility period because of medical reasons; and, accelerated payment of educational allowance under specified conditions.

On the other hand, as the program progressed, certain safeguards and limitations were written into the law: some of these pertained to training institutions (e.g., the school must have been in operation at least two years, must have at least 85% nonveterans in its student population, and must show at least a 50% placement rate for graduates); others pertained to courses (e.g., certain prerequisites for flight training); still others applied to individual veterans (e.g., limitations on the number of changes of program and discontinuance of benefits for unsatisfactory academic progress). Throughout the GI Bill program, educational and vocational counseling has been available to veterans on request. Under certain conditions, such as unsatisfactory academic progress, it is required. In 1977 Congress mandated (PL 95-202) intensive outreach efforts to encourage veterans to use available educational and vocational counseling services.

The GI Bill educational program will be terminated by 1990 as prescribed by the 1976 Public Law 94-502. This 1976 law also established the post-Vietnam era Veterans Educational Assistance program for persons first entering the Armed Forces after that year. In this program, unlike its predecessors, the participants (while in military service) contribute to their own educational benefits program, with the government matching the individual's contributions on a 2-for-1 basis. In addition, the U.S. Department of Defense may contribute as it sees fit to encourage persons to enter or remain in the Armed Forces. In fiscal year 1978, there were 81,200 contributing service persons in the program.

By May, 1978, almost 17.4 million veterans of WW II, the Korean Conflict, and post-Korean Conflict era had received benefits. As in the case of the vocational rehabilitation program, college-level courses accounted for an increasingly large proportion of GI Bill utilization.

It should be kept in mind that the GI Bills have served service-disabled veterans as well as the nondisabled and those with nonservice-connected disability. In fact, a far larger proportion of the service-connected disabled group has used GI Bill educational benefits than has used vocational rehabilitation benefits. It must be concluded, therefore, that the GI Bills have been a significant factor in veterans' rehabilitation, as well as in their educational and vocational readjustment.

6.6. Programs for Blind Persons

Blindness is legally defined from a critical point in the range of visual acuity. The customary legal definition of a blind person is one who has not more than 20/200 of visual acuity in the better eye with correcting lenses; visual acuity might be better than 20/200 but the person would still be legally blind if the limitation in the field of vision were such that the widest diameter subtended an angle no greater than 20 degrees. This definition is used by the United States Internal Revenue Service in determining if a taxpayer may claim a reduction in income tax for blindness.

6.6.1. STATE COMMISSIONS

Blind people have many kinds of needs. State commissions exist in many states to administer the programs designed to meet their special social, medical, psychological, and economic requirements. Massachusetts organized its commission in 1906, New Jersey and Ohio in 1908; by 1965 36 states had commissions for the blind. These commissions are responsible for the vocational rehabilitation of blind adults and also for work geared toward preventing blindness, advising on medical care, providing instruction to families, distributing "talking books" and other aids to blind people, coordinating the many organizations and programs for blind persons, and administering relief and pensions for them. This work is done by one or more departments of state government—representing health, education, and welfare—when no commission specifically charged with administering services for blind persons exists.

When the federal vocational rehabilitation act of 1920 became law the commissions for the blind in many of the states were already offering many different vocational services to blind clients. At the First National Conference on Vocational Rehabilitation in St. Louis in May, 1922, the directors of the new rehabilitation agencies in some states stated that the commissions for the blind had much more money available to them than could be spent in the vocational rehabilitation of all other disabled people under the state-federal program. Some directors of state rehabilitation programs feared that these programs might suffer because the commissions for the blind were more firmly established.

6.6.2. GENERAL PROGRAM MERGER

The Office of Vocational Rehabilitation, established by Public Law 113 in 1943, provided that the Office would supervise vocational rehabilitation for blind people, regardless of where the operations might be directed in the states. Some organizations for the blind opposed this, believing that a program for blind people should have been separate from other rehabilitation programs. Rehabilitation for the blind is now administered by the general rehabilitation agency in about half of the states. Vocational rehabilitation legislation for veterans (PL 178, 65th Congress, and PL 16, 78th Congress) encompassed rehabilitation of veterans blinded in the military service. It allowed for the expenditure of almost unlimited resources to meet the needs of blind veterans.

The exclusive right to operate vending stands in public buildings was given to blind people by the Randolph-Sheppard Act of 1936; as a result many capable blind persons have been guaranteed an opportunity to operate a small business. They are given advice and assistance by the state agency that directs the wide range of other services available for blind people. The Wagner-O'Day Act, passed in 1938, greatly stimulated workshops for blind workers by requiring the federal government to purchase items made in those workshops under prescribed conditions. Some states provide additional preferences for products made by blind workers. Since 1940 blind taxpayers have been permitted a federal income tax deduction.

Blind people have been separated from others in hospices, asylums, schools, and workshops for centuries. Lowered expectations, performance, and opportunity have resulted from this practice, and while many involved in work with the problems of being blind have long recognized the disadvantages of this segregation, only since World War II has there been a discernible movement to remedy the problem.

The public rehabilitation program and other legislation applicable to the blind population are covered in the next section.

6.7. Public Rehabilitation

Evolving attitudes in Western society brought acceptance of the principle of rehabilitation. Recognition of the feasibility and desirability of both social and vocational rehabilitation had slowly developed over several centuries. In America, workers' compensation legislation as a social responsibility of the state had originated in 1909 in Wisconsin and gradually spread throughout the nation (see 37.4.1 for a history of workers' compensation). Likewise the state governments had initiated other social, medical, and vocational programs (see Chapter 12, Agency Structures). But there was strong opposition by conservative politicians, who used a strict interpretation of the states' rights provisions of the Constitution to disclaim national responsibility and to argue against federal financial participation in human service programs.

6.7.1. THE FIRST PROGRAM

Various types of assistance for war veterans—including welfare and education services and benefits—had been under federal administration since 1808. But, these human service expenditures were defended as a federal obligation to those who had served in defense of the country. Then in 1917 the federal government authorized grant-in-aid support to the states for vocational education. Federal sponsorship of vocational education established a precedent for human service programming. The program was under the administration of the new "Federal Board for Vocational Education."

The 1918 veterans rehabilitation act (PL 65-178) excluded disabled civilians, although the question of this exclusion was debated. Ironically though, the Federal Board for Vocational Education was given the additional responsibility for veterans' rehabilitation.

The civilian vocational rehabilitation program of the federal government began in 1920. Like the veterans' rehabilitation program, civilian rehabilitation administration was to be under the Federal Board. But like vocational education, service to civilians was to be a grant-in-aid program to encourage the states to provide the service through their State Board for Vocational Education.

1920 Civilian Rehabilitation (Smith-Fess) Act: Public Law 66-236

In the discussions prior to passage of the Veterans Rehabilitation Act, several Congressmen had informally agreed to work for a separate act that would provide vocational rehabilitation services for civilians through federal grants to the states. Consequently, on September 4, 1918, Representative William Bankhead of Alabama introduced a bill in the House of Representatives that would authorize such grants, and on September 11, Senator Hoke Smith of Georgia introduced a similar bill in the Senate. This proposed legislation was important not because of its extensiveness—in fact, Dr. Harry Mock, a famous industrial surgeon, insisted the bill did not go far enough. Bankhead's bill was important as it broke new ground in committing the federal government to the rehabilitation of disabled people who did not have the veterans' claim on the government. The House and Senate Committees recommended the bills, substantially unchanged from those initially presented, for passage.

But, the 65th Congress did not act then. The new Congress was being formed in the spring of 1919, with a newly elected Republican majority in both the Senate and the House. The bills for civilian rehabilitation had to be reintroduced and again carried through the legislative processes of the Congress and the Senate. The bill was attacked as paternalistic, socialistic, and visionary, and its constitutionality was called into question. While it was being debated in the House, the Rules Committee was discussing a resolution to investigate the Federal Board for Vocational Education in its administration of the Soldier Rehabilitation Act. Several Congressmen argued against giving the Board more responsibilities when its present effectiveness seemed questionable.

Fortunately, those who believed that disabled people should be rehabilitated, and that the federal government should be involved, fought effectively, again and again saving legislation that ran into one danger after another. A new bill was introduced by Rep. Simeon Fess of Ohio and by a vote of 196 to 105 the Fess bill—which was essentially the same as the Bankhead and Smith bills—passed the House on October 17, 1919. On April 12, 1920, the Senate passed its bill again and sent it back to the House of Representatives; the House accepted the Senate amendments on May 25, 1920, by a vote of 102 to 76. President Wilson signed the bill on June 2, 1920.

The act—the Smith-Fess Act—was identified as Public Law 236 of the 66th Congress. It was a simple and short statute but it evidently reflected the thinking of Congress quite precisely. Unfortunately, however, it was interpreted narrowly by the Federal Board for Vocational Education, which was given the responsibility for its administration. Even the meaning of the term *vocational rehabilitation* and the need for a special program outside of traditional vocational education were questioned.

Implementation of Public Law 236

The Federal Board for Vocational Education, formed in 1917 to administer federal grants under the Smith-Hughes Act, had barely begun to operate when it was charged, in 1918, with the task of overseeing the vocational rehabilitation of disabled veterans. This was a federal program in which the states did not participate. Two years later the Board was given the responsibility for administering the civilian vocational rehabilitation act (PL 236). This would have been a huge undertaking, due to the large number of different operations involved, even if the Board had had a long administrative history.

The early mistakes were serious ones. The law did not explicitly authorize the purchase of medical services, and the federal administrators concluded that such services were not vocational rehabilitation service. As a result clients were trained "around" their disabilities.

One of the first problems was the lack of cooperation on the part of many states. The eight states that already had programs before the federal legislation was passed immediately accepted the federal assistance, but many states hesitated to enter the program. The Assistant Director for Industrial Rehabilitation (subsequently referred to as the vocational rehabilitation division) of the Federal Board had to visit these states, urging their participation in the new federal-state partnership for the rehabilitation of disabled civilians. The greatest difficulty sometimes came from the state departments of education. According to the law, the state board of vocational education, which was usually an arm of the state department of education, would be the operating agency. However, the commissioner of education in many states was less committed to rehabilitation than to vocational education programs under the Smith-Hughes Act.

6.7.2. THE PROGRAM DEVELOPS

By the fall of 1921 the staff of the federal vocational rehabilitation agency—its name was frequently changed—had gained experience that enabled them to formulate some principles of service. It was understood, for instance, that rehabilitation is a process that differs with each individual. It was stressed that counseling and restoration were needed before a person entered training.

It was also recognized that those helping the client with rehabilitation should see the client's situation as one in which all other family members were involved, and making use of the assistance of resources such as charities and churches, groups of employees or employers, and medical facilities was recommended. The importance of matching clients' abilities with jobs was recognized, and it was advised that care be taken not to place people in jobs that were too demanding physically. The federal staff found it necessary to keep encouraging states to enlarge the scope of their services and to make services flexible; on the other hand the Federal Board had ruled that federal money was to be used only for training and occasionally for prosthetic appliances.

By 1922 35 states had agreed to participate in the state-federal vocational rehabilitation program; 33 of those states already had organized rehabilitation services. The federal staff published special bulletins to help the state agencies. In 1923, Bulletin No. 80 of the Federal Board, Vocational Rehabilitation Series No. 7, entitled *Vocational Rehabilitation, Its Purpose, Scope and Methods with Illustrative Cases* was compiled under the direction of John Kratz, Chief, Vocational Rehabilitation Division. Its audience was "the general public, who, experience has proved, are generally uninformed on the work of civilian rehabilitation." According to J. C. Wright, then Director of the Board, the purpose was to promote the necessary implementing legislation in states that had already agreed to participate in the new state-federal program.

A national conference met in St. Louis, Missouri in May, 1922, and another was held in February, 1924, in Washington, D.C. The attendance at the conference in Washington was good. A principal speaker was Senator Simeon Fess of Ohio. He reminded the state and federal rehabilitation workers that the Act was due to expire in June, 1924, explaining that Congress

did not ordinarily set such time limits but that the legislators had viewed this project as experimental and were uncertain about the results. As the time for renewal of the Act drew near, agency leadership, organized through the new National Rehabilitation Association (NRA), started to solicit help, approval, and assurances from legislators and members of the administration.

The enthusiasm of the Federal Board for Vocational Education itself had never been great. Personnel in its Civilian Vocational Rehabilitation Division had fought for the program without much assistance from Board leaders, who did not now work very actively for its continuation. Kratz, almost alone, had to enlist the support of influential persons in Congress for renewal.

From 1921 to 1926 the program evolved. Work was being done to lay a theoretical foundation, set up the mechanisms of administration, reach consensus on definitions, investigate the limitations of operations under the laws, and discuss the methods of rehabilitation. As early as June, 1923 there were 36 states participating. The other 12 states took up to 16 more years to come in. The total outlays of all the states grew to $1,188,081 by 1923 but then leveled off until 1931, when the total went over $2 million. There was a rapid increase in the number of people rehabilitated—up to 5,825 in 1925, and this number was not exceeded until 1934. But until 1930 the federal expenditure remained constant at $1,034,000 a year. Likewise a severe limitation was placed on funding for federal administration from 1926 to 1930.

Authority to administer rehabilitation had been given to boards of vocational education at state as well as federal levels. These agencies, with their experience in vocational education, tended to view vocational rehabilitation as another aspect of this endeavor. Generally they did not see how many different kinds of activities went into rehabilitating a disabled individual, how much professional coordination was needed, and how attitudes toward disability influenced the effort; and they did not fully recognize that rehabilitation is "case work" in nature. In the states rehabilitation workers frequently felt that they were hindered because their programs were under education administrators unfamiliar with rehabilitation. In addition, the decade of the 1920s was conservative in outlook; enthusiasm for governmental involvement in the realm of social welfare was decreasing. Presidents Harding, Coolidge, and Hoover considered the years before World War I as "normal" and could see little need for new, innovative human-help programs.

In 1928 the Federal Board issued *A Study of Rehabilitated Persons, A Statistical Analysis of the Rehabilitation of 6391 Disabled Persons;* this study was directed by Tracy Copp, a member of the federal staff. The report contained a great deal of information about rehabilitated persons: their disabilities, their ages, the origins of their disabilities, and their jobs and wages before and after rehabilitation. The disabilities of 53.6 percent originated in employment accidents, 16.1 percent in public accidents, from disease in 23.6 percent of the cases, and from congenital causes in 3.8 percent. Less than 14 percent had had no vocational background before rehabilitation. One-half of the total were rehabilitated through training. About one-half of them were under 30 years of age. There was no direct cost to the agency in rehabilitating 37.9 percent of the individuals; the average cost for each of the others was about $150. This included only cost of training, supplies, and artificial appliances, not living or maintenance expenses. The study confirmed that disabled people could hold many different kinds of jobs with different mechanical and technical requirements.

The federal staff always attempted to perform two crucial functions in working with the states: to help with the promotional work necessary in the states and in the Congress, and to supply materials and directions that would increase the quality and effectiveness of client services. The Civilian Vocational Rehabilitation Series of bulletins alternated in emphasis from one of these functions to the other. The National Conferences were supposed to fulfill both functions. The federal rehabilitation agency has continued its support of state program improvement and staff development to the present time.

6.7.3. THE GREAT DEPRESSION

The state-federal program was continuously in danger of being discontinued by Congress because of the apparently temporary nature of the legislation. The federal government did not have a permanent commitment to the effort; every few years the original Act had to be reaffirmed and new appropriations had to be enacted. This problem was being faced again in 1930 when the 71st Congress was asked to renew the Vocational Rehabilitation Act of 1920 and to allocate funds for its implementation.

Ever since the government had begun to underwrite state rehabilitation programs there had not been any extensive opposition to the idea that disabled persons should be assisted in regaining economic independence. The opposition to the legislation had focused on the constitutional issue of whether the federal government was taking up a responsibility that properly belonged to the states. In considering the renewal of the state-federal program in 1930 those in favor of it countered the constitutional purists by asserting that rehabilitating disabled persons was in the public interest and promoted the national welfare.

The renewal Act was signed into law by President Hoover on June 9, 1930; it provided for a three-year extension of the program, but the allotments were still very limited. The funds would again prove to be insufficient to develop vocational rehabilitation beyond a token assault on the great task at hand.

With federal support of the program assured for another three years, the staff of the federal rehabilitation agency, working with state personnel, could again give attention to making the work more effective. In 1930 the Federal Board for Vocational Education issued a bulletin on the subject of vocational guidance in rehabilitation service. This document served as a basis for evolving the job description of the rehabilitation counselor. It was one of the first attempts to define what the rehabilitation counselor is and does, and in a sense another attempt to arrive at a better definition of vocational rehabilitation itself. The bulletin was an early effort to lay a philosophical foundation toward promoting professionalization of the personnel and procedures of rehabilitation. It was strongly emphasized that rehabilitation workers who had limited preparation should receive more training.

Forty-four states were participating in the state-federal program in 1930; there were only 143 rehabilitation workers on their staffs, and only 20,394 disabled people were in the rehabilitation process. Between 1921 and 1930 only 45,000 persons had been rehabilitated, and only slightly over $12 million (federal share) had been spent in those ten years.

In 1933 the program was caught up in the great

economic measures that the new Roosevelt administration was taking to combat the depression that was worsening each year following the stock market crash of 1929. In October, 1933, a very important step was taken—linking relief and the vocational rehabilitation programs through the Federal Emergency Relief Administration (FERA). The FERA allocated $70,000 a month for the vocational rehabilitation of disabled persons on relief or eligible for relief. In 1932 Congress had given the President broad authority to transfer and consolidate executive agencies. President Roosevelt, in June, 1933, transferred the functions of the Federal Board for Vocational Education to the Department of Interior, and the Secretary of the Interior in October, 1933, assigned the functions of the Federal Board to the Office of Education within Interior. Thus the Commissioner of Education became responsible for the "Federal Rehabilitation Service."

1935 Social Security Act: Public Law 74-271

In June 1934, President Roosevelt appointed a Committee on Economic Security to study the economic security of individuals and to suggest legislation to enhance such security. Early in 1935 this Committee urged that the state-federal rehabilitation program be continued and that it be coordinated with existing and planned economic security programs. The Economic Security bill that was drawn up, however, contained no provisions for rehabilitation.

The representatives of the National Rehabilitation Association, however, managed to gain their legislative objectives by an amendment of the Economic Security bill. Consequently this bill, which became known as the Social Security bill, contained permanent authorization for annual vocational rehabilitation grants to the states of $1,938,000 and $102,000 a year for federal administrative costs. There was no opposition to these aspects of the bill in the House. In the Senate the Committee on Finance unequivocally approved the rehabilitation sections and they were passed by the Senate, becoming law in the form approved by the House. Thus permanent and substantial expansion of federal support for vocational rehabilitation was accomplished, not by direct amendments of the original 1920 Act, but by inclusion of a Title in the vastly important Social Security Act of 1935.

The Social Security Act established the following federal programs: unemployment compensation, old age insurance, old age assistance, aid to the blind, aid to dependent children, maternal and child health services, services for crippled children, and child welfare services, as well as making vocational rehabilitation a permanent program. Later amendments of the Social Security Act provided financial assistance or insurance benefits, or both, to disabled people along with medical services.

The 1939 amendments to the Social Security Act allocated $3,500,000 for annual grants to the states for vocational rehabilitation. Members of both political parties in Congress had developed a very positive attitude about the program.

Administrative Changes

The federal office that administered rehabilitation had not benefited greatly as a result of being assigned to the Office of Education. The National Rehabilitation Association favored autonomy for the Vocational Rehabilitation Service. President Roosevelt issued a reorganization plan for the Executive Branch of the Government under which the Federal Security Agency was established, effective July 1, 1939. There was hope that an independent rehabilitation office would be established in the new agency, but under the plan the entire Office of Education was transferred from the Department of Interior to the new agency, and the Vocational Rehabilitation Service went with it.

Although the administrative agency for public rehabilitation was under three different jurisdictions from 1920 to 1943, the top supervisory staff remained stable. In October 1921 John Kratz was listed as Chief, Industrial Rehabilitation Division, and he continued in that position until 1943, when the Office of Vocational Rehabilitation was formed and the Division was eliminated. Tracy Copp also continued in the federal rehabilitation agency through all those years.

Placing the state programs under vocational education resulted in too much emphasis on education and training and too little on physical restoration and other services particularly needed by disabled rehabilitation clients. Furthermore, the legal advisors of the Federal Board had always refused to concede that the law might permit funds to be used for medical and surgical services or for maintaining clients undergoing training. So the public rehabilitation program remained essentially educational, administered and evaluated by educators, and limited in its capacity to provide other important rehabilitative services.

6.7.4. THE SECOND WORLD WAR PERIOD

Immediately after the United States entered World War II, President Roosevelt asked the Federal Security Administrator to supervise a study of what would constitute an adequate vocational rehabilitation program during and after the war. Many conditions in 1942 made it imperative that national planning for a comprehensive rehabilitation program move forward rapidly. The nation was at war, and injured and disabled servicemen were already returning. The war production effort was speeding up and workers' injuries were on the rise. It was essential for every available person, including those who were handicapped, to work. Furthermore, the rehabilitation movement had reached a stage of maturity by 1942 at which broader definitions of function and responsibility were necessary. By August of 1942, Senator LaFollette of Wisconsin and Representative Barden of North Carolina proposed legislation that reflected some of the needs in state-federal rehabilitation that had been identified over a number of years and some that were generated by the war.

1943 Vocational Rehabilitation Act Amendments (Barden-LaFollette Act): Public Law 78-113

This congressional action of 1943 made profound changes in the public rehabilitation program. For more than 20 years it had been limited in scope of services, restricted in clientele, and uncertainly and inadequately financed. Many of these problems were either eliminated or reduced by legislation enacted in 1943 and at eleven-year intervals thereafter: 1943 (PL 78-113), 1954 (PL 83-565), and 1965 (PL 89-333). When it became law on July 6, 1943, the so-called Barden-LaFollette Act superseded previous federal laws and authorized major new provisions to broaden the vocational rehabilitation program. The major features of Public Law 113 were as follows: (1) broader clientele—extended eligibility to include emotionally disturbed and mentally retarded persons; (2) expanded services—provided for any necessary services, including physical restoration; (3) increased finances—limitations on the maximum

amounts that could be authorized by the Congress were removed.

In the Barden-LaFollette Act vocational rehabilitation was defined to include "any services necessary to render a disabled individual fit to engage in a remunerative occupation." This definition did not differ much from that contained in the original Act of 1920, but in this 1943 Act many services that had been administratively prohibited were expressly authorized. They included "corrective surgery or therapeutic treatment" to reduce or eliminate a disability; hospitalization up to 90 days in connection with the surgery; transportation, licenses, tools, and equipment; prosthetic devices necessary for employment; and maintenance, books, and training materials to be used in training. These services were to be offered "to disabled individuals found to require financial assistance" on a dollar-for-dollar matching basis between the federal government and the states. For medical examinations and vocational assessment of clients there was no requirement to demonstrate financial need.

Mentally ill and retarded persons could be accepted as rehabilitation clients as well as those who were physically disabled. Administrative expenditures of the states were to be reimbursed in full, including costs of counseling and placement. The Administrator was authorized to make technical rehabilitation studies and to conduct or finance the training of personnel involved in the programs of vocational rehabilitation. There was no limitation on the amounts that could be appropriated for vocational rehabilitation programs.

Public Law 113 brought new horizons to the public rehabilitation program. The Office of Vocational Rehabilitation (OVR) was established by the Federal Security Administrator on September 8, 1943, with Michael J. Shortly as its first Director. The new OVR was not under the U.S. Office of Education. This made new administrative and technical developments possible, at both the federal and state levels.

The entry of the United States into World War II placed unusual pressures on vocational rehabilitation. The supply of workers was critically low and the opportunities to utilize disabled persons in war production were forcing the states' programs into greater activity: in fiscal year 1943 the number of persons rehabilitated doubled—from 20,000 to 40,000. The nature of services to disabled clients was changing. There was more emphasis on locating and counseling disabled persons; rehabilitation training courses were becoming shorter and more intensive; more disabled people were being placed directly in jobs without training.

Newly recruited personnel were assembled for short, intensive courses of instruction—usually given by the Washington staff. The federal office arranged that state agency directors be given additional status by working in rehabilitation on a full-time basis, with new prerogatives and new responsibilities. Their revised relationships to their state boards, encouraged by the enactment of Public Law 78-113, enabled them to move aggressively in program planning and development. In 32 states, the state agencies for the blind that were operating under special rules and administrative formats were given more status and authority under Public Law 113.

In fiscal year 1944, 44,000 disabled persons were rehabilitated into employment at a cost of about $150 for each. In that year, over $4,750,000 in federal funds was certified to the states, and state expenditures were about $2,300,000. But the number of individuals served was always far below what it could have been if all handicapped people had been reached. The federal rehabilitation agency estimated that there were at least 1,500,000 men and women in the United States with physical or mental handicaps affecting their employment, and over 250,000 were added to that figure annually.

6.7.5. EXPANSION IN POST-WAR YEARS

The public rehabilitation program was small and not well known by the general public for 25 years. Even if the financial resources necessary to serve all disabled persons had been at hand, there were not enough qualified personnel or facilities. After World War II Pennsylvania and Louisiana set up rehabilitation centers. In Virginia the Army's Woodrow Wilson General Hospital was turned into a rehabilitation center to serve Virginia and neighboring states.

In 1945 the U.S. Congress enacted Public Law 79-176, which established the "National Employ the Physically Handicapped Week" to enhance vocational opportunities of disabled people. President Truman in 1952 changed it to an ongoing "President's Committee" and in 1962 President Kennedy—who had a deep interest in mental disability—expanded it to the "President's Committee on Employment of the Handicapped."

The federal rehabilitation agency placed a great deal of emphasis on the numbers of persons rehabilitated (i.e., placed into jobs) and on the earnings and the economic impact of the rehabilitated population. Not everyone believed that these were the most important aspects of the program; some thought that this emphasis influenced agencies to select the relatively simple cases for service and to neglect the more severely disabled people who needed help the most.

Congress updated its information on services to physically handicapped persons in 1953, when a Special Subcommittee of the House was established. Mary E. Switzer, who had become Director of the Office of Vocational Rehabilitation in 1951, led the discussion, with convincing answers to a series of questions that the Subcommittee staff had submitted.

Switzer stressed the need for research on rehabilitation, adequately supported by the government, and the need for more and better-trained personnel in the state programs, without whom disabled people could not be served. She emphasized that more rehabilitation centers, workshops, and other facilities were needed, stating that while their development might be speeded up by federal assistance, the basic responsibility for the whole rehabilitation program belonged to local agencies with the states assuming much of the burden for development and support. She singled out voluntary organizations for special praise.

E. B. Whitten, Executive Director of the National Rehabilitation Association, testified before the Subcommittee and gave a well-prepared statement. He emphasized the need for increased federal support, stating that there was much more work to be done and that newly developed techniques could not be applied without more financial help. Because the rehabilitation of disabled people was still a pioneering endeavor, Whitten recommended that substantial federal funds be made available for research, experimentation, demonstration, and training. He spoke of the great need for rehabilitation centers and workshops. The National Rehabilitation Association was opposed to the federal government's directly providing rehabilitation services to individuals. Whitten explained that the Association was also against assigning the federal administration of the program to the U.S. Department of Labor. He pointed out that rehabilitation was more than placement and therefore much more comprehensive than the concerns of the bureaus under the Department of Labor.

In opposing the creation of a Federal Agency for the Handicapped or transferring the functions of the Office of Vocational Rehabilitation to the Department of Labor, Whitten argued against another articulate witness, Paul A. Strachan, President of the American Federation of the Physically Handicapped. Strachan argued that many disabled people were not being given adequate help and proposed a single federal agency to coordinate the many programs currently in existence. He recommended that such an agency be part of the Department of Labor.

Not all of the discussion before congressional committees and subcommittees from 1943 to 1953 was about administration. The House Committee on Education and Labor in the fall of 1944 established a Subcommittee on the Handicapped that held hearings around the nation in response to Strachan's arguments. It issued the first comprehensive review of the needs of the disabled population in late 1947. In May 1946 NRA had filed a statement with the Subcommittee recommending new programs for the homebound, cash benefits for individuals for whom vocational rehabilitation was not feasible, and federal assistance for rehabilitation research, education of personnel, and facilities. All of these congressional hearings were very helpful to those who prepared legislation that was to provide for later expansion of rehabilitation programming.

In 1952 Dwight Eisenhower was elected President and a Republican Administration took over for the first time since 1933. Mary Switzer—because of her ability to handle sensitive problems—was well equipped to head the federal rehabilitation agency at this critical time. Much of her time was devoted to adjustments related to the new Administration, while her Assistant Director, Donald Dabelstein, saw that the essential work of the Office went on without interruption. He was one of those who typically receive small notice in a history because their contributions, involving countless small executive decisions and exhibitions of good judgment, cannot be measured, but Dabelstein's

daily supervision of agency affairs was crucial during the hectic days when a new Administration was crystallizing its policies and decisions.

Personalities, conditions, and events were creating a favorable climate for rehabilitation in the Eisenhower Administration. The result was that the Administration asked the Congress for a greatly enlarged program. Because a large number of people, including many members of Congress, worked hard and intelligently, amendments were enacted that would permit the state-federal rehabilitation program to improve services. President Eisenhower said at the signing ceremony when the new legislation (discussed below) was approved, "This law . . . reemphasizes to all the world the great value which we in America place upon the dignity and worth of each individual human being."

1954 Vocational Rehabilitation Act Amendments (Hill-Burton Act): Public Law 83-565

The vocational rehabilitation bill passed by the 83rd Congress was signed into law by President Eisenhower on August 3, 1954, and was designated Public Law 565. It reinforced the existing state-federal program and provided for its future growth and improvement. By the early 1950s the growth of the program had slowed, partly because of the financing system but also because of the lack of technology, professional personnel, and facilities. A new era for rehabilitation was initiated with Public Law 83-565. The Act had been passed unanimously by both Houses of the Democratically controlled Congress. It provided the base for major growth of the program. The main changes made were: (1) Greater financial support to states with relatively larger populations and small per capita income—revised the federal formula for grant-in-aid for services; (2) Extension and improvement of state programs—provided project grants to states; (3) Research and Demonstration funding—authorized federal support of research for new knowledge and demonstration projects to spread application of better methods; (4) Professional preparation—authorized training grants for the preparation of rehabilitation professional personnel; and (5) Rehabilitation facilities—authorized for the first time the use of federal grants-to-states funds for the establishment, alteration, or expansion of rehabilitation facilities and workshops.

Each type of federal support, however, required some matching. The amounts of the general-support grants to the states were based on populations, per capita incomes, and other factors. The most that any state was required to contribute was 40 percent of the total spent in the general rehabilitation program. The federal government paid for 75 percent of the cost of each project.

Included in the legislation were provisions for financial assistance to enlarge or remodel rehabilitation facilities. To help reduce the shortage of trained rehabilitation personnel, funds were allotted for colleges and universities to expand curricula and to provide traineeships to students.

State agency programs were to remain under the responsibility of the state boards for vocational education, although the state directors of vocational rehabilitation were to have direct access to these boards. The state programs could also be decentralized, provided that the state agency would exercise control. The U.S. Department of Health, Education, and Welfare (HEW)—which had been established in 1953 with the dismemberment of the Federal Security Agency—was required to study and report on vocational rehabilitation and to foster improvement and public understanding of the public program.

More than 10 years would pass before additional significant amendments relating to vocational rehabilitation would be made in the laws. Meanwhile the state-federal program continued to grow. By 1959 the total number of people rehabilitated in the state-federal program was 80,739, or 45 percent more than the number reported for 1954 when Public Law 565 was passed.

Another important contribution of Mary Switzer was her promotion of rehabilitation internationally. In her first Annual Report after taking the position as Director of the Office of Vocational Rehabilitation she discussed "Exporting an American Philosophy." In 1961 the Office of Vocational Rehabilitation was authorized to spend $900,000 (in American counterpart funds) in several countries to support projects for the study of rehabilitation problems. Research permitted inquiry into rehabilitation of persons with leprosy and into the cultural and ethnic causes of blindness, mental retardation, and heart disease.

As a reflection of its growing importance, the U.S. HEW Office of Vocational Rehabilitation (OVR) on January 28, 1963, was designated the Vocational Rehabilitation Administration (VRA). Switzer, the OVR Director, became the VRA Commissioner and reported directly to the HEW Department Secretary.

A decade of development under Public Law 565 could be summarized. The National Rehabilitation Association, through its *Journal of Rehabilitation*, issued a "Report of Ten Years of Rehabilitation Under PL 565" in September, 1964. During those ten years the expenditures had increased from $46 billion a year for health, education, and welfare to almost $108 billion, a growth rate somewhat higher than that of America's gross national product ($363 billion to $600 billion in the same ten years). But federal funds for vocational rehabilitation had increased fivefold under Public Law 565—from $23 million in 1954 to $125 million in 1964. While this was a very small proportion of the federal budget, the significance of the rehabilitation program has always been much greater than its monetary size.

6.7.6. THE GREAT GROWTH PERIOD

At the end of 1963 there was a time when everything else stopped while a stunned nation reacted to the assassination of President Kennedy. The nation surmounted the tragedy as it has before, and a new president took office.

President Johnson

In his January 1965 Health Message to Congress, President Johnson urged the enactment of rehabilitation legislation and in March sent the Administration's bill to Congress. By the time the House of Representatives Education and Labor Committee had reported a vocational rehabilitation bill in May, 1965, the legislative wheels were turning furiously in all phases of health, education, and welfare. The Medicare issue was finally coming to a boil after more than 20 years. In such a context the vocational rehabilitation amendments passed the House in late July and moved through the Senate, conference action, and final passage with remarkable speed. When President Johnson signed the bill on November 8, 1965, he had put his pen to the fifth monument to the progress of the rehabilitation success story. (The most notable prior legislation for civilian rehabilitation in America had come in 1920, 1935, 1943, and 1954.)

The 1965 law provided a long list of improvements for the program, including a new method of allotting federal funds among the state agencies and a uniform federal share of 75 percent of the program costs, elimination of economic need as a requirement for obtaining rehabilitation services, creation of a National Commission on Architectural Barriers, and other steps as listed below to expand and perfect programs [U.S. HEW, RSA, 1970].

1965 Vocational Rehabilitation Act Amendments: Public Law 89-333

The most important rehabilitation legislation within a 20-year period (1954 to 1973) was clearly Public Law 333, the Vocational Rehabilitation Act Amendments of 1965. Major provisions were: (1) Expansion of programs for client services—offered five-year incentive grants for agencies (public and private) to plan and initiate expansion; (2) Rehabilitation facilities—provided federal assistance to plan, equip, and initially staff rehabilitation facilities and workshops (public and private); (3) Experimental projects—permitted federal matching of local public funds to help in the rehabilitation of local residents as contrasted to a statewide operation; (4) Innovative projects—developed state rehabilitation projects for the extension and improvement of rehabilitation services for hard-to-rehabilitate cases; (5) Services to determine rehabilitation potential of disabled persons—permitted federal funds to help provide rehabilitation services for a period of six months to certain handicapped persons whose vocational capabilities could not be predicted as favorable at the outset (this "extended evaluation" could run up to 18 months for certain disabilities); (6) Workshop improvement programs—financed new activities to help improve rehabilitation workshops as resources for the vocational rehabilitation of greater numbers of disabled persons; (7) Research and information—extended the authority to undertake research, studies, and demonstrations and to establish and operate a substantially augmented program of information services.

This 1965 legislation, including the provisions designed to strengthen and make more flexible the administration of vocational rehabilitation in the states, had many important implications for

vocational rehabilitation. Under Public Law 565, passed in 1954, to receive federal funding, programs of vocational rehabilitation had to be administered by a state board of vocational education or an independent rehabilitation agency, although agencies for the blind could be administered in whatever setting state law allowed. The 1965 legislation permitted the state education agency or an agency of two or more major organizational units (each of which administers one or more of the major public education, health, welfare, or labor programs of the state) to administer the rehabilitation program. It also attempted to guarantee the administrative integrity of the state rehabilitation agency.

It was the hope at the time that the financing of rehabilitation facilities would make further unification of effort on the part of state rehabilitation agencies and voluntary agencies inevitable and would make more effective the efforts of both. Encouragingly, greater resources than ever before were available for training the personnel and financing the research and demonstrations that are necessary for even greater heights and accomplishments.

Despite the great progress made with Public Law 333, however, one aspect of rehabilitation was not attended to. The National Rehabilitation Association had lobbied for an "Independent Living" rehabilitation proposal for over six years, but the 1965 Amendments still retained a narrow objective—remuneration.

E. B. Whitten (1966) made this interpretation of Public Law 333 of 1965 and its administration regulations:

In general, it may be said that the law and regulations: free the state rehabilitation agencies from restrictions that may have discouraged the provision of comprehensive rehabilitation services in depth to all the nation's handicapped citizens; offer additional strong incentives to encourage rapid expansion of rehabilitation programs; and say, in effect: We believe that rehabilitation philosophy is sound, that its methods and techniques are effective, and that it can contribute substantially to the achievement of equality of opportunity for our people. We are giving you the authority to do the job you say needs to be done, and we shall give you liberal financial support in your efforts [p. 2].

Legislation for Mental Disabilities

The following is a summary of related legislation from 1963 to 1970. These laws authorized important services for certain segments of the population of persons with disabilities.

Public Law 88-164 of 1963 provided for construction of research centers and training facilities relating to mental retardation, construction and establishment of community mental health centers, research and demonstration in the education of handicapped children, and training of personnel in all areas of education for handicapped people at all levels of preparation—from teacher training to the training of college instructors, research personnel, and the administrators and supervisors of teachers.

The 1965 Amendments (PL 89-105) closed a gap in the original legislation, enacted in 1963, by authorizing grants for staffing community mental health centers. In addition, the 1965 Amendments extended and expanded the existing grant program for training teachers of handicapped children and for research and demonstrations in the education of handicapped children. The Mental Retardation Amendments of 1967 (PL 90-170) extended and expanded the programs under which matching grants were made for construction of university-affiliated mental retardation facilities and community retardation facilities.

The War on Poverty

The Economic Opportunity Act of 1964 (PL 88-452) committed the United States to "war designed to eliminate poverty." This was to be done by expanding opportunities for youth, stimulating communities to initiate local action to attack the roots of poverty, helping destitute rural families increase their incomes, expanding small business activities in poor areas of the cities, improving adult education, encouraging states to use public assistance as an instrument for helping families lift themselves out of poverty, and recruiting and training volunteers to help staff the programs to be developed. Less comprehensive legislation with similar objectives had preceded the Economic Opportunity Act, notably the Manpower Development and Training Act and the Depressed Areas Act of 1962. Much of the budget was assigned to the Department of Labor.

E. B. Whitten (1965a) said:

NRA is sympathetic to the objectives of the new legislation, supported much of it in testimony at hearings and otherwise, and is doing what it can to help

ensure that the programs undertaken will contribute substantially to the objectives of the legislation. We are concerned, however, with how slowly the new programs are relating to permanent programs supported by the federal government and the states, whose objectives are similar to those of the new programs and whose responsibilities are to serve some of the same people . . . .

Although VR programs continue to grow, they are facing greater difficulties in maintaining their rate of growth, and some are brought about inadvertently by the new programs. . . . The higher federal shares in these programs put VR agencies in an increasingly difficult position in competing for state funds to match federal funds available for VR services [p. 2].

Further Amendments to the Rehabilitation Act

Noteworthy legislation in 1967 was the Vocational Rehabilitation Act Amendments of 1967 (PL 90-99). Major provisions were: (1) Deaf-blind youth and adults—authorized funds for the establishment of a national center by arrangements with a nonprofit organization; (2) Handicapped migratory workers—authorized a special system of project grants to the state rehabilitation agencies to pay, from federal funds, up to 90 percent of the cost of providing rehabilitation services to disabled migratory agricultural workers; (3) Continued growth of the federal-state program—from the level of $400 million, which the Act authorized for the fiscal year 1968, the 1967 law increased the amounts for allotment to $500 million in 1969 and $600 million in 1970; (4) State planning for rehabilitation—authorized a final year of federal support of this statewide planning in rehabilitation; (5) Residence requirements—required that all states stipulate that no residence requirement will be imposed that excludes from vocational rehabilitation services otherwise eligible disabled persons who are present in the state.

But more than the law books were changing. In August, 1967, HEW Secretary John Gardner, Undersecretary Wilbur Cohen (long a friend of rehabilitation, a key figure in the 1965 Amendments to the Act, and later to be Secretary), and Mary Switzer were the principal figures in a major organizational change in the Department. A new agency, the Social and Rehabilitation Service (SRS), was created to realign the service-giving agencies in a new approach to the problems of all handicapped people, and Switzer was made the first SRS Administrator. It brought together the rehabilitation agency (re-designated as the Rehabilitation Services Administration—RSA), the welfare agency, the Children's Bureau, and the Administration on Aging. The welfare functions were reconstituted into two units, the Assistance Payments Administration (in charge of welfare payment activities) and the Medical Services Administration (in charge of Medicaid and related medical services).

Now the rehabilitation program faced a challenge of unprecedented size—that of bringing to the problems of poor and disadvantaged people the concepts, the philosophies, and the methods on which vocational rehabilitation had been based, without abating its concern for its physically and mentally handicapped clientele [U.S. HEW, SRS, RSA, 1970].

In 1967 the Council of State Administrators of Vocational Rehabilitation, through its Public Policy Committee, considered future program needs at some length and issued a report, *The State-Federal Vocational Rehabilitation Program Looks to the Future—A Statement of Mission and Goals*. The report resulted from the Council's reflections on the impending changes resulting from the creation of the Social and Rehabilitation Service, and the consequent problems and opportunities involved in broadening the public program to play a more direct and active role in restoring all types of handicapped people. In general, the report found that many of the vocational rehabilitation program's basic characteristics—flexibility in federal and state laws and in the funding arrangements, availability of funds for training staff to carry out counseling for specialized groups, the wide range of services already authorized through the program—indicated a real potential for moving more widely into the complex problems and needs of disadvantaged persons.

Again in 1968 the noteworthy occurrence of the year in the field was the federal legislation enacted. The Vocational Rehabilitation Amendments of 1968 (PL 90-391) addressed a number of areas. Major provisions of the 1968 Amendments were: (1) Grants to states for vocational rehabilitation services—authorized $700 million for allotment among states in 1971, and the federal share was increased to 80 percent, effective fiscal year 1970; (2) Establishment of minimum allotments to states—fixed a base of $1 million; (3) Construction of rehabilitation facilities—allocated funds for new construction

as well as expansion or alteration of existing buildings; (4) Private contributions for construction or establishment of facilities—authorized the use of voluntary funds for construction as well as for establishment of a public or nonprofit rehabilitation facility; (5) Grants to states for innovations—extended the program of grants to states for innovation in vocational rehabilitation facilities; (6) Grants to states for special projects—extended the authorization for specialized projects in the areas of research, demonstration, expansion, and training of rehabilitation personnel; (7) State plan requirements—made a number of modifications in state plan requirements for participation in the vocational rehabilitation program; (8) Evaluation of the vocational rehabilitation program—made provision for ongoing evaluation of the rehabilitation agency; (9) Rehabilitation facilities construction and staffing—extended the facilities program; (10) President's Committee on Employment of the Handicapped—doubled the amount authorized for the work of the President's Committee from $500,000 to $1 million; (11) Vocational evaluation and work adjustment—established a vocational rehabilitation program to serve disadvantaged persons, including persons with behavioral problems or social maladjustment as a result of environmental deprivation.

Extension of Vocational Rehabilitation to Disadvantaged Persons

Whitten [1969] reviewed expansion of services to the non-medically handicapped, which was authorized by this legislation, and its implications for vocational rehabilitation:

The term disadvantaged individuals, for whom services are intended, is defined to include any individual disadvantaged in his ability to secure or retain appropriate employment by reason of physical or mental disability, youth, advanced age, low educational attainment, ethnical or cultural factors, prison and delinquency records, or any other condition which constitutes a barrier to his employment. . . .

It is evident from the legislation itself and the report accompanying it that Congress feels that the state-federal vocational rehabilitation program has been a success. It believes that the methods and techniques developed and applied in vocational rehabilitation should be applied to a broader clientele than that ordinarily served by the state vocational rehabilitation agencies. The legislation mandates the provision of the kind of evaluation services that have been used in working with physically and mentally handicapped individuals for many years be applied in working with other disadvantaged individuals. . . .

Although it cannot be said that state vocational rehabilitation agencies are unfamiliar with the problems of the ghetto, it is very likely that the percentage of the agency's clients that come from such surroundings will be greatly increased. This has great implications for the training of personnel and the delivery of services.

The legislation introduces a new concept in the delivery of services. Heretofore, the state vocational rehabilitation agencies have had responsibility for providing all services needed by a relatively narrow segment of the disadvantaged population, that is, the physically and the mentally impaired. They will continue to have this responsibility, but in addition, they will now have responsibility for providing evaluation and work adjustment services to all disadvantaged individuals, many of whom are not expected to be VR agency clients following evaluation. . . .

The mandate to provide outreach, referral, and advocacy services is more important than the simple words may imply. The agencies administering the program will have responsibility to go into the areas in which the disadvantaged are concentrated, seek them out, and bring them to the service.

The legislation and the report assume that a high proportion of the evaluation and work adjustment services will be provided in rehabilitation facilities. Most of these facilities are operated by voluntary agencies. . . . The state vocational rehabilitation agencies will be better funded than heretofore to assist such facilities in expanding their physical plants and staffs, and through the purchase of services, will be better able to guarantee a steady case load for the facilities [p. 2].

In 1968 the National Citizens Advisory Committee on Vocational Rehabilitation completed two years of intensive studies and issued a comprehensive report. This called for continued expansion of the public rehabilitation program (and private programs as well) in much the same general pattern as existed at that time, but with numerous shifts in emphasis. It stressed the need to devise better ways of using the state rehabilitation agency for those handicapped primarily by social, educational, racial, economic, and other non-medical handicaps: in other words, disadvantaged people. The report called for a new grant program in correctional rehabilitation. It recommended the decentralization and dispersal of state vocational rehabilitation offices in major population centers to provide services in neighborhoods where disabled people live, and the establishment of one-stop, multi-service rehabilitation centers in ghettos and other areas where the incidence of disability is high. It proposed changing the federal law to make clear that rehabilitation services are available to any individual who is under a vocational handicap, regardless of its cause. But the Committee still saw services for those with physical or mental disablement as the major program thrust. It also recommended increased funds for expansion of professional training to produce more qualified rehabilitation workers, and funds for an active research program to assure a steady flow of new knowledge and techniques into the hands of the rehabilitation practitioner. In the main the Committee saw the current rehabilitation programs as being essentially sound and on the right track but in need of numerous adjustments, refinements, and redirections into specialized fields of need in which the program offered great potential but presently was providing little service.

As one outgrowth of the Committee's work, a National Citizens Conference on Rehabilitation of the Disabled and Disadvantaged was held in Washington, D.C. in June, 1969. The conference brought "consumers"—that is, disabled and disadvantaged persons themselves—into active roles in both the planning and the conduct of the meeting, right alongside public officials and representatives of rehabilitation programs, health agencies, professional organizations, and welfare groups. Of the many recommendations emerging from the conference, two appeared as central themes throughout: (1) there must be continued expansion of rehabilitation services to all people in need of them, including both disabled and disadvantaged people; and (2) there must be continuing stress on increased consumer participation and involvement in all rehabilitation programs at all levels of operations. And so there appeared to issue again, from a large and quite different group of people, much the same call for continued growth with basically the same concept and many of the same mechanisms, both with shifts in procedural methods and redirections to reach groups previously bypassed or underserved [U.S. HEW, SRS, RSA, 1970].

Developmental Disabilities Program
Special interest groups representing retarded persons convinced the Congress that the "developmentally disabled" constituted a unique segment of the handicapped population. The Developmental Disabilities Services and Facilities

Construction Act of 1970 (PL 91-517) significantly expanded the scope and purposes of the Mental Retardation Facilities Construction Act of 1963. The new legislation was designed to provide states with broad responsibility for planning and implementing a comprehensive program of services and to offer local communities a strong voice in determining needs, establishing priorities, and developing a system for delivering services.

Covering both construction of facilities and the provision of services to persons with developmental disabilities, the new legislation broadened the existing program to include not only mentally retarded individuals but also persons suffering from other serious developmental disabilities originating in childhood. The term *developmental disability* referred to a disability attributable to mental retardation, cerebral palsy, epilepsy, or another neurological condition closely related to mental retardation or necessitating treatment similar to that required for mentally retarded individuals. In addition, the disability must be substantial in nature and must have originated before the individual reached age 18 and have continued or will be expected to continue indefinitely.

States could use formula grant funds to support: (1) a full array of services required by developmentally disabled children and adults; (2) the construction of facilities; (3) state and local planning; (4) administration; (5) technical assistance; (6) training of specialized personnel; and (7) the development and demonstration of new service techniques. The services provided under the "DD" Act could include specialized help directed toward the alleviation of the disability, or toward the social, personal, physical, or economic development of the individual; examples are: diagnosis, evaluation, treatment, personal care, day care, special living arrangements, training, education, sheltered employment, recreation, counseling for the individual and family, protective and other social and sociolegal services, information and referral services, follow-up services, and transportation services [President's Committee on Employment of the Handicapped, n.d.].

Program Continuation
The Vocational Rehabilitation Act Amendments of 1970 (PL 91-610) simply extended the programs that already were in existence. In fiscal year 1969 some 240,000 handicapped persons were rehabilitated. Moreover, a federally sponsored study showed that the state rehabilitation agencies were planning even more effective program efforts.

Reorganization
Most significantly, Mary Switzer retired in 1970. When she left, the rehabilitation organization and orientation of SRS changed. The new SRS Administrator, John Twiname, appointed three associated administrators whose authority superseded that of older heads of programs. After Switzer's retirement, the SRS reverted to the persuasion of social welfare administration. Joseph Hunt, an official of the federal rehabilitation agency for many years and the first Commissioner of the new RSA, was transferred from his position of responsibility. Edward Newman and later Andrew Adams served as RSA Administrators during the Nixon-Ford era. Interim appointments, however, included Acting RSA Administrators James Burress and Corbett Reedy, both of whom had long-term association with the public rehabilitation agency.

6.7.7. BATTLE PHASE
1970 was the 50th anniversary of the American public rehabilitation program. Attention was focused upon its origins, progress, and accomplishments. But while the history of vocational rehabilitation was being celebrated, stern realities of the day would have a strong impact on the future of the movement. The horizontal expansion of vocational rehabilitation to include the culturally disadvantaged population was abruptly discontinued. Starting with services for public offenders, the program had just begun to show its value when the new Administration caused its discontinuation. President Nixon apparently felt that rehabilitation was not an effective approach in the management of public offenders, and instead instigated stronger law enforcement and other plans for deterring crime in order to reduce the criminal population. Likewise, the SRS administration was not enthusiastic about the vocational adjustment approach to the welfare problem.

Administrative Concerns
By 1971 there was fear that the progressive movement of the public rehabilitation program as it had developed would not be allowed to continue. The executive branch of the federal government was not dedicated to the rehabilita-

tion concept—at least not in its current administrative format. While there was never doubt about government sponsorship of rehabilitation in some form, its visibility, if not its viability, seemed to be at stake.

Whitten warned in 1971:

There has been very little to indicate that those closest to the President have any real understanding of the accomplishments of rehabilitation and its potential in meeting human needs. Manpower and welfare legislation have been sent to Congress by the Administration virtually ignoring the existence of the public and voluntary rehabilitation movement. Administration recommendations of funds to finance rehabilitation programs are far below the appropriation authority for such programs, and the prospects for improvement next year are not good. . . .

The efforts of the National Rehabilitation Association, supported by the current Secretary of HEW, to achieve modest gains for vocational rehabilitation this year, have been impeded by the Office of Management-Budget.

. . . . Often, NRA has found Congress more perceptive of the needs of handicapped people than the executive branch of the government and more receptive of suggestions for improvements [p. 2].

The need for renewal of the Rehabilitation Amendments of 1970 was a crucial issue, according to Craig Mills [1976], state rehabilitation agency administrator in Florida at the time. The statutory authorization of a program provides coverage for a period of time, forming the legal basis for congressional appropriation of funds. In the final year, the executive branch usually submits proposed amendments for a developing program. Despite extension by the Congress of the authorization and the cooperation of NRA and other groups with HEW, SRS, and RSA, the Administration failed to recommend legislation for the continuation of vocational rehabilitation.

Mills later observed:

In the light of subsequent events revealed at the Congressional oversight hearings on the rehabilitation program in 1973, many people in rehabilitation felt that the lack of action on the part of the administration represented a planned and concerted effort on the part of HEW to downgrade or abolish the vocational rehabilitation program for the handicapped in favor of a cash benefits, expanded welfare system [p. 13].

Congressional Support of Rehabilitation

The struggle between the legislative and executive branches concerning vocational rehabilita-

tion continued through the early 1970s. The first point of contention was money. Appropriations for rehabilitation programs were included in a bill that the President signed in October, 1972, the amounts of which had been recommended by the President. Nevertheless, $50 million of the appropriation for the state-federal rehabilitation program was withheld by the Administration. Research spending for 1973 was reduced by $17 million below the original estimate. Most serious of all, the Administration attempted to phase out all SRS training programs.

Vetoes

Continuing difficulties in promoting the best interests of persons with disabilities and the public rehabilitation program were experienced. The efforts of the Congress were thwarted by the executive branch. On October 27, President Nixon vetoed the Rehabilitation Act of 1972. This measure had been initiated by the National Rehabilitation Association and amended by both House and Senate. It was a comprehensive piece of legislation designed to expand and improve services to handicapped individuals and included substantial increases in appropriations authorization. It had been passed unanimously by both branches of Congress following lengthy hearings and tedious staff work. In giving the legislation a pocket veto, President Nixon stated that the measure was another example of "congressional fiscal irresponsibility." In recognition of the lack of administrative support for rehabilitation, the Congress had stipulated in this vetoed bill that the Rehabilitation Services Administration would be a separate agency within HEW. This was one of Nixon's objections.

Congress promptly reenacted the Rehabilitation Act Amendments and the only significant changes were to scale down appropriation authorities. The Senate passed this bill on February 22, 1973 by a vote of 86 to 2; the House passed a similar bill on March 18 by a vote of 318 to 57. Conferees agreed on a bill and sent it to the President on March 22, 1973.

President Nixon vetoed the measure on March 28, using substantially the same arguments he had used when he vetoed the similar bill in October, 1972. This veto was the subject of headline news on radio and television and in the press for over a week. Veteran observers on Capitol Hill said they had never seen as much activity on the part of the Administration on any piece of legislation as in this effort to sustain the President's veto.

The entire machinery of the executive branch was brought to bear on Congress: there were Presidential meetings with the Republican leadership; meetings of freshman members of Congress in the White House; private meetings of congressional minority leaders with Republican members; party caucuses; meetings of public affairs officers of all departments of the government, to whom packets of materials were distributed urging the sustaining of the veto; directions that all speeches by Administration representatives urge sustaining the President's vetoes; the President, himself, appearing on nationwide television; and a swarm of Administration representatives knocking on congressional doors. The Rehabilitation Act Amendments were being used as a test case, a confrontation between Congress and the Administration on legislative policy [Whitten, 1973].

Thirty national groups, of and for handicapped people, organized in a determined effort to secure an override of the President's veto, but their effort failed. At 2 P.M. on April 3, 1973, the Senate sustained the President's veto of the Rehabilitation Act Amendments by a vote of 60 to override and 36 to sustain, a two-thirds majority being necessary to override. As he had the year before, the president stated his objections: appropriation authorizations were too high, the independent living features would divert the public program for vocational rehabilitation from its original objectives, and the requirement that the RSA Commissioner be responsible directly to the HEW Secretary was objectionable administratively.

6.7.8. CONGRESSIONAL ACTION

Although the President's vetoes of recent bills had been sustained, the Congress exhibited new determination as the next round of legislation approached. Great support for rehabilitation continued in both the House and the Senate. Moreover the National Rehabilitation Association, with the voice of E. B. Whitten, was strong, and political support came from many interest groups. Dedicated people were aroused by the deteriorated status of RSA in the executive branch of government. Rep. John Brademas of Indiana was a giant in the development of new rehabilitation legislation. In 1971 he chaired the Select Education Subcommittee of the House Committee on Education and Labor and conducted hearings on the NRA proposals. He even

went further than NRA with regard to its proposal for a restricted Independent Living provision (for deaf and blind people). The monumental 1973 Rehabilitation Act and its 1978 Amendments should bear the Brademas name, but it is no longer customary to name legislation after its authors. Jennings Randolph of West Virginia was a leading rehabilitation spokesman in the Senate at the time.

Congressional Oversight

On August 3, 1973, the Select Education Subcommittee of the House Committee on Education and Labor began "oversight" hearings on vocational rehabilitation. The term *oversight* is customarily given to hearings that are not necessarily related to pending legislation but are designed to get information about the Administration's plans, policies, and procedures in the operation of programs.

Administration witnesses reiterated their support of vocational rehabilitation programs. This testimony was offered despite the Administration's two vetoes of rehabilitation legislation, its recommendations for reducing research appropriations, its intention to phase out federal support of training programs, its withdrawal of support for construction and staffing of rehabilitation facilities, and its holding the state-federal vocational rehabilitation program at its 1972 level of operations [Whitten, 1973a].

These oversight hearings were followed by additional hearings by the Subcommittee on November 30, 1973, when representatives of state agencies and rehabilitation counselor educators were called to testify with representatives of U.S. HEW, SRS, and RSA. This second oversight hearing focused on congressional dissatisfaction with the way the Social and Rehabilitation Service was administering the Act and RSA. Craig Mills [1976] gave a personal account of these hearings:

The testimony of the Council of State Administrators of Vocational Rehabilitation revealed a lack of SRS support for Research and Demonstration, Innovation and Expansion Grant Programs and Training. Concern was expressed about the use of resources under the Rehabilitation Act to further the priorities of SRS to the neglect of the needs of handicapped people. Special concerns were expressed on the way SRS had promoted organizational arrangements in the states which appeared to be in violation of the federal Rehabilitation Act and which diminished the effectiveness of specific programs for handicapped people. . . .

Representatives of the Council of Rehabilitation Counselor Educators presented testimony in favor of the preservation of specialized rehabilitation counselor education programs under the law which SRS had proposed to phase out [pp. 16–17].

The Select Subcommittee called upon HEW and SRS officials to explain and justify the approval of a state plan in a state that appeared to be out of compliance with substantial requirements of the Rehabilitation Act. The response given by the SRS officials that "approval of the state plan was in keeping with Administration policy rather than compliance with the law" served as a basis for Congressional determination to mandate organizational changes in HEW and to direct the removal of the Rehabilitation Services Administration from the Social and Rehabilitation Service. According to Mills, this established the basis for future legislation.

1973 Rehabilitation Act: Public Law 93-112

Finally, the Rehabilitation Act of 1973 became law. This major piece of legislation had substantial impact on the rehabilitation movement. In Public Law 112 Congress provided the Administration with face-saving provisions, the most notable of which was the deletion of the independent living program previously proposed. It was clear that with this and other compromises, the Congress would override another presidential veto—and there was time to do so in that session. Knowing this, President Nixon signed the new Rehabilitation Act on September 26, 1973.

The 1973 Rehabilitation Act placed strong emphasis on expanding services to more severely handicapped clients. The following is a brief summary of the major features of PL 112:

1. Extension of basic grant program: the federal-state grant program for vocational rehabilitation services was extended for an additional two years and set authorization ceilings of $650 million in fiscal year 1974 and $680 million in fiscal year 1975.

2. Service priorities for severely handicapped people: state agencies were directed to give priority to serving "those individuals with the most severe handicaps" in their basic state vocational rehabilitation programs. In addition, state agencies were required to describe "the method to be used to expand and improve services to handicapped individuals with the most severe handicaps."

3. Individualized written rehabilitation program (IWRP): the state rehabilitation agencies were required to develop an individualized written rehabilitation program (plan) on each client served. This client program must be jointly developed by the rehabilitation counselor and the handicapped individual (or parent or guardian) and must spell out the terms, conditions, rights, and remedies under which services are provided to the individual; it must state the long-range and intermediate goals to be attained. Each individual's program must be reviewed at least annually.

4. Consolidated rehabilitation and developmental disabilities plan: states were authorized to submit a consolidated vocational rehabilitation-developmental disabilities plan.

5. Special projects and demonstrations: HEW was directed to give special attention to providing vocational rehabilitation services for clients with the most severe handicaps.

6. Sheltered workshop study: a comprehensive, 24-month study was to be made of the role of sheltered workshops in rehabilitation and employment of handicapped individuals.

7. Coordination of programs for handicapped people: HEW was directed to prepare and submit to Congress a long-range plan for serving handicapped individuals.

8. Organization and administration: By statute, a Rehabilitation Services Administration was established within HEW and delegated to the Commissioner of RSA responsibility for administering all aspects of the rehabilitation program authorized under the Act (previously delegated to the Secretary of HEW); the Commissioner was to be appointed by the President. The Act forbade the Secretary to redelegate any of the Commissioner's authority without the explicit approval of Congress. The Secretary was also directed to ensure that all funds appropriated under the Act were used to support rehabilitation programs.

9. Innovation and expansion grants: Separate existing authorities for innovation and expansion grants were consolidated into a single formula grant program.

10. Nondiscrimination and employment under federal contracts: Discrimination against otherwise qualified handicapped persons in any federally assisted program or activity was forbidden. It also required all federal contractors and subcontractors to take affirmative action to employ qualified handicapped individuals. Complaints

could be filed with the Department of Labor by any aggrieved handicapped individual.

11. Federal interagency committee on handicapped employees: this committee was established to investigate the status of handicapped individuals working for the federal government. Every federal agency was required to submit an affirmative action plan for hiring, placing, and advancing handicapped individuals.

12. Architectural and Transportation Barriers Compliance Board: this Board was created to assure compliance with the Architectural Barriers Act of 1968 and to study additional ways to eliminate architectural and transportation barriers in public facilities.

13. Mortgage insurance for rehabilitation facilities: up to 100 percent mortgage insurance was authorized in order to cover the costs of constructing public or nonprofit rehabilitation facilities.

14. National center for deaf-blind youths and adults: funds were authorized to establish and operate a National Center for Deaf-Blind Youths and Adults under whose auspices new techniques would be demonstrated and research related to rehabilitating deaf-blind individuals would be conducted.

Whitten [1974] commented on the implications for the public program of the 1973 Rehabilitation Act: "In almost every major section of the Act, including sections dealing with research, special projects, and training of rehabilitation personnel, expansion and improvement of services for severely handicapped individuals are stated to be among the objectives of such programs" [p. 2]. The new law, however, did not establish any new program to serve severely handicapped individuals. There were no provisions for providing rehabilitation services to those without vocational potential. The definition of the handicapped individual eligible for services was not changed in any significant way: all clients were still expected to be able to benefit in terms of employability from the provision of services. Moreover, there was no significant change in the concept of employability.

Other Acts

The 92nd Congress did not reach agreement on welfare reform; however, social welfare legislation containing a number of important provisions for handicapped persons was enacted. These provisions related to increasing childhood disability benefits and trust fund expenditures for rehabilitation services, expanding Medicaid and Medicare, and federalizing administration of public welfare cash assistance programs. The federally financed and administered Supplementary Security Income (SSI) program of cash assistance replaced separate state-run assistance programs for aged, blind, and disabled people. This omnibus legislation—the Social Security Amendments of 1972 (PL 92-603)—was signed into law by President Nixon in October 1972. It adopted a definition of "disability" as an "inability to engage in any substantial gainful activity by reason of any medically determined physical or mental impairment which can be expected to last for a continuous period of not less than 12 months." The Wagner-O'Day Amendments (PL 92-28) extended bidding preferences on government contracts to workshops for the severely handicapped. Previously, preferences had been limited to workshops for the blind.

Other legislation enacted by the 93rd Congress had important implications for the field of rehabilitation and for persons with disabilities. Two sets of significant amendments to the Social Security Act were enacted during the first Session of the 93rd Congress. Public Law 93-66, signed into law on July 9, 1973, increased social security benefits, raised the federal SSI payment level, and expanded the SSI program. Public Law 93-233 authorized a further extension plus additional increases in social security and SSI benefits. The National Association of Coordinators of State Programs for the Mentally Retarded published a summary by R. M. Gettings [1975] of the federal laws and regulations of 1973 and 1974.

6.7.9. WATERGATE AND THEN FORD

The American constitutional system faced its sternest test since the Civil War during the term of the 93rd Congress. In the eventful days between April 1973, and August 1974, the nation watched with rapt attention the unfolding of developments that ultimately led to the resignation of the Vice President; then, on August 8, 1974, the President of the United States resigned.

The 93rd Congress had a respectable record of legislative accomplishments. Far-reaching measures relating to the President's war powers, budget reform, campaign spending, elementary and secondary school aid, minimum wages and pension reform were enacted, despite the members' preoccupation during most of the two-year period with the Watergate scandal and its aftermath. The Watergate revelations galvanized the 93rd Congress into action and convinced many national leaders and constitutional scholars of the need for Congress to reassert aggressively its claim to certain powers that had slowly eroded away over the years. Among the signs of this new attitude on the part of Congress was increased specificity in the provisions of laws affecting handicapped people. Distrustful of the Nixon Administration's commitment to social programs generally, and programs for handicapped people in particular, congressional committees tended to include detailed statutory specifications regarding the operation of federal programs. An example of such provisions is the statutory transfer of the Rehabilitation Services Administration from the Social and Rehabilitation Service to the Office of Human Development.

There was also an expansion of the activities of the General Accounting Office (GAO) into the area of programs for handicapped people. During 1973 and 1974, GAO, the investigative arm of Congress, undertook several special studies of programs serving handicapped children and adults, including vocational rehabilitation, education of handicapped persons, and developmental disabilities programs. Moreover, Congress established statutory deadlines for submittal of regulations and requirements for prior congressional review of administrative regulations and policies.

To some extent this new emphasis on congressional oversight may have been a reflection of the partisan split between a Democratic Congress and a Republican President. However, a growing number of Senators and Congressmen recognized that it is not enough simply to pass a law. Instead, to carry out its mission effectively, they believed, Congress must be more intimately involved in the process of implementing laws and evaluating their effects [Gettings, 1975].

Rehabilitation Amendments of 1974: Public Law 93-516

The Rehabilitation Act Amendments of 1974 were sent to President Ford by Congress late in the week of October 14. Congress recessed almost immediately thereafter. On the afternoon of October 29, the President vetoed the legislation. The President interpreted his action as a

"pocket" veto, which is permitted when Congress is in adjournment. Such vetoes cannot be overridden—the legislation has to be passed again. Congress reconvened on November 18, and the President's veto was overridden on November 20. The vote was 398 to 7 in the House, 90 to 1 in the Senate. The President persisted in his point that his veto was a pocket veto that could not be overridden. The bill was reintroduced in the House of Representatives on November 25 and was reported out the same day. It was passed by the House and Senate on the 26th and sent to the President. Since Congress would be in session until about December 20, there was no opportunity for another pocket veto. The President signed the legislation.

Public Law 516 extended appropriation authority for all titles of the Rehabilitation Act through fiscal 1976, amended the Randolph-Sheppard Act to strengthen the rights of blind individuals to operate vending facilities in public buildings, called for a White House Conference on Handicapped Individuals, and moved the Rehabilitation Services Administration from the Social and Rehabilitation Service to the Office of the HEW Secretary. The President's announced objections centered on the organizational features of the legislation.

Administrative Struggle

The most important happenings in the federal rehabilitation agency in 1975 were administrative. On November 25, 1975, HEW issued final regulations implementing the Rehabilitation Act Amendments of 1974. These regulations also clarified certain regulatory provisions contained in the final rules governing the Rehabilitation Act of 1973. Organizationally, the regulations are divided into two sections: (1) the state vocational rehabilitation program, and (2) a variety of project grants and other federally administered assistance authorized under the Rehabilitation Act.

The transfer of RSA out of SRS to the Office of Human Development—a move mandated by Congress under the 1974 Amendments—was a long-sought improvement. Rehabilitation still suffered downgraded organizational status, however, from its earlier days as the Vocational Rehabilitation Administration when its head reported directly to the HEW Secretary.

Also in 1975 a significant step was taken at the federal level to allow the practicing rehabilitation counselor to have input at the policy-making level. At a meeting in Washington, D.C. on May 5, 1975, an RSA Advisory Committee for Rehabilitation Counselors was established by Andrew S. Adams, Commissioner, Rehabilitation Services Administration. In attendance at the initial meeting were: George Wright, President, American Rehabilitation Counseling Association, Chairman; Daniel McAlees, Chairman, Commission on Rehabilitation Counselor Certification; Fletcher Hall, Executive Director, National Rehabilitation Counseling Association; Brockman Schumacher, President, Council on Rehabilitation Education; and Joseph Szuhay, President, Council of Rehabilitation Counselor Educators. Also in attendance from RSA were William Usdane, RSA Assistant Commissioner for Program Development, and Harold Shay, Director of the Division of Manpower Department. The Advisory Committee was established "to serve the RSA Commissioner's Office by bridging the people-government gap—to provide the voice of practitioners for the RSA decision-making process, and to bring information to working rehabilitation counselors" [National Rehabilitation Counseling Association 1975, p. 2].

Rehabilitation Extended but Not Expanded

Since 1976 was the year for extension of the Rehabilitation Act, action toward this end was begun in late 1975. On March 15, 1976, the "Rehabilitation Extension Act of 1976" became Public Law 94-230. The new law extended the existing Act for two years without changing anything but the amounts authorized to be appropriated by the Congress.

"What was significant about this legislation," according to LaVor and Duncan [1976], "was not what Congress did, but what it did not do. It can be said that a conscious decision was made by both Houses of Congress not to change existing law by adding any additional amendments, either minimal or substantial. The Act of 1976 was designed solely to extend only the programs' authorizations for two years. This decision was made primarily to assure the continuation of various programs authorized under the Rehabilitation Act" [p. 20].

A number of legislative actions further refined the process of publicly supported rehabilitation services. Early in 1976 Congress dealt a severe blow to President Ford's plans to place a tight ceiling on social welfare spending by overriding his veto of the Labor-HEW appropriations bill

for fiscal year 1976. On January 27, the House voted to override the veto by 28 votes more than the required two-thirds majority (310 to 113). The Senate followed on January 28, by a vote of 70 to 24. Funds for basic vocational rehabilitation grants to the states were increased by $40.3 million (from $680 million to $720.3 million). In addition, the major portion of Administration-proposed cuts in innovation and expansion grants was restored, and research funding was increased by $4 million.

In late September, 1976, both Houses of Congress voted by overwhelming margins to override President Ford's veto of the HEW-Labor appropriations bill for 1977 (HR 14232). This measure included several significant funding increases for programs affecting handicapped children and adults, including: a $127.5 million increase in appropriations for grants to the states to assist in educating handicapped children, and a $20 million increase in the state-federal rehabilitation program.

Two and one-half years after the enactment of a statutory requirement that federal contractors and subcontractors adopt affirmative action plans for employing and advancing handicapped workers, the U.S. Department of Labor released final regulations implementing the law. The legal requirement, in Section 503 of the Rehabilitation Act of 1973 (PL 93-112), was intended to protect handicapped persons against job-related discrimination. On April 28, 1976, President Ford issued an executive order directing all federal departments and agencies that provide financial assistance to issue rules, regulations, and directives barring discrimination against handicapped individuals.

6.7.10. CARTER YEARS

Jimmy Carter assumed the Presidency in January, 1977, having campaigned on promises for many new human rights and service programs that had long been needed. It was assumed that rehabilitation as a "human obligation" would be addressed in the new Administration.

The White House Conference on Handicapped Individuals

The White House Conference on Handicapped Individuals had been authorized in the 1974 Rehabilitation Amendments. This enormous meeting was held at the Park-Sheraton hotel in Washington, D.C., on June 23 to 27, 1977. It brought together 3,700 people designated "to represent 35 million Americans with mental or physical disabilities" for an assessment of their problems and potentials. It provided a first opportunity—after Governor Conferences at the state level—for persons with handicaps to voice concerns and vote for recommendations to solve problems directly affecting their lives. Henry Viscardi, Jr., founder (in 1952) of Abilities, Inc., chaired the Conference. The Conference generated 420 resolutions but their implementation was retarded for lack of staff, budget and other administrative considerations.

Administrative Issues

The governmental changes in 1977 were essentially administrative in nature, but they did indicate a positive attitude toward rehabilitation and help for disabled people. For example, the Administration agreed to double the number of federal employees who enforce civil rights laws and to take major steps to end discrimination in all levels of education. The agreement covers racial discrimination, sex discrimination, and discrimination against handicapped persons.

In a news release on July 26, 1977, HEW Secretary Califano announced the reorganization of the Office of Human Development (newly named Office of Human Development Services). The plan reduced from 24 to 9 the number of programs and staff units reporting directly to the Assistant Secretary of Human Development.

Five program administrators and four staff offices were established. The five administrations were: Administration for Handicapped Individuals; Administration for Children, Youth, and Families; Administration for Native Americans; Administration for Public Services; and Administration for Aging. The Administration for Handicapped Individuals (AHI) included the Rehabilitation Services Administration (RSA), the Developmental Disabilities Office, the President's Committee on Mental Retardation, the Architectural and Transportation Barriers Compliance Board, the White House Conference on Handicapped Individuals, and the Office of Handicapped Individuals. The Commissioner of RSA was also to be the head of the new AHI. Robert R. Humphreys was appointed Commissioner of RSA on November 7, 1977. Humphreys, an attorney by profession, previously served as Special Counsel to the U.S. Senate Committee on Human Resources.

Administrative organizations were established

for the enforcement of the affirmative action provisions (Title V) of the 1973 Rehabilitation Act as amended. In 1978 the U.S. Civil Service Commission was reorganized and renamed. It is now called the Office of Personnel Management (OPM). The federal Equal Employment Opportunity Commission was assigned the responsibility for enforcing affirmative action concerning federal employment of disabled workers. OPM retains the responsibility for helping federal agencies to implement their affirmative action plans through a new Selective Placement Office.

Rehabilitation, Comprehensive Services, and Developmental Disabilities Amendment: Public Law 95-602

This 1978 legislation is by far the most significant event in the recent history of rehabilitation in America. It provided a whole new dimension to the public rehabilitation structure through its authorization of rehabilitation services for independent living. After nearly 20 years of legislative effort the leadership of the rehabilitation movement achieved federal acceptance of the public obligation to rehabilitate its severely disabled members—even though they may never become wage earners. In the early 1960s Congress debated the need to expand rehabilitation to include independent living objectives, but did not enact such a bill; in 1972 Congress passed such a measure but it was vetoed as too costly.

These Amendments to the 1973 Rehabilitation Act were passed by the Congress after months of work on the part of both House and Senate subcommittees chaired by Representative John Brademas and Senator Jennings Randolph, respectively. It was an omnibus bill to extend and expand rehabilitation objectives, methods, and funding authorizations.

Public Law 602 was signed by President Carter on November 6, 1978 at the eleventh hour before it would have suffered an automatic pocket veto. It was approved only after he had extracted assurances from key members of the Congress that they would delay pressing for full funding of its authorized measures.

The following summary of the Act is taken from a federally prepared statement (U.S. HEW, Office of Handicapped Individuals, 1979).

COMPREHENSIVE INDEPENDENT LIVING SERVICES. This new program was "designed to meet the needs of individuals whose disabilities are so severe that they do not have the potential for [remunerative] employment, but may benefit from . . . services which will enable them to live and function independently." State rehabilitation agencies were designated to administer this program which includes a new set of services designed for independent living objectives in addition to the traditional services for vocational objectives. A percentage of the federal allocation is necessarily passed along to local public or private agencies providing relevant services. New Centers for Independent Living may be established and operated by the state rehabilitation agencies or other public or private organizations. A variety of services are to be provided by the Centers, including: counseling, advocacy, skills training, housing and transportation, referral, health maintenance, group living arrangements, social and recreational activities, and attendant care and training of attendants. An individualized written rehabilitation program must be developed for each person served.

NATIONAL INSTITUTE OF HANDICAPPED RESEARCH (NIHR). This new Institute was established to take over the research-related programs formerly administered by the federal Rehabilitation Services Administration. NIHR administration was stipulated to be independent of RSA with the Director of the Institute appointed by the President. Expansion of the activities of Rehabilitation Research and Training Centers was authorized. Public Law 602 also established mechanisms for identifying research needs and priorities, for long-range planning, and for a federal "Interagency Committee on Handicapped Research" for coordination.

NATIONAL COUNCIL ON THE HANDICAPPED. This fifteen-member Council appointed by the President was established with its own staff office to advise and oversee the NIHR, RSA, and other federal agencies with programs concerning handicapped persons.

INFORMATION CLEARING HOUSE. This part of the Act set up the "Office of Information and Resources for the Handicapped" to provide information about available services, research results, and other data for and about handicapped persons.

PILOT COMMUNITY SERVICE EMPLOYMENT PROGRAMS AND PROJECTS WITH INDUSTRY. The

provision here is for two programs aimed at increasing the employability and employment opportunities for handicapped persons: (1) The "Community Services Employment Pilot Program," administered by the U.S. Department of Labor, provides up to 90 percent of the costs for a program of pilot projects for community employment of persons referred by state rehabilitation agencies (including client training, subsistence, work-related expenses, transportation, and attendant care); (2) The "Projects with Industry" program was expanded (see 33.4.13.).

ARCHITECTURAL AND TRANSPORTATION BARRIERS COMPLIANCY BOARD. The Act expanded the Board's enforcement authority.

NON-DISCRIMINATION PROVISIONS. These provisions included minor revisions and clarifications.

STATE REHABILITATION ALLOCATION REVISIONS. The provision gives more equal emphasis to state per capita income in the federal allotment to states.

DEVELOPMENTAL DISABILITIES. In Title V of the Act the definition and other fundamental implications for this program and its clientele were revised. The shift was to a more "functional" as opposed to "categorical" definition. As defined in this 1978 legislation, a developmental disability results from any (one or more) chronic and severe mental or physical impairment(s) manifested before age 22 and that results in functional limitations in several areas of living. Authorization for the Developmental Disabilities and Facilities Construction program was extended for three years.

U.S. Department of Education Affiliation
A new U.S. Department of Education (DOE) was created by Public Law 96-88, signed into law by President Carter on October 17, 1979. Under this Act all of the federal rehabilitation agency programs (developmental disabilities was an exception) were among the old HEW areas specified to be transferred to DOE. The Act created the Office of Special Education and Rehabilitation Services (OSERS) to be headed by an Assistant Secretary. Relevant functions of the old U.S. Department of Health, Education,

and Welfare were transferred to OSERS. Specifically included were selected programs authorized in previous Acts as amended (Rehabilitation Act, Randolph-Sheppard Act).

Support for the move was based upon the belief that rehabilitation would have more visibility and strength in the smaller organization of DOE. Perhaps the attractiveness of remarriage with education was a reaction to the recent domination of rehabilitation by welfare in the HEW Social and Rehabilitation Service Administration and the current trend in Florida and other states for a general human service agency combining rehabilitation and welfare. Prospects in the new DOE for a return to a strong administration of rehabilitation (as experienced under Mary Switzer) was a consideration; consequently this transfer of rehabilitation to education was formally supported by the National Rehabilitation Association, the Council of State Administrators of Vocational Rehabilitation, the American Coalition of Citizens with Disabilities, and other organizations. Many observers, however, believed that the new goals and the techniques of independent living rehabilitation call for even closer ties with health and social services. It cannot be assumed that the concepts and programs of total rehabilitation will fare well in the new U.S. Department of Education.

State Rehabilitation Agency Integrity
The continuing issue of the administrative integrity of rehabilitation is discussed at the end of this chapter (see 6.8.5). Federal law has attempted to mandate that state rehabilitation agencies operate as a single organizational unit; this federal requirement was ignored by the State of Florida in their establishment of a general human service agency, an organizational merger that has been ruled by federal courts to be in violation of the federal rehabilitation laws. Political pressure, however, continues with legislation now introduced by Florida Congressmen that would give the federal Administration (DOE Secretary) waiver authority in such cases and permit the assignment of state rehabilitation to many uncoordinated units with commingled resource. The problem with organizational merger is that rehabilitation is overshadowed by the larger social welfare component. Services to handicapped people suffer due to changes in agency techniques and goals and reduction in rehabilitation resources.

6.7.11. LEGISLATION CHRONOLOGY
A brief chronological summary of the most important federal legislation relevant to rehabilitation is provided below.

1917: PL 64-347—VOCATIONAL EDUCATION ACT (SMITH-HUGHES ACT). Created the Federal Board for Vocational Education to administer federal vocational education grants to the states through state boards for vocational education.

1918: PL 65-178—SOLDIERS REHABILITATION ACT (SMITH-SEARS ACT). Authorized the Federal Board for Vocational Education to administer a national vocational rehabilitation service to disabled Veterans of World War I.

1920: PL 66-236—CIVILIAN REHABILITATION ACT (SMITH-FESS ACT). Provided vocational rehabilitation services to people "disabled in industry and otherwise" through state boards for vocational education; services were to be administered under the Federal Board for Vocational Education. Signed into law by President Wilson, June 2, 1920.

1921: PL 67-47—VETERANS BUREAU ACT. Established the Veterans Bureau as an independent agency with a director responsible to the President. The veterans rehabilitation program moved out of the Federal Board for Vocational Education administration.

1933: PL 73-2—VETERANS ADMINISTRATION ACT. Reorganized the Veterans Bureau and designated this federal agency as the Veterans Administration.

1935: PL 74-271—SOCIAL SECURITY ACT. Provided permanent authorization for the civilian vocational rehabilitation program and increased its budget. Established these federal programs: unemployment compensation, old age insurance, child health and welfare services, crippled children services, and public assistance to the aged, the blind, and to dependent children.

1943: PL 78-16—WORLD WAR II DISABLED VETERANS REHABILITATION ACT (WELSH-CLARK ACT). Provided vocational rehabilitation for disabled veterans of World War II.

1943: PL 78-113—VOCATIONAL REHABILITATION ACT AMENDMENTS (BARDEN-LAFOLLETTE ACT). Extended public rehabilitation eligibility to include the emotionally disturbed and mentally retarded, expanded service to include physical restoration, removed ceiling on appropriation.

1944: PL 78-346—SERVICEMEN'S READJUSTMENT ACT. Known as the "GI Bill" it provided for the education and training (tuition and subsistence) of men and women whose education or career was interrupted by military service.

1945: PL 79-176—JOINT CONGRESSIONAL RESOLUTION FOR A NATIONAL EMPLOY THE PHYSICALLY HANDICAPPED [NEPH] WEEK. Established an annually observed NEPH week. Passed in August 1945. Truman changed it to President's Committee on Employment of the Physically Handicapped in 1952; Kennedy changed it to President's Committee on Employment of the Handicapped in 1962.

1954: PL 83-565—VOCATIONAL REHABILITATION ACT AMENDMENTS (HILL-BURTON ACT). Provided the basis for future expansion through greater financial support, research and demonstration grants, professional preparation grants, state agency expansion and improvement grants, and grants to expand rehabilitation facilities.

1965: PL 89-333—VOCATIONAL REHABILITATION ACT AMENDMENTS. Accelerated the expansion and improvement of services by allotting 75 percent federal funds to the state agencies, funding state-wide planning for growth, additional provisions for rehabilitation facilities.

1970: PL 91-517—DEVELOPMENTAL DISABILITIES SERVICES AND FACILITIES CONSTRUCTION ACT. Provided broad responsibility to states for planning and implementing a comprehensive program of services to retarded, epileptic, cerebral palsied, and other neurologically impaired people.

1973: PL 93-112—REHABILITATION ACT. Placed strong emphasis on expanding services to the more severely handicapped by giving them priority. It also provided for affirmative action in employment (Section 503) and nondiscrimination in facilities (Section 504) by federal contractors and grantees.

1978: PL 95-602—AMENDMENTS TO THE REHABILITATION ACT OF 1973. Authorized the long-sought expansion of rehabilitation to include "Independent Living," as an objective and established the National Institute of Handicapped Research. Provided employer incentives for training and hiring disabled people. These Amendments extended the Rehabilitation Act for four years; over $1 billion was authorized for 1979 with substantial increases through the 1982 fiscal year.

6.8. *National Rehabilitation Association*

Generally organizations begin when people in groups try to meet their needs or to solve their problems. Usually when problems exist that cannot be resolved by individuals acting alone, group action is taken. Organizing the National Rehabilitation Association (NRA) was no exception to this rule.

6.8.1. VOCATIONAL EDUCATION SPLIT

Leaders among vocational educators could not completely identify the special requirements of a program for the rehabilitation of disabled people. People specializing in the new rehabilitation work became restless and dissatisfied with the status and priority their program was accorded in the states' vocational education administrations. These early rehabilitationists believed that this new movement would have to develop its own identity and leadership. While for many years the need would be felt to remain closely associated professionally and administratively with departments of education in the states, some of the early leaders perceived rehabilitation to be an amalgamation of many disciplines and felt that it must not be unduly dominated by any one. The National Rehabilitation Association (NRA) grew out of these convictions. Created by a group of workers in the state-federal program of rehabilitation, it has emerged as the organization that speaks for the movement in America.

6.8.2. ORGANIZING THE ASSOCIATION

At the December, 1923 meeting of the National Society for Vocational Education in Buffalo, New York, the rehabilitation specialists held a Sectional administrative meeting to talk about the notion of a separate organization. W. F. Faulkes, Director of Vocational Rehabilitation in Wisconsin, arranged a luncheon meeting that was attended by seven members of the staff of the Federal Board for Vocational Education, including J. C. Wright, Director; 16 state rehabilitation directors or supervisors; and C. A. Prosser, former Director of the Federal Board for Vocational Education and in 1923 the President of the National Society for Vocational Education.

At the luncheon meeting Faulkes advocated forming a permanent national organization of people engaged in vocational rehabilitation. Prosser, speaking as an individual and not as a representative of the National Society for Vocational Education, said that although he did not think that the Society would object to the rehabilitation groups' electing officers to preside at sectional meetings, he firmly believed that the formation of a separate national organization would be "disastrous." The discussion remained informal, but it became obvious that some of the people present were definitely in favor of organizing an association that could perform many essential functions for vocational rehabilitation and for the workers engaged in that field.

The issue of a separate organization was not fully resolved at the Buffalo meeting. R. M. Little, director of vocational rehabilitation in New York State, moved that "officers be elected for the Rehabilitation Section of the National Society for Vocational Education." At a later business session of the Rehabilitation Section (December 8, 1923) the nominating committee offered its nominations for that Section's officers, in compliance with Little's motion. D. M. Blankenship, Supervisor of the Virginia Vocational Rehabilitation Division, was elected

Chairman of the Section and J. R. Jewell, Assistant Supervisor of the Nebraska Vocational Rehabilitation Division, was elected Secretary. Present at this meeting were the representatives from the Federal Board for Vocational Education and the directors and supervisors from the state rehabilitation agencies. After a long discussion, the new name of the group, following a motion by Oscar M. Sullivan, Director of the Minnesota Vocational Rehabilitation Division, was selected: the National Civilian Rehabilitation Conference.

The new National Civilian Rehabilitation Conference met in Indianapolis in December, 1924, as a part of the National Society for Vocational Education, but at this meeting there was a sense among members that the group had its own identity. Faulkes was elected Chairman of the Conference, with Jewell as Secretary and Treasurer. Eighteen states were represented by 24 rehabilitation directors and supervisors. The meeting the next year in Cleveland was held in conjunction with the annual meeting of the National Safety Council. Many different types of activities were on the agenda, almost all relevant to vocational rehabilitation. It was at this meeting that the constitution of the new organization was submitted by a special Constitution Committee with Sullivan as its Chairman.

The organization was to be known as the National Civilian Rehabilitation Conference and have two types of membership. Active memberships would be for people working in the vocational rehabilitation of disabled civilians, in the employ of any state government or the federal government. Associate members would be people actively interested in any aspect of the rehabilitation of disabled persons. The Conference was to be quite exclusive—evidently those who voted on the new constitution did not think in terms of an association that would and could represent the wide range of individuals and agencies working in rehabilitation. Many hundreds of able and dedicated professional workers in voluntary agencies, in the Veterans Bureau, in hospitals, and in private practice were classified as associate members.

The purposes of the Conference were listed as:

1. To provide through its meetings a forum in which all phases of vocational rehabilitation of disabled civilians and problems incidental thereto may be discussed.

2. To conduct a campaign of education to bring the general public to an adequate understanding of the importance of the civilian rehabilitation movement.
3. To further so far as possible and desirable agreement upon the principles and practices in the field of civilian rehabilitation and to promote comity between the various agencies.
4. To set up a medium through which expression may be given to the views of the membership upon pending legislation and public policies affecting the civilian rehabilitation movement.

6.8.3. THE EARLY YEARS

At this 1925 meeting in Cleveland W. F. Faulkes was reelected President; M. B. Perrin of Ohio was elected Vice-President; Jewell, Secretary; J. F. Marsh of West Virginia, Treasurer. Registrations at the meeting numbered 90; most of the participants came from agencies and employment that would permit them to qualify as Active Members.

At the meeting in Memphis in March, 1927, the Conference voted that "this organization shall be known as the National Rehabilitation Association and shall be considered as having been in existence without formal constitution since the meeting of civilian rehabilitation workers in Buffalo in 1923." Henry H. Kessler proposed to amend sections of the constitution dealing with membership so that "active" membership would include "all persons actively engaged in any form of rehabilitation work." This recommendation was not accepted, even though Dr. Kessler spoke at some length against making the Association an exclusive organization.

The Fifth Annual Meeting of NRA was held in Milwaukee in September 1928, at which time M. B. Perrin completed his term as President of the Association. It was agreed to amend the constitution to allow those "engaged in rehabilitation work under private auspices" to be invited by the Executive Committee to become active members.

The Association had long been concerned that the Vocational Rehabilitation Act appeared to be a temporary measure. A special committee of NRA met and discussed with President-elect Hoover the question of the exact status of the Rehabilitation Act. The Association, although its membership was very small, was attempting to live up to its obligation to build a solid basis for the rehabilitation of disabled people. At every session of the Congress for the next 36 years, members of NRA were to appear before congressional committees and to talk to individual senators and representatives about the needs of the public rehabilitation program.

6.8.4. POLICY AND PROGRAM DEVELOP

In 1930 NRA took major responsibility for the renewal legislation for the state-federal program. It drafted its own bill and succeeded in getting it introduced in the Congress. When it became apparent that close watch would have to be kept on this legislation, the Association made a special appeal to its members for contributions to a fund to finance sending representatives to Washington as needed to lobby for passage of the required bills. The amount of $3,449 was raised by this special appeal. This was a phenomenal amount, considering that the normal budget of the Association was running at less than $200 a year.

At the 1930 Kansas City meeting the matter of membership was again reviewed and a radical change was made from the original structure. Memberships were to be of four types: individual, organization, contributing, and life. All members could vote, and the individual members were to pay dues of $1.00 a year. This change in the membership structure allowed all to feel that they were functioning on an equal prerogative basis. Any person "interested in the vocational rehabilitation of disabled persons" could become a member. The decision had been made that the National Rehabilitation Association was not to be a "professional" organization in the sense of qualification through training or vocational pursuit. The problem of providing a professional affiliation through NRA was one that was to be considered many years later. With the changes in the membership qualifications the Association would be emphasizing social action and public education rather than professional upgrading and professional standard-making, except as these objectives could be accomplished through special projects sponsored by the Association.

In 1932 NRA was very busy with new plans. Standing committees were formed to deal with planning, legislation, research, promotion, and personnel improvement. However, it was always difficult to secure financial support for the many activities and interests of the Association. In 1932 the problem grew so severe that personal loans were made by Oscar Sullivan, William Faulkes, John Kratz, Harry Hicker, and Marlow Perrin to the Association to cover current expenses. Dozens of fund-raising strategies were proposed. Oscar Sullivan wrote a 100-page booklet entitled *Courage Facing Handicaps,* which he turned over to NRA to sell as its First Yearbook. The depression was at its most severe in 1933, and great ingenuity was needed to keep the organization functioning.

The scope of the Association's concerns and activities continued to increase throughout the depression years of the 1930s. Through the Social Security Act, funding for the rehabilitation of disabled people was substantially increased in 1936 and in 1940. But, it became increasingly necessary to alter the basic provisions of the law under which the state-federal program operated. NRA worked to obtain legislation that would permit the program to grow and develop in accordance with the needs of disabled people. It was also necessary for permanent staff members to work on the publications of the Association, direct the membership campaigns, prepare budgets, and control funds. NRA had developed enough so that it could no longer function effectively by volunteer efforts.

The question of hiring an executive director had been considered at several meetings. In 1941 the Board decided to create the position at a salary of $250 a month, and Walter Chapman of Roanoke, Virginia was employed to head offices in Roanoke. He was provided with a secretary, and a total budget of $9,750 was established for the 1942 calendar year. With staff assistance and a national office, the work of the Association could be undertaken more energetically. The Association participated in the preparation and the passing of Public Law 113 in 1943 and enlarged other activities, including publications. It employed an Editor of the Journal of Rehabilitation in 1945, and in 1946 Leonard Calhoun, formerly with the Federal Security Agency and an attorney, was retained, for a fixed fee each month, to keep the Association advised on federal legislative matters. The Association was growing fast—$21,000 was collected in dues in fiscal year 1946-1947—and a goal of 5,000 members was set by the president, Voyle Scurlock, for the next year.

It was decided to permit the affiliation of "chapters" of persons interested and engaged in vocational rehabilitation. But it was not until the fall of 1947 that the Board of Directors approved the new position of Executive Secretary. The Executive Committee recommended E. B. Whitten of Mississippi for the position of Executive Secretary of the Association. His appointment was approved by the full Board and he began work in Washington, D.C. on July 1, 1948, continuing in the office for 26½ years. Under his leadership NRA became a powerful force. It grew in membership and in the size of its budget. By 1965 there were well over 22,000 members and the income was $220,000.

When Whitten first became Executive Secretary the organization was relatively small and activities were quite limited. But it soon became necessary for him to have help in both the internal and the external administrative and professional tasks for which his office was responsible. The Association created the position of Assistant Director and recruited A. D. Puth to fill it in 1954.

The Association has chapters throughout the nation and has formed several divisions to accommodate specialty interests [Crumpton, 1978]. Its National Rehabilitation Counseling Association has its own Executive Secretary to look after its affairs. The formation of divisions (see 2.2.1) reflects the growing complexity of the vocational rehabilitation movement and the desire of the National Rehabilitation Association to serve and lead it.

Whitten's NRA accomplishments are documented in the rehabilitation legislation advancements of the period described in the previous section.

6.8.5. THE FLORIDA TEST CASE

After Whitten retired as Executive Director of the National Rehabilitation Association on December 31, 1974, Puth, who had served NRA with excellence for a number of years as the second in command, was made Acting Director. Then in August, 1975, Diane S. Roupe was hired as the Executive Director. It was to be a trying time for both Roupe and NRA.

In 1975 the State of Florida reorganized its Department of Health and Rehabilitation Services so that state rehabilitation was merged into a general human services agency. This was not in compliance with the Rehabilitation Act of 1973, which protected the integrity of the rehabilitation service delivery system. The National Rehabilitation Association, recognizing the potential harmful effects on persons with disabilities, challenged the legality of this reorganization in the courts.

The Florida law did not specify a single organizational unit for the rehabilitation program, and the functions of the program were split. The Rehabilitation Program Director had no line authority over the program, its staff, or the delivery of client services [National Rehabilitation Counseling Association—American Rehabilitation Counseling Association, 1975].

LaVor and Duncan [1976] outlined the conflict between the Florida Plan and the requirements of federal law: "Over the past few years, several states (Florida most recently) have attempted to reorganize the departments within their states into comprehensive or umbrella type units which become single human services agencies. States claim this is being done because it will streamline the delivery of rehabilitation as well as other services" [p. 26].

The newsletter of the NRA in May, 1977 defended its intervention in the Florida matter, which it called the "overriding issue." It pointed out that there was no longer an identifiable vocational rehabilitation agency in Florida after reorganization, except for a small office of 33 out of some 700 previous personnel. All personnel were assigned to 11 human service district offices, none of which had administrators with a rehabilitation background or interest.

According to the newsletter, the Association was compelled to respond to the reorganization of the Florida Vocational Rehabilitation program because it would reduce the quality and quantity of services to handicapped people and not only weaken the program in Florida but also serve as a precedent for other states. It reported that the leadership of NRA believed in the necessity of obtaining counsel to represent it rather than relying on HEW lawyers, having observed HEW's viewpoint in Florida and other states. The 1975 NRA Delegate Assembly had in fact voted to commit "all possible resources," and this vote was implemented to the fullest extent. It acknowledged regrettably that communication to the membership did not offer them opportunity to understand fully NRA's involvement in Florida. It denied that the Florida matter required an inordinate amount of staff time or that these efforts were responsible for any problems or delays in other NRA services and activities. Roupe referred to the "Florida test case" as her

"number one objective" for NRA. She resigned at the end of 1976 after this and other administrative difficulties. Amos Sales was the able Acting Director during a difficult period from February 1, 1977 to June 30, 1977.

By mid-1977 Dr. Sales, as outgoing Acting Executive Director of NRA, made this report:

I would like to identify a few of the major problems I inherited upon assuming on February 1, 1977 the Acting Executive Director's responsibility of implementing the Association's program and budget . . . . On the first of February, the staff was confronted with many problems needing solution. Solutions were found, but because of space limitations here, I can only share a few of the more major tasks we had to face. The *Journal* publication was six months behind schedule with the November-December issue not ready for press. Discussions with our publisher indicated that we could not get back on schedule in terms of publication this year. The November-December issue was mailed and, upon approval of the Board, we published a combination January-February, March-April issue of the *Journal* on April 18, 1977. . . . In the last year-and-a-half the NRA national office staff personnel dropped from a high of twenty-four to ten in the middle of May, 1977. The major problem faced was financial. Although major efforts were taken by the Executive Committee during their meeting on January 28–29, and by staff following that meeting, the Association in reality at that time was locked into another deficit spending year. The primary factors contributing to this include over-optimistic estimates regarding membership income and substantial expenditures over contributions relative to the Florida Fund. Once a firm awareness of the total financial picture was obtained, the leadership of the Association found itself in the position of needing to borrow $90,000 to meet outstanding obligations for the 1976–77 fiscal year and to meet cash flow needs through September 1977.

An austere budget was necessary to keep the Association from bankruptcy. Staff and salaries were cut, and the Washington headquarters and other expenses were reduced. Whitten had presented and adhered to conservative budgets in earlier years and had built the reserves of the Association, although budget deficits were foreseeable by 1972. An expensive plan of reorganization contributed to NRA's financial plight. With return to conservative fiscal management the organization resumed its leadership position in search of the solutions of rehabilitation problems of the nation's disabled people.

Richard Oestreich was appointed the new Executive Director by the Board of NRA in

September, 1977, following the resignation of
Sales to return to academic employment. Oestreich brought excellent credentials for the post.
He had been Administrator of the Ohio Rehabilitation Agency and, before that, Rehabilitation Director of Goodwill Industries of
Central Ohio; and he had a graduate degree in
rehabilitation administration.

"You remember the fall of 1975 when, in Cin-
cinnati," Oestreich [1978] reminded the NRA
membership, "we agreed as an organization that
'the buck stops here.' NRA would brook no
such organizational structure as was devised in
the State of Florida for the vocational rehabilitation services. All of the effort and resources
spent between then and now have consummated
in this thorough-going and conclusive judgment"
[p. 1]. The U.S. District Court ruled in March
1978 that the configuration of the Florida vocational rehabilitation services was in violation
of the law. The NRA won a long and expensive
legal battle—but the war over the administrative
integrity of rehabilitation continues.

Oestreich resigned in April 1979 to enter doctoral studies in psychology. Although NRA had
been on the brink of bankruptcy, he left it in a
financially stable position. Susan Eggers, who
had been employed by NRA in various positions
for several years, was Acting Director through
September 1979. Earlier in the year the Association had employed, on a part-time but continuing basis, Jack Duncan as its General Counsel.
This attorney, who from 1969 to June 1979 was
Staff Director of Rep. Brademas' Subcommittee
of the U.S. House of Representatives Committee on Education and Labor, has provided
legislative advice of great value to the rehabilitation movement. David Mills became national director of NRA October 1, 1979. Mills, well
known and highly respected in rehabilitation,
had been the Facilities Coordinator for the State
of Iowa rehabilitation agency.

The administrative and financial difficulties of
the NRA in the decade of the 1970s are directly
associated with the so-called Florida test case.
The underlying turmoil, however, was the
struggle for proper recognition of rehabilitation
as a viable alternative to chronic dependency.
Rehabilitationists feared that the established effectiveness of their approach for restoration of
independency to disabled persons would be disrupted if rehabilitation were absorbed into general human welfare administration. These fears
were reinforced by the Florida case in which the
vocational rehabilitation agency was integrated
into a general agency with a social work orientation. The Inspector General of U.S. HEW at the
end of 1979 released an audit that sharply
criticized the Florida rehabilitation program as
administered by its combined social services
agency: the auditors charged that the total
number of clients rehabilitated fell by 52 percent from 1973 to 1977, and that the case load
dropped by 29 percent; it was recommended
that the state of Florida pay back $2.3 million in
federal funds charged inappropriately to rehabilitation. It is clear that the integrity of the rehabilitation effort may be compromised when administered (at either state or national level) by
other disciplines such as social work, medicine,
or education.

Chapter 7

Public Rehabilitation

The United States, unlike most other developed countries, still clings to a provincial operation of direct human services. Federal administration for civilian rehabilitation was seriously considered by the Congress from 1918 to 1920 when matching federal funds were authorized for the states to administer their own programs. From the start, however, the federal law and administrative regulations have dictated state conformity to nationwide guidelines. Thus, each state rehabilitation agency must provide services as stipulated federally to a defined group and meet certain minimum standards in order to receive matching funds.

While nothing precludes expansion of the minimum scope of rehabilitation services, states generally do not appropriate more of their own money than necessary to receive the allowable federal support. Consequently, rehabilitation service patterns are similar from one state to another. There are some striking differences, however, among states and regions in their interpretation of policy and local needs. Some of the differences in patterns of service are based on regional priorities. For example, many of the states in the southeast and south central regions have spent proportionately more on physical restoration than most northern and western states. This program flexibility accommodates variations in area needs.

Federal expenditures for rehabilitation rose rapidly, from less than $50 million in 1955 to $150 million in 1965 to $550 million in 1970 and over $1 billion after 1975. The 1978 Amendments to the 1973 Rehabilitation Act added new programs and provided authorized ceilings for doubling the appropriations for some activities by 1982.

Nationally the pattern of expenditures and services changes only gradually. Over half of all state rehabilitation funds are expenditures directly for clients (purchased services for individuals). Another one-third of the total budget is for client counseling and placement (agency professional staff salaries). Under 10 percent of the cost is for administration. Of the total amount of money spent in services for individu-

als, the categories and approximate percentages are: client training, 40 percent; physical and mental restoration, 22 percent; diagnosis and evaluation, 16 percent; maintenance, 14 percent; and other purchased client service, 8 percent. In the training category there has been a substantial shift so that college training is now under 30 percent of total expenditure while training for personal and vocational adjustment has gone up to over 30 percent of the training budget; vocational school training is about 20 percent; and business school training is around 6 percent of the budget with miscellaneous training taking the rest.

This chapter will describe the American public rehabilitation system, and the focus will be on the operational level: the state rehabilitation agency.

7.1. State Agency Administration

This overview of the administration and operation of the state rehabilitation agency presents a point of view other than that usually obtained by the practitioner. The kinds of information covered in other chapters—in discussions of professional techniques in the rehabilitation process—focus on the individual client. But a different perspective on the services operation, that of the administrator, is described here.

7.1.1. INTRODUCTION

The term *administration* has different meanings and, used broadly, is virtually synonymous with operation. Strictly defined, administration refers to executive functions at the highest, policy-making level of an organization. *Management* is a related term indicating an executive stratum just under the administration level. *Supervision* refers to the next level, implying responsibility for the organization's operations as carried out by the employees who do the directly productive work—in this instance the rehabilitation counselor. While direct service activities are the central functions of the agency, administrative activities are necessary to facilitate the professionals' work with clients.

A primary function of any administrator is the

formulation of long-range goals and agency policies. In public agencies these goals and policies are structured by higher government authority, that is, the elected officials (e.g., President, Governor) and the lawmakers in the Congress or state legislatures. Still the state rehabilitation agency administrator must interpret and implement public laws and regulations to mobilize organizational resources for an effective rehabilitation service delivery program. While the annual financial allocation of a public agency is decided by higher authority, its specific budget is drawn up by the agency administration. Annual objectives are set according to service priorities and incorporated in the state rehabilitation plan. This plan is accompanied by a budget formulated as a part of systematic program planning and budgeting (PPB) processes.

There are various PPB strategies, but the key is to plan for the period according to selected objectives that are given priority according to criteria consistent with the long-range goals of the organization. Management by Objective (MBO) is a device by which every decision made contributes to the achievement of a carefully chosen objective of the organization. Yet despite this structuring, program development is a dynamic and fluid process responsive to evolving needs and changing resources. Revisions are based upon ongoing program evaluation, systems analyses, and operations research data as well as input from a management team headed by an executive charged solely with this agency function. All state rehabilitation agencies are required by the federal government to prepare detailed program and budget plans in order to participate in federal cost sharing.

Another major administrative function is control over fiscal affairs. The financial management of a state agency is complicated by the varied nature of rehabilitation cases, which have no typical pattern of need, and also by the many kinds of purchased services from various outside agencies and professionals (viz., schools, prosthetic firms, physicians, rehabilitation facilities, and others).

Program performance is the ultimate concern of the state administrator. A criterion of excellence for services provided by the agency to its clients translates administratively to setting, facilitating, and enforcing standards for operations and personnel. Quality service to handicapped people is the goal of everyone in the agency. Administrative personnel are responsible for organizing and coordinating the system for integrated effort and productive teamwork for internal and external programming. Administration also means the execution of daily routine procedures such as issuing and monitoring directives and the surveillance of financial and other management matters. In a healthy managerial environment all employees—state director and other central office administrators, supervisors, and counselors—attend to the growth and productivity of their subordinates in accordance with the team goal of effective client service by the agency. Contrary to popular thought, leading in excellence and enlisting enthusiasm is everyone's responsibility in rehabilitation. Still, leadership, by definition, begins with the chief administrator who is obligated to accept the responsibility commensurate with authority.

The most successful administrators of state rehabilitation agencies are career professionals who started as field counselors and have been gradually promoted through the ranks of supervision and management of the agency. A trend in the 1970s was for some governors to appoint "business administrators," politicians, or severely disabled persons who had neither the agency experience nor the professional preparation needed to head a state rehabilitation agency. Fortunately, many states have civil service or other job descriptions and requirements that stipulate an appropriate rehabilitation background (e.g., several years employment in rehabilitation and a masters or doctoral degree relevant to rehabilitation).

The history of rehabilitation documents the critical role of state rehabilitation agency administrators in obtaining needed federal legislation and administrative policy [Obermann, 1965]. Program expansion and improvement have come about in large measure because of the devotion and influence of these articulate and politically astute state directors. They have promoted legislative action through their contacts with elected representatives and their maintenance of a good public image for rehabilitation. Public relations, however, must be conducted by an enthusiastic staff under the leadership of the agency administration.

Other organizational operations provide for the implementing of administrative mandates. These include: the state plan for federal grant funds, personnel practices, administration of funds, administrative operations, local office supervision, and the administration of services.

7.1.2. FEDERAL GRANT-IN-AID

Before the United States Congress established the civilian program of vocational rehabilitation, it was debated whether the program should follow the model of the veterans rehabilitation program and become a federal agency, or whether it should follow the model of the state-federal program for vocational education and thus be operated by the state governments. It was decided in 1920 to make civilian vocational rehabilitation a state-federal program, a partnership operation of the federal and states' governments, each with a specific responsibility but having a reciprocal obligation. The objectives of the Congress were, through federal financial participation, to stimulate the states to undertake rehabilitation of their handicapped citizens and to equalize the financing of these programs. It was assumed that the national agency would provide leadership through the administration of federal "grant-in-aid" funds for state agencies.

Over the years the federal rehabilitation

agency has furnished leadership to the states, including operations research and administrative guidelines, but not direct services to disabled clients. The state rehabilitation agencies have the responsibility of providing the administration of purchased services and casework necessary for offering rehabilitation to the handicapped individuals within each state. Grant-in-aid did in fact serve as a federal stimulus to all of the states and enlisted their participation and collaboration in the public rehabilitation program.

Vocational rehabilitation is one of the oldest grant-in-aid programs in the nation, although all such programs operate on very much the same principles. Federal public law sets forth the purpose, scope, and duration of the program and authorizes the amount of federal funds to be used and the matching ratio, as well as other financial terms. Moreover, the federal law specifies the general terms and conditions for each state's participation. States participating in a federal grant-in-aid program such as rehabilitation must agree to the terms set forth in the federal law as well as its regulations, thereby ensuring nationwide standards.

Uniform standards for the operation of all state rehabilitation agencies are obtained by virtue of the federal regulations written by the federal government (i.e., officially, the Secretary of the U.S. Department administering the Rehabilitation Act). These administrative regulations interpret the intent of the federal legislation but are more detailed; they stipulate more explicit guidelines for the state agencies participating in the federal funding. For federal grant-in-aid support, the state governments must agree to these guidelines in a legal agreement between the state government and the federal government: this contract between the two levels of government is called the "state plan." The state plan is a detailed statement of the proposed operation and must be consistent with the federal law and regulations. Independent living services administered by the state rehabilitation agency require a separate plan although it may be consolidated with the state's plan for vocational rehabilitation. Each state plan has some features that are mandated by the federal government, but each also has unique features. State options permit variations that respond to individual state needs and preferences.

Of the states' expenditures for rehabilitation services, 80 percent are matched with federal grant-in-aid. This "subsidy" from federal tax revenues has two general conditions: (1) that a currently approved state plan is followed, and (2) that the state government appropriates 20 percent matching funds (i.e., one state dollar for four federal dollars). The amount of appropriated federal funds made available to a state varies according to the individual state's population and needs.

In the organization and administration of the program, the state rehabilitation agency has a number of specific functions. Each of these must be exercised according to the degree of its importance in the program. Some of the principles, methods, and objectives of these functions are discussed later in this chapter.

7.1.3. PUBLIC FUNDS

Because public rehabilitation agencies are operated through tax dollars, it is incumbent upon the administrators and other employees to consider carefully the wisdom and legal appropriateness of expenditures. There is a general assumption that the responsibility for economical and appropriate administration of government funds is even more important than administration of expenditures from private, nonprofit corporation budgets. Another reason for the efficient administration of agency funds is that government appropriations for rehabilitation have never been adequate to meet the pressing needs of clients and would-be clients; reductions in administrative overhead release funds for client services. There are also legal constraints with regard to the manner in which public funds may be spent. Fiscal matters are closely audited by accountants employed by both state and federal governments. Improper use of public funds or equipment by any employee is a very serious offense.

Complex programming and budgeting and other administrative practices are followed by state rehabilitation agencies. As indicated earlier, state rehabilitation agencies must have a federally approved state plan in order to qualify for grant-in-aid. There is always the potential threat that the federal rehabilitation administration will withhold subsidy for failure of the state to comply with federal regulations; in fact, however, even delay in the federal matching funds is rare.

Purchased services for cases constitute the

largest category of expense in the operation of a public rehabilitation agency. Financial reporting controls may be administered at the state headquarters level with computer input for case expenditures and other data. The fundamental responsibility, however, for the commitment of case funds for purchased services is, of course, the counselor's. An audit of these expenditures such as is conducted periodically by accountants may require examination of counselor case records. Consequently, justification for all purchased services must be clearly recorded.

It should not be assumed that recording and accounting are only administrative concerns. Much of the data thus collected is of great value in planning and budgeting for improvement of the agency's operation. This has direct impact upon the expansion and improvement of services for future clients of the agency, since operations analyses help the agency to improve its own practice. Adequate study of the effectiveness of the agency's operation also provides documentation for legislation that is needed for expanding the program's budget to provide new staff, facilities, and services to new clients.

7.1.4. STRUCTURE AND OFFICES

Some understanding of the operations of the public rehabilitation program is obtained from a picture of their physical facilities. The offices of professional staff and the administrative facilities, of course, vary greatly from state to state. In most states, the state agency for rehabilitation, typically a part of a larger department of state government, has been called a "Division" (viz. State Division of Vocational Rehabilitation or DVR). In other states the rehabilitation agency is called a "Bureau", "Department", "Commission", "Office", or "Service". While several state rehabilitation agencies are independent, most are affiliated with the state department of Education or Vocational Education, Social and Rehabilitation Services, Health and Social Services, Labor or Human Resources, or some similarly termed multiservice organization. (About half of the states still have a Commission for the Blind or separate rehabilitation administration for severely visually impaired cases.)

Whatever the administrative aegis, federal legislation and regulations have mandated the administrative integrity of the state rehabilitation agency; consequently, each state has a director explicitly charged with the administration of the state rehabilitation program and must have its own professional staff explicitly assigned to the program's responsibilities. The central rehabilitation office may be physically housed with its administrative agency of the state government (e.g., the state department of education) and is usually located in the state capitol. In some states, however, the central rehabilitation office has been placed in the area of the state where there is the greatest demand for services, as, for example, in the largest city rather than a small state capitol. Such an arrangement is possible because the central office staff is given sufficient administrative authority to conduct its work without constant consultation with the officials of the administrative agency. An important consideration is accessibility to other state agencies that provide workers compensation, health, welfare, education, and employment services.

State rehabilitation agencies vary in the nature of the administrative authority structure. When authority is centralized the state agency maintains a large consulting and administrative staff in the central office. On the other hand, a decentralized system of administration delegates greater authority to district and/or local offices.

The 1978 Amendments to the Rehabilitation Act authorized a federal grant program to enable American Indian tribes to administer the provision of rehabilitation services to handicapped American Indians residing on reservations.

Branch offices of the state rehabilitation agency have been established to bring services closer to potential rehabilitants. As the program has grown over the years, more and more community-based offices have been opened in order to improve service delivery and facilitate "outreach" to unserviced cases [Katz, Wright & Reagles, 1971]. Until the program expansion in the 1950s and 1960s, most states maintained district offices only in larger cities; the professional staff—called "itinerant" counselors—were required to drive considerable distances to remote areas to make contact with clients and cooperating resources.

Rehabilitation offices should be accessible to clients in terms of their proximity and the availability of nearby transportation services. Rehabilitation offices should not have architectural barriers that might discourage would-be applicants or cause clients any inconvenience.

7.1.5. PERSONNEL ADMINISTRATION

Setting and maintaining standards for providing professional services to clients of the agency are a primary responsibility of the agency's administration. First and foremost there must be qualified personnel or the disabled public cannot be properly served. Personnel policies therefore must provide for the selection of the best available professional staff. At one time state rehabilitation agencies were obliged, through state patronage practices, to accept political appointees. Even the federal Hatch Act, which outlawed political activities by public employees whose salaries were paid even in part by federal funds, did not prevent abuses. It was not uncommon for the staff of a state agency to lose their jobs upon the election of another party into state offices. While the federal government attempted to. provide safeguards against purely political appointments, the federal administrators would approve a state plan that provided for "minimum standards" for professional personnel qualifications. Rehabilitation personnel in the early years were at best minimally qualified by virtue of their previous training and experience.

Gradually personnel standards evolved so that state rehabilitation agencies were allowed and encouraged to employ the best qualified people available and to provide them "tenure" assurance. The only justification for dismissal became misfeasance (misconduct in office) or nonfeasance (inadequate conduct) in office.

By far the most important agency personnel development was the advent of the rehabilitation counselor education programs, which provided a constant flow of truly qualified professional rehabilitation counselors. Civil service agencies, which for most state agencies are responsible for recruitment and selection of personnel, normally give preference to individuals with a masters degree in rehabilitation counseling, although in some states otherwise qualified people may be employed as beginning counselors.

The 1954 amendments to the federal Rehabilitation Act authorized not only preservice professional education (the masters degree preparation of rehabilitation counselors) but also expanded the training of counselors already employed by state rehabilitation agencies. Thus, extensive in-service training programs were conducted (by the public agencies) to upgrade the professional knowledge and skills of already employed workers. The state rehabilitation agencies, with federal assistance, continue this development programming at all levels of the agency staff. Counselors can now indefinitely extend the depth and breadth of their knowledge about disability and rehabilitation processes.

Federal funding has been used also for outservice training (training provided at a university or other outside source of instruction). There are regional rehabilitation centers for continuing education in each area of the United States. Also, federally sponsored Rehabilitation Research and Training (R&T) Centers offer specialized instruction in areas such as mental retardation. The federal rehabilitation agency has also participated by sponsoring the development of training materials explicitly for state staff.

On-going training for employed rehabilitation personnel is administered through the staff development or training specialist(s) in each state agency office. Even though the organization offers training through universities and central office training supervisors, the most important duties of the line supervisor should be to train for the professional growth of the staff as well as to keep them informed about agency regulations. Senior counselors can also assume training roles; formal training responsibility is often assigned to experienced counselors for the clinical practice supervision of college students from rehabilitation counselor education programs and also for the orientation of newly hired employees. Moreover, the informal instruction of one's colleagues, through the example of good practice and availability for consultation, is a noteworthy contribution made by any well-qualified rehabilitation counselor.

There are many other personnel management functions that accommodate and stimulate a productive professional staff. These practices include: acceptable procedures for merit increases of staff members' salaries; appropriate fringe benefits (e.g., vacations, health insurance, retirement plans); promotional policies that encourage the career development and productivity of candidates and that select the best qualified supervisors and administrators; opportunity for professional growth and satisfaction of career counselors as professionals without promotion to the supervisory role; accommodation of professional practice, including staff offices with proper privacy, availability of needed equipment, and secretarial and aid services; and the freedom and encouragement to exercise professional judgments in casework and planning services without the bureaucratic agency interference that results from unnecessarily elaborate record-keeping, overly explicit rule books to follow, cumbersome signoff forms, or unduly close supervision.

The public rehabilitation program has traditionally been able to avoid many of the bureaucratic casework procedures found in other public human service agencies, such as public welfare. This freedom of staff action is particularly valuable because of the unique problems that each case presents and the uniqueness of the strategies required for rehabilitation services. Unfortunately much of this traditional flexibility of the state rehabilitation counselor has been eroded away by the installation of accountability reporting requirements that restrict the exercise of independent professional judgment. Professional workers are best able to decide what client services are required, how much casework money needs to be spent, how much time needs to be invested, and what constitutes a satisfactory job objective. It is ironic, therefore, that the exercise of professional judgment was restricted by federal and state regulations during the 1960s and the 1970s when, for the first time, professionally prepared rehabilitation counselors became available and were hired for these responsibilities.

Since the 1973 Rehabilitation Act and other federal and state mandates for affirmative action, the public rehabilitation agencies have made a special effort to employ and promote from among minority groups. This administrative policy is significant in that it includes the employment of black, Spanish-speaking, and other minority members on the counseling staff. There is good reason to think that this practice can result in improved and expanded service to the disabled members of minority populations.

7.1.6. SUPERVISION

"Field" supervisors of a rehabilitation office have direct authority over local operations and professional staff. This supervisor, who often works under a district supervisor, has various responsibilities. The most important activity of any counselor supervisor is to assist the counselor in performing and developing effective professional services to the clients of the agency [Emener, 1978]. The role of counselor supervisor is thus not authoritarian but rather that of a teacher and a consultant for improved professional practice; but a supervisor also has managerial functions, serving as a communication link between the state administration and the practitioner in matters such as agency policies, working plans and budgets, reporting forms and procedures, and the overseeing of the day-to-day operations of the office.

One of the most important functions of any supervisor is the continuing evaluation of the staff and the recommendation for such personnel actions as promotion, discharge, transfer, and pay increases. Direct supervisors also have responsibility for promotion of the program throughout their assigned territory. Working with the counseling staff, the supervisors help to establish satisfactory working relationships with community agencies, thereby taking leadership in public relations. They are also responsible for much of the orientation, and perhaps selection, of new counselors and have a responsibility for assigned activities of the entire staff. State rehabilitation agencies generally have several levels of line supervision, from supervisors in charge of counselors or support personnel to those who superintend supervisors. (The term *line supervision* means direct authority over staff; it is contrasted with *staff supervision*, which implies responsibility over a program function or segment but does not carry direct authority over the operations staff.)

7.1.7. PROVISION OF CASE SERVICES

Strictly speaking, vocational rehabilitation is casework service. The casework method—as opposed to group methods—is necessary because of the individual differences among handicapped applicants, their life situations and goals, and the individual nature of rehabilitation case services. Clients differ in age, sex, physical capacity, mental abilities, economic circumstances, vocational competencies, interests, and rehabilitation needs, to name only a few variables. They cannot be assembled in groups for the purpose of receiving a category of rehabilitation service. All must be served on an individual basis, that is, there must be a unique plan for service based upon the unique needs and resources of each applicant. For this reason, the administration and regulations of the organization should be flexible so as to permit such differentiation of treatment.

There are a number of principles for the provision of case services, the application of which is necessary to ensure that clients receive a maximum of personal, economic, and social benefits as a result of the rehabilitation process. These principles are listed below.

1. The rendered services should be the best services for the individual. Each client is unique and there is no "typical" client. Differential selection of services is based on a profile of client's needs and objectives, and every plan of client service is individualized.

2. The services rendered should be adequate to accomplish the social and economic adjustment of the handicapped person. The goal is not just to get the individual a job, but to attain total rehabilitation. The impact of rehabilitation should not be just temporary, but should be permanent, barring unforeseen eventualities such as further disablement. This means that services should be comprehensive in scope and extent.

3. Services provided by the program should supplement rather than take over the initiative of the client. The principal factor in rehabilitation of a client is the establishment or reestablishment of self-sufficiency and self-reliance. Put another way, it is the purpose of rehabilitation service to help disabled persons help themselves through counseling and facilitating services. This tenet should not be construed to mean that clients who lack initiative can be neglected or "closed out" as "unmotivated." The initial ser-

vice of the rehabilitation counselor is to stimulate initiative and to help the client overcome barriers to motivation.

4. Services must follow through to a satisfactory conclusion. Rehabilitation is an active process requiring follow-through to prevent interruptions in the flow of services. Close monitoring can overcome barriers that surface in the course of implementing even a well-planned rehabilitation program. Continuous contact is maintained by the rehabilitation worker to prevent interruptions in case service and to assure the accomplishment of rehabilitation.

5. The services should utilize community interests and facilities in the rehabilitation plan. Whenever possible the rehabilitation should be accomplished within the client's own community. This is in the interest of future social and economic adjustments. Community involvement is also an expression of the obligation of the community to participate in the program.

6. The services sponsored by the rehabilitation agency must be rendered according to a plan developed by the client with the guidance and concurrence of the counselor. With the sound foundation of vocational assessment and counseling, differences of opinion do not often occur between client and counselor over rehabilitation planning. The agency must abide by what it deems feasible and consistent with its authority. This is determined by the counselor, but within these limits the client makes the choice.

7.2. *Case Management*

Case management and case load management are essential functions of the state rehabilitation counselor. The term *case management* refers to the counselor's managerial activities that facilitate the movement of each rehabilitant through the service process. The counselor as a "manager" of the case process of each individual is responsible for effective activity at each step: case-finding, intake, eligibility determination, assessment, counseling, plan development and implementation, service provision and supervision, job placement and follow-up, and postemployment services. This responsibility depends on the rehabilitationist's professional

abilities coupled with planning, coordinating, and managing skills.

Case load management refers to the responsibility of the counselor for the progress of the whole group of clients who constitute the counselor's case load. It is actually the collective result of the counselor's work with individual clients. Case load management requires such administrative talents as observation, evaluation, decision-making, monitoring, and recording.

7.2.1. REPORTING CASE FLOW

Case flow is the movement of clients through successive stages of the rehabilitation process from application to closure. The federal rehabilitation agency requires the state agencies to report annually their program efforts, that is to say, the cumulative result of the case efforts of their rehabilitation counselors. Every state rehabilitation counselor regularly reports progress with each case. This progress is measured through checkpoints such as the client's completion of a given service, or conversely, regression or suspension of services when service fails or is interrupted. Checkpoints in the process, such as being declared eligible, entering a training program, graduating, and getting a job, have been identified for purposes of recording. Standard numerical codes for them have been established by the federal rehabilitation agency. These case reporting codes are uniformly used throughout the nation and will be described briefly here.

7.2.2. STATUS CODES

The public vocational rehabilitation process is categorized in stages (checkpoints of progress) identified by a series of numbered statuses. Each client status has a two-digit code that is fed into computers for information storage and analysis. These status codes show where every client is in the rehabilitation process at any given time. Status numbers and their meaning for the process are as follows:

00 Referral
02 Application acknowledged
04 Extended evaluation (six months)
06 Extended evaluation (eighteen months)
08 Ineligible (from status 02, 04, or 06)
10 Eligible (from status 02, 04, or 06)
12 Rehabilitation plan completed
30 Unsuccessful closure (from status 12)
14 Counseling
16 Restoration
18 Vocational training
20 Service completed
22 Trial employment
24 Service interrupted
26 Successful closure
28 Unsuccessful closure after receiving some help (from status 20, 22, or 24)
32 Postemployment service

Most of the client services identified by these status categories are discussed in various chapters of this book. For example, ineligibility status 08 is used when medical and other evaluations indicate that the applicant is not entitled to services; it is also used when the counselor certifies that it is impossible to determine eligibility due to lack of cooperation, death, and so forth.

Importance of Procedure

The size and nature of counselor case loads vary greatly. Some state agency counselors will carry as few as 25 clients while other rehabilitation counselors may have 250 or more active cases. The size of the case load depends on state policies, pressures for service, characteristics of the case load, counselor initiative and capabilities, and other circumstances. Similarly, the nature of the case loads varies, with some being especially difficult, time-consuming, and costly. Evaluating and summarizing the overall picture is difficult because of the complexities of and differences between the case loads carried by different counselors.

A general survey of case load data has many values. Collectively at the federal, state, regional, and district levels, case load data is needed for program evaluative comparison—of one area to another or one year to the previous period. Moreover, the pooled reports show trends and gaps that document future needs for new or reallocated funding. The combined reports also permit comparison for incentive purposes, such as, for example, rewarding personnel who have been more productive. Counselors can also compare their case loads with those of other counselors and those of previous periods. In the same way the counselors can inspect the movement of their clients within their case loads. Perhaps the most positive value of such reports is to rehabilitants whose counselor is alerted to the fact that their rehabilitation is not progressing. The counselor's attention is needed when the client does not move from a service status on time.

7.2.3. MANAGEMENT TECHNIQUES

A report of the Third Institute on Rehabilitation Services [U.S. IRS, 1965], edited by John Muthard, discussed case load management for agency staff. Case load management is linked to the concept of case management because both are dictated by the agency objectives for cases. Case load management was defined in the IRS report as "The use of techniques . . . to control the distribution, quality, quantity, and cost of all aspects of case work activities in order to accomplish the program goals of the agency" [p. 12]. Responsibility is at all levels—administrator, supervisor, counselor, and other staff levels.

The objective of case load management is to serve the greatest number of rehabilitants at the least possible cost consistent with the highest standards of quality. It involves the sum total of a counselor's job activities and techniques used in the rehabilitation process.

Principles

Principles of the rehabilitation counselor's managerial activities include the following:

1. Work planning controls the work day; this avoids the necessity of responding to one emergency after another. The work pattern should be diversified, but the daily time schedule is based upon priorities.

2. Decision-making is the critical variable in effective case management. On the basis of the best information available, the counselor makes decisions objectively but in accordance with the informed wishes of the responsible client.

3. Case selection priorities are adhered to as set forth by agency guidelines. Since 1973 the federal mandate has been to serve first the severely handicapped. Before 1973 a "balanced" case load was a public agency principle.

4. Management techniques are employed for directing and facilitating the work of people and processes to achieve desired goals.

5. Authority is used as the basis of management. In this instance the authority is of four kinds: program authority—the authority of the rehabilitation counselor to commit the limits of statutory and executive directions; budgetary authority—the counselor's power to provide public funds for purchased or other agency services representing a financial outlay; personal authority—the counselor's right to organize casework responsibilities and other assignments, to plan time schedules, and (within broad limits) to set case priorities; and professional authority—the influence the counselor exerts on clients and the system by virtue of knowledge, dedication, and skills.

Management procedures can help the counselor become more effective, and consequently more helpful to all clients served. Learning how to evaluate one's own efforts leads to the improvement of those efforts. Guidelines have

been published by Henke, Connolly, and Cox [1975].

Managing Time

Productive workers not only keep busy but also invest their time wisely. Productive activities (e.g., counseling and planning, client assessment, job placement, resource development, interagency teamwork) suffer when the counselor is inefficient or spends too much time on unnecessary travel and paperwork. Research shows that counselors vary greatly in use of their time; some counselors are able to complete required office work expeditiously, perhaps because they do not waste time in long coffee breaks and small-talk with staff and others. Research also shows that the average amounts of time in various categories of activities are linked with training; counselors with a professional masters degree seem to spend their time more effectively.

A good technique for the practicing rehabilitationist is to periodically keep a daily time log in order to reveal problem areas. Categories to log should include counseling and planning, clerical work, recording, placement contacts, contacts with interagency resources, supervision of client plans and programs, public information, travel, professional development, supervisory and management conferences. All types and methods (face-to-face, correspondence, telephone) of activities and contacts (with and about clients) should be informally appraised for their productivity; many professionals set aside a few minutes at the conclusion of each day for such reflection and subsequent planning.

Planning ahead through a daily schedule for every week is useful and need not be a chore. A developmentally compiled "to-do" list provides a basis for scheduling. Sometimes it is best to postpone an activity (a "procrastination basket" collects problems that do not have to be addressed at once and may be resolved spontaneously in time). Long-term projections of needed actions (e.g., rewriting a contract, reviewing a client's progress) require some sort of chronological "ticker file." Desk and/or personal appointment books are essential.

Elements of Work

A principle of scientific management requires appreciation for the elements of work. When the elements of a task are identified it becomes clear how the task can be performed more easily or more quickly, or both. The task may be less cumbersome when arranged or performed differently, or it may be delegated to a clerk or another person. Just rearranging tasks and their elements can reduce the complexity. It is generally advisable to group task activities so that one does not change activities often—efficient counselors engage in a small number of categories of activities in a given day.

Work Simplification

Work simplification is a technique designed to provide better work, in less time, at less cost, with less effort, and greater satisfaction to the worker. It uses management principles to avoid haphazard or nonrational decisions. Seven operations are involved: (1) selecting the work that is to be simplified (improved) or the problems to be solved, or both; (2) obtaining facts (identifying the elements) and breaking down the work; (3) analyzing these facts or elements; (4) developing a method for improvement; (5) testing and evaluating the innovations; (6) installing the improved method; and (7) following up the work.

Several techniques are used in work simplification. Charting work performed in some kind of sampling process is a useful first step in learning how effort can be better directed. A "flow process chart" traces the sequence of work, asking, step by step, the following questions: Why is this step necessary? What is done? When should this step be done? Where should it be done? Who should do it? How should it be done? The "work count" technique involves study of the volume of work produced. "Motion economy" and "lay out" studies are techniques designed to minimize the physical effort of production by determining the simplest motion and the best physical layout for the work. Rehabilitation counselors, in learning work simplification techniques for application to their own work and improved case load effectiveness, also are enabled to better serve clients in the placement phase by their knowledge of the subject.

7.2.4. COUNSELOR USE OF TIME

A number of studies, usually analyses of counselor time logs, have been conducted on the important issue of counselor use of time. Muthard and Salomone [1969] reported, "Counseling and guidance activities are the predominant areas in which the RC [rehabilitation counselor] spends his time, but the data clearly show that he spends about two-thirds of his time performing other duties. That . . . suggests that counselor skills may often be underutilized" [p. 136]. Actually their data indicated that according to their own estimates counselors divided their time roughly into thirds: one-third solely for counseling; one-third for professional growth, reporting, public relations, resource development, travel, and supervisory administrative activities; and one-third for planning, placement, recording, and clerical tasks. While only one-third of the counselor's time is in a face-to-face client relationship, most of the remainder is spent professionally with other people (e.g., family, employers, other professionals) significant to the service process.

The time utilization of rehabilitation counselors varies according to type of case load. Katz, Reagles, and Wright [1973] compared time spent with clients in an experimental project that extended state vocational rehabilitation service eligibility to culturally disadvantaged people. There was no significant difference between the culturally and medically handicapped groups in total counselor time for the case although the latter group took less time in one-to-one counseling. For the physically disabled, the purpose of the counselor activity with and for clients and the percentages of total time were as follows: vocational counseling and planning, 36 percent; supervisory services, 30 percent; intake, 13 percent; purchasing services, 11 percent; placement and follow-up, 9 percent; and other, 2 percent. The distribution of time is somewhat different for emotionally disturbed and mentally retarded, with the latter particularly taking more counseling and planning time than the physically disabled. In another study it was reported that patterns of rehabilitation service vary as a function of client age [Thomas, Reagles, Wright, & Dellario, 1974]. More professional time and more contacts were used in job placement of older (over age 45) than younger (under age 25) clients who were physically disabled.

Rehabilitation counselors rated the importance (as they perceived it) of each of their job functions in a study by Wright, Reagles, and Scorzelli [1973]. On a five-point scale from "not important" (1) to "extremely important" (5), six job functions received an importance rating of 4 or higher: developing a plan of client services, utilizing community resources, vocational counseling, affective and therapeutic counseling, referral of clients for medical or psychological services, and job placement. Next highest were 12 functions rated from 3.5 to 4, meaning that rehabilitation counselors consider these activities important: work adjustment counseling, coordinating client services (case management), job follow-up, determining client eligibility, interpreting psychological tests, community and

public relations, conducting rehabilitation research, group counseling, case finding, vocational evaluation, providing training services, and providing restoration services. The above study of masters degree graduates showed that they were generally satisfied with their preparation for these important rehabilitation counselor functions.

7.3. Clientele

Case load data as presented in this section provide an overview of the work and human outcomes of the public rehabilitation program. Data such as the types of services provided and age of clients do not change much from year to year, and are presented here as percentages of the total number rehabilitated in the public program.

It should be mentioned that because the federal government allows considerable latitude in state rehabilitation agency practices, there is consequently variation from state to state in agency operations. National averages are reported here.

7.3.1. PUBLIC PROGRAM GROWTH

The number of disabled persons rehabilitated into employment has increased at a steady rate every decade since the inception of the public program. Because of the 1973 congressionally mandated priority for acceptance of the more severely disabled there was a numerical decline in case closures; this followed an all-time peak in 1973 and 1974 when over 360,000 people per year were rehabilitated. The annual average for each decade is listed below, and estimations are projected for the fiscal year ending September 30, 1980. The average annual numbers of successful case closures nationally were as follows:

1921–30: 4,338
1931–40: 8,778
1941–50: 41,561
1951–60: 68,485
1961–70: 160,374
1971–80: 300,000

With the exception of the reversal in growth beginning in the mid-1970s, there were yearly increases within the decades after 1933. These and other data for this section are derived from

various publications and unpublished reports provided by the federal rehabilitation agency.

7.3.2. REHABILITANT CHARACTERISTICS

A description of client characteristics at time of case closure provides an understanding of the types of people who are served by state rehabilitation agency counselors. The following data (percentage in each category) are based on national averages covering 1975 to 1979 as approximated with adjustment for trends and rounded:

Age at referral—23% under 20 years of age; 40% age 20–34; 28% age 35–54; and 9% age 55 and over (the mean average age was over 32 years).

Sex—53% were male; 47% were female.

Race—78% were white; 20% were black; 2% other.

Highest grade of school completed—19% up to 8 grades; 25% some high school; 31% graduation from high school (12 grades); 11% over 12 grades; and 14% special education (every client with mental retardation).

Marital status—33% married; 44% never married; 23% other (divorced, separated, or widowed).

Primary source of support before rehabilitation—48% family and friends; 21% public assistance or in institution; 19% current earnings; 12% other (e.g., Social Security benefits, workers compensation, and other public and private sources).

Sources of referral—15% educational institutions; 21% hospitals and physicians; 8% health organizations; 9% welfare agencies (public and private); 18% other public agencies; 3% other private agencies; 15% self-referred; and 11% referred by other individuals.

Major disability—29% mental illness; 12% mental retardation; 19% orthopedic impairment or amputation; 7% digestive system; 3% genitourinary; 4% heart or circulatory conditions; 2% epilepsy; 9% blind or vision impaired; 5% deaf or hearing impairment; 1% speech; 1% respiratory disorder; and 8% other.

Work status at referral—73% not working; 18% wage or salary workers (including sheltered workshop employees); 7% homemakers and unpaid family workers; 2% other.

7.3.3. REHABILITATION PROCESS

The nature of the process with these rehabilitated people—represented in the same format—is of interest:

Type of service provided (this totals more than 100% because many clients receive more than one kind of service)—88% diagnosis and evaluation; 43% restoration; 52% training; 23% financial maintenance; 34% other service to client; 5% service to family.

Training services (client total is 52%, as stated above)—12% college or university; 5% other academic school; 4% business school; 12% vocational school; 7% on-the-job training; 24% personal or vocational adjustment training; 12% other.

Months in training—17% under three months; 39% three to 12 months; 44% over one year of training.

Cost of case services paid for by the public rehabilitation agency (does not include other arranged services)—37% of the cases cost under $300; 18% $300 to $599; 30% $600 to $2000; 15% cost over $2000.

Months from acceptance to closure—27% under six months; 25% from six to 12 months; 25% from 12 to 24 months; 23% over 24 months.

7.3.4. REHABILITATION OUTCOMES

Successful outcomes of services can be reported in the same way:

Work status at closure—73% competitive labor market; 5% sheltered workshop; 3% self-employed; 17% homemaker; 2% unpaid family worker.

Occupation at closure—12% professional (including technical and managerial); 15% sales and clerical; 20% service; 30% industrial; 3% agricultural; 20% other.

Increased earnings—547% mean average increase (pre–post rehabilitation) in weekly earnings.

Unfortunately, many cases are not rehabilitated or are not accepted by the state rehabilitation agencies. Reasons relate to the degree of handicap, client-agency relations (i.e., client failed to cooperate, client refused the services, client could not be located) and other reasons (e.g., death, client institutionalized, transferred to another agency). Unsuccessful cases are as follows:

Cases not accepted—11% handicap too severe (or unfavorable medical prognosis); 14% handicap not severe enough for eligibility; 69% client-agency relations; 6% other reasons.

Cases not rehabilitated—10% handicap too severe; 71% client-agency relations; 19% other reasons.

7.4. *Program Evaluation*

Program evaluation means what an organization does to weigh the effectiveness of its operation, and also to plan for future improvement. This is an administrative matter and is not performed by the practitioner. The rehabilitation counselors, however, are interested in program evaluation results because of their potential impact upon the agency policy and personnel and also for the evaluative information about agency services to their clients. Professionals are as much obliged to know about the effectiveness of the services of their own agencies as they are to assess services of outside resources. (See 10.2.3.)

Either the process or the outcome of client service may be assessed through formal program evaluation procedures. Both qualitative (how good) and quantitative (how many) indicators of casework success are used. At one time the public rehabilitation agency and its counselors were credited solely on the basis of the sheer number of closures (cases "rehabili-

tated") without much reporting about the effectiveness of the process or the quality of the claimed outcome. Far better program evaluation methods have since been developed [Cooper & Harper, 1979].

The Rehabilitation Research Institute of the University of Michigan, directed by Donald Harrison, initiated a publication series on program evaluation by public rehabilitation agencies. Their second monograph, by Ralph Crystal [1978], identified evaluation problems of the state agencies by surveying their 1978 Program and Financial Plans (PFP). The PFP contains extensive data on program issues to develop agency objectives and identify resources for use in planning, administration, and evaluating programs.

The University of Wisconsin-Madison conducted a series of studies on program evaluation methods for state rehabilitation agencies [Wright, 1976]. One monograph in the Wisconsin studies described a specific model of re-habilitation program evaluation by Spaniol [1975]. For another monograph of this series, Chope and McMahon [1975] developed a classification adopted by the federal rehabilitation agency for the technology and literature of rehabilitation program evaluation. Some of the material for this section grew out of those Wisconsin studies. Additional materials are from federally sponsored institute reports on this topic [U.S. IRS, 1972; U.S. IRI, 1974; U.S. IRI 1974b]. Only those program evaluation matters of particular interest to the practitioner will be discussed in this section.

7.4.1. CLIENT OUTCOME MEASURES

Practitioners, as well as program evaluators, use client outcome measures to assess services. The methods described by Kelso [1974], as summarized below, can be implemented without specialized knowledge or large expenditure of time, effort, and funds.

Follow-up Letter

A letter sent to clients after closure is one of the simplest and least expensive methods of determining client outcome. In the letter, the purpose of the follow-up is explained and a self-addressed, postage-paid return envelope is included in which the rehabilitant can mail back the completed questionnaire. Even a low return rate of 25 percent can provide clues to the effectiveness of rehabilitation services. Typical questions that might be asked of clients are:

1. How are you presently employed?
2. Since your rehabilitation, what percentage of the time have you been employed?
3. Are you satisfied with the help given you by this agency?
4. Do you need further rehabilitation services?
5. What additional services do you feel you need?
6. Which rehabilitation services have been most helpful to you?
7. Which rehabilitation services were least effective?

The Human Service Scale

The Human Service Scale (HSS) was developed at the University of Wisconsin Rehabilitation Research Institute by S. Kravetz [1973]. The HSS measures the degree of client change (re-duction of unmet needs) during the rehabilitation process. Because the instrument identifies specific areas of client need—based on Maslow's (1954) hierarchy of basic human needs—it may also be used diagnostically. The HSS contains 80 items pertaining to seven areas of client need: physiological, emotional, economic-security, family, social, economic self-esteem, and vocational self-actualization. The instrument may be administered to each client at the time of intake or referral, and again after each service or upon completion of the rehabilitation or at any specified interval following closure. For planning purposes scores from the initial administration, compared with appropriate national norms, suggest what rehabilitation services are indicated. Results obtained at the time of closure or follow-up can be compared with those from the initial administration to estimate how well rehabilitation services have alleviated specific kinds of client needs. The instrument requires approximately 35 minutes to complete and is machine-scorable.

Consumer's Measurement Scale

The Consumer Measurement Scale (CMS) was developed at the University of Oklahoma Regional Rehabilitation Research Institute by William Hills [1973] to obtain information on the impact of rehabilitation services as viewed by the client. One part of the instrument consists of 28 items designed to measure client satisfaction with rehabilitation services in nine areas: counselor effort in placement; participation in planning; speed of service delivery; personal treatment; medical services; training services; physical facilities; agency policies; and employment satisfaction. This portion of the CMS is given to the client to complete at the time of closure, while a second portion is mailed to the client at some specified later time (e.g., three months, six months). The follow-up portion consists of 17 items designed to reflect employment experiences and satisfaction since the time of closure, services that the client now believes should have been provided by rehabilitation but were not, and the degree of satisfaction with various aspects of services.

Goal Attainment Scaling

Goal Attainment Scaling (GAS) is a well-known method of determining client change during the course of human services. Although the method was developed by Kiresuk, Salasin and Garwick [1972] for use in mental health center settings, it is applicable in most helping relationships, including rehabilitation. The strength of this instrument lies in its ability to provide an individualized client evaluation. The method involves specifying major client problems, either by the counselor alone or with client assistance, and assigning to each identified problem area a numerical value indicating its importance to the client's rehabilitation. For every problem area, the practitioner develops a behavioral description of each of five levels of outcome: an expected level, a more than expected level, a best anticipated level, a less than expected level, and the most unfavorable outcome thought likely. A value of "0" is assigned to the expected level of service outcome, a +1 is assigned to the more than expected level of service outcome, a −1 to the less than expected success level, and +2 and −2, respectively, are assigned to the best anticipated and most unfavorable outcome categories.

The identification of problem areas and possible outcome is best done when services are being planned. At this time an assessment is made of the client's present level of functioning, using the GAS five-point scale. When rehabilitation services are completed, the client's level of functioning is again rated with the same scale. A comparison of level of function scores at the time of plan formulation and at closure provides a measure of gain or loss associated with the rehabilitation process.

7.4.2. COUNSELOR EVALUATION

State rehabilitation agencies have various administrative or supervisory methods for assessing the performance of their counseling staff. Appraisal is necessary because the success of the agency most directly depends upon the counselor's work, which is an expression of his or her motivation, knowledge, skills, and other professional and personal characteristics. The traditional measure of productivity of rehabilitation counselors was the annual number of cases closed as rehabilitated (i.e., "closures"). This single measure is simple and represents a proper goal: successfully rehabilitating as many eligible people as possible. But data on total closures is deceptive: some case closures are easier than others and the temptation is to accept only quick and easy cases while denying applicants who

most need help. Moreover, the quality of the counselor's work is not recognized when only the total number of closures is counted.

Several methods have been developed to take into consideration the quality as well as the quantity of case closures made by the counselor. In one so-called weighted case closure approach, credit is given only for rehabilitants who are closed with earnings over the federal minimum wage [Noble, 1973]. Closures can also be weighted according to client satisfaction with services [Reagles, Wright, & Butler, 1970a, Reagles, Wright, & Thomas, 1972]; client gain from services [Reagles, Wright, & Butler, 1970; 1972]; sustention of rehabilitation [Gay, Reagles, & Wright, 1971]; the reduction of service needs [Sha'ked, Bruyere, & Wright, 1975]; or economic benefit derived from case service compared to service cost [Reagles & Wright, 1972]. J. B. Moriarty, at West Virginia University, suggested another alternative to Noble's simple weighting of case closures; he and R. T. Walls described the "profile analysis technique" [Walls and Moriarty, 1977]. Public agency reporting systems and computer techniques permit various kinds of evaluations for various purposes. Selection of criteria depends upon the goal of the evaluation. Muthard and Miller [1966] studied this in *The Criteria Problem in Rehabilitation Counseling*. In 1977 Rubin reviewed the status of program evaluation in public rehabilitation.

Using the number of closures or appraisal of their level of success (e.g., income at closure) in program evaluation is called an "outcome criterion." Another approach for assessing the work of the counselors is to appraise the quality of their day-to-day work; such evaluation criteria are called "process" measures of performance. A standard procedure for multifaceted assessment of staff is to follow systematically a prepared format that categorizes work requirements as performance criteria. State rehabilitation agencies have developed such aids for line supervisors to observe and report on how well counselors execute their responsibilities at work. These lists of behaviors need not be definitive, but they should represent a sampling or overview of what a counselor does. The following list of items has been compiled as an example of the content of a counselor performance appraisal or evaluative criteria of professional activities:

1. Counseling:
   Maintains a good client-counselor relationship.
   Counseling is effective and focuses on the problems.
   There is maximum client participation in counseling and planning.
   Counseling problems consistent with agency goals.
   Counseling consistent with counselor competencies.
   Counseling assists client positively and efficiently.
   Counselor motivated and behavior is professional and ethical.
   Sessions well-planned and arranged and time budgeted as needed.
   Contacts adequate in number, frequency, and length.
   Clients satisfied with progress and outcome.
   Total time in counseling in balance with case load responsibilities.

2. Evaluation and determination of eligibility:
   Reports and correspondence completed satisfactorily.
   Relevant histories, reports, and other information secured.
   General medical report in the record.
   Specialist examinations adequate and necessary.
   Clients and consultants prepared for the examination.
   Diagnostic data secured according to plan.
   Objectives adequately evaluated and reports utilized.
   Major problems recognized.
   Appropriate action taken after evaluation.
   Eligibility determination properly documented.
   Eligibility (feasibility) and priority decisions sound.

3. Utilization of consultants:
   Case consultant help sought for required information.
   Consultations secured in proper sequence.
   Choice of consultants appropriate and wise.
   Consulting reports used in preparing the plan.
   Case problem and background presented to consultant.

4. Preparing the individualized written rehabilitation program (IWRP):
   Client fully participates in and concurs with the IWRP.
   Realistic and suitable goals established.
   Full utilization made of client's interests and potentials.
   All of client's unmet needs covered in the IWRP.
   Everything covered in the plan for the rehabilitation objective.
   Justification of plan established.
   All parties concerned (including referral source) notified.

   IWRP details specified (e.g., dates, responsibilities, amounts).

5. Determination of financial need:
   Needs statement filed when required.
   Accurate analysis made of financial needs.
   Client's ability to contribute toward cost of rehabilitation explored.

6. Use of community resources:
   Relevant resources informed about rehabilitation services.
   Works effectively with resources in obtaining their service.
   Works effectively with resources in getting case referrals.
   Monitors and evaluates purchased services for clients.
   Makes informed choices and use of service resources.
   Relates well with staff of resource agencies.

7. Placement and follow-up:
   Assesses client assets and interests.
   Assesses requirement of job under consideration.
   Matches client assets with job requirements.
   Helps client develop job-seeking skills when indicated.
   Uses industrial directory and develops job resources.
   Makes contacts with employers and former employers.
   Utilizes other resources (e.g., State Employment Service).
   Follow-up adequate to assure satisfactory job adjustment.

8. Case recording:
   Entries of contacts adequate (descriptive and complete).
   Recording entered promptly and documents casework activity.
   All agency records accurately and confidentially maintained.

9. Planning and implementing services:
   Decisions based on adequate information.
   Client participates actively throughout.
   Assistance sought as needed on difficult problems.
   Prompt and appropriate case actions taken.
   Decisions respect client's rights and wishes.
   Case in appropriate status with information recorded.

10. Case load management:
    Plans work with priorities to maintain a maximum case load.
    Client assumes responsibility whenever indicated.
    Effectively utilizes all relevant community resources.
    Plans balance between field and office work.
    Systematizes activity to keep cases moving toward goal.

11. Public relations:
    Promotes the rehabilitation program locally with good public relations.
    Informs local officials and legislators about the agency work.
    Counselor well regarded professionally in the community.
    Cooperates with community agencies and professionals.
    Obtains good interpersonal relations with agency staff.
    Participates in rehabilitation-related organizations.
    Good relationships obtained with rehabilitants, families, and so on.
12. Office management:
    Letters and memoranda well written.
    Arranges time for uninterrupted periods of office work.
    Spends a reasonable amount of time performing office work.
    Prepares accurate, complete, concise, and current records.
    Has proper and productive relations and roles with staff.
    Accepts supervision and administration rules.
    Manages time to maximize direct service opportunities.
    Prepares essential reports and forms promptly and accurately.
    Interprets and uses reports properly.
13. Professional maturity and development:
    Demonstrates professional knowledge and skill; exercises good case judgment.
    Identifies with vocational rehabilitation professionally.
    Regards the agency and its work positively.
    Performs work according to agency and ethical standards.

Seeks to improve performance by professional development.
Participates in in-service and supervisory training sessions.
Evaluates own performance and growth.

7.4.3. TASK PERFORMANCE ANALYSES

The above criteria for the evaluation by supervisors of rehabilitation counselors constitute a rather gross measure of how well they perform. A much more sophisticated procedure was developed at the University of Wisconsin for the Council on Rehabilitation Education by Wright and Fraser [1975, 1976]. Their Rehabilitation Task Performance Evaluation Scale is a comprehensive list of 294 items that covers most of what counselors do in all of their functions for a state rehabilitation agency. The Scale provides a measure of the counselor's effectiveness on specific job tasks rather than on the outcome of their work through measurement of the benefits achieved by rehabilitants. Other methods for evaluating counselors do not provide a behaviorally specific picture of how well the counselor is doing at various functions. The task evaluation approach, on the other hand, yields a diagnostic profile of the counselor's strengths and weaknesses specific to the actual behavior on the job. Moreover, it provides a comprehensive view of performance since virtually all activities of the counselor are defined on the task evaluation scale [Fraser & Wright, 1977]. Supervisors, therefore, can direct their attention toward job components that require improvement through in-service training and closer supervision.

7.5. Federal Rehabilitation Agency

Administration of the state-federal rehabilitation program is described in various places in this book, so only a brief overview is provided here. Previous sections of this chapter have described the state rehabilitation agency that offers services to handicapped individuals. The federal agency, however, has important administrative responsibilities. Affairs are conducted not only out of its offices in Washington, D.C., but also out of ten regional offices located across the nation.

7.5.1. HISTORICAL BACKGROUND

The federal rehabilitation agency has undergone several changes in name and administrative affiliation. Initially (1920) civilian vocational rehabilitation was administered (along with veterans rehabilitation) by the Federal Board for

Vocational Education. In June, 1933, President Roosevelt transferred functions of the Federal Board to the Department of Interior; there the Secretary of Interior in October, 1933, placed the administration of vocational education and vocational rehabilitation programs in the U.S. Office of Education. Then in 1939 Roosevelt established the Federal Security Administration (FSA), to which the U.S. Office of Education was transferred along with the Vocational Rehabilitation Service as a component. The Office of Vocational Rehabilitation (OVR) was created in September, 1943, as an agency of the FSA, but not under the Office of Education. OVR, along with other human services, was moved into the new U.S. Department of Health, Education, and Welfare (HEW) when it was established in 1953. In January, 1963, OVR was designated the Vocational Rehabilitation Administration (VRA) and the Director of OVR became the Commissioner of VRA reporting directly to the HEW Secretary. In August, 1967, the Social and Rehabilitation Service (SRS) was established within HEW with five major divisions, including the Rehabilitation Services Administration—formerly the VRA. (Mary Switzer, who had previously headed first OVR and then VRA since 1951, retired as the first Administrator of SRS in 1970.) In the mid-1970s, various administrative changes culminated in the dissolution of SRS and resurrection of RSA as an agency separate from Social Service.

In 1980, the federal rehabilitation agency and its related programs were placed in the U.S. Department of Education (U.S. DOE) that had been established by a 1979 Act of Congress. This action completed a full circle of federal rehabilitation administrative aegis from education to health and other human services and then back to education. The original association was with vocational education while the new relationship is with special education (i.e., U.S. DOE, Office of Special Education and Rehabilitation Services).

7.5.2. NATIONWIDE SERVICES

The federal rehabilitation agency administers the program mandates of the U.S. Congress, which enacts rehabilitation legislation that is signed into public law by the President. It also, as described earlier, sets forth federal regulations to which the state rehabilitation agencies must conform; as a consequence, the definition of services is applied nationally.

Public vocational rehabilitation services, federally defined as any goods or services necessary to render a handicapped individual employable, are listed below:

1. Evaluation of vocational rehabilitation potential, including diagnostic and related services incidental to the determination of eligibility for, and the nature and scope of, services to be provided.
2. Counseling, guidance, referral, and placement, including postemployment services necessary to maintain employment.
3. Vocational and other training services, including personal and vocational adjustment, books, and other training materials.
4. Services to family members of eligible individuals when such services are necessary to the rehabilitation of the handicapped individual who is undergoing services.
5. Physical and mental restoration services, including, but not limited to, treatment or corrective surgery, hospitalization, therapeutic recreation, prosthetic and orthotic devices, dental services, eyeglasses and visual services, and treatment for mental and emotional disorders.
6. Maintenance, not exceeding the estimated cost of subsistence, during rehabilitation.
7. Interpreter services for deaf individuals, and reader services for blind individuals.
8. Rehabilitation teaching services and orientation and mobility services for the blind.
9. Occupational licenses, tools, equipment, and initial stocks and supplies.
10. Transportation in connection with the rendering of any vocational rehabilitation service.
11. Telecommunications, sensory, and other technological aids and devices.
12. Management services for small businesses operated by the severely handicapped, including the acquisition by the state agency of vending facilities.
13. Placement in suitable employment.
14. Post-employment services as necessary.
15. Other goods and services as needed.

In addition to all of the above listed services for vocational rehabilitation, independent living rehabilitation clients may be offered these special rehabilitation services:

1. Housing, including appropriate modifications of space used.
2. Therapeutic treatment.
3. Health maintenance.
4. Attendant care.
5. Peer counseling.
6. Recreational activities.
7. Services to children, including the development of communication and other skills.
8. Any preventative services to decrease future needs for rehabilitation services.

Services are provided to eligible handicapped individuals, on the basis of a mutually developed written plan, in order to help such people achieve and maintain total rehabilitation. Some state rehabilitation agencies require that the financial need of a handicapped individual be considered in order to determine the client's participation in the financing of certain services. The state agency must also first consider the availability of "similar benefits" (i.e., the client may obtain the help from some other agency or source) before expending funds for certain services. Consideration of similar benefits is specifically required for medical services and maintenance—the latter refers to subsistence payments while the individual is undergoing rehabilitation services. Another requirement is consideration of similar benefits to pay all or part of the costs of training in institutions of higher education. Neither financial need nor the availability of similar benefits is considered with regard to the following services: evaluation of rehabilitation potential to determine eligibility and the nature and scope of services needed; counseling, guidance, and referral services; and job placement. It is to be noted that consideration of financial need or similar benefits applies to possible payment of all or part of the costs of certain services by the client or a third party, and is not a factor of eligibility.

7.5.3. NATIONAL COUNCIL ON THE HANDICAPPED

The 1978 Amendments to the 1973 Rehabilitation Act established the National Council on the Handicapped. Composed of 15 Presidential appointees, the National Council representing handicapped individuals includes people from national organizations, service and administration, medical and research facilities, and business and labor organizations. At least five members must be handicapped individuals or parents or guardians of handicapped people.

Duties of the National Council are as follows:

1. To establish policies for and review the operation of the National Institute of Handicapped Research.
2. To provide advice to the Commissioner of the federal rehabilitation agency regarding its policies, conduct, and programs.
3. To review and evaluate all policies, programs, and activities concerning the handicapped.
4. To recommend to the Department Secretary ways to improve research, disseminate findings, and facilitate implementation.
5. To submit annual reports to the Secretary, the Congress, and the President on the federal rehabilitation agency and on the National Institute of Handicapped Research.

This Council has defined administrative powers and an authorized staff of technical and professional employees. Council members are compensated for their duties and expenses.

7.6. Research and Training

7.6.1. INTRODUCTION

Prior to the American rehabilitation research initiative there was no scientific foundation for understanding the problems of handicapping or developing techniques of vocational rehabilitation. Rehabilitation client service efforts depended upon the trial and error experience of field workers and scattered attempts to borrow relevant techniques from other fields.

Rehabilitation research and professional training programming was founded and funded by the United States government in 1954. Public Law 565 (83rd Congress), signed by President Eisenhower, ushered in a better era for the disabled in this country by authorizing the administration of federal grants to provide research-based new knowledge and trained personnel for informed service to handicapped adults.

Adaptations from related disciplines and professions suffered from a lack of funds for systematic development and creditable demonstration. There was no organized body of knowledge directly applicable to and tested for rehabilitation until federal research programming stimulated these needed studies.

Even if an explicit and research-based fund of knowledge and skills had existed in the mid-1950s, there could have been only limited utilization because no system had been established for professional preparation of agency practitioners. Rehabilitation counselors were seldom prepared for counseling or any of the other skills needed to help vocationally handicapped persons. The lack of trained personnel was a critical limitation to the growth of services. The training program not only provided the foundation for expansion of rehabilitation to all disabled people, but also improved the quality of services. Research and training also increased capability to serve the severely disabled who had been previously considered infeasible.

Research is the foundation for every profession and so it is with rehabilitation. For the first 15-year period, the federal administration of the research and demonstration program unfortunately failed to screen out many agency applications for client service projects that had no research potential. Moreover many projects were approved that had little relevance. Despite generally poor cost-effectiveness, however, a number of projects with important goals were funded to competent research organizations, and thus the technology of rehabilitation was advanced [Wright & Trotter, 1968]. Beginning about 1970, dictated by administrative procedure, the federal agency started making its own decisions about the problems in the field of rehabilitation and often about who should conduct research, such contracts frequently going to business firms. Funds that should have been invested in research to improve professional technology were diverted for operations research on problems of the federal agency.

The most productive mechanism for rehabilitation research has been programmatic studies (i.e., ongoing research conducted in a university research facility organized to investigate a core subject). Rehabilitation Regional Research Institutes (RRRI) and many Research and Training (R&T) Centers, established by the federal rehabilitation agency, have produced practical

research and trained staff in conducting core research relevant to the public rehabilitation program. Centers were authorized explicitly in the federal legislation, but most of the R&T funds have been designated for medical or engineering research rather than for finding new techniques for vocational and life adjustment.

Even while there were administrative inefficiencies, the substantial federal funds for vocational rehabilitation research and training have been productive. The resulting technology in fact has established the profession of rehabilitation counseling. Other nations are only now beginning to develop university rehabilitation education programs after the American model [Wright, 1969a]. Rehabilitation research-based knowledge and skills thus have become an "exportable" technology—not for profit as with munitions shipped to other countries, but for the good will of people everywhere interested in improving the lot of disabled and disadvantaged persons.

7.6.2. NATIONAL RESEARCH INSTITUTE

The 1978 Amendments to the 1973 Rehabilitation Act created the National Institute of Handicapped Research as an agency separate and detached from the Rehabilitation Services Administration, which had previously administered rehabilitation research and related programs. Authorization of the new Institute included programs such as: the dissemination of rehabilitation research information and educational materials; public information services and professional conferences, workshops, and in-service training programs; and the production and dissemination of statistical reports and studies on the handicapped. Research fellowships were also authorized. Ninety percent of the funds of the Institute were stipulated for grants or contracts with appropriate review by peers (experts in rehabilitation). A long-range plan was requested to identify the problems of the handicapped—especially problems related to employment—and to specify funding priorities, goals, and timetables for activities.

The Institute as authorized has the broad goal of improving the provision of not only vocational adjustment services but also other rehabilitation services. It will continue the support of Rehabilitation Research and Training Centers operated in collaboration with universities. These Centers include basic or applied medical rehabilitation research and research on the psychological and social aspects of rehabilitation, as well as research related to the vocational aspects.

Research endeavors are extended beyond the work age range to include handicapped children as well as people over age 60. Mention is made, too, in this 1978 legislation of telecommunications research and various model projects. A model research and training program was authorized for developing new methods of enhancing the employment potential of handicapped individuals. Authorized (maximum) funding for the Institute was $50 million for the fiscal year ending September 30, 1979, with annual increases to double that amount in four years.

7.6.3. RESEARCH ACTIVITIES

Federal financial assistance since 1954 has been provided to projects for the development of methods, procedures, and devices to increase knowledge and improve the methods of rehabilitation. The financial assistance discussed here is grant support to non-federal governmental units, universities, and other organizations (including profit-making firms).

Key terms are defined below [U.S. HEW, Office of Human Development, 1976].

RESEARCH. Research means scientific inquiry, investigation, examination, or experimentation aimed at the discovery and formulation of new principles or uniformities describing replicable facts, testing of specific hypotheses, revision of accepted theories or better understanding in light of new facts, or practical application of such new or revised theories or understandings to test their general validity.

DEMONSTRATION. The term *demonstration* means the application in new settings of results derived from previous research, development, testing, or practice for the purpose of establishing the reliability or further validation of new rehabilitation procedures, or for determining their cost-effectiveness.

DEVELOPMENT. Research development means the use of available knowledge and technology to achieve a workable prototype of a system, process, device, and so on, the logic and use of which is defined.

GRANT. A grant is money paid by the federal government to eligible organizations to carry out a discrete activity or program, or to assist in meeting the cost of conducting same, authorized by a Federal law with a finite termination date and an approved budget.

PROJECT. A project is a discrete activity with a finite termination date.

PROJECT DIRECTOR OR PRINCIPAL INVESTIGATOR. This is a qualified individual designated by the grantee or contracting organization and approved by the grant or contract-awarding organization to conduct the study, project, or demonstration.

PROJECT OBJECTIVES. The state objectives of a project are the significant, observable, measurble results that are expected to be achieved during the project period.

RESEARCH UTILIZATION. Developmental activities seeking to link research findings to planning, policy-making, program administration, and service practice are called research utilization.

The scope of federally funded rehabilitation research and related projects includes:

1. Medical and other scientific, technical, methodological investigations into the nature of disability, methods of analyzing it, and restorative techniques.
2. Studies and analyses of industrial, vocational, social, psychological, economic, and other factors affecting rehabilitation of handicapped individuals.
3. Studies and analyses of the special problems of the homebound and institutionalized individuals.
4. Studies, analyses, and demonstrations of architectural and engineering designs adapted to meet the special needs of handicapped individuals.
5. Feasibility studies, demonstrations, and developmental projects in any of the above areas.
6. Related activities that hold promise of increasing knowledge and improving methods in the rehabilitation of disabled individuals with the most severe handicaps.

There is also an international program of federally sponsored rehabilitation research of great consequence [McCavitt, 1977].

The R&T Centers established by the federal rehabilitation agency in selected universities have the unique synergistic mission of:

1. Assisting in preparing and increasing the number of research and other rehabilitation-related professional and nonprofessional personnel where manpower shortages exist.
2. Disseminating and promoting the application of the new knowledge resulting from research findings.
3. Incorporating rehabilitation education into all rehabilitation-related university undergraduate and graduate curricula.
4. Improving the skills of existing rehabilitation personnel and the effectiveness of rehabilitation services through seminars, workshops, study groups, and short and long-term in-service and continuing education programs.
5. Conducting programmatic research focusing on a limited number of high-priority core area problems requiring in-depth study and having immediate relevance and application to the rehabilitation of severely handicapped people.

Rehabilitation research funding is most liberal for the whole field of rehabilitation medicine and related medical areas, the narrow topic of rehabilitation engineering, and the broad subject of mental retardation. Comparatively little money is designated for the advancement of knowledge and techniques of the vocational rehabilitation processes (i.e., vocational evaluation, counseling and planning, resource development, and job placement and development). This is despite the fact that there is no other major source of federal research funds for the nonmedical vocational adjustment problems of the handicapped population.

7.6.4. INFORMATION UTILIZATION

One of the brightest areas of the federal research and training programming in rehabilitation has been the promotion of research utilization. There is always an unfortunate time lag in any field between the discovery of new knowledge and its application. Thus, research findings are not translated into practice until potential users are informed. Depending upon the research results, changes may be indicated in professional practice, agency policy, or organizational structure. The prospect of change, however, often meets with consumer resistance, which must be overcome by selling or even modifying the research product to maximize its usefulness.

Procedures of research utilization require far more than mere publication of results. First and foremost the research that is funded and conducted must be utilizable—results must have relevant problem-solving potential. Then there must be a strategy developed for the dissemination of results to target groups who could benefit from them. The transmission of information is accomplished by a carefully devised diffusion plan that must be included on the researcher's application for federal rehabilitation funds.

Information storage and retrieval has become a monumental problem because of the creation of so much new knowledge, attributable in part to federal support of the sciences. Fortunately, computer hardware and sophisticated systems, also underwritten or operated by the government, have facilitated knowledge utilization.

Computerized libraries have been established for mammoth collections of books, journal articles, monographs, and research progress and final reports. Examples include systems operated by the Lockheed Corporation and the *New York Times*. The U.S. Department of Commerce operates the National Technical Information Service (NTIS), a sprawling installation at Springfield, Virginia, which for a small price provides microfiche (or even paper) copies of federally subsidized research reports (including those on rehabilitation). Other computerized information systems are operated by the National Institutes of Health (MEDLARS) and the Department of Education (ERIC). Comprehensive taxonomies (i.e., organizations of topic descriptors) have coded terms to "enter" or tell the computer what subjects are being searched for in a review of the literature. Computer terminals have been installed in strategic locations around the country (e.g., large universities and research centers) for direct access to these master storage computers. References and abstracts may thus be obtained at once.

The federal rehabilitation research utilization program has collaborated with these computerized libraries and has developed its own taxonomy of rehabilitation terms. The rehabilitation research utilization program has also adopted many of the techniques pioneered for

American farmers by the U.S. Department of Agriculture Extension Programs and operated through state land grant universities. One such federal project provided for research consultants visiting state agencies [Butler & Wright, 1975].

7.6.5. TRAINING PROGRAMS

The federal rehabilitation agency makes grants and contracts with states and public or nonprofit agencies and organizations, including institutions of higher education, to pay part of the cost of training projects. This is to increase the number of personnel trained in providing services to the handicapped and in performing other necessary functions. Grants have been awarded in the following fields of training: rehabilitation counseling, rehabilitation medicine, rehabilitation nursing, vocational evaluation and work adjustment, rehabilitation social work, rehabilitation psychology, rehabilitation psychiatry, physical therapy, occupational therapy, speech pathology and audiology, rehabilitation facility administration, prosthetics and orthotics, job placement, rehabilitation recreation, undergraduate education in rehabilitation services, and other fields contributing to the rehabilitation of handicapped individuals.

The federal rehabilitation agency [U.S. HEW, RSA, 1977] stated the following objectives for training grants:

1. To increase the supply of personnel available for employment in public and private agencies involved in the rehabilitation of physically and mentally handicapped individuals, especially those individuals with the most severe handicaps.

2. To improve the quality of professional practice in service to the physically and mentally handicapped, with special emphasis on those who are the most severely handicapped.

3. To ensure the maintenance of basic skills and knowledge of personnel engaged in programs serving handicapped individuals and simultaneously provide opportunities for such individuals to raise their level of competence and broaden their expertise [p. 3].

Grants may be either long-term, for support of basic or advanced professional training offered on an academic year basis, or short-term, for support of nonrecurring training needs in technical matters through workshops and so forth of short duration. Some training grant support is administered by the federal regional offices while other projects are of national scope. Teaching grants are given to defray instructional costs (e.g., faculty salaries). Traineeship grants are awarded to the teaching institution or agency for the support of awards to trainees, thereby attracting better-qualified applicants.

The federal rehabilitation training grants program has been very successful. As a direct result of this program, respected institutions of higher education have initiated and continued viable rehabilitation education curricula. Most notable is the rehabilitation counselor education (RCE) development: while only several small RCE programs existed before grant support became available in 1955, there were about 100 well-established, RCE programs twenty-five years later. A description of professional preparation programs has been given in Chapter 2, The Profession.

Chapter 8

Rehabilitation Facilities

During its first 25 years the public rehabilitation program largely neglected the utilization and development of rehabilitation facilities as a needed resource. Until the 1943 Amendments to the Vocational Rehabilitation Act, federal authorization so restricted the state agencies that rehabilitation facilities were seldom used. The most severely disabled (e.g., the mentally retarded and emotionally disturbed) were generally ineligible; state rehabilitation services were limited generally to training and education (i.e., physical restoration was not provided); and the casework approach was influenced by educational guidance and testing techniques (vs. methods such as behavioral observation and situational evaluations that are used in facilities).

Despite the fact that vocational and medically oriented facilities predated the public rehabilitation program, the two systems were not interrelated until the eligibility, services, and methods of state-federal rehabilitation were expanded in 1943. Even then the fee-for-specific-service-practice by state agencies held down the use and expansion of facilities. Facilities could not be built, staffed, and operated on the uncertain and inadequate income from occasional, individually authorized client fees. Inadequate budgets also curtailed referral of clients by state rehabilitation counselors to the relatively costly services that could be purchased from facilities for severely disabled people.

By 1954 it became apparent that public funds would be needed to support a system of rehabilitation centers and workshops, and the federal Rehabilitation Act was significantly amended again. Grants for private, nonprofit facilities were authorized. Establishment grants provided for the expansion and modification of buildings and provision of new equipment. Expansion and improvement grants to facilities made possible a financing of joint projects with the state rehabilitation agencies. Subsequent federal legislation (notably the 1965 amendments) has continued and improved this relationship. Even greater dependency of government programs on a viable network of rehabilitation facilities emerged from the 1970 Developmental Disabilities and Facilities Act expanding services, the 1973 Rehabilitation Act, mandating greater emphasis on the severely disabled, and the 1978 Amendments to the 1973 Rehabilitation Act, extending the purpose of rehabilitation to include independent living.

The population of people needing the services of facilities is enormous. In a comprehensive service needs study conducted by Greenleigh Associates, for the federal rehabilitation agency in the 1970s, it was estimated that the number of severely handicapped, noninstitutionalized population in the age bracket of 18 to 64 was over four million. One conservative estimate is that at least 20 percent of these individuals could benefit from some form of sheltered workshop service. This does not take into account an additional percentage who may be in need of the service of some other kind of rehabilitation facility [U.S. IRI, 1977a].

A 1971 book by Nathan Nelson and the comprehensive report by Greenleigh Associates [1975] were important sources of information for this chapter. Other books on the subject of rehabilitation facilities include those edited by Hardy and Cull [1975] and Cull and Hardy [1977].

8.1. Introduction

Facilities are to rehabilitation what schools are to education. Rehabilitation facilities (like the school system) constitute programming for an important human service. One should not think of the building because it is the *program* that makes the facility. The rehabilitation accomplishment derives from the staff, techniques, procedures, and resources (including housing and equipment) as they facilitate effective programming.

A rehabilitation facility is defined here as a place (program) that helps handicapped people overcome or adjust to their functional limitations. Within this definition there are four things that distinguish a rehabilitation facility from other types of institutions and agencies: (1) the facility is not merely a "place"—it is a program; (2) a rehabilitation facility helps "handicapped people"—this clientele differentiates it from places that serve other populations (e.g., public schools for normal youths); (3) the goal of a rehabilitative facility is to "correct or overcome" a problem—this goal differentiates it from places that are not intended to rehabilitate (e.g., a custodial or penal institution); and (4) the rehabilitation facility's primary focus is on the "functional limitations" that result from medical disablement—this program emphasis differentiates the rehabilitation facility from medical treatment institutions and agencies (e.g., general hospitals and medical clinics).

In this chapter three prominent kinds of rehabilitation facilities will be described: rehabilitation centers, rehabilitation workshops, and rehabilitation residences. Other rehabilitation facilities not covered here include:

1. Mental (rehabilitative) hospitals.
2. Mental health centers and clinics.
3. University-affiliated retardation facilities (UARF).
4. Training schools for the disabled (e.g., the retarded, deaf, blind).
5. Speech and hearing clinics.
6. Low vision clinics.
7. Mobility training services.
8. Substance abuse clinics.
9. Correctional institutions.
10. Nursing homes.
11. Recreational centers.
12. Centers for independent living.

Center programs for independent living and recreation are described in Chapter 40.

8.1.1. OVERVIEW

For purposes of clarity, a brief overview of rehabilitation facilities is presented before giving a more thorough description in subsequent sections on workshops, centers, and residences. The federal Fair Labor Standards Act (Section 14), which set regulations, provided the definition of "workshop": a charitable organization or institution conducted not for profit, but for the purpose of carrying out a recognized program of rehabilitation for handicapped workers, and/or for providing such individuals with remunerative employment and other occupational rehabilitating activity of an educational or therapeutic nature [Greenleigh, 1975].

A "rehabilitation center" on the other hand, has been defined as a "facility which is operated for the primary purpose of assisting in the rehabilitation of handicapped and disabled persons through an integrated program of medical, psychological, social, and vocational evaluation and services under competent professional supervision" [Allan, 1958, p. 46].

In recent years the differentiation between these two types of facilities has become less clear. Generally, the rehabilitation center provides comprehensive psychosocial and vocational evaluations, medical and physical diagnosis and treatment, social casework, supportive counseling and psychotherapy, work adjustment and vocational counseling, skill training, and placement. Sometimes, however, the program may include paid-work activities; in such cases this part of the program closely resembles that of a workshop. The rehabilitation center clients generally live in the facility (e.g., hospital).

In comparison, the workshop in a community does not house clients and its primary emphasis is on providing rehabilitation services through the medium of work for which wages may be paid as a means of helping vocationally handicapped persons to achieve or maintain their maximum work potential. While many workshops offer vocational evaluation, work adjustment, and vocational training alone to accomplish these goals, medical, psychological, social, and other services are available to clients in many workshops. In these instances, the workshop takes on dimensions of a rehabilitation center.

Rehabilitation residences are still another type of facility. They provide an alternative to or transition from an institution. There are various types, some of which are referred to as "halfway," "quarterway," or "three-quarterway" houses, and others are called "in-houses" and

"out-houses" (meaning "instead of going into" or "getting out of" an institution, respectively). All such residences are rehabilitative in nature, providing services of varying types and intensities to assist in maximizing human potential. While the rehabilitation center may emphasize medical service, and workshops may focus on the benefits of work, rehabilitation residences use the dynamics of socialization to facilitate community adjustment.

In general all rehabilitation facilities are characterized by the following unique features:

1. A protected environment wherein handicapped people can obtain skills, support, and supervision fundamental to their overall development without some of the distractions and tensions of outside society.
2. A team approach by specialists who synchronize their individual services and areas of expertise to meet clients' needs as they progress toward their rehabilitation goals.
3. A program goal of helping individuals move from a dependent to an independent role.

8.1.2. DEFINITIONS

The terms defined below have been selected as particularly relevant to the subject of rehabilitation facilities; other pertinent concepts are described later in this chapter. Additional terms relating to rehabilitation facilities are defined in chapters in the Parts titled Assessment, Counseling, and Placement.

DEINSTITUTIONALIZATION. This term refers to the principles of normalization and least restrictive environment, according to which retarded and emotionally disturbed individuals and other handicapped persons are either moved out of institutions into community living arrangements or prevented from being institutionalized by using alternative community care and training.

RESIDENTIAL INSTITUTION. These are either private or state-supported places designed to provide housing, care, and other services to dependent people.

RESPITE CARE. This is temporary care provided in foster homes, institutions, or group homes in which individuals spend up to two weeks. This provides a period of rest or freedom for their parents, attendants, or guardians.

REHABILITATION RESIDENCE. A community-based living arrangement as a substitute for institutionalization is known as "alternative" or "transitional housing." Retarded, emotionally disturbed, and other handicapped individuals live in halfway houses, group homes, or other residences with varying levels of supervision and kinds of services.

COMMUNITY-BASED FACILITY. A local facility that offers needed services for people living within the area is referred to as a community-based facility.

FUNCTIONAL INDEPENDENCE. This is the level of self-care and self-determination that one's physical, mental, and emotional capacities permit, to the extent that housing, care, and other environmental circumstances facilitate. Satisfactory social goals may be achieved when individuals are brought to functional independence even if remunerative employment is not obtained.

ADULT DEVELOPMENT CENTER. This type of facility teaches severely handicapped adults those skills necessary for daily living. Such skills may include home management, leisure time utilization, grooming, social graces, transportation utilization, work orientation on a prevocational level, and personal and interpersonal awareness.

WORK ACTIVITY CENTER (WAC). A WAC is a facility that provides purposeful work and social, developmental, and recreational programs for a community's severely handicapped adults, regardless of their productivity.

EXTENDED EMPLOYMENT. This term refers to a handicapped person's employment in a protected situation for an indefinite period of time.

SHELTERED EMPLOYMENT. This is remunerative employment supplied under conditions designed to meet the various employment needs of handicapped individuals. The employment may be long-term (extended) in duration or even permanent (terminal).

SHELTERED WORKSHOP. A workshop that provides sheltered employment, this type of facility serves individuals who cannot obtain

competitive employment. It gives them an opportunity to work in a protected environment at their level of functioning.

TRANSITIONAL WORKSHOP. This provides assessment and training services along with transitional employment and work experience to enable handicapped people to become competitive in the open labor market or become otherwise employed.

ACTIVITY PROGRAM SERVICES. These are the rehabilitative roles of various disciplines including art, dance, music, occupational therapy, and recreation.

UNIVERSITY-AFFILIATED FACILITY (OR PROGRAM). This refers to interdisciplinary programs in centers sponsored by the federal government to demonstrate innovative methods of delivering services, to train specialists, and to conduct research in developmental disabilities.

8.1.3. HISTORICAL BACKGROUND

Since an account of the rehabilitation movement and the treatment accorded disabled people has been provided in Chapter 6, History of Rehabilitation, only a supplementary view will be given here. A more thorough record is given in Nathan Nelson's *Workshops for the Handicapped in the United States: An Historical and Developmental Perspective* [1971].

The 1800s saw the rise of public interest in human service and rehabilitation-related facilities. These facilities and their services were, in fact, forerunners of the public program. Massachusetts, Pennsylvania, and New York pioneered efforts. In 1837 the Perkins Institution for the Blind near Boston began the first workshop-type program in the United States. Also in Boston, a transitional care residence was opened in 1864 for women released from institutions. New York attempted to establish a workshop for the blind during this same period, but the effort failed, although a halfway house that did survive was opened in New York City in 1845. In 1874 a workshop for the blind and in 1899 a transitional care facility for offenders were established in Pennsylvania.

These early efforts, while scattered, were followed by others in other states, and the history of facilities had begun. Around the turn of the twentieth century, a number of religious and other groups began establishing workshops. Goodwill Industries, St. Vincent de Paul, Volunteers of America, and the Salvation Army began salvage programs that employed the handicapped—those physically disabled, aged, or alcoholics.

Concurrent with advances in medicine during this same period, the beginnings of the facility that has come to be called the rehabilitation center emerged. In 1889 the Cleveland Rehabilitation Center had begun as a program for crippled children (later for disabled adults as well). The New York Institute for the Crippled and Disabled (ICD) in 1917 and the Curative Workshop of Milwaukee in 1919, were other pioneers. These early facilities provided medical, psychological, and vocational services, thus leading the way to comprehensive rehabilitation programming. In addition, in 1913 the first transitional care residence in the United States for people with emotional disorders was opened in Massachusetts.

Rehabilitation facility services continued to grow throughout the first half of the twentieth century, but at a slow rate. The major thrust began during and following World War II. Professional and public interest and concern were stimulated by several significant developments: (1) the development of a vocational rehabilitation technology, (2) advances in surgical technique and drug therapy, (3) acceptance of armed forces and Veterans Administration medical care and rehabilitation programs, (4) success of vocational services for the returning veteran (disabled and nondisabled), (5) expansion of the public program, (6) increased use of handicapped workers by industry, and (7) development of physical medicine and rehabilitation as a medical specialty.

Expansion of facilities was a natural corollary to the increasing public interest in and understanding of the possibilities of complete rehabilitation for even the most severe physical and mental disabilities. Programs for private citizens in many centers were modeled after those developed by the Veterans Administration after World War II for the war-injured. While generally comprehensive in nature, most of the services offered during this period contained a heavy physical restoration component. Civilian facilities were mostly in metropolitan areas, and, while they served an increased number of individuals, they were not available to many others.

It was not until the mid-1950s, when federal funding for rehabilitation programming expanded, that rehabilitation facilities began to get governmental financial support. In 1954 Congress for the first time allocated funds for rehabilitation facility resource development. This and subsequent legislation initiated the beginning of an era of expansion for the facilities movement in America.

A significant aspect of the 1954 Rehabilitation Amendments was the development of evaluation and work adjustment services for state agency clientele. The significance of the work personality in vocational adjustment received more attention. This type of service by vocational facilities made it possible to rehabilitate clients previously thought infeasible for an employment objective.

Under a special program of the Hill-Burton Hospital Survey and Construction Act, federal funds also helped to build and equip rehabilitation facilities and workshops. Grants were authorized to construct medically oriented rehabilitation facilities, including comprehensive rehabilitation centers.

The 1965 Rehabilitation Amendments further strengthened the government's commitment to facility utilization and program expansion. It authorized new construction of vocationally oriented rehabilitation facilities and sheltered workshops. In addition, it provided funds for initial staffing of any public or private nonprofit workshop or facility. Broad authority was provided for grants to workshops to improve their services through improved staffing, better equipment, and other means. In 1978 Amendments to the 1973 Rehabilitation Act authorized grants for Centers for Independent Living, recreational facilities, and other programs for severely handicapped rehabilitants without a vocational goal.

The financial assistance provided by the government since 1954 has had a phenomenal effect on the number of facilities developed. Raush and Raush [1968], who surveyed a sample of 40 halfway houses, found that of these only three had existed prior to 1954. They cited a fivefold increase between 1958 and 1968. U.S. Department of Labor statistics for 1954 showed 262 certificated workshops serving 15,237 clients, by 1975 these figures had risen to 2,766 workshops serving 116,947 clients [Greenleigh, 1975]. On the basis of informal opinion solicited from informed sources, it can be estimated that if work programs of all types and sizes were included, the number of such facilities in 1980 would approach 6,000.

The American public rehabilitation agencies and their collaborating facilities—the vast majority of which are privately operated—have developed a unique partnership that has lent strength, flexibility, and citizen involvement to rehabilitation, according to Lorenz [1973]. The public rehabilitation organization from the very start purchased services from facilities. Public funds—grants and fees for services—have been provided to private facilities for construction, equipment, staffing, expansion, and operation. While the Veterans Administration has owned and operated its own facilities, state-federal re-

habilitation generally did not. The few notable exceptions are state rehabilitation agencies that have state centers and workshops.

Over the years, then, the private sector has been the owner-operator of American rehabilitation facilities for centers, workshops, and residences. The 1977 U.S. Department of Labor study on sheltered workshops reported three-fourths of the workshops as private corporations and only one-fourth as publicly operated. Their vast expansion since 1954 resulted from the infusion of government funds. There is a striking difference in this respect between the operation of public rehabilitation and public education since school systems directly own school facilities, employ their own professional staffs, and determine their own policies and practices.

8.2. Accreditation

The nation's rehabilitation centers and workshops are held accountable for their performance by an accreditation mechanism as well as other outside pressures. Their accountability is demanded not only by their customers, but also by the government and other organizations that purchase services for clients [Selby, 1977]. Developing people requires the highest of professional operating standards in order for need satisfaction to be achieved and sustained.

8.2.1. CRITERIA FOR EVALUATION
Gellman and Friedman [1965] suggested the following (paraphrased) criteria for evaluating a rehabilitation facility (workshop) as a professional tool:

1. Goals—The goals are consistent with rehabilitation objectives (i.e., evaluating, improving, or maintaining the level of employability of disabled persons or improving social learning capacity).
2. Integration—The workshop is integrated into the rehabilitation process (it is on a coordinated level with other major elements of vocational rehabilitation such as counseling, placement, follow-up, and social work).
3. Approach—The workshop focus is on work behavior and its supporting psychological structures (i.e., process as well as outcome).

4. Mechanics—The psychosocial components of work-activity, the work setting, the professional and interpersonal relations in the workshop, and workshop incentives are flexible, dynamic components of rehabilitation.
5. Supervision—The workshop personnel are professionally trained and capable of understanding and using personality forces to achieve rehabilitation goals, and able to individualize client programs.
6. Modifiability—The elements of the workshop program are modified in accordance with client needs.
7. Assessment—The workshop activities for specific clients are evaluated at regular intervals to determine the effect of the program upon the client.

8.2.2. THE NEED FOR ACCREDITATION
"The need for accountability through the medium of independent accreditation," according to Selby [1977], is made evident "by the apparent inability of statistical data, uniform financial reporting, or other quantified data to fully account for the success-failure outcomes of the multitudinous variables involved in the workshop rehabilitation process." Selby went on to say that the evaluation of a facility "through an

appropriate accreditation procedure, can determine whether those principles, methods, and techniques which have been demonstrated by our industry's past experience to possess the highest probability of positive rehabilitation outcomes, are being adequately utilized by an agency'' [p. 25].

8.2.3. COMMISSION ON ACCREDITATION

The Commission on Accreditation of Rehabilitation Facilities (CARF) was organized to establish standards identifying those facilities that consistently offer high quality services to their clients. Since 1966 CARF has continually examined and upgraded the standards by which it certifies the programs of facilities that apply for accreditation.

The *Standards Manual* of CARF provides a systematized collection of fundamental information—definitions, criteria, standards, interpretations, reference, and resource materials—on the various elements of facility operation.

Central to the establishment of CARF were the two national organizations representing rehabilitation facilities, the Association of Rehabilitation Centers (ARC) and the National Association of Sheltered Workshops and Homebound Programs (NASWHP). Formal planning for the Commission was initiated under the leadership of the National Rehabilitation Association, which originally sponsored a "Planning Committee for Accreditation of Rehabilitation Centers and Workshops." This committee, chaired by E. B. Whitten, was composed of leaders from public, voluntary, and professional groups, as well as the two facility associations. After more than two years of study, the final planning and detailed organizational steps for establishment of the Commission were completed by a Joint Committee on Accreditation of ARC and NASWHP, co-chaired by William Spencer and Charles Higgins. Interestingly, ARC and NASWHP merged in 1969 into a new organization, the Association of Rehabilitation Facilities.

Financial (grant) support and encouragement for all of these efforts for development of standards, planning, and establishing the accreditation organization were provided by the federal rehabilitation agency [Commission on Accreditation of Rehabilitation Facilities, 1978].

The purposes of the Commission as summarized from its bylaws are:

1. To upgrade the rehabilitation facility movement and improve the quality of services provided to the disabled and disadvantaged.
2. To offer to the general public and providers, purchasers, and recipients of rehabilitation facility services, through accreditation, a single means of identifying throughout the nation those facilities that are, in terms of concepts and services, rehabilitative in nature and competent in performance.
3. To develop and maintain relevant standards that can be used by rehabilitation facilities to measure their level of performance and strengthen their program.
4. To provide through the accreditation process an independent, impartial, and objective system by which rehabilitation facilities can have the benefit of a total organizational review.
5. To offer to the facility, the community, and the consumers a mechanism of program accountability and assurance of a continuing high level of performance.
6. To feed back to the facility movement information based upon aggregate findings obtained in site surveys in order to share basic data on common strengths and weaknesses of facility operation.
7. To provide within the voluntary sector an organized forum through which all involved in rehabilitation can participate in standard-setting and program improvement.

The Corporate Members of CARF are: the American Hospital Association, Section on Rehabilitation and Chronic Disease Hospitals; Association of Rehabilitation Facilities; Goodwill Industries of America; the National Association of Hearing and Speech Action; the National Easter Seal Society for Crippled Children and Adults; and the National Rehabilitation Association. The Board of Trustees is composed of two persons appointed by each of the Corporate Members plus At-Large Trustees appointed by the Board of Trustees for their expertise in specific areas. This Board has full authority and responsibility for governing the Commission, including adoption or modification of standards, awarding or withholding accreditation, and approval of basic policies and budgets for operation of the Commission. CARF is financed by contributions from its Corporate Members, fees for accreditation surveys from applying rehabilitation facilities, sales of publications, and grants from public and private agencies for support of its educational, demonstration, and research activities. Its headquarters are located in Tucson, Arizona.

The Commission recognizes that different facilities may place primary emphasis on one or more of the following programs (the primary objective for each program is taken from examples stated by CARF in 1978):

1. Physical restoration: to apply physical restorative services to upgrade physical function and enable the person to achieve a better social adjustment or to obtain employment.
2. Social adjustment: to apply psychological and social services to resolve the person's problems in social living and enable the individual to improve social adjustment or to obtain employment.
3. Vocational development: to apply vocational services, including training or transitional or interim employment, to resolve the problem of unemployment and to enable the person to obtain competitive employment or further education-training leading to employment.
4. Sheltered employment: to provide remunerative employment for an indefinite period of time to individuals who cannot meet the standards of the competitive labor market.
5. Work activity: to provide therapeutic activities, including work, for handicapped persons whose physical or mental impairment is so severe as to make their productive capacity inconsequential.
6. Speech pathology: to apply speech evaluation and therapy and other restorative services to enhance communications skills.
7. Audiology: to apply audiological evaluation and treatment and other restorative services to enhance communications skills.

Facilities can be accredited on one or more programs.

8.3. Rehabilitation Workshops

Rehabilitation workshops have developed in response to a need to provide employment, assessment, training, and other rehabilitative services to handicapped people. The workshop offers a controlled working environment with individualized goals that permit persons with physical, emotional, or mental disability, or with cultural disadvantagement, to work at their own capacity and to be paid or rewarded accordingly.

8.3.1. OVERVIEW

Rehabilitation workshops in the United States are mostly operated by private, nonprofit corporations to serve handicapped people. But a workshop operates both as a human service agency and a business. As a business the shop must raise funds by product sales and other means to cover overhead expenses and provide wages to its regular staff and its client workers. As a human service agency, the shop provides supportive services to its workers as clients and even has the unbusinesslike obligation of trying to find jobs elsewhere for its best qualified client-workers.

Program emphasis—productivity or human service—depends on the needs of the people the workshop is committed to serving. Workshops consequently vary greatly as to services offered, type and quality of staff, number and kind of clientele, sponsorship (public or private), sources and adequacy of funding, type of work performed, and methods of obtaining work for clients (e.g., offering a service, subcontracting work, assembling or prime manufacturing of a product for sale, or salvaging or reconditioning materials). Perhaps the greatest difference is implied by the two different names that can be applied to a workshop. The *transitional workshop* is one in which the emphasis is on transitional employment and vocational readjustment with the objective of reemployment in competitive employment. The *sheltered workshop* is one in which the emphasis is on substantial employment for those who appear unable to return soon (or ever) to work in the open labor market. Many workshops combine these two programs.

Two additional types of facilities are included in this section: the work activity center in which the activity is vocational, but work productivity is financially inconsequential although the experience and supportive services have value to the client, and the avocational activity center in which the activity is avocational and the setting offers day care and meaningful experiences to the adult disabled as an alternative to institutionalization.

All four types of facilities offer constructive programs for client growth that may permit "graduation" to the next level. The goal in each one is rehabilitative. While the developmental levels of the clients in the four types are different, there remains a generic base to programming: client evaluation, adjustment, counseling, advancement readiness services, and advocacy, in addition to the use of work or other activity as a vehicle.

The common element among workshops is the performance of rewarding and useful tasks by handicapped persons. Therapy and socialization are important ingredients in all of these facilities, although this may not be a primary consideration in the more vocationally oriented facility. The workshop is the most realistic substitute for work in industry yet devised to test the ability of handicapped individuals to work, to prepare them for work, to provide income from nonprofit employment, and to assist in maintaining their well-being.

8.3.2. FEDERAL LAWS

The Wagner-O'Day Act of 1938 directed the federal government to purchase workshop products made by blind clients. In 1971 the Javits amendments extended this to other severely disabled people. A presidentially appointed Committee for Purchase from the Blind and Other Severely Handicapped is responsible for implementing provisions of the Act. National Industries for the Blind (NIB), a nonprofit corporation, and the National Industries for the Severely Handicapped (NISH) are designated by the Committee to allocate, among qualified workshops, the federal purchase orders. (See 12.1.3 for a description of NIB and NISH.)

Under the authorization of the Fair Labor Standards Act, certificates of exemption from the minimum wage requirements are provided by the U.S. Department of Labor (DOL) to nonprofit workshops promoting employment of the handicapped. The Wage and Hour Division of the DOL issues certificates to workshops, including work activities centers, if they are performing work covered by the law and if any of their clients are incapable of earning at least the minimum wage. The following five different types of programs may be certificated under the regulations governing workshop certification.

1. Regular Program—This is a workshop program, other than a work activities center or an evaluation or training program, that has a certificated rate of not less than 50 percent of the minimum wage.
2. Individual Rate—This refers to a minimum wage for a particular individual, which is less than the minimum wage for the regular program but not less than 25 percent of the minimum wage, and which must have prior certification from the state rehabilitation agency.
3. Work Activities Centers—There is no minimum wage guarantee, but work activities centers for clients whose physical or mental impairments are so severe that their productive capacities are inconsequential must meet certain objective tests of qualification.
4. and 5. Evaluation or Training Programs—There is no minimum wage guarantee for evaluation of training programs. Such programs are required to meet the criteria of the regulations in order to be eligible for certification and to receive prior authorization by the state rehabilitation agency that the program(s) meet the state agency's standards.

8.3.3. CLIENTELE

Greenleigh Associates, Inc. [1975], a consulting firm, was contracted in 1974 by the U.S. Department of Health, Education, and Welfare (HEW) to conduct a congressionally mandated assessment of the role of workshops in rehabilitation. Their study reports are of great value to everyone interested in the work needs of severely disabled people. A subsequent, largely overlapping study conducted by the U.S. DOL [1977] has served to confirm Greenleigh's findings. The DOL study supposedly focused on utilizing "workshops in training 'disadvantaged,' nonhandicapped persons" [p. i].

Greenleigh (1975a) estimated that over 410,000 persons are served in all workshops annually (not including avocational centers). The total daily caseload averages 174,000, with 140,000 of these clients in attendance. It was also estimated that over 180,000 persons were terminated from these workshops annually.

The clients entering most rehabilitation workshops are severely disabled and have limited employability. The individual most likely to be found in a workshop is a person with a mental or emotional disability. Mental retardation was the primary disability for 53 percent of the clients Greenleigh studied, with mental illness primary for 19 percent and blindness for 10 percent. Nearly half of the clients have some form of secondary disability. Many of them are seriously limited in their functioning; one-fourth are unable to travel independently in the community and a similar number are unable to manage their own food preparation.

Difficulty in employability is also attributed to the limited education and work experience of workshop clients. Nearly one-third of those studied by Greenleigh had attended ungraded special education classes; another 16 percent, had received, at best, a seventh-grade education. Only one-fourth had completed high school or the equivalent. Slightly over one-fourth of the clients studied had been employed in the service occupations or in unskilled or low-skilled jobs. At the time of entry into the workshop, most clients were single and lived with their families; approximately one-fifth lived in institutions or rehabilitation residences and another one-fifth had their own residences. Only one in 20 clients relied on their own earnings for primary support. One-half relied on their families, and almost as many used some form of public benefits as their primary source of support.

For the most part, workshop clients come from low income levels. They are disadvantaged by their handicapping conditions as well as their social environments. Many are dependent on others or on public assistance; many have very low educational attainments. In the main, clients of workshops have had little or no occupational training or employment experience. As potential workers they are unskilled or, at most, slightly skilled.

The rate and degree of progress toward self-sufficiency and economic independence varies greatly among disabled persons. Most of these will never be able to attain a level required for competitive employment. After restoration services are completed, however, those who are able to prepare for outside work can move into the structured environment of the workshop for the vocational phase of their rehabilitation. Here the client is exposed to the demands and discipline of a true work situation.

8.3.4. TRANSITIONAL WORKSHOPS

The program of the transitional workshop concentrates on bringing disabled persons who seek economic self-sufficiency to the highest level of functioning they can achieve. When clients reach this level, they must be moved into an employment situation (competitive or sheltered) consistent with their vocational abilities. Those who are not feasible for employment are referred to a facility that will offer constructive use of time (an activity center) or referred to institutional care. Placement from a transitional workshop is not a final action as all of these facilities attempt to move clients up to a higher vocational level.

According to a handbook published in 1966 by the National Association of Sheltered Workshops and Homebound Programs, to play the role expected of it, a transitional workshop must plot a program for two types of clients, representing two levels of potential achievement:

Client A. This client is a severely disabled person who is capable of understanding and using intensive training and work experience, can and does adjust to the disciplines to be expected in a work situation, develops an acceptable measure of skills and productivity, and is ultimately destined to enter the open labor market.

Client B. This type of client is the severely disabled person who has received rehabilitation services identical to client A, who accepts and uses work experience well, who develops skill and productivity but who, for reasons beyond the person's control, is unable to face the rigors of the open labor market.

The term *transitional* reflects emphasis on movement of the client, whether the destination is competitive employment (client A) or sheltered employment (client B). The transitional workshop is specifically structured as a vocational rehabilitation facility. It offers vocational exploration and intensive training (work tolerance, work habits, work performance) with the focus upon the client's needs for vocational readjustment.

Transitional workshop clients move through the process in a relatively short time as compared to those assigned to sheltered work. Nelson [1971] referred to the transitional shops, short-term in nature, as having objectives achievable in a foreseeable period. These transitional objectives, as formulated by Nelson, are paraphrased below.

1. Assessment of work potential—All workshops do assessments either superficially or in depth as part of their programs, but in some workshops assessments are exclusively their primary purpose. Generally, workshop programs having assessment as an essential purpose can evaluate ability to work in competitive industry or in a sheltered environment, or can determine the services needed to enable the person to work one place or the other. (See 17.3, 18.1, 20.1, 22.1, 23.2, and 27.3.1.)

2. Preparation for employment—The preparation of handicapped and disadvantaged persons for employment is a major goal. Among the workshops in the United States whose objectives are short-term, the primary purpose of the greatest number is to prepare clients for employment in competitive industry; many, however, place their "graduates" in selected jobs in protected environments in industry or public institutions, or in sheltered employment in other workshops. When the primary purpose is employment, the principal programs are the development of work readiness, work adjustment, and occupational skills. (see Chapter 13, Adjustment Training, and Chapter 14, Educational Services.)

3. Development of work readiness—Individuals cannot work until they are ready to meet the work requirements of competitive employment. Unsatisfactory levels of performance result from a variety of factors, including limitation of functions, barriers to motivation, lack of preparation, and so on. The development of work readiness through work experience is probably the most frequent objective in short-term workshops (see 35.1).

4. Work adjustment—Many handicapped people are potentially capable of working at standard norms of productivity but are not acceptable employees because of peculiar behavior. For them, exposure to work is not sufficient to enable them to meet employment requirements. It is necessary to identify their deficiencies. Behavioral deficiencies commonly addressed in work adjustment training, as listed by Bergman [1977], occur in these attribute areas: punctuality, appearance, attendance, dependability, honesty, attention to task, initiative, independence, industriousness, personal habits, cooperation with supervisors, cooperation with co-workers, responsibility, emotional and physical stamina, consistency and perseverance, acceptance of standards, accuracy, work organization patterns and rhythms, understanding of instructions, self-direction, self-confidence, self-satisfaction, adaptation to new work, and adherence to safety rules for self and others. (See 13.3 and 13.4.)

5. Competence in vocational skills—Most workshops provide training in vocational skills. Skill training given in workshops is on-the-job. Many individuals receiving skill training need other services, and the training on the job lends itself to the provision of them (see 14.1.5).

6. Improvement of physical functions—Only a few workshops have as a primary purpose the improvement of physical function. While this was the original purpose of the curative workshops, the workshops that emphasize physical restoration now are usually in rehabilitation centers or hospitals. Their objectives are similar to those of occupational therapy programs, but they differ in that they provide paid work in a production-oriented group setting while occupational therapy programs usually involve the person in medically prescribed individual projects (see 15.5.1).

7. Restoration of mental health—There are a number of workshops with the stated purpose of improving the client's mental health. These are usually associated with mental hospitals or psychiatric clinics, but a few are freestanding facilities. The objective is to restore constructive patterns of functioning directly or to make the patient more responsive to other therapies. (See 5.4, 13.2, and 29.3.1.)

8. Provision of related services—Some workshops operate as "launching pads" from which other services may be started. Their purpose is not primarily to use work in the shop to effect change but to use employment as an attraction

to get persons interested in or more responsive to services that will benefit them. The other services may be of a medical, social, psychological, or educational nature.

These short-term purposes typify the principal emphasis in transitional workshops. The objectives described above, however, are an integral part of the programs of many other types of rehabilitation facilities.

Terminology and program variations among workshops are not as clearly delineated in practice (see 13.1.2). Most workshops have transitional work programs as described above. And transitional shops are often called sheltered workshops even though their emphasis is on rehabilitation assessment and training. On the other hand, work activity centers are frequently housed in sheltered workshops as an integral part of their program. The term *extended employment*, which implies substantial productivity and wages, is often applied to the financially inconsequential work done in activity centers. Confusion further derives from the terms *long-term* and *short-term objectives*. The latter term as used above is associated with the relatively short stay of clients in transitional shops. The extended employment provided in sheltered workshops is appropriately considered to be a long-term program.

8.3.5. SHELTERED WORKSHOPS

The primary goal of the sheltered workshop, as distinguished from the transitional workshop, is to provide long-term or extended employment for producers whose output is less than that of workers in competitive industry. Sheltered employment is for earned income; it is for substantial remuneration for substantial production, although both wages and production are somewhat below competitive business levels. The workers are substandard producers (otherwise they would be placed in regular jobs), but they can and do make a contribution through their work, and their work should enable them to earn enough money for their support. Actually, though, in American sheltered workshops the wages paid are generally insufficient for even a minimum standard of living and must be supplemented by public or private financial assistance.

"Our American society" according to Calli and Smith [1975], "dictates to each of us the importance of work, the inherent values of achieving independence, and the necessity of earning one's own living" [p. 159]. Without this contribution, self-worth is diminished and others see the person as a detriment to society. It is important, therefore, to develop extended sheltered employment situations in order that those who cannot achieve maximum vocational independence in business and industry can have the opportunity to improve or maintain their self-worth, and in some way contribute to society.

Calli and Smith pointed out that one of the values of extended employment is that the handicapped people are employed, earning money, and contributing to their own and family support. Another advantage is that it may lead to competitive employment, even though the process may extend over a period of years. Many clients need between three and five years before they eventually become employable in the open labor market.

Clients should be carefully screened for assignment to an extended employment program. A client should be in the active vocational rehabilitation program of a transitional workshop for several months at least before it is decided that the person is not feasible for outside employment. Many factors must be taken into consideration: physical disability, emotional maladjustment, social factors, economic factors, and environmental factors. An individual is usually recommended for extended employment because of multiple problems that will take a long period of time to resolve. Because sheltered workshops continue to try to improve the worker's performance, they are clearly rehabilitative programs.

8.3.6. WORK ACTIVITY CENTERS

Work activity centers (WAC) serve those persons who are not prepared to enter a sheltered workshop program, but who can still benefit from exposure to activities within the world of work. According to Bergman [1977], the purpose of the WAC is to "provide appropriate and individualized developmental services to the whole person in order to build coping skills and abilities, enhance decision-making processes, foster independent or semi-independent living and develop vocational skills and related behaviors. The uniqueness of the individual will prevail in the program by recognition of strengths, weaknesses and individual personality traits" [p. 5]. Long-term work activity centers have been in operation for many years within pioneering workshops sponsored by parent groups and voluntary health agencies. Government funding increased the number of these facilities and improved the operation of existing shops. In addition to offering rewarding work, these work activity centers also provide social and recreational activities.

The U.S. DOL [1977] study on workshops reported that nearly half of the workshop programs in existence are work activity centers. Greenleigh's study showed that the average daily attendance in WAC's is approximately 35,000 people. Largely influenced by the de-institutionalization movement to get individuals out of institutions into community life, WAC's have become the fastest growing of the workshop programs. The clientele are very severely limited and many are mentally or emotionally disabled people who, a few years ago, would have been permanent patients in state custodial hospitals.

Confusion as to the meaning of *WAC* exists due to the diverse kinds of programs that have that name. On the one hand, there are places called "WACs" that engage in arts and crafts and other "keep busy" kinds of activities; on the other hand, there are places called "WACs" that have a strong work orientation and even do some subcontract work. There is a vocational rehabilitative value even in therapy-oriented activity centers [U.S. IRI, 1977], however. A WAC is the beginning point for many rehabilitation clients—the place where they are introduced to work of any kind.

Activity centers associated with workshops are more effective with vocational rehabilitation clients than freestanding WACs. Nevertheless, WACs do fulfill an important need in the community because the activity and small earnings are important to their clients. WACs are also an appropriate resource for other government agencies with nonvocational objectives (e.g., mental health or retardation agencies).

As Bergman said [1977], the individuals served by work activity centers are likely to be classified as nonfeasible for vocational services by state rehabilitation agencies. They are likely to be retarded and over school age. Additionally, these young men and women usually come to work activity centers with a history of failure, rejection, and neglect by the human service

system. What they have learned from their environment has been negative in nature: "attention-getting" behavior has been reinforced and, Bergman said, they are "emotionally vulnerable individuals who often have excessive dependence on others, and limited individual motivations. They are vocationally inept, and often have poor or negative self-concepts. Most of these people will have to be taught problem-solving skills and decision-making abilities. They will require instructions and experiences to compensate for years of under-development and over-protection" [pp. 11–12]. Bergman further stated that prior to their admission to a WAC, most will have experienced few if any obligations, responsibilities, standards, expectations, or demands. All of these negative learning experiences must be dealt with before proceeding to work activities. WAC clients enter the facility with significant deficiencies, they are especially weak in "work comprehension, work tolerance, perseverance and the need to function as part of a team. They are generally naive about the real meaning of work activities, and must be provided with opportunities which will enable them to develop a sense of self-worth and personal pride" [p. 12].

8.3.7. AVOCATIONAL ACTIVITY CENTERS

Work activity centers were contrasted with avocational activity centers—also called day or adult activity centers—in *A Guide to Establishing an Activity Center for Mentally Retarded Persons* [Bergman, 1977]. The latter activity centers are defined as "facilities with a developmental program of structured training for the most severely and profoundly impaired individuals who are unprepared to profit from the vocational orientation of a work activity center program" [p. 5]. The term *activity program services* as a multi-disciplinary effort was defined above.

The first facilities for avocational activities were established in the late 1950s and the 1960s as an alternative for children who were ineligible for workshop training programs. Parents at that time were beginning to explore activity programs as an alternative to institutional care for their severely disabled children. As a consequence, these centers were often begun by chapters of the National Association of Retarded Citizens or the United Cerebral Palsy Association.

Early activity centers, according to Bergman, were intended primarily to keep mentally retarded persons busy and to provide their parents with some relief. "Essentially, they were an attempt to prevent, or at least forestall, institutional placement" [p. 7].

Adult avocational activities centers, because of their very rapid development, do not have consistent standards. The quality of these programs should be judged, by how well they promote the growth of their clientele and meet its social and other needs. The maturation of this population is often delayed by deprivations experienced throughout the critical formative years of early childhood. This combination of environmental deprivation and physical and mental and/or emotional disability often means that the person's development is profoundly curtailed. Some of this loss is reversible, but this potential can be fulfilled only with excellent services.

The essential component of activity centers, as in any human service, is adequate staff (i.e., qualified volunteers and employees in appropriate proportion to the clients). These workers must have the qualifications and the time to give the expert and intensive attention needed to achieve client growth. Staffing patterns properly vary according to the program and clientele of the center. Facility housing and equipment also constitute an important budget consideration. Basically the effectiveness of the facilities depends upon availability of funding. Administration must be informed—and this depends not only on the paid director but also on the board of the sponsoring agency. A board of directors composed of parents of the clients may not have administrative or professional expertise and may not make decisions objectively.

The quality of many avocational activity centers is unacceptable by any standard. CARF or other accreditation is generally not extended to most of these facilities. Unlike regular workshops these centers have not been monitored by outside funding sources, and they are not generally inspected by public licensing authority (as with day care centers for children). As a consequence many adult centers are in substandard housing and without professional staff. More importantly, many of these facilities have improper programs, for example, they fail to provide vocational growth experience. Avocational activity centers have an even higher supportive service responsibility than other types of workshops. They need adequate outside financing to employ professional personnel to help these most severely handicapped people grow vocationally or at least to maintain their level of independence.

8.4. Rehabilitation Centers

Comprehensive rehabilitation is required for many severely disabled people because of the multiplicity and intensity of their disablements. Each of their problems must be identified, evaluated, and treated, and because disability-related problems do not exist in isolation, they cannot be understood and corrected on a piecemeal basis. The person must be dealt with as a whole along with all of the individual's characteristics. These characteristics may be negative or positive, correctable (or circumventable) or irreversible, important or irrelevant, physical or psychosocial, internal or environmental—but they are always, always, interdependent.

8.4.1. INTRODUCTION

A holistic approach to the rehabilitation of the severely disabled is facilitated in comprehensive rehabilitation centers through an integrated program of medical, physical, psychological, social, vocational, and other services. For many clients, it is essential to give this combination of evaluative and treatment services to obtain vocational or independent living objectives. The mission of rehabilitation centers is to offer an intensive, simultaneous, interdisciplinary rehabilitation treatment environment that will enable the person to achieve a better life.

By definition a comprehensive rehabilitation center has a substantial medical service basis. The basic unit is a medical team headed by a physician who is a specialist in physical medicine and rehabilitation—a medical specialty now referred to in America as "physiatry." (The team members will be described later.) Nonmedical services, however, are also important in comprehensive centers and are not considered as merely supplementary to physical restoration. In some instances, the decisive need is of a medical nature, while in others the need may be for the solution of psychosocial or vocational problems. The center staff is composed so as to provide the expertise necessary to meet the diverse needs of the person, the client, or patient.

8.4.2. PROGRAM SERVICES

Speaking of "the increasing pressure for rehabilitation of the severely handicapped" in 1950, Henry Redkey [U.S. GTP, 1950], an official of the federal rehabilitation agency, discussed what rehabilitation case load-carrying counselors could expect from the "newly developed rehabilitation centers." He said: "Any development of such fundamental importance is likely to have long range effects on the rehabilitation process." But Redkey went on to warn that "A rehabilitation center is not a miracle factory, it is basically and in simple terms a new concept in the organization of certain services essential to rehabilitation, designed to make them readily available in concentrated form at the point of greatest effect on the individual" [p. 62]. His words are still timely and still true. While different rehabilitation centers emphasize different program objectives, the following format of services is generally recognized.

Referral

Redkey mentioned the problem of early referral and it is still important. The continuum of medical-psychological-social-vocational treatment should not be disconnected at any point because interruption not only stops restorative processes but often reverses progress. Patients in general hospitals are too often discharged from the hospital (after the acute medical emergency) without referral to rehabilitation. Too many physicians in general practice and other specializations (e.g., surgery) fail to make arrangements for rehabilitation medicine, the so-called third phase of medicine. The rehabilitation center is the bridge between disability and ability; too often that bridge is never crossed or is arrived at too late—after residual abilities have deteriorated and the neglected handicaps are compounded.

Various reasons exist for the severance of continuity of services. Many physicians do not really understand rehabilitation medicine although medical students are now oriented to it.

The lack of rehabilitation counselors on the staffs of most general hospitals has been another reason that people who need rehabilitation do not learn about their opportunity. Medical social workers who should be responsible for rehabilitation referrals typically are not prepared to understand rehabilitation techniques. However, there is a trend for hospitals to employ staff rehabilitation counselors to provide early counseling to newly disabled patients on their personal-social and vocational adjustment problems and to initiate rehabilitation procedures and contacts. When the person goes directly from acute care to a rehabilitation center, the public rehabilitation agency is virtually assured of prompt referral.

Coordinated Evaluation

The first service performed after referral to the center is screening to determine appropriateness of admission, medical diagnostic study, and related evaluations. Coordination of these evaluations is essential for the planning objectives of assessment. (Much relevant material on this is provided in the chapters found in the part titled Assessment.)

Curative Functions

Restoration of physical abilities or the reduction of functional limitations is the basic service of a comprehensive rehabilitation center. Here the medical services are far more extensive than those of the usual hospital or clinic. They include physical therapy, occupational therapy, speech pathology and audiology, experimental orthotics and prosthetics, and other physical rehabilitation techniques beyond the range of usual medical treatment. Illustrative of these services are training to meet the demands of daily living, instruction in the efficient use of artificial appliances, and work and recreation therapy.

Psychosocial-Familial Adjustment

The rehabilitation center patient's stay is long enough to offer the time and opportunity required for extended counseling and social services. Discussions of this area of severe disability and appropriate counseling techniques are covered elsewhere in the book—particularly in various counseling chapters—and need not be summarized here.

Vocational Services

Vocational services may include vocational assessment, counseling, and training. The multidisciplinary evaluations conducted by the center staff provide in-depth and in-breadth information useful in vocational assessment. Many centers employ psychologists and work evaluators to assist the rehabilitation counselor in helping the client to select an appropriate occupational objective. The counselor is not time-limited and need not be hurried. Tentative notions can be tried out in simulated situations until the client makes a wise vocational choice. Many centers provide training of a vocational nature although it is usually elementary. Often fundamental knowledge and skills may be obtained before discharge and future enrollment in a vocational school. Transitional employment is often provided; in fact, workshops are traditionally associated physically with the truly comprehensive center.

Miscellaneous Functions

These facilities can and should be centers representing the needs of the severely disabled in the community. Through the intimate knowledge of the staff—gained through their intensive and longitudinal associations with disabled individuals—and their professional and client contacts, the center is in a position for community leadership. One of the center services to clientele is indirect in that it is a clearinghouse for authoritative information about issues and needed resources. Because public awareness is vital to progress, the center involves itself in public relations, employer information campaigns, promotion of advocacy, self-help groups, and related community affairs.

Professional development of community rehabilitationists is another center responsibility. The center can help to improve professional services by active involvement in both out-service and preservice training programs—perhaps associated with its own (in-service) staff development programming. Because they accept the obligation to discover better techniques for future cases, centers of excellence also conduct ongoing rehabilitation research. An example of such research is the contribution of the Institute for the Crippled and Disabled (ICD) in its pioneering of the work sampling method for client evaluation: the Testing, Orientation, and Work Evaluation in Rehabilitation (TOWER) system research continues as part of the ICD program.

8.4.3. PROFESSIONAL TEAM

Team collaboration is the mechanism through which the interdisciplinary concept is implemented. The techniques of teamwork in rehabilitation are discussed elsewhere in this book. It suffices to state here that the rehabilitation team operates as a treatment strategy, the components of which are so synchronized that the individual professions behave as a treatment totality.

Physiatrist

The physiatrist is a medical doctor specializing in physical medicine and rehabilitation. Many subject areas are important in addition to medicine: physiology, pathology, biochemistry, pharmacology, and the behavioral and social sciences. Such doctors selectively use the whole range of therapeutic aids including drugs, exercise, mechanical devices, and adaptive techniques. The physiatrist is the chief designer of a comprehensive plan of patient treatment and is legally responsible for these physical restoration procedures.

Physiatrists are employed either in private practice or in rehabilitation facilities (e.g., the director of a medical rehabilitation center). The reason physiatrists frequently practice in a rehabilitation center or hospital is that in their work they draw upon a wide variety of other services and use elaborate and expensive treatment equipment. Sometimes, like other specialists, they serve as consultants for the patients of other physicians; more often, and preferably, they assume complete medical responsibility for their cases.

Rehabilitation Nurse

The contribution of the rehabilitation nurse is critical to patients in rehabilitation centers. This nurse must not only have specialized knowledge but also special perception of the patient's future and special patience in helping patients do what they can for themselves. Rehabilitation nursing encompasses preventive, maintenance, and motorative aspects of therapy. The nursing plan, which is developed from the nursing and other evaluations, reflects the needs of the whole person, and the environment to which return is expected. This specialized nurse is challenged by the extraordinary physical and emotional complications of rehabilitation medicine patients (e.g., pressure sores, chronic pain, communication disorders, emotional disturbance).

The rehabilitation nurse must recognize and utilize the hygiene, nutrition, exercise, elimination, relaxation, recreation, and occupational preparation that contribute markedly toward the highest possible degree of success in rehabilitation. The value of knowledgeable nursing care can be readily distinguished in the medical progress of the people with more severe disabilities. With proper nursing care physical deformity can be prevented by early and correct exercise, bladder and bowel incontinence can be overcome or controlled, pressure sores can be avoided, and amputation stumps can be properly prepared for the wearing of a prosthesis.

The psychological care given by the nurse is likewise important as pointed out by W. Scott Allan [1958]: "Nurses have always been concerned with the psychological reactions of the patient to disease and injury; they have combated discouragement and defeat with reassurance, sympathy, and understanding. In that sense, any nurse dealing with an ill or injured patient finds an opportunity to apply some of the inherent philosophy and practices of rehabilitation" [p. 33].

The three job titles associated with nursing are the registered nurse (RN), the licensed practical nurse (LPN), and the nurse's aid.

Physical Therapist

Physical therapists carry out a physical restoration program to help alleviate disability and pain. These therapists evaluate the patient disabled by illness or accident to determine the extent of functional limitation and plan a therapeutic program in consultation with the patient's physician. The program may consist of exercises to develop strength, muscle reeducation, and increased range of motion. Devices such as pulleys, weights, wheels, steps, and walking rails are utilized. Heat from lamps, paraffin baths, ultraviolet light, ultrasound, water and heat in whirlpool baths or tanks, and massage of injured parts are designed to increase circulation, relieve pain, relax muscles, and make the patient feel better. In addition, the therapist may test and measure for certain diagnostic and prognostic purposes as well as for instruction in daily activities and home exercise routines. Emphasis

is also placed on preparing patients psychologically for treatment, especially those who are emotionally distraught at the prospect of long-range treatment.

Corrective Therapists

Corrective therapy—sometimes referred to as adaptive physical education—is the application of medically prescribed exercises and physical activity in the treatment of the physically (or mentally) disabled. Conditioning exercises develop strength, coordination, and agility to facilitate self-care and other activities. These exercises as well as ambulation and socialization activities are given to the bed, wheelchair, or ambulant patient.

Individualized routines are devised for each patient, or the work may be done in groups. Gymnasium-type facilities and equipment, swimming pools, and gear adapted for bed exercise form the working tools for the corrective therapist. Procedures that have been developed include postural exercises, orthopedic exercises, stump-strengthening, gait-training, and elevation techniques. Corrective therapists may also give driving lessons in specially equipped cars, guide the blind in the initial stages for training for independent moving and travel, and train patients in the use of braces, artificial limbs, and other devices.

Occupational Therapist

The Occupational Therapist (OT) evaluates a patient's current level of functioning and plans a therapeutic activity program with other members of the rehabilitation team. The main purposes of this treatment are to accelerate physical and mental recovery and to develop skills that will be useful after recovery. The activities program may be set up to develop functional skills (use of prostheses, restoration of muscle strength, coordination, range of motion, and so on, through graded activities), daily living skills (self-care, homemaking), educational skills (writing, reading, perceptual training), creative skills (art, music), manual skills (crafts, industrial skills), recreational skills (individual, group), or it may be a therapeutic home program to develop avocational interests as a means of adjustment to disability.

The primary purpose of occupational therapy is to help people achieve or maintain their capacities to function in daily living activities. Occupation here refers to those activities and tasks, as determined by age and role in the family and community, that each individual must perform, including self-care activities (eating, dressing, personal hygiene, grooming, and handling objects), work activities (related to school, home management, and employment), and recreation or leisure (games, sports, hobbies, and social activities). The therapist must be able to analyze daily living performance tasks and determine what is required to successfully carry out these tasks. The O.T. thus serves the individual by evaluating performance capacities and deficits, selecting tasks or activity experiences appropriate to needs, facilitating and influencing client participation, evaluating client response, measuring development, sharing findings, and making appropriate recommendations.

Recreational Therapist

Therapeutic recreation is a specialized field within the recreation profession. The recreational therapist plans and directs recreational activities for individuals recovering from physical and mental illness or coping with disability. Through a program of physical or social recreation activities, the therapist encourages the individual to reach a goal of self-sufficiency. When people do things that successfully utilize their abilities, their self-esteem is enhanced. Activities are planned based on the needs and limitations of the individual. The program can include games, dancing, parties, sports, drama, and special events such as trips. Group interaction, socialization, and exercise are some of the benefits of the therapeutic play activities. In addition to making constructive use of time within the rehabilitation facility, these activities help the individual adjust to community life when at home. (See 40.7.)

Prosthetist, Orthotist, Anaplastologist,
and Rehabilitation Engineer

The paramedical disciplines—orthotics, prosthetics, anaplastology, and (biomedical) engineering—are grouped together because they share a common function of creating artificial portions of the body or utilizing other forms of technology to replace or restore bodily function.

Prosthetists and orthotists work closely with the physician to provide total rehabilitation services for the disabled. The prosthetist makes and fits artificial limbs (prostheses) for the upper

or lower limbs and works in the area of cosmetic restoration. The orthotist makes and fits orthopedic braces to brace or support weakened body parts (i.e., the extremities, the torso, or the spine) or to correct physical defects such as spinal malformations. Both work from the physician's prescription to make devices that will give the patient maximum comfort and function. Their work begins after consultation with the patient and after careful and accurate measurements have been taken. With this information they design a device that will meet the individual needs of the patient, constructing it from various materials such as plastic, leather, wood, steel, and aluminum. The patient receives at least one preliminary fitting, which enables the prosthetist or orthotist to make needed changes before completing the prosthesis (artificial limb) or orthosis (brace). The final step is an evaluation of the appliance, as worn by the patient, by the prosthetist or orthotist and other rehabilitation specialists. The physical therapist and occupational therapist then help the patient learn to use the new equipment.

The anaplastologist constructs artificial portions of the body to replace what has been destroyed or removed. Molds or "moulages" are used to fabricate substitute parts in plastic.

The rehabilitation (biomedical) engineer applies principles of engineering (e.g., electronics, fluid dynamics, optics, radiation, thermodynamics) to human biology and medicine. The rehabilitationist should be aware of the potential of these professionals to develop technology that can benefit clients. For example, rehabilitation engineering has produced devices such as an electronic obstacle detector for blind people and an electronically operated artificial forearm that is activated by nerves or residual muscles.

Home Economist

The home economist in rehabilitation helps disabled individuals manage daily activities in the home; for example, the home economist may help individuals learn how to cook, clean, and handle other activities in the home while confined to a wheelchair. Older people may be helped to continue independent living by training that will show them how to simplify homemaking and make it less strenuous. Other family members are often trained to assume household tasks that are no longer possible for a disabled

family member. The home economist in rehabilitation may serve as a consultant to the rehabilitation team. As a resource person, the
home economist can help the center staff correct
problems in regard to work simplification in the
home, nutrition and food preparation, adaptations of clothing, child care, family relations, furnishings, and interior design.

Speech Pathologist and Audiologist

The speech pathologist or audiologist (despite
the dual title, a unified field) has a Ph.D. or
(E.D.) degree and provides diagnostic and rehabilitative services for individuals (children or
adults) with various organic and functional
speech and hearing disorders. (Some masters
degree level practitioners also use this title.)

Speech and hearing therapists—who may
have only a bachelors or masters degree—
constitute the bulk of the paramedical personnel
in this work. To test and evaluate hearing loss
skill is required in the use of modern acoustical
equipment. These professionals evaluate the
bodily processes employed in speech production
and consider the emotional and psychological
factors related to the behavioral dynamics of
speech and hearing disorders. Clients served include those with such problems as stuttering,
articulation defects, aphasia, postlaryngectomy
problems, voice disorders, delayed speech
development, hearing impairment, and speech
and hearing problems associated with cleft palate and cerebral palsy.

Social Worker

Social workers in rehabilitation centers should
have specialized in what has been called "medical social work." Casework practice with both
clients and their families focuses on the medically related problems. Also, general social work
expertise is applied to the issues of community
reintegration, including full use of appropriate
resources for the personal and social adjustment
of clients. Social casework for personal and
familial adjustment is an essential component of
rehabilitation center services.

Chaplain

The clergy is represented on the professional
staff of a residential facility. While it may be on a
part-time basis, total care of residents includes
attention to their religious or spiritual needs.
Chaplains in these settings may serve in a non-
denominational manner. (See 12.1.6.)

Other Staff

The team extends to every employee, including
nonprofessionals, and also to volunteers who are
elsewhere described. Rehabilitation counselors
and other team members are described in other
places.

Rehabilitation centers most fully utilize the
concept of a multi-disciplinary team. In no other
rehabilitation facility does the disabled person
have a more comprehensive array of professional service.

8.5. Rehabilitation Residences

The rehabilitative role of halfway houses and
other community and group living facilities has
gained general acceptance. These facilities are
recognized by social planners as necessary to
accommodate the purposes of deinstitutionalization—to facilitate independent living for severely physically disabled persons, or to provide
the "transitional care" for chronically ill and dependent persons from custodial treatment institutions. Similarly they are seen as facilities
to prevent institutionalization—to provide an
"alternative living" arrangement in the handicapped person's community. Rehabilitation res-

idences also provide a unique mode of treatment, supplementing the services of other
rehabilitation facilities for the severely handicapped.

Residential care along with other rehabilitative services is one of the major requisites for
community and vocational adjustment of many
severely limited people. Given these requisites,
living facilities offer a setting for a unique treatment service. A residence resembling an extended family setting maintains the essential
basis of emotional support, encourages development of peer group relationships and re-

inforcement, and guides the learning of appropriate social behaviors. The group living experience is designed to produce changes in behavior while affirming the expectation of residents that they will indeed achieve their desired goal of independent living.

The services provided are generally aimed at two client groups. The first is composed of individuals who are entering or reentering society from a highly structured and restrictive environment such as a training school for the mentally retarded, a chronic mental hospital, or a penitentiary. In many instances these people may not have a natural home to return to. Even if a satisfactory family or living situation does exist, such persons may not be ready to return directly to their family. If a transition directly into independent living is not feasible, residential living may facilitate these individuals' psychosocial and personal adjustment. Other members of this group of people who may benefit from such a program are those who require a more structured or controlled environment than independent community life affords. For them a rehabilitation residence facilitates community adjustment in times of stress, crisis, or adjustment. Residential living can offer people like the drug and alcohol abuser and the first offender a healthy alternative environment to institutions, one in which problem-solving, adjustment, and stabilization can occur.

The second group of severely disabled people who may require special or rehabilitation residential accommodations are those with serious mobility limitations or other physical impairment of function. In this category are people needing wheelchairs or various assistive devices, specially designed architecture, and self-help equipment or personal services (e.g., an attendant), or both, in order to live independently. For this group, too, the rehabilitation residence represents an alternative to institutional or nursing home care.

8.5.1. TERMS

A discussion of residential facilities would be confusing without clear definitions or descriptions of the various settings for these programs. It should be noted that in practice many of the terms are used interchangeably, but the most accepted definitions are given below. (Residential facilities for physically disabled

people are described at the end of this section and in Chapter 40, Independent Living.)

QUARTERWAY HOUSES. These provide a residential setting located on institutional grounds but separate from the typical labyrinth of wards. The setting provides a less restrictive atmosphere than the institution due to its access and its programming goals. This type of facility may be the first step away from institutional life.

HALFWAY HOUSES. These are community-located, residential treatment facilities. A halfway house, as used here, is a residence that provides a therapeutic transitional living situation implemented and staffed by trained personnel.

THE PREFIXES IN AND OUT. These are commonly used to denote program direction for halfway houses. A halfway-out house, then, may be a residence that provides programs as a transition from (out of) institutions to independent living. Conversely, a halfway-in house may offer community treatment as an alternative (in) to an institution.

THREE-QUARTERWAY HOUSES. These houses, which are in community settings, offer minimal direct professional treatment contact. Personal programming as well as household decisions are generally the responsibility of the occupants.

GROUP HOMES. These are community-oriented residences that are used both as transitional living and permanent residences. House parents make up the staff and no professional staff or services are provided.

Since the majority of these facilities are commonly considered half-way houses, the discussion that follows will focus on halfway houses. Most generally these comments apply to the other settings as well.

8.5.2. HALFWAY HOUSES DESCRIBED

Residential living facilities are usually located in urban settings. This permits mobility and accessibility to employment and educational and recreational opportunities that are often less available in rural settings. More importantly, in an urban setting the individuals are not isolated from the world around them. This integration with the mainstream of society contributes to normalization. The sites are typically located in residential neighborhoods, further emphasizing a return to normal living.

Certain criteria are suggested for the location of halfway houses. They should be in neighborhoods zoned for business but in or near a residential area; within walking distance of shops, churches, and recreation resources; near city bus transportation to treatment and other resources; having well-lit streets and police patrols; and near food markets.

These facilities are sometimes in rural locations. While such places may somewhat limit community access, it is generally felt that they also have advantages. Raush and Raush [1968] suggested that rural settings often offer a simpler, less fragmented pattern of life than is possible in an urban area. This way of life may enable some individuals to achieve independence who could not tolerate the complexities of city life.

While the majority of the buildings used are spacious old residences that formerly housed large families, buildings are now being constructed specifically to accommodate the massive expansion of these programs. Efforts are made to avoid the dormitory atmosphere and the subsequent lack of privacy typical of many institutions. Bedrooms are either private or are shared with only one other person. In addition to living room and kitchen facilities, there are also usually laundry and recreation rooms. Cooking is usually done in a home-like atmosphere and the food is served family style. Lastly, unlike institutions, there are no internal security restrictions. The ultimate goal of community facilities is to provide a physical setting resembling a typical household as closely as possible. In such quarters the way of life fosters independence and responsible social behavior by the residents.

8.5.3. PERSONNEL AND SERVICES

The staff and services provided to clients in rehabilitation residences vary. Client needs dictate treatment and staff patterns within the financial limits that apply. Staff resources of inadequately funded facilities may be minimal, while other programs provide a full-time, highly trained staff including house parents, psychologists, medical personnel, rehabilitation counselors, and social

workers. Frequently, in the more minimally staffed programs, professionals are available as part-time consultants.

Services provided through rehabilitation residential facilities vary greatly also. Some facilities offer little more than room and board, whereas others offer or even require group therapy, educational programs, and structured recreational activities. An essential feature that distinguishes these residences from other housing, however, is the influence of the group in acting as an agent for change. Actually, the group itself facilitates socialization experiences. Techniques used by the staff may involve a range of treatment modalities including milieu therapy, behavioral modification, and reality therapy [Richmond, 1972].

8.5.4. VARIATIONS BY HANDICAP

Although they are very similar in emphasis, many programs can be categorized by the type of handicap of the clientele.

Mentally Ill Clients

Typically the programs for mental health groups are very supportive in nature. For chronically hospitalized people who are reentering society, this supportive atmosphere allows for the practice of skills required for daily living that were not exercised while the person was hospitalized. This may include doing laundry, preparing meals, and doing housekeeping. They may also receive education and training in community living skills that they did not need in the institution (e.g., dialing a "touch-tone" telephone and using a calculator for budgeting). The major role of professional staff and consultants, however, is that of helping the individual learn the social skills necessary to progress from a passive patient to an active, self-reliant individual. Through manipulation of the informal environment, staff attempt to create an atmosphere through which the individual receives modeling of social behavior and feedback on personal adjustment.

Substance Abuser

Given the nature of the disability, the basic program goals in the facilities for substance abusers are intervention in and elimination of the chemical dependency. Different therapies are used, including medical, spiritual, and psychotherapy.

Group techniques often include educational training and vocational counseling. The program is specifically oriented toward the improvement of social and moral behavior. Following the trend of traditional alcoholism counseling, staff members are likely to be people who were formerly substance-dependent themselves. For these chemical abusers, staff from their own peer group may facilitate change more easily than people viewed as outsiders.

Public Offenders

Residential programs for offenders place an emphasis on emergence from the crime-associated subculture. Weekly group sessions along with individual counseling are characteristic of many programs. Keller and Alper [1970] suggested three types of group sessions (all of which are largely utilized): group counseling, guided group interaction, and psychoanalytic group therapy, descriptions of which follow.

1. Group counseling is largely supportive in nature. It is generally confined to a discussion of problems that arise. Through group discussion the individual may receive suggestions that may solve the person's difficulties, along with learning that others care.
2. Guided group interaction confronts members with the "here and now" of their behavior. When treatment is well established, a group solidarity emerges. This allows people to appraise their life situation and their personal behavior realistically.
3. Psychoanalytically oriented groups attempt to resolve individual problems through exploration of unconscious materials. Using the group as a replica of the original family constellation, individuals work on understanding their behavior by means of reliving past experiences. Groups are staffed by both professionally trained members and individuals trained by professionals. Resident staffs in these programs may consist of ex-offenders.

A major emphasis of residences for offender rehabilitation is on vocational counseling and subsequent placement. Vocational exploration, job-seeking skills, and other rehabilitation services may be needed to establish successful employment for the individual.

Mentally Retarded Clients

Programs for the mentally retarded generally emphasize learning specific techniques necessary for community adjustment. Competencies in self-care skills, management of personal finances, participation in community activities, and independence in cooking and cleaning are typical program goals. In addition, development of the skills necessary to gain and maintain employment (whether sheltered or competitive) is of primary concern. These skills may include learning to take public transportation or learning to read signs.

The role staff members play generally involves teaching the above skills. Behavior management techniques often offer the tools for expanding an individual's repertoire of skills. If emotional problems exist, attention is given to the reduction of dependency or the mastery of unsocial behavior.

Severely Physically Disabled People

Residential programs for these individuals attempt to change the environment to fit the individual rather than vice versa: with the previous clientele (mental, emotional, or behavioral handicaps) the focus is on helping the person adjust. Independent living for the orthopedically, visually, or other (seriously) physically disabled person necessitates removal of architectural, transportation, and other physical barriers and physical restoration of the client. Although emotional or behavioral problems may not be at issue, there may be need, however, for training in the skills of daily and community living because of long-term physical, environmental, and cultural deprivation.

8.5.5. NATURE OF PROGRAM

According to Robinault and Weisinger, in 1978 there were 800 halfway houses in the United States, of which some 200 served the mentally ill with a combined capacity of only about 3,000 people at any one time. They said that this was 3,000 of the estimated 100,000 such persons who might well be able to live in the community, provided there were openings for them in halfway houses or alternative rehabilitation residential settings.

Among halfway house facilities, wide variations from the original Fountain House prototype exist as far as categories of residents served, capacity of house, length of stay, auspices, sources of funding, type of staffing, referral sources, and types of services offered. Robinault and Weisinger reported that only a dozen facilities are truly comprehensive in the sense that they include a combination of residential, social, vocational, and support services. They pointed to Fountain House in New York as a model facility. Established in 1948, by a group who believed that obstacles could be overcome or alleviated if clients could organize to help each other, Fountain House was the first center of its kind in America. Located at present in mid-Manhattan, its six-story building houses one of the largest and most comprehensive programs of this kind. Fountain House apartments are supervised apartment-living situations with a comprehensive community adjustment provision sponsored by rehabilitation agencies. The organization leases some 75 apartment units throughout the city, each with about 150 occupants, usually two in every unit. The unit usually consists of a bedroom, living room, bath, and kitchen. The monthly rent is considered small by New York standards. The public supplies the furnishings through a thrift shop that Fountain House operates as a rehabilitation project; both clients and staff share repair, painting, and decorating chores.

Despite their informal organization, these apartments have much in common with halfway houses. Though every resident has privacy, group meetings are held regularly to discuss their problems and concerns, both of a general and personal nature. Few rules exist. There are no surprise inspections, and discretion governs the use of intoxicants and visitor's privileges. The member can move to another residence or take over the lease when it expires with Fountain House. Through the employment activities of the apartment complex and day programs of Fountain House, and the emotional support it offers current and former members, the discontinuity between transitional residential living and the attainment of independence is reduced [Criswell and Beard, 1975].

The Fokus Apartments in Sweden is a housing system to integrate the disabled into a normal apartment setting. For service reasons the "flats" are grouped in a single building of about seven storeys with one flat on each storey left reserved for the disabled; the others on each

storey are for use by nondisabled tenants. Personal help can be obtained from the service department, which is located on the ground floor. There are specially equipped bathrooms with hoists and rooms for physiotherapy. Both the disabled and nondisabled may use a specially equipped laundry. The flats consist of from one to three rooms plus a kitchen. Moving cupboards, walls, raising or lowering benches, among other alterations, are easy to arrange and special equipment can be installed. Each flat has a signal system to the service department. In addition to special transportation system arrangements, roads, pathways, car parks, and as much as possible, the shops are adapted to the special needs of the disabled. Like everyone else in the community, however, they must depend on hospitals and clinics for health care and medical treatment, although home nursing service is made available.

The benefits of the Fokus Apartments are well-known. One is their low cost: two-thirds as much as accommodation in a nursing home and half as much as a bed in a long-stay hospital. Studies reveal other benefits. Increases in the percentage of employed and married tenants indicate that heightened responsibility and independence has stimulated them to live more normal lives [Brattgard, 1976].

The U.S. Department of Housing and Urban Development announced in 1978 a demonstration project program the purpose of which was "to fund the construction of new facilities or the substantial rehabilitation of existing structures which will provide permanent community-based residential housing for the mentally disabled." Clearly such financial support will be necessary to provide rehabilitation residences of the quality of New York's Fountain House or of the Fokus Foundation in Sweden.

8.5.6. OTHER HOUSING

Other types of accommodations are used by the handicapped. Often they are so inadequate, however, that the handicapped person fails to become independent of institutionalization, or suffers deprivation in an unprotected environment. Still other types of housing are truly rehabilitative facilities.

Elderly and severely disabled persons are frequently housed in nursing homes. Established to serve the physically ill, many of these places are exploitative, unsanitary, and inadequate in other very basic ways. They are rarely staffed and programmed to serve other handicapped groups. While some individuals may, in fact, be in need of the concentrated services that a good nursing home may provide, people should not be referred to nursing homes merely because of a lack of other more appropriate resources in the community. As better residential alternatives become available, the use of unsatisfactory and substandard nursing homes becomes less necessary.

Boarding homes are a source of housing frequently used by discharged patients. These have been criticized repeatedly because of exploitation of residents by unscrupulous landlords, unpleasant and often substandard living conditions, and the lack of coordination with the supplementary community services often needed by ex-patient tenants. There have, however, been effective adaptations of such facilities.

Continuity of care can be ensured in partial hospitalization. The "day hospital" provides daily therapy for people who require intensive or long-term treatment yet are able to stay in their own residence at night. The "night hospital" allows the person to continue work activity and return to the hospital at night.

Foster homes provide care for either children or adults. They are a desirable alternative to institutionalization when selected and supervised by social agencies. The foster family can provide an accepting home to the rejected person. These caretakers need to be carefully screened and trained and should be properly reimbursed for their support of public wards. Respite care is a special kind of foster care arranged for a short time to take a very severely disabled person out of the normal home, thereby giving the regular parents or guardians an interval of relief or rest.

Apartment residence can be useful as one of the final learning steps toward independence. Suitability depends upon the amount and quality of supportive services that accompany the placement. Some apartments are constructed with barrier-free design especially to accommodate the aged and physically disabled. Subsidized apartments such as Horizon House in Philadelphia are supervised by social workers and other services. Cooperative apartments with shared recreational and other facilities and supportive services are a suitable choice for many clients. Various residential and day care schools and centers are under private managements. An example is the Devereux Foundation of Devon, Pennsylvania, which serves children with learning disorders.

For most people the preference is to live as independently as possible in one's own home (house or apartment). This is a viable alternative for the majority of disabled and elderly people—if they have help available in their community. Independent living rehabilitation is facilitated by training in activities of daily living, removal of architectual barriers, provision of assistive devices and self-help equipment, availability of special transportation, and attendant and other personal and household services (see Chapter 40, Independent Living).

Part II

Resources

Chapter 9

Organization of Services

People and governments have organized, and keep in operation, elaborate service delivery systems for rehabilitation. This machinery for helping the handicapped has been constructed through trial and error attempts to address problems, either through systematic social planning or by spontaneous citizen response to an outcry about unmet needs. The resulting organizational structure is complicated and cumbersome—but it is a magnificent monument to humanitarianism.

9.1. Introduction

The elaborate organization of rehabilitation services in the United States, with its mixture of public and private effort, needs to be examined critically for a general perspective of the weaknesses as well as the strengths of the system. There are many issues to resolve: the role of public versus private agencies, the proliferation of organizations that provide rehabilitation services, the interaction of the rehabilitation service system with other major service systems, and the relationship of public and private sectors in rehabilitation. It is necessary to know the service system in order to use it properly.

Appropriate utilization of community resources is an integral part of the public rehabilitation process. This professional function of the rehabilitationist implements the total rehabilitation objective of fulfilling the crucial needs of the client. And these needs are varied (e.g., training, therapy, financial, social, legal). The individualized rehabilitation plan worked out to meet client needs may stipulate services provided directly by the state agency as well as services in the community that can be arranged or purchased. Information about community organizations and guidelines for utilizing these human service resources are discussed in this chapter. The knowledge has immediate practical value to the rehabilitation worker.

9.1.1. DESCRIPTION

In the most general sense, human services are activities and goods to help people cope with their personal environments, influence their own destinies, and exercise freedom of choice in their lives [Demone & Harschbarger, 1973]. A service delivery system is the organization and structure that provides activities and goods to people who need them.

Service may be provided through several types of organizations: (1) a public (government) tax-supported agency, (2) a private (voluntary) association—a not-for-profit corporation, and (3) a proprietary (profit-making) business. The last (e.g., manufacturers of hearing aids) sell products for disabled people, sometimes through purchase contracts with agencies for clients. The individual private and public agencies have specific service programs designed to meet specified needs and assist specific segments of the population. These are the service providers described here.

Service-delivery systems may incorporate a number of agencies with interdependent responsibilities and various services, methods, staff, administration, and funding sources. Human services can be broadly categorized as health care, income maintenance, manpower, education, and also be classified according to other human needs served by agencies.

Rehabilitation as an individualized process requires many kinds of services from many different resources to meet a wide variety of handicapping conditions. The rehabilitation service system, therefore, incorporates programs of a number of organizations in a structure organized to satisfy the multiple needs of disabled individuals.

9.1.2. COMMUNITY FOCUS

By helping handicapped individuals become contributing members of society, benefits are accrued by the rehabilitant's community—its economy and productivity, its labor market, its human services, and its institutions. The community too is involved in the process of rehabilitating an individual. Its participation is essential for all phases of the rehabilitation process.

The community is important, first, in the referral procedure. Many handicapped people do not know that the state rehabilitation organization exists or that they are eligible for its services; therefore, the agency must depend on others in the community to refer handicapped people to it. Physicians, teachers, employers, former clients, and other informed people help in directing handicapped persons to the rehabilitation office. Local institutions and agencies such as the county welfare office, local employment service, the vocational and technical schools, public and private secondary schools, union locals, and hospitals participate in referring to the agency those who need rehabilitation services.

The community is also essential in the rehabilitation process itself. Rehabilitation agencies rely on community resources to provide the disabled client with many of the services and facilities needed. For example, the public rehabilitation agency sponsors and uses community workshops operated by nonprofit organizations for vocational evaluation and training; it contracts for diagnoses and treatment by professional persons in private practice; and it purchases training and treatment services from various local suppliers. The greater the resources for rehabilitation in the community, the greater the number of options available to counselors for their clients. (When a needed service is not available in the home community or state, the public rehabilitation program can purchase it elsewhere though the cost may be considerably greater.)

Finally, the community plays an essential role in ensuring the success of rehabilitation following services. The counselor must consider the types of employment that exist in the community to avoid training clients for nonexistent jobs. In addition, once handicapped persons are prepared for employment, community attitudes toward them influence the outcome. The development and maintenance of a favorable attitudinal climate for the acceptance and employment of the handicapped in the community result from organized effort through continuing public information programs [United Nations, Department of Economic and Social Affairs, 1977].

9.2. Rehabilitation Service System

Human services in most developed countries are provided by a network of agencies and organizations (public and private, national and local) that have a rehabilitative value. The system of rehabilitation service delivery is therefore interlaced with other major systems for health, wel- fare, employment, and education. Interagency linkage for rehabilitation operates through a reciprocal referral process in the provision or use of needed services.

The state-federal rehabilitation program is the focal point of the American system of adjustment services for the disabled population. It works with the other social systems and, within the rehabilitation system, with private and other public agencies. In fact, the state and federal governments mandate cooperation between the state rehabilitation agency and related public agencies, and federal statutes encourage a cooperative relationship with private rehabilitation organizations.

9.2.1. AGENCIES OVERVIEW

An operational description of the state and private agencies in the American rehabilitation system is provided by the following excerpt (not verbatim) from Gellman [1973]:

Federal and state funds are dispersed through the state rehabilitation agencies, which provide direct services for clients and purchase or procure from other public or private agencies such services as are not provided by the state agency. The typical state agency assesses applicant eligibility; accepts clients for rehabilitation services; evaluates rehabilitants for rehabilitation potential (with the aid of medical or rehabilitation facilities and workshops); and provides counseling, training or further education, and job placement either directly or indirectly. State agencies refer rehabilitants to and purchase services from medical institutions and physicians, rehabilitation centers, workshops, and educational facilities. The costs are met (in part) by the government. The private or voluntary sector of the rehabilitation system consists primarily of vocational rehabilitation and guidance agencies, rehabilitation centers and workshops, hospitals, and clinics. The rehabilitation centers provide physical medicine and rehabilitation services integrating the medical, psychological, social, and vocational spheres. The vocationally oriented rehabilitation workshops, of which there are several thousand in operation, use work activity as a methodology to provide vocational evaluation, work adjustment, and sheltered employment services. More than 400 speech and hearing clinics make up another large group providing rehabilitation services.

9.2.2. COMPATIBILITY OF COMPONENTS

Rehabilitation in the United States is based on compatibility between the public and private sectors. In fact, a former federal commissioner of vocation rehabilitation, Mary Switzer, believed that the greatest single accomplishment in the field of rehabilitation during the period 1957 to 1967 was the successful relationship of public and private organizations and agencies [Galazan, 1968].

Vail and Townsend [U.S. IRS, 1973] re-ported, "Traditionally, the non-governmental agency had the pioneering role of breaking ground in new avenues of service for the handicapped. These early programs originated from the interest of one or a few persons who recognized a need and sought philanthropic support to meet those needs. From such meager beginnings evolved many of the large multi-service agencies that exist today. The need for major stabilized financing and the uniform provision of services in a broader area account for the rapid acceleration of public agencies and the concomitant change in the roles of the non-governmental agencies" [p. 35].

The early private and governmental programs for disabled persons were modestly funded. Today both sectors have grown enormously as a result of government funding. The interplay between public and private rehabilitation groups today, in fact, is largely caused and shaped by the massive flow of funds from the public to the private sector. As pointed out by Rusalem and Cohen [1970], government funds have "injected vitality, drive, and purposefulness into many private agencies, enabling them to grow from moribund limited forces in their communities to vigorous service supermarkets that reach into almost every corner of the community to serve disabled people" [p. 35].

Private rehabilitation organizations may earn much of their operating budget by selling services to governmental agencies. Their expanded programs could not be underwritten merely by money solicited from foundations, philanthropic persons, and the public, although the non-governmental income of some rehabilitation facilities is now increasing. Rusalem and Cohen thought that the role of service vendor might be painful for voluntary organizations because state agencies make demands about the nature of services to be purchased and also set standards that vendors must meet. Stress between state and voluntary agencies develops when the services requested for rehabilitation do not mesh well with services offered. In spite of the stress, many voluntary agencies adapt their services and act as vendors to the state agency. The growth of voluntary agencies stimulated by the availability of government money has made much of the private sector overly dependent on public funds.

What the proper mix of public and private efforts should be for a particular nation is not easy to ascertain. The European experience has shown quite varied results with different proportions of the two. Lorenz [1973] reported: "In a few countries, particularly England, the private sector involvement has been maintained at a high level along with government-operated facilities, with a high degree of success in terms of service delivery to the disabled. Those European countries that have gone exclusively with the public sector to provide rehabilitation services have also been successful, whereas France, which has relied almost exclusively on the private sector, has experienced problems" [p. 261]. (Since the mid-1970s England has moved toward government encroachment on the private sector.)

In the United States, the differences between public and private sectors have led to constructive changes in both. For example, governmental insistence upon "hard" data to describe rehabilitation outcomes has led voluntary agencies to adopt more objective descriptions of rehabilitation success. When public agencies, with their realistic, though usually more limited perspective, met the voluntary groups with their more idealistic outlook, both emerged from the encounter with less extreme positions, according to Rusalem and Cohen [1970]. The result seems to be an increased responsiveness of each sector to the other's viewpoint, and an overall improvement in rehabilitation services to the community.

9.2.3. DIFFERENTIAL ROLES

A proliferation of nationwide voluntary organizations in the United States champions the cause of people with almost every known disability and handicapping condition. These private but nonprofit corporations in a capitalistic democracy play a valuable role in providing human services. In fact, they probably represent the best manifestation of the idea of free enterprise. While not designed for personal or corporate profit, charitable associations draw their strength from the individual motivation and work of their own (unpaid) workers and contributors at all levels of the organization. Employees, of course, are reimbursed but they serve at the pleasure of unpaid, elected directors.

The traditional role of private agencies has been perpetuated by the limitations of public agencies. There are some things that govern-

ment administration cannot do or does not do well. For example, private organizations are free to (1) give special considerations to selected groups of people, (2) provide services without delay pending investigation of legal eligibility, (3) accept high-risk cases, or (4) try unproved or unpopular methods. Private agencies, such as parent or patient groups, are closer to the consumer than government agencies and may better represent and respond to the views of the handicapped population.

The charity of humanity accounts for the voluntary movement. For the most part the organizations were started by people who had a personal (or professional) interest from firsthand experience with the problem. And they prosper by providing concerned volunteers and contributors the opportunity to do something personally to help disabled people. Yet even a most generous and affluent society will not even begin to donate all of the money and help needed for complete human service programs. Government funds from general taxation are required. In fact, the state-federal rehabilitation budget far exceeds the combined financial resources raised by contributions to the voluntary organizations. This is not to suggest that the private sector can be charged with tokenism because relatively small budgets of voluntary health agencies do provide benefits unobtainable from public funds.

On the other hand, the leadership role of the public rehabilitation program goes far beyond financial considerations. The federal rehabilitation agency has provided operating standards for nonpolitical administration and professional service delivery in the state agencies. It has programmed universal rehabilitation service for everyone, regardless of place of residence, nature of disability, or type of service required. It has induced broad public acceptance and support for comprehensive rehabilitation programming. It has guided and stimulated a mammoth research effort—the foundation of rehabilitation technology. The public rehabilitation agency, in fact, created the profession of rehabilitation counseling through inducing nearly 100 universities to establish training programs, the graduates of which now staff both public and private agencies all over the United States.

Fundamental differences between public and voluntary rehabilitation organizations, unfortunately, create many areas of conflict. Tensions of this type can jeopardize valuable interactions.

Rusalem and Cohen [1970] have discussed the types of disagreements and stereotype-based viewpoints that mar smooth cooperation among the two sectors of the rehabilitation system.

Funding

Private agencies may tend to view the public agencies as imposing unrealistic controls on dispersal and use of funds, while the private sector is viewed by governmental agencies as being apt to fund clients over excessive periods of time and to use funds for services that were not authorized.

Quality and Delivery of Services

Some private agencies are inclined to view the public agencies (including state rehabilitation agencies) as tending to stereotype clients vocationally and push them toward economically oriented services only, without having sufficient regard for the clients' other needs. Public agencies, on the other hand, are alarmed and annoyed by such alleged private agency practices as operating with an unrealistic view of program goals, overemphasizing psychosocial factors in disabilities, providing services without prior agreement from the public agency, and sometimes providing unnecessary service procedures.

Agency Flexibility

The public sector is perceived by many private agencies as inflexible, unresponsive to individual client needs, and limited too strictly by the rule book. Private agencies are often accused of stretching rules and seeking public funds for clients not ordinarily covered by state or federal funding.

A major constraint of the state agency is that its performance is subject to "audit" or review by fiscally trained personnel who are inclined toward a far different interpretation of the laws and regulations than those professionals trained in providing human services, thus limiting its flexibility.

Communication

Public agencies are often accused by private agencies of referring clients without being adequately informed about either the clients or the receiving agency. Private agencies are often accused by public agencies of withholding information about clients' responses to the ser-

vices that have been provided, of failing to notify the public agency promptly about completed placements, and of constructing evaluation reports so as to justify putting clients into extensive fee-paying programs that are of questionable value to the particular individual. Such conflicts arise from the private agencies' excessive financial dependency on government contract funds.

Personality Conflict

As in any human endeavor, the possibility of personal differences is very real in rehabilitation. When individual differences among workers of the two sectors are in consonance with differences among agency approaches, the resulting personality conflict may unfortunately be elevated to the level of agency conflict. A continuing dialogue is the best way to prevent tensions and improve the relationship between public and private agencies. If there are serious conflicts, it may be necessary to use intermediaries or outside experts to initiate the dialogue, identify sources of difficulty, and make independent evaluations to resolve the conflicts.

9.2.4. INTERACTION WITH SOCIETY

Just as service agencies interact within the rehabilitation system, the rehabilitation system interacts with the other major human service systems of society as a whole. Sieder [1966] fits rehabilitation services into the social fabric by viewing society as constituted of five basic institutional systems that interact to maintain an equilibrium and to preserve the integrity of the community. Sieder categorized society in this way: government provides the means for people to decide on common objectives and arranges ways of achieving them with law and order; the economy provides for the production and distribution of goods and services by which people support themselves; education makes it possible for information to be extended and transmitted; religion supports moral values and meets spiritual needs; and a health and welfare system provides for the maintaining or restoring of people's capacity for healthy and independent living.

In Sieder's scheme, the health and welfare system contains rehabilitation as a subsystem along with other subsystems such as family and child welfare, health services, income maintenance, and employment-related services. Units of a given subsystem interact regularly with units of other subsystems to fulfill the more comprehensive functions of the social system as a whole. "Thus the vocational rehabilitation agency, a subsystem of the health and welfare system, will interact with labor unions, a subsystem of the economic system, and with the legislators, a subsystem of government" [Sieder, p. 27].

The systems of government, education, religion, and economy contribute each in their own way to the rehabilitation of citizens, and rehabilitation services contribute reciprocally to the other societal institutions. An example is the contribution of rehabilitation to the economy and the nation's productivity. This was well illustrated during World War II, when rehabilitation agencies recruited and trained thousands of skilled but handicapped workers who might otherwise have been lost from the war production labor force. Whatever the economic situation, the government continues to benefit from the healthier, stronger, and more productive citizenry that rehabilitation helps provide and maintain. The economic impact of vocational rehabilitation as measured by a benefit-cost analysis has been shown (see 1.1.2).

9.3. *Voluntary Organizations*

Voluntary organizations can be described by means of the following tenets:

1. A group of private citizens with particular interests organize to provide a service.
2. The service is financed through voluntary contributions.
3. The organization has limited responsibility for the general welfare or for interests other than its own.
4. The organization is neither responsible nor accountable to government—except for legal requirements of incorporation and licensing needed to protect its specific purposes and to guarantee service standards.

While these tenets are not adhered to consistently, they reflect a persistent philosophy of American voluntary agencies.

9.3.1. INTRODUCTION

Voluntary organizations and their programs may be national, state, or local in scope. Many nationwide human service agencies operate at all three levels with more or less unified governance, fund-raising, and programming. Quite a large number of these groups are exclusively devoted to rehabilitation; still other agencies have substantial rehabilitation activities. The focus here is upon nationwide agencies with rehabilitation activities. Knowledge of these agencies helps the professional worker to understand the rehabilitation system and to support and use it wisely.

The Private Sector

The humanitarian appeal of help for the disabled attracts the support of an array of citizen organizations. Service clubs such as the Lions, Kiwanis, Optimists, and Rotary, and fraternal organizations such as Masons, Knights of Columbus, Odd Fellows, Eagles, and Elks provide help. Lay organizations of churches and synagogues are allies in the effort as are the civic and social groups of the community. Such organizations may sponsor treatment programs for selected individuals or give financial support for the purchase of needed physical aids. They also may raise funds for treatment institutions or specific types of disability. Some organizations rally volunteers to serve in the treatment process.

Volunteers recruited by private organizations serve as an important adjunct to the rehabilitation team. Some have a special personal interest in the disability. They help in motivating the client to make the effort required by rehabilitation, as well as supplementing the work of professionals in the treatment process itself [Sieder, 1966]. It is a responsibility of the rehabilitationist to enlist the support of lay groups when client services that they can sponsor are indicated.

9.3.2. VOLUNTEER SERVICES

A volunteer is one who contributes personal time and service to an organization as a social service. The volunteered work can be at the international, national, state, or community level for either a public or private agency. A wide range of tasks is performed, depending upon the volunteers' interests and abilities as well as agency needs.

The potential volunteer roles in social welfare, according to Sieder [1971], are the following:

1. Identifiers of human conditions or problems requiring therapeutic or rehabilitative services or remedial action;
2. Initiators and makers of policy in organizations created to prevent, control, or treat these social conditions;
3. Contributors of service based on knowledge, skill and interests;
4. Solicitors of public or voluntary financial support;
5. Spokesmen and interpreters of organization programs and of the problems to which they are directed;
6. Reporters and evaluators of community reactions to the organization's program;
7. Collaborators in community-planning activities to meet changing social conditions;
8. Innovators of new service delivery systems;
9. Advocates of the poor and the disenfranchised;
10. Protesters and political actionists working to change the existing system [p. 1525].

Lewis and Lewis [1977] have said, "At one time, the use of non-salaried volunteers to provide a variety of services seemed necessary because of the limited number of professionals available to deal with multiple problems. It is becoming more apparent that volunteers also have much to offer that is unique to them. Frequently, they can offer a depth of personal involvement, a freshness of approach, and a link to the community that salaried personnel could not duplicate" [p. 88].

9.3.3. USE OF VOLUNTEERS

The potential for volunteer assistance in rehabilitation programs is enormous but not fully realized [Roupe, 1972]. Some specific examples of volunteer activity within rehabilitation are:

1. Interviewing clients and arranging for appointments, follow-up visits, school, training, and placement agencies.
2. Supplying, supporting, and encouraging cli-

ents in training: serving as agency liaison to the client.
3. Visiting clients undergoing long hospital stays.
4. Assisting clients engaged in training similar to the trade skills of the volunteer.
5. Providing families who are uncooperative or uninformed with information about the program and services provided clients.
6. Suggesting job opportunities for disabled people [U.S. IRS, 1971a, p. 99].

The "Volunteers in Rehabilitation" project sponsored by Goodwill Industries of America has provided an extensive series of booklets on the utilization of volunteers in rehabilitation facilities. Excerpts from this series by Levin [1973] are used below.

Levin reported that carefully trained and constructively supervised volunteers in the delivery of rehabilitation services release more time for professional and technical staff members to use for direct client contact. Moreover, a greater variety of services can be made available to clients and they can have more individualized services.

Volunteers can do time-consuming clerical tasks. Also the use of volunteers can expand the range of services a facility can provide, enriching the program. Persons with special talents can be recruited to institute activities that would otherwise be unavailable. As Levin said, "Volunteers often bring unusual skills and devote many hours of service that enrich the total facility program through such projects as personal grooming, music and art, one-to-one educational assistance, an on-the-premises library, social and recreational events, and consumer education. Many of these additional services are of special value to clients as they endeavor to become more integrated into their communities" [p. 6].

Levin also thought that volunteer participation in the rehabilitation process helps clients bridge the chasms between the security of their facilities and the uncertainties of mainstream society. By working closely with people of the community, the citizenry can help handicapped and disadvantaged persons become assimilated into social and economic structures.

Rehabilitation clients need assurance of their personal worth, confirmation that their talents and knowledge are appreciated by other people.

This kind of caring reinforces ego strength and is often therapeutic, yet it cannot be purchased at any price because, as Levin said, "Its essence is imbedded in its being given freely. It can only be extended by people who voluntarily give it, whether they are paid staff or volunteers" [p. 8]. Clients know that volunteers are there only because they care. Their kindness and friendship has credibility.

The connection of the volunteer staff with other community organizations increases public awareness about the rehabilitation facility. Thus volunteers reporting on the values and needs of a well-run agency can have great public relations value. Nor is the public support given by the volunteer limited to the dissemination of information. It can extend to changing societal attitudes and obtaining needed legislative action. Fund-raising efforts are related to the degree of public understanding present within the community and to widespread agreement with the facility's purpose and competency. Positive public and community relations make a better basis for profitable fund-raising.

Finally, Levin believed that volunteer service in a rehabilitation facility benefits the volunteers. The "need to help others" and the "need to be needed" are fulfilled by being a volunteer. In this respect he said, "Rehabilitation facilities offer settings in which people can dramatically and significantly help each other" [p. 10].

The International Secretariat for Volunteer Service (ISVS), headquartered in Geneva, Switzerland, is a worldwide, intergovernmental organization for social and economic development. Organized in 1962, it assists and encourages the creation, growth, and improvement of volunteer service organizations, especially in Third World countries. One goal of ISVS is to transform large numbers of young people into more productive members of their societies by helping them to acquire new skills through work and service projects.

9.3.4. PROGRAMS AND STRUCTURES

Increasing attention is being given to the effectiveness of the administration of voluntary organizations. In the rehabilitation service system there is also growing concern over the coordination of public and voluntary program responsibilities. Funding arrangements are still another issue in service to disabled people. The following discussion on the structure and programs of

voluntary agencies will give a better perspective on these issues.

Roles

Some public service roles are more appropriately assumed by voluntary health groups than by agencies of government. There are several categories of functions, in fact, that obviously belong in the private sector simply because voluntary organizations can perform them better or more appropriately than a democratic government:

1. Serving as the representative of a specific segment of society—understanding their unique problems and serving as their united public voice.
2. Serving individual members of a constituency in an advocate role to help them obtain the full benefits society has to offer and receive essential special consideration.
3. Utilizing the help of volunteers, particularly those with a personal interest, for building organizational strength and enlisting their contributions of service and money.
4. Taking risks in expenditures for innovations such as untried methods of providing immediate service before need is documented, risking public criticism in highly controversial matters, and other such programming that may be contraindicated by government tax accountability.
5. Filling in gaps in government programs by direct client service until these inadequacies can be resolved by legislation and funding from tax sources.
6. Supporting government legislation to authorize and fund a full range of quality services to all who need them; publicly criticizing or independently monitoring the administration of government programs.
7. Raising funds for programs of a level or type beyond government authorization and resources or inappropriate for government action.

Programs

The limited funds of these private organizations must be carefully budgeted by their elected officers and directors. Programs of private agencies, therefore, should not compete with public agencies for the right to operate what should be a tax-supported program service. Consequently, direct client services such as the purchase of expensive artificial appliances or medical treatment should be authorized by private agencies only in emergencies or in instances when the service is otherwise unavailable. Still, the government may be slow in accepting responsibility for some services until the need is well established; in the interim the private agency may be forced to operate such programs, examples of which include recreation for the severely handicapped, client advocacy, and antidiscrimination activities.

General programs of voluntary health agencies include public education about the disability, professional and scientific training, research and demonstrations, monitoring and assessing programs, legislative lobbying, publications, and forums. Money spent for programs of a general nature is likely to have greater total impact and long-range effect than the budget allocated for direct (individual) client services.

Fund-Raising

Raising funds for human service programs by voluntary contributions is far less efficient than collecting money by government taxation. In fact, some private agencies spend a substantial portion of their income paying for their financial campaigns (e.g., recruiting and equipping door-to-door solicitors, postage and materials for direct mail appeals, salaries of agency administration staff). Fund-raising cost-efficiency varies greatly according to the reputation and effectiveness of the organization, the public image of the disability and program, competition, the general economy, the local strength of chapters, the type of solicitation, and techniques or devices used.

Successful techniques of public fund-raising, although coldly executed, are essential to private agencies. Sources of revenue include small contributions from personal solicitations by volunteers recruited in various ways, direct (mass) mail from purchased or cultivated lists, advertising campaigns based upon psychological appeal (e.g., television marathons), fund-raising by collaborating community organizations, gifts solicited from foundations and corporations, grants from government, and memorial donations and bequests from wealthy individuals.

The motivations for contributing, methods of getting names, approaches in asking for money, and follow-up to get even more, are all well understood by professional fund-raisers. These "public relations" specialists know the motivations of potential givers, and they talk about such dynamic syndromes as self-interest, obligation or grief, immortality, social climbing, genuine gratitude, altruism, and so on. Now computer science enhances the technology by the analysis and processing of mailing lists to find untapped sources and increase the amount and continuation rate of donors.

In many countries contributions to incorporated, nonprofit charities are tax-deductible. These gifts may be in cash, real property, stock certificates, or expenses incurred during the volunteered service (e.g., money paid out for transportation). In the United States, some complicated legalistic schemes have been devised for the transfer of property by persons in high-income brackets for substantial tax savings over a period of years. Not only health agencies but also churches, trusts, foundations, fraternal lodges, and other nonprofit organizations use such tax advantages as an inducement for affluent donors.

Ethics

There is opportunity for mismanagement or unethical practice in voluntary organizations although there are formidable checks. These groups are incorporated as not-for-profit organizations and must file public reports based upon an annual audit. The National Information Bureau (NIB), a private nonprofit organization headquartered in New York City, evaluates national charities for the information of the public. The NIB appraisal criteria include: reasonable fund-raising costs, unpaid board of directors, program brochures that are not exaggerated, and "fair" fund-raising techniques (e.g., no telephone solicitation, no unordered merchandise, no paid commissions for fund-raisers). Not everyone agrees with these rather "rigid" standards as mandated by NIB, and many well-known health agencies with good programs do not adhere to the NIB criteria for raising money. In fact, less rigorous criteria are set forth by the philanthropic advisory service of the Council of Better Business Bureaus, which also keeps files on nonprofit groups. Most of the well established national voluntary health agencies are members of the American Public Health Association (APHA).

Organization

Voluntary health agencies are usually organized at several levels (e.g., national, state, local). Governance ranges from the strong central authority of the national headquarters to a confederation of separate groups having local autonomy. In centralized organizations the chartered chapters follow a nationwide format for programming and fund-raising. The confederation model, on the other hand, has loosely affiliated chapters that tend to keep a large share of the proceeds from their fund drives for direct client services and other local programs. A decentralized organization, controlled by local patients and parents, may be reluctant to underwrite the expense of research in far-away centers, the salary of a paid federal lobbyist, the education of scientific and professional personnel, national publications, and other long-range objectives. Conversely, a centralized organization may have a broader and better staff and board of directors, better financial resources, and the stability and leadership to attract and maintain strong local affiliates.

Participation by the Rehabilitationist

Rehabilitationists have an opportunity to contribute to the work of local health agencies in a unique way. They can contribute their professional knowledge and insight into client problems. They can suggest wise program solutions. Local board members with a personal interest in the disorder, such as patients or parents, often will not have this professional objectivity or perspective. The expertise of professional rehabilitation workers can be especially helpful in new program planning for human services.

Becoming active in local organizations is not only good public relations, it also opens up new sources of referral and client assistance. Rehabilitationists appropriately serve as directors or consultants to such groups and have often taken the initiative in chapter-organizing efforts. Moreover, community service of this nature has a humanizing effect upon the professional worker who has volunteered time and ability.

Much of what has been said above about the national voluntary health agencies applies to other nationwide or strictly local nonprofit organizations. Many of these are of interest to rehabilitationists and also warrant volunteered time and support. Rehabilitation workshops are organizationally similar in some ways to so-called health agencies. Some have national alliance, as in the instances of Goodwill Industries of America and the Jewish Vocational Services. Many other rehabilitation-relevant local groups (e.g., halfway houses, drug information centers) do not have effective national structures. However, they are like health agencies in that usually they are incorporated, are not operated for profit, have an unpaid board of directors, use volunteers but may also employ paid staff, and collect and administer money from various sources (perhaps including local community chests or united fund drives). Many such local private agencies derive a substantial income now from public agencies in fees for client services (e.g., day care, vocational evaluation, and training).

Chapter 10

Utilization of Resources

Resource utilization guidelines for the rehabilitation worker are provided in this chapter. The focus here is on maximizing the use of existing help for clients rather than mobilizing or strengthening the community's capacity. Relevant information also comes from other chapters (e.g., information about agencies and social systems, public relations, and communications).

Rehabilitation counseling techniques as described later in the book can also be utilized. The counselor's skills in assessment and relationships, learned for client purposes, can be applied to other personal and professional contacts. Utilization of resources means building working relationships with the professional people who work for other agencies—and this can be accomplished through use of the skills learned by counselors. It is necessary, though, to learn the community dynamics, techniques for identifying and appraising services, mechanisms for interaction, agency and system structures, and planning procedures. The organization of community resources can be studied and manipulated by the counselor for the benefit of clients.

10.1. Identifying Resources

The number of services available to rehabilitation clients has multiplied in recent years until it is often impossible for even experienced professional rehabilitationists to keep track of potential resources, especially in metropolitan areas. The problem of knowing community resources is particularly acute for beginning workers and for professionals who must size up a community quickly after being transferred to a new territory or case load. Workers who cannot provide needed services directly must be able to identify the agencies, organizations, and professionals who can provide those services, and referrals must be made smoothly and effectively to the proper resources.

10.1.1. LOCATING RESOURCES
Accurate information about community services is essential. Rehabilitationists must either have such knowledge or know where to find it.

Personal Contacts
One of the best sources of information on community resources often comes from daily work with other professionals and agencies. Agency co-workers can usually not only tell what ser-

vices are offered by a particular agency but can also give advice about approaching and dealing with that agency's personnel. Interagency personnel contacts also provide information, since it is natural to talk about agencies whenever professional persons meet, even though the purpose of conversation may be more specific than a general exchange of information about agencies. Activities such as reviewing case records, attending professional meetings, talking to clients about their satisfaction with community services, and participating in staff conferences, provide the worker with an experientially based storehouse of information [Bodine, 1976]. Moreover, informal and social contacts in the community can be very valuable.

Local Resource Directories

Because of the increasing number and changing nature of human service agencies, it is not enough to rely on personal knowledge and experience as a guide to resources. Formal, printed matter such as resource directories must also be used. The following list of local community resource directories is illustrative of what is available:

1. Social, health, and welfare organization directories are available in many communities. A *directory of social and welfare services* is available in almost every community of 100,000 people or more.
2. Professional registries in each state will list names of physicians, dentists, and other professional health personnel who are involved in rehabilitation.
3. Business or commercial directories, often available from the local Chamber of Commerce, provide addresses for businesses such as hearing aid suppliers, optical centers, hospital supply companies, and prosthetic manufacturers.
4. Directories of human services list key persons and services for social, financial, or health problems. These are often compiled by fraternal, civic, and religious organizations in the community.
5. The telephone directory and local newspapers should not be overlooked. Various federal, county, and municipal agencies and departments are listed under "government" in the yellow pages of the phone book, and newspapers often carry notices of meetings of the various community organizations.

This list of directory sources is not meant to be inclusive, but should provide ideas about where to look for information. Sources of information for compiling a comprehensive directory of statewide resources have been listed by Long, Reiner, and Zimmerman [1973].

Information and Referral Services

Information and referral services, so-called I & R services, vary in structure from well-staffed, autonomous centers to small service components of larger enterprises such as welfare offices, hospitals, or institutions, according to a description by Long, Anderson, Burd, Mathis and Todd [1974]. Although no universally valid definition of an information and referral service can be given, most of these maintain an accurate file of information on community services and agencies. The following objectives of an I & R service in Maryland, showing the range of services that might be provided in such a center, have been listed by Rutherford [1968]:

1. To maintain an office that will provide information, referral, follow-up, and limited "specialized" services to individuals and agencies.
2. To expedite the process by which services reach the client, the agency, or the community in the shortest possible time and in accordance with each one's real need.
3. To evaluate and determine through follow-up by caseworker whether the individual, agency, or community received the services from the referral agency.
4. To make use of the information compiled to assist public and private agencies to serve the needs of the community—to alert the executive director to gaps in services.
5. To assist agencies (by telephone, newsletters, conference group meetings, seminars, and a directory) [pp. 363–364].

Of the several hundred I & R services operating in the United States, some provide general information, but the majority restrict their information to a specific health or welfare concern, such as alcoholism or mental illness. Below are some of the more prominent information and referral service systems [Long et al., 1974]:

1. The United Way of America (formerly the United Community Funds and Councils of America maintains useful I & R centers in many communities and periodically pub-

lishes a directory of information and referral centers. The original focus of the United Way Centers—to provide information on social welfare resources—has been expanded to include specialized information relating to health and aging.

2. The National Easter Seal Society for Crippled Children and Adults maintains I & R services, and their chapter affiliates attempt to supplement existing I & R systems by providing specialized or general information where needed.

3. Social Service Exchanges maintain confidential files of individuals and families known to social agencies; they make this information known to member agencies that need to find out whether their applicants are known to other agencies.

4. Organizations such as churches, labor unions, and governmental agencies provide services which are described as "information and referral."

Computerized information retrieval systems provide the fastest method of identifying community resources, but to date the number of such systems used by I & R centers is small. Wider use of computerized systems would reduce the need for published directories and resource card files kept by individual agencies.

One of the first such extensive computerized resource files was organized in 1975 at the University of Wisconsin-Madison, in the Diagnostic and Treatment Unit of the Waisman Center on Mental Retardation and Human Development. Operating 24 hours a day and seven days a week, the retrieval system contains information on approximately 2,500 private, public, and volunteer agencies in Wisconsin that provide services to children, adolescents, and adults in the areas of mental deficiency, developmental disabilities, drug dependency, and alcohol dependency.

A noncomputerized system that nevertheless provides fast and specific information is Tie-Line, now in use by the Department of Human Resources in the state of Georgia; it has been described by Gettle and Matthews [1975]. Any person in Georgia who wants information about any state or private agency can phone toll-free (on a WATS line) to the Tie-Line Center in Atlanta and speak to a counselor who commands a microfiche data bank on the more than 10,000 service agencies and information resources in

the state. The telephone counselor will provide the needed information, or, if necessary, will contact the agency on an outgoing WATS line and link the caller to the agency with a telephone patch that allows all three to talk on a conference line. If the caller needs to speak with personnel in another agency, the counselor can break the original bridge and reconnect to the second agency while keeping the caller on the line. Tie-Line may be used by deaf and hard-of-hearing persons by means of a special teletypewriter.

10.1.2. COMPILING A DIRECTORY

To survey community resources by on-site visits to resource organizations and to compile a directory of them would require an estimated "two persons working full time . . . three to six months . . . for a moderate sized community (100,000–500,000 persons)" [Long, Reiner, & Zimmerman, 1973, p. 1]. It is clear, therefore, that the typical rehabilitation worker does not have the time to conduct an extensive survey and maintain a complete and detailed resource file such as those found at I & R centers.

A small personal resource file may be needed if an up-to-date and relevant directory is not available in the community. At any rate, every professional user of resources should keep ongoing notes to supplement a published directory or to contribute information to the office file or directory.

The following suggestions by Lynch and Barr [n.d.] are helpful in organizing a personal resources file. They recommend a two-file system composed of an alphabetized set of resource profiles and an index describing the services provided by each resource organization. The resource profiles can be put on cards and filed in a box, or loose leaf paper can be used and kept in a binder. Each resource profile would be put on a separate card or page; it would consist of the resource name, address, phone number, contact person, client population served, geographic area served, fee schedules, hours, services provided, transportation requirements, architectural barriers, referral procedures, and any other relevant information.

The service categories index is a set of pages or cards marked with grids, with service categories listed in the columns (e.g., health, employment, housing) and resource organizations listed in the rows. As new resources are

found, they can be added to the service categories index and need not be alphabetized.

Revisions are needed periodically to keep any
directory up to date. Questionnaires, phone
contact, or personal contact surveys are all possible. With office or personal files the best way
to update is for the worker to make appropriate
entries whenever given the opportunity to observe agency operations.

An excellent reference for surveying resources, indexing information, and planning resource files is the book, *Information and
Referral Services: The Resource File*, by Long,
Reiner, and Zimmerman [1973].

10.1.3. NATIONAL DIRECTORIES

State and local directories, plus a personal or
office cataloging system, will usually suffice for
day-to-day rehabilitation problems and needs.
There may be times, however, when information on national agencies will be required; for instance, when guidelines are needed for setting
up facilities for a particular service not available
locally. National directories are essential for
such occasional needs. Moreover, information
may be obtained about the local affiliates or
chapters of national organizations.

Some national directories contain information
for particular types of disabilities, such as in
hearing, sight, mental health, and so forth, while
other directories are comprehensive guides to all
types of rehabilitation information. The following annotated list, containing both sorts, includes mostly those directories that are periodically updated.

1. The *Directory of Organizations Interested in
   the Handicapped* is published by the Committee for the Handicapped, People to People
   Program, which is headquartered in Washington, D.C. Listing agencies alphabetically
   by name, the guide gives the following information for each agency: address, phone
   number, staff director(s), programs, purposes, and existing publications.
2. The *Encyclopedia of Social Work* is prepared
   by the National Association of Social Workers. This comprehensive sourcebook is written for all human service workers and contains topical articles, bibliographies, and
   descriptions of agencies and services. It is
   rewritten every six years.
3. The *Directory of Agencies Serving the Visually Handicapped in the United States* is
   published in New York by the American
   Foundation for the Blind. It gives a state-by-
   state listing of services on the state and local
   levels. Also listed are directories to organizations that have a concern for the blind.
4. The *Mental Health Directory* is published by
   the National Institute of Mental Health
   (NIMH), Rockville, Maryland. Prepared for
   mental health planners, administrators, practitioners, and "persons needing 'services,' "
   this guide lists several thousand public and
   private facilities with types of services and
   patients. A separate section gives further information on various departments of the federal government that deal with mental health.
5. The *United States Government Manual* is
   published by the U.S. Government Printing
   Office, Washington, D.C., every two years.
   This book is the official organization handbook of the federal government. It describes
   the creation and authority, the organization,
   the function, and the current officials of each
   agency in the legislative, judicial, and executive branches. It also provides descriptions of
   boards, commissions, quasi-official agencies,
   and selected international agencies.

10.2. *Making Referrals*

The process of referral is particularly important
in the United States and other countries in which
there are numerous autonomous organizations
composing the system of rehabilitation. Here,
referral and cooperation by professional personnel is essential for total rehabilitation services
that meet the comprehensive needs of a particular disabled individual.

Federal regulations now require the state rehabilitation agencies to make information on
service resources and referral assistance available to all of the state's handicapped people who
are interested in rehabilitation and related programs. These 1980 regulations also describe a
federal grant program for community information and referral resources; the concept of a

comprehensive rehabilitation center was expanded to mean not only a single facility but also a consortium of facilities (located throughout a community) which are coordinating their services, or, to mean a facility that provides client information and referral to other resources but does not itself provide direct services. (A comprehensive rehabilitation center as defined in this book is a single facility, usually residential, with multiple services within the center.)

10.2.1. SELECTING RESOURCES

The decision to refer a client to another agency or another resource is presumably based on adequate information on the client's needs. In general, a client should be referred if some other agency can serve the individual more quickly or effectively, or if the client's problems are more properly covered by the policy or objective of another agency.

Once it is established that a client does require a service at another agency or other community resource, the task is to determine systematically which resource is the best. Selecting a resource requires more attention when there are several community organizations providing the same service, but in such cases it will be possible to choose the best from many possible resources. The following selection process, taken from Lynch and Barr's book [n.d.], illustrates one approach that may be taken in choosing a resource.

A review of the resource directory, personal file, or other information source will make it possible to identify the resources that can provide the services needed. Each appropriate resource should then be examined (a resource profile collection is helpful at this point) to identify any potential obstacles that might interfere with a client's obtaining service from a particular organization. Architectural barriers could be an obstacle, or the resource might be located too far from a public transportation route. Although a resource might provide the service needed, a client might not meet particular eligibility requirements. Previous contact on the part of the client with the agency or resource can often be an obstacle, especially if the client was dissatisfied with the services received. A client may have negative feelings about the population served by a resource and might feel more comfortable elsewhere. Cost of services to either the

agency or client is a factor which might prove to be an obstacle.

Once the search is narrowed down to those resources that can unequivocally provide service to the client without obstacles, the next criteria to be considered are convenience and accessibility. It may be desirable to select a single agency at one location if several services are needed.

If the above process produces more than one available resource, the relative quality of service dictates selection. The following description tells how to evaluate the effectiveness of community resources, Past performance is a major consideration in such an evaluation.

10.2.2. ARRANGING REFERRALS

Once an agency or other resource is selected, the next step is to arrange a successful transfer to that agency or resource. The process of referral may seem simple, and the procedures may be well defined, but there are nevertheless some critical aspects of the process that can be too easily overlooked.

Client Involvement in Referral

The process of seeing a client need and selecting an agency for referral may have been done without consultation with the client, or it may have been a fully cooperative venture with the client. In the former case, after identifying an agency for referral, the matter must be discussed with the client, who then has the right to decide whether or not the referral should be effected.

A referral procedure can be readily undermined by casual referrals in which the name, address, and functions of an agency are handed to clients without regard for their perceptions and feelings. Rusalem and Baxt [1970] stated that a more successful approach is to interpret the reasons for thinking about a referral, to describe the nature and application procedure for the agency being suggested, and to provide the client with a chance to express feelings and choices.

Information about clients is relayed in the referral process from one agency to another. There are both legal and ethical considerations when this material may result in biases regarding the client [Bryson, Graff, & Bardo, 1974].

The following additional guides for referring clients are suggested by Brammer [1979], with parenthetical additions from the *Vocational*

Diagnostic Interviewing: Reference Manual [Multi Resource Centers, 1972]. It is usually desirable to discuss the possibility of a referral with the receiving agency before talking about it with the client, to avoid possible disappointment. In discussion with the client, the limitations as well as the possibilities of the resource are explained. It is advisable to be direct and honest about the reasons for considering a referral. "Let's explore some other resources and agencies that might be helpful in this situation," is an appropriate remark for introducing the need for referral. The client's readiness for referral and receptiveness to the service to be provided should be explored.

With clients who are minors or are under guardianship, the parents or guardians should be informed of the recommendations and asked to consent to and cooperate with the referral. Information to any referral source must not be given without written permission or a signed release from the client or a parent or guardian. (All available, released information and records should be transmitted to the receiving agency with the referral.)

Clients should be allowed to make their own appointments for the new service, although a service such as taking the client there the first time might be appropriate to offer. When informing clients about an agency, one gives them a card with the name and title of a person to contact, not just the name of the agency. When arranging for a specific interview at the agency, it is important to make sure that the client is present as this will reduce client anxiety about what has been said. An established counseling relationship with the client is to be maintained until the referral is complete and a new relationship begun.

Establishing the Service Agreement

Once the initial contact has been made with an agency and the decision to refer has been made, there are several points that must be clarified: What services will be provided? How long will the service provision take? What will the cost be? These questions may be covered in a standardized cooperative agreement already established between the agency and the resource. Filling out an authorization form may be all that is required. Otherwise, some sort of contract is required with the resource that is to provide purchased services. Lynch and Barr [n.d.] sug-

gested four key elements to be included in a written agreement before services are provided:

1. Client service needs are explicitly stated on the basis of professional diagnostic recommendations. These needs are then translated in terms of service categories to meet each need.
2. The treatment program is specifically stated along with expected outcomes for the client.
3. The services by the agency are clearly defined in terms of what, when, where, how much and by whom; and
4. Agency reporting procedures are set forth including format, timetable, and the specification of content for progress and final reports [p. 69].

Maintaining Effective Referral Channels

In service agreements with other agencies, the performance objectives should be measurable, language should be clear, and content should not be left open to interpretation. Comprehensiveness and specificity in the service agreement are subsequently reflected in good progress reports from the agency.

The rehabilitationist has an obligation to report to the cooperating agency on the progress of the client in other areas and on final outcome. The failure to report back prevents agencies from sharing in the success or failure of their rehabilitative efforts. Thus they have no way of evaluating their particular contribution to the rehabilitation program, and this gap has a personal effect on the people involved [U.S. IRS, 1973b].

According to Thomason and Barrett [1959], "The development of continuous and adequate referral channels is contingent upon: good inter-agency communication as to the nature of services provided the referred client; use of joint staffing of cases when appropriate; and cooperation among agencies in efforts at public education centered around needs of the disabled" [p. 3].

10.2.3. EVALUATING RESOURCES

To ensure the best possible services for clients, it is good practice to ascertain the effectiveness of the various resources used. The appraisal of resources may be done by the practitioner or may be performed at the administrative level, in which case it is commonly called program evaluation. Knowledge of these evaluative strategies provides insight into how one's own work and the agency may be assessed by others (see 7.4).

Evaluation Defined

Trantow [1970] defined evaluation as ". . . essentially an effort to determine what changes occur as the result of a planned program by comparing actual changes (results) with desired changes (stated goals) and by identifying the degree to which the activity (planned program) is responsible for the changes" [p. 3]. In essence, evaluation involves not only the question as to how one is doing, but also an answer to the question "Compared to what?"

Kelso [1974] reduced such elaborate definitions to the kernel statement that ". . . evaluation is simply an effort to learn . . . what and how a program, service, or person is doing" [p. 1]. Kelso went on to observe that rehabilitation practitioners must evaluate their clients' rehabilitation programs from their initiation. Evaluation of a client's program of services is usually done at the conclusion of service, but its use should not be so restricted. Feedback of evaluative client information at each stage of the process allows the practitioner to determine the impact of successive services and thus permits a detailed step-by-step program evaluation. Such continuing process evaluation becomes the informational basis for changes in the plan if services are less effective than was originally anticipated.

Resource Evaluation by the Practitioner

Rehabilitationists do not have time to conduct methodologically rigorous evaluations of agencies they use, but they must make an informal appraisal in each case. The following list of criteria by Lynch and Barr [n.d] provides a structure for observation of the performance of service agencies:

1. Did the service agency do what was promised?
2. Did the client progress as expected?
3. How responsive was the agency to the goals of the rehabilitationist and to the special needs of the client?

4. Did the resource or service agency follow through on its reporting procedure?

These criteria are objectively evaluated from the agency service agreement (which should stipulate measurable goals) and from the agency's progress reports on the client. Since these observations take place during the service process, the rehabilitationist can take early corrective action if the case service is unsatisfactory.

Progress Reports

Progress reports should be submitted by the resource agency periodically or at certain points in the service plan. The value of progress reports depends on how well they express client progress in behavioral terms. Client performance objectives put forth in the service agreement should explicitly describe final behavior, the conditions under which the behavior will be achieved, and the acceptable level of client performance in the behavior. Each sequential progress report should then show the client's movement toward each performance objective. (The art of writing on behavioral objectives has been described by Mager [n.d.].)

Indicators of poor performance by the resource may surface through an inadequate progress report [Esser, 1974]; alarm signals include failure to use referral information, failure to substantiate recommendations, narrow orientation to the client's needs, and consideration of a limited range of alternatives by the resource.

Personal Contacts

An informal approach in evaluating resource effectiveness is through contact with clients and their friends, relatives, and co-workers, as well as other professionals who have independent contact with the client. Each of these sources has a unique perspective on the client's progress and can provide an overall picture of the effectiveness of the resources used by the client. Gathering information by personal contact may seem to be "snooping" or investigating, activities that have negative connotations. However, it should be made clear that information is not being gathered because an agency's veracity or the client's reports are mistrusted.

10.3. Obtaining Referrals

Utilization of community resources as discussed thus far in this chapter has meant the referral of rehabilitation clients to other service providers who will collaborate in the rehabilitation process. But before the disabled person even becomes a client, some community source must refer the person to the rehabilitation agency. Case-finding by the rehabilitation agency also requires the collaboration of other human service agencies in the community.

The case-finding and acceptance of referrals from other agencies as discussed in this section apply most directly to the public rehabilitation agency. State rehabilitation agencies have traditionally sought out people who need the service it provides. This active "outreach" program (as it is now called) to find people who do not "walk in" and request help for themselves was pioneered by the public rehabilitation program.

10.3.1. CASE-FINDING

The value of any human service agency is limited by its ability to find the people who need and would benefit from its services. Procedures for effective case-finding are particularly important in rehabilitation because people who become disabled should start the process without delay. Therefore, early case-finding is required.

Case-finding, as much as any other aspect of rehabilitation, depends upon a community that is organized for case-finding. This is based upon an understanding within the community of the purposes and principles of rehabilitation. Rehabilitation personnel need to understand the mechanisms of community organization.

Case-finding not only has an importance in the number of persons benefiting, but it also has a bearing on the quality of the service that each will receive. How and when disabled people attempt to avail themselves of rehabilitation services has a definite relationship to the results that may be expected. A disabled person whose job skills and work personality have deteriorated from years of neglect presents a more difficult problem than that which the same person may have had years before.

Since relatively few handicapped persons who might benefit from service apply of their own accord, it is necessary for the state rehabilitation agency to devise ways in which persons who may need service will be reported or referred to it. The principal sources through which cases of disabled persons are brought to the attention of state rehabilitation offices are public and private agencies and organizations of individuals who, because of the nature of the work they do, come into contact with or perform services for the handicapped population. It is hoped that there will be some screening to prevent disappointment on the part of people who are not eligible or feasible for state rehabilitation services. Cooperating referral agencies therefore must be informed about who should be referred and about criteria for age and severity of handicap. Referring agencies, however, should not under any circumstances attempt to make the final decision as to eligibility or to inform prospects that they "are eligible for rehabilitation."

Case referral agencies may be divided into types based upon the immediacy of a client's need to work. For example, a child referred by a crippled children's facility or agency can be assisted in anticipation of a future vocational adjustment without time pressures. An injured worker referred by a state workers compensation agency will not have such a long period of time, but, pending recovery from the occupational disease or injury, there may be opportunity to restore the occupational abilities needed for later self-support. Referrals by the state Employment Service, at the other extreme, may be seeking immediate employment. Greater improvement in employment capabilities as a result of services is related to longer case service time span.

A systematic case-finding program is necessary throughout the state in order to ensure the prompt and complete referral of eligible individuals. There is no central clearinghouse for all handicapped persons and probably there should not be. It is necessary to individually find, investigate, and induct the clients for rehabilitation. There is no single type of case-locating model because effective systems vary according to the referring source. Cooperating agencies should be encouraged to systematize the referral process by flagging all cases who may qualify for such service. An example of this is the procedure used by the Social Security Administration disability determination units through which newly disabled persons applying for Social Security disability benefits are automatically referred by the disability examiner whenever vocational rehabilitation is indicated.

It is not sufficient simply to make contact with local facilities and secure an agreement to report cases. A definite working relationship must be established and maintained at the practitioner level. This working relationship must provide for: (1) the designation of an individual within the agency who is responsible for selecting cases to be reported; (2) the training of this liaison person with respect to the standards or criteria by which cases are selected by the rehabilitation agency; and (3) agreement upon a definite routine and form for making referrals.

Generally speaking, it is bad policy to attempt to identify all the handicapped people in a given locality. Any census or case-finding efforts must be conducted for explicit purposes, otherwise there is the constant danger of unnecessarily labeling individuals as "handicapped people."

Agency publicity, a tool for case-finding, is of some value. The federal rehabilitation agency and the National Advertising Council and similar national organizations also provide ongoing or periodic campaigns to inform the general public of rehabilitation services. These mass media campaigns have a long-range benefit, but they seldom result in many self-referrals of disabled people who learn through such publicity about the rehabilitation program.

Early Case-Finding

Case-finding attempts should focus on obtaining referral of handicapped people as soon after disablement as possible. Extra effort is therefore indicated for primary sources of referral (e.g., physicians, hospitals) as contrasted with secondary sources of referrals (e.g., welfare departments), who often do not see cases until there has been long-term deterioration following the disablement, thus complicating the rehabilitation procedure. In evaluating the case-finding services of an agency, it is important to realize that the greatest improvement can ordinarily be predicted for clients referred soon after the onset of disability. The most effective results are obtained when clients are found before an urgent necessity to return to work limits what may be done to enable them to overcome their handicaps.

It is preferable that vocationally handicapped students be identified before they have finished high school because delay in rehabilitation services tends to increase the scope and intensity of the impacts of disability. Truly effective programming would identify and serve people who possess a potential handicap to employment before they try to enter competitive employment. This view of early case-finding and treatment intervention relates closely to the notion of preventive rehabilitation.

Problems in getting rehabilitation services to handicapped students while they are still in school center around lack of sympathy on the part of school personnel with the philosophy of rehabilitation, their fear of embarrassing the student due to the belief that disability is an unmentionable subject or that rehabilitation is a charity service, and their lack of knowledge about the student's impairment or their failure to perceive the student as having a handicap. The need for a systematic procedure for high school referral to rehabilitation agencies is thus evident. It is not enough to talk with school officials about students, and medical records are often lacking or are incomplete.

A health survey form, to be filled out by the students themselves in their final school year, has been devised to aid in case-finding [Wright, 1959]. Students completing this self-report describe their diseases and limitations and give other clues (extended absences, excuses from school, physical education exemption, medication, physical care) that may suggest handicaps severe enough to require rehabilitation. Experience in using this form with approximately 1,000 students has shown that students cooperate conscientiously and without reluctance in revealing health problems of which the school is unaware. Initial screening of the questionnaires by a state rehabilitation counselor, preferably with the school nurse or other school personnel, consistently revealed that about 20 percent of the students have some degree of impairment. Subsequent interviews with these students identified three groups: (1) those not eligible for or interested in rehabilitation services; (2) those with impairments of doubtful severity or permanence (which can be discussed with a physician before application for services); and (3) those apparently sufficiently disabled and interested in services who might immediately make application and have a general medical examination authorized. About 10 percent of all students were identified, through this self-report, as potentially needing rehabilitation services.

Guidelines

Each rehabilitation agency needs to develop its own referral sources and techniques for case-finding within a community. Listed below are general suggestions for effective case-finding.

1. Maintain an open-door policy for new referrals to the agency to show referral sources that more referrals are desired.
2. Make periodic examination of sources of referrals to assure a continuing flow of cases from all potential community resources.
3. Assign each counselor responsibility for maintenance of contact with certain agencies and potential sources of referrals.
4. Prepare formal referral forms for use by referral sources.
5. Develop prompt and cordial reporting-back procedures to inform referral sources about referrals made.
6. Give prompt attention to referrals to avoid delaying needed services.
7. Maintain a record of referrals—by date of referral, source, and actions taken—for evaluation and follow-up purposes.
8. Provide for preliminary evaluation as a basis for acceptance or rejection of referrals.
9. Advise the client and referral agency or other interested parties of action taken and the reasons.

Sources of Referrals

In every community there exist many sources of referral. The sources from which state rehabilitation agencies receive the majority of new cases are listed below.

1. Health agencies: public and private, general and special hospitals; clinics; mental institutions; physicians; public health service; nursing groups; artificial appliance companies; and so on.
2. Employment and guidance service agencies: public and private employment offices; public and private guidance and counseling agencies such as B'nai B'rith, Urban League, and other voluntary religious, racial, and welfare units.
3. Welfare agencies: public and private assistance and relief agencies such as Red Cross,

Salvation Army, Catholic Charities, and state and city public welfare.
4. Educational institutions: public, private, and denominational schools and colleges, including schools for handicapped children and business colleges.
5. Special interest agencies: crippled children's services, health associations, and other organizations of and for handicapped people.
6. Insurance companies: state workers compensation boards, Social Security programs, and private and fraternal insurance companies.
7. Civic service groups: Lions, Masons, Kiwanis, Rotary, YMCA, and so on.
8. Religious groups: Protestant, Jewish, and Catholic social and helping organizations.
9. Employers: government at all levels, industry, and other business.
10. Labor unions: local affiliates of all union organizations.

The above organizations and individuals are excellent sources of referrals for rehabilitation services if informed of the services available.

"In the final analysis, a continual supply of referrals to rehabilitation agencies from outside sources will be dependent upon how well the agencies have met the needs of the clients who had been previously referred," according to McGowan and Porter [1967, p. 45], who provided many of the above suggestions.

10.3.2. REFERRAL MECHANISMS

No one individual professional person, no one agency, no one service can provide directly for all of the rehabilitation needs of most rehabilitation clients. This is the essential rationale for comprehensive rehabilitation through multiple service resources. The development of concepts such as teamwork and the interdisciplinary approach as well as the construction of rehabilitation centers, comprehensive care units, and multi-service centers fill a recognized need for the comprehensive approach. They represent organizational structures within which special skills of many professional disciplines can be made available for use on a selective basis as a client's needs are identified. As specialization developed, the need for interdisciplinary joint action became critical. Referral is the essential ingredient required to move clients from one service to another.

Referral Considerations

McGowan and Porter [1967] offered a number of helpful considerations that make the referral process more rewarding for all parties.

1. Every disabled person is entitled to know all available rehabilitation services and has the right to be considered for them according to individual needs and interests.
2. Suitable referrals should be based on a realistic understanding of the general objectives and services that the agency is equipped to provide.
3. Referral should be made early in the period of disablement, thus providing for contact when the client is most receptive both psychologically and physiologically to rehabilitation measures.
4. The community referral program needs to be effective and comprehensive in order to keep channels open and referrals flowing from all potential sources.
5. There should be a continual exchange of information among the agencies of the community for good coordination of services.
6. A courteous and effective way to nurture a referral source is to supply "feedback" regarding the progress of a referred individual.

Mutual professional respect is promoted between the rehabilitationist and the professionals of other agencies through effective referral processes.

Community Organization

Adequate referral sources are dependent upon good community organization for rehabilitation. Good community organization is based on (1) formal agreements on areas of responsibility, (2) good interpersonal relationships of staffs, (3) regular interagency visits, (4) joint case staffing, (5) joint training programs, and (6) cooperation in public education and other community activities for the handicapped population.

The referral process functions best when the rehabilitation agency has a communitywide reputation for providing effective services to disabled persons. Good counselor-client relationships also promote the community image of rehabilitation. In the long run, successful rehabilitants offer the best proof of the value of rehabilitation.

The number and quality of referrals from a community agency depend upon the preparation of their staff. These professionals must have accurate knowledge about the type of services provided by rehabilitation and must understand eligibility requirements. This is necessary in order for them to refer only people for whom there is a reasonable expectation that the agency's services will be helpful. Informing the personnel of other agencies about rehabilitation is a continuing effort because of staff turnover and program changes.

10.4. Community Relations

Full utilization of resources depends in large measure upon the building and maintenance of an effective community relationship. This means projection of a favorable agency image. Successful rehabilitants are the best publicity. And the rehabilitationist is the best person to tell the story of rehabilitation success. A full-scale promotional program, however, requires many approaches and the participation of the many concerned persons and agencies.

10.4.1. PUBLIC RELATIONS PROGRAM

Public relations (PR) is directed toward many target groups. Thus it must be a continuing process because new organizations are being constantly formed, new agency officials are appointed, and program needs and characteristics shift from time to time. But the general public relations audience goes far beyond the people who work in collaborating agencies. It also includes government officials, legislators, and various interest groups such as associations of handicapped people and their "consumer" advocates. Public relations extends certainly to those directly affected, not only the families of disabled persons, but also most importantly the central person in the rehabilitation process, the rehabilitation client and potential client.

State rehabilitation agencies employ what they call information officers to handle publicity and related work. These public relations people are trained journalists, skilled in writing and experienced in working with the media (e.g., newspapers, television). The information or public relations officer for a state rehabilitation agency may be responsible for dealing with the press in the instance of unfavorable publicity about some incident or program. More routinely the PR person has a continued duty to get informational items accepted by newspapers and other media in order to inform the general public about the services to handicapped individuals. But, the properly used public relations officer is far more than a publicity agent: PR promotional activities incorporate long-range programming to inform the general public about rehabilitation. The PR program also reaches "special publics" interested in rehabilitation (e.g., medical association members, employers).

10.4.2. METHODS

Promoting the agency may involve printed matter such as specially prepared bulletins and pamphlets as well as agency newsletters. Such informational pieces are effective because of their attractiveness, clarity of expression, explicitness of purpose, and effectiveness in distribution. Brochures are helpful in informing handicapped people of the availability of services and in apprising significant others (such as legislators) about the nature of the program. Public relations personnel may also develop audiovisual aids for presentation to live audiences as well as radio and television sources. Materials like this help the rehabilitationist explain the program services to groups. Thus charts and graphs, slides, and other exhibit material may be prepared to explain or demonstrate the rehabilitation program to a variety of audiences. The public relations officer of the agency is often in charge of an internal newsletter that keeps agency staff informed. This person also may provide materials to other workers in the agency to help them fulfill their promotional responsibility. These might include handout folders containing facts and figures, pictures or graphs, and other available information in an attractive package for group or personal contacts by the staff. Materials may also be prepared for the assistance of others (such as public speakers for organizations of handicapped persons) in "selling" vocational rehabilitation in the community.

A successful rehabilitation program is dependent, to a large extent, upon the interest and support of the public, employers, labor unions,

other units of state government, and the many private groups concerned with disabled persons. There are many interested people and organizations. Their knowledge of the objectives, methods, and accomplishments of rehabilitation helps to secure their cooperation and effective participation in the operation of the program and their support in its legislative requests.

Such broad-based public relations is particularly important to rehabilitation because it is not a self-contained or self-sufficient program. Most of the client services of the state agency, other than those of the rehabilitation counselor, are purchased from other organizations. For example, training is purchased from schools, psychological testing is purchased from psychometrists, work evaluation and adjustment services are purchased from rehabilitation facilities, physical restoration (such as surgery) is purchased from physicians, artificial appliances are purchased from prosthetic manufacturers, and so forth. It has long been the policy of the state-federal rehabilitation program not to duplicate existing services but to utilize community agencies needed in the rehabilitation process.

Public relations for the state agency extends to the entire rehabilitation community. Many of the private rehabilitation facilities in the United States were started with public rehabilitation funds and are partially operated through government financing for special projects and client services. As the programs of rehabilitation in the states were expanded and services extended to larger groups of handicapped individuals, the state-federal organization successfully promoted private agencies, stimulating the development of new facilities, staff, and programs. The need continues for good interagency working relationships, and the strategy for mutual success in the future depends upon constructive public relations efforts.

10.4.3. PURPOSES

In the area of legislation for program growth a positive public image of the rehabilitation approach is essential. Moreover, the promotion of legislation is not just for rehabilitation goals but also for related human service programs. This includes legislation for handicapped children, for individuals who are disadvantaged, for industrial safety and health, for workers compensation, and so forth. Disabled people in America are the unheard minority. For their views to be forcefully presented they must build an effective national organization (or coalition of consumer organizations) of, by and for the disabled population. This association of disabled people would provide membership services (e.g., resource advisement, practical magazine, discounted merchandise, insurance) and mobilize their collective voice for legislative action. Outside (foundation) financial support may be required for a massive effort in membership recruitment and program development.

Chapter 11

Resource Coordination

Since the beginning of the twentieth century and the founding of the numerous private health and social organizations, the field of human services has followed a pattern of specialization in attempting to cope with the complexity of problems. Effective coordination of rehabilitation services today has thus become a challenge because of the many different agencies and professions that serve disabled persons. In fact, rehabilitation today by means of a single service or funding source is virtually impossible. The state-federal rehabilitation system does not directly provide comprehensive rehabilitation; this makes coordination of various agencies essential for effective rehabilitation efforts.

Interagency coordination is a problem because the boundaries and responsibilities of agencies are overlapping and poorly defined. Faulty central administration or legislation therefore results in duplication or fragmentation of services. Poor coordination at the local level is blamed for the confusion, and practitioners are cajoled to cooperate with one another. When jurisdiction is not defined, competition and conflict can result between agencies that feel that others are usurping their area of responsibility. This hodgepodge of rehabilitation services causes delay as clients are transferred from one agency to another in an attempt to meet all their needs.

In spite of the need for professionals to know what services are available in a community, it was found in a study by Levine, White, and Paul [1963] that even agency executives were unfamiliar with at least half of the other health and welfare agency programs in their communities. Ross [1976] pointed out that many workers in service delivery systems are trained to render solos when, in fact, the disabled clients require an orchestra of services, carefully planned and coordinated.

The proliferation of human service organizations has attracted negative public attention. Therefore, the merger of rehabilitation and related human services has been proposed for efficiency (see 6.8.5). The only way a merged organization is made less costly, however, is by the installation of subprofessional "generalists" to supplant professional specialists and by the consolidation of administration. This solution ignores the fact that highly trained specialists are needed more than ever for rehabilitation of severely disabled persons. Moreover, a consolidated administration still must cope with the problem of intraagency coordination. The ultimate solution must involve clear-cut lines of responsibility among and between currently overlapping agency authorities. In the meantime, the rehabilitation practitioner must orchestrate cooperative contributions from the various groups in the interest of the client.

11.1. Cooperation Among Agencies

Reid [1969] has described three levels of organizational cooperation: ad hoc case coordination, systematic case coordination, and program coordination. Ad hoc case coordination implies an informal sharing of information and informal cooperation among agencies with mutual clients. Physical proximity or a co-located site is essential to this type of coordination. Systematic case coordination involves agencies' meshing their services and developing specific rules and procedures to govern coordination (e.g., case conference committees, referral routines). This type of coordination requires a unified monitoring and information system. The highest level of coordination, program coordination, deals not with individual cases but with entire agency programs that can meet clearly shared agency or clientele needs. Roessler and Mack [1975] observed that coordination linkages at the program level include joint funding, joint use of staff, and purchase of service agreements.

11.1.1. INTERAGENCY LINKAGES

When two or more agencies collaborate in designated operations to meet mutual objectives, the arrangement is called interagency linkage. Public agency linkages may be mandated by legislation requiring mutual functioning. Other linkages are made through administrative agreements concerning allocation of staff time, delegation of authority, referral procedures, and communication systems. Still other linkages are effected through the informal contacts and working relationships developed by staff [Baumheier & Welch, 1976].

Ideally, interagency linkages occur because the personnel of rehabilitation and other agencies desire to correlate their services for the maximum benefit of their clients. "They may see, for example, how joint case finding will reach more of the potential users of services being offered. They may see how the merger of the strengths of their agencies can handle a problem which is too large, too complicated, or too expensive for a single agency to handle. They may see how the sharing of expertise and manpower can help each agency to realize its objectives more efficiently," according to the (Sixth) Institute of Rehabilitation Services [U.S. IRS, 1968b, p. 3]. With their focus on client needs, professionals can often overcome faulty delineation of agency authority.

It has been contended, however, that money problems and other crises are often responsible for linkages. Morris [1961] found that agencies tend to work together more successfully when they have been badly shaken by a crisis situation or when their trustees or directors have close relationships. Legislative scrutiny is an effective mechanism for causing public agency collaboration. After reviewing the literature, Cubelli [1965] found that money is the most consistently mentioned agency need and that community planning often takes place when agencies are short of money and need to coordinate with other agencies to perpetuate the quality of their programs.

11.1.2. COOPERATIVE PROGRAMMING

Various types of cooperative program arrangements are common to rehabilitation agencies, especially state rehabilitation agencies. These are described below.

Referral Agreements

Agencies agree to exchange client information as well as to refer clients for specific services at cooperating agencies. The more successful referral agreements have incorporated written agreements, periodic staff meetings, agreement on policy, staff education about purposes and methods, and a system for evaluating the effectiveness of the arrangement. State rehabilitation agencies, for example, have had a longstanding referral agreement with the state Employment Service agency.

Purchase of Service Agreements

State rehabilitation agencies purchase extensive services for their clients through service agreements with rehabilitation facilities, hospitals, clinics, schools, and other service providers. Fees are paid to authorized vendors for medical examinations, surgery and treatment, work adjustment and skill training, and goods from vendors (prosthetics, books, equipment, uniforms, etc.). Money is paid directly to clients for their out-of-pocket expenses (e.g., for transportation, personal maintenance). Service vendors are screened for such qualifications as state licenses, professional certification, and facilities accreditation. Expenditures are made in accordance with state fiscal procedures, which vary from state to state, and in compliance with the state rehabilitation plan that outlines the criteria or standards for facilities and personnel. A uniform and current "schedule" is circulated to show interested parties the amount of money the state agency will authorize for a specific service.

Joint Programs of Services

Joint programming for disabled persons is often established when two or more agencies have services that can be mutually beneficial to their respective clients. Examples of joint programs include placing a rehabilitation staff counselor in a welfare office to evaluate the vocational potential of public assistance clients, or establishing a rehabilitation unit in a mental hospital or correctional institution. Joint programs have the potential for expanding services and developing new patterns of service that can benefit clients at the time they are most needed. "Third party funding"—money for rehabilitation from a private agency or from a government source other than the public rehabilitation agency—is a frequently used method for "capturing" federal matching money for joint programs.

Multi-service Centers

Neighborhood centers may simply be buildings where various human service agencies are located, or they may be facilities that offer varying degrees of integrated services. The co-location of several social and rehabilitation agencies in a center allows for streamlining procedures, developing new working relationships with other professionals, and coordinating agencies on every level. Multi-service centers are usually lo-

cated near the clients to be served, and have hours and styles of service that are convenient and appropriate for the clientele.

Agent Relations

Agent relations is an infrequently used arrangement in which one agency acts as the agent for another agency and operates part or all of the other agency's program. In most states, for example, the state rehabilitation agency makes disability determinations for the federal Social Security Administration. A separate staff and organization are required within state agencies to perform this function [U.S. IRS, 1968b].

Service Merger

The provision of rehabilitation services is not a competitive business; therefore the duplication of equipment and staff is an intolerable expense. The following services and functions are ones that may be combined into a single operation for use by two or more agencies: in-house medical examinations, in-service training, transportation systems, vocational assessment unit, policy advisory council, case management, case review committee, automated client information system, common application form, referral form, client services record file, equipment, food services, meeting rooms, parking and security maintenance, adult basic education, child care service, and emergency financial assistance [O'Toole, O'Toole, McMillan, & Lefton, 1972].

11.1.3. PLANNING BODIES

The growing complexity of social services and the demands of social problems have forced communities to undertake social planning much as they earlier assumed the burden of planning for societal functions such as transportation and industry. Planning bodies play a crucial role by offering direct service agencies two main avenues for improving community services. First, there are planning bodies designed primarily to coordinate or consolidate the services provided by agencies. Second, there are planning bodies oriented toward social action, which can be instrumental in solving complex problems of the disabled population through investigations, legislative action, public awareness programs, and advocacy projects. It is advantageous for rehabilitationists to be acquainted with the different types of planning bodies, their activities, and their areas of contribution.

The planning organizations defined and described below all have a special value in the coordination and planning of rehabilitation services. Most planning bodies have a real potential for stimulating change on which direct service agencies can capitalize. It should be kept in mind, however, that many planning and coordination tasks are the responsibility of the direct service agency alone. Sieder [1966], who published authoritative information on planning bodies, is the basic source of the definitions and descriptions presented here. Although her labels for the various types of organizations are not applied universally, it is still useful to understand these different organizational categories.

Councils

The council, according to Sieder, is an ". . . interorganizational body whose membership includes a cross section of public and voluntary organizations and professional and civic groups, as well as individuals interested in an appropriate field of service (i.e., rehabilitation, health, aging, delinquency). The council's goal is to achieve a comprehensive and well-balanced program of health and welfare services in behalf of the whole community it encompasses (state, region, metropolitan area, etc.)" [p. 159].

Councils offer central services to member agencies through information and referral, consultation of experts, joint purchasing, and volunteer recruitment and training. Councils also coordinate the work of voluntary and tax-supported agencies by setting standards, negotiating operating agreements, and developing referral systems. Moreover, they assess the unmet needs, duplications, and inadequacies of service; and they attempt to correct social ills through the support of housing, recreation, public health, and similar programs.

A council generally has no authority to impose decisions on agencies in the community. Its power lies in its ability to mobilize community action by presenting the facts to those who are in a position to make decisions, move public opinion to action, and exercise influence in the allocation of both public and voluntary funds.

The community welfare council found in many large communities is a common example of this type of planning body. The effectiveness of councils in coordinating rehabilitation services has been demonstrated. Kunitz [1964], for example, described how the Contra Costa Re-

habilitation Council, composed of more than 40 rehabilitation-oriented agencies in that California county, was more effective than any single agency in planning rehabilitation services.

A pattern of legislation has established the "council" mechanism in health planning and the areas of mental health and developmental disabilities. The federal rehabilitation agency has long had an advisory council appointed by the Administration. Federal developmental disabilities (DD) legislation mandated the establishment of state "DD" councils to administer federal grant-in-aid funds. These councils, appointed by the state Governor, may have little or no statutory authority, but such quasi-official bodies can be very powerful in orchestrating a harmonious services mechanism.

Exchanges

This type of organization is represented by the social service exchanges, which date back to 1870 and are intended to facilitate communication between agencies regarding clients and to prevent duplication of services among agencies. Social service exchanges maintain confidential files on families and individuals who have had transactions with social agencies. When member agencies receive an application for service, they can inquire of the exchange about whether the applicant is known to other agencies, and if the answer is affirmative, can obtain supplementary information from other agencies and perhaps coordinate services with them [Williams, 1971]. Although the use of exchanges has decreased in recent years, they remain a useful tool for case coordination in some communities.

Case Conference Committee

This type of committee usually consists of representatives from public and voluntary agencies that provide rehabilitation, medical, and social services. In most localities, the case conference committee has the general function of discussing problem cases. Difficult cases of long standing can often be solved in such committees, as the group focuses on client needs and examines ways in which those needs might be met by specialized services volunteered by the respective agencies. A case conference committee encourages working relationships among the participants and serves as both a planning body and a clearinghouse for agencies involved in rehabilitation. The case conference committee as described by a Workshop on Guidance, Training, and Placement [U.S. GTP, 1953a] was a viable coordination mechanism at one time, particularly in smaller cities.

Citizens' Committees

The citizens' committee is a self-constituted organization of individuals who serve as an autonomous body (i.e., one without responsibility to any parent body or other organization). A citizens' committee may be either a permanent, ongoing structure, or it may be an ad hoc group formed for a limited time to address a particular problem and goal.

Commissions

A commission is an official or quasi-official body created by government for investigation of and recommendations on a specific social problem. The commission report may have considerable influence as a long-range planning document compiled by unbiased citizens.

Associations

An association is formed with a membership of individuals or organizations for such regulatory or promotional purposes as establishing standards, policing activities, interpreting functions and programs, and winning public understanding and financial support. Associations are composed of professional individuals such as rehabilitation counselors, while group associations are composed of units such as rehabilitation centers. Their power and authority derive from the membership, and their basic support is from membership dues and contributions made on a voluntary basis. (See 2.2.1 and 12.1.11.)

11.2. Coordination of Processes

Coordinating the rehabilitation process is difficult because of the many kinds of problems created by human disablement and the complexity of professional and agency involvements. With all this complexity, cooperative agreements fail and the parties involved are not able accurately to explain why. Yet it is this very complexity of linkage between the segments of total rehabilitation that makes coordination essential.

11.2.1. AGREEMENT REQUIRED

Roessler and Mack [1975] reviewed the literature and postulated three general types of "consensus" that seemed essential for interagency linkages to succeed: domain consensus, ideological consensus, and interorganizational evaluation consensus. These three types of agreement result from slow incremental recognition of mutual needs and achieved benefits, rather than from some overall rational scheme aimed at immediate coordination of agencies.

Domain consensus means a clear understanding of each agency's role and responsibility in a cooperative arrangement. If cooperating agencies perceive the cooperative relationship as a threat to their autonomy or as an attempt to consolidate power into a superagency, then breakdown in coordination can occur. Domain consensus can be increased by stating common goals, stipulating membership contingencies, and maintaining good communication among agencies.

Ideological consensus is agreement among the agencies that cooperation and joint programming is in fact worth the effort. This type of consensus is enhanced by a demonstration that benefits will result from such coordination and by identification of the specific agency actions necessary to implement the coordination relationship.

Interorganizational evaluation consensus refers to the necessity that the workers in one agency have a favorable opinion of the work done in the other cooperative agencies. Recommended changes in an agency's activities, for example, can be construed as a negative evaluation of those activities; such recommendations can be detrimental to coordination if it has not been established that workers in all the agencies do in fact respect the work done by those in the various other participating agencies. As changes in agency routine are shown to be effective, however, the tension of interorganizational evaluation lessens.

11.2.2. DEVELOPING RELATIONSHIPS

There are a number of actions and considerations that can enhance the vigor and success of cooperative relationships.

1. The administrative and operational staffs of the agencies involved must understand the others' goals, operating procedures, scope of services, and resources.

2. Personnel in all the agencies concerned must have frequent and meaningful contact with one another in order to increase interaction among agencies. Interaction can be advanced through the organization of councils or rehabilitation agencies and organizations, group meetings, staff meetings, joint planning efforts, utilization of common facilities, exchange visits to agencies, speaking engagements, educational training conferences, and publications.

3. The agencies involved in rehabilitation must agree on the basic goals of their programs and the standards by which progress toward those goals will be measured. Priorities of agencies should be parallel, since nothing can undo the accomplishments of a client in one phase of a cooperative program so much as encountering a different set of priorities in another phase of the rehabilitation process.

4. There should be a definitive, written, cooperative agreement or operational plan, or both, that states the level of mutual understanding each agency has about its respective role, overall program goals, the scope of programs, and operating procedures. Operational staffs should take part in the formulation of agreements since they often, because of practical experience, have keen insight into what is

possible or impossible for agencies working together to accomplish.

5. Programs should be reviewed periodically and evaluated in terms of predetermined criteria for success. Then program areas needing revision can be examined [U.S. IRS, 1971a].

Ross [1976], having referred to the above guidelines, went on to say that the existence of agreements between agencies ". . . will not automatically improve services or minimize delay. Enforcement of agreements and cooperation among agencies is essential" [p. 25]. Rather than on force, interagency agreements depend upon mutual respect and understanding.

11.2.3. PRACTITIONER'S ROLE

Although cooperative programs may be developed by administrative staff, the responsibility for their daily implementation falls on the individual rehabilitation worker. The following are suggestions for practitioners who work within a cooperative arrangement.

First, it is necessary to communicate the rehabilitationist's role and responsibilities for the client to workers in the cooperative program. Case conferences, staff meetings, in-service training sessions, and personal contacts will provide opportunities to clarify all roles and objectives of participating agencies and their representatives.

A commitment to teamwork is vital, and some preparation in group dynamics is good. Professionals from different agencies have different frames of reference that can enrich everyone's understanding of clients. Divergent orientations of other professions and agencies should be respected and discussed with tact. A superior attitude manifested by anyone in the group will disrupt the cooperative spirit. Communication flow is essential in a cooperative program.

11.3. Teamwork in Rehabilitation

An essential skill for any professional involved in the rehabilitation process is to be able to work effectively with other professionals. The necessity for teamwork derives from the fact that comprehensive rehabilitation requires a

variety of specialized help [Harrower, 1955]. Each separate profession focuses upon a single part of the problem with fragmented knowledge and effort. The concept of the "whole person" is implemented by interprofessional teamwork which strives for total rehabilitation of the disabled person.

"No disabled person is less than the sum total of his needs . . .", said Allan [1958, p. 123], who elaborated as follows:

The need of joint effort on the part of the various disciplines involved in the rehabilitation process is important not only to the understanding of the patient and his own concept of the full program, it is also vital to the practical success of the entire effort. The teamwork never becomes a reality so long as the physical therapist does not understand and even resents the supposed encroachment of the corrective therapist, so long as the doctor sees no reason for asking the advice of the prosthetist on limb-fitting problems, so long as any one member of a discipline regards the work of other professional or technical people as unwarranted intrusion upon his or her domain. By the same token, the worker in one field of rehabilitation cannot consider himself an expert in the areas properly handled by others [p. 124].

11.3.1. THE TEAMWORK CONCEPT

Community pressures have made teamwork in rehabilitation inevitable. Margolin [1969] traced the evolution of the physical treatment of the disabled through three basic phases. All three phases exist today whether in isolation from each other or in harmonious relationship.

In the first phase there was only concern for the person's illness or injury. It was the specific illness or injury that was treated. More often than not the individual's needs, fears, and hopes were overlooked. While it was during this phase that medical specialists developed (such as physical and occupational therapists), teamwork was not considered necessary. In the second phase there was concern for the total person because it was recognized that disease or injury had psychological concomitants that affected personality functioning. From this conceptual frame of reference grew the rehabilitation medicine movement with its twofold emphasis: on maintenance therapy and on returning the person to the community as a socially and economically useful citizen. Rehabilitation was defined as an interdisciplinary movement, thus laying the groundwork for teamwork activity. The third phase was classified by Margolin as that of psychosocial medicine. Concern is expressed for the total personality and how it functions in its total setting. There is a recognition that disability affects not only the individual

but the entire family and that treatment of the individual cannot be apart from treatment of the family. There is also concern for the impact of social systems upon the care and treatment of the person. The family system, the work system, the medical system, the welfare system—all have varying positive and negative impacts upon the individual's recovery.

Yet despite community pressures, the multiple needs of clients, professional specialization, and increased emphasis on interdisciplinary cooperation, there is still much confusion as to exactly what "teamwork" means in comprehensive rehabilitation, who does it, and how it is accomplished. For example, according to Patterson [1959]:

Teamwork means different things to different people. To the psychologist it may mean the reporting of certain findings, their interpretation, and the making of recommendations to other persons working with a client. To the social worker it may mean obtaining and contributing certain kinds of information about the client, and working with the client in certain areas so that he may be prepared or enabled to benefit from other rehabilitation services. To the nurse, the occupational therapist, and the physical therapist it may mean carrying out the prescription of the doctor and reporting on the results. And to the doctor it often means the cooperation of ancillary workers in carrying out his plans or prescriptions for the patient [p. 9].

While these conceptions may represent teamwork in a limited sense, they fall short of recognizing the potential of comprehensive, interdisciplinary teamwork. Whitehouse [1976], an authority on the subject, has provided a cogent definition of the kind of teamwork that is most effective in helping rehabilitation clients. "Teamwork is a close, cooperative, democratic, multiprofessional union devoted to a common purpose—the best treatment for the fundamental needs of the individual. Its members work through a combined and integrated diagnosis; flexible, dynamic planning; proper timing and sequence of treatment; and balance in action. It is an organismic group distinct in its parts, yet acting as a unit, i.e., no important action is taken by members of one profession without the consent of the group" [p. 215].

As Whitehouse pointed out, team members must not only be concerned for the welfare of the client, but they also should be stimulated by the intellectual problem to be solved. (A proper combination and balance of these two are essential.) Teamwork provides "postprofessional education," which results in a higher professional performance for all than any one person could achieve alone.

11.3.2. TEAM EFFECTIVENESS

The success of a multi-disciplinary team is dependent upon the composition of the team members, the effectiveness of its organization, and above all, the shared feeling that teamwork will yield beneficial results. The team increases its effectiveness when its membership encompasses a wide range of professionals involved in the rehabilitation process. Ideally, all professionals involved with a client should function as a team. The exceptional rehabilitation team can also be measured by how well it organizes into a unit.

Teamwork depends upon the continuing communication of team members, which is facilitated by frequent meetings. It is naive, however, to view teamwork as taking place only at large regular meetings. Many informal exchanges and submeetings take place during interviewing periods. In fact, cases may not even be discussed at some full meetings that are held to discuss staff developments and exchange the philosophies held by the members of various disciplines.

To be effective the team must be duly authorized and have the respect of agency administration. Personnel and physical accommodations are required for the mechanics of the process. Time must be allocated for meetings, a room that affords privacy should be assigned, and implementation of the work of the team must be facilitated administratively.

Administration members notwithstanding, the professionals on the team determine its viability. As Whitehouse [1976] said: "While structure, regulation, and organization are necessary, a common philosophy about teamwork is also essential; competence and experience are important, as well as a strong desire to serve with dedication. Nothing can help more to preserve the quality of the process and its accomplishments and to ease the inevitable frictions than confidence, trust, and positive feelings toward each other" [p. 218].

11.3.3. ORIENTATION

A multi-disciplinary team works well with democratic leadership and a democratic philosophy.

Typically, leadership in professional groups has been established traditionally—by seniority, by superior occupational status (e.g., the physician), or by personal charisma [Horwitz, 1969]. However, research has shown that groups do not always function well with a single, authoritarian leader who makes all the decisions. "In the usual authoritarian situation there is insecurity among the members of the team—a defensiveness or resistance or, sometimes, dependence and passivity," said Patterson [1959, p. 10]. One way to avoid the problem of choosing a captain of the team is to speak of the client as the leader; however, this is not always practical.

A workable notion called "group-centered leadership" was proposed by Gordon [1955] as a method of creating democratic teamwork. Since in any good organization the team is viewed as a group of professional equals, the leadership may rotate to the team member who has primary responsibility for a phase of the client's rehabilitation process. In any event, to keep the group functioning smoothly, the person who is designated as the leader or who acts as chairperson is not the one person who makes the final decisions.

A democratic, client-centered approach, with respect for clinical freedom, is a general principle of the team concept. The team makes its own rules and feels free to break its own regulations at will. Discussions of the team are based upon a consensus of the group. When clients are concerned, group agreement and concurrence of individual members develop in nonauthoritarian discussion. Formal votes with majority opinion should be unnecessary since they indicate a breakdown of the team process. Instead consensus is facilitated by proper communication and by an understanding of the issues.

11.3.4. TEAM COMMUNICATION

An effective team displays effective communication skills based on respect for all the participating members. The team's discourse should be accepting and open. Members need not be fearful of risk-taking as optimism leads to greater accomplishments. Predictions about clients, however, should not be put forth unless one can give reasons for the conclusion, even if it is only a clinical hunch.

Reports are circulated in advance of the meeting to avoid long verbal reports and to give other members time to think about the material (so-called bombshell reports, those given without prior communication with those concerned, are not tolerated). Thus the team is able to spend its valuable meeting time in clarification and deliberation of the presenting problems.

11.3.5. PLANNING GOALS
Detailed goals that reflect the total team effort should be set if the rehabilitation process is to be successful. The rehabilitation plan is based on comprehensive client assessment. The gathering of evidence continues throughout the planning and may include further investigation of the past history, repetition of previous tests, progress reports on current services, reports on observed changes in client attitudes and behavior, and, with each additional fact, reinterpretation by the team. As Whitehouse [1976] said, ". . . diagnoses and prognoses are fluid, dynamic, working hypotheses, not closed decisions . . ." [p. 224].

Decision-making of this type is not scientific. It utilizes the collective judgment of the professionals on the team, and team members from different disciplines may use different methods, some relying upon objective and quantitative measures, others exercising clinical opinions without "hard" evidence. Despite its complexity this multi-faceted approach to decision-making by the membership of the team increases the validity of processes.

11.3.6. PUBLIC AGENCY TEAM
The above discussion of the rehabilitation team primarily refers to rehabilitation in a facility with a multi-disciplinary staff. The team concept in rehabilitation has two distinctly different viewpoints, depending upon place of employment: in rehabilitation facilities the team is a group of staff people representing different professions and techniques (see 8.4.3); in the state rehabilitation agency the so-called team members are actually outside consultants to the rehabilitation counselor. Most of the literature on team operations assumes an interrelationship of members such as is found in a facility. State rehabilitation agencies do not have a residential staff representing various disciplines and sharing the same roster of clients; as a consequence the team approach is fully applicable only in facility settings.

11.4. Agency Collaboration

The medical, social, educational, and economic nature of rehabilitation means that its client activities are connected with those of other agencies in the state and community. In some instances other agencies attempt to render services that are clearly in the field of rehabilitation service and that could be much more effectively performed through a working relationship with the public agency. Since the principal purpose of all such services must depend upon the needs of the client, harmonious relationships with other agencies must be of primary importance to everyone in human service programs. (See 7.1.7.)

11.4.1. MECHANISMS
Collaborative relationships are not automatic but require careful development and maintenance on the part of not only administrators but also practitioners. The first essential of collaboration is a specific and complete agreement as to the work responsibilities of each agency. Even informal agreements should be written, for example, a letter confirming a conversation about help to be given a client. More elaborate ongoing arrangements between two agencies require a legalistic type of document that is updated periodically and interpreted to the operating staffs of both agencies. This formal agreement should identify reciprocal duties to be performed and should designate specific individuals responsible for the work. A definite procedure or plan of operation is also essential for organized relations.

Working relationships between the state rehabilitation agency and the state workers compensation agency provide an example. Workers compensation (either the agency or the service) has a smaller role in state vocational rehabilitation affairs than was conceived by the architects of the original federal rehabilitation legislation; this stipulated rehabilitation services for "individuals disabled in industry and otherwise," the "otherwise" being an afterthought to include other accidents, disease, or congenital causes of handicapping. Subsequently, however, the public rehabilitation program tended to neglect the workers compensation agency despite the fact that the federal regulations made collaborative agreements mandatory. More importantly, the states' workers compensation agencies have several distinct contributions to make to vocational rehabilitation programming. First, this agency can report potential cases soon after injury and before the effects of deterioration make rehabilitation infeasible or more expensive. Second, the workers compensation agency can contribute to the case procedure by utilizing its funding mechanisms so that settlements can pay part of the cost of rehabilitation services. Third, the strategic position of organizations associated with workers compensation, including insurance carriers, can promote the expansion and improvement of rehabilitation programming in the Congress and state legislatures. (See 37.4.)

11.4.2. MANDATED STATE COLLABORATION

Federal rehabilitation regulations stipulate state agency collaboration with various public agencies in addition to the workers compensation agency. The federal law and regulations further require joint planning and cooperation when a state has a general rehabilitation agency and a separate agency for rehabilitation of the blind. The two agencies must establish reciprocal referral services, utilize each other's services and facilities, plan joint activities to improve services to the handicapped population, and otherwise cooperate for effective services.

The utilization of community resources by a state rehabilitation agency depends upon cooperation with both public and private groups. Cooperative arrangements (including suggested written agreements) are outlined in the federal regulations for over 30 of the cooperating public programs (e.g., state Special Education, Crippled Children, CETA, Employment Service, Public Assistance), fifteen voluntary organizations (e.g., sheltered workshops, rehabilitation or disability groups) and several commercial units (e.g., prosthetic appliance makers, hearing aid dealers, private trade schools, disability insurance firms).

"Similar benefits" (services or financial assistance appropriate and available to the handicapped individual from another agency) must be used to pay the cost of a client's service when possible. Exception is made if this causes significant delay in providing restoration or maintenance services. The 1973 Rehabilitation Act required the state agency to try to obtain client expenditures for higher education from other sources.

Cooperative planning is an administrative function to be conducted under the supervision of the officials of the participating agencies. Implementation, however, of any working agreement depends upon the personal, day-to-day relationships of the professional practitioners. Practitioners are close to their clients and this relationship motivates them to become involved in collaborative programming because more efficient services to the individual result.

Chapter 12

Agency Structures

Through a social mandate to meet the extraordinary needs of handicapped people, a great rehabilitation services delivery system has developed. It involves the coordination of three categories of resources: trained manpower, technical methodology, and financial means. To activate and coordinate these resources a complex organizational structure has been constructed. The structural blocks are the various agencies associated with the rehabilitation system.

The purpose of this chapter is to provide an overview of the delivery system by categorizing service functions through descriptions of representative public and private agencies. Presented in this way—for an understanding of the system's structure—it matters not that the agencies, their names, and their purposes are constantly shifting. Directories (printed periodically) give information about current addresses, services, budgets, and other matters needed by the rehabilitationist to use agency resources. In fact, several of these directories were consulted for this chapter: *Ready Reference Guide*, by the U.S. HEW Rehabilitation Services Administration [1978]; *Directory of Agencies*, by the National Association of Social Workers [1975]; and *Consumer Health Education: A Directory, 1975*, by the American Public Health Association and the Health Resources Administration [1975]. National agencies are categorically described in the sections discussing public (12.1) and private organizations (12.2). International organizations are described in the third section (12.3). (Local organizations are discussed in other chapters.)

Many agencies have multiple purposes, yet an attempt is made here to categorize them in the most meaningful way for understanding the system. Classification of an agency under a given function does not necessarily mean that this is its only or even primary service in terms of budget, members served, or public impact. Moreover, officers of the agency might disagree with its classification, for example, the National Easter Seal Society for Crippled Children and Adults could be shown as a fund-raising organization, despite its invaluable national programs such as research and publication. This is because the Easter Seal Society, as it is also called, conducts the national campaign from which come most of the funds that are used by chapters for programs such as local camps and patient services. (Actually, the Society is listed as a Direct Service agency because of its national leadership in helping handicapped individuals.)

12.1. Private Organizations

There are thousands of private organizations in the United States with some relevance to vocational rehabilitation. Each of these agencies has its own unique purpose and program.

This section provides a categorization and description of outstanding private agencies operating at a national level. It should be emphasized that this is not a directory of organizations interested in the handicapped. There are many such directories that describe agencies in detail and provide information about the use of their resources. Nor is the listing provided here intended to be complete, for at best it can only be representative. Its primary purpose is to provide a classification of organizational goals illustrated by selected national agencies. However, it should be pointed out that most of the agencies included could be classified in more than one descriptive category.

Allan [1958] described the scope of human service agencies in his book, *Rehabilitation: A Community Challenge*. According to Allan, the various agencies could be categorized by their different purposes and objectives. Actually, few agencies have a single purpose, but instead conduct several kinds of programs. Still it is possible to classify agencies according to several fundamental dimensions: program goals, nature of membership or sponsorship, organizational structure, methods of financing, and the level of organization (e.g., national, state, or local).

The organizational scheme used in the present chapter first of all differentiates between publicly and privately supported agencies, and then categorizes them according to the primary purpose. Within this section on private agencies, subsections are set up according to agency purpose. This categorization accommodates a broad range of agencies and affords opportunity to acknowledge many of the most important national groups. It is important to note that the subsection label consequently indicates a primary purpose of the organizations listed.

12.1.1. SPECIFIC DISABILITY

Some agencies, particularly voluntary health groups, are concerned with one and only one specific medical disability. This has been found to be an effective method of organization. It provides a discrete purpose and a unique reason for fund-raising and budgeting. It provides an explicit purpose for which those concerned with the disability can rally behind the organization as volunteers. Thus such agencies are able to assemble board members and volunteers with a personal interest. Moreover, disability focus has proved to be an effective fund-raising stimulus: public contributions are more likely to come for purposes of blindness, cancer, or designated disabilities than they are for a less explicitly named condition or program. Some of these explicit disability groups are identified here; all are national health agencies, but some private health groups are elsewhere categorized.

American Heart Association

Founded in 1924, this association has as its purpose: supporting cardiovascular research and transmitting its benefits to the professional and lay public through community service and education programs; coordinating efforts of physicians and others; informing the public of progress in the field; enlisting financial support. Among the community services developed by chapter affiliates are emergency cardiac care programs, special clinics to evaluate work capacity of heart patients, and stroke rehabilitation. The association also conducts professional and lay education.

Arthritis Foundation

Established in 1948, this foundation is the national agency for arthritis, the nation's number one crippling disease. (Some health agencies use the name "Foundation.") As a voluntary health agency with local chapters throughout the country, the organization supports research to discover the cause of arthritis and to develop preventive techniques or a cure; finances training for young medical scientists and physicians and seeks to attract more medical workers to the field of arthritis; expands community services to patients and their families; seeks to improve treatment techniques and to make better arthritis care available to all who need it; finances studies to develop new ways to prevent and correct disability and to develop and test new drugs; and informs doctors and patients of the latest developments in arthritis care and research.

American Foundation for the Blind

A private, national organization founded in 1921, its stated objective is "to help those handicapped by blindness to achieve the fullest possible development and utilization of their capacities, and integration into the social, cultural and economic life of the community." The agency serves as a clearinghouse for all pertinent information about blindness and services to those who are blind. Ongoing programs include: psychosocial and technological research in the

area of blindness; consultation to private and governmental agencies directly servicing the blind and deaf-blind; manufacture of talking books and aids and appliances for blind persons; public education through all media; maintenance of a special library on the subject of blindness for lending and bibliographic purposes; and legislative counsel and action programs.

Publications include: *Journal of Visual Impairment and Blindness* (published 10 times a year in print, Braille, and recorded form), special monographs and books, and the *Directory of Agencies Serving the Visually Handicapped in the United States*.

American Cancer Society

Founded in 1913, this association's major purpose is to organize and wage a continuing campaign against cancer and its crippling effects through medical research, professional and public education, and service and rehabilitation programs.

The Cancer Society conducts programs of public and professional education along with service and rehabilitation programs at the national and local levels. Rehabilitation programs include: Reach for Recovery, for women who have had breast surgery; International Association of Laryngectomees, for men and women who have lost their voices because of throat surgery; and ostomy programs, for those who have undergone intestinal or urinary surgery for cancer.

United Cerebral Palsy Association (UCP)

UCP, as it is called, is a national organization dedicated in 1948 to a continuing overall attack on cerebral palsy. Its primary function is to seek solutions to the multiple problems of cerebral palsy, with affiliates providing direct services to the cerebral palsied in states and communities.

The organization carries on a program of guidance, instruction, and assistance to affiliates and other community agencies, including: professional service programs; research and professional training; infant care centers; adult vocational and service programs; governmental activities; public information; and field services, including assistance in operations of affiliates, women's activities, youth activities, and affiliates' campaigns and organizational events.

The national office of the organization carries on a program of grants-in-aid for cerebral palsy research, training, and education. The medical activities include development and publication of professional information for use by physicians and medical and technical schools; collection and evaluation of data relative to various methods of treatment; and dissemination of information to parents and professional groups.

National Society for the Prevention of Blindness

This organization has been engaged since 1908 in the prevention of blindness and conservation of vision through a comprehensive program of community service, publications, public information, lay and professional education, and basic clinical and operational research. The agency's principal programs and activities include: support of basic, clinical, and operational research; community services, including preschool vision screening programs, glaucoma detection programs, and health information; and professional education programs.

National Paraplegia Foundation

This association was founded in 1948 with the objectives of: improved and expanded rehabilitation and treatment of those suffering spinal cord injuries; expanded research on a cure for paraplegia and quadriplegia; removal of architectural barriers to the handicapped; increased employment opportunities for the handicapped; and accessible housing and transportation. It publishes *Paraplegia Life*, with articles on recreation, new products, and other helpful news for members.

National Multiple Sclerosis Society

Founded in 1946, this association's major objectives are to: stimulate, coordinate, and support research directed toward determining the cause, prevention, alleviation, and cure of multiple sclerosis and related diseases of the central nervous system; conduct lay and professional education programs concerning the disease; administer patient services through local chapters; and carry out worldwide programs of information and idea exchange.

National Association for Retarded Citizens (NARC)

NARC is a citizen membership organization founded in 1950. Its purpose is to further the advancement of all ameliorative and preventive study, research, and therapy in the field of mental retardation; to develop a better understanding of the problems of mental retardation by the public; to further the training and education of personnel for work in the field; and to promote the general welfare of the mentally retarded of all ages.

Principal programs are public education, family counseling, and clearinghouse activities.

Muscular Dystrophy Associations of America (MDAA)

This voluntary health organization was incorporated in 1950 to foster research seeking cures or effective treatments for muscular dystrophy and related neuromuscular diseases. MDAA programs include the following: patient services, including provision of orthopedic appliances and physical therapy; education of those with dystrophy as well as the general public; recreational programs; transportation; community clinics in larger cities; and research.

Epilepsy Foundation of America

Founded in 1967 after a series of mergers, the Epilepsy Foundation of America is the national voluntary health agency leading the fight against epilepsy in the United States. With a network of affiliates in 50 states, the Foundation speaks for several million people with epilepsy. Defining the myriad problems of these people and devising specific detailed programs to solve them are prime Foundation objectives.

The Foundation supports many categories of programs involving various activities under the headings of medical, social, and informational. This organization, for example (continuing a service of the old National Epilepsy League), provides anticonvulsant and related medications by mail at wholesale cost to members with epilepsy upon their physician's prescription. Annual projects include national Epilepsy Month (November).

12.1.2. FAMILY OF IMPAIRMENTS

As indicated in the above listing, many voluntary health groups are concerned about a specific disability. In other voluntary health associations the concern is less explicit in that the goals embrace a whole family of impairments. These are usually grouped, however, in some functional and logical assemblage of limitations.

National Association for Mental Health

This mental health association, organized in 1950, is a private organization with 1,000 local affiliate chapters. Its aim is to improve attitudes toward mental illness and the mentally ill; to improve services for the mentally ill; and to work for the prevention of mental illness and to promote mental health.

The Association sponsors broad programs of research, social action, education, and service. Special program emphasis is placed on improved care and treatment of mental hospital patients; aftercare and rehabilitation; community mental health services; and services for mentally ill children, including treatment and education.

Sister Kenny Institute

The Sister Kenny Institute, which was founded in 1942, is a nonprofit hospital and prototype rehabilitation center. It specializes in rehabilitation of the disabled for the purpose of restoring patients to maximum functioning ability so that they may return to their homes and community and live as full and productive a life as possible.

American Lung Association

Formerly called the National Tuberculosis and Respiratory Disease Association, the American Lung Association was founded in 1904 for the prevention and control of lung disease. Its principal programs and activities are: the promotion of public and professional education programs on the cause, treatment, and prevention of tuberculosis and other chronic lung diseases; the elimination of cigarette smoking; the elimination of air pollution; the improvement of community health and welfare; and the encouragement and support of professional and technical education, as well as medical and social research in the fields of tuberculosis and other lung diseases.

Its publications include the monthly *American Review of Respiratory Disease*.

12.1.3. PROCESS

A single service phase or component of the rehabilitation process is emphasized by the goals of certain organizations. Such agencies may cut across disability lines. The process-oriented agencies therefore generally extend their concern generically to all handicapping conditions but limit their attention to one aspect of the total rehabilitation process.

National Therapeutic Recreation Society

The National Therapeutic Recreation Society, a branch of the National Recreation and Park Association, was founded in 1966 by merger of the National Association of Recreational Therapists and Hospital Section of the American Recreation Society. Its objectives are to improve and enhance recreation and leisure services for the nation's ill, handicapped, disabled, and other special populations.

The Society's principal programs and activities are workshops, conferences, national registration program, setting of standards, technical assistance, and consultation.

Association of Rehabilitation Facilities

In 1969, the Association of Rehabilitation Centers and the National Association of Sheltered Workshops and Homebound Programs merged, forming the (International) Association of Rehabilitation Facilities. Its purpose is to assist in the development and improvement of services of member facilities in programs appropriate to the goals of the facilities engaged in providing services to the handicapped. (In 1976 "International" was dropped from the name.) The Association encompasses 700 rehabilitation centers and sheltered workshops. The principal programs of the Association are educational seminars throughout the year and an annual conference.

Boy Scouts of America, Scouting for the Handicapped Division

Scouting for the Handicapped is a special program of the Boy Scouts of America, the purpose of which is to: encourage the inclusion of handicapped youngsters in regular packs, troops, and posts; emphasize job preparation for handicapped scouts; see that the handicapped youngster gets full opportunity to share the joys of scouting with his normal peers; and encourage the establishment of packs, troops, and posts at schools and homes for the handicapped whenever it is not possible to include these youngsters in ongoing scout activities. To the extent possible, handicapped scouts engage in the same activities as nonhandicapped scouts: cubbing, scouting, exploring, camping, civic activities, recreation, crafts, and so forth.

Publications include *Scouting for the Deaf*, *Scouting for the Visually Handicapped*, *Scout-*

ing for the Retarded, and *Scouting for the Physically Handicapped.*

American Printing House for the Blind

The Printing House was incorporated by the Kentucky Legislature in 1858 to assist in the education of the blind. It provides literature and appliances for the blind on a nonprofit basis. To achieve its objectives, the American Printing House for the Blind publishes and distributes embossed books, books in large type, recorded materials, and educational aids. It manufactures books and periodicals—both braille and talking books—at cost for organizations that provide literature for the blind, and conducts inquiry and research into the specific problems relating to the selection and preparation of literature and appliances for the blind and near-blind.

Publications include catalogs and informational brochures.

National Association of Jewish Vocational Services

Founded in 1939, the organization is composed of 28 local agency affiliates, namely, Jewish Vocational Service (JVS) agencies. This national organization acts as a clearinghouse and coordinating body for all Jewish organizations engaged in work related to vocational rehabilitation. It was formerly called the Jewish Occupational Council.

National Industries of the Blind (NIB)

NIB is designated to allocate federal purchases for goods and services to qualified workshops for the blind. It coordinates the production of about 100 workshops throughout the nation providing employment to over 5,000 blind clients. NIB recommends new products, devises quality control systems, and assists workshops in various other ways. Sales of NIB associated workshops exceed $100 million in yearly sales about half of which is to the federal government.

National Industries for the Severely Handicapped (NISH)

Incorporated in 1974, NISH has expanded employment for the severely handicapped by using sheltered workshops to produce services and commodities for the federal government [Perlman, 1978]. Along with NIB this agency was designated to represent workshops that supply federal purchases. It is a consortium of central nonprofit agencies: Goodwill Industries of America, Association of Rehabilitation Facilities, National Association of Jewish Vocational Services, National Association of Retarded Citizens, National Easter Seal Society for Crippled Children and Adults, and United Cerebral Palsy Associations. NISH has offices in Washington, D.C.

12.1.4. DIRECT SERVICE

Many agencies attend to the needs of disabled individuals by providing or financing direct services. From a fund-raising standpoint the commitment of immediate and tangible assistance to handicapped individuals is the most attractive appeal that can be made to volunteers with a personal interest and also, for that matter, to the financially contributing public in fund-raising drives.

Properly administered, direct service agencies do not overlap with publicly financed resources when spending privately raised funds. Many of these agencies, of course, subcontract with public agencies for provision of direct services to clients and are appropriately reimbursed.

American National Red Cross

The purpose of the American National Red Cross is to bring together, as Red Cross volunteers, Americans of all ages who share an interest in the health, safety, and well-being of all. An all-volunteer Board of Governors makes policy for the national organization, which is administered by a corporate staff. Locally, volunteers govern the activities of chapters and largely carry out the work of the organizations. More than 3,000 chapters are chartered.

Programs are determined locally, according to community needs. Program offerings may include services to members of the armed forces and veterans and their families, volunteer blood programs, community health and safety programs, community service programs for youth, and emergency relief programs for the victims of disasters of all sorts.

National Easter Seal Society for Crippled Children and Adults

The objectives of the "Crippled Children Society," also well known as the "Easter Seal" Society, are to: assist disabled persons and their families in finding and making effective use of resources that will be helpful to them in developing their abilities and in living purposeful lives; assist communities in developing necessary and appropriate resources for disabled persons; establish and maintain programs and services that are appropriate and realistic; and create a climate of acceptance of disabled persons that will enable them to contribute, to the full extent of their competence, to the well-being of the community.

The Society, which was organized in 1921, conducts a three-point program in service, education, and research at the national, state, and local levels. Programs serving all types of physically handicapped children and adults include:

1. Care and treatment services through diagnostic clinics, comprehensive rehabilitation and treatment centers, preschool programs, sheltered workshops, homebound employment, craft outlets, vocational programs, camping and recreation projects, social services, psychological and psychiatric services, provision of special equipment, transportation, and information referral and follow-up programs.
2. An educational program designed for the public as a whole, for professional personnel concerned with the care and treatment of the crippled, for parents of the crippled and others living with them, and for employers and volunteers.
3. Research concerned with the prevention and treatment of physical and associated disabilities carried out (1) through the Easter Seal Research Foundation, and (2) by supporting research projects in universities and other institutions throughout the United States.
4. Sponsorship of meetings and seminars for professional personnel and the financing of scholarships for study in therapy fields.
5. Distribution of substantial quantities of literature to parents, professionals, the general public, and libraries overseas. Gives assistance to foreign visitors in planning itineraries while on visits to the United States.

Publications of the Society feature an important professional journal, *Rehabilitation Literature*.

Menninger Foundation

The Menninger Foundation is a private foundation that grew out of the Menninger Clinic, opened in 1919. The Foundation's objectives are the treatment of mental illness through inpatient and outpatient clinical facilities, with emphasis on research, education, and preventive psychiatry. The Foundation's principal programs include: clinical services, research, prevention (through community psychiatry office, industrial mental health seminars, and so on), and education in the Menninger School of Psychiatry.

ICD Rehabilitation and Research Center

Formerly the Institute for the Crippled and Disabled, the ICD was founded in 1917 and is dedicated to the improvement of the condition of handicapped persons through rehabilitation treatment and training, research, and professional education.

Principal programs are: patient services (including medical diagnosis and treatment, vocational and social adjustment, and training), research, research utilization, professional education (courses, seminars, symposia, and conferences on techniques of rehabilitation), and professional publications.

Goodwill Industries of America

Founded in 1902, Goodwill and its member local rehabilitation workshops provide vocational rehabilitation services, training, employment, and opportunities for personal growth as a step in the rehabilitation process for the disabled and disadvantaged.

The Goodwill programs for preparing the handicapped for useful living are comprehensive, including: vocational counseling, work testing, work conditioning and training, social and medical evaluation, vocational on-the-job training, and job placement.

EPI-HAB

Founded in 1955 by Frank Risch, EPI-HAB is dedicated to the socioeconomic reintegration of the person with epilepsy through medical control, work training, employment, and placement.

Its principal programs and activities are: conditioning epileptics for job responsibility (i.e., attendance, accuracy, quality, meeting schedules, etc.); training epileptics in a variety of skills (e.g., machine shop operations, electronic assembly, sophisticated packaging); training epileptics for specific jobs in industry with the cooperation of subcontracting firms; and socializing programs (i.e., group counseling, sports, and recreation).

Seeing Eye, Inc.

This nonprofit corporation, established in 1929 in Morristown, N.J., is supported by contributions and a substantial endowment. It trains dog guides and instructs blind persons in their use at a nominal fee.

Helen Keller National Center for
Deaf-Blind Youths and Adults

Established in 1969, the Helen Keller Center conducts various rehabilitation services. It is operated by the Industrial Home for the Blind; federal funds are provided.

12.1.5. PUBLIC INFORMATION

Public information for the benefit of disabled people is an important activity of many agencies. In fact it is the primary program of a few organizations.

The general public or selected "special publics" such as responsible professionals are informed through the news media, pamphlets, meetings, and so on. There are many educational purposes, one of the most important of which is to overcome public ignorance and negative attitudes about disability.

President's Committee on Employment
of the Handicapped

The President's Committee on Employment of the Handicapped was established by the President of the United States in 1947. Since then, every President has given his personal and active support to full employment opportunities for the physically and mentally handicapped. (Although this organization receives government funds for administration, it is listed here because of its reliance on the voluntary involvement of private groups and individuals.)

The objective of the Committee is to help the handicapped help themselves. To accomplish this goal, the Committee (1) conducts national education and information programs designed to eliminate physical and psychological barriers; (2) furthers educational training, rehabilitation, and employment opportunities and also promotes community acceptance of the disabled; and (3) provides leadership and technical support to volunteer Governors' Committees on Employment of the Handicapped in all states.

The Committee is composed of more than 600 organizations and individuals representing business, handicapped persons, industry, labor, the media, the medical professional, rehabilitation personnel, religious groups, veterans, youth, and other concerned groups. It engages in two major activities each year: National Employ the Handicapped Week, the first full week in October, provides an opportunity to focus public attention on the problems and progress of the handicapped on national and local levels; and a national meeting held each spring in Washington, D.C. attracts thousands of professionals and volunteers for a two-day program highlighting the progress of the handicapped.

Public administration of this organization is described below. (See 12.2.9.)

12.1.6. ADMINISTRATIVE COORDINATION

Administrative coordination is the business of some not-for-profit corporations. While not likely to attract general public attention, they play an extremely important role in promotion, policy-making, self-regulation, and other administrative efforts. This is particularly important in view of the unrestricted proliferation of voluntary health agencies and other nonprofit groups.

American Public Health Association (APHA)

APHA was founded in 1872. It is an organization of affiliated societies and branches and individual members interested in public health work. Occupational Health and Safety is one of its 22 sections. APHA's principal programs and activities include the promulgation of standards and the establishment of uniform practices and procedures.

Publications include the *American Journal of Public Health.*

National Health Council (NHC)

Major national voluntary organizations and professional societies in the health field are members of the NHC. Its goals are to improve the health of the public throughout the United States. The Council, which was started in 1921, administratively coordinates programming of most national health associations. It also has a regulatory effect by excluding from membership those that do not meet its standards. It publishes annual reports.

National Alliance of Businessmen (NAB)

The NAB has more than 130 branch offices throughout the country staffed by some 5,000 persons, of whom the majority are business executives on loan from and paid by their companies. The Alliance is a partnership of business, labor, and government working to secure jobs and training for veterans, the disadvantaged, needy youth, and ex-offenders. NAB works with employers to have jobs set aside for veterans and other target groups. It asks employers to list openings with the local state Employment Service. NAB was founded in 1968 under President Lyndon Johnson.

12.1.7. RESEARCH

Research, in the long run, is one of the most rewarding investments of agency resources. It provides the basis for future technology that will overcome disability and handicapping. Intraorganizational research is conducted by the scientific staff employed by the organization, while extraorganizational research is administered through awards to universities and other grantees. Many of the organizations mentioned in this chapter underwrite research, but several agencies are particularly noteworthy in this respect. The research programs of private organizations should not duplicate the massive federal research budget.

National Foundation/March of Dimes

Formerly the National Polio Foundation, this Foundation, founded in 1938 by President Franklin D. Roosevelt, now has as its goal the prevention of birth defects.

The National Foundation/March of Dimes' principal programs and activities include: funding basic and clinical research, funding medical service programs for birth defect victims, sponsoring professional education, and distributing public health information.

Joseph P. Kennedy, Jr. Foundation

The Kennedy Foundation was established in 1946. The Foundation has striven to determine causes of mental retardation through research; reduce its effects by treatment and training; promote programs of physical fitness and vocational supervision for the retarded; train professionals to work in this field; and make the general public aware of efforts being made on behalf of the mentally retarded.

12.1.8. SCIENTIFIC ADVANCEMENT

Most of the organizations listed in this chapter make significant contributions to the advancement of science and improved practice through the dissemination of knowledge. Many such associations limit their membership to scientific or professional participants. An outstanding example in the field of disability is the American Public Health Association, which is listed under 12.1.6. Administrative Coordination, because of its broad interdisciplinary program. The agencies listed below are examples of the many organizations that conduct such valuable programs.

American Association on Mental Deficiency (AAMD)

The AAMD, founded in 1876, is a national organization of over 10,000 professionals, representing a variety of interests and disciplines dealing with many types of developmental disabilities.

The objectives of the AAMD are to effect the highest standards of programming for the mentally retarded, to facilitate cooperation among those working with the mentally retarded, and to educate the public to understand, accept, and respect the mentally retarded.

These aims are achieved in the following ways: serving on panels to develop and evaluate standards for services and facilities for the retarded; planning national educational and informational seminars; attending meetings at the local, regional, national, and international level; supporting legislation concerning the rights of the retarded and services available to them as well as the prevention of mental retardation and related developmental disabilities.

Publications are *Mental Retardation* and the *American Journal on Mental Deficiency*, published in alternate months.

American Congress of Rehabilitation Medicine

This organization exists for the purpose of providing a scientific forum for communication among the many disciplines concerned with rehabilitation medicine. It has a membership of practicing professionals, educators, and scientists who are working actively for the advancement of rehabilitation medicine. It focuses its programs and meetings on research findings and techniques of interest to all professionals in the rehabilitation field.

The roster of current membership in the Congress includes physicians of various specialties, rehabilitation nurses, rehabilitation counselors, speech pathologists, physical therapists, occupational therapists, psychologists, social workers, prosthetists and orthotists, administrators, scientists, and engineers.

Publications include an important journal, the *Archives of Physical Medicine and Rehabilitation.*

American Association for Rehabilitation Therapy (AART)

This Association is a professional member organization of medical rehabilitation personnel and other individuals interested in rehabilitation of the mentally and physically disabled. Founded in 1950, the AART organized into separate sections for each of the adjunctive therapies in the fields of physical medicine and rehabilitation.

Local, regional, and national meetings are held to promote the use of curative and technical modalities within the scope, philosophy, and approved medical concepts of rehabilitation; advance the practice of rehabilitation; establish and advance the standards of education of rehabilitation therapists; encourage and promote research; and cooperate with other organizations in the realization of common objectives.

Publications include the noteworthy journal, *American Archives of Rehabilitation Therapy.*

12.1.9. LEGISLATIVE ACTION

There are federal restrictions on the political activity of nonprofit corporations supported by tax-deductible contributions. Consequently, lobbying as a primary purpose is rarely admitted. Nevertheless, most important agencies do exert influence on government legislation and administration. Agency officers inform the lawmakers of program and budget needs, help to draft legislation, testify at congressional hearings and provide data and informed opinion, communicate the progress of relevant bills to the association's membership, and encourage membership contact with their own legislators at critical times. The political action of many private agencies also extends to the administration of relevant laws. Representatives serve in an advisory capacity to public agencies.

National Rehabilitation Association (NRA)

NRA is the national organization of professional and lay persons dedicated to the rehabilitation of all physically and mentally handicapped persons.

Founded in 1925, the Association strives to increase opportunities for handicapped persons to become self-sufficient, self-supporting, and contributing members of the community and to show that this results in social and economic gains to the nation as well as to the individual.

To achieve its objectives, the Association represents its members before governing bodies concerned with rehabilitation legislation; encourages teamwork as a basic system of rehabilitation through the maximum use of the knowledge and skills of all professions; provides, through publications and conferences on national, regional, and local levels, a forum for discussion of all problems related to the handicapped; fosters research to advance the knowledge and skills necessary to improve rehabilitation services to the handicapped; and promotes professional training for all personnel engaged in work with the handicapped.

Publications include the *Journal of Rehabilitation.*

National Federation of the Blind (NFB)

The purpose of the NFB is the complete integration of blind persons into society as equal members. This objective involves the removal of legal, economic, and social discriminations and the education of the public to new concepts concerning blindness.

Publications include the *Braille Monitor,* which is published in Braille, in print, and on records.

National Association of Hearing and Speech Agencies

A private, nonprofit organization founded in 1919, the National Association of Hearing and Speech Agencies works exclusively on behalf of hearing, speech, and language-handicapped individuals. Principal programs are education and training, field service, liaison services with federal or other agencies, public information and education, nationwide-career recruitment, and legislative liaison.

American Orthotic and Prosthetic Association

This national organization was founded in 1917. Its membership consists of more than 400 facilities dedicated to rehabilitation of the handicapped through the provision of professional orthotic and prosthetic services (i.e., braces and artificial limbs).

The Association fosters its members' interests

by representing them before state and federal agencies (both regulatory and legislative) that are concerned with health care services to the orthopedically handicapped. It also serves as a channel of communication between the basic suppliers of products and services and the facilities that fit orthoses and prostheses to patients on prescription.

Sister organizations include the American Board of Certification in Orthotics and Prosthetics and the American Academy of Orthotists and Prosthetists. Publications include the journal, *Orthotics and Prosthetics*.

Council for Exceptional Children (CEC)

The CEC is the foremost association of professionals concerned with handicapped children. Its emphasis on special education is demonstrated by its comprehensive programs, which have influenced both thought and practice. It was founded in 1922 and from 1941 to 1961 it was a department of the National Education Association. One of its several journals is *Exceptional Children*.

12.1.10. AGENCY ADMINISTRATION

Associations of administrators not only of public agencies but also of various other organizations are formed to share experiences and combine forces for desired actions. This type of association can provide needed administrative consistency between unconnected organizations with little or no mandated uniformity. Such agencies can actually become a "silent" government. The operation of these organizations—and perhaps that of all the others listed above—has been facilitated by modern communication technology and rapid transportation, which permit a continuing sharing of ideas by the heads of similar agencies located throughout the country.

Council of State Administrators of Vocational Rehabilitation (CSAVR)

CSAVR is composed of the chief administrators of the state vocational rehabilitation agencies. These agencies constitute the state partners in the state-federal program of rehabilitation services but officially have no direct relationship with one another.

Founded in 1940 to furnish state input into the federal rehabilitation agency, the Council has, since then, provided a forum in which state ad-

ministrators study, deliberate, and act upon matters affecting the rehabilitation of handicapped persons. The Council serves as a resource for the formulation and expression of the collective points of view of state rehabilitation agencies on all issues affecting the provision of services to handicapped persons. The Council maintains communication with similar organizations in health, education, welfare, and manpower fields since such organizations are related to vocational rehabilitation.

The organization provides a forum to enable administrators of the state agencies to study and discuss relevant matters. It also serves as an advisory body to the Rehabilitation Services Administration. It has an advisory role similar to that of the National Rehabilitation Association.

Council of Organizations Serving the Deaf

The Council is a central clearinghouse and contact point for information and combined action by member organizations. Since 1967, the Council has worked to eliminate social and economic barriers that handicap deaf persons.

American Council of the Blind

This agency, established in 1961, provides consultative and advisory services to organizations and others with regard to legislation, litigation, credit unions, and state programs. It publishes *The Braille Forum*.

12.1.11. PROFESSIONAL ASSOCIATIONS

Professional associations enhance the services provided to the handicapped clients of members in various ways. Standards are guarded by high criteria for membership. The quality of professional practice is further improved by ongoing programs of professional development through regular conferences and journals. There are a number of very important professional associations relevant to vocational rehabilitation.

American Rehabilitation Counseling Association (ARCA)

ARCA, a division of the American Personnel and Guidance Association (APGA), was organized in 1957 as the first professional organization for counselors specializing in rehabilitation. Standards for membership have been high from its inception.

ARCA and NRCA are the two professional associations representing rehabilitation counseling. While attempts have been made for merger, the two groups have distinct roles: ARCA represents professional counseling as a result of its parent association, which includes all areas of guidance, counseling, and personnel work; NRCA, on the other hand, reflects the broader profession of rehabilitation represented by its parent association, NRA. The two groups are thus complementary and represent different sources of support, although their membership and programs do overlap. Professional membership in ARCA requires an appropriate master's or doctoral degree and experience in rehabilitation counseling as well as membership in APGA. Student membership is open to those in rehabilitation counselor education. ARCA publishes the *Rehabilitation Counseling Bulletin*.

National Rehabilitation Counseling Association (NRCA)

The National Rehabilitation Counseling Association is a private organization, founded in 1958, with the objectives of developing standards for rehabilitation counseling, promoting professional training, supporting rehabilitation counseling as it contributes to the interdisciplinary solution of problems in rehabilitation, and fostering research to advance knowledge and skill in rehabilitation counseling.

NRCA's principal programs and activities parallel those of ARCA. These include joint sponsorship with ARCA of the national counselor certification program; recruitment and placement service for rehabilitation counseling personnel; committee studies in ethics, professional standards, training, and research; sponsorship of training institutes; awards and scholarship programs; state, regional, and national conferences; and liaison with federal and state rehabilitation agencies and Congress.

Publications include the *Journal of Applied Rehabilitation Counseling*.

American Occupational Therapy Association

The American Occupational Therapy Association is the professional organization for occupational therapists and occupational therapy assistants. Founded in 1917, its primary objects and purposes are to improve and advance the practice of occupational therapy to ensure that the breadth and quality of services adequately and appropriately meet the health care needs of the society served; improve and advance educa-

tion and qualifications in occupational therapy; establish standards of performance; foster research and study of occupational therapy; and engage in other activities to further the dissemination of knowledge of the practice of occupational therapy.

Publications include the *American Journal of Occupational Therapy*.

American Physical Therapy Association

Founded in 1921, this organization's purpose is to meet the physical therapy needs of the people through the development and improvement of physical therapy education, practice, and research, and to meet the needs of its members through identification, coordinated action, communication, and fellowship. Principal programs include education, professional services, publications, government relations, and national and regional conferences.

Publications include the *Physical Therapy Journal*.

American Medical Association: Department of Environmental, Public, and Occupational Health

The American Medical Association (AMA) was founded in 1847 to promote the science and art of medicine and the betterment of public health. The AMA Department of Environmental, Public, and Occupational Health is one of seven departments included in The Division of Scientific Activities, which in turn is one of seven divisions in the AMA administrative structure. Membership in the AMA totals 200,000 physicians.

The principal programs and activities of this department include advising physicians in industry, studying environmental problems, encouraging employment of the handicapped, and disseminating information to employers and to the general public concerning employment of the handicapped.

American Psychological Association (APA)

The APA was founded in 1892 and has nearly 40,000 members, all of whom are professional psychologists. It publishes many journals of interest to rehabilitationists, including the *Journal of Counseling Psychology* by Division 17 of the Association. Rehabilitation psychologists who are specialists in the psychological aspects of disability are members of APA Division 22, which promotes this aspect of the science and profession of psychology through the annual APA conference, special meetings, and publications.

National Association of Social Workers (NASW)

Founded in 1955 through the merger of seven social work membership organizations, the NASW is the professional social work association. Programs express interest in social policy, social work practice, and professional standards. The last embraces the status and economic self-interests of the practitioner membership. Among its important publications is the bimonthly publication, *Social Work*.

American Speech and Hearing Association

A professional association organized in 1925, its membership is limited to persons meeting specified requirements. Purposes are to encourage scientific study of individual human speech and hearing, foster improvement of therapeutic procedures, and exchange and disseminate information. It publishes professional materials including the *Journal of Speech and Hearing Disorders* and the *Journal of Speech and Hearing Research*.

12.1.12. CREDENTIALING AND STANDARDS

Some agencies are organized to develop standards (recognized criteria for acceptable performance) for professionals, service agencies, and educational institutions, and also to provide credentials (certificates) that attest to meeting a set of standards. This is ultimately a method of consumer protection that helps to assure that the handicapped person will receive service of high quality.

These private organizations exert various pressures to bring about conformity to their uniform standards, but they have no direct legal authority. Only state and other government agencies can issue a license to practice or to operate. In some instances, legal permits are granted to those who have been certified or accredited by the relevant private credentialing agency. Generally there are interactions and ties to the various mechanisms for standards: licensing and other legal enforcements, the accreditation of educational institutions and training programs that graduate professionals, the

certification of professionals who wish to practice, and the accreditation of service agencies.

Council on Rehabilitation Education (CORE)

The purpose of CORE is to improve the quality of rehabilitation counselor education (RCE) by the evaluation and accreditation of RCE programs. CORE is sponsored by several national organizations representing relevant professional, employer, and other groups.

Commission on Accreditation of Rehabilitation Facilities (CARF)

CARF, headquartered now in Tucson, Arizona, provides for the development of standards and accreditation of programs of American rehabilitation facilities. It was established by two national organizations representing rehabilitation facilities, the Association of Rehabilitation Centers (ARC) and the National Association of Sheltered Workshops and Homebound Programs (NASWHP). Subsequently these two associations merged, establishing the (International) Association of Rehabilitation Facilities.

Commission on Rehabilitation Counselor Certification (CRCC)

The purpose of CRCC is to help assure the quality of rehabilitation counseling services by the examination and certification of rehabilitation counselors. It was formed by the National Rehabilitation Counseling Association, along with the American Rehabilitation Counseling Association, National Council of Rehabilitation Educators, Council of Rehabilitation Education, Association of Rehabilitation Facilities, Council of State Administrators of Vocational Rehabilitation, National Association of Non-White Rehabilitation Workers, and American Coalition of Citizens with Disabilities.

National Council of Rehabilitation Education (NCRE)

NCRE was formerly the Council on Rehabilitation Counselor Education (CRCE) until it reorganized to include not only rehabilitation counseling but also other rehabilitation education programs. Individual memberships are for rehabilitation educators or trainers with institutional memberships for training programs and staff. This national organization, which has administrative offices housed in the National Rehabilitation Association in Washington, D.C., also has regional affiliates. The NCRE is active in improving the quality and recognition of rehabilitation education. It has had a significant impact on federal legislation (i.e., the funding levels for federal grants for rehabilitation education).

National Accreditation Council for Agencies Serving the Blind and Visually Handicapped

Established in 1967, this Council administers a program of accreditation for direct service agencies and residential schools for this disability group.

American Association of Workers for the Blind

This national organization was founded in 1895 to improve services to blind persons. It operates a job exchange and certifies rehabilitation teachers and mobility specialists.

12.1.13. UNIONS

For many years organized labor in the United States represented skilled trade and industrial workers to a far greater extent than professional and public employees. Rehabilitation professionals such as counselors in state agencies have organized in various areas for purposes of collective bargaining for wages, job security, seniority advantages, and other rights based on union membership. There is a distinct difference in purpose between unions and professional organizations.

AFL–CIO Department of Community Services

The Department of Community Services of the American Federation of Labor–Congress of Industrial Organizations (AFL–CIO) was organized in 1955 to stimulate active participation by members of affiliated unions in the affairs of their respective communities, and to encourage the development of sound working relationships with local social agencies.

In addition to a full-time professional staff, the Department utilizes a considerable number of volunteers in its activities. It conducts programs in the fields of health, welfare, recreation, and relief, including rehabilitation programs for the mentally and physically handicapped, mental health programs, programs for retired persons, health and welfare institutes, counseling programs, and alcoholism and drug abuse programs.

12.1.14. CONSUMER GROUPS

Many of the organizations that are listed above have been developed through the efforts of dedicated individuals with a personal interest in disability. Often a parent or a disabled person has provided the organizational and ongoing leadership needed to keep a voluntary agency successful. There is an increasing trend for disabled people to organize themselves rather exclusively for the purpose of articulating and promoting group causes. Consumerism has been found to be a very effective tool in overcoming "establishment" prerogatives and obtaining new rights. In naming a national health agency, a clear but subtle difference is implied between an "association for" and an "association of" a designated disability group. The latter are sometimes referred to as "self-organized" or "self-help" groups.

National Congress of Organizations of the Physically Handicapped

Formed in 1958, the Congress (COPH) is a national coalition of the physically handicapped and their organizations. The organization serves as an advisory, coordinating, and representative body in promoting employment opportunities, legislation, equal rights, social activity, and rehabilitation. The Congress has a National Board of Governors, State Councils, and member-clubs.

Some of its principal programs and activities include: organizational, legislative, employment, and community service information to member-clubs; a referral service to clubs needing special assistance; a roster of clubs of the physically handicapped and a listing of publications; and an annual membership meeting. Publications include *COPH*.

Paralyzed Veterans of America

The principal thrust of the national effort by this organization is toward improved programs of medicine and rehabilitation. Its efforts are intended not only for veterans but for all those with spinal cord injuries.

National Association of the Physically Handicapped

The Association promotes the economic, physical, and social welfare of all physically handicapped people. Founded in 1958, the organization has a membership belonging to autonomous local chapters, with Members-at-Large in many states where there are no chapters. Principal programs and activities are administered by specialized committees and include efforts in the areas of legislation, employment, barrier-free architectural design, publicity, housing, education and research, recreation and sports, libraries, transportation, and awards.

National Association of the Deaf

A private organization founded in 1880, this association promotes the social, educational and economic well-being of the deaf citizens of the United States. The principal function of the association is to serve as a clearinghouse for information relating to deafness and the problems of the deaf. To this end, it provides experts on the socioeconomic aspects of deafness for interested groups and organizations, provides a representative body that determines and articulates the point of view of the deaf adult on programs relating to problems caused by hearing loss, and conducts studies and workshops on professional services problems and programs.

Disabled American Veterans (DAV)

Founded in 1920, the Disabled American Veterans is composed of about one-half million veterans of American wars. The DAV's paramount objective is to promote the welfare of disabled veterans with service-connected disabilities and their dependents. It provides a service program to assist them in their claims before the Veterans Administration and other government agencies.

Alcoholics Anonymous (AA)

This association has a membership of nearly one million people in 25,000 groups throughout the world. Membership in AA is open to any alcoholic who wishes to stop drinking. It is a fellowship of people, men and women, who share with one another their experiences, strength, and hope that they may solve their common problem and help others to recover from alcoholic addiction. Their primary purpose is to stay sober and to help others to achieve sobriety.

American Coalition of Citizens with Disabilities (ACCD)

ACCD was formed in 1974 by 150 disabled adults. They had convened in Washington, D.C. to formalize a coalition that had helped in the lobbying effort that resulted in the overriding by

Congress of the presidential veto of the 1973 Rehabilitation Act. The Coalition has since concentrated its efforts upon securing implementation and enforcement of rehabilitation and other legislation to enhance the rights of disabled people. A number of groups listed in this chapter are organizational members of ACCD.

Frank Bowe [1978], the very able director of the Coalition, has written an informative book entitled *Handicapping America*. He makes a persuasive argument for the mobilization of political power. Dr. Bowe's book has appendices on voluntary organizations and federal programs for disabled people.

12.1.15. FOUNDATIONS

A great many nonprofit corporations, generally called foundations, have been established from private gifts and endowments for a variety of human welfare purposes. As a rule these groups focus attention on one or more charitable, scientific, or educational purposes. Well-known examples include the following foundations: Ford (1936), Guggenheim (1925), Field (1940), Rockefeller (1913), and Russell Sage (1907). The Kennedy Foundation is described elsewhere because of its focus on one disability, mental retardation. Listings of foundations are published periodically by the New York–based Russell Sage Foundation, *The Foundation Directory* and, also by Europe Publishers of London, *The International Foundation Directory*.

12.1.16. RELIGION

Belief in one's god can provide the strength to cope with life's adversities. In fact, strong religious convictions often develop after a devastating personal loss. For those who have faith in a spiritual power, the fact of irreparable disablement may be accepted as God's will and from the same source comes the strength to adapt. There is no question about the potential for positive adjustment through this mysterious force of faith. Thus, it can be an invaluable resource in rehabilitation and in adjustment to a handicap. Yet it is taboo today in research and education to consider religion as a variable in rehabilitation success. Inexplicably, it is not discussed in the scientific or professional literature despite the fact that religious belief is a primary motivation in the lives of many people throughout the world.

The professional counselor does not provide

religious instruction or guidance except, of course, in a ministerial role when both client and religious counselor are prepared for the relationship. It definitely does not follow, though, that the rehabilitationist must avoid the subject of religion any more than that of sex or any of life's issues. Religion can be a powerful rehabilitation resource, through an organized church or through personal conviction, as the case may be.

Religious organizations have various programs for the disabled and disadvantaged. In addition to matters of religious faith they are active in social welfare, minority and cultural relations, economic affairs, human rights, medical care, and other problems that affect handicapped people. The many organizations and councils with religious focus will not be listed.

One, however, will be described for its work with the handicapped.

Salvation Army

As a branch of the Christian church, "the Army" preaches the gospel of Christ, but it is a charitable as well as religious movement. Founded in England in 1865 and in 1880 in the United States, the Salvation Army operates on a military pattern in about 100 countries. This organization provides direct services to disadvantaged people who are turned away by others. Its programs include emergency relief such as provision of food and housing, settlements, social service centers, employment, family welfare, missing persons assistance, prisoner assistance, and professional counseling.

12.2. Public Agencies

The agencies described in this section are in part federally sponsored, many jointly with state and local governments. Generally the federal government influence extends beyond mere financial support and gives national uniformity to the various regions and areas of the country in terms of eligibility, services, and standards. Thus, even when state or local governments administer the program and there are unique provisions for area needs and priorities, in these federal partnerships the recipients of services are not discriminated against because of residency location. Still there may be variations according to time and place in how programs are administered. Only an overview of the agencies can be provided here. In many instances an agency associated with the rehabilitation system is discussed elsewhere (see Index).

12.2.1. REHABILITATION SERVICES

Public Rehabilitation

Administered by the U.S. Department of Education, the public rehabilitation organization program is financed by federal and state funds with the state rehabilitation agencies providing direct services to medically disabled people. The disabled person must require adjustment services such as counseling, restoration, training, and/or job placement.

The official journal of the federal rehabilitation

agency is called *American Rehabilitation* (formerly the *Rehabilitation Record*).

A complete description of the state-federal rehabilitation program is provided in Chapter 7, Public Rehabilitation, and elsewhere in this book.

Veterans Administration

The U.S. Veterans Administration conducts many programs that provide substantial benefits and services to disabled veterans. Many services also are available for those with non-service-related disabilities and non-disabled veterans. In some cases a veteran may receive complementary services from both the Veterans Administration and the state rehabilitation agency. There are time limitations after discharge for some of the benefits and some are linked to periods of war.

Benefits for veterans also are provided by other federal agencies. Moreover, the states have varying programs of services to veterans, and each state has a Department of Veterans Affairs. With the exception of insurance, all Veterans Administration benefits are conditional upon a termination of service under conditions other than dishonorable. The following are brief descriptive listings of some of the benefits and programs offered by the Veterans Administration.

1. GI Bill educational assistance. Disability is not a factor in eligibility. Thus, a veteran who is not eligible for rehabilitation services because there is no service-connected disability may still be eligible for this program. In addition, the Veterans Administration has a loan program for use in a course of study leading to a standard degree or toward a predetermined vocational objective.

2. Vocational rehabilitation for the disabled. This applies to veterans with a compensable, service-connected disability. Such veterans are provided with counseling and training. A veteran in an approved vocational rehabilitation course may be furnished necessary medical and dental care, hospitalization, or outpatient treatment.

3. Dependent's education. Within specified time periods, this program provides counseling, educational cash assistance, and loans to the dependents of those veterans whose deaths or permanent total disability were service-connected.

4. Hospitalization. All veterans with service-connected disabilities are eligible and receive first priority. Other veterans may receive hospitalization based on inability to pay elsewhere and on space available. Medical care may be provided to the dependents or survivors of certain disabled or dead veterans.

5. Nursing home care. This is meant for certain veterans who have had active military service and are convalescing or who are not acutely ill and not in need of hospital care yet still need some care.

6. Alcohol and drug treatment. After discharge from treatment, veterans may become eligible for follow-up outpatient care for alcohol or drug dependence.

7. Domiciliary care. The purpose is to provide care on an ambulatory, self-care basis for veterans disabled by age or disease who are not in need of hospitalization or nursing home care.

8. Outpatient medical treatment. This service is available to certain veterans with service-connected disabilities.

9. Outpatient dental treatment. Generally, the eligibility is the same as for outpatient medical care.

10. Prosthetic appliances. Such service applies generally to veterans with service-connected disabilities.

11. Aid for the blind. Blinded veterans entitled to receive some compensation for any service-connected condition are eligible. Included are electronic and mechanical aids and guide dogs. Blind Centers are located at selected veterans' hospitals that have comprehensive blind rehabilitation programs.

12. Spinal cord centers. The federal government operates a network of Spinal Cord Injury Centers in selected Veterans Administration hospitals that provide comprehensive rehabilitation services. Veterans with service-connected disabilities have priority for admission. Other veterans so disabled may be admitted as beds are available.

13. Wheelchair homes. Certain veterans with service-connected serious disabilities who require a wheelchair may be entitled to a government grant to pay part of the cost of building or buying specially adapted homes or remodeling an existing home.

14. Pensions. Wartime veterans who have total disabilities not traceable to service and those 65 years of age or older may be entitled to pensions in a monthly amount based upon other income.

15. Death payments. Certain dependents of servicemen or deceased veterans are entitled to monthly payments.

16. Disability compensation. Compensation means a monthly payment by the Veterans Administration to the veteran because of a service-connected disability. Monthly rates increase by percent of disability.

17. Automobiles and adaptive equipment. Veterans with service-connected loss or permanent loss of use of one or both hands or feet, or permanent impairment of vision of both eyes to a prescribed degree, are eligible. Payment may be paid toward the purchase price of one automobile or other conveyance, exclusive of the cost of necessary adaptive equipment. Amounts for specified adaptive equipment are paid in addition. Payment may be made toward repair, reinstallation, or replacement of adaptive equipment, including that for a vehicle acquired subsequently. (The Veterans Administration has established design and test criteria for safety and quality of automotive adaptive driving equipment, along with certification of products made by specific manufacturers. The federal Rehabilitation Services Administration has adopted the

Veterans Administration criteria and certification lists with regard to the purchase of such equipment by the state vocational rehabilitation agencies.)

18. Other benefits. There are a variety of other benefits from various sources available to veterans, for example, burial benefits, insurance, mortgage life insurance, civil service preference, reemployment rights, home and business loans, social security credits for military service, and so on. (See 6.5 on the history of rehabilitation of war veterans.)

Crippled Childrens Program

The Social Security Act of 1935 provided for federal grants-in-aid to the states to extend and improve services to crippled children and to those suffering from conditions that lead to crippling. The emphasis is on service in rural and economically depressed areas. Services under the program include locating crippled children and providing medical and surgical care and other assistance, hospitalization, and posthospital services for them. The concept of medical care has been interpreted in the broadest possible sense, as the program has evolved to the point at which the state programs may include nearly all categories of long-term or chronic illness as well as most services that might reasonably be expected to improve the individual's health condition.

Eligibility is extended to individuals under 21 years of age who are medically indigent and suffering from a crippling condition that is covered under the state program. Beginning in 1963, the Crippled Childrens Program began to open up to a wider range of disabilities by relaxing definitions and initiating additional services in the coverage. The program is now serving many types of handicapped children, not just those who are crippled. Each state defines what specific conditions are covered. Special demonstration projects are also provided, as is a special contingency fund for mental retardation programs.

Developmental Disabilities Programs

The 1975 Developmentally Disabled Assistance and Bill of Rights Act (PL 94-103) defined developmental disability as a continuing and substantially handicapping disability attributable to mental retardation, cerebral palsy, epilepsy, or autism originating before age 18. This definition of developmental disability was radically broadened in Public Law 95-602, the 1978 Amendments to the 1973 Rehabilitation Act. The redefinition represented a shift to a more "functional," as opposed to categorical, definition; developmental disability now means any severe, chronic disability attributable to a mental or physical, or both, impairment manifested before age 22 that is likely to continue indefinitely and results in substantial functional limitations affecting three or more areas of life activity (i.e., self-care, language, learning, mobility, self-direction, independent living, and economic self-sufficiency), and that reflects the person's need for a combination or sequence of extended services which are individually planned and coordinated.

The Developmental Disabilities Act as amended authorized federal grants for the purposes of: (1) providing services for persons with developmental disabilities, (2) developing and implementing a comprehensive and continuing plan for a system of services, (3) providing construction to house services, (4) training specialized personnel for services and research, (5) developing or demonstrating new or improved techniques of service, (6) providing demonstration and training projects, and (7) renovating and modernizing university-affiliated facilities for the interdisciplinary training of professional personnel. In addition, the Act provided for a mechanism to establish and protect the rights of persons with developmental disabilities and to ensure that they obtain quality services. Under the Act, one or more state agencies may be designated to administer or supervise the administration of the state plan.

The Office for Handicapped Individuals

In 1974 the Secretary of Health, Education, and Welfare announced the establishment of an Office for Handicapped Individuals (OHI) as a coordinating and advocacy unit for its target population. Specific functions authorized were:

1. To serve as the focal point in the Department for the consideration of issues and policies affecting the handicapped and for the development of departmental goals for handicapped programs.
2. To analyze program operations on a continuing basis to evaluate the effectiveness of

all programs providing services to handicapped individuals.

3. To develop means of promoting the prompt use of engineering and other scientific research to assist in solving problems in education, health, rehabilitation, architectural and transportation barriers, and other pertinent areas.

4. To provide a central clearinghouse for information and referral. This includes referral to existing information sources in the handicapped field within the Department as well as the other departments and agencies of the federal government, and private agencies and organizations that operate on a national level.

12.2.2. SOCIAL SERVICES

The 1935 Social Security Act as amended authorized federal participation in funding state and local social services to cash assistance recipients. Purposes were as follows: (1) to achieve or maintain economic self-support to prevent, reduce, or eliminate dependency; (2) to achieve or maintain self-sufficiency, including reduction or prevention of dependency; (3) to prevent or remedy neglect, abuse, or exploitation of children and adults unable to protect their own interests, or preserving, rehabilitating, or reuniting families; (4) to prevent or reduce inappropriate institutional care by providing for community-based care or other forms of less intensive care; and (5) to secure referral or admission for institutional care when other forms of care are not appropriate, or providing services to individuals in institutions. Plans for these services vary among the states under federal grant-in-aid provisions.

12.2.3. EDUCATION

Special provisions have been made by governments at all levels for the education of handicapped persons (see 14.2). While public education has been the primary responsibility of state and local governments, the federal government has had a long and increasing role in special schools and education for the disabled.

Special Education Administration

This agency, in the U.S. Department of Education, assists states, colleges, and universities, and other institutions and agencies in meeting the educational needs of the nation's handicapped children who require special services. Major programs of federal assistance to supplement the state's basic provisions for educating handicapped children are as follows:

1. Education of the Handicapped Children. Under this program, each state has a state plan for education of handicapped children. The purpose of the federal grants is to initiate, expand, and improve educational and related services to handicapped preschool, elementary, and secondary school children.

2. Elementary and Secondary Education. This program of federal assistance strengthens educational programs for handicapped children in state-operated or state-supported schools.

3. Training of personnel. This program of grants to universities and agencies prepares teachers and other specialists to educate handicapped children.

4. Innovative programs. This provision supports local projects designed to demonstrate innovative and exemplary modes of meeting state educational needs. At least 15 percent of the funds must be reserved for special programs for handicapped children.

5. Vocational education. This is a grant program for vocational education with at least 10 percent of the funds reserved for handicapped persons.

6. Handicapped children, early education program. The purpose is to develop model preschool and early education programs for handicapped children. Public and nonprofit private agencies may apply to the U.S. Department of Education for these project grants.

7. Regional resource centers. These centers provide states with technical assistance in the development of appraisal and educational programming for handicapped children.

8. Regional centers for deaf-blind children. These centers are authorized to provide deaf-blind children with comprehensive diagnosis and evaluation; a program for their education, adjustment, and orientation; and consultation services for their parents, teachers, and others involved in their welfare.

9. Programs for severely handicapped children and youth. These programs authorize projects to develop demonstration centers and services for severely handicapped children and youth.

10. Regional education program for handi-

capped persons. The purpose here is to provide support services to handicapped persons enrolled in post-secondary school or adult education programs. Project grants and contracts are given to promote and demonstrate new knowledge in education, physical education, and recreation for handicapped children.

11. Media search and captioned film loan program. The purpose of this program is to maintain a free loan service for the educational, cultural, and vocational enrichment of the deaf as well as to contract for research and to train teachers, parents, and others in media utilization.

Special emphasis is due the Education for All Handicapped Children Act of 1975 (PL 94-142). The purpose of this law was to provide educational assistance to all handicapped children. The program is administered now by the new U.S. Department of Education. Funds are distributed to states according to a formula based on the number of handicapped children aged 3 to 21 who are receiving special education and related services. In order to qualify for funds, a state must have a policy and plan for the education of all handicapped children. In addition, children in need of special education are identified, located, and evaluated. An individualized education program is required for each handicapped child. There is a requirement for education in the "least restrictive environment." There must be coordination with other programs that provide services to handicapped individuals.

Education for the Deaf
Gallaudet College in Washington, D.C. was established in 1864 by the federal government to provide a liberal higher education for deaf persons who need special facilities to compensate for their loss of hearing (see 6.2.1). In addition to its undergraduate program, Gallaudet College has a graduate program at the master's level for preparing teachers and other professional people to work with persons who are deaf, a research program that focuses on problems related to deafness, and a preschool for young deaf children. Under a federal agreement, Gallaudet College operates a model secondary school and the Kendall Demonstration Elementary School. Gallaudet has a substantial commitment to the improvement of opportunities for deaf people in all countries. It sponsors the International Cen-

ter on Deafness. Thus its resources—such as the world's largest library collection on deafness—are universally used.

The National Technical Institute for the Deaf (NTID) is a special technical college for deaf people, federally established and funded. Located in Rochester, New York, NTID is part of the Rochester Institute of Technology. In the enrollment of about 1,000 students is represented almost every state in the country with over 80 percent receiving financial support from state rehabilitation agencies.

12.2.4. MANPOWER AIDS
The enhancement of the nation's manpower resources has been a historic and universal justification of vocational rehabilitation. Sometimes the need to provide labor for purposes of production becomes confused with the obligation to provide handicapped individuals with the need for productivity. Yet the distinction is more an administrative than service distinction. Many U.S. Department of Labor programs are clearly vocational rehabilitation. Manpower agencies such as CETA (Comprehensive Employment and Training Act) are described in Chapter 37, Placement Resources.

12.2.5. HEALTH CARE
Federal sponsorship of a comprehensive health care program in the United States has suffered because of a number of fragmented programs. These are described below.

Health Facilities Construction
The so-called Hill-Burton program is administered by the federal Health Resources Administration. The grants, combined with local funds, may be used for new construction or replacement of facilities, but not for land. Rehabilitation facilities are included.

When the Hill-Burton hospital construction program started in 1946 it was assumed that there would be planning to fill unmet needs. This intent was clarified in the 1964 amendments that created nonprofit corporations to plan for needed hospitals and other health facilities. The Regional Medical Program in 1965 and the Comprehensive Health Planning Program in 1966 emphasized planning and resources development. In 1974, the Health Planning and Resources Act (PL 93-641) implemented the planning and resource development program.

This program pays state and local planning agencies to plan and develop health care services. It does not pay for services. There is provision for very limited funds for grants, loans, and loan guarantees to help build or modernize health care facilities. The primary concern, however, is to establish a structure for planning and regulating resources to make the delivery of health care more effective, efficient, and accessible.

Governors have designated, and the federal office has approved, several hundred Health Service Areas for planning. In each of these areas a Health Systems Agency is established that, when federally recognized, receives basic planning support funds. The Health Systems Agency is the basic planning entity generally responsible for preparing and implementing plans designed to improve the health of the residents in its health service areas; to increase the accessibility, acceptability, continuity, and quality of health services in the area; to restrain increases in the cost of health services; and to prevent unnecessary duplication of health resources. A statewide Health Coordinating Council is appointed by the governor to consolidate the plans of the Health Systems Agency and of the state Health Planning and Development Agency into an overall state plan.

Medicare

This 1965 landmark federal legislation, amending the U.S. Social Security Act, was a breakthrough toward a national health insurance system in the United States. The purpose of these amendments to the Social Security Act was to provide basic protection against costs of inpatient hospital and certain outpatient services, physician's services, and services provided by other suppliers of medical services for those persons aged 65 and older, or certain disabled individuals, or individuals suffering from permanent kidney failure who elect to enroll. It is financed by monthly premiums from enrollees and a matching payment from general revenues of the federal government.

Medicaid

Enacted in 1965 as an amendment to the Social Security Act, this program permitted states to provide medical assistance with federal matching funds to needy families with dependent children and aged, blind, and disabled persons, and to as-

sist such families in achieving independence or self-care through rehabilitation and other services. This medical assistance program was designed to replace all other state programs for providing medical services for public assistance recipients (viz., the aged, blind, and disabled, and families with dependent children). States were authorized to extend coverage to comparable groups of medically needy people (e.g., those with enough income for daily living but not enough for medical expenses, and also to financially needy children under age 21). Most states restricted Medicaid coverage to public assistance recipients [Wilson & Litvin, 1976].

Community Mental Health Centers

A Community Mental Health Center is a public or nonprofit legal entity through which comprehensive mental health services are provided to individuals living in a defined geographic (catchment) area. Authorized initially by the Community Mental Health Centers Act (PL 94) of 1963, more than 500 of these centers are in operation across the country, serving over one million people each year. The federal role, which is carried out by the National Institute of Mental Health (NIMH), has provided construction and operational funds to new centers.

12.2.6. COMPENSATION

Something that recompenses, a remuneration for some sort of loss, is implied in the term *compensation*. Technically, *compensation* means to neutralize an effect. But actually there is no way a person can be paid back for a loss from disease, injury, aging, or death. Still, governments try to compensate or force the responsible parties to compensate for loss.

Workers Compensation

The commonly accepted objectives of workers compensation are: (1) replacement of income lost by workers disabled by a job-related injury or sickness; (2) restoration of earning capacity and return to productive employment; and (3) industrial accident prevention and reduction.

There are workers compensation programs in all 50 states, in the District of Columbia, and in Puerto Rico. (The federal Employee's Compensation Act covers the employees of the U.S. government.) For various historical, political, economic, or administrative reasons, each of these individual state laws has serious gaps and other faults. Workers compensation legislation is covered in Chapter 37, Placement Resources.

Along with industrial safety, medical care, and cash compensation, rehabilitation of workers is recognized as one of the primary goals of the workers compensation system. At present the most widespread benefits offered through workers compensation laws to restore a worker are the special maintenance benefits authorized in about three-fifths of the states. These benefits usually are paid (sometimes in addition to the regular disability compensation) for various training and other services designed to aid the injured person to return to work.

Some states directly operate rehabilitation facilities under their workers compensation program, and some insurance companies also have in-house facilities for the rehabilitation of disabled workers. However, the main source of rehabilitation for injured workers in most states is the state rehabilitation agency. Cooperative arrangements between the state rehabilitation agencies and the state workers compensation agencies vary greatly. Each state is unique in coverage, in the type of benefits and the amounts paid under workers compensation, and in the rehabilitation provisions and the working relationships.

Liability Insurance

State laws govern liability insurance. Under an automobile liability policy, an injured person may make a claim for loss of wages, medical costs, and other related expenses. However, payments will not be received for these losses automatically. Proof that a person, persons, or company was at fault or negligent and thus responsible for the accident is necessary. The amount of settlement is dependent on the seriousness of the injury, the amount of actual loss, and the state law governing negligence. All states base recovery for losses upon either contributory or comparative negligence. In those states in which no-fault laws have been passed, it is no longer necessary to prove responsibility for an automobile accident before collecting benefits.

12.2.7. INSURANCE

Much of the insurance against risks in the United States, including automobile insurance, is written by private carriers (profit-making companies). There are numerous federal and state insurance programs as well. The most notable social programs derive from the 1935 Social Security Act and its amendments.

Social Security Retirement

There are many and complicated rules for Social Security, but the following program benefits are specific:

1. Monthly cash retirement insurance benefits. Retirement benefits, also called old-age insurance benefits, may be payable to an individual age 62 or over. If between the ages of 62 and 65, the person may choose to receive a reduced amount, or wait until age 65 and receive the full retirement insurance benefit rate. Payments may be reduced or stopped if the person earns over the exempt amount. Other benefits may be due to spouse or children.

2. Survivor's benefits. An unremarried widow or widower of a fully insured worker may be entitled to benefits if age 60 or over, or if he or she is between age 50 and 60 and disabled. A surviving dependent child under age 18, or 18 through 21 and a full-time student, or age 18 or over and under a disability, whose worker-parent was either fully or currently insured at death and who meets other requirements may be entitled to benefits. An unremarried widow or "surviving divorced mother" may also be entitled to benefits.

Social Security Disability Insurance

The SSDI program is a later addition to the social security retirement and survivor's programs for disabled workers under retirement age and their dependents and disabled children. It not only pays continuing monthly income benefits due to total disability, but also defrays all vocational rehabilitation costs under certain conditions so that the disabled recipient can engage in substantial gainful employment.

To be eligible for disability benefits, an individual must: (1) be under 65 years of age; (2) have a physical or mental condition that prevents doing any substantial gainful work and which is expected to last (or has lasted) for at least 12 months, or is expected to result in death; and (3) have certain work credits (time worked) dependent upon age at the time of disability. Someone disabled by blindness does not have to meet the requirement of covered work. An individual is considered legally blind whose vision is no better than 20/200 with glasses or who has a limited visual field of 20 degrees or less.

The benefits and services to a person who qualifies for social security disability insurance are as follows.

1. Monthly disability benefits based upon average earnings under social security over a period of years.
2. Eligibility for Medicare after being entitled to disability payments for 24 consecutive months.
3. Payment of vocational rehabilitation costs in order to work in substantial gainful employment, if the individual meets the selection criteria for this part of the program.
4. Continuation of benefit payments during a trial work period, in which wages are received, of up to nine months to test ability to work, and for an additional three months if able to engage in substantial gainful employment.
5. Benefits to certain family members. These include unmarried children under 18; children aged 18 to 22 if unmarried and attending school full-time; unmarried children 18 or older who were disabled before reaching age 22 and who continue to be disabled.

The social security disability program encourages people to return to gainful employment whenever possible; and when application is made for social security disability benefits, pertinent information from the file is reviewed to determine rehabilitation potential and referral to the state rehabilitation agency.

12.2.8. INCOME MAINTENANCE

A great many schemes have been proposed and a great many have been tried to deal with the problem of financial poverty. Often the procedure and amount of "dole" depended upon the reason for impoverishment. Generally poverty is considered a dishonorable state to be discouraged by disincentives such as humiliation. Several of the recent American plans for welfare assistance are described here.

Supplemental Security Income (SSI)

The SSI program established for the first time in the United States is a wholly federally financed and administered program of aid for the aged, blind, and disabled. People with limited income and resources who are totally disabled for a year or more and who lack social security insurance coverage are eligible. The new program, effective January, 1974, provides a federal floor of monthly income for eligible aged, blind, and disabled persons in the 50 states and the District of Columbia. Nationally uniform eligibility requirements replaced the multiplicity of requirements that existed in the federal-state welfare programs for the aged, blind, and disabled that were previously administered by state and local agencies. In most states, a person who is eligible for supplemental security income is also eligible for Medicaid and social services provided by the state.

Eligibility for SSI payments based on disability depends on the severity of the applicant's condition. To be considered disabled a person must be unable to engage in substantial gainful activity because of a physical or mental impairment that has lasted (or is expected to last) for at least 12 months or that can be expected to result in death. Blindness under the supplemental security income program is defined as central visual acuity of 20/200 or less in the better eye with the use of a corrective lens or visual field restriction of 20 degrees or less.

As can be seen, SSI and SSDI are basically the same in the federal enabling legislation in respect to federal administration, federal financial control, and eligibility and payments provisions, as well as uniform national policy and guidelines. Conversely, however, they are different on a number of principles: the federal authorization for SSI (unlike the SSDI program) does not depend upon Social Security insurance coverage but instead requires a financial means test for qualification; funding for SSI is by general tax revenues rather than employer/employee contributions to the Social Security Trust Fund.

Aid to Families with Dependent Children

The purpose of AFDC is to provide for the care of dependent children in their homes or in the homes of relatives by enabling each state to furnish financial assistance, rehabilitation, and other services to needy dependent children and the parents or relatives with whom they are living. The major objective of this program is to help maintain and strengthen family life, and to help such parents or relatives to attain or retain a capacity for self-support. The program is authorized by the Social Security Act. Federal funds are available under matching financing formulas (states are required to participate in financing; local participation is optional).

Agencies administering AFDC programs are required to provide social services to help recipients achieve employment and self-sufficiency. Medical services are available to all AFDC recipients under Medicaid. Food stamps are available in virtually all counties if all persons in the household are public assistance recipients.

Food Stamps

The purpose of the food stamp program is to improve the diets of low-income households. The state agency responsible for federally aided public assistance programs submits requests for the food stamps program to the U.S. Department of Agriculture on behalf of local political subdivisions. Individuals apply to local welfare offices. Eligibility is based upon income and family size.

General Assistance

General assistance is a state and local service that provides financial assistance to needy individuals who do not qualify for one of the federally aided income transfer programs. It is administered and funded at the state and local level with no federal funds involved. This form of assistance does not exist in every state or even in all counties within a state. Generally the assistance is used in emergency situations pending the entitlement of the individual applicant for federal or state categorical programs such as AFDC, SSI, or SSDI. The services provided and the method by which they are provided vary significantly. In general, local limitations are imposed on the amount and duration of aid. Assistance is given in either money payment, vendor payment, or food orders issued by the county or city welfare agency.

Need is the basic eligibility factor; all income of all members of the immediate family living in the household of the person applying for assistance is taken into account. The applicant must not be eligible for other federal-state categorical assistance programs. Residency requirements vary, although the applicant usually must presently be in the state and intend to remain. Nonresidents may be aided in an emergency situation only and pending return to place of legal residence. If employable, the applicant may not refuse to accept employment available. Gen-

erally, property limitations are the same as for the federal-state public assistance programs. Other conditions on eligibility may be imposed.

12.2.9. JOB SERVICES

Categorization is difficult for the "job service" area. Certainly the public vocational rehabilitation program has the job objective throughout all services for a client. Moreover, job placement is an inseparable function in the vocational rehabilitation process. Also it is noted that the public employment service under the federal administration of the U.S. Department of Labor (i.e., the state employment service agencies) are essentially "manpower" programs and could be listed under that category.

State Employment Service

A national system of public employment offices is known as the United States Employment Service (USES) of the Department of Labor. The system is charged with placing persons in employment and serving employers seeking qualified individuals to fill job openings. The USES operates through state employment service (sometimes referred to as job service) agencies.

Every local office is required to designate at least one staff member to help the more severely handicapped find training or employment, and to make sure all handicapped persons receive service. Applicants are considered handicapped if they have physical, mental, or emotional impairments that constitute an obstacle to their employment. The employment service (see Chapter 37, Placement Resources) seeks to provide handicapped persons with: equal opportunity for employment and equal pay in competition with other applicants, employment at the highest skill permitted by physical abilities and other occupational qualifications, satisfactory adjustment to chosen occupations and work situations, and employment that will not endanger others or aggravate a person's own disabilities.

U.S. Civil Service Employment

The Office of Selective Placement Programs implements the federal government's policy of promoting the hiring, placement, and advancement of physically and mentally handicapped persons, including disabled veterans. Knowledge and technologies are developed to enhance employment and advancement of all disability groups. Technical assistance is provided to federal agencies in the development and implementation of their affirmative action programs. While most handicapped people will be employed through the regular competitive hiring process, special qualifying procedures are available for certain severely disabled individuals. These are:

1. The 700-hour trial employment authority (about four months full-time) for applicants who are severely physically handicapped, including severely disabled veterans or those who are mentally retarded.
2. The "excepted employment" authority for severely disabled veterans and severely handicapped persons who (1) have successfully worked under a temporary trial appointment, (2) meet the minimum qualification standards, and (3) have been recommended for permanent employment by the Veterans Administration or state agency.
3. The excepted employment authority for severely disabled veterans and other severely handicapped persons who have not served a trial employment period. They must have been certified by the Veterans Administration or a state rehabilitation counselor as being qualified to perform the duties of a specific position.
4. The excepted employment authority for mentally retarded persons. This appointment requires certification of employability for a specific job by a state rehabilitation official. The certification is a substitute for the usual Civil Service examination required under the competitive system.
5. Unpaid work experience under a rehabilitation program arranged by the state rehabilitation agency or the Veterans Administration.

The President's Committee on Employment of the Handicapped

This agency was established by Congress in 1945 to facilitate development of maximum employment opportunities for physically and mentally handicapped people. It cooperates with Governors' committees and local committees across the country and develops public education and promotional programs and materials. A significant force in a national effort to eliminate architectural and transportation barriers, cur-

rently much of its effort is directed toward affirmative action and nondiscrimination in employment of the handicapped and their equal participation in services programs as required under the 1973 Rehabilitation Act. The program is administratively located in the U.S. Department of Labor. It publishes the journal, *Disabled U.S.A.* (formerly *Performance*).

Employment Standards Administration

In addition to responsibility for compliance with affirmative action requirements, this agency becomes involved with handicapped workers subject to the Fair Labor Standards Act who cannot earn at least the minimum wage because of their handicap. The Act allows for subminimum wage certification when necessary and for the shortest period necessary to prevent curtailment of opportunity for handicapped individuals. State rehabilitation agencies are authorized by the Department of Labor to issue temporary subminimum wage authorization for on-the-job trainees sponsored by such agencies. Subminimum wage exceptions usually apply to sheltered workshops.

Occupational Safety and Health Administration (OSHA)

OSHA, which is administered by the U.S. Department of Labor, was created by the Occupational Safety and Health Act of 1970. The purpose is to encourage employers and employees to reduce hazards in the workplace. Just about all employers are covered under the Act. OSHA conducts workplace inspections, usually without advance notice. Employees may make complaints about safety conditions to OSHA. OSHA does not have special standards for handicapped employees; apparently, however, employers sometimes misinterpret an OSHA standard and cite it as a reason not to employ a handicapped person. The error may be in emphasizing the means rather than the general safety principle and therefore ignoring alternate means that may be applicable for a handicapped person.

12.2.10. HOUSING AND TRANSPORTATION

Integration and equality for people with a disability are often blocked by the barriers of housing and transportation. The man-made environment has been designed for the "normal" person. Recently government has intervened to counter those practices that shut out handicapped persons and preclude normal living.

Housing and Urban Development Programs

Housing assistance for elderly or handicapped people is authorized in the Housing Act of 1974 (PL 93-383). The program provides mortgage insurance to assist in producing new or rehabilitated rental housing. Space within the dwelling can then be provided for health and other supportive services. Funds usually go to profit-oriented sponsors. Independent living rehabilitation services also include housing provisions.

Congregate housing is assisted by provision of mortgage insurance. These units may have community kitchens, common dining areas, and other shared facilities. Assistance is also provided by interest reduction and rent subsidies. A direct loan program is also authorized.

The U.S. Department of Housing and Urban Development (HUD) also conducts and supports research and demonstration projects to promote the use of technology in order to allow the handicapped person integration into the environment by elimination of barriers.

Highway Traffic Safety Administration

This agency, along with the U.S. Department of Transportation (DOT), provides assistance to states for traffic safety under the 1966 Highway Safety Act. Funds may be used to support driver education programs in schools. Attention is also paid to uniform licensing programs. Many states use federal funds for projects to benefit mentally or physically handicapped persons, mostly in the form of driver education. The law provides for licensing standards to ensure that only persons physically and mentally qualified will be licensed, and at the same time to prevent the needless taking away of a citizen's opportunity to drive. Moreover, each state must have a system providing for medical evaluation of persons whom the licensing agency has reason to believe have mental or physical conditions that might impair their driving ability. (This agency also sets standards for truck drivers in interstate commerce.)

Federal Aviation Administration (FAA)

The FAA of U.S. DOT has a responsibility to make efforts to obtain more equitable treatment of physically handicapped persons traveling by air. Studies and evaluations are made to determine the effects of the presence of physically handicapped people aboard an aircraft during an emergency evacuation. The objective is to develop uniform criteria for the air carriage of handicapped people.

Urban Mass Transportation Administration (UMTA)

The UMTA of DOT makes special efforts to assure the availability of appropriate transportation for elderly and handicapped individuals. Federal assistance is conditioned upon the provision of special planning, design, and facilities that will allow utilization by the elderly or handicapped. UMTA conducts or supports research and development programs on accessible transportation. Provision is made in the Urban Mass Transportation Act of 1964, as amended, for capital grants to private, nonprofit associations for transportation services for the elderly and handicapped.

Federal Highway Administration

The Federal-Aid Highway Amendments of 1974 declared that it is national policy that the elderly and handicapped have the same right as other persons to utilize mass transportation facilities and services, and that special efforts shall be made to accommodate their needs in any program or project receiving federal assistance. The Highway Safety Act of 1973 required provision for adequate and reasonable access across curbs to be constructed or replaced at all pedestrian crosswalks. That Act also required that bus and other facilities be planned and designed so they can effectively be used by elderly and handicapped persons.

General Services Administration (GSA)

The GSA has the following programs and responsibilities relating to handicapped people.

1. Assurance that certain federally funded buildings are accessible to physically handicapped employees and visitors; enforcement of standards in the leasing, construction, and alteration of buildings.
2. Concession stands for individuals who are blind (Randolph-Shephard Act). GSA provides space and services such as electricity and water in the establishment of vending stands in buildings operated or leased by

GSA. The GSA plans and designs the business space and offers technical assistance to the state agency involved (in almost every instance, the state rehabilitation agency for the blind).

3. Disposal of surplus real property for health and education purposes.
4. Donation of surplus federal personal property to any state for purposes of education, public health, or civil defense; and,
5. Issuance of the federal procurement regulations regarding the purchase of products and services of blind and other severely handicapped individuals (Wagner-O'Day Act). It serves on the President's Committee for Purchase of Products of the Blind and Other Severely Handicapped. Such products are usually made in sheltered workshops.

12.2.11. SERVICES FOR BLIND PEOPLE

Federal and state legislation for special benefits to people who are blind has a longer history than that for other disabilities. There are several programs by which blind people are also served that can be mentioned in addition to the state-federal rehabilitation program.

Randolph-Sheppard Act

This Act, amended by Public Law 93-516, December, 1974, provided a priority for blind persons in the location and operation of vending facilities on federal property. The programs in each state are managed and supervised by a licensing agency, which is the state rehabilitation agency serving blind individuals. Various arrangements are possible for the conduct of the vending business. Equipment and initial stocks and supplies may be provided. Under certain conditions, ownership of the equipment may be vested in the blind vendor. Proceeds from vending machines may be dispersed to the state licensing agency, which in turn may distribute the funds to blind operators in the state, and/or set aside part of the funds for maintenance of equipment and other purposes. In each state, a Committee of Blind Vendors serves as an advisory body and carries out other responsibilities with respect to the licensing agency.

It should be noted that there are also laws and other arrangements for the operation of vending facilities on state government property. Also, there is a growing establishment of such businesses on private property.

Library of Congress

As provided for by Congress, the Library of Congress offers library services to blind and physically handicapped people. Included are talking books for blind people, books in braille, and talking book machines. There are 54 regional libraries and 96 subregional libraries in the United States, with a collection of approximately 15,000 titles in recorded and braille form and 37,000 music scores in braille, large type, and recorded form. Users of the materials must have a certificate of inability to read or to manipulate conventional printed material (from a physician, optometrist, rehabilitation center, or health and welfare agency).

Javits-Wagner-O'Day Act

Under the 1971 amendments to the Wagner-O'Day Act (PL 92-28), provisions for the purchase of certain products by the federal government from blind workers was extended to other severely handicapped individuals. The [Senator Jacob] Javits amendments also created the Committee for Purchase from the Blind and Other Severely Handicapped. This Committee has responsibility for determining which products and services are suitable for purchase from qualified workshops serving the blind and other severely handicapped, and for establishing the price that the government will pay. A workshop must be capable of producing the commodity or service at a fair market price. It is also required that the addition of the commodity or service to the Procurement List will not have a serious adverse impact on the current or most recent contractor.

The Committee has designated two national nonprofit agencies to facilitate the distribution of government orders among the various workshops. These are the National Industries for the Blind (NIB) and the National Industries for the Severely Handicapped (NISH).

12.2.12. MISCELLANEOUS PROGRAMS

Despite the array of programs described above, there are still unmentioned a number of important relevant federal agencies and services. Several examples are given below.

Administration on Aging (AoA)

The AoA was established by the Older Americans Act of 1965 to provide a focal point within the federal government for addressing the concerns and needs of older persons and for coordinating federal programs and policies that affect older persons. There are over 35 million Americans aged 60 and older. This age group has the highest prevalence of handicapping. AoA's efforts are primarily directed toward the low-income and minority elderly. Both its nutrition program and the development of community service systems are aimed at preventing the institutionalization of this group, as well as of other older people in the community who are physically and mentally impaired.

Alcoholism and Drug Abuse

Under federal drug abuse and alcoholism grant programs, the states have central agencies (usually within the Health Department) that prepare plans and coordinate and conduct projects for drug abuse or alcoholism prevention and treatment. Any public or private treatment facility in a state that receives federal assistance must meet the standards of such agencies. Drug or alcoholism treatment facilities may be operated by private concerns or the federal, state, county, city, or other governmental units. The federal administrative responsibility is located in the National Institute on Drug Abuse, or, as appropriate, National Institute on Alcohol Abuse and Alcoholism.

Small Business Loans

Under the Small Business Act, Handicapped Assistance Loan Program, financial assistance (through loans and loan guarantees) is authorized to public or private nonprofit sheltered workshops, or any similar organization, to enable them to produce and provide marketable goods and services. At least 75 percent of the employee hours used in direct production must be accounted for by handicapped individuals. A parallel program in the Handicapped Assistance Loan Program provides for loan assistance for the establishment, acquisition, or operation of a small business concern wholly owned by handicapped persons. (See Chapter 39, Small Business Enterprise.)

National Center for Law and the Handicapped (NCLH)

Funded by the U.S. Department of Education, Office of Special Education and the Reha-

bilitation Services, Administration NCLH was established in 1972. Its goal is to insure equal protection under the law for all handicapped individuals through legal assistance, consultation, and related programs. Their bimonthly publication, *Amicus*, monitors legal developments related to the rights of handicapped persons.

Office for Civil Rights

This federal office has the responsibility to implement and enforce Section 504 of the 1973 Rehabilitation Act as amended. Section 504 prohibits discrimination against handicapped persons in federal and federally assisted programs. It also publishes guides for understanding Section 504 regulations.

Office of Federal Contract Compliance Programs

This U.S. DOL Office sets policy, investigates complaints, and monitors compliance with Section 503 of the 1973 Rehabilitation Act as amended and also Section 402 of the Vietnam Era Veterans Readjustment Assistance Act of 1974. These Acts require contractors and subcontractors of the federal government to provide affirmative action and equal opportunity for handicapped persons and disabled veterans seeking employment or already employed. Public awareness material, technical assistance, regulation guides, and other materials are distributed.

Architectural and Transportation Barriers Compliance Board

This Board was created by the 1973 Rehabilitation Act to enforce the Architectural Barriers Act of 1968, which guarantees handicapped individuals access to and use of all facilities built or leased by the federal government.

12.2.13. RESEARCH

Much of the knowledge that this country has in various areas of science and technology derives from the substantial investment of the federal government in research and development. This is spent in various ways: competitive contracts for specified work, grants to nonprofit institutions from unsolicited applications, and studies conducted by federal employees in government research facilities.

National Institutes of Health (NIH)

NIH conducts or grants funds for a gigantic medical research investment. Federal expenditures for NIH, headquartered outside the District of Columbia in Bethesda, Maryland, were approximately $3 billion in 1978. There are 11 Institutes: Cancer; Neurological, Communicative Disorders, and Stroke; Heart, Lung, and Blood; Eye; Allergy and Infectious Diseases; Arthritis, Metabolism, and Digestive Diseases; Child Health and Human Development; Dental Research; Environmental Health Sciences; General Medical Sciences; and Aging. A part of NIH is the National Library of Medicine, the world's largest depository of medical information; their computer-based information retrieval system is known as MEDLARS.

National Institute of Handicapped Research

The 1978 Amendments to the 1973 Rehabilitation Act authorized this new Institute to take over the former research and demonstration program of the Rehabilitation Services Administration with a director appointed by the President. The independent Institute program was expanded to include not only vocational rehabilitation research but also nonvocational problems and populations. University-affiliated Research and Training (R&T) Centers were expanded. The periodical publication, *Informer*, is the house organ of the federal rehabilitation research program.

12.3. International Organizations

There is world-wide humanitarian and economic interest by people and their national governments in the rehabilitation of handicapped people. The nature and quality of programs vary from nation to nation but international organizations are helping in program building everywhere.

12.3.1. COUNCIL OF WORLD ORGANIZATIONS

The best evidence of international interest in rehabilitation is the list of about 40 members of the Council of World Organizations Interested in the Handicapped (CWOIH) [Rehabilitation International, 1974]. This council of nongovernment agencies directly interested in the handicapped was established in 1953 for consultation and coordination with the United Nations and its specialized agencies. Many member agencies of CWOIH are the international representatives of national health associations for a specific disability (deaf, blind, multiple sclerosis, cancer, etc.) or for professional groups (medicine, social work, teaching, and so on). Still other members are affiliated with the Red Cross, Salvation Army, churches, or veterans groups. The Secretariat for CWOIH is provided by Rehabilitation International.

12.3.2. REHABILITATION INTERNATIONAL

Rehabilitation International is the worldwide catalyst for national organizations for the handicapped. It was founded in 1922 as the International Society for Crippled Children; in 1939 it became the International Society for the Welfare of Cripples; and in 1960 it became the International Society for Rehabilitation of the Disabled, the name being shortened to its present one in 1969. It is a nongovernment federation of organizations carrying out programs for disability prevention and rehabilitation. About 100 national associations, agencies, and boards (government and voluntary) are members. Several international groups are also associated with Rehabilitation International.

This influential organization of organizations is headquartered in New York. Norman Acton, as the Secretary General of this vigorous worldwide group, has developed programs to implement its founders' ambitious goal to "promote the rehabilitation of the disabled throughout the world." Purposes include exchanging information, organizing international meetings, encouraging research, promoting prevention of disability, developing and assisting organizations, encouraging legislation, providing technical assistance, and cooperating with other international organizations for these purposes. Rehabilitation International membership consists of national organizations and associates. It works with the United Nations and government and nongovernment rehabilitation agencies, and offers valuable information services and technical assistance to individuals and organizations.

Standing Commissions of Rehabilitation International are maintained on various aspects of rehabilitation—medical, educational, social, and vocational. Their International Commission on Technical Aids, Housing and Transportation operates a splendid information service out of its Swedish headquarters [Montan, 1969]. The Commission publishes *ICTA Inform*.

Information services also include distribution of selected materials, a professional journal, *Rehabilitation Research*, and their bimonthly magazine, *International Rehabilitation Review*. Technical assistance is provided to countries developing rehabilitation programs, and regional meetings and expert seminars are held. The World Rehabilitation Congresses organized by this association every fourth year are the only such meetings for all interested disciplines and groups. Individual memberships and subscriptions are available.

Rehabilitation International sponsored the design (announced in 1970) of the international symbol of access—the familiar "stick" person in a wheelchair on a blue background—and has made it available for use throughout the world to identify facilities without barriers.

12.3.3. RIUSA

The American affiliate of Rehabilitation International is called Rehabilitation International U.S.A. (RIUSA) and is also headquartered in New York City. RIUSA was founded in 1971 to offer the expertise and service of the American rehabilitation community for the benefit of the handicapped worldwide. It has the guidance and support of the major national voluntary health agencies. Other organizations and individuals are eligible for membership. In addition to its international programs, RIUSA distributes publications to its membership, including a journal of news and information, *Rehabilitation World*.

12.3.4. UNITED NATIONS

The United Nations, founded in October, 1945, and dedicated to world peace and human dig-

nity, has in New York an active Rehabilitation Unit that was long under the leadership of Esko Kosunen. All of the global goals of the U.N. through its 135 member nations need not be explained, but its rehabilitation-relevant programs are described below. The First General Assembly of the U.N. adopted in December, 1946, the social welfare recommendations of its Economic and Security Council covering rehabilitation of handicapped people and making technical assistance available to governments. Thus, since early 1947 experts, fellowships, equipment, and conferences and study groups have been sponsored. Studies and publications are also ongoing program projects of the U.N. Rehabilitation Unit for the Disabled. Other agencies of the U.N. are also concerned with rehabilitation.

International Labor
(Labour) Organization (ILO)

The ILO was established in 1919 as an independent affiliate of the League of Nations and in 1946 became the first specialized agency of the U.N. The Organization has three units: the International Conference of national delegates; the Governing Body; and the International Labour Office, its headquarters in Geneva, Switzerland. The Office serves as a world information center and issues the *International Labour Review*. The ILO works to improve working and living conditions in the world. Although some of its resolutions have been politically motivated, ILO was awarded the 1969 Nobel peace prize. The Vocational Rehabilitation Section of the ILO has been ably directed by Norman Cooper. Responsibilities of this section cover all vocational aspects of rehabilitation. Programs include: vocational rehabilitation standards, technical cooperation, meetings, research, and publications. The ILO concerns itself generally with occupational health and safety, vocational guidance and training, worker protection and conditions, and social security.

United Nations Children's Fund (UNICEF)

UNICEF is an organization of the U.N. (not a specialized agency) to assist developing nations to improve the conditions of their young people and to prepare them to contribute to society. In the rehabilitation field, UNICEF provides imported equipment and supplies for governmental treatment and rehabilitation of handicapped children. Some money has been used for professional staff development in rehabilitation. Relatively low priority, however, is given to rehabilitation because of UNICEF's large-scale measures to prevent disablement by combatting disease and malnutrition.

United Nations Educational, Scientific and Cultural Organization (UNESCO)

UNESCO is a specialized agency of the U.N. Located in Paris, its activities in the rehabilitation field began with war-handicapped children. Its comprehensive program on special education was begun in 1966. UNESCO presupposes that the various aspects of rehabilitation programs should be closely coordinated.

World Health Organization (WHO)

WHO is a specialized agency of the U.N. headquartered in Geneva. The highest possible level of health for all people is its objective. Health is defined as a state of complete physical, mental, and social well-being, not merely the absence of disease and infirmity. WHO maintains an advisory panel of experts on rehabilitation, which it defines as a continuous process beginning with the onset of diseases or injuries and continuing until the disabled are "resettled" in society.

Organization for the International Year of Disabled Persons (IYDP)

International concern for the world's physically and mentally disabled people was expressed by the United Nations. The U.N. General Assembly in 1976 proclaimed 1981 as the "International Year of Disabled Persons" (IYDP). Worldwide objectives are to help disabled persons adjust to society, to encourage public efforts to provide work and social integration for disabled people, to encourage rehabilitation research studies, to inform the public about the rights and abilities of disabled persons, and to promote prevention of disability as well as the rehabilitation of disabled persons. Its goal is full utilization of knowledge about the rehabilitation of disabled persons. Many of the U.N. member states designated an agency or official to facilitate exchange of information and to provide liaison with the secretariat of IYDP and its 23 member advisory committee. A symposium of experts was also authorized to discuss rehabilitation technological advancement for application in developing countries.

12.3.5. OTHER ORGANIZATIONS

There are numerous organizations of American sponsorship with international rehabilitation programs. Rehabilitation International, U.S.A. was described above. Selected others must be mentioned because of their outstanding contributions to international rehabilitation efforts.

World Rehabilitation Fund

The World Rehabilitation Fund, a nonprofit corporation, was founded in 1955 through the inspiration of Dr. Howard Rusk of New York University (NYU). It sponsors foreign nationals for training (e.g., rehabilitation medicine, prosthetics, and orthotics) at NYU and elsewhere, preferably near their local geographic area. Over the years it has supplied more than one million artificial limbs and braces, and it has trained thousands of technicians, therapists, and physicians in rehabilitation. Fellowships through the Fund are also available to American rehabilitation professionals and educators.

People to People Committee for the Handicapped

In 1956 President Eisenhower founded the People to People Program to further communication among the peoples of the world; the People to People Committee for the Handicapped has participated with private, voluntary efforts to exchange information and to collect used but usable artificial limbs and other devices for overseas distribution. This Committee, headquartered in Washington, D.C., effectively promotes international rehabilitation efforts through gift and grant support and membership fees. Executive Director James Burress, a former head of the federal rehabilitation agency, has been particularly active in conducting an extensive organizational service project for developing African countries.

Pan-American Health Organization (PAHO)

PAHO provides assistance to governments in the medical aspects of rehabilitation of the physically disabled. It is headquartered in Washington, D.C.

International Rehabilitation Medicine Association (IRMA)

IRMA has a direct membership of physicians and surgeons who have a special interest in rehabilitation. It has liaison with other organizations including the International Federation of Physical Medicine and Rehabilitation. Both of these medical organizations sponsor world conferences every several years. The publication of an official journal, *International Rehabilitation Medicine*, was announced in 1979 by IRMA.

Helen Keller International
This agency provides technical equipment, consultation, and other services to agencies for the blind in other countries. It also conducts blindness-prevention programs.

Partners of the Americas
Partners is a private organization with people to people projects that promote human development. Chartered in 1966 and headquartered in Washington, D.C., rehabilitation is a primary interest of this organization along with education, public health, rural and community development, and emergency relief. "The poorest of the poor" is seen as an "unhappy distinction" of the "387 million persons in the world with significant disabling conditions." American rehabilitationists such as John Jordan have been active in this extensive hemispheric effort to improve the quality of life of the "more than 75 million disabled persons in the Americas."

Goodwill Industries International Council
Formally established in 1971, this organization shares Goodwill's experience in the establishment of sheltered employment workshops for handicapped persons in America with other nations. Activities include professional training of leadership, program development, technical assistance, and liaison with world-wide rehabilitation organizations and resources. Special emphasis is placed on vocational training and job creation through the establishment of cooperative workshops and small industries. The headquarters are in Washington, D.C.

Chapter 13

Adjustment Training

The preparatory activities of personal-social adjustment and work adjustment services, vocational training, and educational services described in hierarchial order here and in the next chapter are truly basic resources for rehabilitation. Training and education correct or compensate for handicapping. Enablement counterbalances limitation.

13.1. Introduction

Training and education for vocational and other goals are essential rehabilitation tools. Personal adjustment training as described here can be provided for either occupational or independent living objectives. With the latter, however, it is more often needed. Adjustment services are also discussed in Chapters 8, Rehabilitation Facilities; Chapter 28, Personal Adjustment; and Chapter 40, Independent Living.

13.1.1. BACKGROUND

When it began, vocational rehabilitation was practically synonymous with "re-education." The initial federal Rehabilitation Act (Public Law 236, 1920) specifically authorized only two kinds of purchased client service: vocational training and instructional supplies. Even the administration of the rehabilitation program at both federal and state levels was by Boards for Vocational Education. While supporters of a broader rehabilitation program thought there was implied legal authority in Public Law 236 to provide other rehabilitation services (e.g., prostheses, physical restoration, maintenance while in training), the Administrator of the Federal Board for Vocational Education nevertheless restricted rehabilitation service to retraining. Most "prospects" for rehabilitation were given vocational training, but federal funds were not allocated in the early years for the full scope of rehabilitation services. State rehabilitation agents were required to "train around the disability."

The plan for rehabilitation training had to be toward a "specific employment objective," according to the first federal "Case Procedure" regulations [U.S. Federal Board for Vocational Education, 1921]. The client could receive either: (1) "employment training" for acquiring manipulative skill or technical knowledge in actual employment conditions, (2) "general education" in an institution or school where conditions were similar to employment conditions, and/or (3) "tutorial training" for private instruction—perhaps with correspondence course work.

Subsequent federal legislation and administrative regulations have broadened vocational training to cover any type of training that may be necessary in order to rehabilitate a disabled person. Training services can be provided by the public rehabilitation agency for nonvocational objectives. The most notable advance came with the 1978 Amendments to the Rehabilitation Act, which authorized services for independent living such as services for children of preschool age for the development of language and communication skills.

State rehabilitation agencies provide prevocational (basic knowledge and skill) training, personal-social adjustment (nonvocational) training, as well as vocational training (including occupational preparation in college). Moreover, the trainee of the public rehabilitation program may now receive whatever supplementary services may be necessary for the successful completion of the training services: the state rehabilitation agency may provide maintenance funds for the client to pay living expenses while in training, transportation costs for the client (and attendant, if needed) to and from the place of training, the wages of a reader and "talking books" for blind students, training materials and supplies, and tools and equipment. The federal rehabilitation administration allows these services to be provided without regard to financial circumstances, although most state rehabilitation agencies require the client to participate financially if able to pay part of the cost from expendable resources or income.

13.1.2. NOMENCLATURE

The federal rehabilitation agency has used the term *training* in a generic sense to denote any type of instructional service, including education and training programs. It is desirable, however, to understand the conceptual difference between *education* and *training*. Both are concerned with human learning and preparation, but there is considerable difference in purpose and often in setting. In the vocational context, training is role-specific in that it is directed toward preparing a person for a certain occupation; education, on the other hand, is associated with the goals of the individual more than those of the employing organization. *Adjustment services* are described in this chapter as subsumed under training in a generic sense. This terminology and classification overlaps with adjustment counseling and other services that are not entirely pedagogic.

The various kinds of adjustive techniques employed in rehabilitation are operationally described in this chapter. Selected terms are defined below as an overview of these training alternatives.

ADJUSTMENT SERVICES. This term has reference to those services that facilitate individual personal, social, and vocational adaptation to life and its activities. In the broad interpretation of rehabilitation this incorporates not only work activities but also "activities of daily living" (ADL).

SOCIAL REHABILITATION. Social rehabilitation is that part of the rehabilitation process aimed at the integration or reintegration of a disabled person into society by helping that person to adjust to the demands of family, community, and occupation, while reducing any economic or social burdens that may impede the total rehabilitation process.

SOCIAL ADJUSTMENT. This term means the degree to which an individual is able to meet and conform to personal and social responsibilities and standards set by the community. Such behavior requires "social adaptation," which may be accomplished through "social adjustment services," a structured program designed to assist the client to interact with individuals and groups in an acceptable manner.

PERSONAL ADJUSTMENT SERVICES. This term refers to training, counseling, and other programs for helping a disabled person understand, accept, and remedy conditions or attitudes that interfere with rehabilitation; it is a professional process of improving a client's behavior and developing habits, attitudes, motivation, tolerance and understanding, and interpersonal relationships.

WORK ADJUSTMENT SERVICE. This service provides an individualized, closely supervised, remedial work experience designed to promote the acquisition of satisfactory work habits, to increase physical and emotional tolerance for work activity and interpersonal relationships, and to modify attitudes and behavior that inhibit the satisfactory performance of work. Work adjustment training is conducted in rehabilitation facilities that simulate industrial employment; this helps the client form a satisfactory "work personality," which includes self-control, appreciation of employment conditions and requirements, self-confidence, ability to get along with the supervisor and fellow workers, good work habits, and work tolerance.

WORK HABITS. Work habits are ingrained behaviors such as attendance, punctuality, hygiene, social relations, teamwork, effort, initiative, perseverance, dependability, meeting of work schedules, acceptance of supervision and constructive criticism, housekeeping, neatness in work, care with materials and property, cooperation, and safety awareness.

WORK CONDITIONING. The development of work tolerance, including the ability to sustain work effort for a prolonged period and to maintain a steady production at an acceptable rate and quality, is known as work conditioning.

PREVOCATIONAL TRAINING. Prevocational training introduces a person to the meaning of work in society, the responsibilities and opportunities at work, and the range of occupations and lines of training. This prevocational experience may acquaint the person with different machines, tools, settings, procedures, and requirements of groups of occupations in order to help facilitate the choice of a career. Prevocational training is thus an adjunct to vocational assessment, counseling, and training. Prevocational training is an orientation, and the word should not be used as a substitute for "work adjustment" service, which is a broader process.

Other adjustment terms and other types of training (e.g., homebound programs, on-the-job training, compensatory skill training) are explained elsewhere.

13.2. Personal-Social Adjustment

The role of adjustment services in rehabilitation is quite varied because the term *adjustment* takes on a variety of meanings depending upon the specific situation or program (e.g., adjustment to disability, adjustment to work, personal adjustment, social adjustment). Dunn [1974] said, "Adjustment simply refers to the behavior of a person in a situation: the person is 'adjusted' if he behaves as we expect him to behave in the situation and 'mal-adjusted' if he behaves differently. This can be determined by observing what the person does within the situation" [p. 3].

The term *adjustment services* refers to broad objectives such as adaptation to the work situation or improved social functioning. Baker [1972] went so far as to say: "The general purpose of all adjustment services should be to bring about changes in client behavior including

all behaviors that interfere with the client's attempt to become a functional, independent member of his community" [p. 29].

13.2.1. PERSONAL ADJUSTMENT SERVICES

The most common cause of job loss among rehabilitation clients, as reported in the literature, is unacceptable personal behavior at the place of work [Wright, Butler, & Aldridge, 1968]. Problems in personal adjustment may be caused by the frustrations of the disability and handicap, feelings of inferiority, rejection by society, disuse of social skills, negative attitudes, and so on. But whatever the client problems, the rehabilitation plan should not be allowed to fail because of the lack of personal adjustment services. These services are frequently provided in rehabilitation facilities, although they can be rendered in public vocational rehabilitation offices, hospitals, schools, institutions, prisons, or wherever a program of rehabilitation exists.

Personal adjustment relates to any personal problem that impairs the ability of the individual to deal effectively with others. Such problems may involve physical or mental limitations, attitudes, or simply a lack of information. These problems are treatable by understanding and dealing with the direct cause. Psychotherapy or extensive, in-depth counseling may be quite unnecessary.

As Sankovsky [1971] explained, an individual with a speech impediment has a disability that may be remedied by a speech therapist, but it is important to recognize that this limitation can mold the individual personally so as to hinder the ability to work with others and ultimately to affect the adjustment to work. He continued the analogies to other physical conditions: "Observe the individual who literally 'stinks.' This may be a physical problem, as in the case of an individual with a colostomy or one who is catheterized. Frequent and appropriate cleaning and the selective use of a deodorizer may be all that needs to be stressed from an informational standpoint. But what about the individual who refuses to take a shower or brush his teeth? Certainly information on grooming and hygiene are an essential part of his personal adjustment program" [p. 9]. But just providing information may not be effective. Other methods used in personal adjustment programs include thorough evaluation of personal problems, counseling, classes in personal affairs such as grooming and hygiene, and behavioral techniques to modify inappropriate behavior.

13.2.2. SOCIAL ADJUSTMENT SERVICES

Personal and social adjustment are differentiated for the purpose of discussion—it is convenient to think of one following the other. Actually, the dynamics (causal relationships) and interactions between the two are complex and make the distinction between them simply that of apparent manifestation. In any event, this discussion excludes those individuals who have lost contact with reality or whose adjustment problems require therapy by a psychiatrist or a clinical psychologist.

Clients with social adjustment problems have underlying emotional conflicts that must be recognized from their behavior. Clients who act out their aggression are readily identified, but those who have poor communication skills or an unnatural dependency are often overlooked.

A basic problem in the social adjustment of the disabled results from long-standing naiveté, a lack of information or experience. For the handicapped individual made overly dependent by a sheltered home life, entering a rehabilitation facility can itself be disturbing. Such clients may be very homesick and unable to cope with the situation without emotional support from the staff. Another problem stems from sexual naiveté and a lack of experience with members of the opposite sex. Many clients who enter a rehabilitation facility are not sophisticated in sexual matters. These individuals cannot respond appropriately (or perhaps they overrespond) to the coeducational setting, and they need guidance in their orientation.

Social adjustment services look beyond the need of a person to function for an eight-hour work day; attention is devoted to preparing these individuals to live adequate lives after working hours and in other social contexts. Classes and instruction in recreation, social skills, sex education, dating, communication, and related topics help the disabled person start a cycle of self-perpetuating personal adjustment throughout life.

This section is relatively short because the subject is covered elsewhere. The reader is referred to the chapters in the part entitled Counseling.

13.3. Work Adjustment

Work adjustment programs provide a variety of experiences to assist disabled persons who lack the skills needed to succeed in the labor market. Work adjustment helps individuals develop self-confidence, self-control, work tolerances, skill at interpersonal relations, an understanding of the work world, and a "worker attitude"—all of which help them handle the day-to-day demands of a job. Some agencies may describe work adjustment services as work-habit training, work-readiness training, or work hardening, although these are mere fragments of the process.

The term *prevocational training* is also commonly used as synonymous with *work adjustment,* but actually the former term refers to only a preliminary step.

Personal and social adjustment training may also be subsumed under the rubric, work adjustment. Pruitt [1973] observed: "Many facilities operate on the premise that all work is therapeutic and therefore, work adjustment training is no more than providing the client with some type of work activity. Other facilities have well-defined procedures and curriculum to effect the work adjustment program" [p. 20]. Wainwright and Couch [1978] have pointed out the potential for work adjustment services in vocational rehabilitation. While professional expertise and resources are not yet fully developed, they believe that work adjustment can become "the single most important rehabilitation service entity available for handicapped individuals" [p. 40].

The need for work adjustment service can result from a failure to learn acceptable patterns of behavior during adolescence, the need to recover skills that were lost at the onset of a disability, or the necessity of changing jobs, which requires a substantial modification of behavior as well.

In the case of the educable mentally retarded, for example, there may be an elementary lack of knowledge about how to travel in a city, how to get to work on time and leave on time, how to punch a clock, how to behave on the job with respect to others. The individual with pronounced neurotic trends may be fearful of failure or unable to control feelings of anxiety or hostility. The epileptic may have all sorts of real and imagined fears as to the consequences of a seizure while at work. The handicapped person without work experience may simply be unable to handle the manifold and novel experiences of the work situation. The deinstitutionalized post-psychotic patient, unable to return to former employment and fearful of unaccustomed new work, may be unwilling to give up the dependency role of the patient.

Young adults entering the labor market are not automatically employable because they have attained physical maturity. Employability is a learned attribute, culminating from a socialization process that began at birth. The family originally provides the behavioral patterns and motivational systems that induce the children to achieve and become productive. The school experience continues the process of learning the responsibility of work and relationships with peers and authority figures away from home. Household chores for normal children are assigned early in life. Later on, after-school and summer employment succeed household chores. The child gradually is prepared for the pressures and tensions of a formal work life as an adult. In this way a work personality is developed, and career adjustment is facilitated.

But, as Gellman [1961] has explained, handicapping conditions may result in disruptions in this maturation in work roles. He contrasted the situation of the normal to that of the impaired child.

The disabled child is deprived of the complex of family chores and responsibilities which develop a sense of productivity and work satisfaction. The birth of a child with an apparent disability induces parental attitudes of over-protection or rejection which limit independent activities. School brings segregation or isolation. Lower standards for the handicapped diminish the achievement drive. Prejudice against disabled persons restricts opportunities for summer or after-school work. As disabled young adults, they lack the knowledge and experience which underpin a work personality. Having learned how not to work, they see themselves as unproductive and unable to work [p. 108].

A somewhat similar process occurs when adults become disabled by accident, injury, or a psychotic episode. Incapacity or institutionalization separates disabled persons from a work routine. As patients they lose their productive orientation in an environment that leads them to expect assistance. Prolonged disablement without a planned work program may render people unable to fulfill a work role.

Vocational adjustment in a workshop program results from alterations of both behavioral and attitudinal components of the personality pattern through the work experience. The objective is an adequate work personality. Employability is based upon motivation toward work and adaptability to its demands and tensions. The shift in the vocational pattern today toward greater conformity to occupational expectations augments the probability of a client's being both satisfied and satisfactory in life's work. The goal of the work adjustment service is the client's continuing ability to adjust on the job through work orientation, including developing a positive self-regard and interpersonal attitudes and relations [Gellman, Gendel, Glaser, Friedman, & Neff, 1957].

13.3.1. REFERRAL CONSIDERATIONS

The Tenth Institute on Rehabilitative Services [U.S. IRS, 1972a] discussed client referral for work adjustment services the basics of which are reported here. These criteria are important because inappropriate referral may cause great personal harm to the client. The rehabilitationist must know when work adjustment services are appropriate. Two general questions can be helpful: Is this client's functioning or behavior such as to cause serious adjustment problems in the labor market, even with selective placement? Does it appear that this functioning or level of behavior can be changed? The objective of the referral to work adjustment will be to facilitate the transition to employment by improving the client's ability to secure and hold appropriate employment and adapt to the job or to function more effectively on the job. The facility staff works with the client in a work situation to: (1) identify and study the problems in vocational behavior and functioning, (2) make realistic plans and decisions about vocational and related behavior change and functioning, and (3) initiate changes that will promote a client's employability and job satisfaction.

Adequate referral information about a client referred for work adjustment will save time and help the client to attain or maintain a high level of motivation to improve. Referral information should include as much of the following information as possible:

1. Description of functional limitations and emergency medical information.
2. Psychological assessment information describing intellectual, verbal, performance, emotional, achievement, and aptitude patterns.
3. Social information describing educational, home, school, and vocational situations that may reflect on work performance.
4. Work evaluation information describing interests, motivations, skills, problems, behaviors, and effective change techniques.

Acceptance criteria varies with the facility, depending upon its objectives, staff availability and competence, current case load, and work availability. Some general client entrance criteria are:

1. Reason to believe that a client cannot function or adjust adequately in suitable employment because of physical, psychological, social, cultural, or vocational problems. This information comes from the referring counselor.
2. Vocational and related social problems that are not amenable to other less expensive approaches in vocational problem-solving such as vocational counseling.
3. Physical problems that have reached a point of stability such that a client is able to look beyond immediate physiological needs toward physical and/or behavioral growth needs.
4. The expectation that clients having unstable or medical problems will be under medical supervision.
5. Control of social behavior such that a client will not disrupt programming for other clients or be a danger to self or others.

Screening for work adjustment will occur over a period of time during work evaluation and even during early work adjustment. Acceptance involves identifying client problems and determining if the facility staff can help the client solve these problems. While identification of client problems occurs primarily during the client's work evaluation, the referring counselor should report already identified problems from contacts with the client, previous employers, and the client's family. Specifically, client problem areas that can be handled effectively in work adjustment include:

1. Anxiety or discomfort under supervision or difficulty communicating with supervisor.
2. Difficulty accepting and profiting from instruction or criticism.
3. Difficulty understanding, accepting, or acting in the role of a worker.
4. The quality of work below minimum industrial standards.
5. The quantity of work (the amount and steadiness of production) below minimal industrial standards.
6. Inappropriate response to unpleasant assignments or unpleasant aspects of job.
7. Difficulty in organizing work effectively.

8. Interpersonal relations (with co-workers) inadequate or inappropriate.
9. Failure to present a good self-image to others [U.S. IRS, 1972a].

13.3.2. THERAPEUTIC MILIEU

The work setting found in the rehabilitation facility represents a work adjustment technique in and of itself. The client becomes oriented to work since the workshop is patterned after industry and has adjustment situations similar to those the client will encounter in industry. According to Campbell and O'Toole [1970], the industrial atmosphere of the shop helps the client fit into the structure and functioning of a company. Like industry, the workshop has production teams under a supervisor, requiring learning and practicing role relationships with co-workers and supervisors. Products are produced for industrial use, necessitating that quality and quantity standards be met, that job procedures be followed, and that contracts be completed on schedule. Subcontract work provides a variety of job situations to be learned. The rehabilitation shop is the place where the worker's role can be learned, practiced, and tested, yet it is a "sheltered," nonpunitive setting in which client interests are paramount and professional help is available. Still, the client must learn the importance of appropriate behavior and work habits. It is a flexible situation that uses decreasing permissiveness as clients mature as workers.

The shop also provides the first real opportunity for many clients to learn to get along with other people, to enjoy people, and to express personal feelings. Being with other people helps to relieve the sense of isolation that many clients have; observing the problems of others and their successful efforts sometimes inspires clients. The shop staff provides close supervision, with consistent rewards and impartially enforced rules to help clients accept work authority and structure. Times for beginning and ending work are firmly set so that promptness and regular attendance are required. Conditioning for competitive employment is the goal at every step.

For some clients, a gradual exposure to an industrial type of environment is all that is necessary to learn the role of a worker and develop the skills and tolerances necessary for a regular job. For others, a more sophisticated program is required. The most unique and important aspect of the work setting in a rehabilitation facility is that it provides the framework in which techniques such as behavior modification and work conditioning can be carried out. It becomes the clay with which the rehabilitation team can shape and mold a program that fits the individual needs of each client.

13.3.3. MANIPULATION OF WORK SITUATION

A technique of work adjustment, as described by Gellman [1961], is manipulation of the work activity and work environment. Work programs are changed as the client needs change. Programming can be individualized according to the type of work, working conditions, job satisfactions, wages, work pressures, the degree of success, supervisory attitudes, and relations with other clients. Changing the work conditions permits the staff to observe a particular client's work behavior and functioning capacity. Thus it is possible to learn what client characteristics are facilitating or inhibiting employability.

Manipulation of the job situation is useful for both evaluation and therapy. Behavior is changed through manipulation of the environment to increase the client's tolerance for desirable work activities and to decrease inappropriate work behavior. Lustig [1970] explicitly describes how the client's behavior is manipulated through changing the time, position, rate, interpersonal relationships, and quantity of the work.

1. Time. Time refers to the duration of an event or activity. The amount of time devoted to a particular activity in the work situation can be increased or decreased. The frequency and duration of the activity can be controlled to accommodate the client's needs and level of tolerance.
2. Position. Position refers to the worker's location in relation to the components of the work environment. The distance between the worker and other people and the size of the work area can be changed. These variations range from close to distant and from a small to a large area. The distance between people affects how they communicate and participate. The size of the work area affects the kind of activity used. A small area requires use of fine movements whereas a large area allows greater use of expansive or gross movements.
3. Rate. Rate refers to the speed of productive

activity. The speed requirements of the job can be varied from fast to slow and can be modified by personal and other "nonpersonal" factors. These rate variations produce a range of situations for the worker as illustrated below:

a. Slow-personal (e.g., working as part of a team of slow producers or being asked by the boss to work carefully rather than fast).

b. Slow-nonpersonal (e.g., working at a slow-moving conveyor belt job without supervisory intervention).

c. Fast-personal (e.g., working with a team of high production workers or being asked by the boss to work quickly for piecework pay).

d. Fast-nonpersonal (e.g., working on a fast-moving conveyor belt job without directions from the boss).

4. Interpersonal relationships. Workers relate on a hierarchial basis to: those above them (supervisors and bosses), those below them, and those equal to them (co-workers). Since clients who come for help are rarely involved in relationships with people below them, Lustig omitted that description. In their relationships with those above them, workers can be modified by the following characteristics that the authority manifests: attitude, which ranges from positive to negative, and the nature of control exerted, which ranges from laissez-faire to democratic to autocratic.

5. Quantity. Quantity refers to the number and kind of stimuli to which workers relate. Number can vary from few or none to much or many. Kind can be personal or nonpersonal. Lustig subdivided "personal" as follows: sex differences (male, female); age differences (younger, older, equal); and status and historical differences (work experience, educational level, economic position, ethnic or cultural affiliation). He also subdivided "nonpersonal" according to: involvement, which can vary from direct involvement (e.g., use of hands or hand tools) to indirect involvement (e.g., use of machinery); resistance of the material (very resistant to nonresistant); size of material, which can vary from small to large; and, constancy of the work, which can range from repetitious to varied.

Lustig [1970] further said, "There are numerous possibilities for combining these factors. The client who is unable to concentrate on a work task for more than a few minutes can be assigned to a station requiring direct involvement with small materials, and the time and frequency of the activity can then be gradually increased. The withdrawn client who prefers to work in isolation may be forced to change tasks often in order to prevent his becoming preoccupied with a small set of nonpersonal stimuli" [p. 42].

In addition to the components discussed by Lustig, the *types* of work tasks should be subject to variation for several reasons. Dunn [1971] pointed out that the continual assignment to work tasks lower than a client's perceived occupational competency can result in lowered self-esteem and regression of performance level. Leshner and Snyderman [1962] went on to say that in order to achieve acceptable work adjustment it is necessary to use work related to the vocational goal. Anderson [1968] commented on the need for real, meaningful work in order to assess properly the progress and work adjustment of clients. They also thought that it was necessary to have supervisory and other aspects of the work adjustment shop resemble as closely as possible the community job situation (particularly in the latter phases of the client's program in the shop). The point these authors have raised is that the progress and/or success of the individual client may hinge on the type of work performed while in Work Adjustment.

Work geared to a client's competency and interests will provide better work adjustment information, but there are a number of problems presented by this. As Campbell and O'Toole [1970] have noted, much staff effort is already expended in finding and securing contracts or other work activities for work adjustment programs. It is often difficult to obtain any type of work. In most work adjustment programs, the work experience is determined by what work the shop has to offer rather than the client's interests and competencies. Larger budgets and staffs would be necessary to gear work to each client. Moreover, the needs and interests of the clients served also vary, and it would be difficult to maintain appropriate work stations with a consistent flow of clients.

13.4. Techniques

The following three programs, presented by Gellman and Friedman [1965], represent modifications of work adjustment services that are possible in a rehabilitation facility to meet the specialized needs of clients:

1. The "work identity program" is intended for persons who have lost their "work life" and their identity as productive persons because of disablement or hospitalization, or because they have adopted the role of "patienthood" or of a handicapped person. Although they have undergone a normal process of vocational development, they are psychologically deactivated and unable to see themselves as capable of working. The treatment plan introduces stress in manageable proportions to enable ego forces to deal with the demands of reality under tension-producing conditions.
2. The "vocational development program" is designed for persons who have never achieved an adequate level of functioning in achievement-demanding situations or who lack a productive orientation and are characterized by "paralysis of achievement" (e.g., the schizophrenic and the retarded). It is directed toward the formation of a work personality for persons who, because of congenital or early disability, have deviated from the normal process of vocational development.
3. The "acculturation program" is used with persons who can work but are industrially inept. They may be characterized as persons who have the ability to achieve but lack knowledge of (or contact with) a technologically advanced culture (e.g., socially disadvantaged youth, immigrants, or persons coming from an agricultural or nonindustrial community). The program concentrates upon the client's learning how to learn to work, the acquisition of acceptable occupational stereotypes that facilitate job placement or job maintenance, and the development of job skills.

13.4.1. JOB PERFORMANCE AIDS

A work adjustment technique similar to manipulation of the job situation is the use of job performance aids. Instead of training clients to adjust to a work situation, job performance aids are used as prosthetic devices to help those who cannot meet competitive employment standards through training alone because of functional limitations. Probably the most common job performance aids are "jigs," or devices that help clients perform a specific task. A jig might be something as simple as a clamp on a worktable to hold objects steady while they are being worked on, or it might be a complex electronic device. The use of job performance aids can also be referred to as work simplification or job restructuring. While job performance aids are very useful, both client and rehabilitationist should be forewarned that successful competitive employment depends not only on the client's learning how to work with these aids, but also on the rehabilitationist's convincing an employer to allow the use of aids within the competitive job situation.

Job performance aids that can neutralize a wide variety of limitations have been described by Dunn [1974]. For example, if there is a memory problem, a simple printed time schedule may ensure that the person performs all of the necessary requirements of a job. A model board may be displayed at the work station, showing how each subassembly fits together and displaying the assembly sequence as a whole.

In the case in which a worker is very distractable, Lindsley [1964] suggested the use of a rate switch as a "prosthetic response." The rate switch is simply a device that must be repeatedly activated to keep a machine operating or a signal from sounding, thus heightening the level of attention required of the worker in performing the task. An artificial or "prosthetic" response is substituted for the client's natural response so that the individual performs the work at an appropriate speed.

Another prosthetic approach is to increase the "response topography." When the physical features or relationships inherent in performing a task are changed, a functional limitation such as inaccurate finger movement is no longer a barrier. A number of devices are available for expanding response topographies. Independent personal care is facilitated by substituting Velcro (adhesive-like) fasteners for the more commonly used buttons, zippers, and laces, thus enabling a person with poor hand and finger control to dress without help. Macroswitches (large contact panels) are installed on a machine so that a worker with cerebral palsy can operate the machine.

Jobs are also restructured to provide a proper schedule of reward reinforcement. In a therapeutic environment it is common to reinforce the client on a fixed schedule, such as for a given number of units produced or with periodic regularity (once every hour or once every day basis) or every time the individual demonstrates a particular behavior. Normally, however, reinforcers follow variable schedules and this is useful for maintaining high, even response rates. Unfortunately, some people have trouble with variable reinforcement schedules, particularly if lengthy gaps occur between reinforcers. These workers may require a prosthetic contingency such as an automatic reward dispenser to maintain a desired behavior. Regular statements of support by the supervisors also may provide the needed reinforcement.

Chalupsky and Kopf [1967] developed the following guidelines for the use of job performance aids according to seven task variables:

1. Speed of task performance. Tasks requiring particularly rapid performance, such as emergency first aid, suggest training rather than procedural job aids.
2. Task complexity. Tasks that are particularly complex and that include many choice points suggest the use of job performance aids. Simple tasks, quickly learned, may not justify the costs of elaborate performance aids.
3. Frequency of task performance. High-frequency tasks indicate a training approach; conversely, infrequently occurring tasks imply the use of job aids to offset the retention problem.
4. Length of work cycle. Lengthy tasks lend themselves to performance-aiding in preference to training. The short-cycle tasks may not justify performance-aid costs because of the speed with which individuals are able to perform from memory.
5. Task stability. Tasks remaining stable over long periods of time suggest the use of performance aids, while short-lived tasks incur problems of performance-aid modification.
6. Task flexibility. When established task se-

quences are critical, procedural job aids are necessary. Freedom to vary the order of task performance reduces the necessity of procedural aids.
7. Task precision. Tasks requiring extremely close tolerances imply consideration of job performance aids. Tasks in which extreme accuracy is not a requirement may not warrant application of aids.

Workplace design and job restructuring techniques are important not only for preemployment adjustment programs but also in permanent and competitive job placement arrangements. The elimination of barriers at the place of work and other techniques and devices to optimize job performance are thus essential components of rehabilitation technology. Goodwill Industries of America has published a manual on the subject [n.d.].

13.4.2. WORK CONDITIONING

Physical stamina as a problem in the work adjustment of clients unable to work a full day was discussed by Campbell and O'Toole [1970]. (Debilitation and associated problems are also described in Chapter 5, Functional Limitations.) Physical capacity for work must be carefully assessed to avoid reprimanding the client unjustly for what may be symptoms of weakness. Medical attention for these persons is indicated, with a prescribed schedule of gradually increased work hours to build up tolerance. This process is known as "work conditioning" or "work hardening."

When clients are limited in the length of time and amount of energy they can expend, work conditioning can increase their tolerance to a level that will allow industrial standards to be met without ill effects or medical relapse. Nelson [1960] reported that some rehabilitation facilities provide work conditioning services as part of an occupational therapy program, but most shops do not provide conditioning therapy of the sort carried out in medical settings. Instead, a facility typically assigns clients to a limited work schedule on supervised ongoing projects, with perhaps an occupational therapist to serve as a consultant to supervisors during such hardening processes.

In medical treatment, occupational therapy, or physical therapy programs, on the other hand, work adjustment and work conditioning mean developing physical tolerances and capacities, and only secondarily do they involve development of work skills or work personality. An initial goal of sitting tolerance, for example, would be achieved by having a client spend successively longer periods of time sitting; work samples or work tasks would be performed during those times only to keep the client meaningfully productive. Tasks would be completed, and a work personality developed in these cases, of course, but the thrust of the program would be to develop physical tolerances [Sankovsky, 1971].

It is not always easy to identify candidates for work conditioning. Most people, especially men, do not wish to discuss their weaknesses and some may not recognize that they are not up to par physically. Mental patients and people who have been hospitalized for a long time are often in a weakened physical condition.

A lack of physical stamina and resulting fatigue on the job often result from living habits such as staying up late to watch television. This condition can also be related to drug or alcohol abuse. Counseling is required when unhealthy habits contribute to the client's inability to work full days all week. Improper diet is a common cause of chronic fatigue. This is due not so much to poverty as to lack of knowledge about proper food and regular meals. Complaints of dizziness and weakness are meaningful signs for the dietitian.

Poor environment and poor living habits may be responsible for inadequate performance on the job. Thus, inadequate housing and off-the-job circumstances must be attended to before considering job placement.

Campbell and O'Toole [1970] pointed out that some clients become accustomed to thinking of themselves as sick, and that concern for their physical comfort takes precedence over anything else. The slightest pain may assume great importance. These clients must be taught to differentiate between minor discomforts and symptoms of serious physical problems. Otherwise, they do not realize that a headache or an occasional back pain is not reason enough to stay home or to leave work early.

13.4.3. BEHAVIOR CHANGE TECHNIQUES

Behavior modification procedures in one form or another are an effective technique of work adjustment. A commonly used method is to reinforce clients for appropriate behavior. Reinforcers include staff praise and attention, money, and, within certain realistic constraints, nearly anything the client finds rewarding. When it is not practical to give a particular reinforcer immediately, tokens may be substituted that can later be exchanged for the rewarding activity or object. The use of tokens as described by Esser [1977] is a common behavior modification procedure that, when used systematically across an entire program, is referred to as a "token economy." For behavior modification programs to be fully effective, they must be expertly planned and implemented.

The effectiveness of behavior modification as a work adjustment technique derives from the reinforcement principles of general learning theory. Psychologists have described the method as manipulating the environment according to reinforcement principles to increase, maintain, decrease, eliminate, or teach new behaviors. The basic premise of operant conditioning is that almost all behavior is learned, and that a given behavior can be strengthened if rewarded or diminished if negatively reinforced.

The mechanics of operant conditioning within a sheltered workshop, according to Weiss [1975], involve: (1) identifying a behavior that is detrimental to job success, (2) describing a "target behavior" that would be more suitable, (3) recording the frequency of both behaviors, (4) determining the consequences of the unsuitable and target behaviors, and (5) modifying the events that follow the unsuitable behavior. Experience shows that this method can effectively change behaviors that hamper employment, including low productivity, inappropriate work behavior, and so on.

Token reinforcement was mentioned above as commonly used in behavior modification. Initially, the tokens (e.g., poker chips, check marks on a card) should be given immediately after the desired behavior is exhibited, but later, as the client develops more self-control, the period between the behavior and reward is lengthened. Tokens are given then at the end of the work day for something the client wants, whether it be money, food, clothes, recreation, privileges, or something else. Eventually, the rewards of a regular job, a weekly paycheck, the satisfaction of doing a job well, and the pleasure of being independent replace the need for tokens.

The evidence that is available does indicate

that progress in a number of areas can be made using token economies. After a literature review, Molski [1976] cautioned, however: "It needs to be remembered that most of the studies have used psychiatric or mentally retarded populations. Since they have been institutionalized in many cases, they have a captive population where tokens may be of value. Little research has been done on a more mobile population in a community Work Adjustment setting. There is no research indicating the transfer of learning from a token economy into a community job setting" [p. 36].

Operant conditioning techniques have been criticized as dehumanizing and as dealing with symptoms rather than causes. But, proponents of this form of behavior modification counter with the claim that since all behavior is influenced by some form of external control, it should be uniform and systematic. Esser and Botterbusch [1975] presented further information and studies on token economies. Behavioral techniques is the subject of Chapter 29.

13.4.4. THE ROLE OF TEACHING

According to Esser [1977], some type of instruction in independent living skills, social adjustment, job readiness, and so on is found in most adjustment programs, either in a classroom setting or on an individual basis. The teaching method should be based on an overall plan that has identified client needs and objectives.

There are various forms of instruction. Ehrle [1968] described "identification" as a type of learning situation that involves the client's identifying with, then imitating, or "modeling," the behavior of a staff member. Identification and modeling can be effective mechanisms for changing behavior during the work adjustment process, although they are more difficult to use than less subtle teaching methods.

Many clients need some form of instruction. Particularly, retarded and socially deprived people may have had limited exposure to vocationally maturing experiences. Living a sheltered childhood, the young adult has not developed vocationally and consequently does not understand the world of work (i.e., why people work, the role of the supervisor and worker, and the generally accepted rules and regulations of employment). Deficiency in these areas suggests that a teaching approach to work adjustment can be used.

13.4.5. INDIVIDUAL COUNSELING

Individual counseling has proved effective in work adjustment programs. In fact, one of the key factors in an experimental work adjustment project at Vocational Guidance and Rehabilitation Services in Cleveland was the role of the work adjustment counselor, according to Campbell and O'Toole [1970]. They stated that, "The counselor, who acts as a milieu therapist, assesses client behavior and deals with problems as they arise in the workshop" [p. iii]. The counselor suggests alternate patterns of behavior and selectively reprimands and rewards the client toward behavior that is appropriate to the role of the worker. Also, the counselor guides clients' interactions with supervisors and peers and utilizes individual and group techniques.

Ayers [1971] believed that individual counseling is of particular significance when a client first enters a work adjustment program. At this point the counselor is responsible for the development of a total vocational plan. Moreover, the counselor should supply information regarding vocational, educational, and social history and provide tentative goals in the work adjustment program. More specifically, according to Ayers, the counselor in a work adjustment program can: (1) orient the client to the new work setting, (2) interpret adjustment and employment goals to the client, (3) help the client adapt to working conditions similar to those in a competitive work setting, (4) interpret standards of work behavior and production goals to the client, (5) counsel the client regarding problems of adjustment in the work setting, (6) recommend to shop supervision specific work tasks and experiences that may produce client growth, and (7) participate in planning further services that would enhance the client's vocational adjustment.

Having a counselor available in the work adjustment setting has numerous advantages. The counselor can help the client to deal with personal problems and can present and/or interpret information to the client. This arrangement also offers an opportunity for a meaningful client-counselor relationship to develop, and it provides a mechanism to integrate observations of the individual's work performance with other evaluative information.

13.4.6. GROUP COUNSELING

Ayers [1971] also described how group counseling can be utilized extensively in work adjustment programs. In fact, he said, "The group itself is the therapeutic instrument" [p. 33]. The group provides acceptance and support for its members as new feelings of independence and responsibility emerge; old values and behavior can be reexamined, reevaluated, and changed, if the individual members so desire; biased and unrealistic perceptions may be subjected to reality testing by group interactions; and feelings of self-confidence and self-worth may be enhanced by group acceptance. As Bass [1969] emphasized, the specific goals of a vocationally oriented group should reflect the purposes of the work adjustment program. Each member should develop a realistic self-concept as a worker, become aware of the values and standards of worker behavior, and develop effective social skills. Also, Ayers said that in such a supportive milieu, inappropriate interpersonal behavior in the workshop can be treated as a learning situation with minimal threat to the group members. (See Chapter 30, Group Counseling.)

13.4.7. VIDEOTAPE TECHNIQUES
The process of videotaping samples of the client's behavior in the work adjustment program is called "video-counseling." This process can be of great value in enhancing the effectiveness of counseling by presenting the client with realistic feedback about recent behavior. Through selective playbacks clients can see their own behavior as others see it. The playback may be either immediate or delayed, and it is easy either to stop or repeat the viewing for appropriate emphasis. Ayers [1971] thought that the most significant aspect of the process is that the actual behavior of individuals in interaction with others is recorded in the group session. Thus, there is the unique opportunity for these individuals to see themselves dealing with people. In a study by Moor, Chervall, and West [1965], hospital patients who saw themselves on videotape showed more improvement in appearance, attitude, and interaction with others than those patients who had not had the opportunity. DeRoo and Haralson [1971] found that just giving clients the opportunity to view themselves working, without any further discussion, led to significant production increases.

Video-counseling can be employed in at least three areas of work adjustment: improvement of performance, development of personal-social skills, and facilitation of attitude changes, as has

been pointed out by Ayers. Two types of problem clients are candidates: those who are not consciously aware of their behavioral problems and those who deny exhibiting the behavior. In both cases, *showing* clients the behavior rather than just telling them about it will be more effective and more likely to be acknowledged. This technique is well geared to the "low-verbal" client who has difficulty with traditional individual counseling. There are some drawbacks to video-taping, however. Perhaps the most significant is economic [Sankovsky & Knight, 1971]. The equipment is expensive, training is required for the staff to learn to operate it, and valuable staff time is involved when the equipment is being used.

13.4.8. LEVELS OF PROGRESS
Hansen [1972] has provided a four-tier description of client progress in a work adjustment program. Use of his reporting system gives the sponsoring agency a more comprehensive understanding of the client's progress. Moreover, the hierarchical classification identifies those clients who need maximum supervision on a work station. An outline of the Hansen Work Adjustment Reporting System follows.

LEVEL 1. At the lowest level, Level 1, clients need maximum supervision in all work areas. They show poor self-control; their work tolerance is poor; they may not be able to handle interpersonal relationships; and they have not developed self-confidence. If clients continue at Level 1 for a long period of time, it is doubtful that they can benefit from sheltered workshop services and they should be considered for placement in an activity center. Clients unable to develop past Level 1 may never have the ability to adjust to a work environment, but this could also indicate that they are not developmentally ready for a program of work adjustment.

LEVEL 2. At Level 2 clients need less than maximum supervision in all simple, repetitive jobs. Essentially these clients are demonstrating the ability to adjust to work but at a very low level and at jobs that call for little or no judgment. They are showing some degree of self-confidence, self-control, and work tolerance; some degree of handling interpersonal relationships; and are beginning to develop a "work personality." Many Level 2 jobs within the work adjustment program are dependent upon contract operations dealing with simple, routine, repetitive tasks.

LEVEL 3. At Level 3 clients still need supervision in their work, but they are now working at jobs calling for a greater degree of tolerance, approaching the normal work limits; have a fair to good degree of competence in handling interpersonal relationships; exhibit self-confidence; and generally have a work personality.

LEVEL 4. At Level 4, the top level, clients are demonstrating a high degree of self-confidence, self-control, and high work tolerance; they handle interpersonal relationships in a mature fashion; and understand the world of work. These clients demonstrate an ability to work at all jobs within the workshop and may be considered ready for specific training or perhaps for competitive employment.

13.4.9. COMPENSATORY SKILL TRAINING

Compensatory skill training was described by Nelson [1960].

When a client suffers amputation or loss of function of a body member, he is taught to compensate by developing special or substitute abilities. A client may be taught to use a prosthesis for specific work tasks. He may be helped to develop ways of substituting for a non-functioning extremity. At times special assistive devices or special tools may be developed by the shop personnel. In other cases the client is helped in reorganizing tasks to compensate for functional deficiencies" [p. 6].

"Lip reading, speech training, gait training and mobility training for the blind," according to descriptions by Jarrell [1972], "are illustrative of training in very specific skills which may be needed if the client is to enter and receive maximum benefit from a formalized training program or to re-enter the competitive labor market" [p. 231].

Compensatory skill training is closely related to work adjustment services and is considered as such in many rehabilitation facilities. However, a distinction is indicated in that compensatory skill training deals with training in very specific skills, rather than with the broad range of behavioral changes that are frequently dealt with in work adjustment services. Nevertheless, the subject involves essential adjustment processes rather than vocational training, which is discussed next.

Chapter 14

Educational Services

While education is only one of a comprehensive array of public rehabilitation services, it is still fundamental to the concept of complete rehabilitation. Vocational rehabilitation, whenever possible, is intended to restore the competitive position of a disabled person in getting and performing work. This means that, compared to nondisabled workers, rehabilitation clients may need equal or superior preparation in the face of employment prejudices or in the event that functional limitations offset their qualifications. A high level of occupational abilities through educational and vocational training services can compensate for the handicap.

Rehabilitation should result in permanent vocational adjustment, a career rather than a job for the moment. Ideally, it is a one-time, nonrecurring effort. To obtain this goal, the disabled person must be fully prepared to get and retain employment despite competition and fluctua-

tions in the labor market. In addition to other restorative services, training often provides the margin of competency needed for career security (i.e., employment without further placement assistance).

Educational programs can also contribute to clients achieving personal adjustment to disability. Self-confidence may be regained by the demonstration of ability through success in a well-chosen course of study. These achievements are viewed by the client as tangible steps toward a specified vocational goal, and thus training is the basis of continuing motivation and satisfaction.

It is essential, of course, that the objectives are suitable and desired by the client. The rehabilitationist is responsible for monitoring the progress of the preparation program and for continuing counseling as indicated. Nevertheless, it should be understood at the outset that the client must accept the obligation for successful completion of the effort.

The public rehabilitation agencies provide a wide variety of education or training—in public and private colleges and universities, proprietary business or trade schools, state institutions and rehabilitation facilities; with staff instructors or other tutors whenever convenient to the client; through correspondence courses at home or hospital; in rehabilitation workshops and community vocational schools; and on-the-job training in factories and shops.

14.1. Vocational Preparation

Vocational training and vocational education impart the knowledge and skills necessary for a specified occupation. This is different from the types of training services covered in the previous chapter in that it provides specific preparation required for a specified occupational objective.

14.1.1. VOCATIONAL EDUCATION

Most high schools in the United States offer several vocational education options. The two oldest programs are vocational agriculture and vocational home economics, which have expanded to include a number of related endeavors (e.g., agribusiness, clothing management). A variation is the "cooperative" or "work-study" program in which pupils attend school part of the day and work at a job for the remainder. These programs usually involve office or retail sales work and automotive repair or mechanical work, although a number of other occupations are suitable for such instruction. The "learn and practice" approach is applicable to practically all occupations for which post-high school education is not necessary. Some public schools have introduced "exploratory programs" before high school. Others offer the option of a full-time job during the senior year, which is planned and monitored by staff for credit toward graduation [Tolbert, 1974]. Vocational preparation in public school is especially valuable for handicapped youths who have had limited opportunity for work experience.

14.1.2. VOCATIONAL-TECHNICAL SCHOOLS

"These institutions," according to Tolbert, "may offer career preparation somewhat like that of the community college. There is often a tie-in with the public schools, and high school pupils sometimes take related training at the vocational technical center" [p. 106]. Although such schools primarily offer post-high school educa-tion, applicants without diplomas but with potential are often admitted. The lengths of programs range from several months to two years. Typical courses include air conditioning, refrigeration, and heating technology; automotive technology; and carpentry.

Private vocational schools often specialize in preparation for business, trade and technical jobs, cosmetology, and barbering. Many students prefer private vocational schools because the courses, which emphasize skills, have a special appeal to the less scholastic. The rehabilitation counselor has the responsibility of helping interested clients evaluate prospective schools and make an informed choice that fits their needs. For older clients it is noteworthy that many private vocational schools accept students who have not completed high school and that they provide good training opportunities for older unemployed persons.

According to Jarrell [1972], vocational or trade schools are "particularly desirable for occupational advancement in instances where disability requires that a skilled worker transfer to an occupation in which his former skills can be utilized" [p. 232]. This is due to the supplemental nature of the training, which permits the student to build upon an existing skill. Too often, however, completion of a trade school course provides only minimal requirements for employment in nonentry occupations and skills that are not readily transferable. Moreover, the value of the skills learned in trade school may be particularly limited by changing conditions of employment.

14.1.3. CORRESPONDENCE COURSES

Home study courses range from kindergarten through college and vary widely in completion time, difficulty, quality, and cost. Colleges, trade associations, and proprietary schools offer mail study courses.

Correspondence study must be chosen with discrimination and the method is not suitable for many people. But it can be effective, and sometimes "learning by mail" is the only alternative when residential or other instruction is not available. In selecting correspondence study one must consider the ethics of the school, the relevance of the material, and the potentiality and motivation of the student. Correspondence study is most effective when it is considered as supplemental to other rehabilitation training. It takes much persistence to complete such courses without supervision. Consequently, it is good practice to arrange for the help of a regular tutor (e.g., a local school teacher) to explain difficult material.

The rehabilitation facility counselor can readily monitor a client's progress in completing correspondence study, but this is a difficult task when the client returns home. Self-study through correspondence courses consequently is more practical in a residential setting.

14.1.4. APPRENTICESHIP PROGRAMS

Apprenticeship programs commonly provide training in carpentry, masonry, machining, and other crafts. There are approximately 350 "apprenticeable" occupations with about a quarter of a million trainees in the United States. Training periods range from two to five years and the typical entering age is about 17 years.

Apprenticeship programs are available in many of the occupational areas taught in trade or vocational schools. The choice between trade school and apprenticeship program will depend on factors such as the client's age and educational attainment and the community availability of apprenticeship training. A consideration is that apprentices earn a wage, starting at about half of the skilled workers' rate of pay. The apprenticeship method of vocational training—learning under formal supervision, usually while on a job—is particularly appropriate for individuals who are unsuited to classroom situations. Moreover, apprentice training is conducted in many skilled trades for which there are no available school facilities. According to Jarrell [1972], "Ordinarily, arrangements of this type come under careful scrutiny in labor union contracts; however, labor is usually cognizant of the needs of the disabled individual and willing to make special provisions for his entrance into apprenticeship programs" [p. 233].

Many workers get enough experience to become qualified in occupations designated as apprenticeable without serving a formal apprenticeship, either in a union or otherwise. The rehabilitationist might find it easier to set up an on-the-job training program rather than to see to it that the client is registered and trained as an apprentice. However, there are advantages in apprenticeship training and placement, such as written outlines (facts regarding the training received) and the Certificate of Completion of Apprenticeship that is provided as evidence of qualifications for journeyman employment and pay. (Apprentice placement is discussed in Chapter 36, Securing Employment.)

14.1.5. VOCATIONAL SKILL TRAINING

In addition to providing various adjustment services and other specialized programs for people who are handicapped, rehabilitation facilities often sponsor work-skill training as part of their overall program. These skill-training programs may involve routine production tasks (e.g., operating drill presses and other machinery) or may focus on training areas such as building maintenance, food service, clerical work, upholstery, and radio-television repair. Some shops provide generalized trade training while others train clients for specific semiskilled jobs in industry. The advantage of training in rehabilitation facilities is that the programs are tailored to the needs of those who are severely handicapped. Professional staff and time devoted to solving problems help ensure that the client has learned appropriate work adjustment behaviors and compensatory skills. Teaching strategies for severely retarded and other handicapped clients of sheltered workshops have been developed by Marc Gold [1975] and by Bellamy, Inman, and Horner [1977]. Both methods are based upon an analysis of the elements (tasks) of a job.

The rehabilitation facility may also have the flexibility to provide long-term, intensive training, whereas vocational training programs in other settings are subject to a set length of time (e.g., a semester). In some localities rehabilitation facilities have established cooperative arrangements with vocational schools to share equipment, curriculums, and staff involved in vocational training.

Nelson [1971] has described several vocational training programs offered in rehabilitation facilities. This list is not all inclusive, and the terms and programs differ among facilities. However, the following program descriptions give an overview of the types of training ordinarily available in rehabilitation workshops.

Production Training

This type of training consists of teaching a client the specific skills necessary to accomplish the production work of the shop. The level of skill varies with the particular subcontracts, reconditioning jobs, or manufacturing products produced by the shop. Tasks may involve simple routine operations such as packaging, sorting, or assembling, or complicated operations such as cable harness assembly and other jobs in electronic or similar industries.

Trade Training

Trade training is designed to teach clients specific skills, knowledge, and abilities necessary to carry on a recognized trade or occupation. Few workshops provide all the skills necessary for the master level in many trades. However, in certain trades such as upholstering or small appliance repair, the training may be comprehensive.

Vestibule Training

This training consists of teaching a client a specific production skill job for which there is a demand in local factories. The shops may have at times a subcontract from a firm and the client may perform the work well enough to be ultimately hired by the plant that gave the workshop the contract. At other times a job is found with another company that does the same kind of work. Sometimes the client may be taken into the workshop as a permanent employee. The principle of vestibule training is to train intensively for a short time for a production job for which there is demand in industry or in the shop. (*Vestibule training* is a term also used in industry.)

14.1.6. ON-THE-JOB TRAINING

The most common procedure for training new workers in business and industry is on the job, referred to as OJT. New employees learn the routine and tasks of their assigned job from a supervisor or experienced employee or from a trained instructor employed by the company. Conducted at the actual work station, this type of instruction is quite effective, particularly for learning job skills.

Rehabilitation placement workers sometimes persuade employers to hire handicapped clients for OJT with the promise of continued employment, assuming successful training. It is more common, however, for the rehabilitation agency to pay the firm for providing OJT with or without paying the client for any incidental production while in training. Moreover, the contracting firm may or may not be obliged to hire the client upon completion of training, regardless of its success. OJT may be the only possibility where trade schools are not available (e.g., rural communities) or when formal courses are not offered for the client's job objective.

OJT is practical in that it offers a wide range of preparational opportunities. This type of informal but effective training may be purchased from skilled workers and from small businesses for common job objectives (e.g., florist, auto mechanic, cabinetmaker). The training plan is adaptable to the unique needs and abilities of the client. Rehabilitationists must monitor such training closely, but when good trainers and OJT programs are found, this becomes a rewarding rehabilitation resource for future clients.

Employers of OJT clients have the opportunity to instruct them in accordance with their particular needs. Under the progressive wage scale feature, employers pay the client-trainee from the start and throughout the training period only for the services that the client can perform. Chapter 36, Securing Employment, describes OJT as a tool for job placement.

14.1.7. WORK EXPERIENCE PROGRAMS

One method of facilitating an informed occupational choice is to provide the client experience in real work situations. Work experience programs have been described by Campbell, Walz, Miller, and Kriger [1973]. As they pointed out, work experience programs can help clients explore vocational possibilities, expand vocational aspirations, and make tentative vocational choices. While there is no assurance that such programs will accomplish these goals, they have been particularly effective in motivating clients. These programs increase the person's feelings of worth.

Several different types of work experience programs provide the opportunity to work in real work settings. These include cooperative education programs and work-study programs. Unless carefully planned, such programs may have the disadvantages of providing a limited view of only one occupation and of introducing only the more routine activities associated with it. There is also danger of creating negative rather than positive attitudes toward work because of poor relationships with people in the work setting or the negative attitudes of individual workers.

Programs of planned part-time work alternated with part-time study in a formal class are known as cooperative education programs. They are sometimes distinguished from work-study programs since the latter may provide pay for the time spent in the work setting. In either case vocational counseling during the program helps people to interpret their on-the-job experience.

Work-study programs are usually designed for special populations (e.g., disadvantaged, school dropouts, and chronically unemployed). Moreover, they are more often found in junior college, technical, or vocational schools or in specially established centers than in secondary schools. Some state rehabilitation agencies have developed work-study programs with the public school system. Another approach is the volunteer arrangements made by human service agencies for people who cannot obtain competitive employment.

14.1.8. GOVERNMENT JOB PROGRAMS

Government job programs are described here as examples of innovations designed to help potential workers who may be disadvantaged and handicapped. These manpower programs are administered through the U.S. Department of Labor (DOL) and do not have the traditional stability or assumed permanence of the federal rehabilitation program.

There is considerable confusion among handicapped clients and their human service workers at the local level about the overlapping vocational rehabilitation programs administered under various departments of the federal government. Many of these DOL projects are indistinguishable from programs of the state-federal vocational rehabilitation agency in the provision of services to handicapped people. This lack of boundaries has placed heavy expectations for informal cooperation upon local professionals to prevent waste of service money and time. Fed-

eral delineation of departmental authority is needed. Former lines of responsibility recognized DOL as a manpower agency charged with utilizing America's work force for greater productivity, not as a human service agency charged with helping individual citizens obtain a fulfilling life. Until such time as the central government can provide a clear-cut departmental structure for federally financed human services, it will be necessary for local practitioners to cope with a hodgepodge of overlapping rehabilitation job services.

Tolbert [1974] has searched various DOL publications and provided the descriptions given below for each of several selected programs.

JOB OPPORTUNITIES IN THE BUSINESS SECTOR (JOBS) PROGRAM. This program involves a commitment by the business community to hire disadvantaged persons and train them on the job. DOL recruits job applicants and pays the extra costs of employing those with special problems and needs. The National Alliance of Businessmen (NAB) has the responsibility of developing business support and finding job openings. The Manpower Development and Training Act (MDTA) program, utilizing both on-the-job training and classroom work, was originally established to retrain those with out-of-date or obsolete skills. Its major current emphasis is on training the disadvantaged. One may contact the local office of the state Employment Service to learn what kinds of opportunities the program offers. An applicant may qualify for training if he or she is underemployed, displaced from a job, disadvantaged, or hard to train.

THE JOB CORPS. The Job Corps provides job and personal development training for school dropouts between the ages of 16 and 21 who have poor school achievement records and are out of work. Founded in 1965, the Job Corps makes referrals for specific training to other programs such as MDTA.

NEIGHBORHOOD YOUTH CORPS (NYC). NYC helps school-age and older youths from low-income families either remain in school or find work. The emphasis is on providing academic and prevocational training for those aged 16 and 17, and on guiding those 18 and over who are ready for employment to other programs, if additional training is needed.

WORK INCENTIVE PROGRAM (WIN). WIN is aimed at helping those employable individuals receiving financial assistance to become economically independent. The Employment Service provides vocational testing, counseling, occupational placement or training, whichever is needed.

PUBLIC SERVICE CAREERS PROGRAM. This program arranges for disadvantaged persons to be hired and trained by government service agencies. The program also enables those in "dead-end" jobs to qualify for advancement. Other federally funded programs, such as Operation Mainstream and Special Impact Program, are similarly designed to provide help for disadvantaged people.

Still other DOL job programs have provided vocational counseling, training, placement, and other services for handicapped populations.

14.1.9. HOMEBOUND TRAINING

For various reasons, some severely handicapped individuals are unable to leave their homes to participate in vocational training or other rehabilitation programs. There is a great need to involve these people in meaningful activity.

"Meaningful activity," as Towne [1972] has said, "sometimes becomes the difference between home or institutionalization. Not infrequently we find an individual whose isolation has taken a great toll. His separation from society may be vast, sometimes even to the extent that he scarcely identifies with the outside world. This almost schizophrenic situation is a manifestation of monotony and loneliness" [p. 2]. One of the goals of a homebound program is to reestablish the client's contact and identification with the real world.

Experience deprivation suffered by homebound individuals may reduce their levels of intellectual, social, and vocational functioning. If left unchecked, such deprivation can produce irreversible psychosocial consequences, rendering the person unresponsive to almost any rehabilitation intervention. Rusalem and Cohen [1975] stated that: "Extended homeboundedness deprives the individual of the capacity to respond to, and use constructively the rehabilitation services that are made available to him. For example . . . as the period of a person's homeboundedness lengthens, scores on intelligence measures decline progressively, motivation to reverse homeboundedness declines inexorably, and readiness for life skills instructions withers away until the affected person cannot benefit substantially from rehabilitation counseling and instruction" [p. 201].

Homecrafters Program

Crafts programs for homebound disabled people are well known in the United States and other countries. Training and related help are given to the homebound person to produce a marketable item. The Wisconsin Division of Vocational Rehabilitation has one of the first and largest "homecraft" programs. Homecraft teachers are employed by the agency, which purchases equipment and initial supplies for the "homecrafter" and also has arranged to market the products through sales programs. Adrian Towne [1972], who was the director of the Wisconsin agency, indicated that it seems to work out best in nonmetropolitan settings. While substantial earnings are occasionally possible for homecrafters, Towne believed that this is not a realistic goal in most instances. Personal satisfaction stands out as justification for the considerable training cost since the homecrafter creates from raw material a finished product of value to others.

Caution is advised before settling on homebound training and thus closing the door on outside employment. Being confined to a single environment in itself does serious psychosocial damage to the already disabled person. In fact, prolonged isolation at home often has more serious effects than the medical impairment that originally precipitated the confinement. This may occur even when the home environment is physically attractive and the social atmosphere is loving and accommodating. In such sheltered situations there may be a lack of challenge to develop through one's own effort. The resulting experience deprivation can render the strongest person unable to respond to real life. Thus, coping skills and the motivation to improve may progressively deteriorate over time, making rehabilitation infeasible. Prompt action is advised in beginning homebound services. There are homebound "derelicts" whose long and pervasive deprivation of experience leaves no hope for reversal through rehabilitation. Final determination of infeasibility sometimes requires extended evaluation with a trial period.

Herbert Rusalem and Milton Cohen [1975], with the New York Federation of the Handicapped, described alternatives to homebound rehabilitation as suggested by their programmatic research. They found that out-of-home service is feasible for more than 80 percent of all homebound persons referred to a state rehabilitation agency. In fact, they reported, "It is not the severity of the disability nor the medical contraindications that restrict the individual. On the contrary, the deterrents for homebound people ordinarily are geographical remoteness, inadequate transportation resources, architectural barriers, family discouragement of client attempts to become more independent, and clients' emotional responses to severe disability . . . . many homebound persons are actually less severely disabled than other equally limited individuals who are engaged in regular community based employment" [pp. 201–202].

It is concluded that resurrection of homebound people is equivalent to deinstitutionalization. Helping these people to become "nonhomebound" is the preferred course of action, that is to say "home-based services" are usually the last resort for severely handicapped clients. Their rehabilitation, however, requires an intensive and early effort, using the many rehabilitation resources in the community to overcome the physical, environmental, and emotional or motivational barriers.

Subcontract Model

The subcontract model, sometimes referred to as "industrial homework," involves the homebound person in working on subcontracts from private industry obtained either directly with employers or through the mediation of a rehabilitation agency. As Towne said, there is no merchandising problem since the products are on order from cooperating industry. Furthermore, production is not so subject to the peaks and valleys of demand found in the crafts. There will be many homebound clients better suited to an industrial rather than a homecraft program. The person who has no creative needs and who enjoys repetitive manual tasks will find an industrial setup preferable to making handcrafted items. Unfortunately, most subcontract work calls for good hand dexterity and often requires substantial space—factors that rule out some clients. Moreover, there is a need to en-

sure that clients in such employment are paid fair rates (comparable to those of factory workers).

Business Enterprises for the Homebound

While their work is spectacular when successful, most homebound people do not have the characteristics needed to operate a business enterprise in their homes. (The administrative and other talents required of the entrepreneur are not well distributed throughout the population, disabled or not.) Consequently, small business enterprises tend to suffer a high mortality rate. As a result, as Rusalem [1967] pointed out, "Great care must be exercised in selecting the homebound person for self-employment and the product or service that he will offer for sale" [p. 212].

An interplay of facts and events seems to militate against the homebound physically handicapped person in modern business. Perhaps many homebound aspiring entrepreneurs in "culture shock" would not survive business demands in this era of pervasive nonpermanence. Importantly, according to Shworles and Tamagna [1973], ". . . physical immobility may be a primary disadvantage to the homebound person in more highly competitive business environments" [p. 82]. There are the many contraindications, they said, yet there is a "panoply of circumstances and conditions if properly sequenced and integrated motivate towards the goal of small businesses for the homebound or severely handicapped person. Encouragement comes from the simple fact that homebound persons have a history as business entrepreneurs. In the past decade, *Rehabilitation Gazette* has reported many examples of ingenious and highly motivated persons employed from their homes" [p. 82]. Furthermore, the public rehabilitation program record of supporting handicapped people in businesses is well established.

A checklist of planning information should cover the various requirements for establishing the business: capital needed, physical capacities required, an analysis of the work tasks, and other factors. Rusalem [1967] gave the "minimum essentials" for effective performance in business enterprises: (1) a knowledge of the business, (2) adequate capital, (3) willingness to work hard, (4) knowledge of the needs and habits of people in the market, (5) sales ability, (6) ability to study and learn from others, and (7) interest in people, business activities, responsibility, and management. A guide for helping clients start a small business is provided in Chapter 39, Small Business Enterprise. Training can be a critical service for successful business operation.

14.2. *Special Education*

The role of special education services to young handicapped individuals is crucial in their early development as well as during the time when they must learn to adapt to adult life and formulate plans for leaving the school system. Consequently, the provision of educational services for disabled children is an important public program. It is estimated that roughly one out of ten children in the United States is handicapped— has a speech, hearing, vision, or orthopedic problem; is learning-disabled or mentally or emotionally disturbed; or has a serious impairment of one of the body systems so that functioning is limited. Many of these children need special education to prepare for, or even to qualify for, vocational rehabilitation services later.

Special education is a program for children with particular needs that the major segment of the school population does not have. This includes curriculum adjustment, special classrooms, consultation, therapeutic teaching, clinical services in psychology, speech training, and special equipment or facilities for children with specific physical, mental, or psychosocial needs. Education for exceptional children is provided in conventional public schools as well as in public or privately sponsored special schools, including local or regional residential centers. There were about 300,000 specially qualified teachers of the handicapped in American schools by 1980. Through the expertise of these special education teachers, handicapped children are enabled to achieve the same kinds of objectives sought for all children. Donlon and Burton [1976] have written a book on the teaching of the severely handicapped that addresses their social interaction. (Louise Burton is a rehabilitation educator).

Switzer [1955], while she headed the federal rehabilitation agency, provided a succinct description of the relationship between vocational rehabilitation and special education. "Special education provides physically and mentally disabled children and youth with the broad foundation for maximum mental, physical, and emotional adjustment to disabling conditions that is consistent with the individual's abilities and capacities; upon this solid base vocational rehabilitation erects the superstructure of preparation for, entry into, and adjustment to an appropriate occupation, and assumes terminal responsibility with the disabled individual for such refinement and strengthening of his mental, physical, and emotional attributes as may be necessary" [p. 346].

Cooperative efforts between rehabilitation and special education programs are broad and varied. Rehabilitation counselors are sometimes assigned to case loads of handicapped clients of school age. Another approach has been to assign special education teachers to work with clients in rehabilitation facilities. In some states, schools have provided instructors and facilities for personal adjustment training conducted after regular school hours [Rose & Shay, 1972]. Cooperation at its best is achieved through the close working relationship of the special education faculty and the assigned rehabilitation counselor.

Both legislative and judicial action has upheld the educational rights of handicapped children. Up to 1971 only 16 states had enacted mandatory education for handicapped children. That year the now famous test case, *Pennsylvania Association of Retarded Children vs. Pennsylvania*, was won. The PARC case, as it is known, established for the first time that children who were mentally retarded—regardless of the severity—had the right to an appropriate education at public expense. In the 1972 Mills case, the federal court ruled that not only retarded children but all handicapped children had a right to education. Then in November, 1975, the Education for All Handicapped Children Act (PL 94-142) sharply increased federal funding to assist states in educating of children with handicaps. It was mandated that by 1980 the states must provide education for all handicapped children between the ages of three and 21.

Two terms that the rehabilitationist is likely to hear when dealing with special education services are *mainstreaming* and *the least restrictive alternative*. The *least restrictive alternative* means that among all alternatives within a general educational system, handicapped children should be placed where they can obtain the best education at the least distance away from the mainstream of society. Whenever handicapped children are sent to a restrictive environment, such placement should be aimed at their eventual integration into an appropriate public school.

Mainstreaming is still not adequately understood and should not be viewed as a rigid notion that implies integration of the handicapped at any cost. On the contrary, mainstreaming necessitates the selection of the most facilitative, but also least restrictive, programs available to meet the specific requirements of each handicapped child. Children should be in the most normal circumstances possible, but with recognition of their need for specialized attention for the purpose of ameliorating specific limitations. Opportunity to choose the most facilitative environment requires that a continuum of services be available to meet differing needs. These include regular classrooms, special classes, specialized schools, group homes, and residential institutions [U.S White House Conference on Handicapped Individuals, 1976]. Needed rehabilitative services, including counseling, must be available, however.

The Educational Facilities Laboratory [1974] described the "continuum" or "cascade" of services. The cascade system, first introduced in 1962 by Maynard Reynolds of the University of Minnesota and subsequently adopted by the Council for Exceptional Children, is a model for special education that provides a wide variety of services in a number of alternative settings. The system begins by assuming that the greatest number of handicapped children can be absorbed into ordinary schools with little change in existing programs. Gradually, with each modification of the normal classroom setting, a smaller number of students is provided with a greater number of resources and services, until in the residential hospital (the highest level of care) the fewest children use the most expensive resources. Between everyday classroom and residential hospital, the cascade system defines various additional levels of care and treatment on a progressive scale.

Most states recognize seven or eight different areas of concentration in special education including speech impaired, educable mentally retarded, trainable mentally retarded, learning disabled, emotionally disturbed, and hearing, visually, and orthopedically impaired. Special education programs generally are consistent with these categories, although there has been a move to more generic training, which combines a number of competencies and which increases the teacher's ability to work with a variety of handicapped groups. Classifications are only arbitrary labels used to describe persons with similar disabilities, but for discussion purposes these areas of concentration will be used. Much of the material for this section came from the journal *Exceptional Children* and other publications of the Council for Exceptional Children [1969], the national association promoting the professional efforts of special education since 1922.

14.2.1. MENTAL RETARDATION

Children who are mentally retarded may be divided into two major groups for educational purposes: educable and trainable. The educable child is mildly retarded and can benefit from special education, which includes academic, social, and occupational subject areas. The trainable child is moderately retarded but can benefit from special educational experiences, which include self-care, social adjustment, and economically useful activities in a sheltered environment.

Most mentally retarded children can be expected to achieve success after school age when they have a good special education program. In fact, many "retarded adults" (i.e., people who were considered mentally retarded when they were school age) so prepared are indistinguishable in society and achieve essentially "normal" patterns of social and vocational adjustment. If a special program is unavailable or inadequate, however, the problems of the retarded person are compounded.

A fully adequate program for meeting the educational needs of these children requires the efforts of many people: psychologists, social workers, physicians, and nurses as well as the parents. They work as a team concerned with the total well-being of the child. The team's ultimate goal for educable retarded children is to help them toward a social adjustment for independence in the community. Although some degree of supervision may be required, many of these people, after rehabilitation, are able to support themselves in adult life.

The services of special education for educable retarded children center around their deficiencies in academic achievement. Bender [1976] said: "Although it has been stated that many educables attain the grade level equivalent of a fifth or sixth grade, in reality many never attain more than second or third grade educational skills. It must be emphasized that the educational objectives and goals reflect the rate at which these children learn, which is one-half to three-quarters of a normal child" [p. 245]. Most educable retarded students are placed in a structured, self-contained special class. Some may also be mainstreamed into regular classes for most of the day and receive necessary educational support in a separate classroom.

The trainable mentally retarded child requires a totally different curriculum with functional self-care and socialization goals geared to their developmental levels. They may also need help with communication and fine and gross motor skills. Severely and profoundly retarded children are totally dependent, and for most of them vocational rehabilitation effort is not feasible.

14.2.2. LEARNING DISABILITIES

Children may present all degrees of learning deficiencies and many such children can be properly diagnosed as retarded: educable, trainable, or severely and profoundly retarded. Others, however, have "learning disabilities" and should not be classified as retarded children. Many committees, formulated with the goal of generating a working definition of learning disabilities, have engaged in fruitless arguments. Children with learning disabilities generally exhibit some type of discrepancy between expected and actual academic achievement in areas including speech, reading, or written language, and perhaps mathematics and spatial relations.

Although the components of a working definition are complex, they are clarified by Bender [1976], who said, "An overall statement many educators have agreed upon is that a learning disability may be a result of one of more deficits in the essential learning process. These children have normal intelligence, no gross visual or au-

ditory deficits, no severe emotional handicaps and no major organic problems" [p. 242]. Children with such disabilities require teaching techniques over and above those provided in a regular classroom. There appears to be no major consensus what remediation approach works best with these children, according to Bender, who believed that the learning disabled child may be placed in a self-contained learning disability class or in a regular class receiving remedial help in a resource room.

14.2.3. BEHAVIORAL DISORDERS

Students with behavioral disorders are classified either as emotionally disturbed or socially maladjusted. The behavior of the emotionally disturbed student, according to Young [1969], may be inappropriate to the point that it is both distracting and disruptive to the rest of the class, placing undue pressure on the teacher and intensifying the pupil's own problems. Socially maladjusted students are often known as truants, predelinquents, delinquents, and incorrigibles.

Both the emotionally disturbed and the socially maladjusted children have in common an unusual amount of difficulty in dealing with people. Responses are usually in extremes: they worry too much or too little, they are too excited or too calm, they are oversensitive to others or very self-centered, and so on. Seldom is a happy medium found, and the individual with behavioral disorders is seldom at peace with self or others.

Educational programs for disturbed children are available in various types of settings. When children are so seriously disturbed that the home or school cannot cope with their behavior, they are placed in institutions having specialized staff who can give close supervision and treatment. Children live in such settings the year round and go to school within the institution. Children who are less seriously disturbed and do not require constant care may live with parents or in a foster home while attending a public school where both special and regular education programs are available. In such school situations, the children may stay in a special room for the entire day or may go to the special class for part of the day and spend the remainder of the day in regular classes. Some large communities have special schools attended only by children with behavioral problems.

14.2.4. VISUAL IMPAIRMENT

For educational purposes the visually impaired population is classified into two groups: the blind and the partially sighted. Blind students have little or no vision; therefore the senses of touch and hearing must be substituted for sight when teaching them. Aids and devices for instruction include reader services by a sighted person, braille devices, recorders for taking class notes, books in braille, and records. Partially sighted students are able to utilize some remaining vision for learning. Special materials (enlarged print) and instructional procedures (verbal rather than blackboard illustration of lectures) and other special conditions accommodate the learning resources of these students.

Services of special education for the visually impaired group are provided in a variety of organizational arrangements according to the severity of loss of vision. The partially sighted students are integrated as fully as possible into regular school programs with special teachers and resource rooms available when necessary. Blind students are often brought together in publicly supported residential schools where the preparation for possible return to the community is intensive. Today, however, most children with visual handicaps are successfully attending regular local public schools with seeing children. In some local school programs, children who are visually handicapped are enrolled in designated classes with special teachers. In other arrangements, they are enrolled in regular classrooms in their neighborhood schools, and a special teacher periodically travels from school to school to visit them and their regular teachers.

14.2.5. SPEECH AND LANGUAGE DEFECTS

Speech is considered defective when attention is drawn to its deviation from average speech. Major categories of speech defects are articulatory disorders, vocal disorders, stuttering, delayed speech, and speech disorders associated with physical disabilities such as cleft palate, hearing loss, or cerebral palsy.

Young [1969] reported that about 80 percent of the speech cases in schools are articulatory disorders that involve substitutions ("wight" for right, "yeth" for yes, "yeow" for yellow, and so on), omissions (consonants dropped), distortions (whistling the *s* sound), and additions ("on-a" the table). Speech correction services,

he said, are usually concentrated in the following ways: 75 percent in grades K–2, 19 percent in grades 3 and 4, and 7 percent in grades 5 through 12. Speech therapy may be with the individual or in very small groups. The therapy sessions are usually given twice a week for about 30 minutes per session.

Although speech therapy is conducted in various surroundings, the majority of children with speech or language disorders are served in the schools. In addition, there are clinics in hospitals, universities, and community centers; some children receive help on a private-practice basis. With help based on their needs, most children with defective speech perform satisfactorily in a regular class. When this is possible and help is provided in their schools, they have scheduled sessions with the therapist and spend the remainder of their time in the regular classroom. Other children whose problems are more severe must attend a special school or a special class in a regular school.

14.2.6. HEARING IMPAIRMENT

Students who have impaired hearing are also classified into two groups of educational purposes: the deaf and the hard of hearing. When the sense of hearing is nonfunctional for ordinary purposes, the student is considered deaf. The extent of the limitation is partly based on the time when loss of hearing occurred— congenitally deaf (born deaf) or the adventitiously deaf (born with normal hearing but losing functional hearing due to illness or accident). Defective hearing may be considered functional, either with or without a hearing aid.

Deaf and hard of hearing children are educated under many organizational plans, particularly those utilizing resource rooms, itinerant specialists, and special classes. Many cities and states operate special residential schools for severely hearing impaired youngsters.

In all special education programs for the hearing impaired, the teaching depends upon the needs and assets of the children. A group of specialists assists in evaluating the child and works with the teacher as part of a team. The evaluation team includes an otologist or ear specialist who diagnoses and treats the medical problem; an audiologist who evaluates how the hearing is functioning; a psychologist who studies the child's learning abilities; a social worker who helps the teacher understand the influence of the child's family and community; and a specialist in the educational problems of hearing-impaired children.

14.2.7. OTHER PHYSICAL DISABILITIES

Students identified as physically disabled have functional limitations in motivity and mobility because of muscular and neuromuscular conditions. These disabilities include cerebral palsy, muscular dystrophy, multiple sclerosis, paraplegia, amputations, and skeletal deformities. Other students have limited strength, vitality, and alertness for school work due to chronic health problems. Debilitation can occur from heart or lung conditions, rheumatic fever, nephritis, infectious hepatitis, mononucleosis, asthma, hemophilia, leukemia, and diabetes. Epilepsy and anticonvulsant medications may cause limitations in consciousness.

The learning characteristics and degree of handicap determine the kind of program and educational setting the child needs. Many children who are mildly limited in function can and should remain in regular classes. Attention has been focused on the elimination of architectural barriers in existing public schools and the designs of new buildings. Older multi-level buildings precluded the unassisted attendance of physically handicapped children who were con-fined to wheelchairs or who used crutches. Efforts have been made also to prepare and assist regular classroom teachers to work with handicapped students. Some children, however, are so physically handicapped that they require the services of a specially prepared teacher in a special class setting. Related programs of physical, occupational, and speech therapy are either offered as a part of the total school program or are readily accessible. Ordinarily, a special class or unit is located within a regular school building so that those children who have disabilities can participate in regular classes as much as they are physically and academically able to do so.

Still other children who must be hospitalized over prolonged periods of time or who suffer from conditions that make them homebound may be offered individualized bedside instruction—homebound and hospital programs, which can incorporate educational TV, radio programs, home-to-school telephones, and various teaching machines. There are also children who are so severely disabled that they need the comprehensive educational, social, and medical services that can best be obtained in a residential school. It is hoped that after intensive care and treatment, these children can return to their home communities.

14.3. Adult Education

A description of adult education has been provided by Knowles [1971]:

Adult education is a complex field of social practice. It cannot be neatly symbolized, as can other elements of the national educational enterprise, by an elementary school, a high school, or a college. Adult education takes place in factories, living rooms, libraries, settlement houses, hospitals, church basements, military bases, grange halls, YMCAs, hotels and motels, and every other kind of facility used by adults, as well as in classrooms. Indeed, adult education cannot even be considered a subdivision of the educational enterprise, for it is also a part of the business enterprise, the health enterprise . . . and every other kind of enterprise [p. 48].

14.3.1. RELEVANCE TO REHABILITATION

In terms of the handicapped population, adult education classes represent a valuable community resource. Many communities have pro-grams in vocational schools, rehabilitation facilities, or other agencies that provide high school equivalency training, skill training, recreation, and special interest or hobby instruction within classes that are designed for handicapped adults. Rehabilitationists use these community adult education resources for their educational, vocational, and social development benefits to handicapped clients.

14.3.2. RESOURCES AND SERVICES

Most communities have many resources that can be used for the adult education of the handicapped. Some of these resources and their services are listed below.

Public Schools

Most public schools offer evening courses in vocational subjects, hobbies and recreation, home and family life, public affairs and citizenship, driver training, personal development, and academic subjects. Clients who dropped out of high school can receive diplomas through accelerated "equivalency" programs. Urban school systems usually have extensive programs of basic adult education for functional illiterates. Evening classes are given for working men and women who want to better themselves through more advanced courses or trade training. Public school courses are usually given free of cost or offered at nominal fees for registration, plus cost of materials.

Colleges

Community colleges provide academic studies for completing the first two years of college as well as training for jobs in nursing, retailing, and so forth. In the face of decreasing enrollment and because of community awareness, many colleges and universities have expanded their extension and regular courses to make continuing education attractive to everyone. Land-grant and other universities operate extension services with agents in each county who conduct individual and group educational activities in agriculture, home and family life, youth work, and community affairs.

Libraries

An important resource in either formal or informal public education is the public libraries. They provide books, films, and learning materials as well as advisory services.

Public Agencies

Government agencies at all levels conduct educational services. These include in-service training for employees; educational and informational services for special populations (e.g., veterans, prisoners); and informational services to the public in areas of general concern (e.g., health, education, welfare, conservation, public safety, recreation, race relations, consumer education).

Business Organizations

Knowles [1971] said, "Business and industry has been dubbed by educational economists as the third major educational system in our society. It is estimated that corporations spend as much on the education of their employees and their families, dealers, and customers as do all the colleges and universities in the country combined" [pp. 49–50]. Although much corporate education is job-related, growing emphasis is being placed on the development of well-rounded personnel through general education to increase the quality of life.

Labor Organizations

Labor unions also sponsor important educational activities. Most unions have membership programs on union history, collective bargaining, stewardship training, political action, and internal matters. Unions are also active in providing enrichment programs for their members in cultural subjects, leisure skills, economics, and general personal development.

Religious Organizations

Religious institutions provide general educational programs through informal courses, lecture series, and group activities. Content includes such secular concerns as home and family living, leisure skills, public affairs, and personal development, as well as religious and moral subjects.

Social Agencies

Social agencies operating in the areas of health, welfare, youth work, and community action provide a diversity of educational services. Examples of such programs are found in the neighborhood social centers and settlement houses, YMCA and YWCA buildings, and the local Red Cross headquarters. Educational opportunities are also provided to the adults of a community by such institutions as museums and art institutes, by the mass media, and by a wide variety of voluntary clubs and associations.

14.4. Higher Education

"Higher (or tertiary) education" covers post-secondary school levels in a university or equivalent college preparation program, usually toward a degree or diploma for professional and administrative occupations. All of these formal programs of preparation may be supplemented by tutorial instruction, reader services, typing, and other special assistance to make such education feasible for disabled students.

14.4.1. SPECIAL PROBLEMS

All schools of higher education are attempting to accommodate severely disabled students. This has required modification of physical plants to eliminate architectural barriers and also establishment of specialized student services to help disabled staff and students. Issues to be resolved for the severely handicapped individual going to college include architectural barriers, transportation, difficulty in attending extracurricular activities and "educational lag."

"Educational lag" was defined by Fasteau [1972] simply as "not keeping up with the progress of the class, missing some of the essential steps in mastering basic skills, subject matter, or both" [p. 268]. As Fasteau used it, educational lag does not include mental subnormality since it occurs in even the most intellectually capable handicapped student. He says the primary cause for the lag is absence from class due to medical necessity (e.g., surgery, therapy). Another difficulty in keeping up scholastically may stem from poor health because of a lower tolerance to disease and infection, from immobility during inclement weather, or from the necessity of spending extraordinary time attending to their physical condition and prophylactic aids. Another educational difficulty may arise from disability adjustment problems (e.g., depression, social rejection, economic losses). Learning becomes harder when concentration and attention are consumed by the task of adjusting to the social or physical impact of disability. On the other hand, despite the many obstacles, experience demonstrates that extraordinary motivation and effort can compensate for serious handicapping.

14.4.2. PROGRAMS AND ACCOMMODATIONS

The more than 1100 community colleges in the United States are excellent for educating handicapped students. Advantages of the community college system for those who are handicapped were listed by Rizzo and Shworles [1975]: close-to-home availability, an open-door policy to all members of the community, program flexibility, low cost, and a wide array of courses in liberal arts, occupational fields, adult and continuing education, and paraprofessional education.

The City Colleges system of Chicago (CCC) is a good example of efforts by a community college to integrate the handicapped into its student body, to "mainstream the handicapped student into its every component and resource." Shworles [1976] described this program.

Mainstreaming means no steps between the biology laboratories and the mobility impaired student. Mainstreaming means acceptance of alternative examination techniques on behalf of students who have the answers but who cannot write or who are motor-sensory-wise slowed down. Mainstreaming means the abolition of teachers' fears of those blind students with dogs at the front of their classroom or teachers' fears of the cerebral palsied student manifesting different kinds of motor behavior. Mainstreaming means the abolition of "special" and segregated courses for handicapped students [p. 9].

Another accommodating program at Edinburo State College in Edinburo, Pennsylvania, has been described by McComb and Rice [1976]. Included in the program are such things as a pre-college acclimation program for blind students, emotional and social counseling, academic aides, van transportation, volunteers, and a unique system of residential care that replaces the need for the individual to have a personal attendant. Students are carefully evaluated to determine what level of care they require: students needing total care in the dormitory, for example, have almost all activities carried out for them—dressing, bathing and toileting, feeding, wheelchair pushing, academic aid (note-taking, library aid, etc.), laundry, and so forth. The program is flexible and institutionalization is minimized.

There are many innovations and adaptations that enable the handicapped student to adjust to a college setting. To begin with, the campus should be physically accessible to students with physical disabilities of all kinds. The day has passed when the handicapped are segregated in a few scattered "wheelchair campuses" or in special segregated classes. Classroom procedures are readily altered to fit the handicapped without disrupting the rest of the class. Alternate examination procedures can be used for students who cannot write or who are slow because of motor or sensory problems. Off-campus, initial learning experiences provided for in the plan can help students make a smoother transition to the college environment. The mainstreaming experience in college and other schools has demonstrated that faculty and fellow-students learn to truly accept and sincerely appreciate students who are different.

14.4.3. INFORMATION ABOUT COLLEGES

Counseling of the college-bound student includes providing information as to the suitability of the physical features of the campus and the instructional program of the institution. Naturally the college must have a strong curriculum on the client's vocational objective, but there are many colleges to choose from and various kinds of information help the client make an informed opinion. For example, most schools have scholarship funds available that would supplement financing—but these college grants have a different set of qualifications. While the college advisor will help prepare the client's plan of study, the rehabilitation counselor must know enough about the course offering at the college of choice to fulfill case management responsibilities. There are various commercially published training directories, one of which the counselor and client should have available in choosing a college. *The College Blue Book,* published by MacMillan Company, describes about 3200 colleges and includes information for students with a physical handicap.

Both public and private schools of higher education were affected by the 1973 Rehabilitation Act (PL 93-112) and its amendments since most of them receive various forms of federal assistance, grants, or contracts. Section 503 of the Act calls for affirmative action programs in hiring handicapped staff and Section 504 prohibits exclusion of the handicapped from programs and activities. The federal Architectural Barriers Act of 1968 and similar laws in every state are supposed to prevent architectural barriers in new campus buildings. Most college administrations are renovating inaccessible buildings and sponsoring programs to accommodate disabled students and employees.

Chapter 15

Medical Services

Medicine is the first phase of rehabilitation, with the physician and the paramedical team responsible for the therapeutic services aimed at curing or ameliorating the patient's acute illness or injury. The next stage begins when the medical treatment has been partially successful (i.e., the patient survives but with functional limitations). Restoration to reduce the functional limitations of the disablement requires a medical rehabilita-tion team that may include a physiatrist (medical doctor specializing in rehabilitation and physical medicine), prosthetist (artificial limb maker), physical and occupational therapists, and other professionals and technicians. When residual limitations will cause a permanent handicap, readjustment to life is the final strategy in the full rehabilitation course of action.

15.1. Introduction

Rehabilitation is broadly defined as "restoration to a former (positive) state." A more basic definition is "overcoming a present (negative) state." The negative state that is changed is a disability or, more accurately, the primary or secondary effects of a disability. The concepts that follow were discussed in Chapter 4, Impact of Disability, and Chapter 5, Functional Limitations. They are restated here in condensed form for a perspective on medical conceptualizations.

15.1.1. CONCEPTS

Refinement of the rehabilitation nomenclature is needed for conceptual clarity. Thus, the following definitions have been proposed and used in this book.

DISABILITY. Disability is a medically described disease or disorder that is diagnosed and treated by the medical professions (e.g., paraplegia, double hip disarticulation).

FUNCTIONAL LIMITATION. A limitation in function is the primary effect(s) of the disability that restricts the function of the individual (e.g., mobility limitation).

HANDICAP. Handicap is the ultimate effect(s) of the disability that derives directly from limitations imposed upon the individual in various life areas (e.g., getting employment, performing required job tasks).

The goal of rehabilitation as viewed in this context is to:

1. Treat the disability by physical or mental restoration, such as medical treatment, surgery, or psychotherapy.
2. Reduce or eliminate the limitations caused by the disability by providing adaptive services such as mechanical aids and enhanced physical function.
3. Circumvent or compensate for any handicap(s) caused by the functional limitation through rehabilitation services such as counseling, adjustment training, selective job placement, attendant care.

Medicine is clearly the first phase of rehabilitation when the medical "disability" is treated (1. above). Other rehabilitation personnel, including physiatrists, cope with the residual "limitation" in the second phase (2. above). The third phase of rehabilitation dealing with the "handicap" (3. above) is nonmedical, involving rehabilitation counselors and other vocational or social rehabilitationists.

Most presentations on medical information for rehabilitation counselors follow the physician's taxonomic organization according to body systems. Texts on the subject look at one disability after another, from pulmonary to circulatory diseases, and examine the medical pathology, etiology, diagnostic methods, prognoses, and preferred treatment. A more beneficial orientation for the instruction of rehabilitation counselors is to focus upon the effects of disablement rather than medical phenomena.

Rehabilitation counselors are primarily interested in functional limitation or, conversely, functional abilities. The question is what can the client do; in other words, what activities and conditions are not counterindicated by functional limitation. This is a positive approach. It avoids typing the client with a medical label (e.g., cardiac case), which is not only prejudicial but also imprecise and which provides little understanding of what this particular person can or cannot do. Nevertheless, the rehabilitation counselor requires survey knowledge about the medical aspects of disability.

15.1.2. MEDICAL INFORMATION

The rehabilitation counselor needs a more detailed knowledge of medically related aspects of handicapping than is afforded in this book. (A course on Medical Aspects of Disabilities is required in rehabilitation counselor education programs.) While only a small part of the rehabilitationist's time is spent in analysis of medical information, the information is vital in the choice of suitable objectives. It is not necessary, however, to learn anatomy, physiology, diagnostic methods, pharmacology—in fact, a little knowledge may be dangerously misused. Nevertheless, the counselor should know about health care personnel and systems, selected medical nomenclature (including affixes and root terms), general sources of deviation, the relationship of physical and mental states to functional limitations, and the potential for restoration. Rehabilitationists also need a general understanding of the role of medicine in the diagnosis, prognosis, treatment, and management of disability.

Medical information is generally organized according to the various body systems (i.e., a set of organs with a functional relationship). Body systems that are particularly important for the rehabilitation counselor to know about include cardiovascular, neurological, respiratory, skeletomuscular, and sensory systems. Medical reference books and texts for rehabilitation have been listed in Chapter 4, Impact of Disability (see 4.2.1).

15.2. Medical Consultation

The rehabilitation counselor has responsibility for the client adjustment process but does not personally perform all of the services. Services by other professionals and organizations are authorized by the counselor as a part of the whole rehabilitation plan. This necessitates a working knowledge of all rehabilitative procedures, including physical restoration. Perhaps medical knowledge is the most difficult for the counselor, yet it is essential for work with disabled people—thus the value of medical consultation.

For their medically related responsibilities, rehabilitation counselors should have access to a consulting physician. Moreover, the rehabilitationist needs to know how to relate to the medical consultants and their respective roles and functions. Guidelines provided here are derived from the public rehabilitation agency but are generally useful to the rehabilitation worker in private agencies.

15.2.1. COUNSELOR RESPONSIBILITIES

Counselor duties and responsibilities of a medical nature revolve around the following activities:

1. Identifying persons with disabilities and preliminary screening of candidates.
2. Obtaining background information from applicants for medical diagnostic study.
3. Authorizing medical examinations of applicants by physicians or obtaining medical records.
4. Interpreting and certifying the medical findings for agency purposes (e.g., case priority, eligibility and feasibility determination).
5. Determining client's functional capacities and limitations.
6. Helping the client to understand this functional appraisal for purposes of rehabilitation planning.
7. Counseling the client regarding health, disability, and limitations as considerations in life adjustment.
8. Arranging for further diagnostic study by means of records, specialist examination, hospitalization, and so forth.
9. Establishing the feasibility of alleviating or removing the disability and resulting limitations.
10. Counseling and arranging for physical or mental restoration services for the client.
11. Appraising the results of medical services on client rehabilitation and also evaluating medical personnel and facilities.
12. Maintaining a working knowledge about and collaborative relations with the medical community.

The above duties reflect the functions of the rehabilitation counselor as a facilitator of the medical phases of the rehabilitation process. The counselor needs special preparation to perform medically related duties. Medical reports must be analyzed for vital information to be interpreted for functional inferences and implications for client planning. While the counselor becomes adept at interpreting medical information, it is desirable to have a medical doctor available for direct consultation and assistance. However, physicians typically are not qualified—by either training or experience—as vocational experts. Rehabilitation counselors are responsible for the vocational decisions of their clients, but medical knowledge is involved because the choice of a suitable job is partly based upon interpretation of the person's physical condition. Rehabilitation counselors and members of the medical profession quite naturally have reciprocal respect for their complementary roles with disabled people. This relationship is abetted by their knowledge of each other's expertise and respect for their separate functions and responsibilities.

15.2.2. AGENCY MEDICAL CONSULTANT

State rehabilitation offices as well as many private rehabilitation agencies employ physicians on at least a part-time basis as consultants to other professional and administrative personnel. Rehabilitation counselors are encouraged to ask these agency consultants for help with medically related duties. Office or field medical consultants assist counselors by: (1) sharing their knowledge of the medical aspects of rehabilitation; (2) explaining concepts and terminology; (3) clarifying reports from outside physicians and hospitals; (4) advising further medical actions such as the authorization of a specialist's reports or medical treatment; and (5) providing liaison between the counselors and outside physicians. They do not serve in an administrative capacity. Their function is maintaining a facilitating relationship with the counselor, the supervisor, the agency, and the community. Specifically, their duties range from interpretation and advisement to education and public relations.

A medical consultant for the Ohio Bureau of Vocational Rehabilitation, O. L. Coddington, M.D. [n.d.], prepared an (unpublished) state manual of medical information in which he described his role. The following statement is paraphrased from Coddington.

The medical consultant (MC), utilizing a special knowledge, has the major duty of interpreting to the counselor the medical data available in individual cases. In interpreting the medical findings to the counselor, the MC assists in the responsibility of determining vocational and medical implications and, if necessary, recommends other medical diagnostic procedures required for this determination.

The MC alerts the counselor to the need for further medical service in cases in which it has not been provided, and continues as an active adviser in such problems. From a wide knowledge of various medical specialties and resources, the MC recommends to the counselor the specialty or resource to be used on individual problems.

The MC will be better equipped to determine the type of information needed from the specialist and will, in all probability, not ask for a "routine evaluation" in a specialty but for something specific. A medical evaluation depends entirely on what it is wanted for; for example, if the matter is one of evaluation of a middle-aged executive with an orthopedic problem, it is important to know not only about this orthopedic problem but also about the cardiac status. If the person smokes, a chest X-ray is indicated. Alcoholic consumption suggests that certain liver function tests might be done. If the client has a family history of diabetes as well as some other disorders, appropriate blood tests would be made.

15.2.3. USING CONSULTATION

The agency's consulting physician, who has intimate information on available facilities and personnel in the medical community, can assist the counselor in determining suitability of purchased services to meet the client's medical needs. Moreover, the consultant, understanding the rehabilitation process, can eliminate useless or inadequate studies and medical actions. The consultant's responsibility may be further ex-

tended to help the agency establish and enforce standardized and equitable fee schedules for medical services.

Rehabilitationists can learn much from the interpretative functions of the medical consultants. In conversations between counselor and consultant on clinical problems, there is continual opportunity for learning the nature of diseases, symptoms, treatment, and limitations in function. The counselor can also help the consultant to gain better understanding of vocational issues. Thus medical consultation is an educational function in which ideas are exchanged and new information is shared.

The degree to which a rehabilitation counselor seeks medical consultation varies according to the agency's policies and other factors such as the counselor's experience and training in medical matters, the type of cases served, and the nature of the medical problems. Advice from the medical consultant is particularly indicated when the following are involved.

1. Diagnostic studies requiring hospitalization or special effort.
2. Surgical or medical treatment.
3. Prosthetic appliances.
4. Selection of appropriate medical resources.
5. Interpretation of medical information when it is confusing or inadequate, or when it involves unusual conditions or treatment.
6. Health maintenance planning.
7. Functional limitations and abilities and other medical information are not objectively specified.
8. Important client decisions are influenced by the medical facts (e.g., necessity of physical restoration or large expenditures of time or funds).

Typically, new employees on the professional rehabilitation staff require frequent, face-to-face contact with the medical consultant.

Generally the state rehabilitation agency medical consultant also gives administrative consultation. These activities may involve:

1. Advising the state administrator in the formation of medical policy (e.g., standards for medical diagnostic and treatment services, for selection of qualified physicians and facilities, and for the provision of prosthetic appliances and medical supplies).

2. Providing technical consultation to other medical consultants and employees, including the medical staff of the Social Security Disability Determination Unit of the state rehabilitation agency.
3. Chairing a medical advisory committee and serving as its executive officer for the state agency's administrator.
4. Representing the state agency in community relationships, including medical societies.
5. Studying and evaluating the effects of medical services and suggesting program improvement.
6. Training staff in formal programs of instruc-

tion, including the orientation of new counselors.
7. Developing proposed fee schedules for medically related services (state rehabilitation agencies often follow payment schedules set by other agencies).
8. Advising the agency on restoration policies and procedures, including examination and authorization forms, information exchange, and so on.

Despite the value of these activities, however, the medical consultant's primary function is the review of individual cases and consultation with the rehabilitation counselor.

15.3. Medical Diagnosis

State rehabilitation agencies provide medical evaluation without charge as a service to all qualified applicants. High standards have been established for applying the medical aspects of case study and diagnosis in the program. It is necessary to assure adequacy of the medical information in each case, not only for purposes of eligibility determination but also for rehabilitation planning. Thus the diagnostic medical study is a fundamental client service.

15.3.1. MEDICAL EVALUATION

The medical evaluation must provide an adequate basis for: (1) establishing the presence of a physical or mental condition that limits the activities the individual can perform; (2) ascertaining the current health status of the individual and any other (previously unsuspected) physical problems; (3) determining how and to what extent the disabling conditions may be expected to be removed, corrected, or minimized by restoration services; and (4) selecting an employment objective commensurate with the individual's capacities and limitations.

A rehabilitation medical study or evaluation includes a complete general medical examination (or record), examinations by specialists in any medical or related field as needed, and whatever clinical laboratory tests, X-rays, and other studies are necessary to establish the diagnosis and medical recommendations. The study indicates the extent to which the disability limits

(or is likely to limit) the individual's daily living and work activities and the probable results of physical restoration services. In addition to all the other evaluation information available on the individual, this diagnostic study constitutes an informational basis for rehabilitation assessment.

While the medical diagnostic part of the rehabilitation process is concentrated in the early period of the case service, the study continues throughout rehabilitation until closure. Further medical diagnostic services may be authorized long after eligibility has been established and rehabilitation services are initiated. Reevaluation may be necessitated whenever there is a change in the client's physical or mental status, the possibility of restoration is proposed, or the medical suitability of the employment or other objectives needs to be reconsidered. Clients receiving services over a long period of time should have at least an annual medical examination that is comprehensive enough to provide accurate information as to the current health situation.

15.3.2. PLANNING

There is a broad range of medical diagnostic services available from the public rehabilitation agency. These are either provided or arranged for by the state agency for an understanding of the needs for restoration or other rehabilitation services. Included in diagnostic services are:

1. Medical and surgical examinations.
2. Psychiatric evaluations and/or psychological evaluations.
3. Dental examinations.
4. Consultations with specialists in all medical specialty fields and other relevant disciplines.
5. Inpatient hospitalization for study or exploration.
6. Clinical laboratory tests.
7. Diagnostic X-ray procedures.
8. Trial treatment (especially in cases of epilepsy, diabetes, emotional disturbances, or for differential diagnosis in other conditions).
9. Other medically recognized diagnostic procedures.

At the point of initial contact with an applicant for rehabilitation services, the counselor begins to make plans for the way in which the medical diagnostic study will be undertaken. A preliminary medical history is taken at intake. The counselor should secure from the applicant information about the disability, its onset, its symptoms, its remission (if any), and the past treatment, as well as information on previous illnesses. Information about the person's current medical supervision may be important (e.g., the treatment being provided, recency of physician contacts, nature of the doctor-patient relationship, outstanding medical debts, and the individual's general attitude toward and knowledge about the condition).

If the person applying for rehabilitation services is receiving medical supervision from a hospital or clinic in the community, it is important to take this into consideration in planning and arranging for medical diagnosis or restoration. In many instances medical data may be obtained or supplemented from resumes provided by cooperating agencies. Existing medical information should be used to the greatest extent possible.

It is not always necessary to obtain medical examination reports to determine whether or not an individual is under a disability and therefore may be eligible for rehabilitation services. In some cases eligibility can be documented with existing records; in other cases a decision to screen out a referral may be made by the rehabilitationist solely on the basis of an interview or reports, so that neither new medical informa-

tion or extensive medical records need be obtained. Eligibility for public rehabilitation must, of course, be thoroughly documented.

The rehabilitation counselor prepares disabled persons for what may be experienced during the medical diagnostic study. An explanation of the agency's medical evaluation requirements helps to enlist the applicant's cooperation in following through on medical recommendations. The fact that the state rehabilitation agency generally purchases medical examinations on a "private patient basis" should be a potent factor in client acceptance of the medical diagnostic study requirements.

15.3.3. GENERAL MEDICAL EXAMINATION

In the general medical examination, a general practitioner takes an overall look at the medical problem of each applicant for state rehabilitation services. This initial examination is of great potential significance in individual case diagnosis and rehabilitation planning. But in most cases it is only the beginning of an evaluation of the applicant's total medical problem. Incidentally, there are some clients for whom a specialist's report on an obvious impairment may precede the general medical examination; for example, occasionally it may be advisable to have a psychiatric or psychological evaluation done prior to the general medical examination.

A good general physical examination covers the applicant's general appearance, weight, height, posture, blood pressure, pulse, respiration, hearing, vision, blood vessels, lymph nodes, extremities, heart, lungs, pelvis, nervous system, and other parts of the body. In addition, certain laboratory tests are considered indispensable (e.g., urinalysis, serology).

Recency of the general medical examination is important. Thus a new examination may be requested even though a resume of medical records is available and otherwise complete; it may be misleading if the information is not current. In most cases, new examinations should be obtained if medical data are older than three months. This may vary somewhat, however, as in cases of diabetes or certain heart conditions for which it may be necessary to have up-to-date information. State rehabilitation agencies generally have their own medical examination report forms, which include the kinds of information necessary for a complete physical evaluation of an applicant. Medical resumes or abstracts on a different report form or in narrative style, however, may be used if they are relevant, recent, and complete.

15.3.4. SPECIALIST'S EXAMINATIONS

Examinations by outside specialists (in addition to the general medical examination) are often authorized by the counselor and paid for by the state rehabilitation agency. These should be obtained when a more thorough study of the particular impairment will provide a better understanding of the client's condition, the possibilities of treatment, or rehabilitation potential. One or more special examinations may be recommended either by the examining general medical physician or by the medical consultant of the agency. If treatment that involves a major decision on the part of the client (such as recommendations for removal of an eye or an organ) is advised, the agency is obliged to secure, if at all possible, examination from two qualified specialists.

Examining specialists should be supplied with copies of pertinent medical resumes and general examination findings that the state agency has secured on behalf of the client. The history of past medical or surgical experiences and the client's current life situation (including psychological and social reactions to the disability) may be of value to the specialist in diagnosis and planning for restorative treatment. The type of information that will be meaningful to the examining specialist depends largely upon the nature of the disability. (Sometimes it is more convenient for the physician and the counselor to convey this information in telephone conversations.) As with all confidential information and counselor activities in behalf of the client, the client should be informed in advance and be agreeable to the action.

The selection of a medical specialist is generally structured by agency practice and standards. In all instances it is necessary to have a qualified specialist. It is often desirable in selecting a specialist to have the recommendation of the family physician and the medical consultant. The latter usually suggests the sequence necessary for securing specialists' examinations and states what supporting laboratory data are needed.

Reports of examinations in specialty fields are sometimes made on special forms devised by the agency and in other instances by a narrative report according to a specified outline. As with a general medical examination, it is incumbent upon the specialist to provide laboratory findings in sufficient detail to substantiate the diagnosis. Moreover, the diagnosis should indicate cause, nature, and extent of the disability. Recommendations should be made by the specialist for further diagnostic work or medical treatment and a prognosis should be specified. It is highly desirable to have the physician specifically describe capacities and limitations in functions including environmental restrictions. These opinions can only be given when the condition has stabilized or has progressed far enough for a definite diagnosis and prediction. Vocational rehabilitation planning is postponed if the prognosis is too uncertain.

15.3.5. OTHER STUDIES

The cost of inpatient hospitalization for diagnostic purposes can be provided for by public rehabilitation funds. Hospitalization is authorized in cases where the diagnostic study requires procedures that cannot be obtained on an outpatient basis. Most state agencies have strict limitations on the number of days that may be paid for inpatient hospitalization for diagnostic purposes. There are also restrictions as to the nature or purpose of diagnostic expense.

Public rehabilitation services also may be used for physical restoration of a dental nature. This includes corrective surgery or therapeutic treatment necessary to correct or reduce the handicapping effects of the dental or associated disabilities. Examples of kinds of dental services that can be furnished if needed are the provision of dentures, bridges, fillings, extractions, oral surgery, treatment for infections of the gums, and treatment for dental conditions that are associated with cleft palate. Dental defects may constitute a direct barrier to employment because of the cosmetic problem, or, in other instances, they may indirectly contribute to an inability to perform certain job tasks. Moreover, many dental conditions affect the general health of the individual, and over an extended period can contribute to gradual deterioration of the ability to work. Other dental defects contribute to specific disease processes.

15.4. Eligibility Determination

Every agency, public or private, has criteria established for the selection and rejection of clients. In private agencies these criteria are determined by the agency purposes and by the policies of the directors. In public agencies the criteria for eligibility are established by public laws and administrative regulations. This discussion focuses upon the principles of determining eligibility for clients of the state rehabilitation programs. Eligibility criteria for public rehabilitation services are in general set forth by federal statute and regulations, so there should be little difference from one state to another as to who is eligible.

A thorough understanding of the case allows the rehabilitation counselor to make a formal decision regarding the applicant's eligibility for services. In cases of severe disability, complicating factors, or vague criteria standards, more comprehensive information and more reliance on interpretation of data may be necessary. However, at the time of determination, the counselor will be required to document in writing the eligibility status of the applicant. Certification of eligibility does not imply that the full range of services has been determined for the individual; it merely indicates that the client meets the standards for service.

The decision and its implications should be carefully explained to the applicant. In cases of ineligibility, the individual must be informed of policies and procedures of appeal and the reasons for the decision must be clearly explained. Individuals who are found ineligible for vocational rehabilitation by the state agency may be candidates for independent living services. Independent living rehabilitation also must be considered for rehabilitants who start but do not successfully complete vocational services and goals. In every case of ineligibility the rehabilitationist should also explore with the individual alternative resources and agencies, assisting in the referral when appropriate.

In cases of severe disability, the decision to accept for service, as well as the formulation of the service plan, necessitates obtaining information beyond basic eligibility data. Such information will usually be secured through more extensive evaluation and case study. Public vocational rehabilitation programs, for example, provide for an extended evaluation period up to 18 months for severely disabled applicants for whom rehabilitation potential is difficult to assess.

Rehabilitation counselors have the responsibility for determining the eligibility of the clients referred to them. In decision-making it is important to keep the best interests of the client in mind. One must be aware of what has been termed "defensive casework": practices that have resulted in elaborate studies and detailed case recordings to explain why an individual could not be served [Whitten, 1965]. Again it is important to focus on functional capacities, which often are overlooked in systems with limited resources and closure requirements for success. Past experience with certain kinds of clients can also influence personnel. Decisions must be made by interpreting all data in the light of established criteria if the agency is to benefit those it was created to serve.

An interim determination of eligibility may be made by a state rehabilitation agency for applicants who have records of disability and demonstrated difficulty in securing employment because of their disability. The agency can then initiate services immediately to applicants because of the likelihood (based on case records) that the person will be found eligible after a formal evaluation is completed. The final determination of eligibility must be completed within 90 days. This procedure recognizes that a qualified rehabilitation counselor is often able to make a determination from clinical impressions and an understanding of the applicant's history of disability and handicap. Delays in beginning services to severely handicapped applicants can be avoided by state agencies using the interim procedure.

15.4.1. FEASIBILITY

Feasibility refers to the question of whether services will increase an individual's functioning level enough to justify a given investment of money and human resources. There is virtually no way to answer this question except through the exercise of human judgment. In deciding whether an individual will receive services, legal feasibility must be considered; this involves the larger question of feasibility in general but usually as a subordinate concern. This approach has been fostered by law and custom. Voluntary organizations may handle the problem of feasibility in a slightly different way, but, because of practical and financial limitations, they also make a determination at this stage.

Bellamy and Snyder [1976] stated that the central issue in client acceptance by rehabilitation agencies now appears to be one of practicality, not feasibility. Monetary resources continue to be insufficient and agencies must always select only some individuals from among all those whom the services could help. The economic cost-benefit ratio philosophy provides the rationale for the feasibility model; according to this clients are looked upon as investments in terms of the relationship between dollars spent and the individual's projected productivity. If the intent of rehabilitation services is to provide disabled clients with the resources that will enable them to become as independent and productive as possible, then exclusion must be dealt with and revisions made to promote the rehabilitation effort.

Whitten [1965] recommended that all rehabilitation agencies reassess their policies and practices with regard to eligibility and feasibility questions, bringing present knowledge and resources to bear on these issues. Agencies should plan their work on the basis of the following principles.

1. All disabled people have the right to the assistance they need in order to become as independent as possible.
2. Policies on acceptance should not be so rigid that they constitute obstacles; instead these regulations should serve to encourage every eligible client's acceptance.
3. People within the agencies must be responsible for opposing regulations that have a deterrent effect.

Provision for independent living goals incorporated in the 1978 Amendments of the 1973 Rehabilitation Act have facilitated Whitten's recommendations.

Priorities—selection policy setting forth which applicant should be given first consideration for service—are a related issue in eligibility deter-

mination. In a situation in which a rehabilitation agency is unable to serve all eligible applicants, Miller and Olson [1971] said that priorities for service should be established. Such decisions typically occur at the federal or state level and reach the local level in the form of guidelines. Such a system specifies in advance, and publicly, the policies and procedures for providing service and allocating funds. For example, in state-federal vocational rehabilitation agencies the first priority is to serve the severely handicapped population. This priority is mandated by the Rehabilitation Act of 1973. This emphasis is to insure that services for this group are not deferred or delayed because of time or cost, or because of complex problems associated with rehabilitating severely handicapped individuals.

The development of priorities does not abrogate or cancel the established eligibility requirements. A priority directive is usually aimed more at the case-finding behavior of the rehabilitationist than at decision-making for eligibility. In theory at least, the worker will seek out persons in a priority category and be more certain that they are considered in the eligibility process, but such people merit no special considerations vis-à-vis the requirements themselves. However, it is probable that the judgment used in establishing eligibility is apt to be more favorable toward individuals in priority categories.

15.4.2. ELIGIBILITY INFORMATION

The following presentation focuses on vocational rehabilitation eligibility. This information on client eligibility for the public vocational rehabilitation program is based on a variety of public documents, including portions of various federal laws and regulations. Other useful information is from a package of training booklets published by Roy C. Farley of the University of Arkansas, Rehabilitation Research and Training Center [1975].

Criteria for Vocational Rehabilitation

One of the day-to-day functions state rehabilitation counselors must perform is assessing referrals and applicants to identify those who qualify. Not everyone is eligible under the federal Rehabilitation Act, which restricts the provision of rehabilitation services to individuals meeting certain criteria. The state rehabilitation agency is delegated as the sole authority for making the judgment as to who qualifies under the federal regulations. Immediate responsibility for deciding which applicants are legally entitled to services is assigned by the state rehabilitation agency to its professional staff and cannot be delegated to outsiders.

The counselor must gather documentary evidence to support the decision of either eligibility or ineligibility. After evaluating the individual and determining eligibility for services the counselor executes a certificate of eligibility. This must be signed and dated by the counselor, certifying acceptance of the individual for rehabilitation.

Documentation for a certificate of eligibility includes proper medical information, showing the presence of a physical disability, or in the case of mental illness, a psychiatric or psychological evaluation, or both. These required medical materials are processed by the medical consultant and interpreted by the rehabilitation counselor. Public rehabilitation services cannot be withheld on the basis of residency requirements or because of sex, race, creed, or national origin of the applicant. There is no upper or lower age limit that in and of itself can result in a finding of ineligibility, but very young people are not often ready for career planning until closer to work age. Medical services for disabled youngsters may be provided through the state programs for handicapped children.

Certification in each case depends upon an evaluation of rehabilitation potential to help determine eligibility. In the event services cannot be provided to all persons who apply and who have been determined to be eligible, the counselor and the state agency must ensure that priority of services will first be given to those classified as severely handicapped.

The counselor formally declares or "certifies" the eligibility of each qualified applicant for state services. In brief this means that there is adequate documentation that the applicant has a disability and that the resulting vocational handicap can be corrected by agency services.

The counselor must thoroughly evaluate each applicant to determine whether the person is under a "physical or mental disability," whether that disability constitutes a "substantial handicap to employment," and whether the individual can benefit from services in terms of "employability." The term *physical or mental disability* means a medically described condition that materially limits, contributes to limiting, or if not corrected, will probably result in limiting an individual's activities or functioning. The term *substantial handicap to employment* means that a physical or mental disability impedes an individual's occupational performance by preventing that individual from obtaining, retaining, or preparing for employment consistent with his or her capacities and abilities. The term *employability* as it is used in this connection refers to a determination that the provision of vocational rehabilitation services is likely to enable an individual to enter or retain employment consistent with that person's capacities and abilities. The concept of employment is broadly interpreted to mean "gainful" work in any of the following: the competitive labor market, the practice of a profession, self-employment, homemaking, farm or family work (including work for which payment is in kind rather than in cash), extended employment in a sheltered workshop, homebound employment, or other work situation.

Errors

Eligibility determination as a critical function of the rehabilitationist requires considerable professional competency. Some applicants who need and would benefit from rehabilitation services are mistakenly declared ineligible. Others, unfortunately, are made eligible when they either do not need service for readjustment or cannot benefit from service and are needlessly exposed to failure. An attempt to study this decision-making process was reported by Nagi [1969].

Errors in eligibility determination are thus of two kinds: (1) an applicant may be judged ineligible when, in fact, the individual legally qualifies for services; or (2) an unqualified applicant may be declared eligible. In statistics these errors are called Type I errors (when the true hypothesis is rejected) and Type II errors (when a false hypothesis is accepted); in medicine, such mistakes in diagnoses are called 1. "false negative" and 2. "false positive" results. Physicians, in order to help their patient, may tend to overstate the disability and its limitations. Thus medical reports for disability determination may screen in ineligible cases with only borderline problems. Rehabilitationists in charge of eligibility certification also tend to rule in favor of the applicant when in doubt—assuming that it is relatively more difficult for an individual, as compared to society, to sustain the economic consequences of an erroneous decision.

Procedures

A preliminary diagnostic study in rehabilitation includes all of the evaluations, examinations, and other diagnostic studies necessary to help the counselor arrive at a decision about the applicant's eligibility or ineligibility for service (or the need for extended evaluation to determine eligibility). In all cases this includes a general medical examination (or record) to determine the current general health status of the individual. In addition, further examination by specialists may be required for mental or emotional disorders; an assessment is required from a properly specialized physician or psychologist skilled in the diagnosis and treatment of such disorders. Visual impairment indicates need for examination by a physician skilled in diseases of the eye (an ophthalmologist). In the case of blindness, and in all cases of hearing impairment, a hearing evaluation should also be obtained from a physician skilled in diseases of the ear (an otologist). In the case of deafness, an evaluation of visual capacity must be obtained. When mental retardation is suspected, there must be a psychological evaluation, which includes a valid test of intelligence, for an appraisal of social functioning and educational progress and achievement.

Special Circumstances

Because the significant assets and limitations of some applicants are not readily diagnosed, it is possible for the counselor in public rehabilitation to delay a decision on eligibility by using a technique known as "extended evaluation." Rehabilitation services may be furnished under this extended evaluation to determine rehabilitation potential when an applicant has a physical or mental disability that is a substantial handicap to employment but the counselor is unable accurately to assess rehabilitation potential because the preliminary evaluation is unclear. Vocational rehabilitation services necessary for the determination of rehabilitation potential may be provided then for a total period not exceeding 18 months. After this period, rehabilitation may be provided only if the counselor decides that the individual qualifies, and at this time the counselor issues a certificate of eligibility. Services

may be terminated at any time during the extended evaluation period if it is decided beyond any reasonable doubt that the person cannot be expected to benefit in terms of employability. On the other hand, the individual may be made eligible any time vocational feasibility is determined.

Regulations for the administration of social security disability insurance and supplemental security income cases stipulate different and more complex procedures for eligibility determination, reporting, and funding. Extended evaluation is used in both cases and financial need requirements are waived.

In all instances of eligibility or ineligibility certification, the applicant must be notified officially and the decision recorded in the case file. Good professional practice also requires the counselor to convey important information of this nature to the client in a personal communication.

*Criteria for Independent
Living Rehabilitation*

The above discussion focussed on eligibility determination for state vocational rehabilitation services. While the same model is followed for the determination of eligibility for independent living rehabilitation, there are differences in the two sets of federal regulations.

The criteria for eligibility for independent living rehabilitation are: (1) The presence of a severe mental or physical disability; (2) the presence of a severe limitation in ability to function independently in family or community; and (3) there is a reasonable expectation that independent living rehabilitation services will significantly assist the individual to improve the ability to function independently. The determination of eligibility for independent living rehabilitation can be based on existing case record information if it is complete, relevant and current; consequently, special diagnostic studies may not be necessary. As with vocational rehabilitation there must be a written certification of eligibility or ineligibility. Order of selection provisions give first priority to those who are not receiving vocational rehabilitation services because of the severity of the handicap and to those for whom deinstitutionalization is at issue.

Independent living rehabilitation has no restrictions on the basis of age. Programs are specified for preschool children with communication limitation and for older blind individuals. The criterion of feasibility is not eliminated: there must be a reasonable expectation that independent living rehabilitation services will result in improvement in ability to function independently in family or community. This improved independence or maintenance of independence is demonstrated in functional and behavioral areas (e.g., self-care, activities of daily living, driving, using public transportation, shopping, housekeeping, communicating, or living more independently). It should be noted that the 1978 legislation and 1980 federal regulations do not clearly sever employment goal consideration from independent living. It is clear that there should be easy transition from one program to the other as the client's goal switches from a vocation to independence or vice versa.

15.4.3. ELIGIBILITY ISSUES

The 1973 Rehabilitation Act and subsequent regulations led to several debatable issues. First, the less severely handicapped were given lower priority for eligibility; the assumption was that they are less in need of service now and for their future and thus do not represent as good an investment of federal funds as the more severely handicapped group. Priority for the severely handicapped (if strictly implemented) only delays rehabilitation for those who do not at first qualify until their conditions worsen for lack of earlier intervention. This policy violates the well-established principle of preventive rehabilitation at a considerable cost in human happiness and additional ultimate expense. Second, the procedure for selection of the more "severely handicapped" was based upon invalid criteria that failed to accurately identify those individuals with the greatest need. The Congress assumed that the level of vocational handicap depended directly upon the type of medical disability and proceeded to list these disabilities. Such a conclusion is inconsistent with years of rehabilitation experience and research on vocational handicapping, which prove that the nature and severity of the medical condition constitute only one of many causal problems, such as lack of education, inadequate personality development, racial prejudices, lack of transferable skills, and advancing age. Nor does it necessarily follow that if a person requires extensive service, the disability must be severely handicapping. These are simplistic and

misleading definitions formulated by the Congress and little improved by rules set forth in regulations issued by the federal rehabilitation agency.

Professional Judgement

If a government cannot finance an adequate rehabilitation program for all handicapped people who need and would benefit from rehabilitation, there is a better method for client selection; if there must be priorities, there is a better answer than complicated bureaucratic regulations governing case selection, which are both expensive and ineffective. Professional counselors can make fair and equitable client decisions with greater efficiency from clearly stated agency guidelines than from detailed regulations. The Congress must decide what groups shall be served and must determine the order of preference or weight given to case selection criteria on the basis of objective data (e.g., greatest benefit-cost ratio, potential contribution to society, reduction in welfare cost, greatest occupation handicap, or, more reasonably, to some combination of criterion considerations). Whatever the agency's eligibility criteria, selection of the included applicants is a complex and important problem that requires professional judgement for final decisions.

Congressionally mandated priorities for the severely handicapped were an outgrowth of criticism of the public rehabilitation program for emphasizing numbers of cases closed as "rehabilitated." Up to the implementation of the 1973 Rehabilitation Act, there had been ever greater national records each year for the total number of rehabilitations reported. This achievement was viewed negatively, and rehabilitationists were accused of "playing the numbers game." It was implied that the federal rehabilitation agency based its case for expansion and increased appropriations on quantity rather than quality of work. Performance of state rehabilitation agency administrators and counselors was evaluated on this narrow criterion of record closures. No assessment was made of the difficulty of the cases or the gains clients made. "Easy" cases counted as much as those of the severely handicapped who perhaps needed more time and money to achieve employability. As a consequence, counselors were subtly encouraged to screen out difficult, high-risk applicants. Moreover, administrative pressures sifted down to the counselors to close cases prematurely. There was, in fact, undue stress placed on closures at all levels.

In 1973 the Congress overreacted against the federal rehabilitation administration's strategy of numbers by mandating stringent priorities, selection criteria, and accountability regulations. Corrective action for problems in case selection might have been accomplished by relatively simple administrative revisions in case statistical reporting and agency evaluation procedures. Evaluative research procedures were already available for assessing and rewarding state rehabilitation counselors for the *quality* of case work performance and good closures. Moreover, by that time the state agencys' staffs included a growing number of trained counseling personnel who were able to exercise professional judgement rather than be restricted by detailed regulations. Such bureaucratic rules lower eligibility decision-making to a clerical procedure. The use of appropriate incentives and professional judgement in case selection could accomplish agency goals more effectively.

Priority and Potential

Severely handicapped individual is a key term. It refers to the employability of a person who has a severe mental or physical disability that seriously limits functional capacities—mobility, communication, self-care, self-direction, work tolerance, or work skills. It is presumed that one is severely handicapped when rehabilitation can be expected to require multiple services for an extended period of time. The federal Rehabilitation Act of 1973 specified a number of severe disabilities that should be given priority by the state rehabilitation agencies. These were: limb amputation; arthritis; blindness; cancer; cerebral palsy; hemiplegia; hemophilia; respiratory or pulmonary dysfunction; mental retardation; mental illness; multiple sclerosis; muscular dystrophy; musculoskeletal disorders; neurological disorders (including stroke and epilepsy); paraplegia, quadriplegia, and other spinal cord conditions; sickle-cell anemia; end-stage renal diseases; or another disability or combination of disabilities determined, on the basis of an evaluation of rehabilitation potential, to cause comparable substantial functional limitation.

"Evaluation of rehabilitation potential" means ascertaining the nature of the client's handicap and determining whether or not there is a reasonable expectation that the individual can benefit from services in terms of employability. An older term meaning much the same thing was *feasibility study*. As appropriate in each case, evaluation of rehabilitation potential may include: (1) a preliminary diagnostic study, (2) a thorough diagnostic study, (3) provision of other goods or services for assessment purposes, (4) referral for further assessment, and (5) extended evaluation by the provision of service for the purposes of determining whether an individual can be rehabilitated.

15.5. Restoration Services

The purpose of physical or mental restoration in the public rehabilitation program is to remove or reduce the client's functional limitations in order to increase adjustment. When client restoration services were authorized by Public Law 113 in 1943, the Congress differentiated between restoration for vocational rehabilitation and health care services to the general population. It restricted rehabilitative restoration services to individuals eligible for the entire range of vocational adjustment services. The public rehabilitation agency was not authorized to provide medical services in order to prolong life, prevent premature death, alleviate pain, or reduce or prevent disease, unless the client's employability or potential employment was involved. In some cases, of course, the only service needed may be physical or mental restoration in addition to counseling in relation to life adjustment. Such cases are clearly within the scope and purpose of the public rehabilitation program, provided that other eligibility and priority requirements are met.

15.5.1. TYPES

Restoration services for vocational objectives are described as those medical and medically related services that are necessary to correct or substantially modify either a physical or mental (including emotional) condition that is stable or slowly progressing. They include: (1) medical or surgical treatment; (2) psychiatric or psychological treatment; (3) dental services; (4) nursing services; (5) hospitalization (either inpatient or outpatient care) and clinic services; (6) convalescent, nursing, or rest home care; (7) drugs and medical supplies; (8) prosthetic and other assistive devices needed for retaining or obtaining employment; (9) physical therapy; (10) occupational therapy; (11) speech or hearing therapy; (12) recreational therapy; (13) physical rehabilitation in a rehabilitation facility; (14) treatment of medical complications and emergencies associated with the provision of physical restoration inherent in the condition under treatment; and (15) other medical or medically related rehabilitation services.

Physical or mental restoration services for independent living rehabilitation may include any of the above named vocational rehabilitation restoration services. But additional services are offered for non-vocational objectives such as self-care and to minimize reliance upon others. These additional services for independent living include health maintenance and various therapeutic treatments.

15.5.2. CRITERIA

The criteria for providing restoration may or may not, depending on the state plan, require the financial participation of the client. Federal regulations, however, require that the clinical status of the client's disabling condition be stable or slowly progressive, and that the restoration service is expected to eliminate or reduce the handicapping condition within a reasonable period of time. Some state rehabilitation agencies have interpreted a reasonable period of time very narrowly, particularly with regard to the services of a psychiatrist or a psychologist.

Restoration services, like other client services, must be part of a comprehensive rehabilitation program individually written and agreed to as a contract by both the counselor, as a representative of the agency, and the rehabilitation client. The purchase of any restoration service by the counselor is normally done only with the concurrence of the state agency medical consultant. Authorization for purchased services is usually in writing, although there are times, in emergency situations, when the authorization may be oral provided that it is immediately recorded and confirmed by a written authorization. The procedure for client restoration authorizations varies from state to state.

15.5.3. PLANNING

The choice of physician, hospital, or other provider of restoration services is an important element in formulating the client's rehabilitation plan. State agency regulations in this matter may take into consideration the cost of services from public hospitals, cost-sharing with other public agencies, and the state expectation of client participation as well as the state agency criteria for economic need. Agency policies and procedures should provide for the client's free choice of an attending physician (whenever that is practicable) from among those physicians who meet the agency's standards of excellence for providing the services required in the case. Continuing counseling is needed to help the client fully utilize and understand the restoration services being provided by the agency. It is also the counselor's responsibility to coordinate the restoration program with other services that are provided concurrently. Most importantly, the counselor must be assured of the client's desire for any type of restoration program.

Chapter 16

Protection and Advocacy

Active intervention in the problem situations of clients is a traditional approach of rehabilitation counselors. This action orientation was not always appreciated by other professionals who thought that "reaching out" and "getting involved" was a demeaning or undignified role. But after many years of this kind of practice, the function of advocacy has been deemed respectable. Advocacy is now viewed as a necessary professional service to help handicapped individuals overcome barriers.

Advocacy is usually informal, taking the form of such action as requesting supplemental assistance or special considerations from a community agency. Such help, however, may actively involve the rehabilitation worker in, for example, court testimony or other direct action to preserve basic rights or to obtain program benefits to which the client is entitled. To handle such contingencies, rehabilitationists need essential knowledge about legal rights, protective services, current legal definitions, legal processes involved with guardianship, alternatives to guardianship, and general understanding of advocacy services.

The importance of protective services and advocacy in rehabilitation has been accelerated by two events. First, there is now a national effort to "deinstitutionalize" individuals and to give priority to severely handicapped people, thereby increasing the number of clients who are likely to need this help. Second, the public rehabilitation program expanded its goals in 1978 to include independent living. The severity of disability and scope of problems have a positive relationship to the level of intervention required of the professional worker.

16.1. Protective Services

Protective services may be needed for either children or adults. Laws protect neglected, abused, and exploited children under the age of 18. Society must also provide legal protection for adults who are unable to protect their own interests and are therefore in danger of neglect, abuse, or exploitation.

16.1.1. HISTORICAL PERSPECTIVE

It has long been recognized that individuals unable to fend for themselves need protective services, as shown by the Roman Law of Twelve Tables, which provided a protector for lunatics. Traditionally, families have been the primary protectors of individuals in need. In modern days, however, so many dependent disabled individuals outlive their parents that the problems of caring for them have become widespread.

In America before World War I, most states had established statutes on guardianship as a way of dealing with dependent handicapped individuals. The principal concern of those original laws, according to Helsel [1974], was to prevent family fortunes from being squandered by incompetent individuals; the basic procedure for establishing guardianship then was similar to what it is today: a petition was filed and a hearing was held for presentation of proof of incompetency. A judge determined whether or not the person was in fact incompetent, then named the guardian who reported the ward's financial affairs at the end of each year. Even under court monitoring, though, the ward's funds were sometimes manipulated for the benefit of the guardian rather than the ward.

Another strategy for dealing with dependent, handicapped persons was to institutionalize them. Superintendents of the institutions were given responsibility for the wards, but this placed an impossible burden on the superintendents. The resulting lack of control allowed flagrant violations of civil and human rights to go unnoticed.

During the 1950s, governmental agencies moved to provide better protection to dependent individuals and to streamline services to them. To avoid costly and cumbersome guardianship arrangements, the Social Security Administration and the Veterans Administration established substitute or representative payees. In many states, public welfare agencies were given the legal right to appoint concerned individuals to accept welfare payments on behalf of clients unable to manage their own affairs. This approach, however, has the potential for abuse. Still more recently a surge of interest in human rights has led to better governmental protective service systems. New laws and an array of private advocacy groups now defend the rights of the handicapped.

16.1.2. SERVICES DEFINED

Traditional as well as contemporary definitions of the term *protective services* have been given by Helsel [1974]:

Historically, protective services for children meant protection from abuse and neglect. For the elderly, where the term protective services has also been used, it meant help with managing money and activities of daily living. . . . For the severely handicapped, the term protective services has additional meanings. There are lifelong dependency needs that must be monitored and assessed for appropriateness as needs and situations change over a lifetime.

The contemporary definition is currently used in the state of Ohio: Protective services are those services undertaken by a legally authorized and accountable agency on behalf of a client who needs help in managing himself or his affairs. These services may be social or legal in nature and may involve counseling, monitoring, follow-along, program auditing, advocacy, legal intervention, trusteeship, guardianship, and protectorship [pp. 23–24].

16.1.3. SERVICES NECESSARY

Unless adjudicated incompetent, an emotionally disturbed or a mentally retarded adult possesses full citizen's rights, powers, and duties under the law. Being labeled mentally ill or retarded through school or professional evaluations has no legal effect. However, for purposes of obtaining such basic civil rights as voting, driving a car, and obtaining a job or insurance, an application form which specifies a mental or physical handicap or some prior institutionalization can be enough to result in denial. Despite the disability, however, a "retardate" has the legal right to dispose of property, enter into contracts, make purchases, give testimony in court, execute legal instruments, marry, vote, and obtain a driver's license; practically speaking, however, many of these legal rights will be denied in many instances. Parents of mentally disabled adults have no legal authority to direct the lives of their children once they attain adult status and are not under parental guardianship; they must rely on influence and persuasion. Every adult is presumed capable by the law and only court action can change that status.

When individuals have the ability to manage their personal life and conduct financial affairs with minimal assistance, there is no need for legal interference. But if mental disability indicates that an individual cannot manage adult responsibilities alone, a court order restricting the rights of the person and delegating powers and duties to another is needed. Partial or limited guardianship and voluntary agreements administered by court order are possible alternatives. The best choice is the least restrictive alternative available to assist people in leading lives as normal as their abilities make possible.

16.1.4. TYPES OF GUARDIANSHIP

When adults have been legally determined to be incompetent to care for their own persons or property, the court appoints a person as "guardian of the estate" or "guardian of the person," or both. Other legal alternatives that may be available are "limited guardianship," "temporary guardianship," and "standby guardianship." The limited guardian is appointed by the court to supervise and guide the ward where assistance is needed, thus recognizing that the provision of help should be as unrestrictive as possible. A temporary guardian is appointed by the court when, due to an emergency, immediate appointment is required. A standby guardian assumes responsibilities for an incompetent adult should the present guardian die or resign.

16.1.5. ESTABLISHING GUARDIANSHIP

Guardianship is defined by statute in each state. Usually it entails the adjudication of incompetency and the appointment of a "guardian" who has the legal power and duty to act on behalf of the incompetent person, known as the "ward."

Parents or an agency, through an attorney, petition to a court of competent jurisdiction, usually the Probate Court, which then conducts a hearing to determine whether or not the disabled person is competent to manage personal affairs. Before the hearing, the petitioner must obtain a statement from a licensed physician or psychologist, or both, declaring that according to professional judgement the subject of the hearing is substantially incapable of managing property or caring for self. Also before the hearing, the court will appoint a guardian ad litem, a neutral attorney, whose duty it is to interview the alleged incompetent and explain the proceedings and the individual's personal rights—including the right to present other evidence. The guardian ad litem also offers an opinion to the court concerning what actions are in the best interest of the proposed ward. A guardian is appointed at the hearing if the judge decides that the reports and testimony offered constitute clear and convincing evidence that the person is incompetent. The court has the power to appoint any citizen as guardian, although generally a family member or friend is chosen.

16.1.6. COURT ORDERED PLACEMENT

At the time a guardian is appointed, the court may also consider protective placement or protective services for an incompetent person. Examples of protective placements are: independent living with either court-ordered or voluntary services arrangements; foster home residence; residential care facilities; or a nursing home offering minimal to extensive nursing care. Protective services consist of the entire range of health and social services, and the court may choose day care, family planning, financial consultant, medical treatment, and legal services.

16.2. Advocacy Services

Advocacy is the act of supporting, defending, or pleading a cause, proposal, or personal need. Being both an alternative and a supplement to protective services, advocacy services range in scope from several neighborhood people informally helping a single individual to large organizations engaging in both individual and system advocacy.

16.2.1. THE ADVOCACY ROLE

A survey of informed people by Chan, Brophy, Garland, Linnane, and Screven [1976] showed marked distinctions between the way protective service and advocacy services were perceived. Protective services were seen to involve formal or legal proceedings that culminate in action by a court of law. Advocacy was seen to be less formal and more speculative, more flexible, and personal. For example, the advocacy process is viewed as one in which the developmentally disabled person might be encouraged to assume more responsibility and authority with respect to decision-making. An interesting distinction made by some respondents to the survey was that protective services might be viewed as reactions to circumstances, while advocacy services might be viewed more as preventive or assertive actions.

In many respects, rehabilitation counselors and other human service professionals have always performed functions that are advocative in nature. Flynn [1975] defined three broad categories of advocate functions: as a facilitator, initiator, and modifier. As a facilitator, the advocate serves as a channel through which clients can make their feelings known directly to those who influence the rehabilitation process. As an initiator, the professional directly influences the provision of services. The third advocate function centers on modification of negative public attitudes toward persons with disabilities; this covers a broad spectrum. In one way it may involve direct attempts to influence legislation and policies of organizations. In a more limited way, informal discussions with people during daily contacts provide opportunities, when appropriate, to discuss attitudes and prejudices concerning various disabilities.

Having listed the three general functions of advocates, Flynn suggested three qualifications that are necessary:

(1) a genuine interest in serving people with a particular disability;
(2) sufficient knowledge of the disability so as to provide facts instead of myths; and,
(3) enough time to put the other two qualifications to use [pp. 1–2].

In other words, the rehabilitationist, in the advocacy role, is a knowing and caring person who takes time to help.

16.2.2. CITIZEN ADVOCACY

As first described by Wolfensberger [1972], "citizen advocates" are volunteers who assume the role of friend or guide to a person who needs help and support. Usually the strategy of minimal advocacy is adopted, allowing persons being helped to do as much as possible on their own. Since advocates of this type receive no pay and

have no bloodline responsibility, their unselfish concern usually provides inspiration and motivation for both parents and professionals. In addition, advocates can have a unique influence on the rest of the community because they are in a position to bring previously negative or neutral people into active involvement with the handicapped person. It is said that this is done by the advocate's encouragement, example, and active persuasion.

Another supposed value of citizen advocates, as described by Zauha [1974], is an ability to make connections that it is thought professionals cannot make: "As citizens, advocates work in ways in which private persons naturally work. For instance, unlike the professional . . . a citizen advocate can contact persons up and down the line in a service delivery system—the counselor, the counselor's boss, or the counselor's boss's boss—or even shift out of the system to contact parents or professionals in another agency" [p. 11].

Citizen advocates can also supplement the function of guardians by helping them seek out and use community services, especially if the guardian lives far away from the ward. (Advocates are often assigned because of their proximity to the ward.) The advocate may also serve as an impartial third-person observer when a guardian-ward relationship becomes unstable and would benefit from the clarification that the advocate can give.

Zauha has described the office that coordinates citizen advocacy programs as usually only facilitating citizen efforts. Independence is promoted among advocates to ensure that they are advocates of their protégé and not of the sponsoring agency. The agency publicizes the programs and screens, orients, and matches participants. Agency staff facilitate meetings between advocates and other consultants, and generally work to steer advocates toward strong, healthy relationships with persons in need. Mediation of formal processes such as guardianships may be a capacity of a citizen advocate program office.

Advocates and those who think they are needed by clients of rehabilitation counselors all too often assume that the latter fail to do what they can. Advocates therefore may demand much time for explanation that could be better used by the counselors with the client in service processes.

The organizations most active in establishing

citizen advocacy programs are the local chapters of the Association for Retarded Citizens.

16.2.3. OMBUDS SERVICES

An "ombuds" is a person who examines complaints and acts on legitimate ones by requiring a service or securing a change in institutional policy. (Although the term *ombudsman* is the more conventional, the term *ombuds* was coined for this book in recognition of women's equal suitability for this role.) The relationship between an ombuds and the individual voicing the complaint(s) is terminated once the need for it no longer exists.

An ombuds program requires a substantial power base inside the system to be successful. Historically, the ombuds was appointed by a top government or institution official to cut red tape on behalf of persons confused by bureaucratic policy and procedures [Linnane, 1974]. It is the ombuds' goal to provide fair treatment for citizens and to give them a sense of participation in the problem-solving process.

Sweden, Denmark, and New Zealand have had the most extensive experience with the ombuds concept. In several places, it is part of their administrative program for the handicapped. The concept itself was born out of a monumental array of governmental bureaucracy in which the client's interests may get lost. Balthazar [1975] said:

Because the individual citizen is often helpless in the face of so much legislative and administrative machinery, the concept of the "people's man" or ombudsman was born. He as an official may be appointed by a legislative body but is to act independently from governmental restraint. His role is to investigate complaints which are formally made to him when these complaints represent alleged mistakes or abuses in administrative authority.

In a particular sense, he is a cost free advocate of the citizen. He is invested with investigative powers and his function is to report and to apply pressure to correct inappropriate decisions [p. 44].

16.2.4. LEGAL ADVOCACY

By definition, the practice of law involves advocacy and, in fact, lawyers are frequently called advocates. Relevant activities of lawyers include counseling, negotiation, persuading, researching-learning, recording-drafting, planning, translating, managing-administering, and investigating–fact-gathering. Hutchison [Goodwill Industries of America, 1975] reported that several of these activities have particular relevance to advocacy for the handicapped.

1. Counseling—Involves pointing out legal problems to clients including possible future problems, and suggesting courses of action. Interviewing and counseling presuppose the ability to pick legal problems out of a client's conversation and to focus on them.
2. Negotiating—Since most legal disputes do not reach trial, this includes a variety of negotiating situations, such as representing clients in civil negotiations, plea bargaining with district attorneys, or negotiating with attorneys with insurance claims and labor disputes.
3. Persuading—Includes not only persuading juries, judges, legislators and those with whom the attorney negotiates, but also may involve convincing his client to do or not do certain things [p. 7].

Although clients may contact a lawyer advocate on a walk-in basis, they are usually referred to a lawyer by some helping agency, organization, or other advocacy program. The lawyer advocate may address the specific legal needs of an individual client or may arrange a class action suit if an identifiable class of persons is involved. An example of the latter would be cases in which legal action is necessary to ensure that laws enacted to benefit the handicapped population actually become a reality.

Among the agencies and organizations that provide legal services and information helpful to advocacy efforts on behalf of handicapped persons, the following are most important to rehabilitationists, according to Benningfield, Reiser, and Richards [1975]: Legal Aid and Defender Societies, which provide legal assistance to low-income people; the American Civil Liberties Union, which is interested in cases involving the violation of rights of people, including those who are physically disabled; and the National Center for Law and the Handicapped, Inc., a federally funded center in South Bend, Indiana, which has nationwide information on court cases involving handicapped persons and which can offer support, information, and service. (Information about prior court decisions could be extremely helpful to anyone considering court action.)

16.2.5. ADVOCATE COUNSELING

This service helps clients develop assertive skills that will enable them to improve their dysfunctional interactions with individuals and institutions. Unlike other advocacy services, advocate counseling emphasizes teaching and helping clients to advocate for themselves. The advocate counselor helps individuals and groups maximize their impact on institutions in such a way that the institutions are pressured to meet the needs of the people they were established to serve.

Using the law as the highest authority, the advocate counseling method teaches the client how to look for discrepancies in the way institution personnel implement policy. Clients are also taught how to use the administrative mechanisms of due process. Most of this instruction is done in an information resource center, which contains primary and secondary source material such as statutes, relevant case law, rules and regulations, administrative memoranda, and operational rules of various institutions. Clients are taught how to use the resource center, how to define their institutional problem, how to assemble their own exhaustive list of alternative actions and consequences, and how to implement the alternative of their choice [Chan, et al., 1976].

Since these behaviors are new for most people, the advocate counseling approach is also geared to handle internal conflicts and changes in thought processes, feelings, values, and other personal insights. Assertiveness training may be especially needed by those disabled people who have little worldly experience or who evidence feelings of inferiority and succumbing behavior.

16.2.6. CLIENT RIGHTS

Beginning in the 1970s there has been an accelerated effort to more actively include the disabled themselves in the affairs of rehabilitation. This has come about through a growing awareness of the general public and also numerous "special" publics (e.g., people with a personal interest in a particular disability) that disabled people should have a voice in matters that affect them. Moreover, through organizations for or of the disabled, these people learned that collective expressions of their wishes did in fact influence the decision-makers.

Handicapped individuals, it is now acknowledged, do have authority over their own destinies. This right of handicapped people as consumers of rehabilitation services has been recognized by legislators. Agency legislation has mandated the involvement of consumer groups in two ways: the advisory groups of public agencies must include consumer representation, and clients of rehabilitation must participate in their own planning for services and must approve of that plan. All of the rights of the disabled population are not fully implemented, but the principle has been accepted by governments and found to be effective.

Declarations of Rights for Handicapped People

A number of conferences involving consumers and the helping professions have drafted a "bill of rights" for the handicapped in an attempt to clarify those areas in which the handicapped need action to obtain basic freedoms that have been denied to them. Probably the declaration of rights that applies to all populations is the universal declaration of human rights adopted by the United Nations. The declaration proclaims that all members of the human family have equal and inalienable rights of human dignity and freedom. With this premise in mind, various groups such as the International League of Societies for the Mentally Handicapped have drafted declarations of rights. Perhaps the most articulate bill of rights for the handicapped was presented at the United Cerebral Palsy Associations Annual Conference in Washington, D.C., on May 3, 1973. Hundreds of delegates signed this bill of rights, which appears to be representative of such declarations and does not limit its focus to one group of handicapped individuals.

16.2.7. ACCOUNTABILITY

What if there is a conflict between the interest of the agency and that of the client? While the question may arise in either a private or public agency, the latter is governed by legal rules regarding the use of tax funds. The issue assumes that the agency is basically concerned with societal good while the professional is primarily concerned with the good of the client. How is this issue resolved when a client wants, even needs, more service or funding than the agency has to offer?

Some proponents of the client advocacy system go so far as to imply that state agency employees cannot always serve clients in a professional capacity because of their conflicting allegiance. While incompatibility between client needs and agency resources does arise, the problem is not insoluble. Nor does the situation preclude professionalism or force insubordination on the part of the agency employee.

Rehabilitation counselors as professionals have a moral obligation to their clients. Proper conduct is stipulated through a code of ethics (covered elsewhere). In the instance of an unalterable choice that forces adherence to agency regulation, with the resultant action harmful to the client, professionals are obliged to resign. This situation is quite rare. Rehabilitation organizations are created to help, not harm, disabled people. Agency programs and goals are designed for consistency with client needs. None of the evidence supports the contention that professional workers as government employees behave unethically.

Legislative Action by Professionals

Perhaps the greatest charge to be made against the advocacy relationship is that the employee of government may not be free to lobby for improved legislation. Purely selfish use of influence by government employees should be prohibited, but there is nothing to preclude rehabilitation counselors and other state or federal employees from expressing their professional views for political action.

The influence of individual rehabilitation counselors on the legislative and administrative process of the public rehabilitation program is often best exerted through the concerted efforts of the associations that represent this profession. Moreover, as government employees, rehabilitation workers may be in a very good position to give policymakers constructive ideas, from first-hand knowledge, about needed expansion and improvements in the service delivery system.

16.2.8. ROLE RESPONSIBILITIES

The rehabilitationist, Stone [1971] said, must sometimes intervene directly with the society to which the client must relate if the goals of rehabilitation are to be achieved. In addition to having skill in community referral and community coordination, the rehabilitationist must also actively work to obtain the facilities and resources in the community that are needed by clients.

Sinick [1977a] asked, "How can vocational counselors responsibly change society? In carrying out what may indeed be regarded as a responsibility of counselors, at least five possible approaches are available. Not mutually exclusive, all or any of them can be used by the same counselor" [p. 245]. The five approaches involve clients, client environments, institutions employing counselors, professional associations, and counselors as citizens. Each of these approaches is explained below.

In the first approach, clients "are assisted in using themselves in a maximally self-actualizing manner that may, in turn, actuate change in society" [Sinick, p. 247]. The successful client is the most powerful agent of change available in rehabilitation processes.

A second method involves various environments that affect clients: their current and future families, their schools, and their places of employment. Counselors can help their clients by working with sensitivity for change in these environments, according to Sinick.

Institutions employing counselors provide the third approach. Rehabilitation agencies need change as much as other institutions. As Sinick pointed out, "counselors' efforts to deal with each individual as a person require parallel efforts to create a conducive institutional environment" [p. 248].

The fourth approach is through professional associations to facilitate change in society. The combined strength of those in counseling is greater than the sum of individual efforts. Professional associations can supplement counselors' efforts toward changing clients, client environments, and the counselors' employing institutions.

Finally, change occurs through the action of counselors as citizens. With the four other methods, counselors exert influence in their professional role. In this fifth approach, however, they move outside their counseling role to act as concerned citizens and add another dimension to their endeavors. Various nonprofit associations consisting of public citizens have been established to promote a common cause. Such associations can be even more effective than professional associations in bringing about needed changes through government action.

Rehabilitationists, as mentioned before, can influence legislation and social policy as individual citizens. They can become acquainted with local representatives in the U.S. Congress and the state legislature as well as others in public office and keep them informed of the need for specific changes that will ultimately benefit disabled people. They can be effective with candidates for public office. These contacts may be in person or by letters. Lawmakers are especially responsive to the informed opinion of professionals such as rehabilitation counselors in their areas of expertise.

Professional people are responsible for promoting the goals of their profession; every rehabilitationist should also work toward creating a good public image of rehabilitation as a public program. Information about public rehabilitation can be communicated personally to the people who determine government programs and budgets. Friendships with legislative staffs and advisors have even greater impact than a barrage of telegrams and letters at crucial times.

The most recent and perhaps the most powerful method of advocacy involves securing client rights through the judicial system and the administrative procedures of fair employment practices legislation. This movement has addressed the constitutional guarantees of the disabled, and this in turn affects social policy. Knowledge of the legal rights of handicapped individuals and correct advice about exercising them puts the rehabilitation counselor in a key position.

Judicial and administrative protection extend beyond employment rights. Transportation and community services are two other areas for intervention on behalf of handicapped persons. Great change has occurred in educational and vocational rights. But, many potential beneficiaries of these new legal rights are uninformed about them or are unable to seek them out without assistance.

16.3. Legal Services

Attorney services are fundamental in many cases concerning the protection of rights of handicapped individuals. While the intervention of legal counsel is by no means limited to financial matters, the focus in this section is on the role of the lawyer in personal injury cases.

16.3.1. MONETARY ENTITLEMENTS

Disablement may entitle a person to monetary benefits or awards from one or more of a variety of public and private sources. Examples of public financial provisions for disabled persons are state workers compensation for job-related injury or disease, federal social security benefits for disabled workers, and supplemental security income for needy disabled people. Private insurance companies sell policies to provide income in the event of incapacity. In still other cases, another person or company may be found liable or financially responsible for impairments that result from negligence or a faulty product. More than one source of recompense may be obtained in many cases and the dollar amounts can be substantial.

The personal injury lawsuit against a business and its insurance carrier is sometimes settled for large sums. Manufacturers are held financially responsible when personal disability is proved

attributable to their faulty product. Likewise, physicians and other professionals and their employers (or insurance company) may have to pay for personal loss due to malpractice. Because state laws covering personal or product liability vary as do eligibility and other regulations of public agencies, the advice of an attorney is sought to assure justice and fair treatment. The legal representative retained by the disabled person counsels in matters of law, evidence, and testimony, and negotiates with the adversary or with the agency involved for a favorable decision.

16.3.2. ATTORNEY SELECTION AND ROLE

Services of a private attorney are often needed to ensure that maximum legal entitlements are obtained. Legal representation may be advisable even in dealings with nonpartisan government agencies such as the Social Security Administration, Veterans Administration, and state workers compensation commissions. A personal attorney is particularly indicated when an unfavorable administration ruling (such as finding the claimant ineligible) is being appealed. Lawyers who are qualified in such matters frequently recover far more money than their fees and legal costs. They often work on a contingency basis (i.e., they charge only if they win the case) and may earn one-third (or less) of the money collected for the client through their legal action. Free legal aid sponsored by a local bar association or community fund is often available for limited services to indigent or low-income people. Moreover, attorneys will sometimes represent hardship cases for a reduced fee or no fee.

Care in the choice of a lawyer is needed to assure competent, ethical services for the person who has suffered a disability. Some law firms specialize in labor litigation or personal injury suits. Such expertise is of great value. Legal advice that unduly prolongs settlement or exaggerates the limitation should be avoided since a client's hope of a windfall settlement is a notorious disincentive for rehabilitation. Disabled persons, while awaiting legal action, are sometimes encouraged, if not coached, to play the role of the helpless invalid. This has ruinous personality repercussions, facetiously called "compensation neurosis."

Rehabilitation workers who advise disabled clients about possible monetary benefits through legal recourse need to know about legal services. In addition to their professional role in this area, rehabilitation counselors are sometimes called upon to testify or give other evidence in court procedures. Also, rehabilitationists may be retained by either side to give opinions as "expert witnesses." These professional issues are discussed in Chapter 3, Role and Functions, and Chapter 4, Impact of Disability.

Part III

Assessment

Chapter 17

Fundamentals

Human assessment is done to make predictions about an individual. It is used in informal ways by each of us every day of our lives. We assess ourselves to change our behavior and assess other people to adjust our response to them. Assessing self and others consequently serves an important function, since it provides the bases of future action. Yet, this type of assessment is generally so unsystematic and haphazard that it is often inaccurate. The assessment discussed here is systematic, scientifically based, or at least intended to be objective.

The purpose of assessment in human service programs is to secure as complete a picture of the individual as needed to deal with that person's problems. Assessment is therefore fundamental in various kinds of professional services. The type of problem, of course, determines the focus of client assessment. Rehabilitation counselors, with their focus on occupational readjustment, are especially concerned with vocational assessment. As a source of understanding for competent rehabilitation counseling and planning assessing is a basic professional function.

Client assessment has long been an essential phase in vocational rehabilitation, with information collected from various sources. Medical examination was always required to establish the nature of the disability. Furthermore, with the earlier focus on reeducation, client school records were considered and psychological tests were routinely authorized. Some sort of case history was obtained in the application procedure with initial interview data recorded. Background material was solicited from family, school officials, and former employers even before the day of trained counselors. In a sense there was more confidence and emphasis then on the evaluation approach than now. Not enough was known, however, about the limitations or the proper application of vocational assessment, and test results were misused. Similarly, clients became locked into invalid but permanent labels attached to them through faulty tests, old records of previous behavior, and biased opinions of other professionals. Moreover, the diagnostic method leading to the selection of a vocational objective and authorization of service to be provided did not encourage client participation in the planning. Assessment and advisement were too often manipulative and authoritarian, based on the assumption that the professional decisions were grounded in sound knowledge. There was what might be termed a *diagnostic-prescription model* that left little opportunity for client input and responsibility. Professional respect and techniques for nondirective client-centeredness in counseling came later [e.g., Rogers, 1942, 1951, 1961].

With greater professionalism, rehabilitation counselors have given more consideration to the democratic process in human relations. The evolution has been from vocational advisement to vocational guidance to vocational counseling. In the 1960s and 1970s, the counseling profession magnanimously proclaimed that clients be accepted as equal partners. Today's client demands complete authority in setting self goals and tactics. In this climate the counselor may emerge as a consultant to the client, conveying and interpreting information. This shift in role can be facilitated by the constant advances in assessment techniques that help clients to make informed decisions.

Despite technical advances, however, the whole notion of assessing people and the term *testing* have taken on a negative connotation in recent years. In many cases people react unfavorably to tests although it is not the test but the way it is used that is the problem. Unfortunately tests are often incompetently chosen, administered, and interpreted. Special arrangements or consideration for functional limitations are often denied handicapped testees (see 20.5.2). Moreover, testing still seems to reinforce an authoritarian role for the counselor. As a consequence, not only the general public but even some professionals naively regard assessment unfavorably, as a "judgmental" act.

Assessment devices, it should be kept in mind, are never used to measure people. What are measured are characteristics: intellectual capacities, verbal skills, self-confidence, and so on. This is distinctly different from estimating how worthwhile an individual is: with this distinction made, client assessment should be accepted as a valuable tool for rehabilitation counselors.

Client assessment, as described in this chapter, is an integral, indispensable, and continuing part of rehabilitation counseling for all clients. It is the complex whole of a series of information-gathering and decision-making steps. The information comes from many sources and includes client records, test results, interview data, professional observations, and so on. The processing of relevant information is called a *case study*. It is convenient to classify the gathering of this relevant information into components such as

medical, psychological, social, and work evaluations. These evaluations may be conducted by various professionals in addition to the rehabilitation counselor (e.g., physician, psychometrist, social worker, work evaluator). Their reports become parts of an emerging information gestalt which is the "picture of facts" used by the counselor and client in planning a vocational (or other) objective and rehabilitation strategy.

A concrete, sequential procedure for using evaluative data for client goal-setting in the rehabilitation planning process has been described by Stanford Rubin and Richard Roessler [1978, 1979]. Proper selection of a vocational objective by the client requires sufficient information. Therefore, the rehabilitation counselor must facilitate client exploration of both self and the world of work. These authors feel that for rehabilitation counselors to make a "proper fit," the determination requires a thorough understanding of the client during the assessment phase of the rehabilitation process. Rubin and Roessler, authors of a popular Vocational Rehabilitation text, call their procedure the "Crux model."

Evaluation techniques and other relevant rehabilitation assessment information are described in part throughout this volume. Chapter 8, Rehabilitation Facilities, describes the transitional workshop in which client assessment is a fundamental program. Chapter 13, Adjustment Training, explains work adjustment procedures used by rehabilitation workshops. Chapters 4 and 5, Impact of Disability and Functional Limitations, respectively, provide the conceptual framework for evaluating the client's handicap. Chapter 15, Medical Services, outlines the whole process of medical evaluation, including the medical consultant's role in assisting the counselor in client assessment. Several counseling chapters are also relevant. Chapter 27, Vocational Counseling, covers the implementation of client evaluation in the counseling and planning process. Chapter 28, Personal Adjustment, describes the psychosocial problems so important in client assessment. Other counseling chapters describe such important techniques as interviewing, observation, and reporting. Many fundamental skills and areas of knowledge about client assessment also are contained in the placement chapters, Part V.

Categorizing material about client assessment, counseling, and placement is misleading, however, because these functions are inseparable in the actual process. The division of professional functions is confused further by placing them in sequential order as if one function inevitably followed the other—or as if all rehabilitation counselors, regardless of their employment setting, always performed this whole range of functioning. Client assessment must be viewed in context with the entire process.

While the focus in Part III, the assessment chapters, is on vocational adjustment, many of these client assessment methods are applicable in independent living rehabilitation (see 40.1.4). The 14 functional limitations presented in Chapter 5 provide the counselor a conceptual framework for understanding the dynamics of a handicap to employment or independent living. In every instance the person's limitation in function must be viewed in the context of an environment that, by failing to accommodate individual differences, creates the handicap. These physical (and social) environmental obstacles must be evaluated along with the client's motivation, self-confidence, coping or survival skills, and other personal characteristics. Assessment for independent living objectives (c.f., vocational rehabilitation) may be more complicated and take a longer period of time because of the number and severity of the functional limitations involved, and long-range nature of some services for independent living rehabilitation. Despite the broad range of client problems, however, assessment procedures and purposes are quite similar for vocational and independent living programs.

A unique acknowledgement is needed at this point. The University of Wisconsin-Stout at Menomonie, Wisconsin, through its Rehabilitation Research and Training (R & T) Center under the leadership of Paul Hoffman, has contributed to the advancement of technology in this whole field. Many of their reports have been used when collecting practical materials for these chapters on assessment. Credit is likewise given to the other leaders of the Vocational Evaluation and Work Adjustment Association (VEWAA) for technical development and publication in this part of the rehabilitation process. Donn Brolin [1976]—whose book, *Vocational Preparation of Retarded Citizens,* provides conceptual organization to vocational assessment —contributed valuable suggestions. Paul Lustig, who is a noted authority on the vocational assessment of the disabled, also gave many constructive suggestions.

17.1. Principles

Vocational assessment is an application of science, a method for dealing with the occupational growth of an individual entering the world of work. It is a decision-making mechanism that helps people with the problems that stem from their vocational handicaps, a process of producing rational life decisions; various practical determinations are made: what will be done for an individual, how, and to what effect. It includes the establishment of criteria to measure the progress of the client [Dawis, 1976]. It is concerned with the future.

Evaluation and assessment in rehabilitation address the concerns that are significant to a particular client at a given point in that person's life. It focuses on the individual's needs and also utilizes the specific capacities of the helping personnel involved and the resources at hand. This is an endeavor for which a humanistic belief is essential—the concept that people are capable of constructive growth and that organizations are designed for people rather than technological ends. When it is not based on this belief, vocational assessment is far less creative; when linked with the idea that a human life can evolve and change, it is a way of helping those with problems to make the most of their capacities [Gellman, 1968].

17.1.1. DESCRIPTION

The terms *assessment,* and *evaluation* are often used interchangeably, but it is conceptually helpful to consider evaluation as subsumed under assessment. Thus, evaluation data combine into a comprehensive whole known as the case study, which constitutes the information basis for assessment. The purpose of assessment is for planning a course of action. The process is never complete and final because the input of evaluative information and the client and situation are constantly changing. As the overall assessment changes, modifications of the action plan may be indicated. Evaluation and assessment are a major part of the rehabilitation process and essential to client success.

Definitions given below are primarily for conceptual clarity. The reader should know, however, that there is no parallel consistency of terms throughout the relevant literature.

ASSESSMENT. An assessment is based upon a body of information to predict the probability of success of alternative courses of action. This predictive information, from a variety of sources, is collected for the counseling purpose of planning with a client. It represents a complex and continuing series of information-gathering and decision-making steps. Thus judgements are broadly based on a combination of relevant evaluations, counseling, and circumstantial considerations (see *case study*). Inherent in human assessment is a concern for the outcome rather than mere understanding of the data.

EVALUATION. An evaluation is a set of information that describes and projects an individual's level of function in a specific context: physical, emotional, social, educational, vocational. Evaluation is based upon a variety of measurements and other objective observations that yield a comparison with appropriate criteria. Clinical data (i.e., direct observation or measurement of the client) as well as information collected through other means and sources are used in evaluating characteristics of the individual. Thus, multiple components are included in proportion to their composite descriptive value, and both qualitative and quantitative variables are incorporated.

MEASUREMENT. The assignment of numbers representing the amount or quantity of something is called measurement. Expressed in standardized units (e.g., meter or liter), measures provide a comparison of things such as relative length or volume. Measuring then, is the process of assigning numbers (i.e., quantification) that supposedly depict the amount of an attribute. Psychometric measurements are expressed in "standard scores," showing the deviation from the mean average of a comparable group of people.

CASE STUDY. As used in this book *case study* has an explicit meaning (see Chapter 24). It refers to the processing of client information by the counselor from all sources: interviews, observations, references, records, forms, and evaluation reports. All compiled data are screened, organized, and interpreted as an information base for assessment. While in behavioral research the *case study method* makes use of individual case studies to make conclusions about general principles, with the individual case study the clinician (counselor) makes conclusions (assessments) about an individual from the case history and other evaluative materials. (The term *case history* refers to all of the recorded facts about the person.)

Note that the root terms *assess, evaluate,* and *measure* refer to the act, whereas an *ing* suffix refers to the process of doing it. The result of the act is denoted by an "ion" or "ment" ending. Thus, the words *assessment, evaluation,* or *measurement* represent concrete results of the process—the material for a report.

APPRAISAL. As a lay term, *appraisal* means the act or report of estimating, judging, or evaluating something's value or amount. An ambiguous word, it is often used without regard to the precision or method of measurement and refers to anything from a personal opinion or rough estimate based upon casual observation to scientifically objective determinations derived from valid data. *Appraise* therefore is a substitute word for assess, evaluate, estimate, measure, or even an "educated guess" based upon informal perception.

PSYCHOMETRY. Popularly seen as synonymous with testing, psychometry refers to the mathematical aspects of psychological procedures. Just as physical scientists use measurement to describe inanimate objects, behavioral scientists use measurement techniques to quantify human attributes. Thus, psychology, as the science of human mental and behavioral characteristics, has developed psychometrics as the theory and technique for mental measurement. A wide array of psychometric test instruments are now available for measuring learning, interests, personality, abilities, aptitudes, and so on.

DIAGNOSIS. The determination of the causes and nature of a condition is referred to as "*diagnosis.*" The judgement of the condition's duration, course, and termination is referred to as "prognosis." In the medical model, these predictive steps are the bases for the treatment plan. As a parallel in the rehabilitation context described above, p. 338, diagnosis is somewhat like evaluation while prognosis shares the predictive implications of assessment for the purpose of planning treatment.

PREDICTED OUTCOMES. Assessment considers not only predictions but also the consequences of the decisions upon the client in terms of the following outcomes: *false positive* (i.e., success was predicted but failure results); *valid positive* (i.e., success was predicted and in fact occurs); *false negative* (i.e., failure was predicted where success should have occurred); and, *valid negative* (i.e., failure was predicted and would in fact occur). These terms represent the effectiveness of the prediction.

TEST. Any mechanism or procedure used to obtain a measure of trait-aptitude, achievement, interest, and so on. Psychological tests usually produce numerical scores that show the degree to which an individual possesses a particular characteristic or quality like intelligence, mechanical aptitude, verbal ability, gregariousness, and so on.

The terms *assessment, evaluation,* and *appraisal* are particularly troublesome as they are used in different ways. Lay dictionaries indicate that the three words are synonymous. On the other hand, *assessment* and *evaluation* have been differentially defined by an authoritative rehabilitation source: the Vocational Evaluation and Work Adjustment Association (VEWAA). As part of a federal rehabilitation agency grant, VEWAA [1975] published a glossary that gave separate definitions for assessment and evaluation; some of the VEWAA notions were observed in formulating the definitions given above. Most importantly, the guidelines derived from the reports of the VEWAA projects are recounted in various chapters. Unfortunately, however, the VEWAA glossary is lacking in clarity; for example, their general definition of evaluation is the "process of assessment against some criteria."

Despite variations in nomenclature as reflected in the quotations and cited references, an attempt at consistency was made in this book. The term *evaluation* is used here as the description of explicit material, while the broader concept of *assessment* is reserved for the overall context of planning. (Exceptions unfortunately appear in direct quotes where the words are used interchangeably by other authors.) The term *assessment* used in the title of this part is appropriate as this reflects its global planning contribution to the rehabilitation process of a handicapped individual.

17.1.2. THE PROCESS

It is evident that the terms *testing, measurement, evaluation, study* and *assessment* are not as different from one another as might be thought; they refer to distinct but overlapping procedures. Regardless of which term is used, certain considerations are always important. In the first place, the procedure should be selected in accordance with the objective; whether it is labeled a test or an evaluation or an assessment does not matter nearly as much as whether it generates information about the individual relative to goals. In the second place, every procedure used should be reliable with respect to obtained scores or results, since any such device is helpful only insofar as it produces accurate and clearly intelligible information. Unless this is the case, results are useless or even deceptive. Finally, it is of the utmost importance that interpretations of data be as unbiased and objective as possible. When a professional's own personal biases intrude into the assessment process, the facts are distorted.

With the development of many different kinds of evaluative devices, it has become increasingly advantageous to utilize various types of procedures. In gathering a wide variety of information about a person, the material must be interpreted together if the relationships are to be understood. This broad information-based (comprehensive case-study) approach to assessment is valuable because of the highly complex, multiple characteristics of all humans and the special measurement needs and problems of some people who are disabled.

17.1.3. PURPOSES

Crow [1973] noted that assessment is one of many interrelated facets of rehabilitation that usually touch upon and influence one another considerably. Viewing the entire process as a combination of many converging functions permits one to understand assessment better as the crucial ingredient in effective rehabilitation.

Galazan [1961] discussed the role of assessment in rehabilitation in terms of three purposes: prediction, determination of a person's strengths and weaknesses for vocational planning, and discovery of how the individual's potential for vocational adjustment can be enhanced.

Prediction, part of the intake stage, is the most general aim of assessment. According to Galazan, prediction is wholly negative in that its purpose is to reveal which individuals may not achieve rehabilitation. The ideal assessment procedure for prediction is one that eliminates all individuals who will be unsuccessful with respect to rehabilitation. If it eliminates some of the potentially successful individuals as well, this is not a very serious problem administratively, particularly in small agencies that cannot handle all potential cases. In rehabilitation there is a gratifying percentage of successes compared to failures. Moreover, there has always been a large waiting list of unserved people who both need and would benefit from services.

Determining people's assets and limitations in order to help them plan their vocational futures is the second purpose of assessment; this has both negative and positive aspects. The identification of strengths is, of course, positive although these "strengths" may sometimes only reflect relatively lesser weaknesses.

Third, assessment is intended to find out what abilities, traits, or skills need to be strengthened in order for an individual to be able to attain a complete vocational adjustment. This form of assessment is entirely positive in that the results are not utilized to eliminate any choices or services but to identify the kinds of services that are appropriate. The general purpose of this assessment approach is typically to fulfill an individual's potential, regardless of what that potential is.

The purposes of assessment in rehabilitation were dealt with by Meister [1976] in Bolton's handbook on this subject. Meister stated that assessment of rehabilitation clients has as its major purpose the identification and exploration of appropriate life alternatives. When tests are utilized for selection, as in the selection of personnel, the purpose of the evaluation is to reveal which job applicants appear to have a greater chance of success; these people are selected while the less promising candidates are excluded. In the rehabilitation process, evaluative instruments are not administered in order to exclude the less promising people. Instead they are used first to determine an individual's strengths and weaknesses and secondly to serve as a starting point for planning a program that takes advantage of the potentials revealed.

Another important point is that in the context of rehabilitation, assessment is not used merely to classify. Categories from other fields, regardless of how accurate and appropriate they are in those fields, may not apply at all or may not apply usefully to rehabilitation planning with a particular individual. It may be learned, for instance, that a client is schizoid or paranoid, but this information may point to the problem without specifying the solution. The effort to discover and enact a solution encompasses the entire rehabilitation process; the assessment function in the rehabilitation process is that of mapping the constructive client variables.

Assessment is not a pass-fail system, even though it results in selection of certain kinds. What is selected are directions for further exploration. Neither is assessment an inventory of client achievements or skills or personality characteristics, because a list does not reflect the dynamics of client development through rehabilitation. A list cannot convey the client's interacting assets and growth potentials, the outside resources available, or the various elements that together compose a successful rehabilitation. Assessment encompasses all these things as the client and the counselor work together, but the whole rehabilitation process is something different from any one of its parts.

Assessment is used for a number of purposes in counseling. These, paraphrased here, were listed by Goldman [1961]:

1. To provide diagnostic data before counseling; to identify the nature of the individual's problem, the degree of its seriousness, and also the kinds of services that may help.
2. To provide information to be used in counseling; to characterize the individual's capabilities, needs, and so on, for use in organizing the counseling process.
3. To provide data the client requires in order to make decisions. Clients need information as they isolate personal and vocational alternatives and other choices.
4. To enable clients to consider new alternatives by giving them information about themselves that they did not previously have. Discover-

ing such information stimulates people to view themselves differently and to scrutinize possibilities more carefully.

5. To establish a basis for subsequent counseling and decision-making; to involve individuals so that they gain a fuller understanding of counseling as a process in which decisions are made.

17.1.4. STEPS

Crow [1973] described three steps in the assessment process: data-gathering, hypothesis formulation, and evaluative interpretation.

In data-gathering a number of procedures are used: interviews; questionnaires; testing (psychological, dexterity, academic achievement); work samples; interest inventories; job tryouts; situational assessments; and physical, medical, and occupational therapy examinations. A number of dangers are associated with data-gathering and certain cautions must be observed. First, there is a tendency to wait until all the information has been gathered before attempting to make decisions. All those concerned should keep in mind that every decision is necessarily made on the basis of inadequate data. Data-gathering should in itself not receive a great deal of attention; rather it should be thought of as the foundation upon which other procedures are based. Another problem in data-gathering can occur when the final assessment is based only on the collected data. It must be based instead upon both the accumulated data and working hypotheses that have been formed.

Formulating and testing hypotheses is the second step in evaluation, the one most often omitted. Early hypotheses should be tentatively stated as the first data becomes available. As the data-collecting continues, hypotheses continue to be made and tested, with earlier ones frequently being modified. The difficulty with making initial hypotheses is that they can become prematurely fixed opinions. When correctly used, hypothesizing about the client should raise additional questions, which in turn lead to further evaluation.

The last stage in the assessment procedure is interpretation of the information that has been collected and the hypotheses that have been tested. From one point of view the end decision is still actually a hypothesis to be tested and perhaps revised; but if the other steps have been

carried out carefully, the wisdom of the final decision will be confirmed.

17.1.5. THE CLIENT

Underlying the entire mechanism is the client's participation and responsibility in the assessment, and making sure of this individual's own understanding of all the findings is the most significant purpose of assessment. Since it is this individual who is most affected by the results, the client must be part of the assessment team. To assure acceptance and use of the results of the assessment, clients should have as much responsibility as possible for how it is conducted [Genskow, 1975].

Rice [1975] discussed the role of vocational assessment clients, whose feelings and needs should be the principle concern of all rehabilitationists. The degree of a client's responsibility as assessment proceeds will be determined by the philosophy and qualifications of the rehabilitation personnel. If those who are working with the client are confident and capable, they will not make choices for the client but will involve the individual in their work as a team. Clients then are not considered as subjects to be dealt with but are accepted and encouraged to develop and assume the decisive role. When clients are properly involved in assessment, better decisions and plans result.

Crow [1973] pointed out that all clients can participate in the assessment procedure; everyone can make life choices despite disabilities—physical and mental—and despite having been led to believe that decision-making is the province of others. Assessment is not a system in which professionals pigeonhole individuals, but rather it is a way of finding and showing the possible alternatives appropriate to the individual. If it is to do this effectively, it must be thought of not as the charge of an expert but as a collaborative process in which all of the rehabilitation team participate in facilitating the client's decisions.

17.1.6. DIMENSIONS

Assessment as a whole may be considered as the entire effort of collecting, examining, and using data to help clients. With this information a picture of the client is drawn that the client can use, with the counselor's help, when choosing an appropriate rehabilitation objective and planning the services needed to obtain this objective.

Data about a client can be presented at four levels of interpretation: (1) descriptive—a statement about what the person is like presently; (2) genetic—an explanation (based on past development) of how the person became this way; (3) predictive—an inference (based on past and present data) that predicts what the person can become; and (4) evaluative—a value judgement (derived from the data and their descriptive, genetic, and/or predictive interpretations) that leads to a decision about what a person should do.

As presented by Fay Smith [Arkansas Rehabilitation Research and Training Center, 1966], some terms that help suggest the nature of assessment and enable the rehabilitation counselor to view it more clearly are:

1. *Scrutinize*: to consider a situation with care, thought, and objectivity, not only as rehabilitation begins but throughout the process.
2. *Analyze*: to process the information as it is collected.
3. *Synthesize*: to organize the data into an intelligible whole, with the parts in clear relation- ship to one another. This makes it possible to tell the client what has been discovered.
4. *Crystallize*: to produce some sort of plan or idea or a set of guidelines from which the client may make a selection. This is a product of the other steps.
5. *Hypothesize*: to select a direction in which to move. Hypotheses are tentative plans that will be tested as the client implements them. Sometimes a hypothesis will need to be discarded because of a change in the situation or because certain circumstances have been overlooked during previous stages.
6. *Capitalize*: to take advantage of the information that has been collected and the work that has been done in order to produce a plan with substance and validity.
7. *Closurize*: to come to the end of the process, even though in rehabilitation the closure may not be final since clients may return if there are changes in their circumstances.

The dimensions of client assessment encompass the whole rehabilitation process and utilize the full range of the professional responsibilities of the counselor.

17.2. *Definitions*

There are a large number of terms that are related to vocational assessment. Many are also relevant to vocational counseling and job placement, covered in subsequent parts of this book. Since these words cut across several major professional areas, the combined nomenclature is substantial. Consequently, these terms, along with their definitions or descriptions, are presented here is several subsections. (Also see 27.1 and 33.2.)

17.2.1. WORK ACTIVITIES

The terms in this subsection describe what workers do. These descriptions of work activities, categorized below, are necessary for vocational assessment. Definitions reported here are primarily from the U.S. Department of Labor, Manpower Administration [1972] as elaborated by Dunn, Korn, and Schneck in 1976.

ELEMENT. The most fundamental segment of work is appropriately called an "element." An element is described as the smallest step into which it is practical to subdivide any work activity without analyzing separate motions, movements, and mental processes involved. Elements are the basic, individual actions a person makes to satisfy work performance requirements. Elements are described through job analysis or time-and-motion studies conducted by an industrial engineer, job analyst, or other technically trained person.

TASK. Work elements are combined in various manners to perform a work "task." A task, made up of one or more elements, is one of the distinct major activities that constitute logical and necessary steps in the work performed by the worker. Furthermore, these tasks are created whenever human effort, in terms of one or more elements, must be exerted for a specific purpose. With the identification and pattern of job tasks of a specified worker, a position description is developed.

POSITION. A position is defined as a group of tasks performed by one person. There are always as many positions as there are workers in a plant or office. Thus, related tasks that exist within a work establishment or environment are combined to form a position for an individual.

JOB. A job is a group of similar positions in a single plant, business establishment, educational institution, or other organization. One or many persons may be employed in the same job. The positions covered by a single job description are identical with respect to their major or significant tasks, and they are sufficiently alike to justify being covered by a single job analysis.

OCCUPATION. A group of similar jobs found in various establishments is an explicit conceptualization for this term.

In 1946 and 1959, Shartle differentiated between position, job, and occupation as they are defined above. Crites [1969] extended Shartle's definition, noting that occupations are analyzed and described through three dimensions: (1) the tasks performed; (2) the work behavior essential to job performance, for example, critical incidence recording [Flanagan, 1954]; and (3) a worker function description, covering occupationally significant characteristics. The last is especially meaningful to rehabilitationists because it focuses upon functional abilities required for a job and, therefore, what transferable skills of the disabled worker can be utilized. Jobs cluster according to occupationally significant characteristics and are so categorized by the U.S. Employment Service.

It is well to conceptualize these terms—*element, task, position, job,* and *occupation*—on a hierarchy from simple to complex: one or more elements form a task, one or more tasks form a position, one or more similar positions in an establishment can be referred to as "a job," while *occupation* refers to the same job in a number of work establishments.

The study of occupations can thus be used in rehabilitation placement although the direct concern is the description of jobs in local establishments. The description of occupational demands (required tasks as well as environmental situations) based on national data must be verified for specific positions.

17.2.2. NAMES FOR WORK

Words expressing work names and activities are often used interchangeably. It is useful, how-

ever, to think and communicate in more explicit terms. Thus, just as work activities were categorized above, so, too, explicit descriptions distinguish between words referring to work: employment, vocation, career, and so forth.

WORK. Work is simply goal-directed activity for social, economic, or other desired accomplishment or outcome. It always calls for the expenditure of effort, the exercise of physical or mental effort, or both, directed toward a specified end. Whether paid or unpaid, the activity is considered "productive work" if the individual and society consider it socially useful. Work is purposeful mental or physical activity, or both, that produces something of value. The most important thing about work is not remuneration but its activity and product.

WORKER. This term applies to any person who is gainfully employed in manual or nonmanual work, whether or not or however remunerated. It thus includes persons working at all levels and sectors of social or economic activity, including salaried employees and professionals, volunteers, and family workers. (In a more restrictive sense, the word means an employee who does not have supervisory functions, but it is not used in that sense in this book.)

EMPLOY. This is a root word meaning "to hire." *Employing* refers to the process of hiring. Employment is therefore the result of the hiring (or retention) act. To be employed means one has been engaged or is being used for work activities. The word *employment* properly refers to having been hired or retained for work—whether paid or not.

VOCATION. Often used interchangeably with *occupation* or *career, vocation* is a broader term connoting one's life-purpose in a work role. Thus, it refers to the pattern of all of an individual's activities that are purposeful, rewarding, and productive. It is the psychological conception of work as a person's productive behavior. As a "person-centered" word it is more likely to be used by the worker than by the employer who is inclined to think in terms of jobs. Unlike the concept of "career," *vocation* refers to what one does at a given period of time.

CAREER. The sequence of employment throughout one's working life is called a "career." It is the total pattern of vocational events over a person's lifetime: the sequence of jobs engaged in while progressing in an occupational structure or changing from one position, job, or occupation to another.

TRADES. A trade is the category of work that requires special qualifications acquired by several years of practical instruction and experience.

CRAFTS. Craft workers or artisans exercise a craft for the production of goods or services. The work is sometimes of an artistic nature, often done manually with the worker's own tools, and often for the worker's own account through self-management. The terms *tradesman, craftsman,* and *journeyman* are used synonymously in some places with respect to manual occupation.

APPRENTICE. Apprentices are trainee-workers who are learning the skill of a trade or craft through an agreement with an employer who is responsible for the training over a period of time of up to several years.

LEVELS OF WORKER QUALIFICATION. The following distinctions may be made as to level of worker qualification: (1) unskilled worker (one who requires only a few hours or days of instruction on the job to perform the duties); (2) semi-skilled worker (one who has been trained to perform a limited number of skilled functions or operations but who has not the all-round technical skills and knowledge required for a recognized trade or other occupation); and (3) skilled worker (one who has acquired the full qualifications required for the performance of a recognized trade or other skilled occupation).

WORK PERSONALITY. This is the part of the total personality that affects behavior, attitudes, values, habits, traits, and other adjustments to work. It is defined as the set of behavior patterns exhibited in a work situation or the manner in which an individual enacts a work role.

WORK THERAPY. Treatment that uses work experience to change the work personality so that the rehabilitant can function appropriately in a normal work situation has been referred to as *work therapy*. It presupposes the ability to control the work environment and to modify the be-

havior of persons in that work setting in accordance with their needs.

17.2.3. LEVELS OF EMPLOYMENT

The concept of employment level is reflected in a variety of terms. This implied hierarchy does not represent value judgements as to "worthwhileness," as all socially or economically useful work is honorable.

COMPETITIVE EMPLOYMENT. This type of employment covers work for remuneration in business, industry, government, or other organizations that exercise selective hiring practices based upon the qualifications of available applicants. In some countries work in the labor market is called "open employment."

STRUCTURAL UNEMPLOYMENT. This refers to long-term or deep-seated joblessness due to changes in an area, industry, or occupation. It is persistent unemployment resulting from the more massive structural or cyclical shifts in the technology and economy. It especially affects the unskilled, uneducated, and handicapped worker who is less adaptable.

FRICTIONAL UNEMPLOYMENT. In any economic society there is never a perfect or immediate matching of available jobs with available people: in one area jobs may be plentiful, in another scarce, but the unemployed in the depressed area may not know where the jobs are or how to get them. Among the frictional unemployed are untrained, first-time, and young workers as well as those who go from job to job.

DESIGNATED EMPLOYMENT SCHEMES. Schemes of this nature imply acceptance of the principle that certain occupations are especially suitable for the disabled and should be reserved for them.

EMPLOYMENT QUOTA. In some countries a compulsion is placed on every employer (or on those having more than a fixed minimum number of employees) to employ a fixed minimum or percentage of disabled persons. In some countries there is also protection against loss of employment.

SUBSIDIZED EMPLOYMENT. In this scheme some wages of the employee or other monetary considerations are offered to induce the employer to hire or retain workers who are not competitive candidates for the work.

TRANSITIONAL EMPLOYMENT. Work in a selected position is designated by a collaborating company to be occupied temporarily by a handicapped client of a supervising rehabilitation placement agency. It is for purposes of (re)entry into the competitive labor market. The term *transitional* is also applied to workshops, with a similar meaning.

ENTRY OCCUPATION. This is an occupation in which a person lacking previous work experience is employed. It may be the least desirable of jobs in a plant in terms of pay, working conditions, strenuous physical requirements, and low qualifications. Union or management requirements that all new employees—or low seniority workers—must work at entry jobs can preclude employment for some disabled people who must have sedentary work.

EXTENDED EMPLOYMENT. Sheltered workshops use this term to refer to the employment status of a client who remains in the workshop many months (e.g., 18 or more) with marginal possibility of regular employment outside of a sheltered environment. Sometimes this is called *terminal employment*, but efforts are being made to use the term *extended*. (Chapter 8, Rehabilitation Facilities, has a description of work-oriented activities.)

17.2.4. OCCUPATIONAL INFORMATION

Knowledge of a substantial number of occupational information terms is essential in the assessment and placement of handicapped people.

OCCUPATIONAL INFORMATION. As it is used, this term means any and all kinds of information regarding any position, job, or occupation, provided only that the information is potentially useful to a person who is looking for work or choosing an occupation. Occupational information is pertinent facts about jobs and their characteristics and requirements for use in vocational assessment, counseling, and placement. Closely related to occupational information is information about educational and training opportunities, referred to as *educational information*. Other types of information that may be

used with counselees are social, personal, and recreational.

DICTIONARY OF OCCUPATIONAL TITLES (D.O.T.). The *D.O.T.* is published by the U.S. Department of Labor, Employment and Training Administration [1977]. It provides standardized occupational titles with descriptive information on most jobs in the American economy—2100 occupations with over 20,000 job definitions. Also provided is a classification structure under which these occupations are arranged according to interrelationships.

OCCUPATIONAL OUTLOOK HANDBOOK. This handbook is published biennially by the U.S. Department of Labor, Bureau of Labor Statistics [1980]. It describes nearly 1000 occupations and major industries. The descriptions include the nature of the work, places of employment, training, other qualifications, advancement, employment outlook, earnings, working conditions, and sources of further information.

OCCUPATIONAL CLASSIFICATION. This scheme gives: a systematic grouping of jobs according to significant factors involved in the job or group of jobs; the process of determining a title and *D.O.T.* code number to be assigned to an application or job order; and the title or code of a job or group of jobs for which an applicant is qualified.

OCCUPATIONAL LEVEL. Occupational level refers to the amount of prestige associated with an occupation, the size of the income typically earned, the degree of authority wielded, the freedom of action involved, the amount of education required, the amount of intelligence required, and similar, although not perfectly correlated, variables.

JOB DESCRIPTIONS. A job description is organized information that identifies, defines, and provides a detailed picture of the duties, responsibilities, and qualifications of a job. It is used largely for hiring new workers, and the items the interviewer should take into consideration in the selection are clearly stated.

JOB FAMILY. This term identifies a cluster of jobs grouped together on the basis of common job or worker characteristics. The grouping may be based upon work done; tools, machines, or other work aids used; materials worked with; knowledge and skill required; and worker characteristics needed for successful performance.

WORKER TRAITS. The significant characteristics required of the worker to perform the functions of an occupation are called worker traits—aptitudes, general educational development, vocational preparation, physical demands, and personal traits. These are reflected in: training time, aptitudes, temperaments, interest, physical demands, and environmental conditions.

PRODUCTION WORK. This type of work refers to any manufacturing or processing in which many units of a similar kind are produced. This kind of work ordinarily lends itself to division of labor and can be seen in both competitive industry as well as rehabilitation workshops.

PRODUCTION WORK EVALUATION. This evaluation approach is a method of evaluating handicapped clients through the use of actual industrial work brought into the evaluation facility. It is possible for the evaluation staff to vary all the customary conditions of the real job in an effort to discover difficulties that might prevent the client from working effectively in competitive employment.

SIMULATED WORK. Artificially developed standardized work activities carried on under control situations are used as a means of evaluating the handicapped person's ability to perform work and function in a work situation.

SITUATIONAL EVALUATION. This term covers observing, recording, and comparing a workshop client to a realistic standard of essential worker characteristics (e.g., habits, attitudes, skills).

SIMULATED JOB STATION. This term refers to a work setting that has the following characteristics: replication of the tasks and other aspects of a job or work process, control by the evaluator, and a location within an evaluation facility. Pay to the client is not necessarily a component of the simulation.

RESIDUAL WORK CAPACITY. A disabled person's remaining physical and mental work potential and capacity is known as *residual work ca-*

pacity. It can be considered when determining suitable employment, whether sheltered or competitive.

SELECTIVE PLACEMENT. Selective placement is a process used for placing disabled people in employment suited to their age, experience, qualifications, and physical and mental capacities. It requires comprehensive vocational assessment of the assets and needs of the disabled person. It also requires complete job descriptions. This is the final stage of rehabilitation and includes three distinct processes: knowing the worker, knowing the job, and matching the worker to the job.

17.2.5. PHYSICAL DEMAND OF WORK

The International Labor Office, as well as the U.S. Employment Service, categorizes the physical demands of work according to a hierarchy, from sedentary to very heavy, of five levels.

SEDENTARY WORK. The demand is lifting 10 pounds, maximum, and occasionally lifting and/or carrying such articles as dockets, ledgers, and small tools. Although a sedentary job is defined as one that involves sitting, a certain amount of walking and/or standing is often necessary—or permitted—in carrying out job duties. Jobs are considered sedentary if walking and standing are required only occasionally and other sedentary criteria are met.

LIGHT WORK. The demand is lifting 20 pounds, maximum, with frequent lifting and/or carrying of objects weighing up to 10 pounds. Even though the weight lifted may be only of a negligible amount, a job is in this category when it requires walking or standing to a significant degree, or when it involves sitting most of the time with a degree of pushing and pulling of arm and/or leg controls.

MEDIUM WORK. The demand is lifting 50 pounds maximum with frequent lifting and/or carrying of objects of up to 25 pounds.

HEAVY WORK. The demand is lifting 100 pounds, maximum, with frequent lifting and/or carrying of objects weighing up to 50 pounds.

VERY HEAVY WORK. The demand is lifting objects in excess of 100 pounds with frequent lifting and/or carrying of objects weighing 50 pounds or more.

17.3. Comprehensive Assessment

The unique character and much of the effectiveness of the rehabilitation movement, Hardy and Cull [1969] pointed out, can be attributed to the fact that services are individualized. One of the principal reasons for this emphasis is the rehabilitation worker's traditional concern with thorough assessment. The necessity for comprehensive and more effective assessment has become stronger as the variety of services has increased and the problems with which rehabilitation is concerned have become more complicated. Vocational and life adjustment will be only minimal unless rehabilitation assessment is done well.

17.3.1. DISSECTING ASSESSMENT

It is unwise to stress only one part of the assessment, to view one element against another. Total assessment is what gives rehabilitation its effectiveness; it is the foundation of the whole process.

Assessment can be dissected only theoretically and for the purpose of discussion. In practice the process is not divisible. Assessment concerns not just medical evaluation, not just work evaluation, not just psychological evaluation. Rather, it is a process that deals with whole human beings.

17.3.2. DIMENSIONS

In determining the handicapping effect of disability on an individual, an analysis of the following dimensions is necessary:

1. Medical or biological. What limitations in function are imposed by the disability?
2. Functional limitations. What vocational and other problems result from these limitations in function?
3. Psychological. What problems are self-imposed by the individual (i.e., are the result of personality characteristics)?
4. Sociocultural. What problems are imposed by societal forces, particularly those in the immediate environment (i.e., family, peers, community)?
5. Educational. What problems are imposed by deficits in education and training or marketable job skills?
6. Vocational. What problems are imposed by circumstances in the labor market.
7. Personal independence. What problems interfere with living independently in the community?

By considering the effect of the disabling condition on the functioning of the individual, as well as the environmental variables operative in the situation, it is possible to determine the degree and types of handicap(s) impinging on the individual [U.S. IRS, 1973b]. More importantly, it is possible to plan strategies for countering these handicaps.

17.3.3. THE TOTAL BEING

The basic requirements of an individual are inextricably intertwined; people do not have distinct physical, mental, vocational, and financial needs. An individual is a combination of all these and much else and must be treated as a whole [Parham, 1977].

While comprehensive assessment may vary in details from one individual to another or from one place to another, a number of fundamental evaluations must be carried out if one is to put together a complete picture of a severely handicapped person. Most important are the medical, psychological, social, educational, familial, cultural, and vocational components. All are significant in the context of the individual's environment for determining how a handicapped person will adapt.

17.3.4. CLUSTERING PRINCIPLE

Within the context of rehabilitation it is important to remember that pathological conditions tend to come in clusters, as evidenced by the high incidence of multiple congenital abnormalities. Physicians who see one anomaly in a newborn infant routinely examine the baby carefully for other evidences of defect and frequently find one or more other abnormalities. The clustering principle is operating when trauma involving one system of the body is associated with or followed by problems in other systems. Research in social pathology has shown how conditions such as poverty, unemployment, poor education, delinquency, crime, and mental illness occur in clusters. In a family a problem such as severe illness or behavioral maladjustment is inevitably attended by disturbances in the health and welfare of the whole group [Straus, 1965].

17.3.5. HOLISTIC CONCEPT

As characterized by Straus, the holistic concept of behavior emphasizes the relationships among conventionally separated aspects of human behavior: they are not separate but continually affect and depend on one another. Therefore, whenever one wishes to understand one facet of behavior one must take into account the nature of human biology and the limitations it imposes on behavior. One must consider as well the components of a personality—its typical modes of feeling, thinking, and so on; the physical surroundings—natural, geographical, and man-made; the social nature of human beings and the influence of the social context on an individual; the quality of a culture and the influence it exerts; and a person's relationship to time as a way of organizing behavior.

The holistic point of view is in large part a protest against the tendency toward fragmentation that typified much scientific and humanistic endeavor during the first half of this century. (See 1.2.1.)

Chapter 18

Assessment Processes

Vocational assessment is a broad field involving various professions and utilizing a variety of evaluative techniques. Its applicability is not limited to people who are disabled, since medical (disability) evaluation is only one of several assessment considerations. However, limitations in functions so complicate the normal problems of vocational adjustment that comprehensive assessment is often indicated. As a consequence rehabilitation has pioneered in the development of work evaluation for severely disabled clients.

Traditional vocational assessment methods were generally restricted to psychological testing, school grade reports and other records, occupational information, and vocational guidance. School guidance and employment service counselors still use these methods satisfactorily with many of their clients. Rehabilitation planning, however, has always included more extensive evaluation, for example, house calls by the rehabilitation counselor and medical examinations authorized by the rehabilitation agency. Work evaluation is a still further expansion of the rehabilitation assessment process. While comprehensive assessment is not conducted with every rehabilitant, extensive information is usually required for severely handicapped people who have few or undetected or underdeveloped vocational attributes.

Traditional assessment and counseling did not have much access to evaluative observations and data based directly upon the client's work behavior. While there were tests to measure vocational aspects they were administered in a office rather than a work setting. The use of work itself in real and simulated situations, under professional observation and with norms to estimate client performance, is relatively new. The technique is called "work evaluation" in this book. *Vocational evaluation* is a more popular label and seems to be preferred by many rehabilitationists engaged in work evaluation, although they do use the two terms interchangeably. The title *vocational evaluator* became established in the 1970s and appears throughout the rehabilitation literature.

Vocational evaluation as a rehabilitation term is internally inconsistent: the word *vocation* has a broad meaning while the word *evaluation* has a narrow meaning. Evaluations contribute information components that are required in assessment as a planning function of vocational counseling. Choosing a vocation—particularly for a handicapped person—requires various kinds of evaluations (i.e., medical, educational, social, psychological, and work). As an investigatory process, each component is properly referred to as an evaluation; but, the integrating and planning process is the assessment phase of vocation counseling (see 27.3.1). In public rehabilitation the counselor is legally responsible for vocational planning. In fact, the assessment-planning function is so basic to vocational counseling in any setting that it cannot be delegated.

Rehabilitation counselors are professionally

trained to assemble and interpret the various components of evaluative information in order for clients to make informed occupational decisions; while they may not personally conduct all of the evaluations, they have the ultimate responsibility for the adequacy of the data (i.e., the accuracy, relevancy, and sufficiency of planning information). While evaluation information may be compiled by other professionals and specialists, rehabilitation counselors coordinate and interpret to the client the total evaluation in the planning process (see 3.2.2.). In some areas (e.g., psychological testing) the rehabilita-

tion counselor may assume full responsibility or may delegate the collection of data to a team member. While work evaluation is quite reasonably viewed as an inherent function of the rehabilitation counselor, it is frequently assigned to a specialist. These specialists (work evaluators)—usually employed in rehabilitation facilities—are not, typically, professionally educated counselors but many are trained in work evaluation (see 2.4.1). Views on these issues were stated by Sink and Porter [1978] in a publication jointly sponsored by NRCA and VEWAA.

18.1. Strategy

Collecting information and making decisions in sequence is a fundamental strategy in assessment. It is necessary to determine what decision must be made and to establish whether the information that has been gathered is adequate for the purpose. If adequate information is available, the decision is made; if not, enough additional data is collected to make it possible. This method is efficient and easy to apply to most human service situations; it is used in rehabilitation with a five-level assessment process.

The first rehabilitation assessment level is a screening phase; it consists of a study that establishes that a person is medically disabled, is functionally limited, is handicapped, and requires a service offered by the agency. In this preliminary case study the interview is the fundamental tool; the rehabilitationist weighs heavily the things clients say about their condition and life experiences. One also uses the kind of referral information routinely conveyed by the referring agency, such as reports from testing and physical examinations.

The second level of the assessment process is comprised of an in-depth collection of diagnostic data over a broad range of conditions relevant to adjustment: medical, psychological, social, occupational, and so on. The rehabilitation counselor and client collaborate in identifying information needed for planning and then proceed to answer their questions. Answers are sought through diagnostic examinations, records and reports, and counseling. This is often called the

clinical stage because it is characterized by thorough counseling. (Actually, though, all of the five levels of assessment involve much direct client contact of a counseling or other "clinical" nature.)

The third assessment level, work evaluation, consists of direct observation of the client's work habits, ability to learn particular work skills, and capacity to acquire the attitudes, tolerances, and behaviors needed for effective work performance. Actual and simulated work situations are used so that the client can be appraised and a plan devised to help the person to adapt successfully to employment. The environment is controlled and the client is observed, usually for several days, so that interpretation of the client's work-related characteristics can be incorporated into the evaluation. Work evaluation is appropriate when it is not feasible through more efficient methods to determine what level of vocational functioning an individual has currently or can be expected to achieve through work adjustment or other rehabilitation services. While this level may be skipped with many clients, it is often required for rehabilitants who have functional limitations that are multiple, severe, and poorly described. A variation of work evaluation may be used with independent living rehabilitation cases (see 40.2.2).

Planning for adjustment is the fourth level assessment process and is always a part of rehabilitation service. It is determined in this phase that adequate data have been gathered for informed decision-making. The rehabilitation counselor helps the client to understand the information in order to decide upon a wise course of action. Counseling is crucial to this phase for the plan to be of the client's own making. The individualized written rehabilitation program is the product of this assessment process.

The fifth level of assessment occurs throughout adjustment or other rehabilitation services (e.g., job training, starting a business, placement) and continues until the case is closed. Client evaluation techniques are applicable while the client is in job training, job try-out, and employment follow-along or follow-up by the counselor. Additional sources of evaluative information—trainers, supervisors—are routinely checked and previous evaluations (medical, psychological, and so on) may be expanded or updated if indicated. (In the early years of rehabilitation counseling this fifth level of client assessment was known as "supervision of services.") With successful case closure this is the culminating level of rehabilitation assessment.

Assessment that proceeds through these five levels is comprehensive, cost-efficient, direct, economical, and effective. The strategy moreover respects the individual's right to make a decision on the basis of valid information and with professional counseling. Every client who participates is ultimately responsible for self-determination within the framework of agency eligibility and service provisions, but by virtue of the assessment and counseling strategy, the client's decisions are information-based.

18.1.1. ASSUMPTIONS

It is necessary for rehabilitationists to be knowledgeable about theories of vocational psychology and human behavior (see 25.3 and 27.2.2). But theory cannot fully explain the nature of vocational choice and the meaning of work. Consequently practical experience in the world of work is also needed.

Certain assumptions are fundamental to rehabilitation client evaluation. From a theoretical standpoint evaluation can be considered a way of obtaining data about handicapped individuals. As an empirical procedure evaluation specifies what client characteristics are to be measured and identifies the elements that contribute to vocational adjustment. The theoretical elements

related here, from the discussion of Gellman and Soloff [1976], are some of the considerations that affect client evaluation.

The Work Sector

In an industrial culture the work sector is separated from other aspects of life such as the domestic and educational realms. The work sector is comprised of a number of components such as productive activity, work-related endeavors, and by-products of work. It is distinguished by purposeful behavior that is geared toward achievement and that utilizes learned behavioral modes and skills; it has various kinds of rewards for the worker, which may or may not include financial remuneration. But whether or not wages are paid, all productive activities are economically useful for society.

The Work Personality

A person's work personality is the configuration of responses that are revealed by the person in a productive situation. The work personality is a combination of attitudes, behavioral modes, concepts of value, incentives, and capabilities; it is needed if an individual is to function appropriately in a work setting. These personal qualities influence satisfactory function while choosing and preparing for a job, seeking a job, and performing it.

Development Aspects

The work personality is a product of growth; its formation begins very early in life and its development normally continues during childhood and young adulthood. People growing up in an industrial culture get their motivation and their desire to succeed from the family; the knowledge and training needed in order for an individual to live up to the family's standards come from educational experiences and extracurricular activities. Usually children are able to do family and self-care chores—assuming a productive role—at an early age. Most young adults learn about the responsibilities and rewards of competitive employment through summer and part-time jobs. An individual's introduction to the work sector culminates with the first full-time job, in which the work personality matures. When functional limitations prevent or delay this sequence of developmental experiences and introduction to the work sector, one's work personality is retarded.

Work Roles

The term *work role* refers to the behavior deemed appropriate for the work. The appropriate role varies according to expectations of the culture, the period, the occupation, the tasks assigned, the job setting, the interpersonal environment, the remuneration or other rewards for productivity, and the employer. It is somewhat influenced by the employee's work personality —to the extent that the worker can mold job expectations. But generally one's work personality is typed for appropriateness to standards of the work role under consideration. There may not be much flexibility in the pattern of work personality that fits a specified work role. But fortunately there is as wide a variation in the roles of the environment of the world of work as in the work personalities of workers in the population.

Job adjustment and *work environment* are two terms that relate to the concept of work role. The degree of job adjustment to a work environment depends upon the extent of the compatibility between the work personality of the disabled individual and the work role requirements of the work environment. The work environment consists of three elements: (1) the work itself, with its requirements for various worker attributes; (2) the physical surroundings with their demands; and (3) the social interrelationships between workers and employers. The employee's work roles must correspond, on at least a minimal level, with the qualities and behaviors considered appropriate to the given work environment.

Work evaluation, the estimation of future work behavior in a client, is based on the premise that the work personality has a degree of continuity. It is assumed that the work personality that is revealed in a transitional workshop will be like the work personality in real work situations. The forces that molded the work personality of the younger person for a particular set of employment situations influence the work patterns of the mature individual. However, work personalities can also be changed. People are likely to change when they encounter a drastically different situation, such as moving from a state of dependency to a work setting.

Evaluation therefore must be considered as a way of finding the forces, both external and internal, that may alter development of the client's work personality.

Employability, Work Evaluation, and Adjustment

The relationships among employability, work evaluation, and adjustment were discussed by Dunn [1971a]. Work adjustment training focuses principally on the way an individual relates to the work environment. Work environments were characterized by Lofquist and Dawis [1969] as demanding and reinforcing certain capacities. These researchers described the work personality as a mixture of capabilities and needs. The relationship between the work environment and the personality of the worker provides material on which forecasts of tenure and effectiveness can be based.

The "general work environment" is a set of requirements (e.g., attending and being on time) and reinforcing elements (e.g., pay and promotion) common to all work environments. The general work environment can also be said to require particular minimum ability levels and minimum levels of responsiveness to reinforcement. These minimum requirements mean that there are certain critical vocational behaviors such as regular attendance and promptness, appropriate interpersonal conduct, productivity, and meeting standards of work quality. The critical behaviors also include responsiveness to reinforcers such as monetary payment, social rewards, and the personal importance of being useful.

Employability depends upon the correspondence between the work personality and the general work environment. The critical vocational behaviors delimit employability; to be employable an individual must demonstrate each and every one of the critical behaviors required in the general work environment. Work adjustment training is aimed at altering the unemployable individual's work personality so that it bears enough relationship with the work environment to warrant a prediction that the person will be able to perform a job at an acceptable level of effectiveness and with a needed amount of satisfaction. Employability is achieved when those elements of the work personality that were inconsistent with the work environment are sufficiently altered.

18.1.2. GUIDELINES

Gellman [1968] presented a number of principles to serve as guidelines for vocational assessment. Underlying them was the assumption that this endeavor has as its foundation a set of theories about the work personality, the work sector, and the objectives toward which vocational rehabilitation must be aimed. The following guidelines are substantial revisions from Gellman's list.

1. The perspective of vocational assessment is toward the future in order to forecast vocational growth and behavior.
2. Vocational assessment is individualized.
3. The findings of vocational assessment are formulated as if-then statements.
4. A treatment (service) strategy is part of the plan.
5. The client's progress and the accuracy of predictions are monitored as a continuing assessment measure.
6. It is assumed that clients' behavior can and does alter as a result of rehabilitation treatment.
7. The rehabilitationist involved in vocational assessment must have comprehensive knowledge of the resources that can aid a particular client with a particular problem.
8. The goal of vocational assessment is to help clients select and adapt to a suitable work environment.
9. Familiarity with the demands of the labor market is necessary for vocational assessment.
10. Vocational assessment originates with the need for rehabilitation and goes on throughout the entire process. It ends when rehabilitation is complete, when the client is placed and is performing a job at the level believed to represent the individual's best ability.
11. Vocational assessment incorporates the expertise of people from every relevant professional field for multi-faceted evaluation components.
12. The usefulness of vocational assessment is a function of the usefulness of the questions it raises for rehabilitation counseling. It entails

two phases: one in which working questions are framed and their relevance to the client tentatively established; and one in which the earlier questions are revised in accordance with findings from the first phase.

18.1.3. GOALS

The goals of vocational assessment were characterized by Gellman and Soloff [1976]. The ultimate goal is to make it possible for handicapped people to gain in productivity so that they can adapt effectively to work environments, whether financial reward is involved or not. Through observation of the work personality, evaluators can establish what an individual can and cannot do and the kind of relationship a person can be expected to form with various work environments.

Prediction is a second goal. Because vocational assessment is instrumental, it must focus on the future. It must attempt to characterize a client's future work personality on the basis of a work setting that functions as a kind of laboratory, and it also anticipates how the client will evolve vocationally. From workshop observations, evaluators try to picture what alterations will take place, keeping in mind a number of questions: whether the individual will be capable of working, what kinds of work will be possible, how the client will adapt to future work environments, and what training or other rehabilitation treatment is appropriate. All these questions involve the usual concerns of evaluation with skills, abilities, interests, and physical tolerances. In order to predict, however, the evaluator considers expected changes in work behavior as well as present characteristics.

Third, assessment is intended to identify modes of behavior and measure adjustment levels as the client responds to different work environments. Predictive equations, or expressions of the client's responses in a work situation, are used to do this. The equations take the form of if-then statements, expressing what the client will do if certain conditions are present; they are formulated on the basis of client characteristics and portray the individual's responses to changing aspects of the work setting. At the basis of the equations are hypotheses that can be validated in a quasi-experimental way in the workshop and in actual employment situations.

The fourth goal of vocational assessment is to design a treatment strategy, which becomes a guide for choosing the programs that will enable the client to learn appropriate work behaviors. The strategy is based on an understanding of the individual's work personality and its potential, appraisal of how the limitations will influence the work personality, estimation of the likelihood that the client will learn to compensate for the limitations, prediction of the client's (future) vocational capabilities, examination of ability to benefit from training, and descriptions of the work environments suitable to the individual's possible occupations.

The techniques used for vocational assessment depend on staff, agency, and client variables (e.g., needs, competencies, goals). Whatever techniques are employed, evaluation produces a characterization of the work personality, forecasts of work behavior, a prediction about the extent to which the client can alter this behavior, and a statement about how well the client is able to adjust to different work environments. Four basic methods are used. Work behavior is appraised by observing the client in a work setting. Learning ability in a work environment is estimated by means of situational techniques, on the basis of the client's ability to solve problems and alter behavior as necessitated; the ability to learn skills is measured by tests. Finally, the psychological and social effects of a work situation on the work personality are examined by means of observation of the client's responses to the work environment and to other people within it [Gellman, 1968].

18.2. Interpretation

Some human characteristics can be measured, but most psychological characteristics must be evaluated through inference from behavior because they cannot be directly observed. Nevertheless the understanding of these psychological characteristics is essential in vocational assessment. Most important for vocational assessment are those long-term, stable characteristics referred to as "traits." Interpretation is the evaluator's bridge from abstract data to meaningful reality.

18.2.1. MAKING INFERENCES

Kelly [1967] discussed the steps involved in making inferences about traits from observation of behavior. It is assumed that behavior depends upon people themselves and the circumstances to which they are reacting. In observing variations in behavior among individuals in the same circumstances, one can reasonably conclude that the differences result from disparities in traits. To evaluate, one observes behaviors in standardized situations and infers the status of each individual with relationship to various traits.

Verbs in our language are used to depict behavior. A person "discusses" a problem, "smiles" at co-workers, "helps" a stranger cross the street. Adverbs or adverbial construc-

tions are used to depict the behavior in more detail: the person discusses the problem "intelligently," smiles "warmly," "voluntarily" helps the stranger. The adverbs modify only the activity expressed by the verb; they do not imply qualities in the individual's personality.

But the next step is to make such an inference. Because of the intelligent discussion, one infers that the person is intelligent; from the smile the inference is that the person is warm or friendly. When this step is made and the transition from adverbs to adjectives is completed, the process of evaluation has begun. The last step is to use nouns instead of adjectives. This person is said to possess intelligence, warmth, and so on. It is important to notice that the trait is wholly a construct, that it has not itself been observed; its existence is something inferred.

18.2.2. TYPES OF INFORMATION

Many different forms of data are gathered in the assessment process. Much of it is expressive, that is, it has been communicated by the client in interviews. Data can also be manifest; this is information about what the client has done.

Test scores that can be related to some kind of criterion are a legitimate source of information upon which to base predictions. In the same way the kinds of facts sought are those that can be used to make predictive estimations. For instance, research has shown that students with a high score on the Miller Analogies Test (MAT) are more likely to succeed in graduate study in fields such as rehabilitation counselor education (RCE). The MAT score consequently is one type of information that can be used to screen RCE applicants.

Regardless of what the origin of information is, the principle obtains. If a fact is to be incorporated into an interpretation, one must know that there is a relationship between the fact and the conclusions one is drawing. Basically, data that does not come from tests must be verified in the same way as information obtained from tests [Goldman, 1971].

Cronbach [1970] dealt with classification of tests, in terms of form, objective, content, and other such characteristics. He divided tests into two categories, those designed to determine maximum performance and those intended to measure typical performance. The former are used when it is desirable to find out what an individual's potential is; these are called ability tests. The other kind of test is used to find out what an individual will characteristically do under certain circumstances. Personality and interest tests are of this type, since descriptions like "lacking in self-confidence," "interested in music," and "anxious when uncertain of others' expectations" are typical responses.

18.2.3. ASSUMPTIONS

A number of assumptions underlie vocational assessment and particularly the evaluations made in rehabilitation counseling and planning.

1. Clients have the right to make decisions about their own future based upon adequate information about themselves and their options.
2. Clients are able to develop plans with properly interpreted assessment information through counseling.
3. Dynamic observation is more accurate than static examination: a set of observations that have been made over an extended time period, ideally in a continuous manner, is preferable to a single examination or a couple of separate examinations.
4. Observation of the behavior of an individual is best made in a real-life situation.
5. The instruments must be chosen with the in-

dividual in mind because functional limitations, age, sex, education, cultural background, and other such considerations may influence test accuracy.
6. Prediction is best based upon material from past evaluations of similar people.
7. The most effective evaluation takes into account the person as a unique individual with a pattern of strengths and weaknesses, a particular history and present situation, and a unique combination of needs and drives.
8. Assessment is most effective when evaluations are done by a team of people from various fields contributing information.
9. The assessment of severely disabled individuals—because of the special problems involved and the time needed to observe development potential—may be a prolonged process.

18.2.4. TREATMENT OF THE DATA

There are several rather drastically different methods of treating and interpreting data.

Statistical Treatment of Data

Objective procedures are required to link test scores with human qualities or behaviors. Bolton, Lawlis, and Brown [1976] discussed the procedures by which test scores are interpreted. The raw scores obtained from psychological tests are almost always used in conjunction with other kinds of information about how the test was designed and how other people have performed on it. The three major ways in which test scores can be interpreted are the criterion-referenced method, the predictive method, and the normative method.

Criterion-referenced tests take a sampling of the characteristics or abilities needed to accomplish an objective. The interpretation, then, depends upon the a priori assessment by experts of the appropriateness of the test. Educational achievement tests and occupational trade tests are especially suitable for criterion-referencing.

The predictive interpretation of scores involves verifying the test results by determining how closely the test scores and later performance in the relevant area are related. For instance, statistics suggest how probable it is that a respondent with a particular score will finish a training program in automobile mechanics.

The normative method is the most frequently

used. Raw scores are translated into standard scores that show how the respondent's results compare to scores among a norm group (people with known characteristics).

Clinical Treatment of Data

The clinical approach is mostly subjective and less precise, and according to some research the mechanical approach of relying solely on test data is just as effective. However, the clinical method usually is necessary because the issues are so very complex that statistical prediction tables are unavailable. The vocational counselor of course draws upon a store of knowledge that is the basis for clinical prediction. Thus the interpreter using the clinical method performs mentally some of the statistical operations upon which mechanical interpretations are based.

Types of Interpretation

The various kinds of interpretation are characterized by the questions appropriate to them. In descriptive interpretation, one asks what kind of person the man or woman is. How well does this person grasp spatial relations? How does this woman feel about the responsibilities of motherhood? How does this man's verbal skills compare with his nonverbal skills? How does this individual like to spend leisure time?

When interpreting data genetically, the evaluator asks how the person got this way. Is a person's reading deficiency a result of physical or emotional problems or a lack of skills? Does an individual's distaste for work with the hands originate in the attitudes of parents or failure experiences or is it just a matter of preference?

Predictive interpretation seeks to forecast how well a client will do in a given education or training program or other endeavor, how fulfilling contrasting occupations would be for this person, and so on. In evaluative interpretation, the counselor tries to find answers to questions relevant to a preferred course of action, such as the selection of a school or occupation.

Essentially, as one moves away from descriptive toward evaluative interpretation one's distance from the facts increases. The only objective of the descriptive approach is to portray the individual at the present time. In interpreting genetically and predictively the perspective is away from the present but toward the past in one instance and the future in the other. An evaluative estimation incorporates judgmental

statements with other forms of interpretation and verges on decision-making [Goldman, 1971].

18.2.5. APPROACHES

The interpretation stage is one of the most critical phases of evaluation, according to Goldman [1964], whose discussion of the subject is related here. When data about an individual have been gathered, they must be reshaped to express probabilities about the person's future. This means that all data interpretation contains an element of estimation and therefore may be inaccurate. Descriptive interpretations, such as a statement that an individual is energetic or that a person likes music, are actually no more than expressions of probability derived from limited observation.

Interpretation is as yet in the early stages of development as an art. Even expert interpreters are severely hampered by the fact that there are few established connections between test scores and future criteria. There is not much predictive data upon which to build accurate and reliable interpretations. This is equally true of nontest information such as avocational pursuits and how they relate to vocational outcomes.

The evaluator must bridge the gap between the data, whether test or nontest information, and interpretation. This involves, with test results, finding out what the scores mean in a context other than the test, for instance, what the score implies about the person's effectiveness in an occupation or training program. In descriptive rather than predictive terms the test might indicate some of the individual's characteristic feelings or behavior. The score does not actually measure potential success or personal characteristics but measures the individual's reactions to certain stimuli in a particular situation. Any conclusion drawn from the test scores necessitates the making of inferences—going beyond the test data. For such generalization, descriptive or predictive, there must be a demonstrated relationship between the test data and the interpreted characteristic or behavior [Goldman, 1971].

The various steps and the order in which they occur are similar for statistical and clinical interpretation. The first step in both is to choose information relevant to the assessment question, the information needed by this client to develop a rehabilitation plan. The second step is quite different for the two methods, as this is the stage at which the statistical interpreter refers to a formula or table and finds equivalent values. The clinical interpreter, however, must assimilate information from a number of sources, sorting out inconsistencies and deciding how much weight to place on each type of information; the problems involved in making this decision may account for the relative popularity of the statistical method. Vocational assessors frequently do not place proper weights on their data; they may put too much emphasis on one type of information, they may be influenced unduly by the source of information, they may be biased by extraneous characteristics of the client, or they may fail to consider all of the accumulated facts, having made prejudgments from initial reports and impressions. Recency of information may also unduly influence the final decision. When using the clinical method it is necessary to perform mentally those operations that are done in statistical interpretation through computation. For example, the relative importance of spatial visualization ability, mathematical achievement, and fine finger dexterity for a given occupation must be estimated so that the appropriate weight can be assigned to each. In addition, other kinds of information about the person and the occupation must be considered.

In the third step the two methods differ also, because statistical procedures produce a quantitative expression of probabilities and the clinical technique yields a qualitative expression that is subjective. The interpretations that result from the two methods, it is important to note, vary in the extent to which they can be reproduced. The statistical interpretation is always the same, but the clinical interpretation is something that will vary according to the evaluator, the time, and the client, even when the information is basically similar. The element of variability is sometimes an advantage of the clinical approach. It may be that a particular client is unusual enough to lead the interpreter to take an unaccustomed step. Or the interpreter may have learned about a new local resource and decides to reject a prediction now outdated. While the statistical prediction is not subject to the errors in judgment of clinical prediction, the vocational assessor may have far more information available to make clinical interpretations.

The last stage of clinical interpretation can take two different forms. A picture of the client can be compared with a schematic representation of the typical effective worker in a given occupation. Alternatively the interpreter does not compare two descriptive pictures but attempts to estimate how this individual would respond to the challenges and opportunities of the given occupation.

More work needs to be done if the interpretation process is to be more completely understood. At the present time the statistical method has limited application, for the principal reason that the predictive procedures that have been devised have been applied to so few occupations, preparation programs, and institutions; interpretation would be better however if the available techniques were completely utilized. The limitations of the clinical method, on the other hand, stem from the failings of evaluators, from lack of familiarity with people and the techniques for learning about them, from illogical thinking, and from poor vocational and educational knowledge.

There is need for a combined approach, using statistical predictions whenever available and appropriate, but also for employing well-qualified counselors to interpret both statistical and clinical material.

Correlational Approach

Developing and interpreting tests have been primarily the domain of correlational methods, which seek to evaluate people in order to select appropriate schools, occupations, and so on. Mainly the object is to determine which of a number of possible alternatives will probably prove most suitable. The client is told what can be expected in terms of the amount of effort that will be required and the likelihood of success among various occupational choices. Vocational assessors rely on description and correlation. They draw a portrait of the client, look for relationships between personal characteristics and the requirements of different occupations, and make the most suitable match.

Experimental Approach

In contrast to the correlation method, the experimental approach deals less with the variations among people than with the ways in which divergent courses of action will tend to influence people. Assumed is the notion that people's surroundings can be altered so as to improve their opportunities to adapt more satisfactorily. The effort is to control the elements of the environment—the equipment, the rewards, the tasks—in order to find out what variables increase adaptation in the clients. The approach has implications for the rehabilitationist who can try out different environmental circumstances to determine what is most suitable for the client. Also one can see how a particular job could be altered so that it could be performed by the disabled worker.

Synthesis of Approaches

These various approaches can be used in combination to enhance the quality of evaluation. On the one hand clients can receive evaluative information identifying suitable work preparation programs and suitable jobs. On the other hand, changes can be made to help clients fulfill more of their potential in a modified environmental situation. Finally, it may be possible for clients to generate some of these changes on their own by a better understanding of self and environmental relationships.

18.2.6. THE PREDICTION TASK

For the client to formulate occupational plans entails predicting what the individual's response to a given occupational or educational situation will be. This sort of appraisal is very difficult, since it involves envisioning what the person will be like at some future time and in different circumstances. Imagining how a given occupation may change in time complicates the problem.

Dailey [1971] distinguished passive prediction —in which outcomes in an individual's life are anticipated based on the assumption that there will be no professional intervention—from active predicting, which anticipates how the individual will respond to a variety of alternatives.

It is obvious that, because of the multiplicity of changes that are likely to affect the client and the client's situation with the passage of time, vocational assessment, however valuable, can offer people only rough estimates of the results of their future occupational and educational endeavors. This does not mean that the assessment endeavor is not worth the effort; rather it suggests that awareness of the limitations of all predictive procedures is always in order.

Prediction Using a Trait Model

American and British psychology for the last half century has relied primarily on the trait model. The first efforts to predict occupational performance utilized work samples, but by the 1920s predictions utilizing traits—hypothetical elements seen as the basis of performance— became dominant. A multitude of trait tests were widely used in occupational guidance situations.

Traits and trait tests still dominate the field of psychology, but methods of predicting occupational effectiveness based on traits do have a serious disadvantage: traits do not very accurately forecast occupational performance.

Prediction Using the Behavior-Consistency Approach

Dunn, Korn, and Andrew [1976] discussed the advantages and disadvantages of prediction based on the concept of behavioral consistency. According to this concept the way an individual has performed in the past is the best indication of future performance; the notion was that the accuracy of job predictions could be increased if past behavior resembling the behavior that will be required in the future is scrutinized.

While there is much to be said for the behavior-consistency concept, there are potential problems in using it in vocational assessment. A particularly serious problem is that the occupational effectiveness of disabled people seems to be less subject to prediction than that of nondisabled groups—perhaps because the disabled population is underdeveloped. The accuracy of predictions based on behavioral consistency has not been established in the industrial context or in rehabilitation. Any notion that people do not change and adapt runs counter to rehabilitation principles. Meister [1976] took the position that the history of an individual may not best predict the future, that rehabilitation may actually be considered as a concentrated effort to alter or even overturn this kind of pattern. But, he noted, the lives of all people are unique; this influences the attempt to find characteristic tendencies in a life as well as the modification of these tendencies.

18.3. Decisions

From the earliest stages of work with a client until the case comes to a close, data is collected and hypotheses are formulated and tested so that the client learns to make choices, with the help of the counselor and finally, it is hoped, independently. Decision-making on the part of the client is a product of the evaluation process. Rehabilitation has as one of its major objectives the client's self-sufficiency with regard to participating in the assessment and the making of choices, in other words, improving the individual's ability to assume responsibility. The goal is to change a client's dependency and help make it possible for that person to function without the help of the rehabilitationist.

Another objective of assessment is to help those responsible for rehabilitation applications arrive at an important decision, that is, whether the individual needs and would benefit from services [Karan, 1976].

The rehabilitationist must determine what traits are to be evaluated: the type of inquiry that is being conducted or the nature of the decision that has to be made with reference to the person being evaluated. It is not possible to evaluate everything about an individual and it is not practical or economically feasible to try to evaluate a person with equal attention to every trait. Therefore, the evaluator first determines what traits have a bearing on the problem and then selects the methods that can yield the most useful evaluation of these traits [Kelly, 1967].

18.3.1. ELEMENTS IN DECISION-MAKING

Effective decision-making is based first on sufficient data and second on a satisfactory method of examining, arranging, and synthesizing the data. The elements of a decision theory model serve to elucidate this. Researchers from many disciplines, including psychology, economics, political science, and education, have scrutinized decision-making as a whole and have produced models to represent it. While there are minor differences among these models, they share a number of basic characteristics:

1. Decision-making is defined as the selecting of alternatives from among a number of possible alternatives.

2. Every alternative has several possible consequences.
3. Each consequence has a certain chance of happening.
4. There is a certain value for each consequence.
5. The value of every alternative can be ascertained through an examination of the probabilities and values of all the possible consequences of each alternative.
6. The alternative that has the highest anticipated value is the one that should be selected.

Someone facing a decision, therefore, needs to know what all the possible alternatives are, their possible consequences, and the probabilities and values of these consequences. The effectiveness of the choice is likely to be a function of how much of this information the individual has [Mehrens & Lehmann, 1973].

18.3.2. VOCATIONAL CHOICE

The "square pegs in square holes" approach to vocational guidance, Tyler [1964] stated, is unworkable. As a substitute, a method in which individual differences are taken into account and the idea of decision is emphasized may solve some of the problems. A system like this was devised by Cronbach and Gleser [1965], who separated selection decisions from classification decisions. For those involved in vocational counseling, such a differentiation is important. A selection decision relates to such questions as whether a particular individual has the qualifications needed for a given job or program. A classification decision involves considering which of a number of different vocational circumstances might best suit a person. These latter decisions are more complicated and harder to make than selection decisions and more important in vocational rehabilitation. It is necessary to keep the distinction in mind because evaluative instruments that would help in making one type may not be useful in making the other.

It is also useful in vocational counseling to differentiate between decisions made about an individual and those made by the person, Tyler stated. During the past decades in counseling, more and more emphasis had been placed on decisions by the person. Therefore counselors now feel that their mission is not to select the most appropriate among various vocational alternatives for a client but instead to help the person form alternative plans and arrive at intelligent decisions. In order for people to do this, Mehrens and Lehmann wrote, they must have sound knowledge of themselves. Aptitude and achievement tests and evaluations of interests and characteristics yield important information that can help counseling clients develop more accurate images of themselves.

Tyler suggested that there are two questions that an individual must pose at any point in life at which a decision must be made. Ask, first, what alternatives are really feasible, and second, which of the possible alternatives one really wants. In choosing a vocation different types of information are needed to deal with these two questions. For the first question the data that comes from ability appraisal is the most useful. Basically, the question of whether a given occupational alternative is possible can be answered yes or no.

Obtaining the answer to the second question—that of the individual's true preference—is made easier with information that comes from interest tests and other indications of incentive patterns. In thinking about occupational preferences, people must anticipate how they would feel in various vocational circumstances. This requires a great deal of information and fine discrimination.

These are the two processes that occupy the client making vocational choices and those who are attempting to help. Experience and research in counseling and vocational assessment continue to reveal the complexity of both of them (see 27.5).

Chapter 19

Occupational Information

Vocational assessment is a way of enabling clients to correlate their characteristics as workers with the characteristics of occupations. A necessary component is to help clients form an accurate characterization of their vocational traits and then to compare this with various occupations. When people do not know how to make decisions about their capacities and limitations or do not recognize the significance of past activities or achievements, as is frequently the case, the rehabilitation counselor helps them increase their self-knowledge and decision-making facility. The choice of a vocational objective in all cases depends upon knowledge of suitable occupational alternatives. Yet it is difficult to convey appropriate occupational information because of the complexity of the information clients require for a decision and the large number of occupations they have to consider. The systematic collection and classification of occupational information provides orderly access to an otherwise chaotic mass of information covering thousands of occupations.

The focus of this assessment chapter is on obtaining occupational information, while its utilization is addressed in Chapter 27, Vocational Counseling.

19.1. Classification Systems

Any extensive collection of objects or information must be organized in a systematic way in order to be used effectively. Classification systems, which delineate the likenesses, differences, and relationships among objects, are as necessary to understanding the world of work as any other sphere of knowledge. Information must be classified so that people entering the work world can gain a full and realistic picture of the potentialities within it and also choose effectively from among many alternatives. Those involved in vocational counseling are enabled through the classification of information to deal with a large amount of complex material and to pass information on to clients in such a way that they can understand it.

Various systems of classifying occupational information by industry and by other common characteristics have been devised. The *Dictionary of Occupational Titles*—referred to as the *D.O.T.* [U.S. DOL, Employment & Training Administration, 1977]—uses an industrial classification method. Occupations can also be grouped together in relation to their social status, the personal characteristics and training they require, and earnings. Several major classification systems, as related by Norris, Zeran, Hatch, and Engelkes [1972], are discussed in this section. The 1977 *D.O.T.* (4th edition), as well as supplements, will be described separately and in more detail.

19.1.1. CLASSIFICATION BY INDUSTRY

The systems that classify occupational information by industry, developed for use in the federal government, enable both clients and professionals to become familiar with the occupational world. It is common for clients to choose vocational goals after examining general occupational areas, but they may also do so after selecting one industry; in a community where there is only one industry, people may feel they must select occupations within it.

Industrial classification systems, especially the Census and Standard Industrial Classification, can be used to explain statistical data on various industries and also to assess the occupational opportunities in a given geographical area. These systems are also used as a way of filing occupational information.

The Standard Industrial Classification System (SICS)

The U.S. government devised SICS as a means of gathering and organizing information about industries. The system is explained fully in the *Standard Industrial Classification Manual* [U.S. Executive Office of the President, Office of Management and Budget, 1972]. The 1972 edition was the first extensive revision in 15 years. It contains an alphabetized list of the major products, processes, and services of industries; a listing of Standard Short Titles that have been used to name industries; and a comprehensive procedure for identification and classification.

SICS is intended to categorize establishments according to the nature of their activities. Establishments are separated into two classes: those that make products or offer services, and those that manage or provide administrative services for other divisions of the same organization. Through use of the system it is possible to gather, tabulate, set forth, and examine information about establishments and also to foster consistency in how the statistical information gathered by government agencies, state agencies, and trade and private organizations is represented.

Divisions and Major Groups

The Standard Industrial Classification System is composed of major divisions that are subdivided into principal groups. These in turn are divided into groups of related industries and finally into single industries. The major classifications are Agriculture, Forestry, and Fishing; Mining; Construction; Manufacturing; Transportation, Communication, Electric, Gas, and Sanitary Services; Wholesale Trade; Retail Trade; Finance, Insurance, and Real Estate; Services; Public Administration; and Nonclassifiable Establishments. This system permits the recording, analysis, and presentation of information on the basis of Division (alphabetical code), Major Group (2 digits), Group (3 digits), and Industry (4 digits), at the appropriate level of detail.

19.1.2. CLASSIFICATION BY OCCUPATION

Typically a number of diverse occupations compose a single industry. As is true with industries, occupations must be classified in order for information about them to be readily intelligible. Useful data about some 23,000 occupations can be presented by grouping them in a classification scheme or taxonomy.

The International Standard Classification of Occupations (ISCO)

ISCO was developed by the International Labor Office, Geneva, Switzerland. The system was revised in 1968. The classification structure of the U.S. Bureau of the Census served as a basis for the system used in the *International Standard Classification of Occupations*. This international system can be used for comparison of occupational data among nations and as a classification plan for those nations that have not prepared their own.

The ISCO Groups

Classification is based on the type of work performed. The system consists of major groups subdivided into minor groups. The minor groups are further subdivided into unit groups, which in turn are divided into about 1,500 occupational categories.

The major groups represent very broad fields of work rather than specific types of work performed. The major groups are: Professional, Technical, and Related Workers; Administrative and Managerial Workers; Clerical and Related Workers; Sales Workers; Service Workers; Agricultural, Animal Husbandry, and Forest Workers; Production and Related Workers; Transport Equipment Operators; and Laborers, Workers Not Classified by Occupation, and Armed Forces. Minor groups cover a broad range of occupations.

The unit groups are clusters of occupations related to one another by similarity of characteristics of the work they entail. Homogeneous unit groups may be based on kind of work performed, similar equipment used, or subject matter.

19.1.3. AMERICAN CENSUS SYSTEM

In accordance with provisions in the American constitution, the Bureau of the Census has collected demographic information once every decade since 1790. Since 1820 occupational information has been collected. At present occupational data are obtained from everyone at least 16 years old who works or is looking for work; information about the unemployed

pertains to the last job the person had. The Census Bureau gathers information about the type of work an individual does. A classified index was developed by the U.S. Department of Commerce, Bureau of the Census [1971], primarily to define the industrial and occupational classifications adopted for the census data.

The Occupation Classification System

The broad categories in the occupational classification of the Census Bureau are: (1) Professional, Technical, and Kindred Workers; (2) Managers and Administrators (except farm); (3) Sales Workers; (4) Clerical and Kindred Workers; (5) Craftsmen and Kindred Workers; (6) Operatives (except transport); (7) Transport Equipment Operatives; (8) Laborers (except farm); (9) Farmers and Farm Managers; (10) Farm Laborers and Farm Foremen; and (11) Private Household Workers. These broad categories are broken down into three-digit occupational codes.

Utilizing the System

The Census system is the most comprehensive tabulation of employees with respect to numbers, age, sex, and ethnic backgrounds. It displays relationships among industries and suggests developments that are taking place by indicating changes during a 10-year period. It is easy to use this system in collecting information about local occupations for comparison with national data.

The three digit code used in the Census classification is broadly correspondent with three of the nine digits of the *D.O.T.* code. There are also close relationships between the Census system and the Standard Industrial Classification (SIC) System, and the SIC code is incorporated into the Census report when appropriate.

19.1.4. OTHER SYSTEMS

Several other systems for classification are worthy of mention before describing the American *D.O.T.* Variations in conceptual order are noteworthy.

Canadian Classification and Dictionary of Occupations (CCDO)

The Canadian Department of Manpower and Immigration [1971] publishes the *CCDO* in two volumes: *Classification and Definitions* and *Occupational Qualifications Requirements*. This classification system was intended to be used in manpower studies, surveys, census work, the preparation of educational and training programs, counseling and placement, rehabilitation, endeavors pertaining to the movement of employees, personnel, and other facets of business and industry.

The type of work is the major criterion for classification in the *CCDO*, although other elements were considered so that the occupation could be more precisely defined: material or equipment or product, criteria, background of workers, work setting, services, and relation to other jobs. The *CCDO* differs from other classification systems in the large number of general occupational categories it uses. Dividing occupations into 23 groups instead of the usual nine results in closer similarity among the occupations in the various groups.

In the *CCDO* certain special groups of occupations—for instance, supervisors, foremen, inspectors, laborers, managers, technicians, and technologists—are categorized separately. Certain kinds of information are included for each occupational definition. There is a unique code number, a code reflecting environmental qualities, physical tasks, training period, and worker functions with respect to data, people, and things.

The *CCDO* incorporated certain elements of the U.S. *D.O.T.*: the data-people-things components, training-time measurements, and designations for personal characteristics. It borrowed the organization relating occupational definitions to classification from the *International Standard Classification of Occupations*. Because of this structure the relationship between one occupation and others in its group can be readily viewed.

Classification of Occupations and Directory of Occupational Titles (CODOT)

CODOT is a classification of all occupations in Great Britain [Great Britain, Department of Employment, 1972]. Because occupations are treated separately only when the differences are important for the purpose of employment or compilation of statistics, only about 3,500 distinct occupations and a number of residual occupations are listed. The occupations are classified mainly according to type of work. As jobs were grouped into occupations and occupations into broader fields, elements such as materials, equipment, products and services, and substitution and promotion were taken to reflect the type of work.

The 3,500 occupations are placed into groups at three levels: 378 unit groups, which are basic groups of closely related occupations in which the principal work is quite similar; 73 minor groups, which are similar in that the tasks carried on are alike or in that one type of corporate activity is reflected; and 18 major groups, or collections of minor groups. All the occupations are arranged on four levels that reveal various amounts of detail. The code numbers are spaced so that more numbers can be added to express subtler relationships between occupations or groups without disturbing the entire system.

19.2. Dictionary of Occupational Titles

The U.S. *Dictionary of Occupational Titles, D.O.T.,* published by the U.S. Department of Labor (DOL), is an outgrowth of the needs of the American public employment service system for a comprehensive body of standardized occupational information for purposes of job placement, employment counseling and vocational guidance, and for labor market information services (see 27.4). In order to implement effectively its primary assignment of matching jobs and workers, the public employment service system (see 12.2.9 and 37.2) requires a uniform occupational language for use in all of its offices. They need this information to compare and match the specifications of employer job openings and the qualifications of applicants who are seeking jobs. Rehabilitationists also use the *D.O.T.* in vocational assessment.

Most of the material presented in this section is paraphrased from U.S. DOL publications on the *D.O.T.*

19.2.1. BACKGROUND

The need for descriptive occupational information was recognized in the mid-1930s, within a few years after the passage of the Wagner-Peyser Act that established a federal-state employment service system. As one facet of public employment service operations, an occupational research program was initiated, using analysts located in several field stations scattered throughout the country to collect the information required. Based on these data, the first edition of the *D.O.T.* was published in 1939.

That first edition contained a total of almost 17,500 concise definitions presented alphabetically, by title, with a coding arrangement for occupational classification. Blocks of jobs were assigned 5- or 6-digit codes, which placed them in one of 550 occupational groups and indicated whether the jobs were skilled, semi-skilled, or unskilled.

The revised second edition, issued in March 1949, combined the material in the first edition with its supplements. It also included new occupations. Material included information relating to occupational classification of entry applicants with no previous work experience. Under that coding structure, an applicant's vocational readiness and preference were indicated.

The third edition, published in 1965, eliminated the previous U.S. DOL designation of certain occupations as being skilled, semi-skilled, or unskilled, and substituted a classification system based both on the nature of the work performed and the demands of such work activities upon the workers. These indicators of work requirements included eight separate classification components: training time, aptitudes, interests, temperaments, physical demands, working conditions, work performed, and industry.

The 1977 edition of the *D.O.T.* was the result of continued research on the changing occupational structure of the American economy conducted by the U.S. Employment Service and job analysts in affiliated state Employment Service Occupational Analysis Field Centers throughout the country. This fourth edition was based on more than 75,000 on-site job analyses conducted from 1965 to the mid-1970s, and on extensive contacts with professional and trade associations. These activities were designed to re-verify and reevaluate the job content and definitions of the occupations listed and to identify new occupations. As a result of this program, over 2,100 new occupational definitions were added and some 3,500 that appeared in the third edition were deleted. Many thousands of other descriptions were substantially modified or combined with closely related definitions to eliminate overlap and duplication, and to reflect the consolidation and restructuring of some occupations.

This fourth edition contains approximately 20,000 definitions, about 1,800 less than in the third edition. It also includes new and more detailed occupational information, incorporating material formerly published in four separate publications. It eliminated age and sex references in both definitions and job titles. A supplement to it is designed for use by the Social Security Administration as a guide to possible new careers for disabled workers and to the determination of benefit eligibility by a description of selected characteristics of occupations (physical demands, working conditions, training time).

19.2.2. CODE AND DEFINITION

Work is organized in a variety of ways. As a result of technological, economic, and sociological influences, nearly every job in the economy is performed slightly differently from any other job. Every job is also similar to a number of other jobs. In order to look at the millions of jobs in the American economy in an organized way, the *D.O.T.* groups jobs into "occupations" based on their similarities and defines the structure and content of all listed occupations. Occupational definitions are the result of comprehensive studies of how similar jobs are performed all over the nation. The term *occupation*, as used in the *D.O.T.*, refers to this collective description of a number of individual jobs performed, with minor variations, in many establishments.

There are six basic parts to an occupational definition in the *D.O.T.* Each definition presents data about a job in a systematic fashion. The parts are listed below in the order in which they appear in every definition:

1. Occupational Code Number.
2. Occupational Title.

3. Industry Designation.
4. Alternate Titles (if any).
5. The Body of the Definition—which includes the lead statement, task element statements, and "May" items.
6. Undefined Related Titles (if any).

Occupational Code Number

The first item in an occupational definition is a nine-digit occupational code. In the *D.O.T.* occupational classification system, each set of three digits in the nine-digit code number has a specific purpose or meaning. Together, the numbers provide a unique identification code for a particular occupation that differentiates it from all others.

The first three digits identify a particular occupational group. All occupations are clustered into one of nine broad "categories" (first digit), such as professional, technical and managerial, or clerical and sales occupations. These categories break up into 82 occupationally specific "divisions" (first two digits), such as occupations in architecture and engineering within the professional category, or stenography, typing, filing, and related occupations in the clerical and sales category. Divisions in turn separate into small, homogeneous "groups" (first three digits); 559 such groups are identified in the *D.O.T.* The nine primary occupational categories are listed below;

0/1 Professional, Technical, and Managerial Occupations.
2   Clerical and Sales Occupations.
3   Service Occupations.
4   Agricultural, Fishery, Forestry, and Related Occupations.
5   Processing Occupations.
6   Machine Trades Occupations.
7   Bench Work Occupations.
8   Structural Work Occupations.
9   Miscellaneous Occupations.

The first of the nine digits always signifies the occupational category. For example, in a code number starting with 652 the first digit, 6, indicates that this particular occupation is found in the category, "Machine Trades Occupations." The second digit refers to a division within the category. For example the divisions within the Machine Trades Occupations category are as follows:

60   Metal Machining Occupations.
61   Metalworking Occupations, n.e.c. [i.e., "not elsewhere classified"].
62/63 Mechanics and Machinery Repairers.
64   Paperworking Occupations.
65   Printing Occupations.
66   Wood Machining Occupations.
67   Occupations in Machining Stone, Clay, Glass, and Related Materials.
68   Textile Occupations.
69   Machine Trades Occupations, n.e.c.

In the example, the second digit, 5, thus locates the occupation in the Printing Occupations division.

The third digit defines the occupational group within the division. The groups within the Printing Occupations division are as follows:

650 Typesetters and Composers.
651 Printing Press Occupations.
652 Printing Machine Occupations.
653 Bookbinding-Machine Operators and Related Occupations.
654 Typecasters and Related Occupations.
659 Printing Occupations. n.e.c.

The third digit in the example, 2, locates the occupation in the Printing Machine Occupations group.

The middle three digits (i.e., the fourth, fifth, and sixth digits) of the *D.O.T.* occupational code are the worker functions ratings of the tasks performed in the occupation. Every job requires a worker to function to some degree in relation to data, people, and things. A separate digit expresses the worker's relationship to each of these three groups. The fourth digit signifies a function pertaining to data which are coded as follows:

0   Synthesizing.
1   Coordinating.
2   Analyzing.
3   Compiling.
4   Computing.
5   Copying.
6   Comparing.

The fifth digit pertains to people, coded as:

0   Mentoring.
1   Negotiating.
2   Instructing.
3   Supervising.
4   Diverting.

5   Persuading.
6   Speaking-Signaling.
7   Serving.
8   Taking Instructions-Helping.

The sixth digit indicates the primary function of the occupation that has to do with things:

0   Setting Up.
1   Precision Working.
2   Operating-Controlling.
3   Driving-Operating.
4   Manipulating.
5   Tending.
6   Feeding-Offbearing.
7   Handling.

Worker functions involving more complex responsibility and judgment are assigned lower numbers in these three lists while functions that are less complicated have higher numbers. For example, "synthesizing" and "coordinating" data are more complex tasks than "copying" data; "instructing" people involves a broader responsibility than "taking instructions-helping"; and "operating" things is a more complicated task than "handling" things. As an example, the occupation Gambling Dealer (as with dice, roulette, or cards) is coded 343.467-018, with the middle three digits indicating function: the data function is coded 4 for computing; the people function is 6, meaning speaking-signaling; and the work with things involves handling, coded 7. As noted above, the worker functions code indicates the broadest level of responsibility or judgment required in relation to data, people, or things. These functions are numbered and listed in decreasing order of complexity, one function encompassing all those above it. It is assumed that, if the job requires it, the worker can generally perform any higher numbered function listed in each of the three categories. The hierarchy is more precise in the data and things lists than in the people list.

The last three digits of the occupational code number indicate the alphabetical order of titles within six-digit code groups. They serve to differentiate a particular occupation from all others. A number of occupational titles may have the same first six digits, but no two can have the same nine digits. If a six-digit code is applicable to only one occupational title, the final three digits assigned are always 010. If there is more than one occupation with the same first

six digits, the final three digits are usually assigned in alphabetical order of titles in multiples of four (010, 014, 018, 022, and so on). The full nine digits thus provide each occupation with a unique code suitable for computerized operations.

Occupational Title

Immediately following the occupational code in every definition is the occupational "base title." The base title is always in upper-case boldface letters. It is the most common type of title found in the *D.O.T.* and is the one by which the occupation is known in the majority of establishments in which it is found. Some titles are classified as "master titles"; these are designed to eliminate unnecessary repetition of tasks common to a large number of occupations. Master titles define the common job tasks having a wide variety of job variables and a wide variety of titles. An example is the title "SUPERVISOR (any ind.)." Each individual supervisory occupation has its own separate definition in the *D.O.T.* in which its unique duties are described, but at the end of the definition the reader is referred back to the master definition (in this case, by a sentence reading "Performs other duties as described under SUPERVISOR (any ind.)." By referring to this master definition, the user will learn about the typical supervisory duties that any individual supervisor also performs.

Another type of *D.O.T.* title is a "term title." These include occupations with the same title but few common duties. Since neither master nor term definitions are occupations, they are not coded in the occupational group arrangement but are found in separate sections of the *D.O.T.* Other major types of titles used in the *D.O.T.* include "alternate titles" and "undefined related titles." An alternate title is a synonym for the base title but is not as commonly used. Alternate titles are shown in lower-case boldface letters immediately after the base title and its industrial designation. A particular occupation may have a large number of alternate titles or none at all. Alternate titles carry the code numbers and industry designations of the base title. Undefined related titles, if applicable, appear at the end of the occupational definition, in all upper-case letters and preceded by the phrase, "May be designated according to . . ." (or a similar phrase). This type of title is for an occupation that is really a variation or specialization of the base occupation. It resembles the base enough to accompany it, but differs from it enough to require an explanatory phrase and its own unique title. An alternative title or an undefined related title takes the same code as its base title. These titles are also listed in the Alphabetical Index of Occupational Titles according to the nine-digit codes of their base titles.

Industry Designation

The industry designation is in parentheses immediately following the occupational base title. If often differentiates between two or more occupations with identical titles but different duties. Because of this, it is an integral and inseparable part of any occupational title. An industry designation often tells one or more things about an occupation, such as location of the occupation, types of duties associated with the occupation, products manufactured, processes used, or raw materials used.

While a definition usually receives the designation of the industry or industries in which it occurs, certain occupations occur in a large number of industries. When this happens, the industry is assigned a cross-industry designation. For example, clerical occupations are found in almost every industry. To show the broad, cross-industry nature of clerical occupations, "clerical" is an industry designation in itself. Occupations that occur in a number of industries, but not so widely as to warrant their own industry designation, are given the designation of "any industry" (any ind.).

The Body of the Definition

The body of the definition usually consists of two or three main parts: a lead statement, a number of task element statements, and a third part known as a "may" item.

The first sentence following the industry designation and alternate titles (if any) is the lead statement. It is followed by a colon (:). The lead statement summarizes the entire occupation. It offers essential information such as: worker actions; the objective or purpose of the worker actions; machines, tools, equipment, or work aids used by the worker; materials used, products made, subject matter dealt with, or services rendered; or instructions followed or judgments made. From the lead statement, the user can obtain an overview of the occupation.

Task element statements indicate the specific tasks the worker performs to accomplish the overall job purpose described in the lead statement (e.g., "Turns handwheel . . ."; "Turns screws . . ."). They indicate how workers actually carry out their duties. Many definitions contain one or more sentences beginning with the word "May"; they describe duties required of workers in this occupation in some establishments but not in others. The word "may" does not indicate that a worker will sometimes perform this task but rather that some workers in different establishments generally perform one of the varied tasks listed.

The definition also contains a number of additional information elements designed to assist the user. Among these elements are:

1. Italicized words. Any words in a definition set in italics are defined in the Glossary of the *D.O.T.*; they are technical terms or special uses of terms not ordinarily found in a standard dictionary.

2. Bracketed titles. A bracketed title indicates that workers in the base title occupation perform some duties of the bracketed occupation as a part of their regular duties; to learn more about this particular aspect of the occupation, the user can look up the bracketed occupational title.

3. Unbracketed titles. Unbracketed titles are used for occupations whose workers have a frequent working relationship with workers in the occupation being defined.

4. Roman numerals. Several somewhat different occupations with the same job title may be found in the same industry. In this event, a roman numeral follows each title and industry designation. There is no necessary connection in the sequence of these numbers with the level of complexity of these occupations or the frequency with which they occur.

5. Statement of significant variables. Another element found in some definitions is a statement of significant variables. It appears near the end of a definition and shows the possible variations in jobs that a particular definition can cover. This eliminates the need to include a large number of almost identical definitions in the *D.O.T.* The statement begins with "Important variations include . . . ."

19.2.3. ORGANIZATION

The 1977 *D.O.T.* is a single volume with 1,371 large pages. It is organized according to the following major headings of sections as described below:

INTRODUCTION AND SUMMARY LISTING. This section includes a short discussion of the *D.O.T.*, including its purpose and history. It gives a brief explanation of its use and lists occupational categories, divisions, and groups.

MASTER TITLES AND DEFINITIONS. Master title definitions describe work duties that are common to a number of jobs. Occupations in which these common duties are an essential part of the job refer the user to the master definition in order to save space and avoid unnecessary repetition of the common duties. Clues to classification of jobs utilizing master definitions are provided.

TERM TITLES AND DEFINITIONS. Term titles are titles commonly used for a number of jobs that may differ widely in job knowledge required, tasks performed, and job location. Term title definitions broadly indicate the jobs that are known by the titles and provide information helpful in finding appropriate specific titles and codes.

OCCUPATIONAL GROUP ARRANGEMENT. Definitions are numerically arranged by the nine-digit codes according to occupational category (first digit), division (first two digits), and group (first three digits). Code numbers indicate areas of technology in which the occupations are found.

GLOSSARY. The glossary defines technical words that are italicized in *D.O.T.* definitions. Technical words are listed alphabetically.

ALPHABETICAL INDEX OF OCCUPATIONAL TITLES. This section arranges titles and codes in alphabetical order and gives complete nine-digit codes for all titles. Titles with two or more words are treated as a single word.

OCCUPATIONAL TITLES ARRANGED BY INDUSTRY DESIGNATION. In this section titles and codes are arranged according to industries. Industries are identified by the abbreviated industry designations found in occupational definitions, followed by the complete industry title. It lists titles and codes found in a particular industry or industries.

INDUSTRY INDEX. This section lists in alphabetical order all industries that are identified in *D.O.T.* occupational definitions and indexes this material by page numbers.

APPENDIX: EXPLANATION OF DATA, PEOPLE, AND THINGS. The significance of worker functions ratings are interpreted according to involvement with data, people, and things.

19.2.4. LOCATING TITLE AND CODE

The occupational classification system in the *D.O.T.*, with its homogeneous arrangement of occupational titles within a given technology and in order of complexity, offers an overview of the total occupational structure in America. It can assist in the identification of career ladders and possible skill transfers vertically within an industry or horizontally among closely related technologies. The structure of the *D.O.T.* also indicates basic kinds of information to collect in vocational assessment. Occupational definitions are the bridge in the process of helping people identify suitable jobs. Knowing how to use it, consequently, can be of great value to the rehabilitationist in client assessment and placement. Moreover, many agencies require use of *D.O.T.* codes for client recording purposes (e.g., to identify the job obtained when the case was closed).

Occupational titles and codes in the *D.O.T.* are based on the type of information presented in the lead statement and task element statements. To use the *D.O.T.* it is best to have the following information about the work:

1. Worker tasks or actions (e.g., operates machines, writes reports).
2. Purpose of the work (e.g., to shape metal parts, to inform employees).
3. Machines, tools, equipment, or work aids used (e.g., punch press, electric typewriter).
4. Materials, products, subject matter (academic discipline), or services involved (e.g.,

granulated ingredients, plastic products, accounting, child care).

5. Instructions followed and the amount of independent judgment exercised (e.g., follows oral instructions from supervisor, applies general knowledge).
6. Location of the work (e.g., outdoors on a farm, indoors in an assembly area).

The more complete and comprehensive this information is about the tasks performed by a worker or required by an employer on a particular job, the easier it is to determine the appropriate code.

There are three different arrangements of occupational titles in the *D.O.T.* as mentioned above: the Occupational Group Arrangement, the Alphabetical Index, and the Industry Arrangement. All of these can assist in identifying and classifying jobs.

Occupational Group Arrangement

In the fourth edition, the primary method of identifying or classifying jobs is by use of the Occupational Group Arrangement. For job placement and referral purposes, this is the preferred method for finding an occupational title and code if one has obtained sufficient information. The other two arrangements of titles are supplementary and should be used in conjunction with the Occupational Group Arrangement. Using this group arrangement saves time by eliminating the extra step of referring to other sections of the *D.O.T.*

To use the Occupational Group Arrangement:

1. Obtain all the relevant facts about the job.
2. Find the one-digit occupational category that seems most likely to contain the job.
3. Find the most appropriate two-digit occupational division of the category.
4. Find the best three-digit group within the division.
5. Examine the occupational definitions under the group selected and choose the most appropriate title. If it does not correspond closely with the information collected, repeat these steps to find the most appropriate classification.

In the process of choosing the appropriate occupational category, division, and group, one develops information about the job that will be helpful in classifying it. It should be remembered that jobs requiring more responsibility and independent judgment have lower worker functions numerals and will be found near the beginning of the group, while those requiring less responsibility and independent judgment have higher numbers and will be found nearer the end. The Occupational Group Arrangement should also be used when one is interested in knowing about closely related jobs.

Alphabetical Index of Occupational Titles

If only the title of a job is known, a search through the Alphabetical Index of Occupational Titles can provide a lead to an appropriate classification. This may require assumptions about the nature of the job that may be incorrect. Therefore, this method should be used only if it is not possible to obtain sufficient information to use the Occupational Group Arrangement.

To use the Alphabetical Index follow this procedure:

1. Look through the index for whatever title of the job is known. If it is found, write down the nine-digit code to the right of the title. Using this code as a guide, find the definition for the title in the occupational grouping. Read the entire definition before deciding whether it is the most appropriate classification.
2. If the title cannot be found, or the definition appears inappropriate, look for another title. Several procedures may be helpful: (1) Invert the title (e.g, from maintenance carpenter to carpenter, maintenance). (2) Contract the title (e.g., from rubber-belt repairer to belt repairer). (3) Find a synonym (e.g., *car mechanic—automobile mechanic*). (4) Consider other factors: job location (e.g., parking lot attendant, storeroom clerk), machines used (e.g., punch-press operator, machine feeder), materials used (e.g., log loader, plastic-tile layer), subject matter (e.g., accounting clerk, credit analyst), services involved (e.g., cleaner and presser, broker), activity performed (e.g., teacher, inspector), or job complexity (e.g., machine setter, welding-machine tender).

When there is information on several of these factors, however, it may be more appropriate to use the Occupational Group Arrangement.

Occupational Titles Arranged by Industry Designation

The Industry Arrangement of titles may be useful if there is limited information about a job. One may know the industry in which the job is located, but have little or no information about such things as products made, materials used, services rendered, and other essential data. The Industry Arrangement can also be of assistance if a person wants to work in a particular industry, or if the rehabilitationist needs to learn more about related jobs in the industry.

To use the Industry Arrangement:

1. Look through the industry titles and read their definitions. Select the one most likely to contain the job.

2. Survey the occupational titles listed under the selected industry. Choose the title that seems appropriate to the job, and write down the nine-digit code to the right of the title. Using this code as a guide, find the definition in the Occupational Group Arrangement. Read the entire occupational definition before deciding if it is the most appropriate classification.

How to Obtain Titles and Codes for Unlisted Occupations

There are occasions when *D.O.T.* users are unable to locate titles, codes, and definitions in the volume. This could occur for one of several reasons:

1. The user may be unfamiliar with the structure of the *D.O.T.*
2. The *D.O.T.* contains most jobs found in the American economy but not all of them.
3. New jobs are continually being created as the result of technological change and other labor force pressures.
4. The user may be seeking very specific information, whereas *D.O.T.* definitions are composites of jobs.
5. The user's job information may be broader than that covered in just one definition.

Users who cannot find the occupational information they need in the *D.O.T.* should contact the nearest state Employment Service office for assistance.

19.3. Obtaining Information

The problem with occupational information is to express definitions functionally so that an accurate determination of the relationship between an individual's qualifications and the demands of the occupation can be made. The first step is to specify the basic trait requirements of the job including aptitudes, interests, temperaments, physical capacities, working conditions, and training time. These requirements of an occupation have been described for vocational counseling and placement information.

19.3.1. COMMON JOB CHARACTERISTICS

The U.S. Department of Labor, Bureau of Labor Statistics [1975] has listed 25 common job and personal characteristics and requirements that can be matched with occupations. The 25 job characteristics are:

1. High school degree generally needed.
2. Technical school or apprenticeship required.
3. Junior college (Associate in Arts degree).
4. College degree (B.A. or graduate work or first professional degree).
5. Jobs widely scattered (found in most parts of the country).
6. Jobs concentrated in certain localities.
7. Works with things—usually necessitates manual skills.
8. Works with ideas—intellectual skills needed.
9. Helps people.
10. Works with people—usually a pleasant personality needed in addition to the ability to get along well with other people.
11. Able to see the physical outcome of work —tangible product.
12. Chance for self-expression, expression of one's own ideas.
13. Work as a part of a team—interaction with other employees necessary.
14. Work independently—initiative, discipline, and organization needed.

15. Work closely supervised.
16. Directing others' activities.
17. Generally confined to work area.
18. Overtime or shift work necessary.
19. Exposure to weather—outside work or work in temperature extremes.
20. High level of responsibility—making of important decisions required.
21. Requires physical stamina—for extensive lifting, standing, and walking.
22. Work with details—technical or written material handled continuously.
23. Repetitive work.
24. Motivates others.
25. Competitive.

This list permits the important personal characteristics of interests, capabilities, preferences, and educational accomplishments to be paired with the characteristics typically associated with an occupation or a group of occupations.

19.3.2. OCCUPATIONAL EXPLORATION

The *Guide for Occupational Exploration* was released in 1979 by the U.S. DOL Employment and Training Administration [1979]. It serves vocational counseling in that it groups thousands of occupations by interests and by traits required for successful performance. It also provides a convenient crossover from occupational information about a client to potentially suitable occupational groups. The *Guide* facilitates counselor use of the 1977 *D.O.T.* by coordinated vocational exploration using the U.S.E.S. Interest Inventory and Interest Check List and the General Aptitude Test Battery (G.A.T.B.), which are published by the U.S. DOL. Results from the administration of the G.A.T.B. to a client are translated with a set of Occupational Aptitude Patterns (O.A.P.) based on work groups in the *Guide*.

The occupational preferences of the client—derived from the interest tools, G.A.T.B. and interview—serve as entries to the 12 Interest Areas in the *Guide for Occupational Exploration*. The interests and their definitions are as follows:

1. Artistic. Interest in creative expression of feelings or ideas.
2. Scientific. Interest in discovering, collecting, and analyzing information about the natural world and in applying scientific research findings to problems in medicine, life sciences, and natural sciences.
3. Plants and Animals. Interest in activities involving plants and animals, usually in an outdoor setting.
4. Protective. Interest in using authority to protect people and property.
5. Mechanical. Interest in applying mechanical principles to practical situations, using machines, hand tools, or instruments.
6. Industrial. Interest in repetitive, concrete, organized activities in a factory setting.
7. Business Detail. Interest in organized, clearly defined activities requiring accuracy and attention to details, primarily in an office setting.
8. Selling. Interest in bringing others to a point of view through personal persuasion, using sales and promotion techniques.
9. Accommodating. Interest in catering to and serving the desires of others, usually on a one-to-one basis.
10. Humanitarian. Interest in helping individuals with their mental, spiritual, social, physical, or vocational concerns.
11. Leading-Influencing. General interest in leading and influencing others through activities involving high level verbal or numerical abilities.
12. Physical Performing. Interest in physical activities performed before an audience.

Each interest area is delineated (and coded) further by several work groups and then by several subgroups. For example, all artistic interest areas are coded 01. The work group the Visual Arts is 01.02, a subgroup of which is Commercial Art coded 01.02-03.

Each of the 66 work groups (which have a total of 348 subgroups) contains descriptive information and a listing of jobs (with *D.O.T.* codes). Jobs in a work group are similar in terms of required adaptabilities and capabilities. An appendix to the *Guide* lists all nonmilitary occupations, providing a bridge from the *D.O.T.* to interest subgroups. The work groups in each interest area usually start with the group that requires the most preparation and experience.

The *Guide* can be used by an intelligent and motivated client for independent occupational exploration. Instructions have been prepared for this purpose as well as for use by vocational counselors.

19.3.3. FUNCTIONAL INFORMATION

The U.S. DOL Employment Service over the years has developed functional methods for presenting occupational information and have been described in supplements to the *D.O.T.* These publications of the U.S. DOL, Employment and Training Administration have special value in rehabilitation counseling.

General Educational Development

General educational development refers to both formal and informal training that enhances the worker's ability to think and follow directions and to use the basic linguistic and mathematical skills.

General educational development as described by the U.S. DOL has three components on six levels. The components of development are reasoning, mathematical, and language. Reasoning development ranges from applying common sense and understanding simple instructions to the top level of applying principles of logical or scientific thinking. Mathematical development ranges from simple arithmetic to the highest level of applying advanced mathematical techniques. Language development likewise is characterized on a scale from simple to advanced levels of comprehension and expression.

Specific Vocational Preparation

Vocational training is obtained in a school or college, in military service, through paid or volunteer work, in an institution, or through an avocation. A number of situations can provide specific vocational preparation: vocational education in high school shops, technical and art schools, and some college programs; apprentice training; in-plant training provided by an employer in a formal program; on-the-job training in which the individual learns the job through instruction by another worker; and/or essential work experience (i.e., the performance of jobs that serve as prerequisites for other jobs). A U.S. DOL time chart outlines nine different levels of specific vocational preparation:

1. Short demonstration only.
2. Anything beyond short demonstration up to and including 30 days.
3. Over 30 days up to and including 3 months.
4. Over 3 months up to and including 6 months.
5. Over 6 months up to and including 1 year.
6. Over 1 year up to and including 2 years.
7. Over 2 years up to and including 4 years.
8. Over 4 years up to and including 10 years.
9. Over 10 years.

Aptitudes

Aptitudes are the particular capabilities that an individual needs in order to learn or accomplish a task with competence. The following are U.S. DOL definitions of specific aptitudes with the designated letter code.

G   Intelligence: General learning ability; the ability to "catch on" or understand instructions and underlying principles, and to reason and make judgments.

V   Verbal: Ability to understand meanings of words and ideas associated with them, and to use them effectively.

N   Numerical: Ability to perform arithmetic operations quickly and accurately.

S   Spatial: Ability to comprehend forms in space and understand relationships of plane and solid objects; frequently described as the ability to "visualize" objects of two or three dimensions.

P   Form perception: Ability to perceive pertinent detail in objects or in pictorial or graphic material and to make visual comparisons.

Q   Clerical perception: Ability to perceive pertinent detail in verbal or tabular material.

K   Motor coordination: Ability to coordinate eyes and hands or fingers rapidly and accurately in making precise movements with speed.

F   Finger dexterity: Ability to move the fingers and manipulate small objects with the fingers rapidly or accurately.

M   Manual dexterity: Ability to move the hands easily and skillfully.

E   Eye-Hand-Foot Coordination: Ability to move the hand and foot coordinately with each other in accordance with visual stimuli.

C   Color discrimination: Ability to perceive or recognize similarities or differences in colors, or in shades or other values of the same color.

The degree of aptitude a job demands in order to be performed on an average level is coded numerically, with average demands indicated. The amount of aptitude is reflected in terms of the aptitudes of the employed population. Code number 1 represents the top 10 percent of the population; 2, the highest third, exclusive of the top 10 percent; 3, the middle third; 4, the lowest third, exclusive of the bottom 10 percent; and code 5, the lowest 10 percent.

Interests

The U.S. DOL Employment Service revised its 1967 Interest Check List in 1979. This new edition is described elsewhere (see 19.3.2 and 20.3.2).

Temperaments

With relationship to the gathering of occupational information, temperaments refer to the adaptability demands that a particular jobworker situation imposes on the individual. Temperaments became components of occupational analysis as a result of the observation, based on placement situations, that effectiveness in a job is frequently a function of the individual's temperament. In other words, ineffectiveness or discontentment with a job may result not from inadequacy in performing it but from failure to adapt to circumstances of the job.

In selecting workers, employers usually want information about personal characteristics, which have to do with temperaments, in addition to other qualifications such as background and training. It is common for employers to stipulate which personality traits are desirable and which are not. These traits can be tentatively evaluated through interviewing, testing, and analyzing work histories. By looking at the demands that certain job-worker situations make on the individual, one can link traits to jobs. As described by Dunn [1971b], ten "temperaments," or personal traits, needed by a person in particular job-worker circumstances, are as follows:

1. Adaptability in accepting responsibility for the direction, control, or planning of an activity.
2. Adaptability to situations involving the interpretation of feelings, ideas, or facts in terms of personal viewpoint.
3. Adaptability in influencing people in their opinions, attitudes, or judgments about ideas or things.
4. Adaptability in making generalizations, evaluations, or decisions based on sensory or judgmental criteria.
5. Adaptability in making generalizations, evaluations, or decisions based on measurable or verifiable criteria.
6. Adaptability in dealing with people beyond giving and receiving instructions.
7. Adaptability in performing repetitive work, or to performing continuously the same, according to set procedures, sequence, or pace.
8. Adaptability in performing under stress when confronted with emergency, critical, unusual, or dangerous situations, or situations in which working speed and sustained attention are make-or-break aspects of the job.
9. Adaptability to situations requiring the precise attainment of set limits, tolerances, or standards.
10. Adaptability in performing a variety of duties, often changing from one task to another of a different nature without loss of efficiency or composure.

Physical Demands

The physical activities that an individual must engage in at work are formulated as variables that can indicate both the requirements of a particular job and the specific physical capacities that the employee must have. In other words, "depth perception" denotes a physical requirement of a number of jobs and also a particular ability that many individuals have. The worker must have at least the physical capabilities demanded by the job. There are six basic physical variables, developed to supplement use of the *D.O.T.*

Variable No. 1, strength, refers to lifting, carrying, and pushing and/or pulling. Usually an individual who can do one of them can do the others. There are five degrees of strength. Sedentary work requires the lifting of 10 pounds and the ability to carry small objects infrequently. A sedentary job usually demands some walking and standing. Light work requires being able to lift 20 pounds, and lifting or carrying objects that weigh a maximum of 10 pounds is frequently necessary. A job is in this classification if it requires considerable walking or standing or when the worker, while most often sitting, must push and pull arm or leg controls. Medium work demands that the worker lift 50 pounds and be able to carry or lift up to 25 pounds with frequency. For heavy work it is necessary to lift 100 pounds and frequently carry objects weighing 50 pounds; and for very heavy work, it is necessary to lift objects over

100 pounds and often lift or carry objects that weigh over 50 pounds.

Variable No. 2 involves climbing and/or balancing. No. 3 includes stooping, kneeling, crouching, and/or crawling.

Variable No. 4 involves reaching, handling, fingering, and/or feeling. Handling is defined as work with the hand but not the fingers, while fingering does not involve the hand or arm. Feeling entails the perception of physical characteristics in objects, such as size, shape, temperature, or texture, typically through use of the fingertips.

Variable No. 5 consists of talking and hearing; No. 6 is seeing. This variable is subdivided into the functions of far and near acuity, depth perception, field of vision, accommodation, and color vision. Far acuity is clear vision at a distance of 20 feet; near acuity is vision at a distance of 20 inches or less. Field of vision refers to the space that can be viewed up or down or to the side while the eyes are focused on a particular point. Accommodation, particularly important in near-point work at different distances, is the adjustment of the lens to focus on an object.

Environmental Conditions

There are seven variables that compose the physical surroundings of a job. Variable No. 1 relates to whether the job is performed inside or outside. Inside conditions are defined as those in which the worker is not exposed to weather conditions but may be exposed to changing temperatures. In outside conditions there is no protection from the weather. A job in which the individual is inside at least 75 percent of the time is defined as an inside job; an outside job is one in which the worker is outside about 75 percent of the time. A job is categorized as "both" if it is carried on inside and outside in roughly equal amounts.

Variable No. 2 refers to extremes of cold plus temperature changes, extremes of cold being defined as a temperature low enough to result in definite physical discomfort unless the individual has special protection, and temperature changes being defined as those that produce marked physical reactions. Variable No. 3, extremes of heat plus temperature changes, is analogous. Variable No. 4 is wetness and humidity, and No. 5 is noise and vibration that are noticeably distracting or physically harmful. Variable No. 6

consists of hazards; No. 7 includes fumes, odors, toxic conditions, dust, and poor ventilation, to any extent unpleasant or harmful.

Worker Functions

Studies by the U.S. Department of Labor suggested that any job necessitates the worker's performing with different degrees of relationship to data, people, and things. From this premise three hierarchies were constructed according to increasing levels of complexity, or worker functions. The labels for the worker functions are standardized *D.O.T.* terms that briefly sum up what is done in a job. Data functions include comparing, computing, and synthesizing; people-related functions range from serving to negotiating and mentoring; and, functions related to things are described as handling, tending, and operating. The *D.O.T.* chart that displays these hierarchies is called the *Structure of Worker Functions*.

Job descriptions can be formulated in terms of data, people, and things by selecting from each hierarchy the uppermost level relevant to effective conduct of the job. The result is a reflection of the level of complexity of the job as a whole when carried out successfully.

Machines, Tools, Equipment, and Work Aids (MTEWA)

Four categories of devices needed for the performance of particular functions—machines, tools, equipment, work aids—are defined. A machine is a device that includes a number of mechanical components and the structure within which they are contained. Constructed so that it will exert a force to perform work, move something, or process information, a machine may be started by human force or an external power source.

Tools are operated by hand. In addition to the ordinary hand tools there are those that, while operated by a person, get their power from some external source, such as pneumatic hammers or electric screwdrivers. Equipment is defined as those devices that produce power, transmit signals, or alter material through the use of light, heat, chemicals, and so on. Nonprocessing devices (e.g., weight scales) also belong to this classification.

Other needed instruments are called work aids. These are things like jigs and clamps, micrometers and tapes, and graphic instructions of various kinds.

Materials, Products, Subject Matter, and Services

These terms—materials, products, subject matter, and services—refer to the material worked on (wood or metal for instance), the items produced, the things involved, and the services (for instance, dentistry or hair care).

19.3.4. OCCUPATIONAL INFORMATION SET

An occupational information set encompasses all the data about jobs and occupations that provide a standard by which to measure an individual's vocational attributes during evaluation. Such sets contain what is usually referred to simply as "occupational information." There are two basic types, primary and secondary. They differ mainly in origin. Primary occupational information comes from direct observation of people at work, and secondary information comes from sources outside the work environment or is inferential in nature.

The type most satisfactory for the purposes of vocational assessment is primary information, because it is firsthand. For the same reason, however, it is difficult to obtain. Primary information is typically derived from job analysis, which is the best source of information about job requirements, but this takes a considerable amount of time and no rehabilitationist would be able to be informed personally about all of the occupations that exist in any locality. The D.O.T. is a relatively satisfactory substitute for firsthand job analysis information since this is the type of data on which it is based, and it is comprehensive and easy to use. When, however, it is possible for the rehabilitation worker to analyze a job as part of work with a client, this is the preferable approach.

The D.O.T. has proved to be very helpful in work evaluation [Colvin, 1973] because it delineates the ability requirements that workers in each occupation must meet. These occupational requirements and worker characteristics are framed as behavioral descriptions. In addition the D.O.T. characterizes career ladders and indicates, for each occupation, what preparation is needed and how entry is gained. Consequently it is possible to derive from the D.O.T. a comprehensive set of behavioral characteriza-

tions for each occupation; this constitutes an occupational information set for client evaluation.

Occupational information is vital for planning the vocational assessment of a client. It is through particular occupational information sets that the client's vocational characteristics and various jobs and occupations can be matched [Korn, 1976].

19.3.5. INFORMATION SOURCES

Hoppock [1976] discussed the various kinds of occupational information and suggested various ways in which each can be obtained. His recommendations are related here.

Supply and Demand for Workers

The best source of information about worker supply and demand is the state Employment Service. These agencies have the latest information about community labor market conditions and predictions (see 35.2.2). They collect and analyze data on the local employment picture, which is not necessarily reflective of national conditions. The *Occupational Outlook Handbook* and reports from the Occupational Outlook Service, U.S. Bureau of Labor Statistics, Washington, D.C., are good sources of information about national supply and demand trends.

Nature of the Work

The *Encyclopedia of Job Descriptions in Manufacturing* [Ross, 1969] contains information about what different types of work are like. Firsthand knowledge gained from visiting work sites is even better. It is also a good idea to ask workers to describe in detail what they do. (See 27.3.1.)

Work Environment

It is advisable to learn about the work environment by visiting places where clients might want to work. Work sites will differ in various places within one occupation, so hasty generalizations are to be avoided. Information on working conditions is contained in *Sociological Studies of Occupations*, published by the U.S. DOL, Manpower Administration (see 34.2.4).

Physical Demands

A definitive statement of requirements of jobs is part of the client planning process. Estimates must be accurate—neither overly restrictive nor understated. Local employers and employees may be able to give valid information on physical demands, but it is best to base conclusions on job analysis data or the personal observations of the trained and experienced rehabilitationist (see 34.2.3).

Aptitudes

The worker trait sections in the *D.O.T.* contain this type of information. Information that comes from employers is likely to be so general that its utility in terms of choice of an occupation is limited; qualities like "reliability" and "honesty" are desirable in workers in all occupations (see 20.3.2).

Interests

Information about the relationship between scores on an interest test and effectiveness in given occupations is provided by the test's instruction manual (see 20.3.2).

Tools and Equipment

Local employers, workers, and unions have facts about tools and equipment. While this is important information, it is subject to change with advancing technology.

Legal Requirements

Licensing boards at the city, state, and federal levels have information about the legal requirements of various jobs. One should not assume that a license is not needed until these offices have been checked, as license requirements increase every year. There are jobs licensed by some cities or states but not by others. There are many jobs in which workers must have licenses in some or all sections of the country, including airplane mechanics, apprentice seamen, architects, auctioneers, barbers, boxers, cement-block manufacturers, chauffeurs, cosmetologists, dealers in firearms, dental hygienists, food handlers, service station attendants, ice-cream manufacturers, journeyman electricians, landscape gardeners, morticians, motor-vehicle dealers, parking-lot attendants, real estate salesmen, structural welders, among a large number of others.

Unions

Administrators in local unions can supply information about requirements and about the fees connected with joining a union. Unions and employers have facts about closed-shop arrangements and the number of workers that belong to unions. While the union regulations will contain no mention of discrimination in the admission of members, a union local may in fact discriminate against a handicapped person just as employers do. (See 38.3.)

Educational Requirements

In addition to the *Occupational Outlook Handbook,* the Bureau of Labor Statistics publishes the *Jobs for Which* Series, which provides information on the amount of education and other specialized training usually required for various jobs. Regrettably for handicapped and other disadvantaged workers, the amount of formal education or training required by employers is often more than is actually necessary to satisfactorily perform job functions.

Apprenticeship

Facts about apprenticeship can be obtained from people involved in vocational education in the schools, from employers, from union personnel, and from the state Employment Service. The Bureau of Apprenticeship and Training, U.S. Department of Labor, Washington, D.C., can supply addresses of apprenticeship agencies.

There are now more than three hundred occupations for which apprentice training is provided. Some of these are aircraft engine mechanics, auto mechanics, boat-building, bookbinding, bricklaying, cabinetmaking, carpentry, commercial photography, dental mechanics, engraving, painting, pattern-making, photoengraving, plumbing, printing, radio and television repairing, refrigeration and air-conditioning mechanics, sheet-metal work, stonemasonry, tool and die-making, and watchmaking. (See 36.2.5.)

Earnings

Material on earnings in all kinds of occupations is published by the U.S. Bureau of Labor Statistics, and also by the professional, trade, business and union organizations. The local branch of the state Employment Service may be able to supply data on the prevailing wages in an area.

The College Placement Council's *Salary Survey,* which is sent to everyone who subscribes to the *Journal of College Placement,* reports what salaries are being offered to college seniors by various companies in various industries.

Number and Distribution of Workers

The Bureau of the Census, U.S. Department of Commerce, will indicate, in response to any request, which of its publications contains the information desired. Material that has been tabulated but is not available in print can be obtained in transcript form at cost. It is also possible to arrange for other tabulations at a cost. The Census Bureau provides information on the number of people working in various occupations in any area in the country by age, race, and sex.

Stability of Employment

Various conditions affect the stability of a given occupation in particular, beyond their impact on the total labor market. These variations may be of short- or long-term impact. Conditions such as the seasons, the weather, strikes, and so on, cause short-term fluctuations in some jobs. Long-term trends in an occupation also occur for various reasons: technical progress derived from new inventions and industrial methods; population changes resulting from the birth and death rates or immigration; age pattern in a particular occupation; natural resources supply stemming from depletion, discovery, or trade; the general economy of the nation and its trading areas (e.g., depressions); available capital for financing growth of industries relevant to the occupation; employment policies affecting hiring requirements (e.g., preparation level, personal characteristics); supply and demand of products or services involving the occupation; production policies and methods; governmental regulations of business and labor (e.g., minimum wages, workweek); and wars or other calamities. The *Occupational Outlook Handbook* contains relevant information on anticipated changes. (Also see 37.5.1.)

Hazards

Employers, employees, professional organizations, and unions have information about accidents and diseases associated with various occupations. Another source of this data is the *Accident Prevention Manual for Industrial Operations* of the National Safety Council [n.d.] (See 34.2.5.)

19.3.6. PUBLISHED INFORMATION

Occupational information comprises a job description and a listing of the requirements needed to perform the work effectively. The information consists of characterizations of the work, the training needed, selection factors, hiring policies, working conditions, physical demands, and job stability. It also includes facts about the opportunities for members of special groups, the limitations on such groups, the employment outlook for the future, wages, chances for advancement, licenses required, working hours, and types of equipment needed.

A number of methods of securing occupational information have been developed. Reading published occupational information, making observations and visits to job sites, and job analysis are the major methods of obtaining this data.

Printed occupational information comes from profit-making publishing companies, manufacturing and other business firms, unions, professional agencies, associations, trade organizations, and government agencies (see 27.4.2). The information is presented in many different ways designed for various purposes and toward various audiences. It may refer to one or to many occupations, may reflect the present or predict the future, or may relate to local or national conditions.

Among the occupational information compiled by the United States Employment Service are State Industry Surveys, Occupational Guides, and the *Job Guide for Young Workers*. Various states have published guides and surveys of occupations and industries that can be obtained from the state Employment Service. The U.S. Employment Service has a bibliography, *Guide to Local Occupational Information*, which names all the job guides prepared by the states and cross-indexes them according to state and occupation with *D.O.T.* codes.

19.3.7. OBSERVING JOBS

For direct knowledge about the meaning of work and job requirements and satisfaction, there is no substitute for personal experience. The firsthand or direct methods are discussed below.

Visits to Job Sites

The technique of leaving the desk to visit and observe at the work site is traditional in rehabilitation counseling and vocational guidance. The information that is obtained through visits to employers and people at work comes partly from observation and partly from discussion. One questions the employer and the workers, but with great care, since discussions could disrupt production and questions could be counterproductive to placement goals. The right question at the right time can elicit information that adds to what is observed or what is already known about the employment situation. It is also a method of validating what has been learned indirectly.

Direct observation itself, however, is the principal purpose of the job site visit. Because there is much to see, some method of organizing the information is necessary. Sinick [1970] devised an outline that could be used for this purpose by graduate students in counseling. The items can be arranged or modified for other purposes. Sinick's "Outline for Reporting Observable Aspects of a Business or Industrial Firm" has six main headings:

1. "The business or industry." The basic facts (name, address, products or services, major operations) are listed.

2. "Physical features of the environment." Includes transportation to and from the job; mobility at the job site (location of various buildings, kinds of space); lighting, heating, and so on; sanitation; noise and vibration; hazards; and other physical elements.

3. "Psychosocial features of the environment." A list is made of the characteristics of the workers by age, sex, membership in minority groups or among the disabled; interpersonal relationships (whether people work by themselves or with others, whether they have the opportunity to talk to one another, how close the supervision is); and other such features.

4. "Physical demands of work performed." Noted are the stance, limbs used, visual acuity and other sensory requirements, dexterity, weights lifted, and so on.

5. "Psychological demands of work performed." The requirements relevant to intelligence and other mental capacities, precision, repetitiveness, adaptability, and the like are noted.

6. "Psychological rewards of work performed." Autonomy, responsibility or lack of it, initiative, service, and other psychological benefits are noted.

Informal Job Analysis

In a visit to a work site the rehabilitationist who is trained in the techniques of analysing jobs can analyze jobs in a quick and informal way. Job analysis as a technique is a major source of data about jobs, and a procedure that those involved in vocational rehabilitation should know (see 34.2). There are many purposes the more formal or elaborate analyses serve: placement, training, the development of tests and work samples, job classification, the development of pay scales and advancement structure, improvement of work methods, planning, and others. Job analysis relates to many aspects of the work world: the nature of the business or industry, the physical environment, the work force, work factors, and treatment of employees. It can present a picture of a job in its context and enable someone not familiar with a particular kind of work to understand what it is really like. It is analogous to the individual analysis that emerges through various techniques of appraisal, bringing to light previously obscured potentials in an individual. Hanman [1951] devised a list of items a simple job analysis should include:

1. Title, code, and location.
2. Description of the work; what is done, how, and why; what equipment and materials are involved.
3. Definition of the requirements, in terms of skills, knowledge, degree of precision, and the like.
4. An assessment of the personal abilities and characteristics needed by the worker.
5. The physical and environmental requirements.
6. The amount and type of training required.
7. The psychological tests that might be used to select employees.
8. Information about where workers come from and what relevant apprenticeship guidelines are.
9. Explanation of the relationships between the given job and others; statement about the promotion rate and structure.
10. Explanation of how much supervision is involved.
11. The terms of employment: earnings and hours, equipment the worker must supply.
12. Special conditions (e.g., obtaining a license, membership in a union).

Job Analysis Information

When precise descriptions of specific jobs are needed, a formal job analysis is indicated. According to Andrew and Dickerson [n.d.], job analysis is the examination of what a worker does, why it is done, how it is done, and the skill needed. Determining what, how, and why produces a clear image of the work performed. Determining what skill is utilized provides additional information and suggests how complex the work tasks are.

What the worker does encompasses the various processes that are performed. Physical operations include carrying things, cutting, bending, joining, preparing, taking down, regulating, cleaning, finishing, or in some other way altering the state of the work by the use of physical energy. Planning, calculating, and judging are among the mental operations that direct the physical operations. A worker performs both physical and mental tasks. The analyst determines how wide the entire range of the job is and takes into account all the operations it encompasses and then describes all the tasks so that a total characterization emerges. The description can be organized according to a time scheme or a division that groups tasks together by type, whichever provides the most coherent picture.

How the work is done relates to the techniques used. Physically this means the various types of equipment that are used (machines, tools, and other devices), the procedures that are required, and the pattern of movement that the worker follows. Mentally this implies primarily the knowledge that is necessary for the accomplishment of the work.

To determine why a worker does a job is to identify its objective and to show the relationships of its various tasks. The job analyst identifies and states the reason for each element of the job in order to define the general objective.

Determining the skill required allows for a statement about the difficulty of the job. This section of the job analysis is a listing of the manual skills, knowledge, abilities, and other necessary worker characteristics. The material is divided into two types of information: about the work itself and about the qualities of the worker. The work entails worker functions, work fields, and materials or products or services. The worker traits include extent of preparation, aptitudes, temperaments, interests, and physical demands and external conditions.

There are a number of effective methods of job analysis. The procedure utilized by the U.S. DOL is characterized in the *Handbook for Analyzing Jobs* [U.S. DOL, Manpower Administration, 1972]. When this procedure is used with information specific to the locale, the resulting characterizations and data will be congruent with those in the *D.O.T.* The DOL's "task analysis technique" is appropriate when there are indications that a local job situation is like one described in the *D.O.T.* and the rehabilitationist wants to ascertain this without conducting a job analysis. Task analyses utilize checklists for information in the *D.O.T.* This procedure is outlined in *Task Analysis Inventories, A Method for Collecting Job Information* [U.S. DOL, Manpower Administration, 1973].

19.4. Occupational Outlook Handbook

The *Occupational Outlook Handbook* has been considered a standard reference work for many years; it is a useful guide for clients looking into career possibilities as well as a storehouse of objective information for the rehabilitationist working with these clients. The U.S. DOL, Bureau of Labor Statistics puts out an updated version every several years. The *Handbook* describes only several hundred of the thousands of occupations in America, but it discusses most occupations requiring long periods of preparation—95 percent of all sales workers; 90 per-

cent of professional, craft, and service workers; 80 percent of clerical workers; 50 percent of all operatives; and a smaller proportion of managerial workers and laborers. Following are suggestions about how to use the *Handbook* and brief descriptions of the contents.

19.4.1. INTRODUCTION

All of the occupations in the *Handbook* are arranged in "clusters" of related jobs: industrial production; office; service, education; sales; construction; transportation; scientific and technical; mechanics and repairers; health; social science; social service; and art, design, and communication occupations. Most career clusters in the *Handbook* describe a variety of jobs in a single field of work. (Training and skill requirements within a particular cluster often vary greatly). Specific occupations and industries are listed alphabetically in the index. In addition to occupational outlook material, the outlook for industries is covered.

The U.S. DOL Bureau of Labor Statistics has prepared pamphlets, based on information in the *Handbook*, that classify and describe selected occupations by the type and length of training required. An example from this series is *Jobs for Which a High School Education is Required*.

For those who are interested in working for a specific industry, the *Handbook* has descriptions about the outlook for the different jobs in that industry and their varied training requirements and earnings potential. There are 36 industries discussed in the *Handbook*, classified according to major divisions in the economy: agriculture; mining and petroleum; construction; manufacturing; transportation, communications, and public utilities; wholesale and retail trade; finance, insurance, and real estate; services; and government. An explanation is provided of the kind of information that will be found in each job description. Following most of the job titles are numbers within parentheses; these are *D.O.T.* code numbers. Information about each occupation follows the same format in order to facilitate comparisons. After each occupational title and *D.O.T.* code there are several sections, as described below.

19.4.2. NATURE OF THE WORK

In the first section of discussion about any occupation, the principle duties of workers in the occupation are described. While each job description is based on the occupation as typically performed, the particular duties will differ from one employer to another because of variations in the size of the business or industry and in location. Individual workers do specialized tasks in some occupations, while in others they do all the tasks associated with the occupation. Obviously the duties of a job change because of technological improvements; new processes are devised, and products or services undergo changes. In the preparation of the *Handbook* the effort is made to keep the information as up to date as possible, but because of the speed with which change

takes place, the publication is not always completely current. A periodical, *Occupational Outlook Quarterly*, reports recent developments.

19.4.3. PLACES OF EMPLOYMENT

The *Handbook* presents information about the number of people who work in a given occupation and shows how they are dispersed over various industries or over different geographical territories. An individual looking for a job needs to know the size of the occupation because large ones, even when their growth is not rapid, have more openings than smaller ones due to the number of workers who retire or die.

19.4.4. QUALIFICATIONS AND ADVANCEMENT

The *Handbook* points out the preferable method of entry with relation to each occupation, and for many occupations it lists the various ways in which a person can become trained. It is important to remember that the amount of training an individual has had frequently determines the level of entry and the rapidity of advancement. All states have certain requirements for some occupations in order to ensure that workers are sufficiently well qualified.

The *Handbook* allows the reader to match a set of personal characteristics with the characteristics of a job.

19.4.5. EMPLOYMENT OUTLOOK

Prospective job opportunities are discussed in the *Handbook* in separate "employment outlook" sections, most of which begin with a prediction about the growth that is expected through the next several years. An occupation is characterized as likely to grow at about the average rate, faster than average, or slower than average. The employment opportunities in a given occupation are usually good if the employment is growing at least as fast as the economy in general, while opportunities in occupations that are staying about the same size or decreasing are more limited, since the only openings result from turnovers.

The expected demand-supply ratio is the basis for discussion of prospective job opportunities in the *Handbook*. The outlook is labeled "excellent" when demand is expected to exceed supply by a great deal and "keenly competitive" when it is expected that supply will be greater than demand.

19.4.6. EARNINGS

The *Handbook* addresses a number of the questions that people selecting a career are likely to ask: whether the income will be enough to enable one to maintain a certain standard of living and to justify the cost of training; whether earnings will increase with increased experience; whether in certain parts of the country or certain industries earnings will be higher in the same occupation.

It is not easy to discover which jobs offer the best financial reward, because accurate information is available only for wages and salaries, and for certain occupations it is not possible even to determine wages and salaries. However, the *Handbook* does contain comparisons of earnings among some occupations, usually showing whether the earnings in one field are greater or less than those of workers in private industry who do not have supervisory positions.

19.4.7. WORKING CONDITIONS

Since people differ markedly in their preferences about working conditions, this factor can affect job satisfaction a great deal. Some people would rather work indoors, others outdoors; some prefer the routine quality of a 9-to-5 job to the variety of shift work, and so on. The *Handbook* covers different types of working conditions in relationship to various occupations.

The environment refers to work settings, which range from clean offices to dirty, stuffy places. People who recognize their preferences in settings can often avoid those they dislike. Outdoor work means the exposure of the employee to all kinds of variations in the weather. There are individuals who feel that this type of setting is more healthful than indoor environments.

Hazards and physical demands are two other types of working conditions dealt with in the *Handbook*. In some jobs the worker is exposed to the possibility of receiving burns or cuts, of falling or getting injured in other ways; care in following safety regulations is essential. The physical demand category refers to whether the job requires standing, stooping, or heavy lifting. People working in occupations in which these activities are necessary must be certain that they have the physical capacities required.

Chapter 20

Psychological Testing

Psychological tests are widely used in educational, rehabilitative, health care, governmental, and business settings by people who have found tests to be efficient and useful tools for sampling present behavior in an attempt to predict future behavior or the behavior of an individual in other situations. In rehabilitation, tests provide a basis for the psychological evaluation phase of client assessment. The rehabilitation counselor often conducts or requests psychological testing to help in the evaluation of assets, limitations, interests, adjustment problems, and other relevant characteristics of clients.

The purposes of psychological tests include: (1) description or diagnosis of the client's characteristics (e.g., mental retardation), and (2) prediction or estimation of expectancies of outcome if the person is placed, at a future time, in a specified situation. Tests generally measure amounts, not kinds, of behaviors or traits and are rarely used to make pass-fail decisions. While diagnostic tests can identify deviations from specified normal behavior standards, they should not result in labeling or stereotyping people.

Since there are many types of tests it is important to be specific about what is meant by a psychological test. Cronbach [1970] defined a test as "a systematic procedure for comparing the behavior of two or more persons" [p. 21]. Noll [1965] defined psychological tests as a standardized measure:

A standardized test is one that has been carefully constructed by experts in the light of acceptable objectives or purposes; procedures for administering, scoring, and interpreting scores are specified in detail so that no matter who gives the test or where it may be given, the results should be comparable; and norms or averages for different age or grade levels have been pre-determined [p. 5].

Standardized tests as used in psychological evaluation differ from classroom examinations, which usually have less systematic procedures for administration, scoring, and interpretation.

The usefulness of psychological evaluations to rehabilitation counselors was described by Sindberg, Roberts, and Pfeifer [1968].

20.1. Definitions

The field of psychological evaluation, testing, and measurement has many relevant terms with explicit meanings that sometimes vary from the lay definitions. Some of these words are listed in this section in several categories that roughly parallel the order of discussion in the chapter.

20.1.1. GENERAL CONCEPTS

Listed here are general and miscellaneous terms of fundamental importance.

PSYCHOLOGICAL EVALUATION. This refers to the service performed by a psychologist in testing and evaluating a client's intelligence, aptitudes, abilities, interests, adjustment, and other psychological characteristics.

PSYCHOMETRY. This is the science of measuring mental and psychological characteristics, including psychopathological components.

PSYCHOMETRIST. A person who administers, scores, and interprets intelligence, aptitude, achievement, and other psychological tests is called a psychometrist.

TEST. A test is a type of examination given to an individual or a group to measure a particular behavior or characteristic.

STANDARDIZED TESTS. These tests follow established or prescribed methods of administration and scoring and include norms for measuring performance. Such tests have been carefully tried out.

MENTAL MEASUREMENT. This general term refers to the use of the psychophysical methods and is also used for mental or intelligence testing.

AUTOMATED SCORING. For a test to be scorable this way it must be an objective instrument requiring explicit response from the testee, and it

must use a printed answer or response sheet that is coded so that the marks can be read by mechanical, optical, or electronic means.

OBSERVATIONAL PROCEDURE. Observation is an organized method of recording, for the purpose of appraising behavior, what a client does.

RATING SCALE. Scaled ratings present a list of descriptive words or phrases that are checked by the observer or the rater.

MENTAL SCALE. A series of mental tests is called a scale when arranged—usually in order of difficulty—to give measurement of the level of mental development in terms like mental age, intelligence quotient, or percentile rank.

BATTERY OF TESTS. Several tests administered separately but in a series for a coordinated purpose are called a battery.

PSYCHOLOGICAL PROFILE. A graphical representation of an individual's standing, or level, in a series of tests, measuring various aspects of mentality or other psychological characteristics, is known as a profile.

20.1.2. TEST CONSTRUCTION

The statistical concepts given here will be more completely described in later sections of this chapter.

RELIABILITY. Reliability means the consistency of the scores of a test.

VALIDITY. Validity means the extent to which a test measures what it is intended or purports to measure.

SCORE. A score is the quantitative value assigned to the response to an item or to the whole series of responses in a test. A "raw score" is the performance before statistical weight or correction is applied.

AVERAGE. Average is a general term applied to measures of central tendency. The three most widely used averages are the arithmetic mean (M), the median (Mdn), and the mode (Mo). The arithmetic mean is the sum of a set of scores divided by the number of scores. The median is the middle score in the distribution, the 50th percentile, the point that divides the group into two equal parts with half of the group of scores falling below the median and half above it. The mode is the most frequently occurring value in a series—the peak, or peaks, in a frequency curve.

NORMAL DISTRIBUTION CURVE. This is a frequency distribution that has the shape of a bell-shaped curve.

STANDARD DEVIATION (SD). The SD of a distribution of scores is the square root of the mean of the squares of individual deviations from the mean in the series.

PERCENTILE RANK. A percentile (%ile) score is the position of a value in a series arranged in order of magnitude, calculated by the percentage of scores falling at or below that position.

QUARTILE. This refers to one of three points that divide the scores in a distribution into four equal groups: the 25th percentile, which sets off the lowest fourth of the group; the 50th percentile, or median; and the third quartile or 75th percentile, which is exceeded only by the highest fourth.

STANDARD SCORE. A standard score expresses an individual's distance from the mean in terms of the standard deviation of the distribution of scores of a specifically designated group.

INTELLIGENCE QUOTIENT (IQ). IQ is an arithmetical figure, a numerical expression of intelligence that is derived by dividing mental age (determined through psychological testing) by chronological age (of the testee) and multiplying by 100. It indicates one's intellectual performance compared to the statistical norm for one's age group. An IQ of 100 is average.

DEVIATION IQ (DIQ) SCORES. DIQ scores are a type of standard score expressed as the test's standard deviation above or below a mean of 100.

NORM. This is a statistical measure based on a specified sample and used in the interpretation of raw scores. Norms represent the test performance of a specified group comparable with the client or client goals.

20.1.3. HUMAN CHARACTERISTICS

Many human characteristics can be measured by today's tests. A number of these characteristics are given below (a later section will describe relevant instruments).

INTELLIGENCE. There is no universally agreed upon concept for intelligence; consequently several definitions are needed: stage of mental development, problem-solving ability, ability to adapt rapidly and appropriately to environmental demands and new situations, ability to apprehend abstract interrelationships, or, ability to learn from experience. The intellect is the mind in its cognitive aspects—the higher thought processes involving perceiving, knowing, and understanding.

LEARNING. Learning is the facility with which knowledge is acquired as a function of experience.

MEMORY SPAN. This involves the number of individual items (usually digits or syllables) that an individual can reproduce correctly and in order immediately after a single presentation.

ACHIEVEMENT. Usually indicating academic activity, an achievement test is one designed to measure level of knowledge attained in a given area such as reading or arithmetic, but it may refer to manual, personal, or social success.

ABILITY. Abilities are powers possessed by an individual whether physical, mental or social; inherited or acquired; general or specific. The word *ability* (as distinguished from *aptitude*) implies that the task can be done now without further training.

PRIMARY MENTAL ABILITIES (PMA). PMA refers to hypothetical units, various combinations of which constitute all distinguishable abilities: verbal comprehension, word fluency, number computation, space perception and visualization memory, perceptual speed, and general reasoning.

APTITUDE. Aptitude is the potentiality for acquiring proficiency after appropriate training and experience. Aptitude facilitates learning in various tasks: academic (activities involving classic learning), verbal (comprehending and using words and associated ideas in language), numerical (performing arithmetic quickly and accurately), spatial (comprehending geometric forms in space and visualizing their dimensional relationships), and mechanical (dealing with machines).

PERSONALITY. Personality in the narrow sense, as used in testing, relates to affective or nonintellectual aspects of behavior. It can include characteristics such as emotional adjustment, interpersonal relations, motivation, attitudes, and interests.

ADJUSTMENT. This is a dynamic process in which one becomes better acquainted with one's inner self, goals, other persons, the environment, and ways of meeting life's crises. It is not a static state.

INTEREST. Positive feelings about subjects, objects, situations, or processes are called interests. Expressed interests are verbal expressions of preferences; manifest interests are expressed in actions, through participation in activities. Inventoried interests are estimates of interests based on responses to a large number of questions concerning likes and dislikes or preference of activities.

MOTIVATION. Motivation is an aroused, incited response to one's environment that is not controlled by external pressure.

ATTITUDE. An attitude is a predisposition with regard to one's actions or thoughts. Attitudes dictate the response—positive or negative—readiness that one has acquired by experience and that consequently influences one's ideas, opinions, beliefs, prejudices, values, purposes, interests, and behavior.

MANUAL DEXTERITY. This refers to the ability to move and coordinate the hands easily, rapidly, and accurately in placing and turning motions used to accomplish elements of manual work.

MECHANICAL ABILITY. The knowledgeable application of the principles of mechanics and skill in the use of tools and the operation of machinery is known as mechanical ability.

TRADE TEST. Trade tests are designed to measure proficiency in a specified skilled occupation. The format is usually a series of tasks involving the performance of definite pieces of work in that occupation, and/or technical information with regard to the occupation.

20.1.4. TYPES OF INSTRUMENTS
Terms for several major types of tests and measurement techniques are given below:

INVENTORY. In the field of evaluation, an inventory is a device (e.g., questionnaire) in which subjects mark a list to indicate whether certain kinds of behavior characterize them or not, and to reflect how they would react to certain imaginary situations.

PROBLEM CHECKLIST. This is a type of self-report inventory in which clients are asked to check personal concerns. The Purdue *Handicap Problems Inventory* is explicitly related to rehabilitation [Wright & Remmers, 1960].

QUESTIONNAIRE. This is any instrument composed of a series of questions that is used to furnish a cross-sectional view of the respondent in terms of certain characteristics of the person.

DIGIT-SPAN TEST. This test is a method of determining memory span by the number of digits the person can repeat in order, after a single hearing.

VOCABULARY TEST. This type of mental test aims at the determination of an individual's store of understood words. It is given by presenting the subject with a standard list of words to define or to pair.

PERFORMANCE TEST. This is a type of mental test in which the subject is asked to do rather than say or write something. The requirement of using language or symbols is greatly reduced or eliminated.

NONVERBAL TESTS. These are intelligence or other mental tests that do not employ verbal material, or, sometimes, that can be given without employing words (e.g., to deaf or culturally different individuals).

CULTURE-FREE TESTS. Tests like this attempt to measure certain aspects of the individual without distortion in the final results due to cultural or sociological biases that favor one group over another.

SITUATIONAL TESTS. In this technique the person is placed in a testing situation closely resembling or simulating a real-life situation.

PROJECTIVE TEST. "Projectives" are relatively unstructured tests in which ambiguous stimuli are presented to the testee. Responses are assumed to reflect the underlying personality patterns or dynamics of the individual.

20.2. *Test Construction*

Psychological tests are constructed through sophisticated psychometric procedures. The research effort of the test author does not stop with the completion of a sound instrument for the measurement of a human characteristic; the author who publishes a psychological test is obliged to prepare a manual for the instruction and understanding of potential users. The American Psychological Association [1974] has published *Standards for Educational and Psychological Tests and Manuals*. The evaluation of a test to determine its uses and limitations can continue long after its initial publication by the test's author and by other researchers. Further study contributes to improvement and revisions for future editions.

20.2.1. STANDARDIZED TESTS

The psychological tests described in this chapter are standardized instruments. The term *standardized test* signifies a measuring instrument with the following characteristics, as summarized from Adams [1965]:

1. There are detailed instructions for administering the test, typically including the words the examiner will use in giving directions and stating time limits.
2. There are specific instructions for scoring, usually including a key that the scorer uses. All the scorer has to do is compare test answers with the key. In some instances samples are included.
3. Norms are provided for scores to help in interpretation.
4. There is data by which the usefulness of the test can be evaluated. Research is done to establish the reliability and validity of the test before it can be purchased.

5. A manual comes with the test that describes its construction, purposes, and uses; explains how it should be administered, scored, and interpreted; provides tables of norms; and summarizes results of research on the test.

Standardized tests are constructed first by selecting items (questions to be answered or tasks to be performed) that appear to measure a particular behavior or knowledge. The items are then presented to groups of people to determine which items differentiate people into individuals who do well on the item and individuals who do poorly. Items that do not differentiate people into two such groups are discarded and new items are generated to replace them. Eventually a set of items is found, all of which differentiate the test group; these items become the test instrument.

20.2.2. STATISTICAL CONCEPTS

In taking a test, people score points by answering the questions in a certain way or by performing the task correctly. The total number of points obtained by a testee is known as the "raw score."

When a large group of people take a particular test and a set of raw scores has been obtained, the test population can be analyzed through certain mathematical manipulations on the raw scores. Perhaps the most visual way of seeing how a group performed on the test is to plot a graph of the raw scores, with the horizontal axis listing the raw scores and the vertical axis showing the number of times a particular score was obtained in the group of testees. Such a graph of scores versus frequency of occurrence is known as a frequency distribution.

Although frequency distributions will vary in

shape for different tests and test populations, most psychological and mental tests result in a frequency distribution of the same general type, known as a normal distribution. The graph of a normal distribution is a symmetrical, bell-shaped curve centered on the mean raw score. The mean score, the arithmetical average of a set of scores, is obtained by summing all the scores and dividing the sum by the number of scores.

In a normal distribution, the number of scores above the mean is equal to the number below it, with most scores being concentrated near the mean. Frequency of occurrence decreases as scores depart further from the mean, according to a precise mathematical equation. The assumption that tests produce scores with a normal distribution is usually made and has been very useful in test development.

The standard deviation (SD) is a measure of the variability of scores around the mean; in other words, the SD characterizes the distribution of scores. A distribution with scores clustered tightly about the mean has a small standard deviation, and thus does not differentiate well between testees because most of the test population responded the same way to the items. In a normal distribution, 34.13 percent of the scores are 1 SD above the mean and 34.13 percent are 1 SD below it; 68.26 percent of all scores are within 1 SD (plus or minus) of the mean, 95.44 percent are within 2 SD of the mean, and 99.72 percent are within 3 SD of the mean.

Raw scores alone are meaningless, because their interpretation depends on the number and difficulty of test items. A raw score of 10, for example, represents good performance if the items were difficult and there were only 10 possible points, but represents poor performance if the items were easy and there were 100 possible points. Raw scores have meaning only when compared to scores of other persons taking the test, a criterion of mastery at the assigned task, or to norm group scores (norms) provided in the manual of a standardized test.

20.2.3. NORMS AND NORM GROUPS

A norm group is a specified group of people who have taken the test and who have been selected by the testmaker for certain specific characteristics that define the group (e.g., age, education, geographical location, or occupation).

Establishing norms is an important part of the process of standardizing a test because a person's raw score is understood through comparison with norm group scores. Depending on the test the norm score may be expressed in terms of the number of correct answers, the time needed to finish the test, the number of errors, or another objective measure.

The norms indicate the testee's relative performance or deviation from the average [Anastasi, 1976]. Norms then provide the basis for comparing performance. As Mehrens and Lehmann [1969] emphasized, norms and standards are not the same. Norm information describes people's actual performance; it does not express how they should perform.

Types of Norms

The comparison of a test score can be based on national norms, local norms, or specific group norms. National norms are obtained by testing a very large number of people representing both sexes, all age ranges, major geographical areas, and all or most educational and socioeconomic levels. These norms supposedly represent the scores of the general population.

Local norms are obtained by testing a large number of people living in a particular community, county, or state. This group may or may not have characteristics similar to those of the national norm group. In many cases, local norms are preferred to national norms because the former may reflect local tradition, culture, educational standards, and social characteristics, and therefore mirror local reality more accurately than national norms do.

Specific group norms result when people from an appropriately identified group are tested. These groups are often defined by membership in a vocational or disability group, such as musicians or educable mentally retarded adults, respectively. These norms are applicable when general population (national or local) norms are inappropriate for comparison. The choice of norms to use for comparison depends on the availability, appropriateness, and recency of the norms.

Perspectives on Norms

It is possible to interpret norms in a meaningful way only in relation to a reference group: a sample of all the 10-year-old children in a given community, for instance, or a sample of all educable mentally retarded adults in the country. The reference group is selected in accordance with the types of decisions being made; one reference group would be necessary for choosing students for vocational study and another for choosing students for college.

20.2.4. EXPRESSION OF NORM SCORES

Norm scores are commonly expressed as percentiles, standard scores, normalized standard scores, transformed normalized standard scores, and grade equivalents.

Percentile Scores

A percentile score is a number that represents the percentage of persons in the standardization sample (norm group) whose scores fall below a given raw score. A percentile is not a percent score. A percent usually refers to the number of correct items, whereas a percentile refers to the relative standing of a person's score within a group of scores. For example, someone successfully answering 75 out of 100 questions has correctly answered 75 percent of the test items, but the raw score may be at the 65th percentile, which means that the individual's score is above 65 percent of the scores of those (in the norm group) who have taken the test. Percentiles are easily computed and understood so they have been widely used for expressing intelligence, multiple aptitude, interest, and adjustment test scores [Downie, 1967].

Standard Scores

Increasing use is being made of standard scores. They express the testee's distance from the mean in terms of the standard deviation of the distribution. A linearly derived standard score is computed by dividing the difference between a raw score and the mean by the SD of the normative group. A shortcoming of this method arises when the distribution of the test group is not normal but skewed (lopsided); in this case the test's scores would not be comparable to scores from another, normal, test distribution.

Normalized Standard Scores

Comparability of scores from dissimilarly shaped distribution is facilitated through nonlinear transformations, the scores arranged to fit a normal bell-shaped curve. Normalized standard scores can be computed by reference to tables giving the percentage of cases falling at different SD distances from the mean of the normal bell-shaped distribution. A continuing an-

noyance of using standard scores (even if normalized) is that they are expressed as plus or minus values above or below zero (the mean.)

Transformed (T) Standard Scores

Standard scores (whether or not normalized) can be further transformed to avoid negative values. T scores are obtained by multiplying the normalized standard score by ten and then adding the resulting number to 50. T scores have a mean of 50, a standard deviation of ten.

The deviation intelligence quotient is a transformed standard score having a mean of 100, a standard deviation of 15 or 16, depending on the specific intelligence test. Major intelligence tests use deviation intelligence quotients, although some older and seldom used ones report intelligence quotients as the ratio of mental age to chronological (actual) age.

Grade Equivalent Scores

Achievement test scores are commonly reported as grade equivalents, which indicate the testee's academic level of achievement in each achievement area tested, such as reading, spelling, and arithmetic. The test manual provides achievement norms that have been determined by testing pupils in grades K through 12.

20.2.5. RELIABILITY AND VALIDITY

Before it can be assumed that a test is adequate for use, its measurements must have two critical characteristics: reliability and validity.

Reliability

The repeatability and precision of a measurement are referred to as reliability. When a measure is completely reliable, any change in the test score reflects a change in the attribute being measured. A test is unreliable to the degree that its scores are influenced by extraneous factors. These sources of error can be both systematic and random.

Repeatability of scores represents the stability of the measurement. This form of reliability is estimated by the test-retest method (i.e., the same test is administered on two or more occasions and the results correlated).

Precision of scores represents the consistency of the measurement—the agreement between two measurements taken simultaneously. This form of reliability is estimated by various internal comparison methods (e.g., slit-half, alternate form, interitem correlation).

The reliability of a test may be expressed in terms of the standard error of measurement (i.e., standard error of a score). This measure can be more useful than the reliability coefficient in the interpretation of individual scores. Computation of the error of measurement provides a prediction of the range of fluctuation likely to occur in a single individual's score as a result of irrelevant, chance factors. Conditions that are irrelevant to the test purposes represent error variance. For this reason the psychometrist or test administrator maintains uniform conditions (the environment, instructions, timing, rapport, etc.) whenever the test is given. No test score, however, is perfectly reliable.

Error results from five principal factors: insufficient sampling of content, insufficient number of items, subjectivity in scoring, inadequate standardization of directions and other aspects of test situation, and changes, during a short period of time, in characteristics of people being tested. The reliability coefficient is best calculated when as many of these sources of error as possible are taken into consideration.

Reliability is necessary for validity but is not enough in itself. Unreliable measurement cannot yield useful results; on the other hand, many highly reliable methods do not yield results that are meaningful in any real sense [Nunnally, 1970].

Validity

Simply stated, a test's validity means the accuracy of its measurement—it measures what it is supposed to measure and nothing else. The issue of validity places responsibility on the test user to know the nature of the phenomenon being studied. A test's name only identifies the instrument; it is necessary to study the manual, evaluative reports, and other research and clinical experience for an understanding of proper uses and interpretation of a test.

Several types of evidence of validity are recognized:

1. Content validity. This refers to the completeness of coverage of the range of behaviors the instrument is designed to measure. Estimating this type of validity involves a systematic examination of the test content to determine if the entire domain is sampled proportionately. Content validity is determined by the development and choice of appropriate items in the early stages of test construct. Content validity is often confused with so-called "face validity," which has nothing to do with what a test actually measures and so is not properly termed *validity*. Face validity only means that the test looks valid to the testee and other untrained observers; this is actually a desirable feature of a test for reasons of client rapport and public relations.

2. Concurrent and predictive validity. The criterion measures against which test scores are validated may be obtained at the same time as the test scores or after a stated interval. Both concurrent and predictive validity depend on the relation between the test scores and on this independent criterion, whether it is of the present or of the future. Concurrent comparisons may be similar tests, judges' ratings, or behavioral observations presumed to measure the same thing the test does. Predictive validation involves the relationship of the test score to a future behavior (e.g., graduation from school).

3. Construct validity. Construct validity of a test is the extent to which it measures a theoretical construct or trait. Examples of constructs include intelligence, mechanical aptitude, verbal fluency, and anxiety. Because this is an abstract description of behavior, understanding it is more difficult and time-consuming. Factor analysis, a statistical procedure for identifying psychological traits, is one method used.

20.3. *Classification of Tests*

This section describes the purposes for which standardized tests are designed. It will also provide further understanding of the concepts of psychometric measurement.

20.3.1. BASIC DIMENSIONS

A number of fundamental differences or dimensions of tests are described below.

Maximum Performance vs Typical Performance

Maximum performance tests elicit a person's best performance and therefore measure top natural ability, learned ability, and motivation as integrated into the behavior sampled in the test. In contrast, typical performance tests elicit a person's usual performance, as it might be demonstrated in daily living.

Speed vs Power

Speed tests measure a person's quickness in answering many easy items. Such tests may not require much analytical ability because the items may be so easy that all could be correctly answered if there were sufficient time. Some special ability tests such as clerical speed tests are examples of this type of test.

Power tests measure a person's analytical and reasoning abilities by presenting a few, very difficult items in an untimed test. Although some abstract reasoning tests are examples of power tests, there are in reality few tests that are purely speed or purely power tests; most tests are a combination of the two.

Objective vs Subjective

Objective tests are characterized by systematic procedures for scoring that make the score independent of scorer judgment and expertise. Almost all standardized tests are objective tests. A few, however, are regarded as standardized in spite of the fact that they lack systematic scoring procedures and rely on the evaluator's personal judgment and values. The Rorschach is such an example of the subjective standardized test.

Verbal vs Nonverbal

Verbal tests require verbal or written responses to verbal or written questions. Nonverbal tests require physical performances, such as manipulations of an object, in response to presented directions, pictures, figures, forms, and other objects. Intelligence, multiple aptitude, achievement, interest, and personality tests can be verbal or nonverbal; most contain elements of both.

Criterion vs Norm-Referenced Test

Criterion-referenced testing uses a specified content domain as the frame of reference for interpretation; norm-referenced testing uses a specified population (i.e., an individual's score is interpreted by comparing it with scores obtained by others on the same test). In criterion-referenced testing the focus is on what the individual knows and can do—not on how this person compares with other people. Criterion examples are vocabulary size, reading comprehension level, and areas of arithmetic mastery. Scores may be interpreted in terms of expected performance, as in a training program or on a job. Expectancy tables show the relationship between the test score and the criterion (e.g., grade in a course of study).

Individual vs Group

Administered to one person at a time, individual tests are used for (1) evaluating people with suspected or known mental retardation or sensory deficits, (2) stimulating maximum performance, interest, motivation, and effort, and (3) observing and evaluating the testee's behavior. Group tests are administered to several people at a time and are used when group members are free from sensory deficits and retardation, and when there is insufficient time to test each group member individually. All group tests can be individual tests, but not all individual tests can be group tests. The Wechsler Adult Intelligence Scale is an individual test that cannot be administered to a group.

20.3.2. TEST CONTENT

The most common way of classifying standardized tests is according to their content (i.e., what they measure). Even this scheme is not perfect, however, because there is often a looseness between what is measured and how it is interpreted, and thus a given test may be classified into more than one content area because it can be interpreted to measure different aspects of personality. These ambiguities will be discussed as the test categories are described.

Standardized tests can be categorized in a number of ways in terms of administrative methods (e.g., individual or group administration, oral or written directions). Most frequently they are classified according to what they measure: (1) intelligence and aptitude tests; (2) achievement tests; (3) interest, personality, and attitude inventories.

The first two types are frequently regarded as tests of maximum performance and the third type as tests of typical performance. According to another categorization, intelligence, aptitude, and achievement tests are cognitive measures while interest, personality, and attitude inventories are noncognitive measures. Some term the noncognitive measures as inventories because answers are not objectively right or wrong; and use of the term *inventory* may also minimize the apprehension of the person taking the test. However, these measures are standardized tests as described above, regardless of whether they are called tests or inventories.

Intelligence Tests or Tests of General Ability

These tests all measure intelligence as it is defined by the particular test's author. There is, however, no universally agreed-upon definition of intelligence, a fact that is important to keep in mind when interpreting intelligence tests.

Intelligence tests mirror different conceptualizations of intelligence. Some contain only verbal material and others have nonverbal items; some emphasize problem-solving and others, memory; some produce one score and others, a profile of scores. Because of these and other disparities, results differ; if one person takes two kinds of tests, it is probable that two different scores will be obtained.

Defining and measuring intelligence is a complicated problem. Many people have the mistaken notion that intelligence tests measure a capacity, either inborn or acquired in some way during childhood, that remains the same throughout an individual's lifetime. But intelligence is a highly complex phenomenon, and tests do not measure it fully. Because past learning influences performance on these tests, achievement rather than intelligence is sometimes reflected in the scores.

Mehrens and Lehmann [1969] discussed the difference between intelligence tests and aptitude tests. The differentiation between the two is based on whether a test yields a general measure or not. Tests that do are considered intelligence tests, while those that measure multiple or specific factors are called aptitude tests. Both of these types of test measure aspects of personality that are influenced by hereditary and environmental factors.

The individual tests of mental ability that are most widely used are the Wechsler Adult Intelligence Scale (WAIS) and the Wechsler Intelligence Scale for Children-Revised. The WAIS, which takes about 45 minutes, is considered the most effective measure of adult intelligence so far developed. As defined by David Wechsler, intelligence is the aggregate or global capacity of the individual to act purposefully, to think rationally, and to deal effectively with the environment. The WAIS yields three scores from six verbal and five performance subtests: Verbal IQ, Performance IQ, and Full Scale IQ. The verbal subtests consist of General Information, General Comprehension, Arithmetical Reasoning, Similarities, Digit Span, and Vocabulary. The performance subtests are Digit Symbol, Picture Completion, Block Design, Picture Arrangement, and Object Assembly.

A number of other tests of human intelligence are commercially published. The Stanford-Binet test, with several American revisions, is the oldest device of its kind; it was first developed for use with children. A more thorough coverage would also include: California Test of Mental Maturity, Columbia Mental Maturity Scale, Cognitive Abilities Test, Culture Fair Intelligence Tests, Goodenough-Harris Drawing Test, Henmon-Nelson Tests of Mental Ability, Kulmann-Anderson Intelligence Test, McCarthy Scales of Childrens' Abilities, Otis-Lennon Mental Ability Tests, Peabody Picture Vocabulary Test, and Raven's Progressive Matrices.

Specific or special aptitude tests are selectively listed below. The classification was suggested by Nunnally [1970].

Psychomotor Aptitude

These measures include visual-motor speed and coordination (manual and finger dexterity). Dexterity tests do not correlate well with one another and frequently measure very different abilities. Despite this psychometric fault—or perhaps because of this characteristic—motor tests have been found to be of considerable value in the vocational assessment of disabled people. They are also useful in industrial selection, particularly for work that is uncomplicated, that utilizes a particular group of motor skills, and that depends a great deal on speed. Routine production-line assembly, sewing machine operation, and packaging are examples of this type of work. The motor tests that have highest validity are job samples, which reproduce the equipment used on the job.

Performance tests in general are described in Chapter 23, Work Evaluation Techniques. A number of dexterity tests are described (see 23.1.2).

Mechanical Aptitude

Mechanical aptitude tests include psychomotor, perceptual, spatial, and mechanical reasoning aptitudes. Such tests are useful in predicting vocational or trade school success and performance at skilled mechanical type jobs.

Mechanical work is not based on any single kind of test function to the degree that performance in school is related to general intelligence tests; therefore, a combination of tests is needed in order to make predictions about a given type of mechanical work. Various sets of tests are used for different types of work (e.g., mechanical comprehension, perceptual skills, and spatial relations). General batteries of tests are not easy to design or employ for the purpose of vocational counseling because the range of skills needed for different mechanical jobs is so great. Therefore there are test batteries designed especially for choosing people for particular kinds of work; for instance, assembling electronic equipment.

Clerical Aptitude

While the term *clerk* applies to people in many different jobs, for example, the grocery clerk, the court clerk, as used here the word clerical relates to the office clerk who handles records and paper. The prediction of clerical performance depends especially on perceptual speed, which is used in tasks like proofreading, scanning, and alphabetizing. The Minnesota Clerical Test exemplifies those that depend heavily on perceptual speed; it contains two sections that are timed individually, Number Comparison and Name Comparison. The Clerical Speed and Accuracy Test of the Differential Aptitude Test (DAT), the Clerical Perception Test of the General Aptitude Test Battery (GATB), and parts of the General Clerical Test all measure perceptual speed for clerical aptitude.

While clerical work necessitates perceptual speed, it relies on other attributes also. Verbal comprehension, particularly a command of spelling and grammar, is often important; because some arithmetic is frequently necessary, a test of numerical facility is sometimes indicated. Certain dexterity tests are useful when the work involves accounting or other office machines.

The DAT measures a number of verbal and arithmetical abilities as well as perceptual speed; and the General Clerical Test, with nine short subtests, yields clerical, numerical, and verbal scores.

Artistic Aptitudes

The measurement of artistic aptitude evolves into several components. Most painting requires the ability to make line drawings, to combine colors, and to achieve properties of "balance." In musical ability there are the basic sensory skills of tonal memory, sense of pitch, and recognition of rhythms, which to some extent cut across different kinds of musical production.

Multiple Aptitude Tests and Achievement Tests

These two types of test are very similarly constructed in that they both contain items related to specific academic subject areas, such as arithmetic, or specific academic objectives. The primary distinction between multiple aptitude and achievement tests is the use to which the results are put: multiple aptitude test information is used to predict future learning and performance, whereas achievement test results are used to assess present knowledge, skills, and performance. In different situations, the same test may be used to measure aptitude and achievement.

Vocational aptitude batteries are an important tool in vocational rehabilitation. The GATB (in conversation, pronounced "gat-bee") was produced by U.S. DOL, Bureau of Employment Security and is generally administered by the state Employment Service agencies. Nine factors are measured by the GATB: verbal, numerical, spatial, form perception, clerical perception, motor coordination, finger dexterity, manual dexterity, and general mental ability (the last score results from a combination of three other scores).

The DAT battery is commercially published by The Psychological Corporation. Its subtests are verbal reasoning, numerical ability, abstract reasoning, space relations, mathematical reasoning, clerical, and language. (See 23.1.3.)

Sensory Tests

Although they are not specific aptitude tests, sensory tests are often so classified. Many senses may be tested, but the two most important to vocational success are vision and hearing. Visual modalities that may be tested are visual acuity (blindness), depth perception, color discrimination (color blindness), and eye muscle strength and balance. Hearing modalities include pitch, loudness, level of noise that causes pain, and auditory discrimination (deafness). Some vision and hearing tests measure all of the respective modalities; others measure a few of them.

Personality Tests

Sweeping and vague definitions of personality have been formulated by some psychologists—"the total functioning individual interacting with his environment" is an example. These definitions take in all aspects of ability, which have been separated from personality here.

A consideration of personality involves two general questions: what people are like at any particular time and how they came to be that way. When personality is measured, the emphasis is on the first question, and the aim is to characterize a person with respect to attributes such as aggression, extroversion, and the like.

Tests of personality attributes, like tests of abilities, focus largely on individual differences. There are four general categories of human attributes with which personality tests deal: (1) social traits—the individual's typical behavior in relation to others (e.g., honesty, gregariousness, hostility); social traits are frequently regarded as the outermost personality level, how a person seems to others; (2) motives—a person's "needs" or "drives," especially those considered "nonbiological" (e.g., the need for accomplishment, aggression, affiliation); (3) personal conceptions—one's sense of self and view of the world (e.g., interests, values, self-esteem); (4) adjustment/maladjustment—an individual's degree of freedom from serious emotional problems or the tendency to engage in disruptive behavior.

Types of Personality Tests

These instruments measure emotional, motivational, interpersonal, and attitude characteristics. Personality tests can generally be identified as self-report tests or projective tests.

Self-report tests elicit from a person self-descriptive information that supposedly represents typical behavior or reactions. They are objective in the sense that they provide structural questions, elicit forced choices from a few provided answers, and may have keys or scales to detect faking, malingering, and socially desirable responses. (Socially desirable responses are answers that represent what the testee thinks is the socially "good" response and do not represent the testee's true feelings, thoughts, or behavior.)

Projective tests elicit perceptions, stories, or actions from testees that represent their fantasies, reactions, or behavior. These tests are subjective in the sense that testees respond to ambiguous inkblots, words, or pictures, and may make an unlimited number of responses. Theoretically, testees do not know the meaning of revealed information and therefore do not know how to fake or give socially desirable answers. Projective tests have low reliability and validity, when these characteristics can even be demonstrated, but nevertheless clinicians have found them useful. The Rorschach and the Thematic Apperception Test are examples of projective tests.

Personality Inventory Measures

Printed tests that ask people to describe themselves are much more frequently used to measure personality than any other test method. Personal conceptions emerge from self-inventories, which are often employed to test social traits, motives, and adjustment; but, while there is some common ground between personal conceptions and the three other elements of personality, they do not coincide completely.

The Minnesota Multiphasic Personality Inventory (MMPI) is the best example of a self-report test of personality in terms of sound construction and wide use. There are many years of extensive research behind the MMPI and its modification. Moreover, its utilization has been described in hundreds of articles. The MMPI indicates the presence or absence of eight forms of mental illness and also measures masculinity and femininity interest and social introversion.

1. Hypochondriasis (Hs): Excessive concern with physical functions and imagined illness.
2. Depression (D): Intense despondency and sense of worthlessness.
3. Hysteria (Hy): The evolution of physical malfunctions (blindness, paralysis, vomiting) as a way of avoiding emotional difficulties.
4. Psychopathic deviate (Pd): Someone with-

out a "conscience," with little concern for others, frequently in trouble.

5. Paranoia (Pa): Suspiciousness so intense that the person imagines intricate plots.
6. Psychasthenia (Pt): Intense apprehensions and compulsions.
7. Schizophrenia (Sc): Bizarre thoughts and behavior, lack of communication with the rest of the world.
8. Hypomania (Ma): Overactivity, extremely low ability to concentrate.
9. Masculinity-femininity (Mf): The proportion of male to female interests.
10. Social Introversion (Si): Shy, introverted, not extroverted.

In addition to the mental-illness scales available on the MMPI, four so-called validity scores are used. These provide information about the test-taking attitude of the subject and the relative honesty with which responses were made.

Another test that is administered fairly frequently, though by no means as widely used as the MMPI, is the California Psychological Inventory. While it has many items like those of the MMPI, its primary scales gear the test more toward the normal personality.

Other personality inventories include the Adjective Check List, Edwards Personal Preference Schedule, Eysenck Personality Inventory, FIRO Scales, Gordon Personal Inventory/Profile, Guilford-Zimmerman Temperament Survey, Mooney Problem Check List, Tennessee Self Concept Scale, and the Thorndike Dimensions of Temperament.

Projective Techniques

A different approach to the measurement of personality is provided by projective techniques. Instead of describing themselves, as required by the self-description inventories, subjects characterize or explain other things. Underlying these techniques is the assumption that people's reactions to an "unstructured" stimulus are affected by their inner drives, motivations, and attitudes. A structured stimulus is one that has a meaning publicly agreed upon. An unstructured stimulus has no such public meaning and therefore provides much room for subjective interpretation of it.

The Rorschach method produces an estimate of personality based on responses to a set of 10 different cards that all have one meaningless inkblot, some of which are in color. Comprehensive guides for scoring by clinical psychologists have been published.

The stimuli on the Thematic Apperception Test (TAT) are more structured than those on the Rorschach test. There are 29 cards with indistinct pictures on them and one blank card. Most pictures are of one or more persons, doing something the observer cannot see clearly; the testee is asked to tell a story about the scene. This test supposedly produces a comprehensive characterization of personality based on content, social relationships, ideas and fantasies, attitudes and feelings, needs, tensions, and conflicts. The premise is that the stories that are told reflect the personal ideas, experiences, desires, and values of the testee.

Other projective techniques include various word association tests, self-expression (Draw-A-Person-Test), and toy tests.

Interest Tests

Interest tests measure a person's liking or dislike for a wide variety of specific activities, objects, or types of persons encountered in daily living. On that basis, interest tests may be used to predict how well a person will fit with a specific vocational group.

Bingham [1937] defined an interest as the proclivity to become absorbed in an activity and continue in it, and an aversion as the opposite tendency. Five pairs of interest factors would therefore suggest that a preference for one element of a pair implies a dislike of the other element of the pair. Interest factors for jobs were expressed as "a preference for" each of the following:

1. Activities dealing with things and objects vs. activities concerned with the communication of data.
2. Activities involving business contact with people vs. activities of a scientific and technical nature.
3. Activities of a routine, concrete, organized nature vs. activities of an abstract and creative nature.
4. Working for the presumed good of people vs. activities that are carried on in relation to processes, machines, and techniques.
5. Activities resulting in prestige or the esteem of others vs. activities resulting in tangible, productive satisfaction.

In analyzing a job for interest factors, the choice of one factor presumably results in the exclusion of its opposite. Thus, to state that a job necessitates a preference for activities of a routine and organized nature implies that it does not demand a preference for activities that are abstract and creative. (An obvious limitation of this perspective is that many jobs involve a preference for both types of activities.)

The Strong-Campbell Interest Inventory (SCII) occupational scales have been normed on criterion groups of people employed in various occupations. In general, these criterion groups included people who were successful, persistent, and satisfied with their individual occupation(s). It also includes Basic Interest Scales (e.g., Mechanical, Mathematics, Nature) as well as Holland's Vocational Types (e.g., Realistic, Investigative, Aesthetic, Social, Enterprising, and Conventional). It was especially designed for mature high school and college students and adults who are interested in high level occupations and assumes a high level of reading ability.

The Minnesota Vocational Interest Inventory (MVII) was designed specifically to measure the interests of people 15 years of age and older in nonprofessional areas. It is especially useful for noncollege students. It is empirically keyed, using a criterion group such as store clerks or machinists, with a reference group of "tradesmen" in general.

The Kuder Occupational Interest Survey assesses individual preferences, likes, and dislikes for activities and compares them with those of other persons in a wide range of occupations. The manual for this Kuder test has an extensive list of occupations grouped according to their major interest area(s).

The Interest Check List of the U.S. Employment Service is a nonscorable interviewing aid designed particularly for use with persons who have no well-defined vocational interests. This instrument, as revised in 1979, consists of 210 sample tasks which have been keyed to the 66 work groups in the 715 page *Guide for Occupational Exploration* published by the U.S. DOL Employment and Training Administration [1979a]. Responses are reviewed with a counselor.

20.4. Selection and Interpretation

Since there are hundreds of tests published and available for use, volume alone prevents the psychometrist from becoming equally familiar with each test and making assessments based on personal experience with each test. Consequently, the user must rely on the test manuals and test reviews for information about a test's items, norms, reliability, validity, strengths, and weaknesses.

Experienced test users eventually develop repertoires of favorite tests that they feel comfortable administering, scoring, and interpreting. Different users, therefore, might select different but equally reliable and valid tests to administer to a given person. The choice of test(s) for a particular person (with a particular set of needs) will depend on the referral request, the referral background information, practical considerations, and interview content.

The referral request to a psychometrist presents the purpose(s) for the testing, the specific information desired, the eventual uses of that information, and usually a request for alternatives or recommendations. This permits the range of tests to be narrowed to those that can provide the needed information and give a basis for the recommendations.

The referral background information presents the client's personal characteristics (e.g., age, sex, race), specific disability information, and other details pertaining to the purpose for testing. This background enables the psychometrist to narrow the choice of tests to those that have norms consistent with the client's characteristics and are appropriate for the existing disability. Practical considerations, such as the tests available and the time allotted for testing, can be decisive in determining which tests are actually administered.

The interview content may reveal information or behavior that is relevant to the choice of tests. Information elicited from the client during the interview may bring to light other functional limitations or client characteristics affecting test selection or interpretation. Behavior during the interview may indicate the client's motivation and attitude toward testing, level of anxiety, and ability to comprehend instructions and directions. The interview content may indicate alternative or supplementary evaluation procedures. This is especially true when new information about the referred person and observed behavior strongly suggest that the envisioned tests will not provide sufficient information to satisfy the referral request.

No matter which tests have been selected, the psychometrist must be sure that their reliability and validity have been demonstrated for the disability and cultural group of which the testee is a member.

20.4.1. USER QUALIFICATIONS

The misuse of tests is reduced by the requirement that they be administered and interpreted by qualified psychologists; obviously, however, there are different levels of qualifications for different kinds of tests. In order to learn how to administer individual intelligence tests and the majority of personality tests the psychologist must receive comparatively intensive training, while many educational achievement or vocational proficiency tests can be given by people whose special training is quite limited.

The qualified psychometrist selects tests in accordance with the objective of testing and the individual characteristics of the client. Knowledge of a test's technical value in relationship to norms, reliability, and validity is also needed. While conducting tests, psychometrists are aware of all the circumstances that may influence the client's performance. When it is time to interpret results or offer recommendations based on test results, other relevant information about the person is integrated. Most importantly, an understanding of human behavior helps the examiner avoid making unfounded inferences while interpreting results; when assistants or individuals in other disciplines conduct psychological tests, a qualified psychologist must be consulted for interpretation. Frequently heard criticism of psychological tests, and misuse of test results, arises largely from lack of knowledge.

20.4.2. TEST INFORMATION SOURCES

The number of tests that have been devised is vast. Consequently, it is essential to know how to obtain information about a given type of test and how to evaluate its scores. This task is made more difficult in that tests are periodically revised. Among the sources of this information are: texts [e.g., Anastasi, 1976; Bolton, 1976; Cronbach, 1970; Thorndike and Hagen, 1977] and reference books in specialized testing areas; the *Mental Measurements Yearbook* [Buros, 1978] and their supplements; test reviews in professional journals; publishers' test catalogues; the test per se and its manual; journal articles reviewing the general area of psychometric measurement; and educational and psychological abstract and index series.

The *Mental Measurements Yearbook* series edited by O. K. Buros and published periodically by the Buros Institute of Mental Measurements, is the single most valuable source of information about testing. Monographs prepared by Buros on more specialized topics such as reading, intelligence, vocational, and single school subject tests supplement the Yearbooks.

The purpose of the *Yearbooks* is to list and present critical reviews of every newly published standardized test. The reviews come from a large group of authorities, all of whom appraise two or three tests in fields in which they are especially well versed. The *Yearbooks* also provide facts that would be necessary for a user to know: author, publisher, publication date, cost, time to administer, appropriate grade levels, number of forms available. There is also a cumulative bibliography of the publications in which each test has been discussed.

The *Yearbooks* are made more useful by two other Buros supplements, *Tests in Print* and a monograph series. *Tests in Print* is a listing of every test in English that is available commercially. The monographs collect complete data on specialized subjects—personality tests, reading tests, vocational tests, and others. Using the monographs makes it unnecessary to look through all the *Yearbooks* to compile complete information on a specific topic [Thorndike & Hagen, 1977].

20.4.3. TEST INTERPRETATION

Test interpretation is the complex art of translating test information into meaningful statements about a person. The talent for this art is acquired through training and experience.

On a shallow level, interpretation is the mere translating of percentiles, quotients, normalized standard scores, and grade equivalents into descriptions of present performance and predictions of future performance. On this level, interpretation is usually insufficient and rarely helpful.

On a deeper level, interpretation is a synthesis and evaluation of test information that gives an understanding of clients, their disabilities, and their life situations. Such understanding is crucial before judgments are made about client adjustment, potential, or limitations. Interpretation at this level permits a synthesis of material that reveals aspects of the total person and satisfies the purposes of testing.

Although evaluators all have their own methods or styles of interpreting test material, there does exist a general sequence of interpretation, consisting of the following steps:

1. Assessing the influence of the test, evaluator biases, and testee behavior and disability on test performance. A test samples behavior, and different tests will sample behavior differently and to different degrees. The evaluator must ascertain that the test administered did sample an adequate spectrum of relevant behaviors. Evaluator bias can significantly color the interpretation and must be taken into account. Testee behavior during testing, such as poor motivation or high anxiety, can influence the quality and quantity of test performance and must be considered when the evaluator is deciding whether or not the test information is representative of the traits that were supposedly measured.

2. Synthesizing test information with other relevant information. Interpretation is made more accurate and meaningful when test information is considered in the context of the testee's personality, history, disability, and current situation.

3. Deciding what that information means and how it is specifically relevant to the person tested and the reason for testing. Test information is sometimes ambiguous or contradictory to other test results or the testee's history. Alternative interpretations of the same information are often possible. Interpretation is a skillful resolution of ambiguities, selection of the most reasonable explication of the data, and specification of which daily life circumstances and traits influence the client's adjustment, motivation, or performance.

4. Effectively communicating precisely what the test information warrants. The psychometrist's contribution is to interpret the test, and the

counselor then works out the relationships between the interpreted test information and the individual case history. This division of responsibility is appropriate since the rehabilitation counselor has a total view of the client that comes from both test information and other data that have emerged or will come to light during counseling. It is through this integration of information and the counseling relationship that test results are communicated to the client.

20.4.4. COUNSELING USE

Learning how best to use the results of tests in counseling rehabilitation clients is more a matter of experience than anything else, but there are a number of general rules that can help considerably. These recommendations to counselors (paraphrased) were made by McGowan and Porter [1967]:

1. Before explaining what the scores mean it is well to give the client a brief, clear explanation of what the test is for and what significance the results have. Then, during the interpretation period there should be no question about this and it will be possible to focus on the client's reactions to the scores.

2. The test information must be made relevant to the client's behavior in the past and the present, and as it is expected that the individual will act in the future.

3. It is important that the client does not associate the scores with the interpreter. The information should be explained so that the individual can deal with it—skeptically, positively, or negatively—without involving the counselor.

4. It is a good idea for interpreters to have thought about how they themselves do on tests and to have come to terms with the subject; this will usually enable them to explain scores to clients in an objective manner.

A number of more specific recommendations for interpreting tests were suggested by McGowan and Porter. The interpreter should have faith in a client's ability to solve problems; female clients should hear about career alternatives and homemaking plans both; various options should appear as positive alternatives, not as last resorts; new educational and vocational opportunities should be mentioned and explored, not cut off; test information should be discussed in connection with other aspects of the client's life; if a client rejects low scores, these feelings should be reflected—poor performance should not be unquestioningly accepted; the client should participate in the interpretation; the objectives of the test should be explained in practical terms, not in "psychological jargon"; the terms *interest* and *aptitude* should not be used interchangeably; test scores are one element of a large picture and not ends in themselves; results should be used in planning with the client, not used diagnostically; before any conversation about a particular test, the client should be reminded of it; the tests should enhance the client's self-understanding and not seem to yield some magic number; low scores or information that will be unwelcome should be explained directly but in their true context; the explanation of scores should be simple, without sophisticated statistical terminology; it is important to have in mind the client's expressed and manifest interests, not just inventory scores; the client should be permitted to summarize and organize the information frequently; the client, not the interpreter, should summarize the interview as a whole; and, the session should conclude on a positive key, even if part of it has been negative.

Goldman's 1971 book *Using Tests in Counseling*, has a thorough treatment of this subject, including test selection, administration, interpretation, and reporting. Of particular value for rehabilitationists is a 1976 text by Bolton, *Handbook of Measurement and Evaluation in Rehabilitation*.

20.4.5. TEST REPORTS

The written test report is the vehicle for transmitting information from the psychometrist to the rehabilitation counselor. Because it should not be merely an account of the test results, it is preferable to regard this as a "psychological evaluation."

The psychological evaluation, along with other evaluations, provides the basis for the counselor's case study for vocational assessment. Decision-making is simplified when the psychometrist includes only meaningful information in the report, for then time is not wasted in searching for significant results, and there is less danger of the reader's missing information or drawing it out of context. Generally, information is most meaningful when it (1) describes the person rather than test scores, quotients, or percentiles; (2) relates to the functional limitations and their consequences; (3) substantiates conclusions, recommendations, and alternatives; and (4) is relevant to the reason for testing. The counselor may ask that all other information be included in the psychological evaluation report.

The psychological report should also include statements about (1) the client's relevant history and present life situation; (2) the client's behavior during testing or any functional limitations that might have influenced the test performance; (3) specific problems of test administration and interpretation related to the client's disability; (4) answers to the referral requests; and (5) supporting and documentary conclusions, recommendations, and alternatives. Moreover, the psychologist's report to the rehabilitation counselor should be clearly written (not too technical), realistically applied to the actual circumstances, reasonably comprehensive (e.g., four pages), explicitly addressed to the individual tested, adequately interpreted (use of norm scores), vocationally oriented, and promptly provided (one or two weeks).

20.5. *Measurement Issues*

Psychological tests do not give complete answers or completely accurate information. But, they can contribute valuable additions to the assessment bases—when properly employed. Rejection of psychometry arises out of misuse or misinterpretation. Some of the issues are briefly discussed below, and more thoroughly, by Thorndike and Hagen [1977].

20.5.1. TESTING MINORITY PERSONS

The utilization and interpretation of tests with people from minority groups and people from backgrounds that are atypical in the predominant culture, is a problem that has given rise to great criticism. The point is made that it is not good practice to give tests designed for average middle-class white males to members of these other groups.

Questions on this issue are based in part on the fact that achievement tests are designed to evaluate the skills an individual has acquired, while the educational goals for minority students may not be the same as those for the typical American. Other questions have to do with the actual test content, which is intended to reflect basic skills. Finally there is discussion of the attitudes of minority students toward tests taken in the schools. It is possible that these students have developed negative feelings about testing because their experiences with tests in the past have not been successful, and, as a result, motivation and effort are poor.

Those concerned with the development and improvement of tests must discover what inferences are legitimate for people whose backgrounds are not typical.

20.5.2. TESTING DISABLED PERSONS

Functional limitation of various types can change test performance. Particularly notable are the following.

Visually impaired people may be unable to read as rapidly or as accurately as the competition or norm group in various kinds of tests (e.g., speed, intelligence, or ability tests). Hearing-impaired clients may not understand the verbal instructions [Levine, 1960]. When it comes to manipulative tests requiring eye-hand coordination, people with movement defects (motivity limitation) in the upper extremities, may be penalized, even in using a pencil and turning pages.

There is also a more subtle but perhaps more serious and frequently overlooked problem in that the disabled person may get scores on personality tests that for physically normal people would indicate maladjustment. For example, physically disabled individuals who are emotionally quite well may answer items designed to measure preoccupation with health matters (hypochondriasis and hysteria) objectively and

truthfully, but the score may indicate that they have these problems.

20.5.3. INVASION OF PRIVACY

The issue of invasion of privacy has come into the foreground recently; the question is what types of information people should be asked to reveal and in what kinds of situations. Testing is only one of many areas concerned with this problem. There is concern about the kinds of records that should be retained and who should have access to them.

Not only the data itself but the purposes for which it is being collected are subject to question. It makes a difference whether material is being gathered because the person has asked for help with personal concerns or for purposes of documentation. When people ask for help, it is assumed that they agree to the utilization of necessary information. In these instances, the notion of invading their privacy is not an issue so long as the material is used to benefit the individual. Generally this is the purpose in rehabilitation assessment.

20.5.4. NORMATIVE COMPARISONS

Comparing one individual's performance on a test with norms that reflect the typical performance of a sample, is another practice that has received much attention. Critics have argued, with increasing vigor, that the purposes behind tests are not served and are, to some extent, defeated, by such comparisons. They convincingly argue that what needs to be determined is the person's ability to do a specific thing.

The American Personnel and Guidance Association [1978] has published an extensive policy statement on the subject of the responsibilities of users of standardized tests.

Chapter 21

Work Behavior Analysis

Behavior is a function of the person, the environment, and an interaction of the two. In order to predict behavior, evaluators should study the situation in which the person will be functioning with the same effort and attention as they study the person. It is futile to try to predict how well a person will do on a job without considering how the job situation will affect performance. Competency to perform the tasks of a job is a necessary but not sufficient indicator of acceptability as a worker. Dunn [1973a] pointed out that to be acceptable, a worker must not only meet minimal production expectations but also must conform to the social expectations of employers and co-workers in a particular job setting.

Work behavior analysis uses the job setting to evaluate behavior in relation to both social and production expectations. Because a job setting is a behavioral setting, it is possible to describe the behaviors required of the worker in that particular environment. To evaluate the appropriateness of a client for any job setting, one must determine behavior patterns that are typical of a satisfactory worker in that behavioral setting. Just as job analysis sets forth tasks to be performed by the worker, the behavior analysis provides a means for the evaluator to identify behaviors expected in the physical and social environment of the job.

21.1. The Meaning of Work Behavior

The term *behavior* is used here as any observable action of an individual. In this sense, behavior applies to objectively observable actions made by a person—exclusive of internal (e.g., glandular) reactions that are not directly displayed. Vocational assessment is concerned with behaviors that must be exhibited by indi-viduals in order for them to be employed. These behaviors can include anything the individual may say or do in a work setting.

Planning for vocational rehabilitation requires two areas of behavioral evaluation: work performance and personal-social interaction. Work performance refers to the observable actions of an individual in relation to a work task, including the functional abilities and skills of the person. The evaluation of work performance includes the determination of the individual's dexterity, coordination, and tolerances at work. In observing work performance the evaluator considers the client's ability to handle materials, to follow directions, to learn from demonstrations, and to coordinate body movements. Physical abilities such as lifting, bending, or stooping are considered. The focus of work performance observations is on the functional abilities and skills needed to complete assigned tasks successfully.

Personal-social interactions are observable actions of an individual in relation to the social environment of work, including various personality manifestations. The focus of observation of personal-social behavior is on expected worker conformity to the interpersonal circumstances of a work environment. These and other ideas for this chapter were expressed by Korn, Ranney, Schneck, and Schober [1976] in a publication of the Stout Vocational Rehabilitation Institute.

21.1.1. WORK ENVIRONMENTS

Judgments and predictions about a client's function within a vocational context depend on information about work environments. This information about work settings can be classified into two major categories: activity demands and environmental circumstances. Analysis of these factors helps the work evaluator to identify behavior patterns and conditions required for a worker to perform adequately in a work environment. The suitability of a client for functioning on a job cannot be accurately predicted without knowing what the requirements of the setting are in relation to production and social expectations. [Korn, et al, 1976].

Specific information related to production aspects of a job setting is found through an analysis of the work tasks—activity demands —that are required by the job. The most widely used procedure for developing this production-related information is called "job analysis." In addition to the tasks performed, a job analysis describes various worker qualifications needed and the environmental conditions of the work.

The second major category of information used in analyzing a work environment is the work behaviors required for acceptability— environmental circumstances. The work environment as a behavior setting is made up of three factors: the worker behavior that occurs; the physical context in which the behavior exists; and the social context in which the behavior exists.

Behavior setting analysis identifies the typical pattern of behavior among workers and the physical and social characteristics of the setting in relation to these behaviors. It is necessary to have information about minimum production requirements (e.g., units per day) and the maximum scrap rate acceptable.

A major component in the analysis of a job setting is a description of the physical and environmental characteristics of the setting. There are six components of a work setting that relate to its physical and social characteristics: rules and customs for the job, work tasks, social or interpersonal situation, physical environment, time and place, and relationship of behavior and setting.

21.1.2. DEMANDS OF WORK

Competitive employment requires the worker to be able to cope with a variety of behavioral demands. Walter Neff [1976], in a discussion about vocational potential, has described what he called the demand characteristics of work situations. Demand characteristics include not only the know-how required by specific work tasks, but also an elaborate set of attitudes, opinions, beliefs, and feelings referred to as the "work personality." Successful adaptation to work presupposes an appropriate interaction between these two sets of demands.

The demand characteristics of work environments include both structural aspects and interpersonal aspects. Under structural aspects, there are several important features of most work settings that can present major problems for the handicapped person. First, there is the necessity for required abilities such as the function of mobility. Most paid employment requires travel to the place of work. Many jobs require mobility while at work. Second, there is the problem that most work is public, that is, it is carried on under the almost continuous observation of supervisors and co-workers, and perhaps the general public. Third, the typical work situation is relatively impersonal; that is, intimacy is both discouraged and inappropriate. This may place heavy burdens on those who have strong needs for more intimate relations:

the immature, the dependent, or even the emotionally disturbed. Another structural aspect of most kinds of work, Neff said, is the degree to which they are bound by time. The time structure of most jobs sets them off rather sharply from the environments of home or play.

The interpersonal features of work settings, Neff went on to say, are at least as important as their structural features. Here are two issues: the demands of supervision and the relationships with work peers. After an initial period of close supervision, workers are expected to be more or less self-regulating, but the degree to which they can really work on their own has fixed limits, which vary from job to job. Clients who are rendered so fearful or so angry by ordinary supervision that they cannot work effectively are destined for early discharge. Similarly, the ability to get along with work peers is an indispensable requirement for adaptation to work. Immature or disturbed people may demand too much attention from their fellow workers and find them indifferent to personal problems.

As in other sectors of society, the work situation has specific customs and rules of conduct. Probably as many people are discharged or resign from their jobs because they cannot behave toward their colleagues in expected ways as because they lack the requisite work skills. Adaptation to work is a process of acculturation comparable to that required of an immigrant who comes to a new country.

21.1.3. VARIABLES

The types of variables in a behavioral analysis have been referred to by the acronym *SORC*. This indicates the focus on situational antecedents (S), organismic variables (O), response dimensions (R), and consequences (C) [Goldfried, 1976].

Situational Antecedents

The evaluation of situational antecedents of behavior differs radically from traditional approaches to assessment. A detailed account of specific situations is made to identify the components that elicit various forms of emotional response and other undesirable behavior of the individual. Information about these situational antecedents is needed not only for placement evaluation but also to develop a treatment plan (e.g., behavior modification).

Organismic Variables

These variables involve an individual's physiological characteristics—including activity level, stamina, substance dependency—all of which can serve as important determinants of behavior.

Response Variables

Response variables refer to the dimensions of various behaviors. These include frequency, strength, duration, and latency of response.

Consequences

The fourth class of variables involves the consequences of certain behaviors. This class is important because of the well-established principle that so much of what one does—whether the behavior is deviant or adaptive—is maintained (reinforced) by its consequences [Skinner, 1953]. Even when a given course of action has a mixed payoff, in the sense of having both positive and negative consequences, the fact that the behavior continues to persist is frequently explained by the immediate positive, as opposed to long-range negative, consequences that ensue.

"In focusing on each of the SORC variables," Goldfried said, "it should be apparent that the analysis of problem behaviors in such terms has clear implications for therapeutic intervention" [p. 316]. Whenever maladaptive behavior exists by virtue of conflicting incentives in the environment, however, the appropriate corrective action is toward environmental and not individual modification.

21.1.4. CATEGORIES

The three categories of behavior information as identified by Korn and his colleagues are specificity of behavior, frequency of behavior, and duration of behavior. To avoid becoming confused when interpreting information resulting from the three categories, it is important to understand the rationale behind each and the useful role each can play in behavior identification and analysis.

Identification of Specific Behavior

In work evaluation and adjustment services, specific behaviors can be separated into two subgroups: client assets and client liabilities. Client asset identification is particularly important because it provides information about client behavior and performance needed to help clients see themselves as productive workers and to choose and obtain appropriate preparation and employment. Identifying client liabilities that are critical to vocational success is also important. On the basis of this insight, remediation strategies can be designed to maximize client change with regard to the problem.

Frequency of Behavior

Frequency of behavior or performance refers to the number of times it occurs within a fixed period. Frequency counts are used in establishing baselines and in documenting client liabilities as well as assets. Often, however, there is need to know the duration of the behavior as well as its frequency of occurrence.

Duration

Duration is the length of time over which a behavior or performance occurs. It is recorded through the measurement of the total time each behavior consumes in relation to the work day.

Factors that precipitate the behavior should also be identified and recorded. For example, it may be noticed that certain interactions with the supervisor are followed by acting out behavior. Moreover, it may be noticed that the behavior is curtailed by certain types of interventions. Records should be kept of these dynamic factors for an informal treatment plan.

21.2. Behavioral Observation

Nothing deserves greater thought than choosing the type of information to be sought, since, obviously, the planning based upon evaluation is limited by the relevancy of the data. Assessment is also structured by the data format. Since the possibilities of what to record are virtually endless, selectivity is required.

21.2.1. TYPES OF DATA

Formats for observational data are of three general types: narrative, checklist, and rating. Each type of record has particular strengths and limitations. (See 32.3.1.)

The narrative type report records all information about behavioral events in much the same fashion and sequence as in their original occurrence. The narration may or may not include interpretation. While narrative accounts could be exact reproductions of behavior, in practice not everything that happens can be recorded, nor is it necessary or even advisable to preserve all details.

Observational data also may be reported by making notations on a checklist. Checklist data are limited in scope to those specific aspects of behaviors and situations that can be anticipated and on which observers can readily agree. Whereas narrative recording calls for minimal structuring by the observer, the checklist represents maximal observer structuring. Items to notice in a behavioral situation are listed ahead of time. They are selected and presented for quick and objective answers. The behaviors are recorded with checks or other marks to code them into predefined categories. They give information about which behaviors occurred or how often or how long they occurred during the period of observation. The checklist is used for noting static qualities like sex, race, and family membership as well as for recording action and interaction. With both types of data, observer interpretation is minimal or nonexistent. Other observers (even without training) would classify similarly.

Ratings or rankings constitute the third type of data. In contrast to the reporting formats already mentioned, ratings specifically call for observer interpretation. The information recorded represents the observer's judgment of what this behavior signifies.

21.2.2. OBSERVATION TECHNIQUES

The goal of behavior identification and analysis is to be able to observe, record, compare, and make accurate judgments about clients in a work evaluation or adjustment services program. Korn, Ranney, Schneck, and Schober [1976] described the specific steps included in the process of making behavior (or performance) observations. First, the evaluator forms ideas about what behavior pattern is to be expected of a worker in a certain work environment. This provides a list of relevant behaviors to observe and criteria against which to compare the observed behaviors. Then an appropriate work setting, real or simulated, is selected.

Analysis of these data includes categorizing the behavioral information for comparison with expected patterns. The client's behavior pattern can be compared to that which is expected of a worker in selected work settings. This approach is particularly helpful to rehabilitation counselors because the information can be used to set up specific behavior treatment plans for the job objective.

A number of techniques are available for making behavior observations. Selection of an appropriate technique is based on the type of information desired, ease of usage, amount of information collected, compatibility of information with other data collected, and numerous other considerations. Some of the behavior observation techniques include: time sampling, counting-timing, interval recording, critical-incident recording, event recording, point sampling, and anecdotal sampling. Different techniques may be used to develop a pattern of the client's behaviors.

Time Sampling Technique

Time sampling involves scheduling and conducting a given number of observational periods over a specific time span (a workday, a week). The observational periods may be specified as two minutes, five minutes, or longer—but they are always the same length. The times at which observations are made vary in random time sampling but are predetermined in systematic time sampling. In the latter, observations may be set for particular times, such as after each break.

Counting-Timing Techniques

This simply means the recording of only those client behaviors that can be counted or timed. The counting-timing behavior observation technique provides the observer with all three categories of behavior information: identification of specific behaviors, the frequency at which the behavior occurs, and the duration of these behaviors.

Interval Recording

Interval recording is a simple procedure to collect data about specific behaviors, the frequency of those behaviors, and the approximate duration of behaviors. As with any other observation technique, interval recording requires selection of specific observation periods. These observation periods in this type of recording are broken down into short intervals (e.g., ten seconds, one minute) and the particular behavior or behaviors to be observed are specified. Operational definitions are written for each behavior and then listed on the recording sheet. Observations are recorded at the end of each interval. Codes are used to facilitate recording.

Critical-Incident Recording

Critical-incident recording uses a method that groups specific behaviors and performances of clients into two separate categories: client assets and client liabilities. Assets are defined as behaviors that contribute significantly to getting and keeping employment. Liabilities are defined as behaviors that restrict the client's overall potential for getting and keeping employment.

Critical-incident recording is not concerned with the recording of any one specific behavior but rather reports on any behavior or performance displayed that is either an asset or limitation. This type of recording is most useful in work activity programs, extended (sheltered workshop) employment, or long-term adjustment services programs. The need for clear and distinct documentation of client assets and limitations is a major reason for using critical-incident recording.

The evaluator's judgment as to whether or not a behavior is critical is the most important aspect of this recording technique. In using critical-incident recording, the observer must recognize that for a behavior or performance to be critical, it must be either something the client does that relates directly to success or something the client does (or does not do) that results in problems [Korn, et al, 1976].

Event Recording

Event recording deals primarily with specific types of behavior that have been previously identified as requiring further identification or analysis. This method is designed primarily to determine how frequently behaviors occur. Data is collected that assists in determining whether or not the behavior occurs to the extent that it requires remediation in order to increase the client's employment potential.

Point Sampling

In point sampling observation the evaluator determines the observable behaviors (events) to be recorded and sets a time interval between observations. Each time an observation is made, the evaluator observes the individual just long enough to code the observed behavior by placing a tally mark into the proper category on a record sheet. This process is continued at specified time intervals throughout the day. Then the tallies in each category are counted into percentages that indicate the relative proportion of time the person engages in each behavior. Practiced evaluators can make point sample observations of individuals in several seconds.

Anecdotal Recording

Anecdotal recording is a brief narrative of an event. This technique is used to describe the event and to explain the situation in which it occurred. In most cases anecdotal recording is used when an unanticipated behavior was observed that requires explanation.

21.2.3. INTERPRETATION

It is well to distinguish carefully in all observation between the literal description of the behavior itself and the interpretation of the behavior by the observer. Observers will vary, however, in even their literal descriptions of behavior because of the subjectivity they bring to the situation. Robert Overs [1973] has provided much of the material related here on observations.

Rationale Behind Behavior Observation

Observations by rehabilitationists are used in the assessment process for various reasons.

1. Many aspects of a person's vocational functioning cannot be measured by tests or work samples. Tests or work samples do not reveal how a client interacts with co-workers or supervisors, whether or not a client is punctual in getting to the job setting, or what clients do while they are working.
2. Case history materials from outside sources (e.g., letters of reference from former employers) may be inaccurate through bias, omission, or obsolescence.
3. The most direct way to gather information about people is to observe what they actually do

in a real situation. Evidence shows that such observation is best for determining what a person does typically. [Korn, Ranney, Schneck, and Schober, 1976].

Scope of Observations

The scope of the behavioral event being observed influences the interpretation of the content. An aggressive act may be understood as occurring because of an internal hostile reaction associated with paranoid thoughts, because of a normal reaction to being forced to do something inconsistent with one's disability, or because of cumulative rejection and insult from inconsiderate people.

Behavior may be analyzed on at least four levels of abstraction: behavior unique to the individual, behavior as an interaction process between individuals, behavior of the group to which the subject belongs, and behavior accounted for by the values, norms, and expectations derived from the larger society that both clients and evaluators bring to the situation. Of primary interest is the degree to which the client's behavior is consistent with rehabilitation goals.

Observed Behavior Versus Inferred Attitudes

In work evaluation reports, Overs said, it is important to differentiate between the behavior actually observed and the inferences attributed to it. If a client yells at another, does this represent hostility or horseplay? The observer's own attitudes toward the incident will influence interpretation of the behavior; for example normal lower-class behavior frequently appears aggressive to middle-class people. Plausible inferences based on observed behavior are extremely important for an understanding of the client.

Klopfer [1960] broke down information about the client into what he called three levels of communication:

1. Public communication: e.g., what parents will tell the evaluator about the client.
2. Conscious perception: e.g., what the client will admit in a counseling interview or in filling out a personality inventory.
3. Private symbolization: i.e., material that the client does not care to admit or that is not within the level of awareness.

Even the private symbolization level may be inferred from careful observation, however.

The interpretation of behavior is influenced by the professional training and the orientation (or biases) of the observer. Behavior is much more meaningful when interpreted in terms of an appropriate theory [Overs, 1973]. Relevant theories are discussed in the chapters on counseling.

21.2.4. ERRORS OF OBSERVATION

There is danger of error in any observation process. But observation many times is the only way to gather needed information about individuals during their work evaluation. Many of the errors that occur in making decisions about people are due not to a lack of available information but rather to the way this information is interpreted. It is this human element that is most often responsible for making incorrect decisions.

A list of common errors to avoid in observing work performance follows.

1. Decisions are only as good as the information on which they are based. Assumptions are never as good as information directly recorded about the client. For instance, a work evaluator might incorrectly assume that an individual is good on all assembly tasks because that person had a high production rate on one specific assembly task.

2. First impressions are often misleading. The small sample of the total behavior of the individual based upon a single first observation is probably not a good indication of the behavior patterns that are typical of the person. An individual's behavior in a work setting on the first day is usually different from that person's behavior two weeks later in the same situation. Only repeated observations over a period of time and the gathering of additional facts can establish a typical behavior pattern.

3. Maintaining an open mind controls the tendency to generalize about people on the basis of one or two characteristics. Preconceived ideas about people based on physical, racial, or group characteristics leads to stereotyping individuals.

4. Oversimplifying gathered information often leads to a false or incomplete conclusion. The evaluator should not attempt to make judgments about individuals based solely upon one or two traits.

5. Personal biases and prejudices of the observer should be recognized. Observers may be favorably impressed by individuals who flatter them as contrasted with the troublemaker who is difficult to get along with.

6. Information or opinion from other people may influence the evaluator's judgment. Making objective decisions from behavior observations is more difficult when one is confronted with strong opinions about or attitudes toward the client from others. However, decisions about clients should be made on the basis of facts rather than predetermined attitudes and biases of others. While it is important to consider history and the judgment of other people, the final conclusions should be based on all of the objective data. Evaluators should also refrain from making premature decisions because of pressure from other people [Korn, et al, 1976].

21.2.5. RECORDING

Observations made by the work evaluator are a primary source of information about the client's ability to function in a work situation. But the usefulness of observations depends upon the evaluator's ability to record these observations in a clear and concise manner and with sufficient detail to permit later analysis of the client's behavior (see 32.3.3). Dunn [1973] has stated basic guidelines for recording observations; these are paraphrased below.

1. Describe behaviors in observational terms. The essence of good behavioral observation reports is that they use descriptive terms that enable a reader to recognize the behavior when it is seen. Many reports are actually interpretations or impressions of behavior and not descriptions. For example, the term *unmotivated* provides the reader with an understanding of what the evaluator thought about the behavior, but it does not convey what the evaluator actually saw.

2. Describe the situation in which the behavior occurred. Behavior is the product of the interaction of the person and the environment. Because the behavior and the setting in which the behavior occurs are linked, both must be described to interpret the client's behavior. If, for example, the record only indicates that the client was frequently observed talking with co-workers, it cannot be concluded that this is a problem behavior. Talking with co-workers is an appropriate behavior during breaks but an inappropriate one during working periods on jobs requiring a high degree of concentration. Additionally, information about where and when the behavior

occurs is particularly useful in specifying situations to be avoided in placement of the client.

3. Describe what happened—not what did not happen. Instead of saying "didn't return from break on time," the record should state "was five minutes late returning from break." A description of the behavior that actually occurs provides an indication of the magnitude of the problem and sometimes indicates activities that the client finds rewarding.

4. Describe the behavior's frequency, rate, or duration whenever possible. Many common work behaviors can be described in quantitative terms. For example, talking with co-workers can be described in terms of how many times per hour and how long. In many instances the vocational problem is not a behavior but the frequency or duration of a behavior. This information is particularly helpful if the client is to be considered for referral to an adjustment program since it provides meaningful baseline information.

5. Begin the description with an action verb. Action verbs describe observable activities, for example: *selects, uses, drops, stops,* or *leaves.* The evaluator can save time when writing observational records by beginning with the action rather than the client's name or a pronoun.

6. Use a terse, direct style of narration. The composition should impart information concisely. Words that have only one meaning or connotation are preferred when recording observations.

7. Record observations as soon as they are made. Behavior observations should be recorded immediately on a form specifically used for such recording. Many important behaviors are so subtle that by the end of the day the evaluator may not be able to adequately recall certain details. Additionally, if the evaluator delays recording observations, there is a tendency to emphasize events that occur later in the day rather than giving even coverage to all events.

Whereas a single observation record provides a description of client behavior in a specific situation or work task, Dunn pointed out that a series of behavior observations provides the evaluator with a set of cues to more accurately analyze recurring patterns of work behavior. These observations facilitate better understanding of the client's ability to function successfully in a work situation.

21.3. *Rating Behavior*

This section describes various instruments or "scales" for rating behavior. Behavior rating scales provide structure for a predetermined series of judgments to be made about the degree or extent of some human characteristics. These characteristics are assumed to vary with each individual and in different situations. A behavior rating scale is a device for systematically recording an observer's judgments about an individual's behavior. Rating scales consequently provide a quantitative measure of the degree to which some quality is present.

Observations using the behavior rating scales provide a common base for comparing individuals in terms of similar behaviors. In work evaluation, the purpose of observation is to measure (quantify) those behaviors that are relevant to employability. The behavior categories selected for the rating scale should be relevant, behaviorally stated, and directly observable (e.g., attending to task, talking to co-workers).

Rehabilitation is concerned not only with a person's acquisition of job performance skills but also with the development of other behaviors that will enable the individual to find and keep employment. People more often lose jobs because of deficiencies in personal-social behaviors than lack of job skill. Many rehabilitation clients have not developed appropriate interpersonal conduct at work due to social deprivation or vocational inexperience. These rating instruments provide data about those social behaviors that are critical in determining a person's success at finding and keeping employment.

21.3.1. PURPOSES

Rating instruments serve a number of purposes in rehabilitation assessment. Some of the major uses as stated by Esser [1975] are paraphrased below.

1. Rating scales are useful for identifying

specific work behaviors, both positive and negative.

2. The structure of many scales calls attention to important areas that might otherwise be overlooked.
3. Information from scales serves as a basis for formulating goals for client adjustment programs.
4. They may be used as tools to determine, periodically, an individual's progress within a program.
5. Rating scales may be used to evaluate a program's effectiveness in bringing about client change.
6. In some instances, rating scales have been used as predictive devices.

Like any tool, the value of rating instruments depends upon how they are used. Even a well-designed instrument will not be effective if improperly used. The evaluator must have a specific purpose in mind for using a particular scale.

21.3.2. RATING SCALES

There are five broad categories of rating scales: numerical, graphic, standard, cumulated points, and forced choice. These are described below.

Numerical Scales

Numerical rating scales generally consist of a number of traits that are rated according to numbered labels or cues such as:

0 Never
1 Seldom
2 Sometimes
3 Usually
4 Always

The highest numerical value is assigned to the response that appears to be most desirable, although this could be reversed.

Because numerical rating scales are relatively easy to develop and administer they are used frequently. Moreover, the data from these scales are easily tabulated for study or research purposes. Unfortunately there are various problems associated with this type of instrument, stemming mostly from the fact that they are prone to error in design and bias in application. But, if numerical scales are carefully constructed and administered, these problems are minimized.

Graphic Rating Scales

These instruments consist of a series of statements that describe a trait. The format may be either horizontal or vertical. In the following vertical format the scale is on "tolerance for criticism" as a trait:

1. Falls apart when criticized; cannot take any negative comments.
2. Can only take criticism if sugar-coated and gentle.
3. Occasionally disturbed by criticism.
4. Rarely disturbed by criticism; nearly always responds positively.

Numerical values, as in this example, are usually deleted because they may distract the rater.

Standard Scales

The so-called standard scale provides the rater with a set of standards by which to evaluate something (e.g., handwriting). Establishing predefined scale values is so difficult that standard scales are seldom used in work evaluation.

Cumulated Points

The checklist is the most common rating approach in this category. Generally the rater is supplied with a list of traits with instructions to check those that apply to the individual.

Scale values are often assigned to checklist items, the most common method being that of arbitrarily assigning a +1 value to positive traits and a −1 value to negative traits or a value of 0 (zero) as a neutral category. More sophisticated statistically derived weights are preferred. Checklists are popular because they are easy to use and require a minimum degree of discriminative judgment by the rater. These devices are prone to response bias, however.

Forced Choice Ratings

In this method the rater is "forced" to select a statement, from paired or grouped statements, that is most representative of the rated individual. While this type of construction was designed to eliminate the problems of rater bias, it generally fails to do so.

21.3.3. ERRORS IN RATING

The use of ratings is based on the assumption that the rater is capable of making observations with precision and objectivity. Many sources of bias, however, reduce the accuracy of judgments reflected by ratings on scales. Some of these limitations are described below.

The Error of Leniency

Evaluators tend to rate a person they like or know well higher than others. The opposite is also true as the rater is influenced by negative feelings about a person; this phenomenon is called "negative leniency."

The Error of Central Tendency

Raters hesitate to express extreme judgments and thus tend to give ratings in the direction of the group average. This is more likely to happen when the rater does not know the individual.

Halo Effect

This well-known phenomenon is the tendency to be influenced by the general impression that the evaluator has of the individual. If the impression of an individual is generally favorable, the evaluator is more likely to give that person a better rating on any given trait. While the halo effect is quite similar to the errors of leniency, halo errors are an unconscious tendency; errors of leniency result from definite likes and dislikes on the part of the rater.

Proximity Error

Proximity error results from the tendency of raters to give similar ratings for traits that are close together in space or in time. As a consequence, ratings for traits located next to each other on a rating form are likely to have a higher correlation than nonadjacent ones.

Logical Relation Error

Traits that seem to be logically related in the mind of the evaluator are likely to receive similar ratings. This is true regardless of the position of the items on the scale.

Contrast Error

The rating of others in an opposite direction from ourselves is known as contrast error. This is probably most prevalent in peer ratings and may not be a common source of error in evaluator ratings of clients. In fact, there may be undue leniency accorded clients of another race.

There are various ways to minimize these errors. Knowledge of the various types of errors is itself a preventive measure. Training in the use of the particular rating instrument through practice and group discussions also helps to reduce error. Evaluators should have the opportunity to observe individuals in the actual situations in which the traits are manifested. When ratings are obtained in a work setting the evaluator should be familiar with job requirements. Providing an adequate amount of time for rating is also important.

Independent ratings on client behavior should be obtained from several observers. These ratings on client behavior should be comparable when the conditions have been the same.

21.3.4. ERRORS IN SCALES

In addition to the limitations described above, there are other inadequacies in behavior rating scales. One of the most obvious weaknesses in a rating scale is the ambiguity of terms describing traits. Precise definition of human behavior is difficult because of varying cultural interpretations. To have a full understanding of the behavior to be rated, the evaluator needs clear and concise descriptions on the form. Words such as "motivated" or "cooperative" are not precise. It is better to use behavioral statements.

The following criteria were suggested by Esser [1975] as general guidelines for selecting or developing rating scales:

1. Persons using the scale should agree on the meaning of the terminology in the scale.
2. Statements on the scale should be concise and unambiguous.
3. The scale should cover only those traits and behaviors that can be observed.
4. General terms (e.g., *often, superior, average*) should be defined so that they convey identical meaning to all persons using the scale and its findings.
5. Behaviors should be specifically expressed and distinct from one another in order to show exactly what is being rated.
6. Scales should avoid terminology that has religious or moral connotations and social value judgments.
7. Each trait should be defined to assist the rater in describing a person's behavior according to that trait.
8. Good cues apply to a point or very short range on the scale. There should be little

doubt about the position of one cue in relation to others.

9. Traits should be rated on the basis of present, observed behavior rather than what is considered to be future performance.
10. Scales should include opportunity to indicate "don't know" or "no opportunity to observe" although such categories can be misused by nonchalant raters.

Despite the various problems and cautions, rating scales have advantages that account for their wide use. They not only require much less time than many other information-gathering procedures, but they are also interesting to use (particularly when graphic scales are utilized). Moreover, rating scales can be used in a variety of settings for many types of behaviors. And they can be used by subprofessional personnel after training in use of the instrument is provided.

21.3.5. REHABILITATION SCALES

The rating scales mentioned below have been selected on the basis of their general availability and suitability for use in a wide variety of rehabilitation settings. Included are most of those reviewed by Esser [1975]. In several instances scale items are selected and paraphrased to illustrate client behaviors of interest to the rehabilitation worker.

Staffing Preparation Form

This instrument was designed by the Chicago Jewish Vocational Service (JVS) to assist floor supervisors in improving their observational skills and the inferences that are made on the basis of these observations. The instrument is intended to facilitate learning which client work behaviors are acceptable or not acceptable in a competitive job. A manual provides information about critical work behaviors along with suggestions on how to recognize and evaluate such behaviors. Advantages include the fact that it puts supervisors' observations on a more systematic basis. Also, communication among staff members and other agencies is enhanced because of consistent terminology about behaviors.

This scale has 12 behavior categories that are organized into six more basic behavior dimensions: supervision, quality and organization, acceptance of work role, productivity, relations with co-workers, and self-preservation. A definition is provided for each of the 12 work behavior categories, including a list of concrete behaviors (cues) to aid floor supervisors in recognizing and categorizing client behaviors. Each of the 12 areas is rated on a five-point scale in order of relative performance. These client behaviors are as follows:

1. Comfortable and not anxious with supervision.
2. Follows through on instructions and applies them to work.
3. Work is done correctly and carefully.
4. Recognizes work as different from school, home, or recreation.
5. Productivity is consistently high.
6. Spends time appropriately with co-workers.
7. Works well with others on joint tasks.
8. Appropriate interpersonal relations with supervisors.
9. Accepts unpleasant tasks when assigned.
10. Open and clear in communication with foreman.
11. Work organization is good.
12. Next, alert, and involved.

Opposite statements anchor the other end of each behavioral statement.

San Francisco Vocational Competency Scale

This is probably the first rating instrument relating to vocational rehabilitation to be published commercially. Developed by Samuel Levine and Freeman Elzey of San Francisco State College, it was published in 1968 by The Psychological Corporation and has widespread use.

The purpose of this scale is to measure the competence of mentally retarded persons participating in sheltered workshop and vocational training programs. It consists of 30 items relating to four areas of vocational competence: motor skills, cognition, responsibility, and social-emotional behavior. Each item is rated according to one of four or five statements or terms.

Behavior Identification Format

This was not designed as a rating scale but rather as a tool to be used in observing, identifying, and recording work and work-related behaviors that may limit or enhance employment opportunities for rehabilitation clients. The emphasis of the format is on teaching rehabilitation personnel how to describe in writing specific behaviors as clearly and concisely as possible. Its 22 behavior categories are as follows: hygiene, grooming, and dress; irritating habits; odd or inappropriate behaviors; communication skills as related to work needs; attendance; punctuality; ability to cope with work problems (frustration tolerance); personal complaints; vitality of work energy; stamina or eight-hour work capacity; steadiness or consistency of work; distractibility; conformity to shop rules and safety practices; reactions to change in work assignment; reactions to unpleasant or monotonous tasks; social skills in relations with co-workers; amount of supervision required after initial instruction period; recognition-acceptance of supervisory authority; amount of tension aroused by close supervision; requests for assistance from supervisor; reactions to criticism and pressure from supervisors; work method and organization of tools and materials.

The Behavior Identification form also contains space for recording specific behavior observations. After a problem behavior is described, it can then be rated according to one of three rating classifications: A—Acceptable; B—Selective Placement; and C—Change Needed. It does not yield a numerical score.

Work Adjustment Rating Form (WARF)

WARF was developed by James Bitter and D. J. Bolanovich at the Jewish Employment and Vocational Service in St. Louis, Missouri. The scale was designed to provide an objective measure of the concept of "job readiness" as it relates to retarded clients in workshops. The authors defined the concept of job readiness as the attainment of performance patterns that will conform to those required by a work environment.

The Work Adjustment Rating Form contains 40 items belonging to eight subscales. These subscales include: the amount of supervision required, realism of job goals, teamwork, acceptance of rules and authority, work tolerance, perseverance in work, extent trainee seeks assistance, and importance attached to job training. The WARF yields a numerical score that is the sum of all positive responses.

Chapter 22

Work Evaluation Essentials

Work evaluation as a component of vocational assessment is unique in its emphasis on real (or simulated) work. It directly addresses the vocational characteristics of the client as a would-be worker. It appraises the person's work habits, attitudes, aptitudes, skills, and interests as well as physical, social, and psychological traits under work conditions. It shows how fast and how well the person works and how much the individual wants to work. It identifies barriers to vocational success such as lack of motivation or proper incentives, difficulty in getting along with co-workers or supervisor, immature work personality, improper job placement, and lack of training or education.

The essence of work evaluation is its use of the situational approach to make sample observations of the individual at work. The evaluator actually sees how the person behaves in a simulated or real job situation. Most importantly this work experience allows the client (as well as the evaluator) to understand personal adequacies, inadequacies, and needs for vocational adjustment. An excellent overview of work evaluation was published by Paul Hoffman [1973].

22.1. Tools of Work Evaluation

Each of the many methods and techniques for work evaluation has unique strengths and weaknesses; they are therefore used selectively. A particular procedure is selected according to the characteristics and problems of the client, the proposed service, the resources available, the client's employment prospectives, and the work setting [Gellman, 1968].

Tool has the conventional meaning of an instrument that is used in the performance of a task or needed in the conduct of an occupation; tools are, for example, an attorney's law books, a teacher's chalk and board, a florist's greenhouse. In the case of rehabilitation, tools are the means and media by which rehabilitationists conduct client evaluations. There are many different types of evaluation tools, both formal and informal; it is difficult to divide them into classes because they evolve as need arises rather than as parts of any predetermined plan [Vocational Evaluation and Work Adjustment Association, 1975].

22.1.1. SITUATIONS AS TOOLS

The ultimate purpose of any evaluation is to help clients gain self-understanding and the informa-

413

tion necessary for them to make better vocational and life choices. Work evaluation is unique in that it often uses actual situations to appraise a person's abilities. Various kinds of situations are used as work evaluation tools: job sites, production workshops, simulated job stations, various sampling methods, test administration, trial training or employment, and job placement follow-up.

Situations as tools identify a client's work habits, interests, abilities, and potentialities. Situational techniques also disclose the individual's motivation, maturity, self-image, physical and emotional endurance, growth potentiality, ability to relate to supervisors and other workers, and many other characteristics that influence employability. The work situation can be manipulated (e.g., changing the tasks assigned, varying the supervisory approach) for exploratory purposes.

The work evaluator also uses other tools; these may include job analysis, occupational information, audiovisual materials, interviewing techniques, techniques for recording and reporting, and procedures for using client information. Most important and pervasive in the work evaluation process, however, is the indispensable tool of observation.

22.1.2. ON-THE-JOB METHODS

On-the-job evaluations are the most realistic of the various tools of the work evaluator; actual work environments within rehabilitation facilities and outside present a variety of situations for the work evaluator. In cooperation with local companies many rehabilitation facilities have organized different kinds of on-the-job evaluation (OJE) and on-the-job training (OJT) programs; large rehabilitation facilities are able to conduct evaluations in many types of employment within their own walls. Job site situations, production work situations, trial training, and simulated job station situations are variations of OJE.

Among evaluation sites, the actual work situation is the most accurate tool since the measuring device is closest to the object of measurement in this instance. However, the client must usually be prepared to engage in that level of work activity or the experience might be counterproductive. This technique is generally most effective when the client has been screened for employability following prevocational evalu-

ation. In this case then, OJE serves as a cross-checking mechanism to verify the accuracy of other evaluation methods indicating placement readiness. (See 23.5.)

22.1.3. PRODUCTIVE WORK

Production work situations involve the evaluation of clients doing actual work that is brought to the rehabilitation workshop; prime manufacturing in a workshop is used in the same way (see 8.3.4). The evaluator observes how the client behaves in performing this work and thus learns about what the individual can do. On-the-job and production work situations differ in that with production work the typical features of the actual job are varied so that the client's problems in working are revealed. Some sheltered workshops do not simulate the real situation closely enough or make the regulations strict enough to resemble competitive employment. The production method also may have the disadvantage of contracted work that does not represent the whole labor market or all jobs in the community suitable for the disabled served.

22.1.4. TRIAL TRAINING

In trial training situations a set training plan is followed, and the training personnel provide the supervision and participate in the evaluation. The client does not inevitably enter the training program after the trial. As with other methods, the aim of placing the client into the trial training situation is to help the individual vocationally. (See 14.1.5.)

Clients enter into this type of evaluation so that their capacities to perform in the training setting and their suitability for the subject matter of the program can be determined. Frequently they have been selected through evaluation in a prevocational situation. The trial training takes place either inside the rehabilitation facility or outside; it is comprised of adjustment, daily life activities, remediation, or other training content. The training can be in any type of work and involves acquisition of all the related information. After the client has participated in the trial, the teaching personnel evaluate the client's chances of effectiveness in the training program.

22.1.5. SIMULATED JOB STATIONS

Simulated job stations replicate all the features of a particular work operation as realistically as possible except that remuneration may not be involved. The stations, which are controlled by the evaluator, are inside the evaluation facility. The principal components of simulation are the tasks of the work itself and the major physical and interpersonal conditions of the job. This is the difference between simulated job stations and work samples: work sampling concentrates on the performance of the work tasks whereas job simulation involves realistic working conditions.

The use of the simulated job station as a tool has been applied by the armed services and some industries especially to measure people's effectiveness subsequent to training. The Army has simulated tanks to evaluate the performance of a whole crew; typical situations that necessitate the crew's cooperating and functioning as a unit are replicated. In the air travel industry, crews are tested at intervals in simulators that can present them with emergency situations.

While a work sample can show that a client is effective in doing a certain operation within the evaluation program, it is possible that the same person may not be able to do it successfully when also exposed to the external conditions that are associated with the job—noise, high temperatures, and the like. By means of the simulated station one can evaluate client responses to circumstances in which a combination of traits (e.g., endurance and coordination) is necessary if the job is to be performed satisfactorily. Many demands and circumstances typical of actual jobs are not appraised while fragmented and partial evaluations are being conducted.

An assembly line can be duplicated so that a group of people can be evaluated. Different factors can be controlled and their impact on the workers observed; for instance, a slow worker and a fast worker could be placed next to each other. The fact that the simulation can be manipulated in this way by the evaluator makes it an extremely useful technique.

Simulated job stations are attracting attention, partly because of increasing sensitivity to the impact of external conditions on people's work performance. This technique is a way of measuring such influences. A disadvantage of job simulations, however, is their costliness, since they need to be closely supervised.

22.1.6. WORK SAMPLING

A job or work sample is the basic tool of work evaluators. It is a sampling of the activity and other demands of a real job or occupation. The sample is devised according to an analysis of the work in order to simulate all performance requirements of the work, including the mental and physical skills and the use of equipment and materials. (See 23.2.)

Every sample should be representative. In designing a work sample, the evaluator makes sure that all components are as close as possible to those of the real job. Client performance on this simulation of a job is observed by the evaluator in order to predict suitability for the actual job. Clients also learn about themselves as they experience samples of various jobs and learn what work they like and do well; work samples also provide the client opportunity for interesting and efficient vocational exploration.

22.2. *Facilities and Personnel*

As the scope of the public rehabilitation program widened in the 1970s, eligibility was extended to clients with more severe limitations. Frequently these people had less contact with the world of work and their employability was less apparent; many times they were in effect imprisoned by their handicaps and did not know how to discover what they could do. In contrast to rehabilitation clients of the preceding years, many had not generated vocational interests, and some did not understand their capabilities or the rewards of productive labor.

Extensive efforts were made to find out how these people could be helped vocationally through rehabilitation services. The vast expansion of rehabilitation workshops in the 1960s facilitated services to this new clientele of severely disabled people. The rehabilitation facility trend contained the roots of present work evaluation and work adjustment systems. Because the general rehabilitation counselor could not conduct the entire evaluation, facilities and specialists in evaluation evolved so that the kind of case study information that the state rehabilitation counselor and the client needed could be obtained [Crow, 1973].

Rehabilitation facilities—described in Chapter 8, Rehabilitation Facilities—vary in purpose and clientele but many have evaluation units [Couch, 1973]. Rosenberg [1973] listed the four objectives with which work evaluation units are concerned:

1. Establishing, by means of work sample testing in principal occupational categories (e.g., clerical, skilled, and service), the individual's present functioning level, work habits, interests, and capabilities.
2. Evaluating the client's attitudes, motivation, and vocational objectives through observation of the person at work over a period of time.
3. Evaluating the individual's social behavior in interactions with others, including work supervisors and instructors.
4. Helping the person learn appropriate work behavior, work tolerance, and self-assurance through experience in a simulated work setting.

The methods, orientation, and goals of work evaluation endeavors vary according to the needs and resources of the clients being served, the composition of professional staff, and the information asked for by referral sources.

22.2.1. PROCESS ORIENTATIONS

The *process* of work evaluation denotes the method in which vocational data are dealt with. D. J. Dunn [1975], whose discussion is related here, distinguished between two major orientations toward process: information gathering and information processing.

Information Gathering

When this approach is taken, the data that are needed for vocational decision-making are collected by the evaluator and given to outside consultants. Evaluation then becomes essentially clinical; the function of the evaluators is to gather vocational material about the client. While they do interpret the data in order to recommend particular decisions, they frequently have only a portion of the relevant information about the client. As a result their findings may be lacking in validity or significance.

Often, evaluators whose work is based on information gathering do not develop extensive working relationships with their clients. They talk to the client enough to ensure that the individual performs satisfactorily in the program but do not inform clients of results or talk about the meaning of a person's performance during the program. Because counseling is not a part of this orientation, these interactions may not have much effect on the way the person responds as evaluation proceeds.

Evaluation based on the information gathering approach is of limited direct value in helping clients to make choices. It is not a process that results in changes in the client; rather it is intended to produce complete and correct vocational data for the use of rehabilitation counselors in formulating future decisions and plans with clients.

Information Processing

According to this approach, work evaluation is a tool through which clients learn. They can gain knowledge about the world of work, greater self-understanding, and decision-making skills. In contrast to their function in information gathering, rehabilitation professionals who view evaluation as information processing will assume an instructional role. They give the client specific work tasks so that learning about occupations can take place; they report results to enable the client to gain greater self-knowledge; and they form working relationships with clients to allow the client to make decisions and try them out without being harmed by failure. Through actual experience the client is taught how to assimilate and interpret vocational data.

One benefit of this approach to evaluation, as in information gathering, is the data generated. Another advantage relates to the client, whose perception of self, ability to deal with occupational information, and skill in making decisions are increased. These results have a long-lasting influence on the client in terms of vocational growth.

Comments

The degree to which occupational data, feedback to the client, and counseling are used in a program is what characterizes it as an information gathering or an information processing effort. The orientation taken by the evaluation program relates to the requirements of the particular client or group, the requirements and practices of referral agencies, and, crucially, the professional qualifications of the evaluators. The information processing (cf, case study) approach requires preparation in rehabilitation counseling with post-masters specialization in work evaluation. Information gathering may be assigned to a trained work evaluator without credentials in professional counseling.

As a practical matter, selection of the work evaluation approach to be used cannot be based only on the needs of the client, however desirable this might be. Outside agencies and personnel determine what clients come into a program, and the staff within the program have their own viewpoints and attitudes. Personnel in state rehabilitation agencies, for instance, are usually counselors who examine, bring together, and utilize evaluation information; they sometimes see information processing by others as an encroachment. On the other hand, agencies without their own professional counseling staff are quite receptive to information processing being done by facility staff. Because the requirements of the client, the practices of the referral agencies, and the qualifications of the evaluators are all interconnected, combinations of the two orientations are common.

22.2.2. CONTENT ORIENTATIONS

The content orientation is an expression of the subject of the vocational information that is produced through the work evaluation of clients. Dunn [1975], whose discussion is followed here, described the three principal orientations toward vocational content: individual characteristics, specific jobs, and occupational clusters. Because content is intertwined with the methods used in evaluation, a discussion of content orientation includes mention of evaluation techniques.

Individual Characteristics

When the work evaluation orientation is toward information on individual characteristics, the program generates data about the personal qualities needed for effective work performance. These vocational characteristics in the client are measured and scores are correlated with information about the demands of various occupations. The client then is matched with a suitable occupation. This person-job matching method has predominated in the vocational counseling field since early in this century.

This orientation is used by almost every work evaluator to some degree. Its major advantage is that, theoretically at least, evaluation of just a few characteristics can be used to determine the individual's suitability to many different kinds of work. For instance, an individual evaluated for major groups of characteristics as given in the *Dictionary of Occupational Titles (D.O.T.)* [U.S. DOL, Employment and Training Administration, 1977] can be looked at with respect to the demands of thousands of occupations so that the best matches can be determined. This method obviously has great economy.

Most standardized tests, including the General Aptitude Test Battery and several commercial work sample systems are based on individual characteristics. While work evaluators frequently criticize standardized psychometrics, this does not reflect so much the trait and factor premises (see 25.3.5) that underlie many tests as on the fact that they involve a "paper and pencil" technique.

Specific Jobs

Evaluation using the specific-jobs approach for its information content has as its subject matter the particular employment or training opportunities that are available locally. Job analysis is used extensively to produce job samples; these simulate real employment environments—using actual equipment and duplicating actual standards—that exist in particular places of employment [Experimental Manpower Laboratory, Mobilization for Youth, Inc., 1970].

The specific-jobs approach is used quite frequently in work evaluation. Internal employment stations as well as job sites are used in the evaluation program.

The major strength of the specific-jobs orientation is that it is a convincing demonstration of the client's ability to perform a certain job. Information predictive of an individual's effectiveness at a given job is obtained when the evaluative criteria are those of the job itself.

Occupational Clusters

In this information orientation, jobs or occupations are considered in large groups according to elements that they share: for instance, product, materials, or content. The premise upon which this approach is based is similar to that underlying the individual-characteristics orientation. The work tasks typical of various classes of occupations are listed, and during the work evaluation process clients are evaluated in terms of their performance of these tasks.

There is only one clustering system widely adopted in work evaluation: the one used in the *D.O.T.* to group occupations together by means of coding (see 19.2.2). Another system devised by the Office of Education has 15 main groups of occupations classified according to subject matter or knowledge content. This system is not as coherent or as detailed as the other, however, and its use is generally limited to educational and training purposes.

There are other classification systems, but none have been widely adopted in work evaluation. Two of these, the Bureau of the Census system and the industry-occupation matrix of the Bureau of Labor Statistics, contain a great deal of material about workers' characteristics and earnings. The extent of their usefulness for evaluation is still unknown, however.

The occupational cluster approach is not utilized as frequently as the other two, but evaluators do refer to it to formulate suggestions in terms of large groups of occupations like clerical work. This orientation is advantageous because it allows for the fact that many people are able to do or be prepared for a variety of occupations.

Comments

As is true with the process orientations, external factors affect selection of a particular content approach. Since the concept of individual characteristics is so common, there is a tendency to rely on this orientation. But the vocational decisions that need to be made also influence the selection of a content approach, and these decisions depend upon the qualities and requirements of the client. Most frequently, younger people in school or just out of school are dealing with career choices in terms of occupational clusters; older clients are choosing from among particular jobs. For disabled clients, who may have changed in personal characteristics since the onset of disability, it is very useful to be familiar with the present characteristics. Generally, when evaluation services are for one type of client, a single content orientation is adopted; when the clients are different in age, limitations, vocational development, and potential, all of the approaches are useful.

Content orientations also relate to the material an agency or program has available, although in many instances adaptations can be made so that the material at hand can be used for new purposes. For instance, the General Aptitude Test Battery (GATB) [U.S. DOL, Manpower Administration, 1970] measures nine aptitudes (individual characteristics). Aptitude profiles for small groups of occupations can be drawn through the use of scores on specific groups of aptitudes for each group. Moreover, by means of combinations of individual subtests from the GATB, Specific Aptitude Test Batteries can be devised to evaluate people in terms of specific jobs. Other evaluation materials now in existence do not have this flexibility. (See 20.3.2.)

22.2.3. CARF STANDARDS

The Commission on Accreditation of Rehabilitation Facilities (CARF) sets standards for (work) evaluation and work adjustment (see 8.2). To receive accreditation in this service area, rehabilitation facilities must meet CARF standards. At the same time many referral organizations like state rehabilitation agencies require that clients be referred only to accredited facilities. The standards are formulated with a subcommittee of the Vocational Evaluation and Work Adjustment Association (VEWAA).

Piccari [1976] discussed several of the important CARF standards [CARF, 1976, 1978]. The first, nicknamed the "Laundry List" by the Standards Committee, reads as follows:

Vocational evaluation services shall be provided on a systematic, organized basis for the purpose of determining individual vocational objective(s); assets, limitations, and behaviors in the context of work environments in which he might function; and specific recommendations which may be used in the development of the individual's rehabilitation plan. The range and scope of the evaluation services shall be sufficiently comprehensive to assess or obtain information concerning at least the following: a. physical and psychomotor capacities; b. intellectual capacities; c. emotional stability; d. interests, attitudes, knowledge of occupational information; e. personal, social, and work history; f. aptitudes; g. achievements (e.g., educational, vocational); h. work skills and work tolerance; i. work habits (e.g., punctuality, attendance, concentration, organization, interpersonal skills); j. work related capabilities (e.g., mobility, communications, hygiene, money management, homemaking); k. job seeking skills; l. potential to benefit from further services, which are specifically identified; m. possible job objectives; n. the individual's ability to learn about himself as a result of the information obtained and furnished through the evaluation experience.

This list was made up on the basis of the services most typically offered by work evaluators in the country as a whole, to describe the "range and scope" of services. The Standards Committee stressed the idea that in order to be evaluated completely and accurately, a client must be evaluated in all these categories. Some of the information will be produced by evaluators themselves, and some may come from the referral agency or other sources. The professional evaluator synthesizes all the data into a coherent whole, according to the VEWAA view.

Evaluators reporting to the Standards Committee emphasized that while specific material is needed before an individual evaluation plan can be constructed, a referral agency frequently simply asks that a client be evaluated without supplying any information. Typically the client then goes through a standardized process, and the results do not fit that person's unique requirements. The Standards Committee, in order to pave the way for more individualized evaluation, agreed upon providing for a written evaluation plan. This would allow the client to take an active role in the evaluation, help evaluators organize the program to fit the particular client, and better enable referral agencies to recognize the nature of evaluation. In other words, the evaluation is organized around the individual client; the evaluator must have data from interviews and tests and questions from the referral agency so that a program suitable for the individual can be devised. The CARF standard that provides for this is as follows:

Based on referral information, the initial interview, and determined objectives, a specific written evaluation plan for each individual shall be developed. This plan shall: a. identify the questions to be answered through the evaluation; b. indicate how these questions will be answered; c. where appropriate, specify persons (staff, family, etc.) who will be involved in carrying out the plan. There should be evidence that these individuals are aware of their role in carrying out this plan; d. be periodically reviewed and modified as necessary.

The Standards Committee also took up the subject of instruments and techniques unique to work evaluation. The Committee stated that four tools are the most important to this type of evaluation. This standard was formulated:

The vocational evaluation service shall assure that a variety of work settings and tasks are available sufficient to meet the evaluation needs of individuals being served. A vocational evaluation service shall use two or more of the following techniques:

If psychometrics are used: the selection, administration, scoring, interpretation, and reporting of all psychological and psychometric tests shall be under the supervision of a person who meets the qualifications as defined by state law and/or the American Psychological Association standards.

If work samples are used: a. the vocational evaluation service work sample's resources shall be representative of realistic competitive worker skills; b. the work samples shall be established by an analysis of job tasks or traits related to a specific area of work, and be standardized as to materials, layout, instructions, and scoring; c. competitive norms or industrial standards shall be established and used.

If simulated job stations are used, the individual's job performance shall be evaluated against competitive industrial standards (e.g., quality, quantity, physical demands).

If on-the-job evaluation is used, each job site shall be evaluated as to its appropriateness with regard to: a. adequate supervision; b. appropriate safety; c. physical accessibility; d. transportation accessibility; e. competitiveness of work tasks and demands.

According to the Standards Committee, each of these tools is significant in itself but a service that employs only one of them is not vocational evaluation. The standard does allow supplementary methods to be used, but at least two of the listed techniques must be used.

22.2.4. WORK EVALUATION SPECIALIST

Professionalization in rehabilitation has been discussed previously (see 2.1). The rehabilitation counselor in the delivery of vocational rehabilitation service is comparable to the physician in medical practice. In both professions there is an increasing need for specialization as the fund of knowledge expands. So in medicine there are psychiatrists, physiatrists, orthopedists, surgeons—and even subspecializations (e.g., neurological or cardiac surgery). Specialization in rehabilitation counseling is described in 3.4.

It does not matter much whether the central professional person in rehabilitation is called a "counselor" or "rehabilitationist" (an often-used general title in this book). The important issue is to prevent splintering of the profession in order that services to all rehabilitation clients in all settings and phases can be given with the highest possible level of expertise. Rehabilitation counseling is the long-established title for this field—which is a good reason for its continued use—but, more importantly, counseling is the pervasive function of the (vocational) rehabilitationist's role. Vocational assessment is a necessary function of all rehabilitation counselors, and some counselors specialize in it. Ideally all work evaluators should first be trained in rehabilitation counseling.

There has been confusion about the role and functions and the professional status of work evaluators. Their relationship with rehabilitation counseling is still not well defined (see 2.4.1). Until the 1960s some rehabilitation counselor educators took a very narrow view of appropriate responsibilities, thinking that counseling was more demanding than rehabilitation functions such as job placement and work evaluation. (Experienced rehabilitation counselors have always understood that in the state agency their responsibilities were broader.)

In the 1960s when the rehabilitation workshop movement dramatically expanded, there were few available rehabilitation counselors with the professional masters degree, and the salaries were not competitive with those paid by state rehabilitation agencies. Moreover, most of the rehabilitation education program masters degree graduates did not have special training in work evaluation (and still do not). Consequently workshops hired and trained nonprofessionals to do work evaluation. Federal funds subsequently have been made available for several preservice training projects for work evaluators. Still, few qualified rehabilitation counselors specialize in vocational assessment or do work evaluation in rehabilitation workshops.

Many work evaluators belonged to the National Rehabilitation Association (NRA), which is not a professional organization and does not require any professional credentials for membership (see 2.2.1). In 1965 a group organized as the American Association of Work Evaluators. Then in 1968 the leadership in this field established the Vocational Evaluation and Work Adjustment Association (VEWAA) as a division of NRA. Robert Couch described VEWAA in 1973.

The report of a task force of an extensive project of VEWAA acknowledged that vocational (work) evaluation is not a profession but a function. What is important is not who performs the evaluation or the method by which it is conducted. What matters is the result: the client should obtain information that will enable the individual to make specific and constructive vocational plans. Client responsibility in rehabilitation planning was explained by Kenneth Shaw in 1976.

22.2.5. TARGET CLIENTELE

Work evaluation is not a routine component of vocational assessment. In fact a sound vocational objective and preparation plan could be developed in many cases through counseling with little information from sources other than the client. With disabled applicants for public vocational rehabilitation services, however, counselors always obtain substantial outside information (e.g., medical reports, referral information, psychological reports, educational or work records, family observations) for eligibility determination or planning purposes. Still only selected cases require work evaluation.

Clients with a variety of special problems—retardation, emotional disturbance, vocational immaturity, cultural difference, social hostility or alienation, motivational difficulty, illiteracy, or other severe limitations in function—may require work evaluation, over and above other evaluation methods, for adequate vocational assessment. People with severely handicapping characteristics are more likely to need evaluation in a work-like setting, particularly if they have multiple limitations. The rehabilitation potential of such cases and the way they can solve barriers to employment may not become apparent without work evaluation. They may not even believe in their own capacity to become productive, or they may not appreciate the personal value of work. Perhaps they are moved only by the pleasures of the present moment, unable to make the effort for delayed rewards. While it is frequently said that these individuals do not have the desire to work and belong to society, this is contradicted by the evidence: through the experience of work the gratifications are learned as well as the techniques.

Another characteristic of severely handicapped individuals is a tendency to stay where and how they are; in other words, they do not come to the rehabilitation agencies and therefore the service agencies must find ways of going to them. In order to involve clients from these groups in services, those who design them must make the programs seem relevant. Evaluation and other rehabilitation services for a vocational objective must be seen by these people to relate to their needs. Disincentives of a financial nature are built into welfare systems: legislation is needed to reward even partial self-support.

According to Pruitt and Longfellow [1970], many people who need work evaluation have the same kinds of problems: developmental, attitudinal, and readiness problems. The developmental problems stem from a disadvantaged or insulated childhood during which the individual did not have the customary vocational experiences needed to learn the work role. As the child must crawl before walking, so a person must pass through various developmental phases before being able to operate competitively in the work world. After a problem like this is diagnosed, the individual will usually be recommended for a work adjustment program before a concentrated work evaluation is conducted.

Attitudinal problems are of two types. Some people, out of a sense of alienation, reject the social meanings of work; others function in a way that is safe. The latter have strong security-dependency feelings that outweigh the necessity of working. If an unemployment or welfare check represents security and working seems to threaten security, this individual will choose not to work. A person who has failed many times in educational and vocational efforts will tend to "play it safe" by refusing to get involved with any employment situation. Generally, attitudes such as these are formed under the influence of people important in the individual's life or through actual experience.

Some clients have readiness problems; they function satisfactorily during the vocational skills developmental phases but have not settled on their goals. Or they have conflicting feelings about employment or their employability. Yet another group, some disabled people, have not learned how to accept their disability or adjust their perceptions of themselves as needed to assume the role of self-sufficiency.

In all three categories the focal point is the person's inability to take on the role of worker. The problem, which is treatable, can be identified through work evaluation.

Chapter 23

Work Evaluation Techniques

An individual's work potential can be appraised and future performance in job training and employment can be predicted more accurately with the use of a combination of work sample and psychological tests, along with other assessment and counseling procedures. The major assumption underlying this comprehensive approach to vocational assessment is that evaluation that uses work observation provides otherwise missing data and a global understanding of the severely handicapped client.

Work (job) sampling techniques have developed with the growth in the number of rehabilitation workshops—particularly the transitional workshops, which conduct extensive work evaluations. Work sample evaluation is also used in conjunction with the prevocational ef-forts of occupational therapists and the simulation techniques used in military and industrial training programs. Self-help evaluation techniques are described in Chapter 40, Independent Living.

The present chapter discusses a wide range of devices for the evaluation of work performance, beginning with traditional psychometric tests of performance typically administered by a psychologist. The focus in the chapter, however, is on the work sampling approach associated with work evaluators.

Ideas and material for this chapter have come from many sources. Most noteworthy are publications of the University of Wisconsin-Stout. Robert Overs of the Curative Workshop of Milwaukee and his writings are also notable.

23.1. Performance Tests

As work sample techniques were devised and refined, many concepts—standardized administration and norming, for instance [Neff, 1966]—were borrowed from psychological testing. But even though they have this relationship, work samples and psychological tests are different in kind. The performance types of psychological tests and the work samples that assess particular traits best display the resemblances between the two.

Generally, performance tests require one to handle objects; paper and pencil are very little used. Nonlanguage tests, administered by means of demonstration, gestures, and pantomime, do not require either the examiner or the person taking the test to use language. The Army Examination Beta, used to test foreign-speaking and illiterate recruits during World War I, was one of the first nonlanguage group tests. Usually groups taking a test have some facility in a given language so that some language can be used to conduct it; in other cases it does not affect the nature or difficulty of the test to give brief instructions in two different languages. But no nonlanguage tests necessitate use of written or oral language by the examinee.

Nonverbal tests, more precisely termed "nonreading tests," do not require any reading or writing but depend on oral instructions and explanations by the examiner. Nonreading tests are appropriate for preschool and elementary school children, people from minority groups who use a variation of English, functionally illiterate people of all ages, and those with sensory and other functional limitations. Verbal comprehension, reflected in the understanding of language, is estimated by means of pictures and spoken instructions.

23.1.1. MANUAL DEXTERITIES

It has been customary in personnel work, vocational counseling, and psychology to speak of manual dexterity as though it were a single ability. If it were, people would be able to become equally adept in all manual activities and a single test could reveal all these abilities. But it is now recognized that there are a number of manual dexterities. The term *dexterity* is a general designation for a large number of specific aptitudes that involve principally the use of the upper extremities and the eyes. Two very important types of dexterity are finger dexterity, or the ability to make skillful, controllable manipulations of small objects mainly through finger movement; and manual dexterity, or the ability to make skillful, well-controlled arm and hand movements to manipulate large objects within certain periods of time.

Standardized tests of manual dexterity take much less time to administer than work sample tasks and are more accurate because of design and development; however, they do not allow for as much observation as that for clinical appraisal of group factors such as those involved in intellectual functioning. A number of major factors related to manual dexterity have been identified. They are described below:

MULTI-LIMB COORDINATION. The ability to utilize, together, gross movements that require use of more than one limb at once.

CONTROL PRECISION. The ability to adjust muscles in a highly controlled and precise manner (needed in order to quickly and accurately operate with the hands, arms, and feet).

RESPONSE ORIENTATION. The ability to choose the appropriate response quickly (appraised in complex coordination tests in which various groups of signals demand various choices of controls and movement direction).

REACTION TIME. The speed with which one can respond to a stimulus—this is independent of the nature of the response and of the stimulus (i.e., auditory or visual).

SPEED OF ARM MOVEMENT. Speed of gross arm movements (regardless of degree of precision).

RATE CONTROL. The ability to make continuous motor adjustments in anticipation of changing speeds and direction of a moving target (common factors in pursuit and tracking tests).

MANUAL DEXTERITY. The ability to use arm-hand movements with skill and control to handle fairly large objects under speed conditions.

FINGER DEXTERITY. The ability to manipulate small objects with skill and control primarily through use of the fingers.

ARM-HAND STEADINESS. The ability to move arm-hand positions precisely.

WRIST-FINGER SPEED (TAPPING). Measured by paper-and-pencil tests that require one to tap the pencil in relatively large areas.

AIMING. Measured by paper-and-pencil tests in which the subject places dots quickly and accurately in a number of small circles.

There are other factors in the gross motor category, measured by physical fitness tests, such as: static strength (continued exertion of force up to a maximum), dynamic strength (muscular endurance requiring repeated exertion of force), explosive strength (mobilization of energy for bursts of muscular effort, as in sprints and jumps), trunk strength, extent flexibility, dynamic flexibility (repeated, rapid flexing movements), body coordination, gross body equilibrium, and stamina (capacity to sustain maximum effort). The abilities called into play by motor tests may change with practice.

Tests of different types of dexterity often have very low correlations. It is therefore important to identify the required dexterity for measurement when attempting to predict success. In fact, different criteria of performance on the same job may call upon different tests. For example, tests predicting quality of work are often poor predictors of speed. Consequently, the worker who would be superior in a shop stressing quality of output might rate no better than average in a shop emphasizing quantity.

23.1.2. DEXTERITY TESTS

A number of well-designed tests of dexterity have been published and are available for use in assessment. Measures of dexterity are particularly important in rehabilitation because many clients suffer limitations in motivity. Motivity —which means the power or ability to move something else—has been operationally described in Chapter 5, Functional Limitations.

Crawford Small Parts Dexterity Test

Designed to measure fine eye-hand coordination, this individually administered apparatus test takes about 15 minutes to complete. It makes use of a board containing 42 holes on the left and right bottom portions and three bins for pens, collars, and screws across the top portion. Tweezers are used to pick up one pin and place it in a hole on the board; in the second part a small screwdriver is provided for screwing 30 screws through a plate. Time scores for each of the two parts are compared to the appropriate table of norms. Percentile norms based on the time needed for completion are available on unselected applicants, appliance factory applicants, and other male and female groups.

O'Connor Dexterity Tests

These tests were designed to measure the ability of the person to rapidly manipulate small objects. The tests are individually administered in about 10 or 15 minutes each. The O'Connor Finger Dexterity test requires placing 1/16" pins, three at a time, into 100 3/16" holes. The O'Connor Tweezer Dexterity test presents a similar task, only instead of placing the pins in the holes with the fingers, one uses tweezers. The time to complete the placements is recorded for the scores.

Purdue Pegboard

This dexterity test was designed to aid in the selection of employees for industrial jobs requiring manual dexterity. It measures dexterity for two types of activity: one involving gross movements of hands, fingers, and arms, and the other involving "fingertip" dexterity. Five separate scores are obtained: right hand, left hand, both hands, right hand plus left hand, and assembly. The pegboard contains two rows of 25 holes into which pins are inserted. At the top of the board are 4 cups containing pins, washers, and collars to be assembled. No tools are required. A raw score is the number of pins placed in the board within the time limits and is converted to a percentile score using a table of norms. Percentile norms are given for ten groups of male and female industrial workers and others.

Pennsylvania BiManual Work Sample

This test combines finger dexterity of both hands with manual dexterity, providing an indication of the individual's ability to coordinate both hands. This test is individually administered to seated examinees in less than 15 minutes. Both assembly and disassembly scores are obtained. The client turns a nut on a bolt and then places this in a slot in the board. There are 20 practice trials followed by 80 timed assemblies. The examinee then disassembles the 100 pieces and the time in minutes and seconds for doing so is recorded.

Time scores for each are compared to norms of employed workers of both sexes, students, and also employed and unemployed blind persons.

Bennett Hand-Tool Dexterity Test

The purpose of this test is to provide a measure of proficiency in using ordinary mechanic's hand tools; it reflects a combination of aptitude and achievement based on past experience in handling tools. This individually administered apparatus test takes between five and 18 minutes to complete. A sturdy work table 34 inches high is required for mounting the apparatus frame. The examinee stands during this test. Three different sizes (4 each) of nuts, bolts, and washers are removed from one side of a hardwood frame with the aid of three wrenches and one screwdriver. The nuts and bolts are then fastened and tightened through the holes on the other side of the frame.

One time score in minutes and seconds to completion is obtained and this is compared with norm tables. The percentile norms are given in the manual for the following groups: male job applicants in a southern plant, male adults at a vocational guidance center, airline engine mechanics, apprentice welders in a steel company, electrical maintenance workers, employees of and applicants to a manufacturing company, boys at a vocational high school, and high school dropouts in a metropolitan center.

Stromberg Dexterity Test

The Stromberg test was developed as an aid in choosing workers for jobs that require speed and accuracy of arm and hand movement. It is an individually administered apparatus test that can be given and scored in about ten minutes. The client stands at a steady 30-inch table for the test. The materials are 54 round red, blue, and yellow discs and a durable board containing 54 holes on one side. Both sides of the disc are painted.

The client receives four trials; trials 1 and 2 are practice and are not scored. The numbers of seconds needed to complete trials 3 and 4 are added to obtain a final score; this final score is compared to the various norm tables representing trade school students, male and female applicants, male and female workers, and others.

23.1.3. SPECIAL APTITUDE TESTS

The professional demands of personnel selection and vocational guidance and placement workers stimulated the development of tests to measure mechanical, clerical, musical, and artistic aptitudes. Tests of vision, hearing, and motor dexterity have also found application in these areas. Thus a strong impetus for the construction of all special aptitude tests has been provided by the urgent problems of matching job requirements with the specific pattern of abilities characterizing each individual.

The concept of special aptitudes originated at a time when the major emphasis in testing was placed on general intelligence. Mechanical, musical, and other special aptitudes were thus regarded as supplementary to the description of the individual in IQ terms. With the advent of factor analysis, however, it was recognized that intelligence itself comprises a number of relatively independent aptitudes, such as verbal comprehension, numerical reasoning, numerical computation, spatial visualization, associative memory, and the like. Several of these traditional special aptitudes, such as mechanical and clerical, are not incorporated in some of the multiple aptitude batteries. This topic is covered in Chapter 20, Psychological Testing.

23.1.4. MOTOR FUNCTIONS

Many tests, discussed above, were devised to measure speed, coordination, and other characteristics of movement responses (see 5.14). Most are concerned with manual dexterity, but a few involve leg or foot movements that may be required for the performance of specific jobs. Some measure a combination of motor and perceptual, spatial, or mechanical aptitudes, thus overlapping with the work sample tests to be discussed in the next sections. Motor tests are characteristically apparatus tests, although several paper-and-pencil adaptations have been designed for group administration. There is little correlation between printed tests and apparatus tests designed to measure the same motor functions.

Motor tests are used in the selection of employees and in the evaluation of work potential of disabled people for job placement. Many are constructed on the principle of simulation or "job miniature." This means that the test closely reproduces all or some of the movements required in the performance of the job itself, not that they are miniatures in the sense of involving smaller movements; on the contrary, the test and the job call for the use of the same muscle groups. The most important point to note in evaluating such tests is the high degree of specificity of motor functions.

23.2. Work Sample

Work sampling, the primary technique of work evaluation, is based on observations of client behavior in the activities of a simulated job (or simulated occupation). A work sample is a defined work activity involving tasks, materials, and tools that are similar to those in an actual job (or occupation). It is used to appraise an individual's physical and mental abilities, interests, and other characteristics relevant to the target job. It can be a simple mock-up of a single work component or the complete reproduction of a job. If the actual job—as opposed to its simulation—is used as the tool for evaluation, all of the job's inherent variables are available for observation rather than only a sample: this tool is referred to as "job tryout" and is not a mere sample of work. Simulation is a procedure that enables the evaluator to reproduce or represent, under controlled conditions, phenomena that are like the actual situation.

The best predictor of the ability to do something is the experience of having done it successfully. Thus, the most accurate work evaluation method is the observation of the worker doing the actual job—the job tryout method or on-the-job evaluation (OJE). The next best approach is to let the person try sample activities of the job, although this is not as accurate because jobs cannot be completely duplicated in work samples. Still these simulated or miniature work situations approximate the tasks of real jobs better than psychological tests.

23.2.1. JOB SAMPLE

The terms *job sample* and *work sample* are often used synonymously in the work evaluation literature although the words *job* and *work* have different definitions. Further confusion develops when the words *job* and *occupation* are used interchangeably. Reference to *work activity* conveys a more general meaning (cf. a job or an occupation), as does the term *work sample*. A job sample, therefore, is a type of work sample. Job samples can be defined as work samples that attempt to replicate a job from an industrial, commercial, government, or other setting.

Actual Job Samples

An actual job sample is a sample of work that has been taken in its entirety from an employment setting and brought into the evaluation facility for the purpose of appraising the client's interests and potential in that particular job. The job sample should contain the complete range of the job's activities—motions, mental functioning, performance and quality demands, operations, materials, equipment, tools, and so forth. When industrial standards for this job are known, the client's performance can be compared directly to the performance of satisfactory employees.

A disadvantage of the actual job sample is that it relates to only one job. The cost of producing sufficient numbers of job samples to cover all of the local jobs is prohibitive; the trend in work sample development is therefore construction of samples that relate to numerous jobs and occupations. Another drawback in the development of job samples is that because of rapid changes in technology that affect jobs, the sample may become obsolete. Also, the environmental elements of the working conditions (e.g., supervision, co-workers, noise) cannot be faithfully duplicated.

Simulated Job Samples

A simulated job sample is a representation of the common critical factors of a job. It differs from an actual job sample in that all the factors affecting the job cannot be replicated. For example, a service station could be built within a facility, but the pressure and environmental factors (such as customer annoyances) could not be duplicated. In some cases, however, enough information might be derived from a client's performance to predict success on the job.

Trait Samples

The concepts of single and cluster traits are also useful. A single trait sample assesses a single worker trait or characteristic. It may have relevance to a specific job or to many jobs, but it is intended to assess a single isolated factor. Such samples are being developed, but not without considerable difficulty. Inherent in trait sample construction is the insidious inclusion of additional traits that contaminate the measurement of the target trait.

A cluster trait sample contains a number of traits inherent in a job or a variety of jobs. It is based upon an analysis of an occupational grouping and the traits necessary for successful performance.

23.2.2. TEST ALTERNATIVES

A major assumption of work sample evaluation is that it is an effective substitute for persons who do poorly on psychological tests. A substantial portion of the population consistently do poorly on standardized psychological tests. Following are some of the more obvious reasons for their poor performance.

1. Most psychological tests are verbal (i.e., test performance is dependent upon the manipulation of verbal symbols). Therefore, the people with low verbal ability (regardless of whatever other potentialities they may possess) tend to perform poorly on standardized tests.

2. Most psychological tests require at least a minimum amount of achievement in reading, writing, and arithmetic. Test results of people with educational deficiencies therefore may reflect their academic deficiency rather than whatever the test purports to measure.

3. Most psychological tests require a minimum intellectual level. Test performance is predicated upon the assumption that the testee can understand, comprehend, and follow the test instructions. Consequently, persons of low intellectual ability may perform poorly because they do not know what they are supposed to do.

4. In testing, the external conditions (lighting, ventilation, noise level) can be standardized, but it is not possible to control the internal factors (motivation, anxiety level, sensory and percep-

tual ability, attentiveness, and the ability to concentrate upon the test task). Therefore, persons who are unmotivated, anxious, or unable to concentrate upon the test task will not demonstrate their true performance potential.

5. Physically disabled people have functional limitations that were not anticipated in the test construction. Therefore, some tests made for the nonhandicapped person may be inappropriate in rehabilitation.

6. Persons who consistently perform poorly on psychological tests are not proportionately represented within the standardization norms of many tests. Therefore, persons who are physically disabled, retarded, culturally disadvantaged, or emotionally disturbed may not be a part of the population they are compared with.

Work samples differ from psychological tests in the degree of relatedness to the criteria (i.e., work behavior and job performance). A paper-and-pencil vocational interest or aptitude test has little direct relationship to the world of work and a performance test has not much more. Work sample evaluation lacks only the overall physical and psychological conditions of real work. The major implication of the relatedness of work sample tasks to real work is in terms of the client's perceptions and conceptualizations of the tasks. Evaluation clients see themselves as performing a work task rather than taking a test. Consequently the work sample is seen as a more interesting and attractive task, resulting in greater client effort to do well. It seems that a more realistic picture of work potential is obtained from work sample evaluation than from psychological testing. This face validity is important in client acceptance and use of the results—both positive and negative—in choosing a job objective.

Work samples not only measure qualitative performance but also allow for the evaluation of such factors as motivation, self-concepts, interpersonal relationships, initiative, ability to accept criticism, concentration, attention span, physical stamina, emotional maturity—in addition to the ability to improve in any of these factors. Moreover, work samples provide information on manifest interest as opposed to the implied interests of psychological tests. This means that work sample evaluation reports can have more immediate application in vocational counseling than psychological reports.

The major advantages of the work sample method were summarized by VEWAA [1975] as paraphrased below.

The work sample is the closest approximation of the "reality of work" that can be achieved within the rehabilitation facility.

It can provide experience in a wide range of jobs.

Its required standard can be performance identical to work.

It not only appraises work skills, but also reveals aspects of the client's adjustment, interest, and attitudes.

Clients respond more naturally to work-related rather than abstract tasks.

It can reduce cultural, educational, and language barriers in the evaluation of work potential.

Work sample performance reports are better received by many prospective employers than predictions based on other sources.

VEWAA also listed some of the disadvantages of the work sample method:

Developing specific work samples for all the jobs in the labor market is not feasible.

There sometimes is limited comparison between the environment in industry and the work sample setting.

Technological change is so rapid that work samples may become inapplicable.

Work sample researchers have rarely used statistical methods to develop reliability and validity information.

It should be added, too, that when validity is reported on work samples the level is typically far below a level acceptable for individual prediction.

23.2.3. DESIGN ISSUES

Work evaluation through work samples is severely and justly criticized because of the consistently low coefficients of validity: work samples do not measure what they claim to measure—at least not very accurately, because much of the information about clients that comes from work samples is intangible in nature and not readily quantified. The picture of the whole person may emerge during the process but no more than a segment of the worker's relevant traits can be measured. This is, incidentally, a compelling reason for the specialist in work evaluation to be trained basically in rehabilitative counseling for an understanding of the psychology of human behavior.

Rehabilitation counselors complain about the usefulness of existing work sample norms. Norms should enable the counselor to compare a client's performance with industrial workers' performances. If the work sample is based on existing work, it is possible to obtain both competitive standards for production quality and quantity. The norms can then be used in comparing the client's productivity with that of employed workers. It should be noted, however, that the industrial norms are based on the performance of persons who have had experience doing the task. To compensate for this clients should practice the work sample for as long as necessary to demonstrate whether or not they can achieve a competitive level.

Instructions for administration are a part of standardization. It is often necessary to give clients a period of time to grasp the essentials of a work sample. This learning period is distinctly separate from the formal evaluation phase. Clients are given ample time, prior to the timed performance, to practice using tools and apparatus and to understand fully what they are supposed to do. The evaluator assists them until it is agreed that the clients understand the work well enough to be timed.

When a client does not perform adequately following standardized industrial instructions, the evaluator should find other methods to facilitate understanding of the task. While some clients may learn through repeated instructions or demonstrations, others learn by imitating the evaluator's example at each step. Evaluation of the client's ability to learn and to retain also is an integral part of the process. Successful performance on a work sample shows that the client understands.

Every individual should have the chance to be retested because existing industrial norms are based on experienced rather than entry-level workers. Also there is need to learn about any positive and negative changes in the client's functioning. This includes changes in: speed, accuracy, or quantity; reactions to new situations (including initial testing and retesting); adjustment to the environment; potential for further improvement; job readiness; memory; transfer of skill; and interest.

The appropriate criterion is also a problem. Outcomes on individual work samples are usually stated as a performance score. This score is often reported in two major dimensions: time necessary to complete the required task or tasks, and the quality of the product. This score is supposed to portray all the knowledge, skills, and other abilities that an individual possesses or lacks. But, this raw score is meaningless unless it is related to some sort of norm score. That is, the client's performance must be compared against those of a larger group of people such as individuals with the same limitation or workers who are successful in this job. Another point of view is that comparison should be intrapersonal, not interpersonal (i.e., the strengths and weaknesses of the person should be considered rather than how that person compares with other people).

Some commercial evaluation systems list specific aptitudes and abilities necessary for performance of their work samples. These are similar to the criteria used in publications of the U.S. Department of Labor (U.S. DOL): the *Dictionary of Occupational Titles (D.O.T.)* [Employment and Training Administration, 1977], *Manual for Use of the U.S.E.S.: General Aptitudes Test Battery* [Manpower Administration, 1970], or *Handbook for Analyzing Jobs* [Manpower Administration, 1972]. Although these worker functioning requirements are listed with reference to specific work samples, their relationship to the performance norms being used and their relationship to each other are not generally established.

23.2.4. WORK SAMPLE DEVELOPMENT

The development of work samples may be a time-consuming function. It involves a number of steps and a manual for use of the sample by evaluators is prepared. The steps as suggested by Korn [1976a] follow.

Determination of Need

Establishing that a need exists for a new device is the crucial first step in work sample development. It is an important decision since the cost of a facility-developed work sample is high—particularly in the personnel cost. Usually determination of the need for a work sample is based upon labor market demands in the agency's area and current and projected client vocational functioning and special placement needs. Mechanisms for documenting whether or not additional devices need to be developed are program evaluation data, labor and employment

market surveys, data from job development projects, information derived from previous work evaluations, and job placement and closure records.

Determination of Work Sample Intent

This second step involves deciding what the sample will be used for. Work samples can be used to accomplish a number of things, including changing a client's "attitudes" or "ideas" about a particular type of work or providing an opportunity for clients to experience success, but individual work samples should never be designed to solve all problems. Other solutions that may be more appropriate (e.g., on-the-job evaluation or a psychological test) need to be considered.

Description of Evaluation Task

The third step involved in work sample development is to describe the task(s) to be evaluated. Work sample development is traditionally based on job analysis or direct use of occupational information resources although alternative procedures can be and are used.

Development of Pilot Work Sample

The fourth step in developing a work sample is the making of a pilot version, in view of the disastrous effect that poor sample design can have on factors such as standardization, reliability, and maintenance of the sample, as well as the ability of the target clientele to complete the sample components. During the fourth stage of sample development, a pilot manual is drafted, with particular emphasis on sample administration, instructions, and scoring.

Field Trial and Modification

The objective of this fifth step is to determine if the pilot model of the work sample is adequate for daily client use and what can be done to improve it. Modification of the sample's instructions, client orientation, and the observational and scoring system should be made during the field trial and modification stage, if required.

Development of Technical Support

This sixth step need not be completed for all work samples, but must be carried out for work samples that purport to predict, for samples based upon constructs, and for samples that are normed. Procedures for adequately defining the predictive or constructional relationships of samples and for the construction of norms require knowledge of psychometric theory and techniques.

Dissemination and Usage

At this final stage an adequately developed sample should be capable of being used or replicated by any other evaluator in any agency. The Materials Development Center at the University of Wisconsin-Stout has a work sample clearinghouse to which completed work samples can be submitted for review and possible free dissemination.

23.3. Commercial Systems

Work sampling began in 1936 with the development of the so-called TOWER system by the nonprofit New York Institute for the Crippled and Disabled (ICD). Subsequently other systems have been devised. Recently a number of profit-making firms and companies have been selling systems complete with elaborate machines. A number of these commercially available work evaluation systems will be described in this section.

23.3.1. TOWER SYSTEM

The acronym *TOWER* is for Testing, Orientation, and Work Evaluation in Rehabilitation. The system, which is based on job analysis, is designed for the physically and emotionally disabled; it is also applicable for use with the retarded in some occupational areas or with modifications. Continuing research and development on TOWER is being done by the ICD Rehabilitation and Research Center.

The TOWER system used 110 work samples to appraise the vocational potential of the disabled person in 14 occupational areas. These broad areas of work evaluation are: clerical, drafting, drawing, electronics assembly, jewelry-making, leather goods, lettering, machine shop, mail clerk, optical mechanics, pantograph engraving, sewing, workshop assembly, and welding. While the numerous work samples are being taken, the client's work personality is observed. A five-point rating system is used.

TOWER (the complete battery) takes about three weeks, but clients seldom take all work samples in the system. Clients are exposed to those samples felt to be within their functional abilities. Prior medical, social, and psychological evaluations are conducted along with continuing rehabilitation counseling. This preliminary screening is emphasized for planning purposes. The choice of the TOWER areas depends upon the evaluation plan consistent with client interests. Client involvement is through the ongoing counseling and team approach.

ICD publishes a printed manual bound in a looseleaf folder and a separate book, *TOWER*. The purposes and procedures are clearly described, including all tools and materials required. Instructions to clients are mainly written and supplemented by evaluator explanation and demonstration as needed. Clients do not begin until they understand the task and readministration is encouraged to upgrade performance.

The client is exposed to many different kinds of occupations in the vocational-training exploration. The TOWER manual has specific occupational information that is given during the administration of the work samples. The scope of tasks in each occupation is presented in a graduated sequence from simple to complex, with frequent demonstrations in the use of hand tools.

Scoring of time taken and of errors made is explained in the manual. Equal weight is given to the time and quality of the client's finished product. Work behaviors and personality characteristics are also rated. Over the years several hundred evaluators have gone to ICD in New York City for training in the use of TOWER.

23.3.2. SINGER SYSTEM

The Singer Vocational Evaluation System (VES) is sold to a wide market, including schools, manpower programs, and rehabilitation facilities. The system uses an audiovisual (teaching machine) approach to present programmed instruction to a handicapped person on what to do in the work evaluation process. Separate work stations are outfitted with a variety of industrial tools appropriate to the occupation. Each work station has its own audiovisual presentation that is completely controlled by the client for self-pacing. An occupational exploration segment helps the client to determine interests by describing the actual jobs related to the work stations.

Over 20 work samples are contained in the entire system: sample-making; bench assembly; drafting; electrical wiring; electronics assembly; plumbing and pipe fitting; carpentry; refrigeration, heating, and air conditioning; soldering and welding; sales processing; packaging and materials handling; needle trades; masonry; sheet metal; cooking and baking; small engine service; medical service; cosmetology; data calculating and recording; filing, shipping, and receiving; soil testing; photo lab technician; production machine operation. Work samples are independently housed in a self-contained carrel. (It is not necessary to purchase all units.) About three weeks, on the average, would be needed to administer the entire system but the work stations are usually administered selectively (the average number is 5 to 7 per client).

The Singer system is intended to help clients and their evaluators determine the client's work tolerance, aptitudes, and interests. It is for the physically, mentally, or emotionally disabled, including those who have a poor work or educational history.

There is much personal interaction between the evaluator and the client, including joint ratings of the client's overall performance on standardized forms. An extensive amount of occupational information—mostly in the skilled trades—is provided the client for the choice of vocational placement or training. Interest measures are also provided. Even though performance is timed, the emphasis is on quality of performance.

23.3.3. JEVS WORK SAMPLES

This system bears the name of the Jewish Employment and Vocational Service (JEVS) of Philadelphia where it was developed in the 1960s under a contract with the U.S. DOL, Manpower Administration. The basis of the JEVS system is the "Worker Trait Group Organization" of the U.S. DOL. While it was originally intended for the disadvantaged, adaptation has been made for disabled people. It consists of 28 individually packaged work samples covering 20 different work areas within 10 worker trait groups. The worker trait groups are: handling; sorting; tending; manipulating; checking and recording; classifying, filing, and related work; inspecting and

stock checking; craftsmanship; tailoring and dressmaking; and drafting. It requires about two weeks.

The system uses extensive observations: for each work sample, defined work factors are required and summarized daily. Many of these work factors are rated on a three-point scale. Because each work sample is individually administered, the evaluator is able to observe and report on a wide variety of work personality characteristics (e.g., reaction to supervision, ability to follow directions, attention span, initiative, punctuality, grooming). Standardized forms are used for reporting. Scores indicate the kind and quality of performance and behavior required for competitive employment.

The JEVS system procedure is well standardized, but the emphasis is on accurate observation and recording as opposed to imparting information to the client. The abstract nature of many of the work samples offers little opportunity for a client's vocational exploration. Moreover, evaluation results are reported in the technical format of *D.O.T.* worker trait groups. For these reasons the JEVS system is probably more appropriate for the procedures of state Employment Service personnel.

23.3.4. VALPAR SYSTEM

Designed for the evaluation of industrially injured workers, the Valpar Component Work Sample Series is marketed by the Valpar Corporation of Phoenix. The system is keyed to the *D.O.T.* worker trait arrangement and uses a trait-factor approach based on task analysis.

The 12 work samples are intended for use as individual components. They are: small (mechanical) tools; size determination; numerical sorting; upper extremity range of motion; clerical comprehension and aptitude; problem-solving; multi-level sorting; simulated assembly; whole body range of motion; tri-level measurement; eye-hand-foot coordination; and soldering. These samples are not grouped as a system and are self-contained. The order and number of work samples administered are left to the discretion of the evaluator with little client involvement.

The time needed to complete the entire system is generally over 10 hours. Total time for each task is converted to percentile scores. The evaluator also uses a five-point scale to rate clients on each of 17 worker characteristics.

Norms are available on employed workers as well as sheltered workshop employees. The samples are well designed, appealing to clients, and easily administered and scored.

23.3.5. WREST

The Wide-Range Employment Sample Test (WREST) is a short battery of 10 work samples marketed by Guidance Associates of Delaware. The samples are: single and double folding, pasting, labeling, and stuffing; stapling; bottle packaging; rice measuring; screw assembly; tag stringing; swatch pasting; collating; color and shade matching; and, patternmaking. These are short, low-level tasks that appraise manipulation and dexterity abilities. Their very simple nature is of little use to a client in job exploration. Moreover, the scores are not clearly related to the competitive job market for use in vocational counseling.

The entire battery can be administered to groups of three to six persons in only two hours or to an individual in even less time. The short administration time, precise instructions, and industrial norms are distinct strengths. The tasks, which are given in order from 1 to 10, resemble a formal psychological situation and allow little client involvement. Nor are there systematic instructions to structure the evaluator's observation reports on work behavior. Perhaps WREST is useful in a preliminary evaluation stage to identify potential work tasks for new clients.

23.3.6. MC CARRON-DIAL SYSTEM

The McCarron-Dial Work Evaluation System developed by psychologist Lawrence McCarron is available from Commercial Marketing Enterprises of Dallas. For the chronically mentally ill and retarded it is based on five neuropsychological factors: verbal-cognitive; sensory; motor abilities; emotional; and integrating-coping. Seventeen separate instruments are used, including the Wechsler Adult Intelligence Scale (or Stanford-Binet) and various other tests, scales, and tasks.

The work evaluation begins with a preliminary screening through interview and referral information. Administration of the work sample process starts with factor one and continues through factor five. For the first three factors the setting is one of formal testing, while four and five require a period of placement in a work setting—commonly a rehabilitation workshop. The first three factors may take a day to go through while two weeks of systematic observation are needed to evaluate the emotional and integrating-coping factors.

The system attempts to appraise the client's ability to function in one of these five program areas: day care, work activities, extended employment, transitional workshop, and competitive employment. Emphasis is on training and placement. In this system psychometric instruments of proven value are utilized in combination with performance and behavioral observations.

23.3.7. OTHER SYSTEMS

No attempt has been made here to rank (or even approve) the various work evaluation systems. Nor is the list of systems complete. There are several additional systems that should be mentioned.

Talent Assessment Program

This system was developed by Talent Assessment Programs of Des Moines, Iowa. It is composed of 11 tests that measure characteristics of work in industrial, technical, and service occupations.

Micro-Tower System

Designed by the ICD Rehabilitation and Research Center of New York City, the evaluation consists of 13 work samples. It measures aptitudes required for various low-skill occupations. Micro-Tower uses group discussions, audiovisual presentations of occupational information, and behavioral and attitudinal scales for comprehensive evaluation. It was designed for use with culturally disadvantaged people.

Vocational Information and Evaluation Work Samples

This system of the Philadelphia Jewish Vocational Service was designed for mildly to severely retarded persons. Its 16 work samples evaluate potential in six worker trait groups for jobs that are common in the labor market and suitable for the retarded.

Hester Evaluation System

This system was designed at Goodwill Industries of Chicago for disabled (except blind) people. It is based on the *D.O.T.* groupings of data, people, and things, as well as work trait groups, physical limitations, working conditions, and general educational development and specific vocational preparation (see 19.3.3). It is not a work sample but rather a battery of psychological tests with client scores related to the *D.O.T.*

MacDonald Vocational Capacity Scale (VCS)
The VCS was developed at the noted Mac-Donald Training Center in Tampa. It consists of eight tests administered during a two-week period to predict the vocational potential of young retarded adults. The eight factors are: work habits, physical capacities, social matur-

ity, general health, manual skills, arithmetic achievement, motivation, and the ability to follow instructions.

Comprehensive Occupational Assessment and Training System (COATS)
COATS, sold by PREP, Inc. of Trenton, N.J., appraises general behavior, interest, and performance capability relative to various job situations. It consists of four independent components or "systems": employability attitudes, job matching, work samples, and living skills. This is a very comprehensive system that takes only one week to complete.

23.4. Evaluating the Systems

Installing and operating a work evaluation unit represents a substantial investment for a rehabilitation facility. The purchase of commercial systems as well as the development of work samples deserves careful consideration of the cost in relation to the potential effectiveness or benefits of a work evaluation unit.

23.4.1. CONTRIBUTION

The first consideration in selecting an evaluation system—or even a single work sample—is its contribution to the vocational assessment process. How effective is it in helping the rehabilitation client make and implement wise planning decisions? This is not only a statistical issue of validity and reliability coefficient and tables of norms, though these data are essential for using work evaluation outcomes in the decision-making process. Every bit as important as comparative scores provided by work samples is the insight provided to clients. And this decision-making insight is facilitated through the rehabilitation counseling process. Any evaluation system must be evaluated first and foremost for its value in rehabilitation counseling.

23.4.2. CLIENT POPULATION

Another consideration, according to Botter-busch and Sax [1976], is the client population. Some evaluation facilities are capable of serving clients with all types of mental, physical, psychological, and cultural handicaps. Other facilities serve only those with a single disability or category of limitations. A facility dealing with

clients having many types of handicaps would generally need to have techniques covering the entire range of occupational areas and skill levels within these areas. A facility providing services to a single disability group could limit their occupational evaluation areas. For example, a facility serving only mentally retarded clients could realistically avoid evaluation for occupations that require a great deal of formalized training or higher education. Some work systems claim to have been designed specifically for a particular level of client functioning, but no commercial systems are designed for or have special instructions or modifications for blind or deaf people. The evaluator should be aware of the need to make modifications in the work samples so that they meet the special needs imposed by the functional limitations of these and other clients.

23.4.3. PURPOSE

A third consideration is the purpose of evaluation. Although all good work evaluation techniques provide career information, a particular technique may either emphasize occupational information by providing a hands-on experience or it may emphasize the appraisal of present skills and aptitudes without relating it to career information. Some systems attempt to provide a thorough evaluation of the client's aptitudes and work behaviors; others provide occupational information and experience, often at the expense of a thorough evaluation of abilities.

The relationship between the community and

the vocational evaluation unit is a related consideration in the selection of a commercial system. The evaluator must carefully investigate the types and number of jobs that are available in the local labor market. The small rural rehabilitation facility in a one-industry area will most likely need fewer work evaluation stations than a facility in an urban area. Labor market information obtained through job surveys, local employment offices and agencies, and client placement records provides the basis for intelligent decisions on what type of evaluation tools are needed locally.

Assessment objectives may not be for immediate placement; therefore, it is also necessary to know what training opportunities are available for clients—these should also be reflected in the selection of evaluation tools. The range of occupations widens and chances for upward mobility are increased as a result of training. The presence of an area vocational-technical school, private trade and business schools, on-the-job training programs, apprenticeship programs, and higher education should be reflected in the evaluation indicators. Work evaluation techniques covering a wide variety of occupational areas and assessing the full range of client aptitudes and interests are needed if the facility is in an area in which many employment and training opportunities are available.

23.4.4. ALTERNATIVE CONSIDERATIONS

The final area of concern is basic. Botterbusch and Sax [1976] posed the question, "Why even use a commercial evaluation system at all?" [p. 3]. All of these systems are expensive yet none of them meet all of the individual needs of a facility in terms of community jobs and training, client populations, and purpose of evaluation. A facility can develop its own evaluation unit based on job or work samples taken from local industry and from the subcontracts of its workshop. Work samples designed for local needs can enhance the relevancy of the evaluation program. On the other hand, most jobs in most communities are not unique; work and occupational samples generally have broad geographic use.

Moreover, the development of a work sample is expensive because it takes extra staff time. The development of evaluation tools also demands a working knowledge of job and task analysis, form and report design, behavior analysis, statistics and research design, industrial engineering techniques, and other skills that the evaluation staff may lack. The lack of developmental time and expertise of work evaluators in part accounts for the use of expensive commercial evaluation systems.

The selection of work samples should be based on knowledge of what is needed and not on the cost or attractiveness of the hardware. This requires a study of community jobs and training and consideration of other available evaluation resources. A central or coordinated arrangement for work evaluation in the community will reduce cost by eliminating duplication. The public should not pay for overlapping services among competing agencies.

23.5. On-The-Job Evaluation

On-the-job evaluation (OJE)—a work evaluation experience that takes place in a competitive job or job-training setting—is the most direct method for analyzing all aspects of work behavior (see 22.1.2). The most valid test is the one that most nearly approximates its criterion. In other words, the closer a test is to what it is supposed to measure, the better the measurement. In work evaluation, there is no situation that resembles a job more closely than the job itself. As a consequence, on-the-job evaluations should be an important tool for work evaluators.

During OJE the client is treated by the employer as any new employee. Usually clients work in entry (lower level) jobs requiring little training. While clients are experiencing the work setting and the job tasks involved in the work, the employer or supervisor is observing them and evaluating them as with all new employees.

Many valuable ideas for the following description of OJE programs were gained from an article relating the experience of J. K. Genskow [1973].

23.5.1. DESCRIPTION

The OJE experience is not engaged in with the goal being employment or training at that particular place; hence the employers can be objective, not feeling that they will be expected or pressured to hire or train the client. This type of evaluation can take anywhere from a day to a month or more. It can be done with or without recompense either to the client or to the employer.

On-the-job evaluations are usually most appropriate in the last phases of the evaluation process. They are preceded by other evaluation procedures, such as psychological and work sample testing. Several OJE experiences may be indicated before the client's final choice of training or placement objective.There are other times, however, when an OJE can be used during the evaluation process: it is especially useful as a reality test for a client who rigidly makes unrealistic job choices early in the evaluation process.

The OJE method gives clients a realistic work experience for self-appraisal because it takes place in a competitive work environment entailing specific production and social requirements and the performance of real job tasks. An OJE experience also enhances the client's work personality because it encompasses many behavioral skills that are required by employers, such as getting along with the boss and other employees, knowing when to talk and when not to talk, and showing initiative.

The job site is typically in a community industrial or commercial establishment, although actual work can be done within the rehabilitation facility in accordance with U.S. Department of Labor specifications. Clients are given the chance to perform the particular tasks that constitute a given job, being instructed and supervised as though they were actually employed by the organization. They may not necessarily be paid wages because performing the job is obviously for the benefit of the client rather than the employer. Typically the evaluator does not supervise the client's activity.

The rehabilitation facility retains its responsibility for clients in job-site situations, regardless of whether they are remunerated or not. Insurance is paid for either by the employer or the rehabilitation organization. There is no obligation on the part of the employer or the client with respect to an actual job after the evaluation is over. But clients can be offered jobs after a successful job-site experience.

23.5.2. VALUE

The OJE method increases the efficiency of the work evaluation program. By sending some clients away from the evaluation program's shop area, more clients can be served in the available space at the workshop. An OJE provides a setting that is fully and appropriately equipped to do its work. Hence the evaluation program need not buy expensive equipment. Furthermore, the OJE employers are expert evaluators in their trade or business and therefore provide expertise not found in the regular staff evaluators.

The rehabilitation facility increases community involvement through on-the-job evaluation programs. Clients become representatives of the agency to numerous OJE employers and their employees. Rehabilitation agencies in general find that these programs have the important byproduct of improving public recognition and relationships.

The OJE may lead to on-the-job training (OJT) or direct employment in that setting. Usually, however, after an OJE experience, if OJT is recommended, this training is obtained from another employer. Otherwise the OJE site may be lost for future clients. Sometimes, however, employers are so impressed that they decide to hire an OJE client even though this was not the original intention.

23.5.3. SELECTING THE SITE

OJE projects are time-consuming. Close coordination between the agency and the OJE site determines whether or not an OJE is successful. Usually one staff member maintains a close relationship with the employer. This staff member serves as a consultant to the employer on each client and functions as a troubleshooter to prevent disruptive incidents.

Unfortunately, some employers, especially large businesses, are reluctant to serve as OJE sites. Small business often provides the best opportunities, and working with one person involves fewer coordination problems. Trade schools also make good OJE sites. The question of insurance and wages arises and should be settled before OJE placement. It is recommended that the OJE employer check insurance coverage since an unpaid client is not covered by workers compensation insurance. Perhaps the employer's regular liability insurance will also cover this situation. The state Employment Service office can advise on U.S. DOL regulations covering any exemptions from federal wage and hour laws.

23.5.4. EDUCATING EMPLOYERS

Initially most employers are naive regarding handicapped individuals and tend to treat them differently. This reaction should be dealt with by the coordinating OJE staff member, so that the client is treated as any other new employee. Sometimes a client is even fired, but this is treated as a client learning experience by the agency. With some clients the OJE is their first experience with any employment situation, hence the evaluation agency should keep in touch with both supervisory staff and client.

Different employers evaluate the effectiveness of their employees with different criteria, so the agency staff member must find out how a client will be rated. When a client is rated poorly, this should be interpreted to the client in counseling.

When a client determines a job area to explore, the OJE staff confers to locate a suitable employer in that area. The counselor or staff member who knows the prospective OJE employer calls or visits the job site and describes the evaluation program and goals to the employer.

Chapter 38, Job Development, includes guidelines on employer relations. In large businesses the personnel department may be the first contact unless a company administrator is available. The evaluation staff member should describe the rehabilitation agency and its evaluation program. This leads into the role of the OJE in the program, which then is identified as the purpose of the visit, with an appropriate comment on the possibilities of this company as an OJE site. It is helpful if a specific client can be described, with emphasis on both needs and predicted potential for the individuals doing this type of work. The purpose of the OJE in helping this client should be clearly stated. Often with small businesses the work potential of the client is emphasized, while with large businesses emphasizing the community service aspect may be appropriate.

After an employer to conduct the OJE is located, the client must be prepared through agency and company orientations. Clients should commit themselves to stay a definite period of time, preferably a week, with the option to stay longer if appropriate. The first day or two is a danger period for quitting.

Special effort is indicated with the first OJE effort of new employers so that they will be willing to continue with other clients. One of the serious problems OJE programs have is the effort necessary for recruiting and keeping job sites.

Chapter 24

Case Study

The rehabilitation case study, the processing of information for client assessment, parallels evaluation, the gathering of background information about the handicapped person's potential. This is a vital function of rehabilitation counselors, and when not effectively carried out can result in unsuccessful case closure. An accurate and broad information basis assures development of a realistic objective and feasible rehabilitation plan.

There is probably no more essential aspect of rehabilitation than the compilation of evaluative information for case study and planning. The rehabilitationist, however, must be able to find out how to get information. The following guidelines are recommended.

1. As much material must be compiled as is feasible, since inadequate information leads to mistaken inferences.
2. One should particularly note markedly positive or negative information, for instance, high and low test results.
3. Personal characteristics always must be considered in the context of external conditions.
4. In integrating the pieces of information into a coherent whole, all the data must be regarded as interrelated.

5. Each piece of information should be set beside others so that contradictions between different data can be identified and resolved.
6. The accuracy of each piece of information should be verified.
7. At the beginning of the case study process it is important not to overlook any material that may have significance in client understanding and rehabilitation planning.
8. Case studies should be completed expeditiously in order to avoid delays in the provision of needed services.
9. Financial considerations may indicate, whenever practical, the use of existing records (e.g., a medical resume) instead of authorizing a new evaluation (e.g., a physician's examination).

This chapter focuses upon the rehabilitation counselor's responsibilities in processing and using client information. Client evaluations (e.g., medical, work) may be conducted by other disciplines or specialists on the rehabilitation team (e.g., physician, work evaluator); however, the counselor's compilation, interpretation, organization, and utilization of obtained information is traditionally referred to as the rehabilitation case study. Case study is the information processing required for the planning goals of the assessment function in counseling. These distinctions between the terms *evaluation*, *case study*, and *assessment* are not clearcut in practice. However, it is well to think of the case study as incorporating all forms of client information of value in the assessment process: the counselor's clinical observations and interview material, impressions and facts from the client's family and acquaintances, historical records (educational, medical, social, institutional, vocational), and evaluation reports by other professionals (physician, psychologist, work evaluator). The case study then is the information base for client assessment and both the study and assessment are conducted by the rehabilitation counselor.

24.1. Preliminary Case Evaluation

The preliminary evaluation is the first phase of case study in all state rehabilitation agencies. Its primary focus is on the establishment of eligibility; the decision whether or not the client will be accepted for more evaluation and other services is made on the basis of the information that emerges. At this phase the decision (i.e., whether the individual is eligible or ineligible for service) is arbitrary and perhaps contrary to the wishes of the recipient. Considerations such as legal stipulations, agency policy, and financial priorities must be taken into account, but even with these limitations the evaluation should lead to planning information that will be of benefit to the client.

Important data is typically obtained from the agency that referred the individual before the first interview. This material is used in preparation for the intake interview and is later combined with and checked by other data that becomes available.

24.1.1. INTAKE

The first contact with a rehabilitation counselor should take place as soon as possible after the person has been referred. Wherever it is conducted—in an agency office, the person's home, the hospital, or school—the basic objectives are to (1) find out what the applicant's vocational problems are and whether the person may be eligible for services, (2) make sure that the client wants the services, (3) obtain relevant information, and (4) ascertain what topics need to be investigated further.

During the first interview a primary objective is to learn about the person's reasons for applying: has the individual applied because of a personal interest in obtaining rehabilitation or has there been pressure from the family or some other agency? While it is understood that clients may not be aware of their needs or willing to talk about them at this point, they are urged to explain their own wishes. This information helps to determine the applicant's willingness to participate actively in counseling and in planning services. If someone seems to need service but has a negative attitude toward rehabilitation, the counselor should find out what has impelled the individual to apply for services. Lack of motivation for rehabilitation does not justify dropping the case. By means of subsequent counseling the person can be helped to develop more positive attitudes.

Another important goal in the first interview is to see to it that the applicant knows what the objectives of rehabilitation are and how clients are involved in making and implementing the rehabilitation plan. Agency policies and practices are explained with relation to the individual's needs, and the requirements are outlined clearly. Seeing that the client understands all this is the responsibility of the counselor.

The first interview—if conducted by the counselor assigned to the case—also helps to establish rapport between the client and the counselor. The first interview must encourage people to feel comfortable and give them the feeling that they can talk about themselves. This is a critical stage for the establishment of an ongoing counseling relationship. In many social agencies, however, the intake interview precedes the assignment of the applicant to a professional worker. There is a distinct disadvantage in fragmenting the counseling process by having one person on the staff conducting all "intakes." In most instances, advance information about the referred person's needs facilitates selection of the appropriate counselor before the initial interview. In many cases the first contact is at the referring agency by the counselor assigned to that type of agency clientele.

24.1.2. DATA COLLECTION

Intake, which begins when the applicant comes into contact with the agency and ends when eligibility has been determined, usually takes relatively little time. But, because it involves gathering a large quantity of information, perhaps more than is collected during any other phase of rehabilitation, information-gathering during intake is a very significant aspect of work with the client. The determination of eligibility is only one purpose of the intake stage, however, and therefore information should be processed and selected with more than this issue in mind. As soon as the applicant makes contact with the agency, the entire rehabilitation process commences. Intake launches the first phase of the rehabilitation case study. To process information only in relation to eligibility determination is to use time inefficiently and limit the potential value of communication between the client and the worker.

24.1.3. DATA PROCESSING

Early during rehabilitation a substantial amount of material is collected from interviews, reports and records of various kinds, testing, and other media. The client should be apprised of this information so that greater self-knowledge and decision-making capacities can be developed. However, some material can be intimidating or difficult, if not impossible, for the client to understand and as a result it is not appropriate simply to hand it out. One way of handling this is to gather and arrange the material according to categories. Then the information can be shared with the client in an organized manner.

In all cases information is conveyed to the client in a constructive framework. The counselor is in fact obliged to provide the counselee all knowledge useful for decision-making purposes, and clients are entitled to a meaningful interpretation of everything that will contribute to positive outcomes. However, material that will not help clients make informed decisions does not need to be conveyed to them; examples include invalid test results, reports containing biased views, records with obsolete labels, and concepts that are unintelligible to them. This does not mean that clients are shielded from unpleasant facts about themselves or their situations; on the contrary the interpretation of such information can be the basis for self-understanding and improvement.

24.2. Interviewing for Information

The interview is so important and pervasive a part of the rehabilitation process that it is described in one context or another throughout this book. Interviewing as an indispensable tool in evaluation and case study warrants discussion here. The focus in this section is on the case study aspects of information collection. Professional skills needed for effective interviewing are covered later, in the chapters in Part IV, Counseling.

24.2.1. UTILIZATION

The interview is a tool with many uses. It is an efficient way to get information from an individual; the straightforward way of learning something about a person is to ask that person. Purposes and aspects of the interview and some suggestions about approaching it follow.

1. The interview can elicit information that will not be revealed on a form. (However, since interviewing is comparatively expensive, as much data from other sources should be collected as possible.)
2. The interview can confirm data that has been obtained in other ways. Since there is no one technique by which a complete portrait of a person can be produced, information from

tests and other sources should be correlated with that which emerges from an interview.

3. Through an interview, missing or inaccurate case history information can be supplied or verified.

4. A questionnaire is always limited in coverage and usefulness because it delineates some but not all problem areas.

5. Even when the questionnaire lists all of a person's problems, there is limited provision (space) for elaborating on them, whereas the interview can probe to get these problems out into the open.

6. Nonverbal communication during personal contact may be more meaningful than verbal responses.

7. Because the interview is a two-way conversation, the applicant can receive as well as give information.

8. Interviews provide not only descriptive data but also explanations: what has happened to an individual and the impact it has had are two different things, and the latter is more likely to be revealed during a discussion than on paper.

9. The flexibility of interviewing permits general questions as well as explicit data requests.

After it has been determined that an interview would be appropriate, the interviewer sets up a plan.

24.2.2. TECHNIQUES

Advance planning will make the interview more efficient. The first step is to estimate how much time will be necessary to get the information required. The more facts previously gathered, the briefer the interview can be. Much of the necessary information can be obtained from various written sources such as tests, reports and hospital or school records. However, information that is collected by others may need to be verified.

Interviewers should behave in a natural manner, attempt to go slowly, concentrate on the client, and accept silences when appropriate. They need to be themselves rather than take on some other role. The genuine desire to help, something the client will recognize if it is there, is what one is attempting to get across. When clients feel that the interviewer is really concerned, they will overlook any number of technical mistakes and a good relationship will be established.

It is important to feel at ease and conduct the conversation in a leisurely manner. The client needs time to get involved and participate in the situation. The interviewer must also cultivate the art of listening, focusing all attention on the client and observing the individual's responses, which will reveal feelings about various topics. Silence can be constructive. Sometimes when the listener waits, more elaboration of a subject will follow. Silence can also enable both people to think about the things that are being discussed and synthesize various elements of the conversation.

24.2.3. INFORMATION WORKSHEET

The Individual Assessment Worksheet, developed by the State of Iowa rehabilitation agency [1975], can be used during intake to facilitate the examination of a client's history for material relevant to employability. It can also serve as a guide for analysis and the composition of the record, ensuring that the interviewer will be certain to cover important aspects of the applicant's history adequately.

The Individual Assessment Worksheet lists a number of important categories: disability, family, education, employment, finance, and so on. Each category refers to an aspect of the client's life; when enough information about them has been obtained there will be sufficient material for the preliminary case study. So that the user will be certain to explore all the subjects completely enough, each category is further subdivided into a series of factors. Under Disability, for instance, appear the subheadings stability, treatment, mobility, attitude, and litigation. Questions about these topics will elicit further data pertinent to the individual's disability as it affects the capacity to work.

Other sections of the Worksheet permit the user to indicate whether various pieces of information about the applicant constitute "assists" or "barriers" to employability, or if more information is needed. While professional rehabilitation counselors should not be forced to use a mechanical device like this, it does provide structure for the preliminary evaluation.

The following format and many items are adapted from the Iowa Worksheet, except for materials on functional limitations, which are primarily derived from Chapter 5, Functional Limitations.

Disabilities/Functional Limitations

Areas to cover and suggested questions follow.

1. Stability. Is the condition improving, deteriorating, or stable? Does the condition fluctuate so as to cause absenteeism or reduced performance? What kinds of activities or environments agitate the condition?

2. Treatment. What treatment does the client receive or has the client received: kind, when, where, by whom, frequency or how long, current and future status? Is the treatment schedule adhered to? If medication is used, what are the effects? Are prosthetic devices (properly) used or needed?

3. Limitations in Function. In what respects is the person limited in functions as a result of the disability? What corrections or adaptations have been or could be made to improve residual abilities? How would these functional limitations be described and quantified as to severity? How well does the person compensate for or avoid the limitations?

4. Attitudes. How does the person react to the disability and its limitations (e.g., succumb, deny, overcompensate)? What is the source and duration of maladaptive (or adaptive) reactions? Should the personal adjustment problem be treated and if so, how? Does the person recognize problems and desire to change?

Family

A number of questions about the person's family cover significant members, including parents, spouse, children, or others. The questions are categorized.

1. Stability. What is the relationship between this person and the family?

2. Support. Will the family be supportive of the goals and methods? Do they understand how and why they should cooperate?

3. Relocation. Would the family be willing to make changes in their life style, even to move to another locality? Will the person be allowed to leave home for evaluation and training?

Personal-Social

In this area, too, there are many questions, some of the most important of which are given below.

1. Incentives. What are the person's reasons for applying to rehabilitation? Were there out-

side pressures for or against the application? What disincentives to vocational rehabilitation success are involved (e.g., loss of welfare or health insurance eligibility)? Is the person in litigation for disability benefits (e.g., workers compensation)?

2. Relationships. How well does the person get along with others? Does this person belong to religious, social, or other organizations? Is sexual adjustment satisfactory? Is the person liked and respected by neighbors?

3. Recreation. Does the person have leisure time outlets? Is exercise a problem?

Employment

Again only a sample of questions, at best representative, can be provided here.

1. Work Experience. What is the employment background (e.g., kinds of jobs; how long worked; for whom, where, and when; and why left)?

2. Stability. Is there a stable career pattern or evidence of job-hopping? Are there unexplained gaps in employment? What are the reasons for unemployment?

3. Assets. What vocational skills has the person acquired? Is a good interviewing impression made on prospective employers? How well motivated is this person? Are the work references all right?

4. Potential. Can the person return to the former employer? Are the jobs in the local market suitable?

Education and Training

Questions include: What was the highest grade in school? Why did the person leave school and what kind of grades were obtained? What subjects were liked and disliked? What other training has been taken—in vocational school, on-the-job, in the armed services? What interest and potential does the person have for further vocational preparation?

Finances

Economic considerations are also varied.

1. Financial Means. What are this person's (or family's) financial resources? What is the amount and source of the current income? Are capital funds (e.g., real estate) available for rehabilitation expenses?

2. Financial Requirements. How much will the rehabilitation cost? What are the person's financial needs and income expectations?

These questions and their categories are by no means definitive. Information limited to only these matters would most certainly be inadequate for rehabilitation planning. Moreover, if such an outline were adhered to in an interview, any opportunity for a warm and spontaneous client relationship would be destroyed. Counseling is not merely a matter of collecting bare facts. Nevertheless, the Iowa notion of obtaining comprehensive information at intake is commendable. While the particular method of a list does not suffice for competent counseling, their organization and processing of material has value.

24.3. History-taking

In conducting the interview and taking the case history during intake, one recognizes that while a person's past does not necessarily foreshadow the future, each individual's development is unique and everyone's potential for change is suggested to some extent by this singular history. In this sense a case history is relevant to rehabilitation, which is an effort to alter if not reverse the direction of a person's life.

In rehabilitation case studies, aspects of a client's history are scrutinized one by one and in relation to each other in an effort to understand the person and develop hypotheses from which even greater understanding can be achieved. As an example, one might be taking the history of a client who lost both legs in an accident at the age of 12. The impact of such an event would vary with its relationship to a large number of other circumstances. Such factors as the social adjustment and functional educational level of the person at the time and the attitudes of other members of the family would dramatically affect the way in which the disability influenced the individual. At the same time, however, it is important to recognize that because any interpretation of a person's past is usually based in large part on conjecture, as much information as is available should be brought out to support the interpretation. One looks for confirmatory evidence in the history itself, in counseling with the client, and in evaluations throughout the assessment process.

An informative intake procedure (interviews, examinations, records collection, and so on) and the preparation of the case history are the preparation stage of the case study. The questions raised at this point will set the direction for further investigation during the assessment process [Meister, 1976].

24.3.1. CAUTIONS

There are theoretical and practical precautions about history-taking. Obtaining the information itself can be a mechanical process that overly formalizes the counselor-client relationship. However, the skilled counselor can make it a productive experience in which both interviewer and client achieve greater understanding. The counselor's expression of genuine interest in what has happened to the client can build rapport. On the other hand, most vocational counselors deny the necessity of routinely conducting a thorough, systematic investigation of the way that the client has functioned physically, psychologically, and socially in the past. In most cases a comprehensive account of the individual's life does not need to be given to the counselor for the client to make a wise vocational choice. Much of this argument pertains to the relevance of data; only certain areas of a person's life—present or past—influence vocational issues.

Counseling students in clinical practice sometimes object to investigating a client's background for fear that the information may not be true or may influence their independent judgments and attitude toward their client. Indeed, a little knowledge can be a dangerous thing. Hasty generalization and judgment based on unverified data do occur, but qualified counselors objectively appraise all client information and accept the client as a person whether the history is good or bad, true or false. Each new bit of information should be treated as contributing to a hypothesis to be tested, not as a fact. This stance is crucial in the early case study stages: the initial information about a person tends to have enduring influence and to have greater weight than contrary, even more creditable, evidence obtained later.

The nondirective approach to counseling (see 25.3.3) also spurns evaluative information from outside sources; the notion is that this places the counselor in a judgmental posture. It is true that the use of the diagnostic process, as in medicine, may lead the client to assume that the professional will prescribe a solution to the problems uncovered. Professional counselors, however, are able to maintain client involvement and responsibility in the complete procedure of securing, interpreting, and applying information. Rehabilitation counselors must have vocationally relevant history to help clients plan their future (see 27.3).

24.3.2. INTERVIEW GUIDELINES

While it may not be easy to reconcile the pros and cons of history-taking, these guidelines offered by McGowan and Porter [1967] help the interviewer make history-taking an effective technique.

1. Filling out the application and other data forms is not an end in itself; the focal point in rehabilitation is the client and not the documents.
2. The interviewer should not direct the client's attention away from some element of the past just because that point has been covered for the purposes of the record. Significant revelations may be made if clients are allowed to talk about the parts of their lives that have the most meaning for them.
3. It is important that the client realize the purpose of the history and understand how it may contribute to the rehabilitation process.
4. When the client objects to the history-taking or seems to feel that it violates the right to privacy, the interviewer should accept this.
5. In the event that more information is needed, the client should be asked if it is acceptable to ask relatives, friends, employers, and so on for information.
6. Clients should not be allowed to wander aimlessly in their discussion; the interviewer

should keep it adequately structured to obtain relevant information. (See 26.2.)

24.3.3. COVERAGE

Client history data consists of the following types of material, as explained by McGowan and Porter.

Identifying Data

This includes the client's name, address, birthdate, birthplace, names and addresses of parents, nationality, marital status, children (number, age, and sex), and religion. Noting the sources of this information is useful.

Referral

Referral information should be comprehensive. The referral source should provide a complete reason for making the referral to rehabilitation. The referring agency should also provide copies (with client permission) of all relevant case documents, including the history.

Disability

It is necessary to take a history of the disability, including date of injury or onset of illness and description of functional limitations. The history should also include: the effect of disability on client and family; client's course of action since onset; increase or decrease in severity; client's opinion about possible alternatives relative to disability.

Previous Medical History

This information is valuable in the medical evaluation phase: nature and dates of past illnesses or injuries; client's report of effects and treatment; dates of hospitalizations and the names of hospitals and doctors who have treated the client. The client should sign written permission for release of information from these medical sources.

Personal and Family History

This includes home life, education, work history, present family and economic circumstances, and personality habits. Material of this kind is written in narrative form and in considerable detail. Following are some suggestions for collecting information within each category.

1. Early Life and Home Background. This includes information about the client's parents, parents' occupations, siblings, birth order of the client, relationships among family members, economic status of family, membership in a disadvantaged group, and so on. These facts will tend to come out in any discussion of the client's early life. The interviewer records the information in the appropriate place.

2. Education. Highest grade completed, age at which the client left school, and family educational history are all recorded. Also include the client's vocational training, effect of disability or illnesses on work in school, quality of schoolwork. School and training records (grades, test results, observations) should be obtained if possible; this can help in planning for the client's vocational future and eliminate duplication in testing. The client can give an account of social activities while in school, membership in clubs, and recreational or athletic involvement. Results of psychological tests and school records may suggest intellectual capabilities, but educational accomplishments are also influenced by physical and mental conditions, cultural and geographical factors, and the like. Is the individual's educational history compatible with that of others in the family, the social environment, and the person's own work history?

3. Work History. Record the jobs held, duration of each, client's opinion of own ability to get along with supervisors and co-workers, and why terminated or resigned. What type of work is the individual best at? Where do preferences lie? Is there any suggestion of hostility toward others in work situations? Also note special skills, influence of local employment conditions on client's employment record, desires and ambitions, stability of work record, and attitude toward work.

4. Current Family and Economic Situation. All people are strongly influenced in the way they respond to new life situations by the quality of their bonds with other family members. Adult relationships have as much significance as those formed early in an individual's life. Is the client still close to parents and siblings? What is the person's marital situation? At the present, who are the people in the client's household, what is the economic status of the family, what emotional support do they give to the client? What is the client's position in the household, how does the family stand in the community? Other factors such as a history of welfare dependency or public offense, the family's social life, the internal equilibrium of the family, relatives' willingness to help the client with the problems of disability, the spouse's outlook on the problems, the quality of the marriage and of the relationships among parents and children, and the physical and mental health of the children are also important.

5. Personality and Habits. Information about the personal characteristics of the individual both before and after the onset of disability is needed. The interviewer attempts to learn about the temperament, likes and dislikes, attitudes, and personal habits of the applicant. Is the individual seriously concerned about the disability situation? Participation in social activities, leadership qualities or the lack of them, physical appearance and demeanor, and any responses that suggest the presence of an emotional disturbance should be noted.

These items are merely suggestive of the sorts of questions that should be asked in interviewing for a case history. Typically, additional information will come from the doctors, psychologists, former employers, and social agency personnel who have had contact with the client; by consulting with these people the rehabilitationist can pinpoint special concerns, the knowledge of which will contribute to the evaluation strategy and assessment results.

Finally, the history suggests the environmental context in which the individual functions, including what the disability means to close relatives and significant others. The rehabilitationist attempts to find out about the physical surroundings of the person and tries to see the person at home or work and to talk personally with all of the people involved. Both the physical and social environment of the client have a great bearing on rehabilitation service needs and outcomes.

24.4. Multi-dimensional Study

Case study in rehabilitation incorporates information of various types and from diverse sources. It is convenient to look at rehabilitation case studies as made up of separate components. And in fact different tools and even separate professions are involved in client evaluations and other data gathering. But, the overwhelming fact remains that a human being is a whole that cannot be fragmented in order to be understood.

It is impossible to distinguish clearly among the medical, psychological, educational, social, and vocational components of a case; they are not separate or unrelated. However, in some cases it is necessary to evaluate in one realm more thoroughly than in others. The individual situation—personal and environmental characteristics and goals—suggests what components of a given case need to be emphasized the most and the depth of evaluation that is needed.

In the case study the counselor must arrive at clinical judgments; the pieces of information from all evaluation components are arranged into a logical pattern within which there are a great many interrelationships. Besides establishing what the major evaluation issues in a case are, the counselor must also take related, less important, factors into consideration.

It is the rehabilitation counselor's task to decide how much as well as what kinds of information may be needed for planning in a given case. The accepted procedure is to obtain a certain amount of data in each area and to explore some in more depth as appropriate. There is no feasible way to generalize about the amount of material that should be gathered. Guidelines can be suggested, however.

One tailors the amount of material to the purpose for which it is being obtained. The rehabilitation counselor seeks information for different reasons than do social workers or investigators in other spheres. For the rehabilitationist there are three fundamental decisions to be made:

1. Whether the client is eligible; in other words, whether the client's disability causes functional limitation severe enough to interfere with adjustment (in either vocation or inde-

pendent living or both) so that the individual requires and would benefit from rehabilitation.
2. What the rehabilitation objective of the client should be.
3. What services will help the person reach this goal.

There will be wide variations from one client to another with respect to how much needs to be known in order to make each of these determinations. One may be easy to make on the basis of little information; another will necessitate the amassing of a great deal of material.

24.4.1. MEDICAL CASE STUDY

Medical evaluation was dealt with in Chapter 15, Medical Services (see 15.3). Consequently, the subject requires only a brief review here. (The medical evaluation by physicians is often referred to as a "diagnostic study.")

Purpose of Medical Evaluation

There are four principal objectives of medical evaluation within public rehabilitation:

1. To document the existence of a physical, mental, or emotional disability that substantially circumscribe the person's ability to perform activities. This is one step in the process of establishing eligibility.
2. To determine the person's general physical and mental condition and also to find out whether there are impairments heretofore unknown. This is to find out what the person's functional limitations and abilities are.
3. To discover how and to what degree the disability can be corrected or reduced. This is to provide direction in restoration services.
4. To lay the foundation for choosing a rehabilitation objective that is medically suitable.

It is in the beginning stages that the medical study plays the greatest role, although because of alterations in the client's situation or condition it may be necessary to get further medical information later. Clients whose rehabilitation is taking an extended period of time should have a medical examination once a year.

Disability History

Rehabilitation personnel obtain a variety of data about the client's physical condition and functional limitations from medical records, interviews, and observations. Existing medical records can present a picture of the individual's disablement as well as the diagnosis, the medical outlook, resulting limitations, and suggestions about restorative measures. Information is also secured by means of interviews with the client and the family. This type of information should be shared with the examining physicians as part of the case history.

Choice of the Examining Physician

It is best to obtain medical information from physicians who already know the person, for instance, the family physician. If it seems that the results of a special examination would be helpful, this should be discussed with the family doctor. Sometimes it is appropriate to talk to the individual's doctor about plans for rehabilitation.

Medical histories and resumes should be used for reference when the medical study is being planned, but usually they are not a substitute for information about the current medical condition of the client. In many cases rehabilitation clients get a better medical evaluation than they have ever received before.

Sometimes needed medical information is difficult to obtain, perhaps because the client does not want to be examined or the physician does not want to release the results. More frequently, the medical examination or report is flimsy, even though authorized and paid for by the state agency. These problems are serious barriers since the rehabilitation program cannot begin until complete medical information about the disability has been secured.

The examining physician needs to know what type of medical data the counselor requires in order to appraise the client's physical condition properly. Physicians must provide information relevant to environmental and activity restrictions. For example, if motivity is limited, the physician should report how much weight the person can safely lift.

Scope of the General Medical Examination

The report provides a medical history and results of a comprehensive examination, including information about the client's weight, height, posture, blood pressure, pulse, respiration, hearing, vision, blood vessels, lymph nodes, extremities, heart, lungs, pelvis, and nervous system. A number of laboratory tests are standard in a general physical examination: urinalysis, serological test (for syphilis), and chest X-ray. Others that should be included are a blood count (red and white and hemoglobin) and, for clients 40 or over, an electrocardiogram. The urinalysis for sugar or albumin detects diabetes or kidney disease; chest X-rays indicate heart pathology, tumors, and conditions of the lungs and chest. Besides documenting the disabling condition, the general medical examination should reveal any other health problems related to planning rehabilitation services and objectives.

Acceptance of Medical Resume

A resume of medical care and examination can be substituted for the general medical examination if the resume covers the client's general physical condition (not just one aspect) and provides information that is recent enough to be used as a basis for making rehabilitation plans.

Speciality Examinations

Medical specialists conduct more detailed examinations of specific conditions, for example, a visual or hearing impairment, cardiac disability, or emotional disturbance. Specific information about methods of restoration or the utilization of a client's remaining assets can come from the medical specialist. It is sometimes helpful if the specialist can be advised of the person's provisional vocational objective or, better still, its physical demands and working environment.

Interpretation of Medical Information

Rehabilitationists are bound by professional and legal obligations relating to their use of medical information. They do not talk about the results of a client's examinations with anyone except others involved professionally in the individual's rehabilitation, and even in these instances they make every effort to see that the information is understood correctly and that the client's privacy is not violated.

The rehabilitation counselor does not have the qualifications to explain the medical aspects of examinations to clients, and clients should be told that under no circumstances can the counselor do this. Rehabilitation counselors are trained to interpret functional limitations derived from the medical reports, but they should not let clients see these medical reports directly. The physician alone has the responsibility for telling the person about specific medical findings. It is the counselor, however, who integrates the medical evaluation as a part of the global case study.

24.4.2. PSYCHOLOGICAL CASE STUDY

The psychological case study provides the basis for prediction by an examination of the individual's behavior in the past and present. Over and beyond testing, evaluative information for the psychological case study comes from various reports and records by other people, counseling, and direct observations. Psychological study is needed in all cases for selection of an appropriate occupation and service strategy, but it is particularly important when the client has a mental or emotional problem as well.

Even though psychological testing is the subject of Chapter 20, it is important to understand the use of such tests as an integral part of the comprehensive case study of clients.

Recommended Standards

Unless a client is mentally retarded or emotionally disturbed, it is up to the rehabilitation counselor to decide whether psychological testing should be done and, if so, how comprehensive it should be. In many state rehabilitation agencies the rehabilitation counselor, even though qualified to do testing, arranges for someone else to do it. While an agency specialist or an outside psychologist may conduct and interpret the tests, it is the counselor who is charged with utilizing the results that are obtained so that the client's self-knowledge and ability to make decisions is increased. McGowan and Porter [1967], whose discussion is followed here, presented two lists to specify conditions—according to state agency guidelines—under which psychological testing should and should not be done.

Psychological testing is necessary in certain situations.

1. Testing is needed when mental retardation must be documented for eligibility determination. An individually administered intelligence test and an appraisal of social functioning, educational progress, and achievement are required.

2. Emotional disturbance as either a primary or secondary disability also calls for psychological or psychiatric evaluation, or both.
3. A program of costly training, such as four years of college, should include psychological testing in the assessment process.
4. Uncertain or ambiguous data on the client's abilities, aptitudes, achievements, interests, and personality characteristics suggest the need for psychological test information.
5. Inadequate information on the client's characteristics due to lack of experience in education and employment may indicate testing.
6. Significant assets (e.g., a special aptitude) or limitations (e.g., a reading deficiency) for which there is no other simple measure may be found by tests.
7. Testing is called for when certain suspected disabilities involving the central or sensory nervous system may be revealed.

Psychological tests may not be necessary when the applicant:

1. Has been successfully employed in the recent past and plans to go back to the job as soon as physical restoration is complete.
2. Has been successfully employed and only job placement with slight changes in the kind of work is needed.
3. Has an excellent educational background and does not intend to pursue education or employment in unrelated fields.
4. Needs other types of vocational assessment information (such as situational evaluation) to make planning decisions.
5. Does not want to be tested (counseling should eventually resolve client reasons for reluctance in any phase of the rehabilitation effort).

When Clinical Psychologist Indicated

Clinical study is appropriate for clients with language handicaps, emotional or nervous conditions, mental retardation, serious visual or hearing impairments, cerebral palsy, orthopedic impairment of both upper extremities, and sometimes for long-term homebound or bedridden people. Conventional testing is usually not sufficient as an evaluation tool for these individuals. Counselors usually do not have the qualifications to administer the necessary clinical tests of personality and intelligence or to use projective methods. Some who do have this training do not have enough time. Typically these clients are referred to a clinical psychologist.

Sometimes individuals in the groups for whom conventional testing is normally adequate prove to need clinical testing. Psychiatric consultation is often appropriate in conjunction with clinical psychological evaluation. The mentally retarded person also needs psychological consultation in order to determine the nature and extent of intellectual impairment.

24.4.3. EDUCATIONAL CASE STUDY

An evaluation of the client's general educational and training level—the characterization of the person's particular abilities and achievements —is made on the basis of experiential background. This consists of facts about the schools attended, level completed, grades obtained, and special vocational courses. Whenever the training program or vocational objective that has been selected involves educational qualifications, transcripts of grades and aptitude and achievement test scores from schools attended are obtained in addition to the educational history.

All the material about intellectual and emotional characteristics should validate the plans that have been formulated with the client. The rehabilitation counselor, appreciating the relevance of past educational experiences to future vocational adaptation, attempts to understand why the applicant succeeded or failed educationally and the lasting effects of these experiences.

The specific items that will compose the educational case study are listed below:

1. Academic training; name, address of each school; highest grade completed; year client left school; types of courses; major, likes, dislikes; reasons for lengthy interruptions or major changes in education.
2. Specialized or vocational training: correspondence or night courses, apprenticeship, short-term vocational courses, business college courses.
3. Educational plans and interests: client's own characterization of preferences for training and specific plans already made for training.
4. Educational achievement: grades in high school and college; other indications of performance such as class standing and results of psychological tests taken; information about how disability influenced performance in school, participation in extracurricular activities; social acceptance by peers; study habits.
5. Information from school personnel: factors influencing grades; opinions of teachers and others of client's adjustment in nonacademic terms; their opinions of the usefulness of further training.

The amount and type of information on the intellectual and educational background will vary somewhat from one client to another, although general categories will usually need to be covered. Emphasis is placed on elements that seem to have the most to do with the client's vocational future.

The educational history is more important and should be examined in more detail if the client left school recently. The longer a person has been out of school, the less important the specific information is. The extent of the education is relevant also: for an individual who went only through eighth grade, for instance, the details are less meaningful than for someone who graduated from high school. Sometimes the information is not readily accessible, which is another consideration. In general, the effort to obtain it should be proportionate to the client's interest in further education (see 14.1).

Material from other aspects of the case history may suggest that a careful examination of the educational history is in order. When it seems likely that a person may not be physically capable of going through training, one looks into the record for data on how well the individual tolerated training before. When interviews suggest that the client has family adjustment problems, one looks at the background for adjustment in other spheres. When scores on aptitude tests and vocational interests are inconsistent, one goes over the educational achievements and demonstrated interests.

Caution about the meaning of school grades is warranted. Sometimes the grades of a disabled student do not reflect accurately either potential or actual achievement. As to potential, a person may have been laboring under a scholastic handicap (e.g., problems with vision or hearing), requiring unavailable special considerations in instruction and examinations. Moreover, teachers may not give accurate grades to the disabled child; grades may be either too low because of teacher bias or too high out of pure sympathy.

Educational Considerations

Cundiff, Henderson, and Little [1965] defined educational considerations as those factors directly linked to academic performance, and discussed their vocational significance. Grade placement, they stated, is generally considered as relatively meaningless in terms of educational performance, and it has been overly emphasized in the sphere of employment. Sometimes, however, a high school diploma is used as a screening device for employment. Technological growth in the recent past has resulted in yet greater stress on grade placement as an indicator of educational achievement. Educational achievement tests are reliable measurements of individual mastery in various subjects, and of a person's ability to use these competencies in solving problems related to job performance.

Knowledge of study habits and methods of learning may be important, but there are not many ways to appraise them objectively. Some information may be suggested through a comparison of achievement and aptitude scores and some may be found in school records. Subjective information can come from the client during interviews. Educational potential may not be a consideration in client assessment if vocational training services are not to be provided.

24.4.4. SOCIAL CASE STUDY

The social case study encompasses the person's current social functioning, family role behavior and relationships, and the client's self-image within the framework of interpersonal circumstances. It helps to show who the client is as a social being. It is also used to indicate how rehabilitation can help this client to develop (see 13.2.2 and 28.7).

While social information can be compiled in many ways, the clients' revelations during counseling sessions are probably the most valuable. Their own views of their personal-social problems and of the sort of assistance they need are tremendously helpful.

Besides the information that comes from the client, human service agency records can be useful; other professionals who have served the client should be contacted whenever possible.

Rehabilitation workshops can provide social evaluations (see 8.3.4). When data that does not come from the client is secured, it is placed into the proper segment of the case history with a notation as to its origin.

The counselor must pay attention to the order of life events and note when cause and effect relationships may be implied by the client's story. For instance, did the client's psychosocial condition worsen after the death of wife or husband? Direct questions are usually the best way to obtain a full account of the client's view of life situations.

The Social Component

The term *social components* is a label for the many different elements that compose the client's social evaluation. It is very difficult to estimate the relative significance of these components; how important, for instance, is a woman's attitude toward child care compared to her desire for a good living standard? Nor are these elements, so significant in themselves and with respect to one another, easy to appraise in terms of their importance to the general goal of helping a disabled individual become employed. In fact, the social components may be more challenging to deal with than others because of their subjective nature. For this reason they tend to be deemphasized in the case study process, even though they may hold the key to rehabilitation success. It is easier for the rehabilitation counselor to depend on the medical or the psychological findings and to appraise the employment history than to gauge the impact that reversing family roles would have on the client. In addition, there are not many techniques for assessing social factors.

Specific guidelines have been developed for medical, psychological, and work evaluation. In some rehabilitation facilities, a social worker usually contributes information about the social component gained through case-work contacts with clients and their families. In other settings, such as the state rehabilitation agency, the task belongs to the rehabilitation counselor, whose competence to perform it is based upon specialized knowledge about the impact of disabilities and general knowledge of human behavior.

Home and Family Relationships

Data about the client's home life is gathered through visiting the home, contacting other agencies involved with the client, and talking to the client. The social history contains the names of family members, ages, educational status, and employment. A sense of how the family operates and conducts its cultural life is expressed, as well as how others in the family may have affected the client's interests and goals. (See 31.2.)

Many kinds of information will be revealed by a scrutiny of the family history. One looks for signs of extreme deprivation; insecurity or dependence in the client's past; suggestions of independence, initiative, and the like. One looks at the behavior patterns of the client and other family members. Does the client dominate and the others give way? Do they let the disabled member take the "sick" role? One attempts to find out whether the family has the financial resources and the willingness to participate in rehabilitation, entering into the record the assets available. Some public rehabilitation services may be authorized only to the extent that the client's (or the family's) monetary capabilities do not permit; the state agency requires a study of financial need for such services.

The person's cultural life is another area of the social case history. It includes aesthetic quality of home, books, music, recreation, entertainment. Religious ties may be relevant (see 12.1.16). Contradictory or improper views of the client's rehabilitation and vocational possibilities among family members warrant further investigation. Community adjustment issues are the person's hobbies, means of recreation, membership in social organizations, history of conflict with the law, chronic dependencies, and reputation.

24.4.5. VOCATIONAL CASE STUDY

Vocational information can be considered to have a very general scope or a much narrower one. Generally, vocational information involves any kind of information about a client that would be useful in planning vocational rehabilitation, including medical, social, and psychological data, in addition to records, test scores, work evaluation, and so on. But vocational information can also be considered as material that is strictly pertinent to the client's employment possibilities, in other words, those facts about the client's past activities and preparation that will be useful to the rehabilitationist in helping the person find an appropriate job and perform in it effectively.

The sources of vocational information in the broader sense are in work records, the statements of past employers and co-workers, school records, previous tests, observation, work evaluation, and consultation with others who have been involved in the client's case. It is also necessary to know what employment opportunities exist in the client's locale. After this material has been collected, it is examined with relationship to the general goal and to the medical, social, and psychological data that has been obtained. The individual is guided in terms of positive capacities rather than the disability [Jeffrey, 1966].

Sources of Information

The client and other family members can reveal where the client has worked, and the kind of work that was involved, the length of time the job was held, the client's feelings about the work and the work environment, the earnings, and the reason the individual left the job. Former employers and co-workers can give very useful information about the client's vocational history. Records from schools and training programs compose a third important type of information. These suggest what the client's performance and attitudes were like and reflect test scores and subjects taken.

Observation, consultation with other professionals, and research into the local vocational opportunities are other sources of vocational information. During the interview one pays attention to details that reveal the client's feelings about employers and jobs. Professionals who have known the client—ministers, social workers, doctors—have different viewpoints and may reveal new perspectives. Finally, vocational information also includes material on local opportunities and requirements, the client's ability and willingness to move, and local training opportunities, all of which should be carefully surveyed.

Work Experience Factors

Cundiff, Henderson, and Little [1965] discussed the factor of work experience, stating that, historically, vocational objectives were frequently chosen on the basis of gross relationships between occupational skills and experience and job requirements. Underlying this approach was the assumption that there is considerable uniformity and stability in basic occupations. For severely disabled individuals, job selection may require evaluation in a simulated work experience (see 22.1).

Taking a careful and extensive work history is crucially important for people who have severe employment problems; it is not sufficient for the counselor to list places of past employment. The history must show how long the person held a job and what the characteristics of the work were; how much responsibility and what skills were involved; the reasons the person obtained and then left the job. As one accumulates this information, indications of habits and attitudes emerge.

When the employment record is not extensive, as is often the case with severely disabled people, it is necessary to find out more by examining casual work experience, hobbies and other avocational activities, for example. Evaluation in a transitional workshop is often needed (see 8.3.4). When a person's previous occupation is no longer appropriate because of a disability, this information can be crucially important.

The work history should be examined with former employers and co-workers. Their viewpoints may possibly be prejudiced in some way, but a more accurate case study can be developed if a variety of interpretations is obtained. The client's own view of the employment history may well be biased; people whose experiences have been overwhelmingly negative may be prejudiced against themselves. The opinions of others then help to validate or negate self-reports.

The rehabilitationist's characterization of the client is not complete until the individual's view of work has been pinpointed. It is important to find out what the client hopes for in terms of work and also income expectations. Economic realities are such that it is essential for the client to understand what opportunities actually exist (see 35.2). If the individual does not have this insight, this is something that must be worked on during counseling and vocational exploration (see 27.4.3).

Vocational History

Compiling the vocational history enables the counselor to become familiar with the client's vocational capabilities, skills, and habits along with interests, goals, and motivations. The record of past achievements is still the best indicator of future performance. Each client's vocational history should list all the jobs held, beginning with the most recent. When someone has held a large number of jobs they need not all be listed individually, but the record should show type and duration of employment. The list should contain the employer's name and address, type of business, job title, wages, starting and ending dates, reasons for leaving.

It is necessary to know what level of skill each job involved and whether this level of skill is still adequate. The client's ability to get along with others in the employment situation, punctuality, dependability, and methods of working need to be known. If job changes have been frequent or there have been incongruous shifts between occupations, the reasons should be scrutinized. This is particularly true when there seem to be disparities between the client's preparation and avowed vocational preferences.

The detail in the vocational history depends on the depth and type of the client's work experiences. Those with no work history obviously are not subject to thorough examination, but even in these cases it is well to look carefully at indications of vocational interests. Clients who .have held many different kinds of jobs, on the other hand, can provide information about skills that is probably more significant than that about interests. Past employers' attitudes toward the client, the possibility of different work in the same place, and related work possibilities should be investigated.

Sometimes there are special reasons for an unusually thorough examination of the vocational history. A client, for example, whose vocational aspirations seem to conflict markedly with the results of tests and grades in school would be in this category. Interests and abilities should be carefully assessed. Another instance would be a client whose social adjustment at home and at school has generally been poor. This will tend to prove true at work as well and thus the vocational history should be carefully investigated for what it reveals about social adjustment.

Present Vocational Interests and Assets

Applicable vocational interests can be determined by inquiring into client preferences in terms of working with people, things, or ideas. Clients' characterizations of their aptitudes as commercial, intellectual, mechanical, and so on are also revealing. Avocational interests and activities often show what the person truly wants to do.

It is important to find out what the origins of the client's preferences are, whether they come from experience, reading, observation, false values, or pressure from others. How long the client has had a given interest, how often expressed preferences seem to change, and the actual knowledge that interests are based on, need to be determined. One also attempts to find out whether people believe their preferences are congruent with their capabilities, whether they believe their interests will change, and whether they find vocational significance in their leisure activities.

The rehabilitationist inspects the congruence between a client's avowed preferences and objectively determined abilities and also that between preferred activities and inventoried interests. Additionally it is important to consider whether the interests are realistic in terms of possibilities for work preparation and employment. Special conditions and skills are meaningful: car ownership, union membership, friends who can help with getting a job, special licenses, a good speaking voice, good manual dexterity, typing ability, foreign languages, and avocational proficiencies that might be applied to employment [McGowan and Porter, 1967]. Review of the client's functional limitations and functional abilities in the vocational context should be conducted systematically.

Appraising Vocational Information

Vocational information is appraised with relation to other types of data that have been obtained. One considers not only the client's functional limitations but also the length of time since onset of the disability, recommendations for physical restoration, and other health conditions that may influence the rehabilitation plan.

Social and psychological information is also considered. How do relatives feel about the client's vocational future? Is the client well adjusted socially? What is the desired standard of living? How long can job preparation last without representing an economic hardship? What is the person's self-image, attitude toward employment, intelligence, maturity? What does work mean to the individual?

Evaluation of vocational information in the case history is based on one principle: doing it in terms of the individual person. The client has the right to be guided on the basis of strengths rather than on the disability. Laymen often ask questions like "What kind of job can a quadriplegic do?" There are two kinds of answers to this question. A list of possible jobs is one answer. A far better response is that the question is actually about a person and therefore the answer must relate to that particular individual and a complete assessment of the individual's potential vocationally [Jeffrey, 1966].

An instrument useful in vocational case study, the Vocational Diagnosis and Assessment of Residual Employability (VDARE), has been published by the University of Georgia [McCroskey, Wattenbarger, Field, & Sink, 1977]. The VDARE worksheet provides a systematic way for utilizing a person's work history when one exists.

24.4.6. CASE STUDY INTERPRETATION

A fund of evaluation information about a client has no value in itself until it is sifted, synthesized, and interpreted. This work—the case study—is conducted by the rehabilitation counselor. All the information is arranged into a pattern that has significance. It is a process in logical thinking—the "teasing out" of a consistent pattern of vocational meaning from a mass of relevant and irrelevant facts about the person's significant assets and liabilities.

In short, basic information about the components of rehabilitation case study are obtained from the counselor's interviews, observations, and inquiries, and, from educational, psychosocial, medical, and vocational histories, records, and evaluation reports. Evaluative data from various professionals may be used, but the counselor is responsible for the case study process and the use of the information it provides. Client assessment is not accurate unless the evaluations are interpreted correctly and all the relevant information has been integrated. It will be incorrect if the psychological component is invalid or the medical conditions are not considered, for example. Each piece of information, accurate in itself, screened for relevance, and correctly interpreted, is put into its place within the entire configuration of facts. When the case study is complete, the counselor must explain the results to the client so that the client can make informed decisions.

Part IV

Counseling

Chapter 25

Principles

Since the creation of public vocational rehabilitation, counseling and guidance, along with training and placement, have been fundamental services. While nationwide use of the title "rehabilitation counselor" came later, the function of "counseling"—equated with "guidance" or "advisement"—was used to help the disabled person choose a suitable vocational objective. Unfortunately the counseling function was seen as a discrete activity limited to the planning phase of rehabilitation. Federal rehabilitation regulations still list counseling as only one of the various rehabilitation services. The misleading implication is that it is one of several equal and parallel elements successively provided each client in a series of services. Thus, even the government has failed to recognize counseling as the integrating and facilitating element of rehabilitation upon which all of the other client services depend. It should be recognized that the professional functions of rehabilitation counseling continue throughout the process.

Confusion over the real meaning of the role continued after the term *counselor* came into general use in the 1940s (Dabelstein, 1946). The advent of professional rehabilitation counselor education in the 1950s in fact only perpetuated the problem. Many of the universities that were granted federal funds after 1954 to start masters degree programs appointed counselor educators who promoted relationship counseling as the only professional function in the rehabilitation process. This narrow perspective was strenuously promulgated in journals and texts for several years. Some educators went so far as to equate counseling with psychotherapy. Consequently, the early programs of rehabilitation counselor education generally neglected course content covering the vocational rehabilitation process as a whole. Meanwhile, experienced rehabilitation workers were not very vocal in defending the professional nature and critical importance of counselor activities that are not directly therapeutic. To make matters worse, client assessment, case coordination, and placement procedures for vocational rehabilitation did not yet have a research basis. It was hard to argue, for example, that finding a job for a client was a professional function to be performed by the counselor.

The 1954 amendments to the federal Rehabilitation Act authorized funds for technological research as well as professional training (see 2.3); the impact of this, however, was not felt for several years. Gradually research-based techniques were developed for evaluation, coordination, and placement services, and they gained professional respectability [Bolton, 1979]. Meanwhile, however, specialists in these key counselor functions emerged outside of the aegis of rehabilitation counseling education and professional counseling affiliation (see 2.4). Thus work evaluators and placement employees of rehabilitation agencies now have divergent backgrounds and affiliations. This fragmentation does not change the fact, however, that the rehabilitation worker requires a knowledge of counseling in serving disabled clients throughout their readjustment process. A broad concept of the rehabilitation counselor's role incorporates these fundamental functions as fully professional and substantial services provided within the framework of the counseling relationship for both the development and the implementation of a comprehensive rehabilitation plan (see 3.1).

Considerable material selected for this and other chapters on rehabilitation counseling was originally published in the journal of the American Rehabilitation Counseling Association, *Rehabilitation Counseling Bulletin*. Many of these articles were reprinted in books edited by Bolton and Jaques [1978, 1979]; other books of reprinted journal articles include those by Patterson [1960] and Moses and Patterson [1971].

25.1. Professional Relationship

Counseling is a helping relationship. The concept of human relationships is fundamental for all counselors—this concept is in fact basic for social workers and other rehabilitation professionals who work face to face with individuals. This is because the behavior of each person reciprocally affects the behavior of the other. In these professions particularly, the total self is fully and deeply engaged in the process of helping.

25.1.1. IMPORTANCE

Various counseling theories have centered on the powerful force of a constructive relationship with the client, and techniques have been developed for using and manipulating this force. But the relationship is a delicate one, and the art of capturing or maintaining it is not fully understood. At least 20 relationship characteristics desirable in counseling can be mentioned— caring, warm, permissive, interested, sincere, receptive, accepting, involved, facilitative, nondominating, uncritical, respectful, natural, genuine, empathetic, positive, understanding, attentive, supportive, client-centered. Students of counseling can be helped to develop these characteristics necessary for a successful client relationship. Moreover, applicants for counselor education may be screened for these personal attributes.

The counseling relationship begins on the first contact. It is said in the theater that actors obtain a lasting image from their audience when speaking opening lines. First impressions, however, are not quite so fixed in the ongoing business of counseling, which is rather a dynamic affair that is gradually built and sustained. The nature of therapeutic relationships, in fact, actually changes dramatically as treatment passes through phases. While it will not be as dramatic as in psychoanalysis, even vocational counselors experience notable shifts in client attitude due to stresses and progress in counseling.

25.1.2. METHODS

Counseling should generally create a comfortable atmosphere in which the client feels accepted as a person. The experience of having a friendly, interested person listen attentively to one's troubles—neither minimizing the difficulty nor sympathizing, neither criticizing nor advising—tends to induce a warm response in the client. A bond develops from the sense of being understood for what one is.

Strains are nevertheless put on the relationship during the course of counseling. An example is the transference phenomenon, which must be understood and recognized if it is to be handled properly. Transference comprises the irrational elements carried over from other relationships, particularly from the past, and now displaced upon the counselor. It comes from unconscious motivation and should not be confused with real feelings. The development of transference is used as a part of treatment in psychotherapy but not ordinarily in the goal-limited counseling of rehabilitation.

All that has been written about the fundamental role of relationships might lead some to conclude that changes in behavior can be promoted just by listening to someone talk, encouraging the expectance of change, treating the person with the proper feelings and attitudes, and reinforcing what is positive. Anyone who is a decent, caring, sensitive person can do this. Actually the professional's expertise includes these natural ways but requires training and experience to make them an effective tool. Complete understanding of the varied problems confronted by clients requires education, which enables the counselor to respond in ways that expand the client's self-knowledge and sustain the client relationship. This is why people who would be rehabilitative counselors should be well selected as well as professionally prepared.

Reinforcement effects are a dynamic result of the counseling relationship. The positive response to behaviors and decisions consists of approving comments and bodily communication (e.g., smiling, nodding). No matter how noncommittal counselors try to be, they cannot avoid conveying positive or negative reinforcement to the client. The client's susceptibility to the counselor as a reinforcer or as a model of adequate behavior is largely dependent upon the positive relationship status of the two people.

Interpersonal communication is the key to establishing a helping relationship. The counselor gives the client total psychological attention: this is called "attending behavior," a skill of nonverbal empathy. It is done by eye contact, body posture, and personal warmth and acceptance. "Facilitative listening" is a learned technique that encourages a client to deal with feelings.

There are many techniques alluded to in this book that enhance the counselor's relationship with the client. In rehabilitation the counselor personifies for the client the agency's expenditures in behalf of the individual (e.g., for the purchase of a needed artificial limb, payment of school tuition). These things are very tangible and can help place the counselor in an acceptable position to help.

25.1.3. PROFESSIONAL POSTURES

There are counseling postures that can help in relationship development. The following are examples.

1. Assume the client acts in good faith. People are basically good and honest—at least they are more likely to be when this is expected.
2. Permit the client to be unique. Individuality is great because people should be different. It is not fair to expect other people to share one's own personal or cultural values.
3. Tolerate imperfections and mistakes. People have an innate capacity to change for the better, and this growth often results from the opportunity to experience mistakes.
4. Agree about goals and roles. Some concrete structure, such as who is responsible for tasks, helps to avoid relationship problems.
5. Understand that the responsible client has the ultimate authority. This means that the counselor's relationship is only a helping one.
6. Adopt an attitude of "critical empathy." The counselor understands the client's feelings but participates as an outside observer who, because of judicious objectivity, can make seasoned interpretations of these feelings. Intensive personal and emotional involvement causes perceptual distortion, which interferes with the helping role and can "burn out" the professional.

Counselor-client interaction takes many shapes and has varying strengths. It must be disciplined for effective use. Professional relationships are not just friendly associations formed for pleasure; the contact is for professional purposes. Yet this is one of the problems: clients bring into counseling the feelings and methods of behavior practiced with friends and family. Much of the responsibility for keeping the relationship healthfully structured and productive thus rests with the counselor. The professional is controlled by training and ethics toward the end of helping a client who is dependent upon the counseling service (see 2.2.2). Without this conscious purpose and the imposed structure, the relationship deteriorates, becoming unproductive or even destructive. Counseling relationships and strategies are described in more detail later (see 26.1) and in other books [e.g., Brammer, 1979; Hackney & Cormier, 1979].

25.2. Terms and Concepts

Counseling and clinical psychology share many descriptive terms with psychiatry and social work. This common terminology of adjustment facilitates communication among people in the mental health professions. It also benefits the rehabilitation counselor who works closely with them. A number of the more important terms are defined in this section. Additional terms—referring to concepts more relevant to psychotherapy than rehabilitation counseling—are defined at the end of Chapter 28, Personal Adjustment (see 28.7.5).

25.2.1. COUNSELING TECHNIQUES

A large body of knowledge exists on the technical methods of counseling. When implemented, these techniques become the skills a counselor uses to help clients. These elements of the craft sometimes have rather explicit labels, a number of which need to be defined.

ACCEPTANCE. Acceptance is best described as the psychological atmosphere existing with a person that conveys the right to be a unique person. It does not necessarily signify approval of the client's uniqueness. In counseling, this positive, uncensuring attitude toward the client implies the understanding of feeling and behavior and recognition of the person's worth as an individual, but without condoning antisocial behavior.

CONFRONTATION. This is a technique of counseling sometimes used to move a client forward. Clients may be confronted with the probable consequences of their present undesirable behavior pattern; or they may be confronted with problems of meaning, purpose, and value and be challenged to find answers.

EMPATHY. As an objective, insightful, and understanding awareness of the feelings, emotions, and behavior of another person, empathy is to be distinguished from sympathy, which is subjective, emotionally compassionate, and noncritical.

HELPING RELATIONSHIP. This is a relationship in which the counselor has the intent of and ability

for promoting the client's growth, development, maturity, and improved functioning and coping.

INTERPRETATION. Making an explanation that has not been specifically stated by the client but which can be inferred from the client's speech or other behavior is called "interpretation." It involves explaining to the counselees what their behavior (in the broadest sense) really means.

INTERVIEW. The word *interview* means a conversation directed to a definite purpose, one other than satisfaction in the conversation itself. It may be used for securing information from people, for giving information to them, and for purposes of influencing their behavior in certain ways. Interviewing cannot be considered counseling for it is a distinctly different process and has different goals. An interview is generally an interrogation to gain certain information so that the interviewer can make a judgment about the interviewee. In counseling, the process is introspective, having the goal of an individual's becoming self-sustaining.

ORIENTATION. In a program this means the process of introducing an individual to an agency by providing information regarding agency's program, services, procedures, physical layout, personnel, regulations, and other pertinent information. As a psychological expression, orientation means awareness of oneself in relation to time, place, and person.

PERMISSIVENESS. An uncritical atmosphere in an interpersonal relationship and situation that permits freedom of expression to another person is called "permissive."

POSITIVE REGARD. Positive regard is expressed by a warm and acceptant attitude on the part of the counselor toward the client. The counselor prizes the client as a person, regardless of the client's particular behavior at the moment. It means caring in a nonpossessive way, respecting the other person as a person, and liking without demanding.

PROBING. Probing is leading the client into unexplored areas. The counselor feels it important and in more or less subtle ways insists that the counselee discuss a particular topic more deeply.

RAPPORT. The condition of mutual understanding, respect, and sustained interest between individuals is called "rapport." In a general sense, rapport suggests a relationship based on a high degree of community of thought, interest, and sentiment.

STRUCTURING. This is a statement of the rules of the helping process or an understanding of such rules by clients that is imparted by the way the counselor acts in specific situations. Structuring explains the counseling procedure, the expected outcome, limitations of time, or the responsibilities of the counselor or client. It is usually done early in the initial phases of counseling.

SUGGESTION. Suggestion is a communication process by which one attempts to directly induce an idea, feeling, decision, or action in another person by circumventing the critical decision-making process. Persuasion is employed to change a client's attitudes, behavior, or goals.

SUMMARY CLARIFICATION. This means that the counselor selects those ideas and feelings from a given segment of an interview that seem most important and attempts to feed them back to the client in a more organized and concise form.

SYNTHESIZING. This is the process by which case study information from various segments of counseling and other information sources are combined into a meaningful whole for purposes of understanding and planning.

WARMTH. In a professional relationship, warmth is behavior exhibited by a counselor that conveys both cognitive understanding and feeling for the individual.

25.2.2. MENTAL MECHANISMS

Mental mechanisms as understood here are psychological devises used by people to assist them in dealing with emotional needs (e.g., affection, personal security, self esteem) and stresses (see 28.7.2). Mental mechanisms for defense are un-

consciously utilized strategies for protection against anxiety.

These mental mechanisms for coping and defense are natural human reactions. They are used to a certain extent by most people; it is only when the distortion of reality is excessive or exaggerated that an individual is felt to be maladjusted. Certainly psychological mechanisms are an important part of the reactions of humans seen in counseling.

COMPENSATION. The individual through this process attempts to make up for real or fancied deficiencies.

DENIAL. This is the refusal to face the reality of a situation. It is an attempt to resolve emotional conflict and allay consequent anxiety by denying some of the important elements of experience. An example is refusing to admit the presence or permanence of a disability or to recognize the handicap.

DISPLACEMENT. By this defense mechanism, an emotional feeling is transferred from its actual object to a substitute (i.e., another person, object, or situation), which then becomes invested with the emotional significance associated with the former object.

IDENTIFICATION. Identification is an attempt by an individual to gratify repressions by endeavoring to pattern one's self after another person.

PROJECTION. Projection is an unconscious mental mechanism whereby that which is emotionally unacceptable in one's own self is unconsciously rejected and attributed (projected) to others; in other words, faults seen in others may actually be one's own.

RATIONALIZATION. Through this mechanism, the individual attempts to justify feelings or behavior that would otherwise be intolerable. Excuses for one's motives may reduce guilt or self-depreciation, but such deceit prevents accurate self-appraisal.

REACTION FORMATION. Adopting attitudes and behavior that are the opposites of impulses the individual either consciously or unconsciously disowns is called "reaction formation." The ex-

hibited behavior is rigid and reinforces the repression.

REPRESSION. Repression is the involuntary rele-
gation of unbearable ideas and impulses into the
unconscious. Even while repressed material is
not voluntarily recalled, it may emerge in dis-
guised form.

RESISTANCE. The psychological defense against
bringing repressed material into awareness is
called "resistance." The resistance to the
emergence of repressed (unconscious) memories
into awareness is an important clue to the
dynamic significance of life experiences.

SUBLIMATION. In this mechanism, consciously
unacceptable instinctual (e.g., sexual) drives are
diverted into personally and socially acceptable
channels.

SUBSTITUTION. Unattainable or unacceptable
goals, emotions, or objects are replaced by more
attainable or acceptable ones through this mechanism of the mind.

SUPPRESSION. Suppression is the process of dismissing unpleasant memories, thoughts, or desires from the conscious mind. It is distinguished
from repression by the fact that the effort is conscious and voluntary. Potentially obnoxious behaviors are inhibited.

SYMBOLIZATION. This is the mechanism by
which a person forms an abstract representation
of a particular object or idea.

WITHDRAWAL. Use of this mechanism represents a retreat from reality. There are various
forms of withdrawal: admitting defeat, reducing
ego involvement, lowering aspirations, restricting situations requiring the need to cope, cur-
tailing energy and effort, or becoming apathetic.
Fantasy, an extreme form of daydreaming with
an imaginary experiencing of satisfactions not
obtainable in reality, often accompanies withdrawal.

25.2.3. REACTIONS TO DISABILITY

This important counseling subject—reaction to
disability—is discussed in various chapters on
the impact of and personal adjustment to disability (e.g., see 4.3). Various terms defined

elsewhere in this chapter are also particularly
important in the psychosocial aspects of disability.

AS-IF BEHAVIOR. This refers to the disabled individual who acts "as if" the disability is not
there. It is a type of denial, an attempt to conceal
and forget about the limitation. Impetus for
these actions comes from feeling inferior, feeling
that the disability makes one fall below normal
standards. This reaction is not adaptive since the
individual experiences a great deal of stress in
constantly attempting to "cover up" the problem.

BODY IMAGE. An aspect of the self-concept,
body image is a continuously developing representation of a person's perception of his or her
body. It includes conceptions of appearance to
others, of physical capacities, and of general attractiveness. When the body is disturbed by disease or trauma, its image may be interfered with.
The cultural values of body-whole or body-
beautiful have to be dealt with and the disability
has to be incorporated into the body image.

CRISIS THEORY. A crisis is a devastating event
that forces individuals to utilize all the resources at their disposal to reinstate the unity of
their psychological structure. Rehabilitationists
should be aware of the phases an individual goes
through during a crisis, since the first concerns
of an individual meeting a crisis are safety needs,
and the person may engage in defensive retreat
and denial. Any attempts to counter these procedures may be met by increased retreat. Later
on when the individual again recognizes growth
needs, a therapeutic relationship can be beneficial.

COPING WITH DISABILITY. The individual learns
to struggle successfully with the limitations imposed by the disability. When a person is coping
with a disability, the emphasis is on what the individual can do, and areas in which he or she can
participate are seen as worthwhile. There is an
awareness of the problems caused by the disability. Difficulties are not naively ignored or
denied but realistically judged, accepted, and
coped with.

COVERING. Covering is the practice of many individuals who are disabled to make an effort to

keep the disability from being the focus of attention. The purpose is to make social interactions easier.

MARGINALITY. This refers to the situation of a person attempting to fill two conflicting roles. The disabled individual is caught between the identity of a "normal" person, which is more desirable but sometimes not acceptable to other nondisabled people, and that of the deviant, which is available but certainly not desirable. The options that seem open to the individual are to reject the disability and present the self as normal, or to heighten the handicap and fill what others feel is the role of a disabled person.

MINORITY GROUP STATUS. The disabled population have been likened to minority groups since there is a diminution in their social status by virtue of the fact of their disablement. The individual who is disabled is often evaluated on group membership rather than on any individual characteristics and so is reacted to as one of a category of people.

PASSING. If the disability is not apparent and the individual can hide it, one option open to the individual is "passing," which is ignoring the disabled role, denying the stigma, and attempting to maintain membership in the larger group. An individual may attempt to pass due to feelings of inferiority, social pressures, and the desire to be considered normal.

REINTEGRATION PROCESS. When an individual becomes disabled, it becomes necessary for the disability to be incorporated into the self so that it is perceived as only one aspect of the self rather than the totality. The individual can then define worth in terms of what is possible rather than in terms of what has been lost.

REQUIREMENT OF MOURNING. This is based on the notion that when people feel the need to protect values important to them, they will either demand that those unfortunate individuals who are different from them must suffer or they will devaluate those deviant persons who should suffer but do not. The reasons behind this are that other people want to see suffering as an indication that the values refused to the unfortunate individual are still worthwhile.

RESOCIALIZATION PROCESS. Disability can have a large impact on the individual's total socialization process, from dating and marriage to finding and keeping a job. The individual in effect has to be trained or retrained to deal with the social environment so that the ambiguity of social situations and the stigmatizing effects of the disability are minimized.

SELF-CONCEPT. This is one's conception of one's various personal characteristics and attached values. Interactions with others are of great importance in the development of the self-concept. A healthy individual can integrate new experiences (such as becoming disabled) into the existing self-concept, whereas an individual who already has problems with self-concept ignores, denies, or distorts experiences inconsistent with the way the self is viewed.

SICK ROLE. Illness or disability is a role that an individual acquires and which carries with it certain assumptions and expectations. There is also a disturbance in the individual's ability to carry out expected tasks.

SUCCUMBING TO DISABILITY. This means that the individual gives up to the disability. The total emphasis is on what has been lost and what the individual cannot do, with little attention given to those areas of life in which the person can still participate.

25.2.4. OTHER RELEVANT TERMS
Many concepts relevant to the counseling process are explained throughout Part IV. Still there are miscellaneous terms in addition to those listed above that it will be well to know in advance. While some of the words are used by the lay public, they have a precise professional meaning.

ACQUIRED CHARACTERISTICS AND REACTIONS. These are characteristics and reactions that are developed or learned. They are not congenital or inherent at birth. Attitudes, a predisposition to act, are acquired.

AUTHORITARIANISM. The authoritarian personality is one that accepts widespread beliefs; is intolerant of ambiguity; values strength, authority, and power; is rigid in beliefs; is very dogmatic, reluctant to change, highly ethnocentric, and very prejudicial to all out-groups (e.g., the disabled).

AVOIDANCE. The act or practice of staying away from something undesirable or unwelcome is known as avoidance. For the person who is disabled, this may include denial or withdrawal from acknowledgment of the disability. "Normal" individuals may have a variety of fears, guilt feelings, and negative attitudes toward disability; for them, the easiest way to relieve the discomfort of interacting is to keep away from interactions with individuals who are disabled.

DEVALUATION. The nondisabled may view those who are disabled as lacking something of importance, with the result that their worth is devalued and they are held in lower social esteem. Society espouses the values of independence and self-reliance.

ENVIRONMENT. This is a general term designating all the people, objects, forces, and conditions that affect an individual. Life space includes the person and the environment, which interact to produce a unique living situation for the individual. Community ecological circumstances that determine the disabled person's adjustment include social attitudes, the economy, human service resources, and accessibility considerations (for transportation, housing, and other accommodations).

MOTIVATION. The concept of motivation is used to explain the factors within the individual that activate, sustain, and direct behavior toward a goal. The "motivational" model puts the blame of not improving on the client—the client is said to be unmotivated. It is better, however, to look at the environmental influences (disincentives). The rehabilitation staff has to take some responsibility for providing those positive experiences and expectations that will result in the desire for recovery and independence.

PERCEPTION. Perception is the process of recognizing and identifying external objects and the mental integration of sensory experiences.

SPREAD. When a person is devalued due to a socially defined deviation in physical appearance or performance, the negative opinion may "spread" to other characteristics of the person. A connection is made between an abnormality of the body and an abnormality of the mind. There is a tendency to make inferences according to one prominent feature. Thus, the properties of a single characteristic of an individual are imposed on the total person, even when other characteristics are not actually known; the abilities of the total person are underrated.

STIGMA. A stigma is an identifying mark or characteristic that signifies a deviation from a cultural norm and as such is discrediting to the individual.

UNCONSCIOUS. The unconscious is a part of the mind (i.e., mental functioning) the content of which is only rarely subject to awareness.

25.3. Counseling Theories

A scientific theory is an empirically plausible and systematic analysis of a set of facts, principles, or circumstances and their interrelationship that, while still based upon hypothetical assumptions, provides a basis for inquiry or action. Derived through thought and observation, theories are constructed to explain what might happen in a situation such as counseling, thus leading to the development of new methods in science or professional practice.

Psychologists with different views of personality functioning and behavior change have developed different theories. This section summarizes a number of prominent theories dealing with counseling and psychotherapy. Several counseling theory texts are available [e.g., Patterson, 1973], and other references cited here provide a more extensive description and detailed analysis of theories relevant to counseling. Techniques suggested by various counseling theories are also discussed in other chapters of Part IV.

Theoretical knowledge is essential for an understanding of the counseling process and is consequently fundamental to counselor effectiveness. This body of knowledge, collected over the years from thought and experience and research by many theorists, is the foundation for helping clients. It is also helpful in the counselor's own development; only through a sound understanding of the self can the counselor's full potential for helping others be realized.

A theory has significance for the counselor, the success of whose work depends upon the use and synthesis of information. It helps the counselor to think more clearly, to collect and weigh ideas. It offers a framework within which behavior can be accounted for and modified. It serves as the groundwork for hypotheses that can be tested.

Valuable guidelines are inherent in every counseling theory. Explanations are given for the qualities and attitudes that help clients: empathy, respect, honesty, interpretation. A good theory, therefore, is eminently practical. It is a structure of explanation, a rationale for proceeding, a point of departure for positive action. For every counseling dilemma, theory can provide enlightenment and direction.

As the counselor soon learns, concepts from different theories overlap. In fact, the idea that is found in only one theory is very unusual. What distinguishes one school of theory from another is the emphasis on different strategies. These unique elements fortunately may be applied selectively. Because no one theory is adequate by itself [Berenson and Carkhuff, 1967], effective counseling is usually based upon a combination of ideas from different theoretical frameworks.

Most counselors agree that it is not necessary to accept all aspects of a theory to use one of its elements. The objective should be to select those aspects of various theories that are best suited to the occasion (i.e., the counselor, the client, the problem, and the situation confronted). Selecting ideas from the many different theorists is moreover a process that contributes to the evolution of the counselor's own style. Unfortunately, some counselors, tied to a single school, are unable or unwilling to employ the varied and rich heritage of counseling psychology by orchestrating the alternative selections of theory and techniques.

In actual practice most counselors choose from various theories and techniques according to the circumstances and their own predisposi-tions. The term used for this selection and organization into a comprehensive system of compatible elements drawn from varied theories is *eclecticism*. Eclecticism is to be distinguished from "syncretism," which is an uncritical attempt to combine incompatible systems; some self-styled eclectic counselors, however, actually have simply failed to master any theoretic foundation.

Theory and the art of applying it in counseling are the methods by which the practitioner develops in effectiveness. The theory does not dominate but serves the counselor, who uses ideas from different conceptual frameworks.

25.3.1. TRADITIONAL PSYCHOANALYSIS

Psychoanalytic theory as first and traditionally presented is based on the work of Sigmund Freud, 1856–1939. The principal elements of classical psychoanalysis deal with the development of the personality and the determination of behavior. Dr. Freud believed that human beings are controlled by internal forces over which they are virtually powerless. The best they can do is to learn how to govern these forces through discipline and with help from the environment. These forces and techniques for dealing with them are discussed below.

Unconscious Forces

Unconscious mental forces cause maladjustment and maladaptive behavior, the symptoms of which also come from the unconscious. The objective of therapy is to uncover those circumstances or conditions that bear directly on a person's symptoms and adjustment problems.

Structure of Personality

Behavior is explained by three principal components: the id, the ego, and the superego. The id, the major system, expresses the essential purpose of the individual, which is fulfillment of instinctual needs. The ego mediates between the id and the external world, seeking to decrease tension by finding an appropriate way to satisfy needs. The superego is the conscience; it evolves mainly through a process of identifying with parents. It is an internal force that gradually takes the place of parents in directing behavior.

Instincts

Two different sorts of events result in individual behavior: situational circumstances—or environmental stimuli—and innate instinctual forces. The latter are responsible for much of behavior.

As psychological energy is built up it must be decreased by either a primary process, a secondary process, or a habitual response. The first response category, primary process, has to do with the principle of homeostasis; it is an undirected attempt to decrease tension to a neutral condition, the seeking of pleasure for immediate satisfaction. Secondary process is the attempt to decrease tension in a rational way; the ego is in control and activity is reality-based. The third kind of response, the habitual or repetitive response, serves to account for the fact that some behaviors are not aimed at decreasing tension. They may instead cause greater tension such as that connected with sexual responses.

Aggression

The psychological forces of aggression and the sex drive figure prominently in human behavior. Human beings are therefore controlled to a large extent by inner forces.

Growth Stages

According to Freud, there are five psychosexual stages of development, which are characterized by certain responses. The first year of life is the oral stage in which pleasure is experienced through sucking. Freud related weaning, which ends this period, to an individual's potential to behave sadistically.

During the second year of life, the anal period, the locus of pleasurable sensation changes to the anal zone of the body. Satisfaction is felt in elimination and later in retaining the feces.

The phallic stage begins at about age three and continues through approximately age six. The child is now able to derive pleasure through touching the sex organs. During the later part of the period a boy feels a desire to possess his mother (Oedipus complex) and a girl experiences the desire to possess the father (Electra complex). How the male child resolves the castration complex during this period may have important repercussions later.

The next stage, from approximately age six to the preadolescent years, is the latency period. The child concentrates more on the acquisition of skills at this time.

In the genital stage, which arrives with puberty, there is potential for a number of problems. Biological urges, connected with sexual development, are strongly felt; they must be sublimated if the individual is to conform to cultural standards. This is the last period before maturity.

Techniques

Psychoanalysis uses a variety of techniques, but the principal element of all of them is allowing the patient to talk out. After the patient talks about situations or events that prompt emotional reactions, the analyst concentrates on their possible significance and shows the individual how they relate to current problems. In reacting to the patient's talk, the analyst assumes that alterations in speech patterns can effect thinking. The process of transference, in which the individual's feelings are directed toward the analyst as surrogate parent, is an important part of therapy. By means of free association and dream analysis the unconscious is exposed and the patient's attention is directed to subjects of particular importance. Psychoanalysis is usually a lengthy, time-consuming, and expensive process.

25.3.2. INDIVIDUAL PSYCHOLOGY

Individual psychology, or "Adlerian psychology," was originated by Alfred Adler, a highly reputed psychiatrist born in 1870 in Vienna. While some aspects of Adler's theory are in opposition to psychoanalytic theory, others are based in that school. Adler, along with others, attempted to isolate the actual reasons for maladaptive behavior. Instead of looking for explanations in the past and seeking to show what happened in an individual's life to cause a problem, Adler and his followers proposed that human behavior is attributable in great part to the desire to achieve social status.

Forces Underlying Behavior

Human beings are socially motivated. Inherent in all people is a striving for superiority. Compensation—which can be either constructive or neurotic—occurs when a person attempts to counteract areas of believed inferiority.

Fundamental to individual psychology is Adler's suggestion that abnormal behavior is the result of two principal factors. One comes about as a result of a sense of inferiority that the individual develops in early life; the other results from the individual's attempt to handle these inferior feelings through inappropriate behavior.

The feelings relate to an individual's sense of biological inadequacy and incompetence. These two proposed causes of maladaptive behavior are the two fundamental postulates of Adler's theory.

Postulates

Human beings are basically and innately social, so their behavior comes about as a result of the wish to achieve social status. Although essentially social, they are all unique. This uniqueness allows each person to feel independent and therefore have a sense of pride and importance.

Consciousness, rather than Freud's unconscious, is what actually determines human conduct. People are highly sensitive to themselves and to their environment and therefore are able to govern their behavior. Their actions are responses to their own creative potential and to their underlying need for activities that will increase the effectiveness of their own unique lifestyles.

The theory of individual psychology concentrates upon health and normality rather than abnormal conditions. Abnormal behavior is the result of ignorance, lack of understanding, or inexperience; it is corrected by addressing these deficits.

Behavior is purposeful. It represents an individual's attempt to fulfill a significant need, and usually the purpose relates to the desire to find an appropriate social position. This objective is achieved through self-assurance and a positive self-image, which enable one to undertake activities positively and to acquire the skills necessary to form good social relationships. When a person retreats from social interaction it is frequently because of feelings of inferiority and insecurity. This response forms the foundation for further maladaptive behavior, which then becomes a defense mechanism while arousing hostility in the very people whose approbation the individual needs.

Perceptions are a very significant aspect of behavior, since people tend to conduct themselves according to their perceptions of circumstances. Usually people who feel inferior or insecure have realistic reasons: their size, personal appearance, social status, intellectual limitations, and so on. Regardless of the reason, however, the actuality is not as significant as the individual's perception of it. Misguided perceptions or notions about other people's responses may lead to inappropriate behavior, and this in turn accentuates the difficulties in the situation. Changes in behavior are brought about when the person's self-perceptions or perceptions of the situation are improved.

Competition can contribute to personal development when properly used. On the other hand it may interfere severely with development if it is construed as hostile or unjust.

Disturbing conduct has four principal objectives. It may be aimed at gaining attention, power, or revenge, or it may be used as a means of withdrawal.

Tools

The Adlerian counselor uses a variety of tools and techniques, as appropriate. The objective is to determine what the undesirable behaviors are and then to decide how they can be changed. Both the counselor and the client are involved, but the counselor's role in this process is most influential. The counselor makes specific recommendations about how the behaviors can be changed and what the preferable alternatives are.

Among the tools are consulting, instructing, giving information, advising, and telling. Counselors of this school concentrate on helping clients understand their behavior and on urging them to work hard to change it. Warren Rule [1978] has written about the rehabilitation uses of Adlerian life-style counseling.

25.3.3. CLIENT-CENTERED COUNSELING

Client-centered counseling is so termed because of the position and freedom it gives the client. This method focuses on the client and is designed to place substantial responsibility on the individual. The approach is also termed the *self-theory* because of its indebtedness to phenomenological philosophy and existentialism.

Background

Client-centered counseling—originally referred to as "nondirective"—was formulated by Carl Rogers [1942, 1951, 1961]. Rogers held that all people have inborn capacities for purposive, goal-directed behavior. If free from disadvantageous learning conditions, people develop into kind, friendly, self-accepting, and social beings. Faulty learning causes people to become self-centered, hateful, antagonistic, ineffective.

Client-centered counseling aims to correct this by providing the client with an opportunity to expand awareness of and liking for self. Behavior can be understood only from the person's subjective point of view and can be changed only by the person's own determination to change. Hence the task of the counselor is not to direct or make interpretations, but to create an accepting, nonthreatening atmosphere in which the client can (re)examine the self to form a more positive view and move to more rewarding self-actualizing behavior.

Rogers was especially opposed to the intervention approach in which the client was dominated by the counselor. In his theory he emphasized that the counselor's role should be limited and the client's extensive; the client has freedom in self-expression and takes much responsibility for deciding how to solve problems.

Theoretical Themes

The major themes of the Rogerian approach are affective responses, faith in human nature, the purposiveness of behavior, client responsibility, and observation. Two related conceptions are: first, that all individuals have the innate capacity to comprehend the significant elements in their lives; second, that the abilities and strengths of individuals may be tapped more completely by means of counseling. The principal role of the counselor is to give clients an environment in which they feel free to talk about themselves and to examine their feelings deeply without apprehension or discomfort.

Techniques and Tools

The techniques of this approach are implied by the concepts that form its foundation. As these concepts are brought to bear on the counseling process, the counseling becomes effective [Carkhuff & Berenson, 1977]. The counselor's philosophy and beliefs are incorporated into the techniques.

A number of techniques are basic to this theory and express its important themes. A major procedure is reflecting feelings—restating in a slightly different way, but precisely, the feelings the client has voiced. Another technique is careful listening, which displays real interest in and acceptance of the client. Third, clients are urged to voice their thoughts and feelings fully. And finally, their feelings are given recognition, understanding, and clarification. The objec-

tives of client-centered counseling are attained through the use of these and other procedures. These techniques are supplemented by a climate of friendliness, understanding, and permissiveness.

Some of the basic concepts of the Rogerian approach, discussed below, are philosophical in nature, but practical techniques are implied.

Active Involvement of the Client

Basic to the client's development is involvement in the counseling process. Voicing feelings gives people an opportunity to evolve and participate in a relationship with the counselor. To express felt experience and to examine problems rationally both further growth.

Capacity for Growth

All individuals are capable of perceiving and coming to terms with relevant happenings and situations. Their mental and psychological capacity to handle problems and to learn from past experience is assumed.

Growth through Permissiveness

The relationship between the counselor and the client is friendly, accepting, and permissive. Clients will benefit more from the counseling and apply what they learn if there is little organization and control. When the climate allows for self-expression and freedom, more progress will be made.

Basic Goodness of Human Nature

Human beings are considered as essentially good, their nature positive and dependable. People can reach self-fulfillment and will work harder toward this end when they perceive their own inner potential. Central to this theory is belief in human beings as worthwhile, constructive, and self-fulfilling individuals.

Insight and Change

Complete functioning depends upon one's understanding, which underlies changes in behavior. The feeling of freedom that comes from the counseling relationship facilitates the achievement of understanding.

Independence and Integration

Counseling always has as its objective the attainment of the sense of independence and the coordination of an individual's various traits. To act on one's own is considered a way of gaining in strength and skills.

Focus upon the Emotional or Affective

Emotional elements of problems or circumstances are viewed with much more care than intellectual aspects. The way *the individual* feels is what is significant rather than what another person thinks might or should be felt.

The Therapeutic Benefits of Counseling

Interaction with the counselor and the content of the counseling process both contribute to the individual's development. The setting, the relationship established, and the climate help the person, regardless of the methods used.

Client Responsibility

Counseling helps people most when they become accountable for their own behavior, thinking, and choices. It is this responsibility, not the implementing of the decisions of others, that results in growth.

Counselor Observations and Feelings

The counselor's judgments, founded upon experience and feelings, have an important place in the process. One's viewpoint is not inflicted on the client but is used to help. Objective evidence has some weight but is not as valuable as more subjective information.

Tentativeness and Tolerance

This approach is marked by tentativeness as the client has latitude to think, experience, and take action; the counselor is tolerant, empathetic, accepting, and open in attempting to get the client to voice feelings. The lack of rigid organization enables the client to examine feelings in detail.

The Irrationality of Behavior

When people are behaving in an irrational manner, they will discover this themselves. Expressing feelings enables them to see that their conduct is inappropriate and allows them to recognize the necessity for change. This understanding precedes the conscious attempt to make changes.

Humanistic Psychology

Humanistic psychology, as applied to counseling, is something of an outgrowth of the client-centered method. It is concerned with the uniqueness and wholeness of each individual. Humanism rejects efforts to group people according to traits or labels. The basic problems of living are difficulties in experiencing one's self, inability to find pleasure and fulfillment in one's activities, and failure to make meaningful contact with others. Treatment in the humanistic framework is an experiential process intended to increase the client's awareness of self and the capacity to relate.

25.3.4. LEARNING THEORY APPROACHES

Certain methods are termed *learning theory approaches* because they implement learning concepts that impact on counseling. Because learning is considered as alterations in behavior that result from factors other than maturation, the implementation of learning theory is obviously important to counseling.

The background of learning theory goes back to the 19th century and the classic conditioning experiments of physiologists. Ivan Pavlov [1927] is usually credited with the early development of the theoretical rationale underlying the behavioral approach. He helped establish the principle that learning is a conditioning process. Pavlov, a Russian, showed that dogs could learn to respond (salivate) to a neutral stimulus (bell tone) if they were presented (paired) with an unconditioned stimulus (food); he also showed that lack of periodic reinforcement (food) could result in the extinguishing of the newly learned response. (See 29.1.)

The principles of operant conditioning were put forth by B. F. Skinner [1938, 1953]. He observed that much behavior is not elicited by *antecedents* (as explained by classic conditioning). These "operant behaviors" are a function of their *consequences*. Conditioning or changing human behavior through the systematic use of rewards thus became a practical tool.

Until the 1960s learning theorists generally believed that the classic or operant models of learning were responsible for the acquisition and maintenance of human behavior. Albert Bandura [1969] and others then demonstrated that subjects could acquire new response patterns simply by watching other people modeling certain kinds of behavior. For example, one group of schoolchildren watched a live model being aggressive toward a doll, while another group saw the same model being very gentle and calm with the doll. When members of both groups were later mildly frustrated they reacted aggressively or passively according to their model viewing experience. Later research has shown that this "modeling" effect holds for models seen in other circumstances and in real life.

Dollard and Miller published *Personality and Psychotherapy* in 1950, which attempted to apply the principles of learning theory to the etiology and treatment of abnormal behavior. While that book adhered to psychoanalytic concepts, it initiated the use of behavioral concepts and terms in counseling.

Reinforcement Theory

In contrast to approaches that seek to utilize the principles of conditioning in counseling, reinforcement theory is an effort to combine learning theory, psychoanalytical insights into human nature, and the concepts of social science that deal with the social factors in learning. It offers a view of human mentality according to the principles of learning. A number of elements compose the reinforcement theory.

First, neurosis is acquired through experiences of certain sorts. Individuals develop neuroses by learning modes of conduct incongruent with their needs and with the demands of the environment. Phobias, irritability, and uncertainty, as well as other symptoms of maladjustment, cannot be conquered by effort. Neurotic individuals are able to behave normally but fail to do so because they have learned other behaviors.

Second, the potential for change lies primarily in the capacity to acquire new modes of conduct as alternatives to the undesired behaviors. Altering the behavior is difficult because the present conduct stems from a conflict between two or more forces that cause differing responses. People may find it hard to change behavior even when they understand this, although often they are not conscious of it. Another reason it is difficult to modify behavior is that the symptoms in fact decrease the conflicts, thus promoting the behavior.

Third, the neurotic learns to utilize a symptom in the normal course of events, and the behavior therefore persists. Repression is another acquired behavior.

Classic Conditioning

Classic conditioning has been used for a relatively long period of time; features of this approach have a place in current counseling.

People have been conditioned to certain forms of conduct by the adults who figure prominently in their lives and by external factors. Children are urged to conform and to act so as to satisfy others. Personal difficulties often come about when an individual adheres to strong inhibitions as a safeguard against impulses. Because the perceived necessity for inhibitions in society is at times overestimated, defensive or neurotic conduct can result. Inhibited individuals attempt to make it seem that they are accepted by and accepting of others. Actually, they are really absorbed with themselves and are not the tolerant, friendly people they would like to appear. Their self-concern leads to tenseness and anxiety and they are lacking in forcefulness. They are basically insincere, defensively trying too hard to be pleasant.

The complete fulfillment of potential is impeded by feelings of fear and anxiety. The objective of therapy in this situation is to promote greater relaxation and more uninhibited and constructive behavior. Since inhibition is the problem, there is little possibility for growth and fulfillment until the inhibitions can be decreased or conquered. Verbal conditioning is used to handle symptoms.

Operant Conditioning

Operant conditioning, as devised by Skinner [1953], is like other behavioristic approaches in that its goal is an alteration in behavior through relearning. The premise underlying operant conditioning is that behavior is acquired and that it can be unlearned if preferred responses are used to replace it. The undesired responses are obliterated and the preferred behaviors stimulated by reinforcement. The desired behavior is specified and then the conditions appropriate to it are set up. Positive reinforcement and negative reinforcement are used to encourage the desired response and discourage the undesirable behavior, respectively.

Behavior can be programmed if the counselor and the client can isolate the response that needs to be altered and the client can make the necessary change. Reinforcement of undesired responses is eliminated and reinforcements for the preferred behaviors are devised. After choosing a given behavior, one establishes the situation in which it can be controlled and practiced. The individual can do this independently after learning the procedure.

Behavioral Counseling

The behavioral counseling approach [Krumboltz & Thoresen, 1969] has much in common with the others; it differs in that the procedures are used in a more flexible manner and in that it assumes a wider variety of causes for behavior.

Different responses are acquired as people try to fulfill their needs. They continue those behaviors that seem to produce satisfaction and that bring about desired reinforcement. Inappropriate conduct at times persists only because people find it satisfying in some respect or because they are not capable of changing. Psychotherapy can best help and instruct people to change if it is utilized as a learning theory approach.

Another assumption of this type of counseling is that the variables are very similar to those that characterize other relationships. Reinforcement, extinction, and acquisition influence the process, which is arranged and manipulated so that these procedures work effectively.

Four principal ingredients constitute this approach. First, a counseling objective is identified and established. Second, procedures are utilized as required to meet the client's needs. Third, there is much experimentation with a wide variety of techniques; and finally, techniques are changed whenever new information indicates that this is desirable. The process is made more effective through self-correction, feedback, evaluation, and research.

Reciprocal Inhibition

In this approach one uses the behavioral manifestation of a reaction inconsistent with the response to be extinguished. The idea is to inhibit or do away with former responses by promoting new ones. The person unlearns the undesired reaction and acquires replacement responses through reinforcement and practice [Wolpe, 1969]. Such techniques are now commonly referred to as "desensitization."

25.3.5. THE TRAIT-FACTOR APPROACH

The trait-factor approach has long guided vocational counselors in many kinds of educational and rehabilitation settings (see 27.2). It has served as a contrast to the client-centered approach in several important ways: (1) by emphasizing direct participation on the part of the counselor and giving the counselor substantial responsibility; (2) by stressing the counselor's function as essential in guiding the individual toward suitable vocational and educational decisions; and (3) by placing emphasis on the intellectual elements of decision-making and problem-solving—as opposed to the client-centered approach, which underlines the importance of emotional aspects of a problem.

Background

This approach was founded by Frank Parsons [1909] in Boston early in this century. Parsons believed that young people faced with job choices needed help in the form of guidance. The University of Minnesota was the principal institution associated with the development of the trait-factor approach. Major contributors were Walter Bingham [1937], Donald G. Paterson and John Darley [1936], and E. G. Williamson [1950, 1965].

Major Theoretical Elements

The trait-factor theory deals primarily with the idea of evaluating or measuring to determine a person's qualities and characteristics. The information gathered is used to assist the person in making suitable vocational decisions. Substantially less consideration is given to individual feelings and to alterations of behavior than occurs with other approaches. The emphasis is on assessing traits and then making life decisions with these traits as a focal consideration.

Central to this approach is the concept that human beings have definite traits that can be measured (see 20.1.3), and also that through assessment of these characteristics a set of guidelines can be established to correlate traits with a particular job or profession. It is necessary to have appropriate tools by which to measure the traits and also to set up procedures through which a substantial amount of data about vocations can be obtained.

According to this theory, people are sources of data about themselves that are useful in making choices and plans. The person's environment is also full of data essential for effective decision-making. When using this approach one does not try to change either people or the environment to any great extent but rather to use them as they exist. For instance, in assessing an individual given qualities will be revealed, and in looking at the person's surroundings certain possibilities and limitations will become clear. Decisions are formed with these data as the starting point.

The synthesis of data is an integral feature of

this approach—material from a variety of sources must be organized in an intelligible way. Then the data taken into consideration by the client and the counselor are used in pinpointing and solving difficulties and in making suitable decisions. It is feasible to predict the chances for success in various sorts of educational and vocational endeavors. All choices are made in an objective, systematic way and with past experience in mind.

According to the trait-factor methodology, emotional difficulties are traceable to an individual's inability to make choices and are dealt with as such. The emotions themselves are not viewed as significant because the process of making decisions is emphasized. One assumes that if a person has the ability to arrive at appropriate decisions and carry them out, anxiety or other emotional impediments will disappear.

To work effectively, the trait-factor approach must utilize reliable measuring instruments and sound information about various opportunities. This additionally implies that skilled personnel are available to explain the data to the client.

Techniques

The techniques utilized in this system are clearcut, objective, and logical; they relate to understanding of the client and the feasible alternatives. The counseling strategy is to help the person toward improved self-assessment stemming from the evaluation of personal strengths and limitations relative to goals.

Interpretation assists the client in understanding and utilizing the findings of tests and other data. Advice-giving is appropriate but is done in an objective manner and with the involvement of the client. Reading and studying help the client gain better understanding of self, others, and the external world.

A number of techniques promote effective decision-making, including informal discussion, group counseling, field trips, working, and role play.

25.3.6. DEVELOPMENTAL COUNSELING

Underlying the developmental approach is a broad definition of counseling. As a methodology, developmental counseling focuses on the concept of the developmental process, which is viewed as a pattern of experiences involving changes in the physical, mental, and emotional aspects of personality. These changes are continually taking place in a coherent pattern [Blocher, 1966]. Because people and the world they live in are always changing, adaptation to these alterations is a great task.

Major Theoretical Elements

At the core of developmental counseling is the attempt to help people develop more effectively. It is believed that if people are helped to cultivate and make use of their capabilities they can avoid many difficulties. Because a purpose of counseling is to give people the information and guidance they need in order to go through the developmental process more smoothly, this developmental approach is especially appropriate for use with children.

Process and product are emphasized equally in intervening with behavior. Behavior modes are looked upon as stages through which a child passes rather than as end results. Each new mode serves as a basis for later stages of development; what happens in development serves as a foundation for continuing growth.

Human beings are regarded not only as tension-reducing animals but as creatures who react to a stimulus hunger as a drive to action. People feel motivation to gain control over the external world and therefore govern the origins of its stimulation; they do not merely wish to decrease the stimulation in the environment. Human beings thus manipulate the external world as best serves their purposes.

Counseling is aimed at enhancing self-knowledge, sharpening awareness of one's potential, and providing a methodological structure for making the fullest use of one's abilities. An individual's responsibility for choices is emphasized, as this is the end result of learning about the self and one's potential. Essentially, the counselor and the client are in a partnership, both weighing the problem carefully and selecting a means of approaching it. The individual's latitude in decision-making is substantial; the counselor helps as much as possible with developmental problems. While the approach does not use evaluation as such, it does offer an organization through which a rational decision can be made.

Children are viewed as being engaged continually in the process of evolving a lifestyle, which becomes their way of life. The development of a positive self-image is stressed, as this is necessary in avoiding apprehension and its detrimental effects on conduct. To enable people to live as effectively as possible through helping them develop is the final objective of counseling.

The freedom to make choices, to develop, and to take action is considered an essential aspect of human experience. The counseling is aimed at helping people use all the freedom they have within their own limitations and those of their surroundings. An objective is to avoid or overcome any kind of obstacle to complete development.

25.3.7. RATIONAL-EMOTIVE THERAPY

Rational-emotive therapy (RET) was begun in 1955 by Albert Ellis [1962]. It is widely considered a kind of protest against more traditional methods as well as an effort to do away with some of the complexities of the healing process. At the core of this theory is the sense that irrational and neurotic behaviors acquired in early life continue: the lack of reinforcement does not cause their extinction. Even though the response is not reinforced, individuals in effect reinforce it themselves by continually telling themselves that they are inadequate and worthless. Thus they persist in behaving neurotically as a result of irrational self-judgments.

A number of philosophical elements form the foundation of rational-emotive therapy. If one comprehends these, the theory itself becomes more clearly intelligible and wider implementation in therapy becomes possible. The major concept is that man is rational in a unique way and at the same time irrational in a unique way. Emotional problems are caused by illogical or irrational thinking; they can be resolved if the thinking becomes as rational as possible. Human beings can better their circumstances substantially by means of sound mental processes and self-discipline. It is not necessary for people to remain emotionally disturbed; improvement is possible when a person's inner dialogue becomes rational.

The basic ideas of this theory form an organized pattern. Designated A, B, and C, they express the following: A stands for the individual's behavior, B is the individual's internal verbalization that results from the behavior, and C is the consequence of the act. For instance, a man applies for a job (A); he concludes that he must be incompetent (B), because he does not get the job (C); otherwise why was he not employed?

What is significant is not what happens as a consequence of an act. Rather it is what people tell themselves about the act that creates the problem. When people keep attributing negative qualities to themselves and therefore take on blame, they will keep having emotional problems.

Emotional difficulties are the result of illogical thought processes. The perceptions people have of themselves and the way they see their relationship to a situation cause these disturbances. If people were entirely rational the problems would not occur. But, because emotions and thoughts are so intertwined, they cannot actually be separated and thus are considered as fundamentally the same. The elemental processes of sensation, movement, emotion, and thinking take place together rather than separately. Emotion is a complex operation that begins with perception and appraisal of something. The appraisal results in a tendency to move toward or away from the object according to its appeal.

Irrational thought begins early in life and is promoted partially by a biological tendency toward faulty logic but more strongly by cultural forces. Thought is conducted by means of symbols, the use of which comprises language. Individuals employ this language to tell themselves irrational things about themselves. Continuing negative feelings come about as the result of stupidity, lack of information, or disturbance. They can be corrected by intelligent utilization of information and logic, but the positive thinking must be expressed in words.

Continuing self-verbalizations add to emotional problems. Connected with this is perception of the self and perception of how one relates to a situation. These views are often erroneous and self-deprecatory, and the individual has very negative feelings. Negative ideas and feelings may be conquered if a person is made to articulate positive self-assessments rather than negative ones.

Self-deprecating ideas and feelings may be attacked by a reorganization of perceptions and more logical thinking. Because the problem is exacerbated by false views, valid perceptions should improve the soundness of the thinking. At this point a person can move toward improved adjustment.

Techniques

Those techniques of therapy that seem best suited to altering an individual's thinking are the ones selected. The objective is to enable the person to reason more clearly, realistically, and hopefully. Ellis pinpointed eleven irrational ideas that he maintained promote a detrimental attitude or a neurosis. All of them emphasize the idea that most people do not have realistic or reasonable expectations for themselves or others.

The elements of this theory imply that the therapist uses a comparatively straightforward method—directing, giving advice freely, addressing the problem in an intellectual and very definite way. The techniques are precise; objectivity and reason are important. The client's unreasoning and self-deprecatory verbalizations are identified forcefully and exposed. The therapist shows how these thoughts are producing the problem, pointing out the flaws in the logic of self-verbalizations and instructing the client how to reorganize, question, contradict, and restate thoughts to produce more logical and economical reflections. Instruction is a basic technique, the client being shown how to think and act more effectively.

25.3.8. REALITY THERAPY

Reality therapy originated with William Glasser [1965, 1972], a California psychiatrist who, through work in private practice and as a consultant, became convinced that traditional psychotherapeutic methods were insufficient for modern needs. His theory is to some extent a protest against traditional theories; it represents an effort to evolve more rational methods for helping people to avoid emotional disturbance and to function more satisfactorily in life. His theory stresses the importance of an individual's achieving a certain amount of success. It is thought that if people feel good about themselves and about their interpersonal relationships, they will be able to cope with the majority of problems.

The main elements of the theory form a set of tenets organized to give experience a sense of meaning and purpose. Part of the pattern is the need that all people have to feel that they are worthwhile and able to conduct life and solve problems satisfactorily. It also emphasizes the idea that people must be accountable for themselves. The theory does not include the idea of neurosis as usually defined. People who have problems have behaved in an inappropriate manner; they are not ill.

It is of the utmost importance for people to believe that they are successful and for them actually to achieve some degree of success. Accomplishment depends on a deep sense that one can do something well. A person who feels this way will function effectively, and efforts to shore the person up, which do not work anyway, will not be necessary. The objective of therapy is to launch individuals into demanding and meaningful activities that will give them chances for success. At this point people learn to feel that they are competent and capable of rising to the challenges of society.

The fundamental needs are to be loved and to be able to love others. Loneliness is not a set of circumstances that comes about but is rather the result of personal failure. People avoid loneliness and the difficulties that come with it when they form close bonds with others. These relationships help them gain self-confidence and help decrease the frustration that often causes unhappiness and retreat.

While emotions play a vital role in human experience, it is reason and logic that are necessary for appropriate conduct and success. Emotions can mislead people and make failure likely. In fact, feelings stem from behavior, so behavior must be rectified if unwanted emotions are to be avoided.

Frequently maladjustment stems from people's inability to meet their needs, with the manifestations usually receding when the needs are satisfied. Another cause of inappropriate behavior lies in a sense of inadequacy and incompetence with respect to facing problems. When the two fundamental needs—to love and be loved and to feel self-worth and feel useful to others—are not fulfilled, people feel inadequate. This feeling is overcome when they learn how to fulfill needs.

In order to live successfully, individuals must feel responsible for themselves and for the things that they do. Responsibility entails the capacity to meet one's needs.

25.3.9. GESTALT THERAPY

As developed by Fritz Perls [1973], gestalt therapy established an appropriate vocabulary and a useful conceptual framework. Perls, Goodman, and Hefferline [1951, 1965] formulated the background and organization for gestalt therapy. Emphasizing the application of gestalt psychology, gestalt theories on the structure of perception have served as a foundation for viewing mental disturbance. Psychopathology is considered a disturbance of figure-ground formation, with the figure the focal point of the individual's perceptual attention and the ground forming the background of the perceptual field. What the figure is may change quickly, according to the individual's perception.

Gestalt psychology developed basically as a reaction against other multi-faceted and analytic psychologies. Its principal theme has been that the whole is something very different from the parts in isolation. The entirety of an individual must be considered if the individual is to be understood; and only after the whole is comprehended can the parts have significance.

Gestalt therapy has three tenets: (1) a person structures experience as a whole, integrated organism; (2) individual experience consists of "gestalts" that are configurations of "figures" (what is being attended to) and "grounds" (what is being ignored); and (3) the person must have initiative to choose some gestalts and break up others for the adaptation of personal needs with the environment. Inability to choose or shift gestalts produces personality limitations.

According to gestalt theory, then, ineffective behavior is a sign that two aspects of a psychological process are in opposition. To improve the situation the disharmonious elements must be exposed. After facing these and disclosing one's thoughts, conduct can be improved. Awareness is emphasized as the origin of change; awareness of the self and the current situation moves one toward development. The entirety of a person is interacting creatively with the environment. Counseling is aimed at reorganizing a person's sensory capabilities; this is accomplished through a confrontation with the therapist or with other people who provide incentive for recognizing feelings. The chance for discovery of the self is thus central to this approach. When the individual can change in perspective and awareness, alterations in behavior become possible.

Main Concepts

In gestalt therapy that which exists in the present, current reality, is what is most significant. Treatment is therefore focused on the entire person and the individual's entire situation. From the unity of the organism-environment flows the quality of the individual's relationship to the environment. When an element of the surroundings is inappropriate or discordant, then the attempt is made to modify the environment so that it is more suitable to the individual.

People change for the better only if they are totally, actively involved and if all functioning is brought into play. Fundamental to all behavior is the quality of interaction between the individual and the environment. People operate as totalities if they are completely organized and integrated in themselves.

The individual as a social and cultural being connects with the physical environment in a field of interaction. As a result of positive interaction with others in experiences that have emotional significance, people become capable of altering or abandoning their manifestations of maladjustment or illness. The core of the healing process is in one's relating to others. At times the interaction comes about as a result of games or exercises in which there is interpersonal confrontation. Growth depends upon one's awareness that the field of interaction exists and comes about as a result of the individual's contact with surroundings.

Techniques

While the techniques of therapy are basically the same as those utilized in other approaches, in gestalt theory more confronting, telling, questioning, and instructing are used. The counselor's bearing is one of self-confidence and knowledgeableness, and the client is told abruptly and unhesitatingly what is best. The therapist's task is to reorganize the client's personality to its gestalt or whole; explanation, instruction, persuasion, and analysis are the means. The aim is to get the client to act, and this response is then assessed and a plan devised.

25.3.10. CRISIS INTERVENTION

The theoretical formulations of crisis intervention were developed by Gerald Caplan [1964]. Crisis theory centers on a concept called "homeostatic equilibrium," which means a state of relative psychosocial balance (i.e., a state in which coping and adaptive techniques are operating to handle daily problems). A crisis situation occurs when a person faces an obstacle to important life goals that is insurmountable, at the time, by means of the customary methods of problem-solving. The obstacle becomes emotionally hazardous when it is perceived by the person as an unmanageable threat. It is an internally experienced, acute disturbance resulting from the individual's inability to cope with what are seen as ominous events. The crisis is typically followed by disorganization and confusion, with ineffective attempts at problem solution. The outcome may take several weeks.

Various techniques have been devised to cope with the unique problems of a human crisis. The clinical process in crisis intervention has these immediate goals: to relieve the person's present anxiety, confusion, and feelings of hopelessness; to restore the person's previous level of functioning; to help the person's family and friends to learn what personal actions are possible and what community resources exist; to understand the relationship of the present crisis to present and past problems; to develop new attitudes, behaviors, and coping techniques for this and future crises. (See 28.4.)

25.3.11. EXISTENTIAL ANALYSIS

A number of modern theories have their foundation in the conventional psychoanalytic or behavioristic theories. Existentialism is considered as a kind of third influence in psychology and as a segment of contemporary philosophy [May, 1969]. As such, it has had an important influence on counseling and psychotherapy.

Existentialism has dealt more with the premises underlying therapy than with methodology. Its assumptions about human nature therefore contribute ideas to therapy but they do not deal with techniques. One assumption is that human beings are capable of self-awareness and of sensitivity to the environment. Another is that conduct is meaningful only if viewed in relationship to the result toward which it is aimed.

Existentialism is the result of the formulations of famous twentieth-century theologians and philosophers concerned with human nature.

Theoretical Elements

Existentialism is founded on an effort to understand people as they actually are within their own realities and to perceive and understand

their surroundings as they do. This idea has special meaning in counseling as a process within which the needs of individuals must be understood and people must come to greater self-knowledge. Among the major elements of this philosophy are the idea that man is a meaningful totality whose state of being is to be always engaged in the process of becoming. To comprehend man fully is therefore a consistent objective of existentialism.

According to existentialism, the human being is at the center of existence. People's continual efforts to become express their need to feel significant and to attain status. The environment should adapt to human beings rather than coerce them into conforming with the false expectations of other people. Because man's being is vague and the world is indistinct, people must concern themselves preeminently with their own welfare.

Another tenet is that it is necessary to recognize and accept guilt and anxiety, the latter defined as the experience of the likelihood of imminent nonbeing. As one works to fulfill oneself, one feels anxiety, probably due to the apprehension of failure.

Time is meaningful but not as traditionally understood. Because people are always becoming, they cannot be defined at any given time. The alterations they are undergoing or constructing make them slightly different all the time. People can transcend present time and look at the future; this is a unique capacity that can be utilized. The ability to transcend the present enables one to imagine what one would like to be and what one would like to obtain from future experience.

Freedom is an important concept, since people are viewed as capable of choosing and of acting upon these choices. In existentialism man is frequently considered the creator of culture and not its product. Determinism is not denied, but it is not seen as directly relevant to human life. While individuals operate within the norms of their own culture, they govern or rise above them rather than being controlled by them [Arbuckle, 1965].

Human beings are considered as responsible; the element of responsibility in human nature, as defined by existentialism, is strong.

Chapter 26

Interpersonal Communication

Sharing information is a basic human activity. People exchange information with each other for many purposes and in various ways. Information is shared for personal or social development, protection, pleasure, and other purposes throughout daily life. Meaningful messages are sent with words and signals of all sorts. American Indians used a universal language of hand signals to stand for ideas or things. And a well-developed sign language denoting letters and concepts has been standardized for the deaf.

"Man has developed a host of different systems of communication which render social life possible," observed Cherry [1966]. "Most prominent among all those systems of communication is human speech and language. The development of language reflects back upon thought, for with language, thoughts may become organized and new thoughts may evolve. Systems of ethics and laws have been built up. Man has become self-conscious, responsible, a social creature" [pp. 3–4].

Communication and interviewing skills are essential in any kind of counseling. Expertise— over and beyond a natural lay level of conversation—can be learned. Practical guidelines are given in the two sections of this chapter.

26.1. Communicating

Without communication and understanding between counselor and client, no helping relationship could exist. It is therefore a primary goal of counselors to facilitate communication throughout the rehabilitation process and to overcome the obstacles that impede, distort, or complicate the understanding. By using seven basic skills—listening, leading, reflecting, summarizing, interpreting, informing, and confronting—the counselor enhances the quality and effectiveness of verbal interchange. Sensitivity to clients' nonverbal behavior and to their special communication problems is also essential.

Personal communication skills involve sending and receiving messages that can be clearly interpreted. Different persons, however, attribute different meanings to the same message, according to semanticists. This phenomenon, which is called "perceptual distortion," occurs because any stimulus is interpreted under the influence of a person's past experiences. Expert counseling, therefore, requires not only interviewing skills but also knowledge of the dynamics of the communication process. This section describes certain techniques that have been developed to facilitate the process of sharing information and feelings. (Also see 30.3.)

Brammer [1979], Carkhuff and Berenson [1977], and Egan [1975] have described the counseling techniques that facilitate understanding. These communication skills, described here, are further explained and illustrated in Brammer's book, *The Helping Relationship: Process and Skills*. Further guidelines are described in Chapter 32, Written Communication.

26.1.1. LISTENING

In counseling listening is a very active process. It involves suspending judgment and focusing upon the client in order to hear the content, the feeling, and the reason for the feeling in the client's expression of his or her experience. Listening provides the counselor with the cues needed in order to respond to the client's inner experience [Carkhuff & Berenson, 1977]. Brammer [1979] said that listening skills are demonstrated when the counselor can answer in considerable detail the question, "What is going on in this person right now and in his or her life space?" [p. 69].

Listening is the basic skill upon which paraphrasing, clarifying, and perception-checking are based. To use all these skills successfully, the counselor must want to understand and communicate with the client and to build a relationship of trust and acceptance.

Paraphrasing

The paraphrase is a brief restatement of the client's basic message. It involves responding to the content, feeling, and meaning of the client's expression of his or her experience. The counselor learns to create an interchangeable base of communication so that both counselor and client can be sure of the accuracy of the counselor's response. Counselors use paraphrasing primarily to check on their understanding of a message, secondarily to let the client know that they are trying to understand.

Without introducing any additional ideas, the counselor attempts to express the client's meaning simply and precisely. This requires constant concentration on the speaker's thoughts and feelings. One should enter in during a natural pause and look for a sign from the client that the paraphrase is accurate. As with other listening skills, the paraphrase can become overly stylized. To prevent this the counselor should avoid using repeated responses such as "I hear you saying . . . ."

Successful paraphrasing gives the client a sense of being understood; it may also help elucidate and organize disconnected thoughts. (It is particularly important in talking with brain-injured clients who have a communication disorder.) Finally, it gives the client encouragement to continue talking.

Clarifying

Clarification is used in counseling to bring vague material into sharper focus. When paraphrasing is difficult because the counselor feels confused (for any reason) about the client's basic message, clarifying can help. The counselor may say, "I'm not sure if I'm with you, but . . . ," or can ask the client to restate things, perhaps in more detail. Clarifying should not shade into interpretation of the client's message or criticism of the manner in which it has been presented. The counselor avoids appearing critical by admitting confusion.

Perception-Checking

To test and promote clarity of communication between listener and speaker, the perception-check is used. After hearing a series of statements, the counselor paraphrases what has been said, asks the client whether the restatement is accurate, and asks to be corrected if it is not. The process is one of both giving and receiving feedback in order to elicit what the client really wants to say. The counselor may observe, for instance, that the speaker seems irritated and then ask if this is the case. Perception-checking helps keep the lines of communication clear and gives the client a feeling of being understood.

26.1.2. LEADING

Leading, which is especially appropriate in the early stages of a counseling relationship, helps the client explore and express feelings, respond more easily, and take an active part in the helping process.

Indirect Leading

A method of giving the client responsibility for the direction of an interchange is to use the indirect lead. A deliberately general question such as "What would you like to talk about?" at the beginning of an interview encourages the client to select the subject; a lead like "How do you feel?" can be used at other times to keep the conversation going, but again, along lines of interest to the client. While this kind of opening is occasionally threatening, it more often has an encouraging effect.

Direct Leading

By means of the direct lead the counselor helps the client look at a subject more closely and thus come to sharper awareness of its significance. The client will usually follow specific suggestions to elaborate or illustrate. "Tell me more about your accident" would elicit detail that should enhance the client's perception of the event. While the counselor has a definite purpose in giving the lead, the client has freedom in deciding how to respond.

Focusing

In the earlier stages of counseling especially, the client's conversation is likely to be rather aimless. Sometimes the counselor's indirect leading has encouraged wandering. After the topics that most concern the client have been aired, however, further rambling may become confusing. At this point the counselor uses focusing. This technique pinpoints one topic for further discussion and helps the client concentrate on an important idea or on emotions hidden beneath the surface.

Sensing that the discussion has become too diffused, the counselor asks the client to select a focal point and pursue it further or to isolate and name feelings. Feedback from the client helps establish the importance of various subjects. "Again, the ultimate expected outcome is more meaningful verbalization, and eventually, increased understanding" [Brammer, 1979, p. 77].

Questioning

The form of a question either inhibits or promotes responsiveness. Instead of attempting to obtain information or using questions that can be answered with Yes or No, counselors ask open-ended questions that will bring out the client's emotional reactions. "What were your feelings about your job?" would prompt a fuller answer than "Did you like your job?" The purpose of questions generally, it should always be remembered, is illumination for the client.

26.1.3. REFLECTING

Reflecting expresses the counselor's attempt to recognize a client's feelings, experiences, ideas, and view of the world.

Reflecting Feelings

In reflection of feelings, one expresses differently the feelings another person has verbalized or implied. It serves to concentrate on feelings, clarify them, and help the person acknowledge them. To use the technique successfully counselors must be sensitive to their own feeling states and those of others.

Reflecting is superfluous when the client is expressing obvious emotions. Instead it should be used to identify or call attention to subtler feelings that are not being addressed. The counselor might say, "You feel guilty that your handicap is a burden to your wife." If the reflection is accurate, the client may confirm it and may benefit from the insight. Insight is not always therapeutic, however, and may be dangerous until the disturbed client is able to handle unacceptable emotions.

Reflecting Verbal Content

This is similar to paraphrasing, and it may help the client learn to articulate more easily. The listener repeats in compact form ideas the speaker is having difficulty expressing.

The basic reflecting skills tend to coalesce because how the client says something is as important as the statement itself. While paying careful attention to both, the counselor decides whether reflecting content or reflecting feelings would be more helpful and places emphasis accordingly. The result of skillful reflecting is the client's having a sense of the counselor's understanding and ultimately improved insight into the self and others.

Reflecting Behavioral Cues

Sometimes nonverbal language is more revealing than spoken words. When noticing expressive behavior such as a clenching of fists, changing postures, staring, or flushing, the counselor can reflect the client's total experience by first mentioning the observed behavior and then reflecting feeling.

Common Errors in Reflecting

Reflecting is often marred by stereotyped responses, poor timing, overreaction, and inappropriate language. The listener should avoid relying on one or two phrases such as "You feel . . . ;" this rut in style produces an insincere effect. It is also important to pace reflections so that they neither interrupt the speaker constantly or come so seldom that understanding is diminished.

The counselor may tend to go beyond the client's statement, reflecting deeper feelings than the client is experiencing or willing to admit. Reflecting responses should be in keeping with the intensity of the client's statements. The expression of too much depth of feeling, even if the reflection is quite accurate, may be rejected until the client is ready and often retards the counseling progress. Finally, the counselor's language must be appropriate to the client's cultural experience. Academic terminology would be unfamiliar to an educationally handicapped person and therefore inappropriate. On the other hand, speech should sound natural.

Even if a counselor does make mistakes in reflecting, the client will usually appreciate and respond to the sincere desire to help. And a correcting response from the client can produce elucidation and progress even after an inaccurate reflection.

26.1.4. SUMMARIZING

In summarizing, the counselor brings together disparate ideas and feelings that the counselee has voiced during a session or over a period of time. The summary is also a review of the process that has been going on and an evaluation of what has been accomplished.

From everything that the client has said, the counselor selects the main threads and without adding any new ideas attempts to tie them together. If the client has expressed feelings of anxiety, the counselor might summarize, "As you've talked about your health, your family, and your job you seem to be quite worried about all of them." In the summarizing process the counselor points out what the discussion has produced (e.g., recognition or greater perception

of a problem) and suggests what course it might take next (e.g., examining possible solutions).

Summarizing can serve many purposes, such as starting or ending a session, testing the counselor's understanding, encouraging the client to elaborate, and terminating the counseling. But the most important purpose is giving the client a sense that progress has been made. If the counselor can get the *client* to summarize, this is a good test of understanding.

26.1.5. INTERPRETING

In interpreting, the listener explains the speaker's message. The immediate aim is to cast new light on the speaker's experience; the final goal, to teach people to interpret without help. With interpretation the counselor's own viewpoint comes into play.

The counselor must determine that at a given point another perspective would be useful to the client. The first step in interpreting is to identify the underlying message and paraphrase it. Then the counselor explains, perhaps in accordance with some theoretical framework but certainly in terms appropriate to the client's own level of intellectual sophistication, what it may mean. The interpretation should be offered in a tentative manner ("Do you think maybe . . ."), and the counselor should try to get the client's reaction. If the new perspective is valid, the client's understanding should be deepened. The goal of all interpretive effort in counseling is self-interpretation.

26.1.6. INFORMING

Sometimes simply sharing information is more useful than anything else the counselor can do. However, advice-giving, a special kind of informing common in counseling, is quite controversial.

It is important to distinguish between providing factual information and the advising done by rehabilitation counselors who have information that their clients need in order to make wise decisions. This expertise about disability, occupations, testing, training, getting employment, and so forth is the counselor's primary attraction for the rehabilitation client. One must be careful to apprise the client of the probable accuracy of imparted data (e.g., the prediction of success in a desired training course). This means the effective rehabilitation counselor must have, and be able to share, a broad storehouse of practical information and sources of information.

Counselors sometimes go beyond the informing function and get into advice-giving merely because their clients expect it of them. But the technique has many limitations and should be used, even when appropriate, with great caution. Even those who do not condemn advice-giving in counseling have drawn attention to several problems connected with its use. The major limitation is that clients asking for advice do not usually follow it. Frequently they do not really want suggestions but are merely expressing feelings of dependency. Here the counselor's job is to discern the difference and address the feelings first. Critics have also maintained that giving advice impedes the client's progress toward independence. Yet another drawback is that the advice may be wrong.

With these potential pitfalls in mind, suggestions may usefully be offered when based on accurate information about alternative courses of action. In specific situations such as hospitalization, advice may help clients make immediate, practical choices. While the counselor should not advise a client on a major personal decision, suggestions can be offered in a tentative, nondirective way that does not shift the responsibility for self-determination.

26.1.7. CONFRONTING

Confronting, Brammer [1979] believed, is a combination of skills that may "threaten or thrill, depending on the timing and the readiness of the helpee to be confronted with feedback honestly offered" [p. 83]. It involves informing clients of a discrepancy between things that they have been saying about themselves and things that they have been doing [Gazda, Asbury, Balzer, Childers, & Walters, 1977].

Recognizing Feeling

To respond to a client's feelings one must first be sensitive to one's own inner experience. Tenseness, sweating hands, jerking muscles, and fluttering eyelids reveal the counselor's own anxiety, guilt, anger, pleasure, or pain. These client feelings during a counseling session should be recognized and sometimes explored.

Describing and Sharing Feeling

The expression of feelings can be of great value; it may relieve pent-up tension (i.e., be an emotional catharsis). This "ventilation," however,

must be cautiously provoked and only by a qualified counselor.

Self-disclosure of information about the counselor, if it is appropriate or relevant to the client's problem, can lead to greater closeness between counselors and clients. If the counselor has had a concern similar to that of the client and has found a solution to the problem, this can be reassuring to the client. Furthermore, the client's solution may even be similar to the one that was used by the counselor. The success of Alcoholics Anonymous and other self-help groups is related to this dimension of self-disclosure [Gazda, et al., 1977].

Expression of the counselor's own feelings is sometimes useful, mainly as a model. Clients frequently fail to understand the value of expressing feelings, and there is also a tendency to avoid felt expression through rationalization. But, describing feelings brings relief and satisfaction, and the counselor by example can help the client to do this. Sharing feelings with the client also helps build trust in the relationship.

The revelation of feelings does have limitations, however. While occasionally the articulation of felt experience is a goal in itself, it is more often only a step in the process of problem-solving. Also, clients may occasionally reveal more feeling than they are able to handle; consequently, one should be cautious about encouraging expression of deep feeling in a client known to have severe emotional problems or difficulty in handling these problems. Strong resistance in the client, any question as to the counselor's own qualifications to help disturbed people, and the availability or nonavailability of support services are some of the other factors that should be taken into account before the technique is used.

Feedback and Opinion

There are times when the counselor's reactions and opinions can help the client achieve clearer self-knowledge: reactions from others help to establish our identity. A number of things govern the use of feedback in counseling: (1) the client must be ready for it; (2) the counselor should give opinions rather than hand down judgments; (3) feedback is helpful only if it concerns something the client is capable of changing; (4) only a small amount of feedback should be given at one time; and (5) the response should be prompt and relevant to current behavior.

It should be clear that an individual is ready for feedback. In the absence of a direct request the counselor asks if the client would like comments. Describing the client's behavior before expressing an opinion keeps responsibility for the opinion on the counselor, where it belongs, since these are personal reactions for the client to take or leave. Distinguishing between an individual's behavior and the individual as a person keeps opinions from entering the realm of judgment. "The way you keep repeating yourself is beginning to irritate me" focuses on the client's manner, not basic characteristics. It also points to something within the individual's power to change.

It is well to avoid giving too much feedback at one time, since, in quantity, it does not have a chance to sink in. It is also important to focus on the present rather than dredging up material from past discussions. Finally, the counselor asks whether the feedback was helpful.

Repeating

Repeating something has the effect of self-confrontation when something the client says appears to carry special emotional significance. Noting this, the counselor asks the client to keep repeating the statement in simple form. The flow of conversation stops suddenly and the emotion surfaces, to be discussed or allowed to well up further. Brammer suggested that the value of this kind of confronting is that the counselor can tap feelings obscured behind long sentences and constant topic changes.

The counselor's task is to decide when repeating will help the client release important feelings. Gestures that seem to signal strong emotions can also be repeated. Time should be allowed for analysis of the feelings that emerge from the process of repeating.

Associating

Associating also facilitates the "loosening" of feelings. The counselor urges the client to leave the realm of rational, structured discourse and talk about anything, however vague or meaningless it may seem. Or one selects what appears to be an emotionally significant word and asks the individual to say all the other words that come to mind in connection with it. Associating can result in further exploration of feelings and then explanations.

26.1.8. NONVERBAL COMMUNICATION

If the counselor is sensitive to the nonverbal language of clients, the entire communication process will be much more effective. A speaker's voice, body position, and gestures transmit messages that may alter the meaning of what is said. Brown and Parks [1972], whose ideas are related here, stated that this is especially important in rehabilitation counseling, ". . . since nonverbal behavior is often the primary mode of communication for some groups such as the mentally retarded, speech handicapped, and certain other clients whose handicaps have caused unsatisfactory experiences with people" [p. 176].

Eye Contact

One of the most important forms of nonverbal communication is eye contact. It is used to obtain social feedback, to indicate receptiveness to feedback, to hide feelings (by means of avoiding eye contact), and to seek recognition. While eye contact from a client is usually a positive sign, the reverse is not always true. Lack of eye contact may signal the client's negative self-image rather than poor communication. It is necessary to observe this behavior as an indication of the client's responses during a discussion, but also to recognize that it is only one of a number of expressive activities.

Gestures

Smiles, head nods, gesticulations, self-manipulation, and other gestures convey information about a client's emotional states; this information should be absorbed and utilized. Restricted hand movements and exaggerated trunk and leg movements, for example, may indicate stress. Gestural behavior has special significance for the rehabilitation counselor, who must consider the client's handicap and its effect upon body language.

Distance

Distance is the space that separates two speakers. Cultural norms dictate acceptable distances, but generally the closer the participants are, the more positive their communication. Eye contact and apparent listening convey attention and psychological closeness. There should be no physical barrier such as a desk between the counselor and client.

Body relaxation, position of the torso, and changes in distance may also have psychological significance. The counselor conveys a positive attitude by leaning forward to decrease distance. Again, in interpreting a rehabilitation client's use of space, one should consider that the individual's physical characteristics or handicap may influence distance.

Interpretation

To interpret the totality of a client's behavior, the counselor must be aware and take into consideration that certain nonverbal behavior in a disabled person may be the result of medication, reaction to the disability, and the like. Specific nonverbal behaviors, especially in combination, may indicate a positive or negative "counseling climate." Such behaviors as a high eye blink rate, little eye contact, movements of the lower body, back body lean, and negative head nods may be signs of a negative climate, while the opposite behaviors indicate a positive atmosphere. When observing the negative indicators, the counselor should attempt to determine the source of what the client appears to consider a threat.

Observation

Self-training in observation is useful to all human service workers. Simple exercises to develop the powers of observation can be practiced. One such exercise would be to look at a picture, preferably one with several human characters in action, for several moments. The observer then looks away and reconstructs the scene—what the people were doing, how they were dressed, how old they appeared to be, and what their facial expressions were like. Someone doing this exercise over and over with new photographs, television scenes, and real-life street views will find the technique becoming a habit.

Rehabilitationists must be perceptive in order to understand their clients. Perception, of course, is based not only on sensory input (e.g., seeing and hearing) but also on knowledge of human behavior. It is not enough to be interested in people; rather one must be interested in persons. Someone concentrating on personal needs is neglecting the client.

To be an accomplished observer it is necessary to: (1) have a true interest in other individuals, (2) have a knowledge of human behavior, (3) have developed techniques of observation and recall, and (4) be able to integrate sensory input with prior knowledge for meaningful implications.

Continuing uses and satisfactions result from being a trained observer. For example, a client has a violent epileptic seizure; the information that comes from a careful observer can be very helpful to the physician (e.g., the side on which seizure symptoms appeared first). How can anyone objectively report the turmoil of a grand mal convulsion? A simple device is to mentally describe (in words) the event as it happens, as if reporting it at the moment, and then to record these verbatim descriptions soon afterward.

26.1.9. COMMUNICATION LIMITATION

The rehabilitation counselor must be aware of the ways in which a disability may limit the function of communication. Individuals with hearing and speech impairments are most likely to have difficulty expressing themselves. Certain forms of cancer as well as neurological disabilities such as cerebral palsy may result in a speech defect. Clients who have suffered a stroke or brain injury often have a communication problem. Of course, ethnic and cultural backgrounds are also likely to affect a client's capacities to communicate.

It is the counselor's obligation to discover each client's most effective channel of communication (verbal, auditory, written, and so on), to motivate the client to self-expression, and to gear the interchange to the client's own level. As Sheets [1973] pointed out:

Language is a tool whose need lies dormant until you have something of value to communicate to the handicapped individual and he has something to say to you. This concept is of particular importance to the severely involved person who speaks only at the expense of great physical effort. If there is nothing to say which will justify the effort, he will likely remain quiet. Part of your responsibility will be to make the task of self-expression a satisfying and rewarding process [p. 4].

The counselor's delivery should fit the client's needs. A slow, relaxed pace may be the most appropriate. The professional can formulate questions so that they can be answered simply. In general, after assessing the "language deficit" in a client, one can facilitate communication by adapting vocabulary and sentence structure, as well as the pace of the dialogue, to the client's capabilities (see 5.2).

Because the counselor serves as a model it is well to exhibit personable behavior and animated speech. The "spark" in the counselor's voice not only assures interest and attention but may also inspire vigor in a client who has lost spirit.

26.2. Interviewing

An interview is a conversation that has a definite purpose besides satisfaction in the discussion itself. The interviewer and interviewee communicate back and forth in a variety of ways, using facial expressions and voice tones, gestures, postures, and so on. The words take on varying meanings when spoken with different inflections and used in different contexts. All these elements together—the words themselves and the various communicative behaviors—compose the interview, the conversation in which meanings are purposefully exchanged. Many of the ideas related here are from *Clinical Interviewing and Counseling: Principles and Techniques* by Edinburg, Zinberg and Kelman [1975], and *How to Interview* by Bingham and Moore [1959] or were presented by Miller and Obermann [1968] in their *Inservice Training Program* series. One of the best books on the subject is *Interviewing: Its Principles and Methods* by A. Garrett [1972].

The ability to interview effectively stems from no single trait but rather incorporates a number of attitudes, skills, and techniques. An interviewer becomes adept only after much study and practice. Learning to interview should be supervised for the protection of the client because in the learning process the student must experiment and make mistakes. It is so with the trained professional, too, for interviewing is not a science but an art.

The practitioner can always use individual initiative, new ideas, and fresh combinations of old methods. Just as the accomplished interviewer cannot be constrained by a set of rules, there is no prescription that can guarantee that a beginner's work will be successful. But there are a number of accepted general guidelines that may help any interviewer avoid errors, learn how to work efficiently, and establish productive relationships with interviewees. Successful interviewers must learn and coordinate many different skills in order to establish carefully the goals of a given interview, organize it intelli-

gently, and execute each of the various steps effectively.

Sharing information with clients is a basic function of all rehabilitationists. Therefore, the focus here is on the counseling interview.

26.2.1. PREPARATION

Preparation begins even before the interview takes place. As with any plan, it is necessary to have knowledge of pertinent facts, a set of objectives, a strategy, and arrangements.

Deciding What Is to Be Accomplished

Usually the client will come to the interview with definite expectations and goals in mind. However, the interviewer should also have specific objectives and a clear sense of what should be accomplished. It is probably a good idea, especially for inexperienced interviewers, to write out a list of objectives, possible problems, and appropriate modifications.

Knowing the Interviewee

It is advisable to learn as much as possible about the client before the interview. Information about applicants can be found in school and company records, test profiles, social service reports, and other sources. Previous files should be reviewed for reopened cases. Even before application the referring agency will provide information. Although different kinds of information will prove useful in different cases, it is well to be informed as fully as possible in advance.

Making Appointments

Setting up the appointment in advance will save time and ensure the client's convenience.

Providing for Privacy

Privacy is of critical importance for a productive interchange. A good working relationship between two people is complicated when others are involved. If the discussion will deal with subjects that are highly personal or may be embarrassing, it is necessary to make sure that other people are not present or within earshot. Confidentiality is an ethical issue that has practical consequences for interviewing success; for example, when privacy is lacking, the interviewee may feel self-conscious and withhold information.

Time

Interview sessions are generally planned to begin and end at predetermined times. The duration of a session varies according to its purpose and other considerations (e.g., client fatigue, the counselor's work schedule). A counseling period is customarily limited to an hour; in state rehabilitation, however, the contact time is often only a matter of minutes. Whatever the setting, the full day of any counselor should not be devoted to relationship counseling.

Practicing Taking the Interviewee's Point of View

As preparation for all interviews, the worker should, in imagination, take the client's place: try to think, react, and feel as the client might during the session The capacity to see things as others see them and enter into the other person's feelings—empathy—is essential in a skilled interviewer. It is an ability that to some degree can be acquired, or at least cultivated.

Knowing One's Own Personality

Every individual is committed to certain opinions, values, and attitudes, to an extent unrealized by most people. Everyone has conscious or unconscious prejudices, maintains some stereotypical ideas, and makes certain prejudgments about individuals and groups. Probably the truly open mind, wholly unclouded by preconceptions and wholly receptive to new ideas, does not exist. But people can become aware of their preconceptions and can reduce or eliminate irrational modes of thought.

26.2.2. INITIAL INTERVIEW

In many respects the first interview is the most difficult. From the very beginning, sincerity, acceptance, and understanding must be demonstrated to the client. Since it is desirable to become familiar as quickly as possible with this person's special ways of communicating, sensitive listening is especially important.

The initial interview serves as the major source of contact between client and agency. The individual becomes acquainted with the agency—its ways of operating and its purposes—and learns what services might be helpful.

The first interview is all the more crucial when it is the only one, as is sometimes the case. An example is an applicant who is ineligible but should be referred to another agency for needed services. When, on the other hand, the initial session is to be followed by one or more other interviews, it serves to set the tone and pattern for the whole interaction. In any case, it is certainly important that the first interview be a productive one.

Establishing Rapport

The first task in the initial meeting is to establish rapport: to create an atmosphere in which the professional and client can work together harmoniously. If established at the beginning, such a climate will usually prevail during subsequent sessions.

Acceptance, very important throughout interviewing, should be demonstrated to the client as soon as possible. Communicating this attitude may take a few minutes or a number of hours, but it is fundamental to effective counseling. Acceptance can be expressed early in the initial interview through the creation of a hospitable atmosphere—arriving on time, giving warmth to the situation, starting the conversation, and being attentive.

Clients will respond to the way they are treated as they come through the door. Personal introductions should be arranged for when possible. Whoever first sees the client, perhaps a receptionist, should have a friendly greeting and preferably introduce the person by name to the interviewer. Being on time is important; frequently, having to wait gives a person the feeling that no one cares. Another simple way of expressing acceptance is through the appearance of the office—it should not be austere or forbidding. Small gestures such as showing a person where the coatrack is and offering to get coffee contribute to an atmosphere of hospitality. Finally, the interviewer should find a relevant topic of conversation to acclimate the client to the unfamiliar situation. This involves picking up on clues to what the person is interested in.

Once a helper-client relationship has been established, it is usually quite difficult to change.

Therefore, whatever relationship is formed in the very beginning will probably continue as the model of interaction throughout the entire process. Unpleasant topics as well as agreeable ones may emerge, and the client who feels relaxed and accepted during counseling is able to cope better with the problems that must be solved in the course of achieving adjustment.

Gathering Information

During the initial interview it is necessary to obtain information about the client. This is usually required by the agency for its records, but the information also serves as a starting point for the client's rehabilitation planning. Various types of information may need to be obtained during the first interview, depending on the agency or work setting.

Some agencies—particularly those with a social work orientation—have an intake worker take applications and do the preliminary work-up of applicants. The person is then assigned to a caseworker. This has several advantages, including the opportunity to selectively assign the client to the professional most competent in the area of the presenting problems and other circumstances (sec. 3.4). In many rehabilitation agencies case loads are fixed according to geographic territory or other arbitrary assignment procedure; in such agencies counselors usually see their clients from the outset, at the time of referral.

Certain cautions should be observed when the rehabilitation counselor is charged with collecting information. If the attempt has been made in the beginning of the interview to establish rapport and lay the foundation for a working relationship, a definite change in style will be necessary as the business of data-gathering comes up. It would be appropriate to explain that the interview up to this point has probably typified future discussions but that before it continues, agency requirements should be gotten out of the way. Asking whether the client is willing to shift into data-gathering for agency records is probably a good idea.

Information-gathering can sometimes be streamlined by exercising forethought during the first phase of the interview. Required information may come to light as rapport is being established, and noting it will save a question later. Generally, creating a sense of rapport and gathering mandatory information, two primary

functions of the first interview, can be ordered and combined as appropriate to the situation.

There are a number of ways, Miller and Obermann [1968] mentioned, in which the interviewer can go about acquiring information from the client. Many think the straightforward approach is as economical and effective as any, but a less direct method can also be used. If it is necessary to find out how long the client has been disabled, asking just that would tend to elicit the information quickly. On the other hand, the same information would probably come out after a leading comment like, "I know you've found it somewhat difficult to adjust to living in a wheelchair." (See 24.2.)

Outcomes of the Initial Interview

When the initial interview has been successful, the client leaves with a sense of satisfaction. This stems from feeling that there has been an opportunity for self-expression and that together the client and the counselor will do everything possible to solve the problems that have been mentioned. Rapport has been established; the individual is beginning to feel free to talk about personal concerns and also to express negative feelings such as hostility, fear, or inadequacy, without worrying about the other person's reaction.

Clients often ask for opinions during the initial interview, and when they do, it should be explained that it is not the counselor's function to pass judgment. Clients must understand that it is *their* job to examine their situation so that they can make informed decisions about their lives.

Because counseling is a learning experience for the client, it is important to be aware of the probability that early in the interview the client will begin to "learn" what responses are expected. Miller and Obermann suggested that the initial interview should be structured so that techniques that work at this point will be equally useful as the counseling continues.

26.2.3. ENVIRONMENT

When it is feasible, interviews should be conducted in a proper office setting. In rehabilitation counseling, however, this is often not convenient or even possible. Clients sometimes must be interviewed in their home, in a hospital bed, or when they are working. There may be noise, distractions, and intrusions. But even outside the office the counselor still strives to obtain a satisfactory atmosphere, as described below.

Seating Arrangements

It is a good idea to make sure there is adequate seating and to arrange the chairs in the office before the client enters. While some interviewers feel comfortable at a desk, others are most at ease in a less formal situation; it is up to the individual to make this choice. The desk can represent a barrier; it can also be used to create a sense of distance when appropriate. It has been felt that sitting behind a desk is a way of maintaining distance and a professional manner, but in fact this is not necessarily true. Today many counselors arrange their office furniture in a casual manner, with the desk out of the way. A compromise is to place the visitor's chair beside the desk. If the interview is skillfully conducted, any seating arrangement will be satisfactory, but clients tend to feel that there is interest and concern when the office space is thoughtfully organized and the chairs are comfortable. Edinburg, Zinberg, and Kelman [1975] discussed this and other aspects of the interviewing atmosphere as well as further interview considerations: technical elements, unpredictable situations, concluding the interview, and termination.

Entering the Office

Usually clients will select a chair upon entering the office, but some hesitate to do so and ask for direction. An answer such as "Wherever you wish" allows the client free choice and also indicates right away that the counselor's authority does not extend to everything. In contrast, selecting a seat for the client may suggest that the counselor's function is to tell the client what to do. Once in a while, extreme anxiety really prevents an individual from making this choice. Then the only option is to point out a chair.

The counselor may show the client where coats and hats can be put, but occasionally people will strongly prefer to keep their coats on. After the initial suggestion the choice should be up to the individual. But it should be recognized that someone who wants to sit bundled up in a coat is probably anxious and apprehensive at the thought of any kind of self-exposure.

Appearance of the Counselor

The counseling relationship may be affected by the worker's personal appearance. A client may question the maturity and thus the professional competence of a young counselor whose dress is extreme. A flashy or provocative appearance might focus attention on the person as an individual, interfering with the counseling objective of concentration on the client.

To some extent fashion dictates what clothing and hair styles are acceptable, but some people mistrust individuals with a nontraditional appearance and might be unable to relate to someone who carries any style to an extreme. Sometimes it is necessary to make a compromise between personal taste and the conventions of the work setting.

Addressing the Client

Traditionally, any client in late adolescence or older has been addressed as Ms. Jones or Mr. Smith. A notable exception is often found in medical facilities in which even older patients are often called by their given names by the staff. The formal address underlines the professional nature of the counselor-client relationship. It also points up the fact that the counselor thinks of the client as an adult and expects adult behavior.

Sometimes people ask to be called by their first names. When this happens, the reasonableness of the request should be acknowledged. There are several ways in which it can be handled. It is possible to choose to go along with the client's wishes, to discuss the subject further, or to decide (and explain) that the use of last names seems preferable. Any decision, however, may be viewed as tentative; the subject can be discussed later and another agreement arrived at if appropriate.

26.2.4. TECHNICAL CONSIDERATIONS

Every interview is different, which makes interviewing interesting. But the trained interviewer is prepared for unexpected events. These technical considerations are often neglected in formal counseling instruction; experience, however, helps the counselor to cope smoothly with all situations.

Personal Information

Generally the disclosure of personal information should be avoided even though clients frequently ask personal questions. It is important to find out what the client who asks such a question really wants to know. Sometimes mere curiosity is the motive. In other instances interviewees are trying to get closer to the counselor, or to perceive the counselor as an individual, or to change the subject.

Usually the client who asks "Are you in school?" or "Are you a psychologist?" is concerned about qualifications. Such a question may express the fear that the counselor will not be able to provide sufficient help, and one should try to get at this fear by asking what the client is concerned about. Immediately answering the question instead might suggest a lack of forcefulness. But even though it is important to guard against revealing personal information too readily, the general principle of withholding it is not to be viewed as an ironclad rule. In the event that it appears reasonable to answer a personal question, the response should be brief and pointed. Then the counselor should steer the conversation with a sentence like, "Let's go on talking about you." This will return the focus to the client, where it belongs.

Sometimes clients want to know if the counselor has personal knowledge of their problems. There are ways in which it can be explained to clients that one can understand someone else's situation without having experienced it. Analogies from medicine can be used: the ability to deliver children or to do surgery does not come from having a baby or undergoing the operation. Likewise, the clinician's expertise in understanding a problem does not come from experiencing it. It is important for the client to see that intellectual understanding, not personal knowledge, is the crucial ingredient.

Telephone Calls during the Interview

It is common to get telephone calls during the day from rehabilitation clients, sometimes because it has been suggested that those in need of extra support call between visits. When a client calls during an interview, the best response is to listen carefully in order to decide whether there is enough urgency to warrant continued interruption. If not, another call can be arranged. Of course, in an emergency everything else is dropped (see 28.4).

In general, it is best to try to avoid receiving telephone calls during counseling appointments. They are a distraction and may give the client in the office a sense of being slighted.

Emergency Phone Calls

The greatest difficulty in an "emergency" is deciding whether it is a true emergency or not. On receiving an emergency call from a client, it is necessary to try to determine whether the individual is actually in a state of crisis or is merely responding, because of extreme anxiety or agitation, as though the situation were an emergency. The decision must be made with the caller whether or not circumstances justify such an extreme reaction. Usually if the client explains the problem in detail, the degree of its seriousness becomes sufficiently clear. Of course, if both parties conclude that the situation is a true crisis, immediate action must be taken.

It is best if the client handles the situation even if some guidance is necessary. Occasionally it becomes evident that the individual is incapable of dealing with the problem or is bent on self-destruction (see 28.6.1). Then intervention is necessary.

Lateness

When a client is habitually late, it is important to find out why. There may be a practical reason, in which case a better appointment time can be arranged; it may be, however, that the lateness is a way in which the client is dealing with a continuing emotional conflict. Asking about the reason for lateness encourages the individual to become aware of and scrutinize possible causes, such as feelings of reluctance or opposition (see 28.2). Discussion will reveal whether the client is late for everything or just to counseling sessions. "Chronic" lateness is an indication of how a person relates to other people, and this subject should not be explored too soon. It is not a good idea to suggest possible explanations such as the client's wish to antagonize people or a deeper desire to harm others by making them wait. This kind of exploration is appropriate only when the client sees that the lateness may have a meaning. Counseling is most effective when geared to the client's capacity for conscious awareness. Frequently someone who is habitually late is not aware of the pressures that account for this tendency.

One does not try to squeeze an explanation out of such an individual. If the person is late only to counseling appointments, discussion can begin with mention of the client's feelings about counseling. It can be suggested that the individual try to notice what feelings are associated with coming to the sessions; this will help indicate what is really going on. After it has been revealed, either directly or indirectly, that the client is apprehensive about counseling or perhaps feels hostile toward the counselor, further elucidation can take place.

If the counselor is late for an appointment, the client may feel slighted or rejected. After apologizing it is important to make every effort to be on time in the future.

Cancelled Appointments

Occasionally a counselor has to change an appointment because of illness or a schedule conflict. When this happens it is important that the client not feel uncertain either about why the appointment is being cancelled or about when another one will be scheduled. Because ambiguity is inherent in the counseling situation, it is always a good idea to explain when purely practical considerations affect it. It is appropriate to tell the client generally why the change is necessary but not helpful to explain the situation in great detail. Another definite appointment time should be established instead of making a vague promise to get in touch. To set up another appointment as close as possible to the original will reflect continued interest in the client.

Clarification is also a good idea when the client cancels an appointment; one should find out whether the change is necessary or whether the client is experiencing some emotional conflict. Avoidance behavior is not unusual at any stage of the rehabilitation process, but it is usually better to get this information indirectly than to ask outright. When the reason for the cancellation seems fairly clear, the subject can be brought up at an appropriate point.

Extra Appointments

It may be helpful to suggest an extra appointment when a client seems especially disturbed during an interview or appears to be going through a period of crisis generally. Such a suggestion demonstrates interest in the individual.

Motivation should be looked into when the client asks for an extra session. It may be that the additional time is really needed, but it is also possible that the individual is testing the counselor's concern or permissiveness. Whether choosing to make the extra appointment or not, whether for clear reasons or not, it is important to be prepared to explain the decision to the client.

Physical Contact

The client may offer to shake hands when entering the office, and the interviewer responds. Usually this does not happen past the first interview.

Sometimes a client will want to touch or hold hands during an interview in order to get a feeling of closeness or achieve unrealistic ends. The counselor should not initiate physical contact; hugging or otherwise touching an individual may seem threatening or sexually provocative (see 31.3.6). The very rare exception is when a client is violent and in danger of self-injury, in which case physical restraint must be used.

Note-taking

The basic rule on the subject of note-taking is that the object of concentration should be the client rather than the notebook. While inexperienced interviewers tend to wonder how they will remember what has been said, they usually find that when they give their full attention to the client this is not at all difficult. There is no need to remember details like dates and addresses; these can be noted in the records for reference purposes. The interviewer pays close attention to the speaker; if the client asks why few notes are being taken, it is explained that such a procedure would distract attention from the client's statements, responses, and feelings. It should be frankly stated that after the meeting some details will be forgotten but that the basic outlines of the client's thoughts and problems will remain clear.

In order to focus on the client, then, the counselor should minimize note-taking. It is helpful, however, to devote a few minutes immediately after each interview to summarizing it. To write down the principal topics of discussion is a fundamental part of the counselor's work (see Chapter 32, Written Communication).

Tape Recording

A tape is a much fuller record of an interview than any written account, as Benjamin [1969] pointed out in his discussion of the subject. A tape preserves completely what has been said, and in the case of a videotape, also what has been seen. The principal uses of taped interviews are for student training or research. There is also no better device for showing counselors objectively what they are doing and how they are doing it. The fact that an interview is being taped should not be concealed. Saying something like "I am recording this interview to learn from it afterward and it will be kept strictly confidential" is usually satisfactory to the client. If the individual does object to the taping, these feelings should be respected.

Counselors at all levels of professional development can benefit from listening to tapes of their interviews. They can often acquire deeper appreciation of the seriousness of the discussion, clarify its purpose, and obtain significant insights. Tapes can promote learning on the part of clients as well (see 35.4.3).

Recordkeeping

It is generally understood that agencies must have records containing identifying data and general summary material (see 32.1). Usually recordkeeping is taken for granted and clients seldom bring it up, but occasionally they do ask to look at their records, in which case it is appropriate to explain that this is disapproved by the agency. Other clients, although they do not ask to see the record, want to know what it says. When a particular client is unusually preoccupied with the records, discussing this concern may reveal the extent of the individual's apprehension or mistrust. Possibly the concern is related to some legal issue such as divorce, guardianship, arrest, or commitment; if legal considerations are involved, it is important that the record be objective and nonjudgmental. If agency records may have any bearing on matters of such complexity, agency policy is a guide and supervisors should be consulted.

Since the primary purpose of agency records has to do with accountability to clients, the client's interest should be used as a guideline in determining what to put into the record. Interview notes that are put in the official record should differentiate fact from interpretation and explicitly label the counselor's opinion as such. Notes kept for personal use only are locked up or destroyed when they have served their purpose.

Agency policies about confidentiality are strict; clients can be told this. Even a client who wants the record sent to requesting agents must sign a written consent form. The individual and the counselor talk about what should be included. When records are subpoenaed, however, the administrative officials of the agency or institution handle the matter. (See 2.2.2.)

Invitations

It is not unusual to get invited to special occasions in clients' lives: weddings, bar mitzvahs, graduations, and the like. It is up to the counselor to decide, as Edinburg, Zinberg, and Kelman [1975] said, whether to accept such invitations. The relationship with the client and the goals of counseling should be considered. Also, the professional and the client should talk about what accepting the invitation would mean and how the counselor would be introduced to friends and relatives present, since the professional would tell the truth if questioned. It would be necessary for the client to realize and assent to the idea that the counselor's presence would probably lead to revelation of personal information. For this and many other reasons, one should think carefully before accepting this kind of invitation. New clients rarely extend social invitations; when they do, it is easy to refuse. Invitations more typically present difficulties after the relationship has developed over an extended period of time.

Very seldom does a client suggest to the rehabilitation counselor that they do something together such as have a drink or dinner or go to a movie, unless the individual is trying to personalize the relationship, perhaps on a romantic or sexual level. One can reject this kind of invitation most easily by just stating that it is not possible to accept. If the client keeps on making these overtures, the question must be raised as to whether the counselor's behavior is provocative in any way. When experienced professionals encounter this kind of situation with a client, they ask the individual casually what is going on. Questioning the client about the behavior may lead to a better understanding of what the purpose of the counselor-client relationship should be.

Gifts

People give gifts to their counselors for a number of reasons, and it is important to understand what the reason is before deciding in a given case whether or not to accept a gift. When the client is motivated by the hope of making the relationship more personal, it is not a good idea to accept. In refusing the gift, one can go into this explanation or simply cite agency policy on personal gifts. A client who is especially insistent can be referred to a supervisor.

It is not usual for counselors to give gifts to

their adult clients, although those who work with children frequently send birthday cards or give birthday presents. Someone who has worked with an individual for a long time may mark a special occasion such as graduation from college with a relatively impersonal gift like a book, however. Cards or notes are appropriate for special occasions like weddings, the birth of a child, and so on.

26.2.5. CONTINGENCIES

The course and circumstances of every interview are usually planned. There are instances, however, of unpredictable events or situations. The counselor needs to know how to cope with unanticipated problems.

Crying

It is not unusual for clients to cry during an interview in which strong emotions are being aroused. They will sometimes apologize, feeling either embarrassed or afraid that crying shows they are weak. The counselor chooses whether to say nothing or make a comment. It may be appropriate to ask why the client feels bad about crying or what it is that the client feels so disturbed about. If the individual has been talking about an unhappy experience such as a loss, crying is very natural, and this can be pointed out. But frequently the person will not know clearly what the reasons for crying are. It can be brought about by various emotions: anger, fear, and anxiety, as well as sorrow.

Once in a while a client's crying will get out of hand; the aim then is to help the client get back in control by stopping the conversation. Comments like "Try to pull yourself together" are not helpful; instead the individual should be made aware of what is causing the crying by comments like "You seem so disturbed about your illness" or "You seem to be afraid you will never be able to work again." Conscious or unconscious problems have led to the loss of control; the point is to replace the emotional turmoil with more rational consideration. Sometimes someone "lost" in a disturbed world can be brought back to actuality by a question like "Are you feeling that this is happening now?" If the reasons for the disturbance seem unconscious, the individual can be helped to identify them through questioning by the counselor; if the crying continues, possible explanations can be suggested. It is certainly appropriate to offer

a box of tissue handkerchiefs to wipe the tears and ease the tension.

The counselor may at times be very deeply affected by a client's emotions, and a beginning interviewer in such a situation may lose self-control. If the counselor cries, however, the therapeutic relationship is jeopardized. Such a response would mean that identification with the client had gone too far and neutrality of the relationship had been upset. It would also inhibit free expression on the part of the client in the future, since the individual would probably hesitate to upset the listener. Empathy is very important, but it should be critical—as if one were outside looking into the dual counselor-client relation. The counselor who becomes too involved through emotional sympathy should discuss the situation with a supervisor. (See 25.1.3.)

Client Extending the Period

Sometimes clients attempt to prolong a session by starting on a lengthy, intricate story as the interview is supposed to come to a close. Usually the motivation is either anxiety about the interview ending or unrealistic expectations about its results. It is best, for the client, not to allow the interview to run over. If the individual's problem is anxiety about the session coming to an end, an extension would only postpone facing the problem and, in actuality, prolong the anxiety itself, since obviously the interview must end sometime. If on the other hand the client is motivated by excessive expectations, continuing the interview would reinforce the client's hope that the counselor has a kind of magical power to solve problems. When the solutions do not materialize, though, the client feels let down and disenchanted. The client should not be interrupted crudely, but it must be recognized that ending the interview at the appointed time is in the client's best interest. The subject of ending sessions can itself be incorporated into the counseling process.

When the client does not respond to the observation that it is time to leave, the problem can be brought up. Asking whether the individual feels reluctant to leave, suggesting that they talk about this at the next session, and stating that it is important to understand the problem, will probably help the client. To say these things will place the issue into its proper framework, the therapeutic process, and minimize its significance as a point of contention. This approach will also provide the client with a chance to leave with dignity. If an even more decisive measure seems necessary, the counselor can walk to the door. Only rarely and when a situation is especially critical, should one plan—with the client's agreement—to continue the session overtime.

Client Unable to Sit Through the Session

Sometimes people are so nervous or apprehensive during a counseling session that they cannot sit still. They walk around the room, leave to get a drink of water or go to the bathroom, and so on. While it would probably be better for such people to have a seat and talk about what is making them anxious instead of working off all this energy, the client cannot be made to sit down. Rather the aim is to try to encourage the individual to become aware of what this continuous activity may mean. One method is the direct question, such as "What is making you so anxious that you can't sit still?"; there are many others. Always conscious of the idea of a counselor-client relationship being a working partnership with different tasks to accomplish, the counselor asks the questions and makes the observations that will help clients examine their behavior.

Clients Wanting to Leave Early

It may happen that feelings of anxiety, uneasiness, or anger make a client want to cut an interview short. The individual may even get up to leave the office. Such situations are usually avoidable. Noticing that a client seems uneasy or anxious, the counselor asks the client about what is causing this reaction and together they examine the situation. It would be useful to point out that this sense of uneasiness is something that can be looked at and discussed so that it becomes understandable. If the individual seems concerned that someone else could never understand the problem or if the anxiety seems out of control, it is desirable for the client to stay and gain insight into the situation.

Some clients hide their urge to terminate; acting bored or indifferent, they say there is nothing more to discuss. In this instance the individual needs help in order to recognize and examine the true reasons. Saying something like, "It seems as though you're really angry or uncomfortable; maybe we could talk about it,"

may indicate these reasons. Another approach would be to point out that avoiding negative feelings will not resolve them, that discussion would be more helpful. It could also be pointed out that what the client feels and what the client does are two different things: "Just because you feel like breaking off our discussion doesn't mean you have to do it. You can understand the feeling without acting on it."

Client Does Not Want Further Contact

Sometimes an individual refuses to make another appointment. The counselor asks why the client does not want to come back and the two of them discuss the reasons. If the client has felt angry about how things have been going and has concluded that further work together would be useless, this sort of response—and any other negative reaction—must be looked into.

In other cases clients try to terminate counseling by telephone; they phone to cancel one appointment and do not make another one. Or they simply fail to come to the next scheduled session. The client should be called so that another appointment can be arranged. Clients who repeatedly fail to show up should be contacted.

It is not uncommon for inexperienced counselors to have clients want to quit or to switch to someone else. Possibly the individual had a mental image that this counselor does not fit, in terms of age, sex, or apparent expertise. It is not a good idea to try with either warnings or promises to force someone to come back. Sometimes even though one does everything possible to explore the reasons someone wants to leave, the attempt fails. It must be remembered that there is no way to force a client to continue, and the limitations of both people involved must be accepted.

In rehabilitation agencies as well as other settings, counselors sometimes experience these unpleasant prospects of discontinuance with a client. When the counseling relationship is severed the counselor should transfer the case to a colleague in order to salvage the rehabilitation prospects of the client.

Client Brings Someone to the Interview

Once in a while a client will bring someone along to the interview. It should be determined whether the motivation is positive or negative —usually through discussion of the matter with the client—before a decision is made on whether to let the other person stay. When in doubt, the best idea is probably to include the third person and evaluate the decision while the interview is going on. Elements of the situation that need to be taken into account are the counselor's feelings, the goals of the interview, and the interests of the client and those of the other person.

Other Contingencies

Counselors do not have to give clients their home phone numbers since most agencies have a screening system for emergencies and contact the counselor when necessary. Some such agencies do not allow personnel to give out their numbers.

The rehabilitation worker often has occasion to visit a client who is hospitalized. If there is an opportunity to discuss the subject in advance, this is a good idea; a mutual decision can be made as to whether the counselor should make a hospital visit. Hospitalized people are usually in fairly severe physical condition; preoccupation with medical problems could interfere with counseling. On the other hand, a rehabilitation counselor's visit to the hospital often provides special support and demonstrates concern to a client, even in a short call.

Sometimes people requiring hospitalization become extremely anxious. Rehabilitation counseling can prevent anxiety about the future that might interfere with recovery. While the counselor must avoid compounding medical problems by hindering the hospital regimen in any way, the rehabilitation connecting process should be started early after the onset of disability and continued through physical restoration without unnecessary interruption. Staff rehabilitation counselors are employed by many general hospitals.

26.2.6. CONCLUDING THE SESSION

The time allowed for a counseling session has practical limits that necessitate ending the interview period promptly. Starting and finishing sessions on time also provide consistent structure to the relationship.

One should begin to anticipate the end of the interview about ten minutes before it is over. It might be useful to ask if there is something the client would like to talk more about. It is not always necessary to fully summarize what has been discussed if other sessions will be scheduled, but a brief outline of the main points is advisable for planning. It will also remind the client of the problems that require special attention, both during interviews and in between them. The counselor paces time in order to talk about the need for future sessions. The meeting can be ended by mentioning that the time is up and noting when the next appointment is scheduled. It is polite to get up and show the client to the door.

26.2.7. TERMINATION

Preparation for fulfilling the need for counseling begins in the initial session when goals are discussed. The degree of success in reaching these counseling goals influences the decision to terminate and its timing.

Emotions Surrounding Termination

When a close relationship has been established, both counselor and client probably experience various emotions upon conclusion. There may be anger, a sense of rejection, or guilt; feelings of relief and pleasure or pride in accomplishment may be noticed. Such repercussions are greater at the conclusion of personal adjustment counseling than they are after vocational counseling.

The counselor's attitude toward termination will vary according to how the work has gone with a particular individual. Sometimes it is difficult to end the relationship with a client who has been especially rewarding to work with, who has responded to the experience in an extremely positive way; in such instances one may tend to prolong it further than really necessary. On the other hand, when the sessions do not seem especially productive or good rapport with an individual has not been established, it may be tempting to terminate too early. In both kinds of cases a way should be found to handle conflicts.

Sometimes clients feel defensive and refuse to acknowledge the significance of termination or any feelings associated with the experience. In such instances it is important to help the client express feelings by asking what the whole experience has meant to the individual and what has been accomplished. Usually people who receive counseling expend considerable energy on it, whether the duration is short or long; they tend to be quite involved, even though they may not admit it, in this special self-scrutinizing process. Those who have been in counseling for long periods of time usually have stronger feelings about termination; perhaps weeks may be needed to sort out and resolve these feelings.

Termination after Brief Counseling

People may get counseling for crisis intervention or for treatment over a period of one to three months. Typically this is done on a limited-time basis so that both the professional and the client know from the beginning when termination will come. It may become the main topic during the counseling, but more typically issues relative to termination are dealt with only for portions of the last few sessions, and the discussion revolves around the client's coping mechanisms and plans for the future.

Resistance to Termination

Frequently clients regress in some way toward the end; regression is a response to the termination process. Unconsciously trying to perpetuate the counseling, these individuals may introduce new problems that need attention or old problems that they have neglected to mention before. The counselor, noticing this resistance, explains this reaction to the client. If the termination has been planned and agreed upon by both, it is not a good idea to continue counseling, but it is permissible to arrange for an appointment later as a follow-up measure.

Termination by Mutual Agreement

Mutual agreement is the best way to decide on termination. Both parties conclude that much progress has been made and that what work remains can be done by the client without professional help. Either can suggest that the time for termination has come, but usually the worker picks up on cues that indicate the client's self-understanding and readiness to deal indepen-

dently with problems. When this happens, it is time for the two of them to summarize what has been accomplished, what must still be done, and what the client feels the future will be like.

Termination Provoked by a Disagreement

A difference of opinion is sometimes the immediate cause of termination, suggested by either party. A counselor who does not feel the work is proceeding well may suggest termination for clinical reasons. The client may leave out of disappointment or because of a feeling that the counseling will not help. To a dissatisfied client one can recommend a consultation or consider a referral. If a client denies needing help by claiming suddenly to be well, there may be little the worker can do but go ahead with termination while at the same time urging the individual to come back if this later seems desirable.

Termination Due to Outside Factors

External factors like relocation can make termination necessary; it is a common problem with clinical practice students temporarily placed in a counseling agency. Without careful preparation, the discontinued client may feel some anger or have a sense of being abandoned. In turn the counselor may feel some guilt about leaving someone in need. But, a transfer to another counselor need not be traumatic if a good relationship has been established.

A Positive View of Termination

There are many positive ways to look at termination, even though it does mean that a good working relationship will come to an end. The client has learned to view the world in a better way and has learned to think and operate more independently; these are continuing resources for the individual.

Chapter 27

Vocational Counseling

Vocational guidance and counseling as a professional field is usually considered to have begun with the work of Frank Parsons. A noted lawyer concerned with the work problems of underprivileged youths, Parsons offered vocational counseling at the Boston Civil Service House. In 1908 he opened the Vocational Bureau of Boston to help youths choose a career. The posthumous publication of Parsons' 1909 book, *Choosing a Vocation*, led to the first national conference on vocational guidance in 1910.

According to Parsons the goal of vocational guidance was the selection of a vocation, sufficient preparation for it, and the achievement of vocational effectiveness. He considered three factors necessary for a systematic occupational choice: (1) a sound knowledge of one's personality, abilities, and limitations; (2) understanding of the demands and rewards of various types of work; and (3) a clear conception of how these two sets of data are related. (See 25.3.5.)

This concept of vocational decision-making prevailed, Patterson [1964] explained, for over 30 years; while different aspects of it were stressed at various times, the basic outlines were not challenged. During the decade from 1910 to 1920, when there were not many ways of measuring people's capabilities and interests, vocational information was emphasized. As testing methods were devised during and after World War I and into the 1930s, evaluation of the candidate became the focal point. In the 1940s interest turned to Parsons' third factor, the relationship between the person and the occupation.

It was not until the post-World War II period that efforts were made to build concepts dealing with the motivations behind vocational decisions and the processes and outcomes of these decisions. At that time a number of people created systems to describe the process of vocational choice, its implementation, and to some extent, its progress through the life-span; Osipow [1976] has provided an excellent review of this work. The theories and techniques of vocational counseling will be briefly described following the definitions listed in the next section.

Descriptions of the theories and technique of vocational choice, with their apparent objectivity, may seem to depersonalize the process. Test scores, occupational information, and other objective data do not, however, overcome the subjectivity involved in choosing a career. In fact, with many people there is no formalized choice or decision-making process; they merely accept an existing employment opportunity. The purpose of vocational counseling is to facilitate a deliberate career choice based upon factual information. Still there are many influences outside of the assessment and counseling strategy: opinions of family and friends, socioeconomic background, age, sex, institutions (such as the client's school and church), geographic area (urban or rural), and local industrial circumstances.

27.1. Definitions

Many of the terms used in vocational counseling are defined in Part III, Assessment and Part V, Placement. Some additional terms, however, are especially relevant to the present chapter.

27.1.1. VOCATIONAL COUNSELING TERMS
The following definitions of terms pertain explicitly to vocational counseling.

CAREER DEVELOPMENT. Referring to the continuous total flow of a person's work experience, this term signifies vocational self-development and encompasses progress in educational and occupational pursuits from the time of choice and entry into work until the person's permanent retirement from the work-force.

CAREER PLANNING. Planning a career is a three-phased process involving: (1) development of an adequate understanding of self, (2) learning about relevant aspects of the world of work, and (3) integration of this knowledge so that effective decisions can be made.

CAREER MOBILITY. This is the act of moving from one occupational level or stage to another. It may involve promotion to a more responsible job, demotion, discharge, moving to another organization, or retirement.

OCCUPATIONAL EXPLORATION. This is a program through which clients search for self-understanding (values, needs, abilities, influences, etc.) and training or vocational information, and learn how to make career decisions.

SECONDARY INFORMATION. The body of facts about a client not directly elicited or observed by the counselor is called secondary information. Such information is obtained from other professionals and agencies, either verbally or through such documents as psychometric reports, school records, medical reports (examination or history), social service reports, and so on. While valuable to have in counseling and planning, secondary information often requires validation by the counselor.

CLIENT BACKGROUND INFORMATION. Pertinent information regarding the client obtained prior to assessment, counseling, and planning can come from professionals (e.g., physicians, psychologists, school counselors, social workers) or lay persons (e.g., parents, former employers, houseparents) and other sources that can provide meaningful information.

VOCATIONAL OBJECTIVE. In vocational rehabilitation this is a specific, work-related, time-oriented statement that is set forth at the beginning of the client's rehabilitation service program but may be modified as the need arises. Set by the client with the counselor's concurrence, it is the basis for the rehabilitation plan (i.e., services needed to reach the vocational objective).

ASPIRATION LEVEL. In choosing life goals and in understanding everyday activities, individuals differ widely in level of aspiration (i.e., in their expectations of accomplishment or in the demands that they make upon themselves). "Aspiration" refers to the degree or quality of success sought and the "level" reflects the difficulty of the achievement for the individual.

JOB SATISFACTION. Significant satisfactions to be derived from work are of three distinct, though related, types: (1) monetary rewards and prestige; (2) intrinsic satisfactions (i.e., the pleasure in a specific activity and in the accomplishments of specific ends); and, (3) concomitant satisfactions such as derive from working in a particular physical environment or with a particular group. Lofquist and Dawis [1975] have provided an operational definition of "job satisfaction" as a characteristic of each worker with reference to the particular job: the degree of correspondence between the individual's vocational needs and the reinforcers or need-gratifiers afforded by the worker's job.

JOB SATISFACTORINESS. A characteristic of each employer with respect to each worker, job satisfactoriness, as defined by Lofquist and Dawis, refers to the degree of correspondence between the demands of a given job and the abilities of the individual performing the job.

VOCATIONAL ADJUSTMENT. This is a dynamic process of interaction of the worker with the work environment. It is related to the aptitudes, interests, abilities, skills, health, education, economic and social backgrounds, and other factors of the worker. It is further related to duties, pay, job security, supervision, hiring requirements, social environment, supply of workers, community pattern, demand for workers, working conditions, promotional possibilities, and many other job factors. Moreover, the vocational adjustment a person makes varies with the imme-

diate job situation and with the social, economic, and political patterns of the time. It is the totality of worker satisfaction and satisfactoriness.

27.1.2. OTHER RELEVANT TERMS
While a number of relevant concepts are described elsewhere, the following terms are so important that their definitions are reiterated.

OCCUPATIONAL HANDICAP. This is the inability to perform at a satisfactory level all of the essential requirements of an occupation. The requirements of an occupation are varied: physical capacities, manual skills, aptitudes, education, personality, interests, credentials (e.g., licenses), and so forth.

EMPLOYMENT HANDICAP. This refers to the difficulty a disabled person may have in getting a suitable job because of discrimination. Here there is no occupational handicap for the job applied for, but the employer is unwilling to hire the person because of misunderstanding and fear surrounding the disability or because of prejudicial attitudes.

PLACEMENT HANDICAP. When the rehabilitation worker has difficulty in placing a client on a job because of the client's occupational or employment (or both) handicap, it is called a placement handicap.

VOCATIONAL HANDICAP. As used in this book this term means any difficulty in adjusting or readjusting to the world of work. It is a general term meaning trouble obtaining, holding, or performing any (otherwise) suitable vocation because of the individual's disability or functional limitation.

27.2. *Theories*

In the Chapter 25 overview of theories of counseling and psychotherapy it was stated that theoretical knowledge provides guidelines to practice. The usefulness of theory in understanding vocational development and occupational choice is now shown in this section. Theoretical structure helps the vocational counselor systematize and analyze the vast amount

of data about the individual and the world of work. Theories tell the practitioner what to look for, where to go, what to expect.

Early theories of occupational choice portrayed people in an economic perspective: motivation for work was seen as largely financial. More recent theoreticians emphasized the psychological and sociological aspects of occupational choice and vocational development. Other conceptualizations of occupational choice and vocational development are to be found in anthropology, literature, and religion. In broadening the conceptual base for vocational psychology, however, most theorists have neglected the economic incentives of work. All existing theories offer only partial explanations of the meaning of work.

References cited in this section were selected for their bibliographic usefulness and include many outstanding books on the subject. Of particular value is a monograph by Joseph Zaccaria [1970] and other books from the Houghton Mifflin Guidance Series.

27.2.1. OCCUPATIONAL CHOICE

The traditional theories of occupational choice are built upon the view of a normal person who progresses through stages of human development. These theories assume that a person selects an occupation, although the theories do differ as to the dynamics of occupational choice process. Moreover, each theory tends to emphasize certain factors from among the many that influence occupational choice. They all stress, however, that the choosing of an occupation is a relatively distinct event.

Trait-Factor Theory

The first well-articulated theory of occupational choice was derived from the psychology of individual differences, also referred to as trait psychology, trait-measurement psychology, differential psychology, the actuarial (or factorial) approach to occupational choice, and trait-factor theory.

Trait-factor theory has been operationalized through the development of psychological tests to measure human traits. Williamson [1973] noted that the individual is organized in terms of a unique pattern of capabilities and potentialities (i.e., traits). These traits are correlated with an explicit set of qualities (factors) that are needed for success in a given job category. Testing (i.e., the objective measurement of traits) is therefore a direct way to predict success in a job.

Katz [1963] summarized the nature of trait-factor theory and its general implications for guidance.

1. Each person is "keyed" to one or a few "correct" occupations.

2. If left alone, the individual would gravitate toward the right occupational choice.
3. Without assistance, however, wasted time and motion and some possibility of choosing the wrong occupation tend to occur.
4. The "key" can and should be learned during early adolescence.
5. The correct or appropriate occupation greatly influences educational decisions.
6. Both the occupational choice and subsidiary decisions should remain constant over a period of time. The final occupational goal then can be selected early and should determine preliminary decisions related to and leading up to that goal.

Parsons [1909] pioneered elements of trait-factor theory in a model of guidance for people who need to make occupational choices. According to his early notions, people have different traits; each occupation demands a particular combination of characteristics in workers; and vocational guidance should match people and jobs. In Parson's characterization of vocational guidance he outlined a similar three-step process of studying the individual, studying occupations, and matching the person with the job. The National Vocational Guidance Association [1937] also identified studying the person, studying occupations, and counseling to match worker and occupation as the principal elements of vocational and educational guidance. This has become the basic framework for application of the methods of psychometric assessment, the development and use of occupational information, and the implementation of various counseling systems.

Need-Drive Theories

The concept of motivation has been centrally important in psychology for a number of decades. Need-drive theories hold that individuals have needs that become the force or drive toward need-satisfying objects, individuals, or activities. The motivation to satisfy needs may be either cognitive or emotional, conscious or unconscious, directly or indirectly expressed. Behavior directed toward fulfilling people's needs is typically described as goal-oriented. According to several need-drive theories, work is a way of satisfying needs.

Although Maslow [1954] did not direct specific attention to occupational choice, implicit in his thinking is the idea that success, satisfaction, adjustment, and so on, are related to the amount of satisfaction that an individual can attain with respect to a basic hierarchy of needs. Maslow described man's need structure in terms of a hierarchy in which low-order needs must be satisfied before high-order needs can be met. His needs structure has become the basic framework for a number of generalized considerations of human functioning such as mental health, general adjustment, classroom dynamics, and marital behavior. Maslow's needs are: physiological needs; safety needs; need to belong and to be loved; need for importance, respect, self-esteem, independence; need for information; need for understanding; need for beauty; and need for self-actualization.

Allport, Vernon, and Lindzey [1960] also developed a way of measuring the relative importance of six basic interests, motives (needs), or evaluative attitudes:

1. Theoretical: characterized by an overriding interest in the discovery of truth and by an empirical, rational, intellectual approach.
2. Economic: emphasizing practical values and closely resembling the stereotype of the average American businessman.
3. Aesthetic: placing the highest value on form and harmony; enjoying and evaluating every experience from the standpoint of its grace, symmetry, or fitness.
4. Social: emphasizing altruism and philanthropy.
5. Political: primarily interested in personal power, influence, and renown, not necessarily in politics.
6. Religious: mystical, interested in the unity of experience and in attempting to understand the cosmos as a whole.

Maslow, as well as Allport and his associates assumed that people make decisions, including occupational decisions, on the basis of their value system (needs) and their general personality orientation.

Psychoanalytic Theory

Brill [1949] has made the major contribution to a psychoanalytic interpretation of occupational choice. The psychoanalytic conception of occupational choice is based on the two major concepts of sublimation and identification. In sublimation, socially unacceptable motives are expressed as (changed into) socially acceptable behavior. Occupations are selected as general or specific sublimations of fundamental instinctual wishes or needs. Through the mechanism of identification, the young male may transform his relationship with his father into an ideology (model) that directs vocational strivings.

Theory of Early Parent-Child Relationships

Anne Roe has developed a theory of occupational choice that is in part psychoanalytic but is broader in scope. She presented a new taxonomy of occupations consisting of eight groups: service, business contact, organization, technology, outdoor, science, general culture, and arts and entertainment. She further subdivided each group into six levels, her final formulation consisting of an 8×6 arrangement of cells into which any and every occupation can be placed.

Her classification system provides the framework for a description of the occupational structure. In order to explain the psychological differences among workers in the various groups and levels, she postulated that three essentially different psychological climates result from early parent-child relations [Roe, 1957]: emotional concentration on the child results in an overprotecting or overdemanding climate; avoidance of the child results in a neglecting or rejecting climate; acceptance of the child results in a casual or a loving climate.

The occupational group an individual selects is determined by the early parent-child relationship; there is a direct causal relationship between the childhood psychological climate and the evolution of the individual's need hierarchy. Thus, warm parent-child relations result in children's learning to satisfy their needs primarily through interaction with other people; later, when making an occupational selection, these people tend to choose person-oriented occupations (e.g., human service occupations). On the other hand, people who experience cold modes of early childrearing (e.g., avoiding, neglecting, rejecting, and overdemanding climates) learn to fulfill needs in ways that do not involve people. These individuals characteristically choose occupations involving objects (e.g., technology), animals (e.g., outdoor), or ideas (e.g., science). Within each occupational group there are six levels of occupations; the level people select is influenced by their need intensity.

Composite View

According to Hoppock [1976] it will take considerable time to gather enough evidence to confirm or contradict existing theories, and more to test new ones. He stated that because there are no ideal formulations but many reasonable theories, a composite theory is indicated. Drawing from several existing formulations, Hoppock presented the following theory:

1. Occupations are selected to meet needs.
2. The occupation people choose is the one that they believe will best meet their most important needs.
3. Needs may be intellectually perceived, or they may be only vaguely felt as an attraction in a certain direction. In either case, they may influence choices.
4. Occupational choice begins when people first recognize that an occupation can help to fulfill needs.
5. Occupational choice is more effective as individuals learn to anticipate how well a given type of work will meet needs. The capacity to anticipate depends upon self-knowledge, knowledge of occupations, and the ability to think clearly.
6. Information about oneself influences occupational choice. It helps people to become aware of what they want and to anticipate whether or not they will be able to obtain what the occupation offers.
7. Information about occupations affects choices. It helps people learn that occupations may meet needs, and it helps them to estimate the degree of fulfillment that may come from various types of work.
8. Job satisfaction depends upon the extent to which the job meets the needs one believes it should meet. The degree of satisfaction is determined by the ratio between what people have and what they desire.
9. Satisfaction can come from a job that meets present needs or one that promises to meet them in the future.
10. It is always appropriate to change occupational choice when one believes that a change will meet needs better.

27.2.2. VOCATIONAL DEVELOPMENT

The salient idea in all the theories of occupational choice is that one, several, or a group of dynamic factors influence the individual and that at some point in life each person chooses an occupation in conjunction with these forces or as a reaction to them. Each individual is assumed to be better suited for certain jobs than for others. It is hoped that people can learn to find and choose appropriate jobs. Counseling and guidance are important at the crucial point when an occupation is actually chosen. People who select the correct occupation become happy, satisfied, successful, well adjusted, and socialized. On the other hand, those who select inappropriate occupations are dissatisfied and unsuccessful and require remedial assistance. In all these theories there is the implication that the individual must find a correct "slot."

In another group of theories, however, the occupational life of the individual is considered very differently, from a developmental perspective. Each person is seen as proceeding through various periods, phases, or life stages, with vocational aspects as only one element in human development. Basically, the individual does not choose an occupation, but instead chooses a series of occupational and occupationally related activities at different life stages that, taken together, comprise vocational development rather than a specific occupational choice. Occupational choice does not take place at a particular time, but vocational development continues over an extended period as the individual works toward vocational and vocationally related goals. People are not designated for a correct occupation; everyone can be successful and satisfied at many jobs. Such theories, emphasizing the element of time and development in people's lives, are known as theories of vocational development. Related methods of helping people vocationally have emerged as developmental vocational counseling.

Historical Antecedents to Contemporary Theories of Vocational Development

Terman [1925] in his classic study of the concomitants of superior intelligence was the first to suggest a developmental approach to work and work-related activities. He discussed educational, marital, and vocational adjustment of intellectually superior people. Because his cross-sectional method studied people of different ages, some notion of development was involved. The details of a theory of vocational development were not offered, however.

Erikson [1950] and Havighurst [1950] presented related discussions of the general course of human development and the role of psychosocial crises (Erikson) and developmental tasks (Havighurst) in it. In essence their formulations are as follows:

1. Individual development is continuous.
2. Development can be divided into life stages for the purposes of discussion.
3. People in each life stage can be characterized by certain general common traits.
4. Most people in a given culture pass through similar developmental periods.
5. Society places certain demands upon people.
6. These demands are essentially similar for all members of the society.
7. The demands change as the individual goes through the developmental process.
8. Developmental crises occur when people become aware of the need to change current behavior and learn new things.
9. In meeting and mastering developmental crises, people pass from one stage of maturity to another.
10. The crisis or task appears in its purest form at one stage.
11. Preparation for meeting the developmental crises or tasks is made in the stage prior to the stage in which the tasks must be encountered.
12. The developmental task or crisis may present itself in a later phase in somewhat different form.
13. The crisis or task must be met successfully before the individual can pass on to another developmental stage.
14. Mastering the crisis through learning the required tasks leads to societal approval, happiness, and success in later stages.
15. Failing to master a task or crisis leads to societal disapproval.

Both Erikson and Havighurst presented the general concepts of psychosocial crises and developmental tasks as well as a general conception of human development on which theories of vocational development could be based. Havighurst [1953] extended his original presentation of developmental tasks; he elaborated upon the sociological, psychological, and biological dynamics of the tasks, further characterized them, and specified the ways in which they are typically mastered. An adolescent, for instance, faces the task of selecting and preparing for an occupation, in addition to the following:

1. Accepting one's physical makeup.
2. Accepting a masculine or feminine role.
3. Establishing relationships with age-mates of both sexes.
4. Becoming emotionally independent from parents and other adults.
5. Becoming assured of economic independence.
6. Developing intellectual equipment necessary for civic competence.
7. Desiring and achieving socially responsible behavior.
8. Preparing for marriage and family.
9. Establishing values congruent with an adequate scientific world-picture.

Havighurst discussed developmental tasks in terms of an advancing pattern of vocational development, synthesizing the notions of vocational life stages, psychosocial crises, and vocational developmental tasks. In encountering and learning to accomplish the critical developmental tasks, a person passes from one life stage to another.

An Approach to a General Theory

Ginzberg, Ginzberg, Axelrod, and Herma [1951], finding existing theories insufficient, attempted to devise and partially test what they stated was an approximation of a theory. Ginzberg's was the first specifically developmental theory and the first theory of occupational choice per se. (Of course when Ginzberg was working on this, the distinction between occupational choice and vocational development had not yet been made.) The study found that occupational choice is a long-term process, that it becomes progressively irreversible, that the final choice is a compromise between the person's ideal and the available realistic alternatives, and that the entire process takes place in a series of rather definitive stages or periods.

Because people must resolve the conflict between subjective desires and the objective limitations imposed by the environment, selecting an occupation is a compromise. In addition, every time an occupational choice is made, many possible decisions are eliminated; thus as time goes on the range of appropriate choices decreases. Over time, the feasibility of access to many occupations is limited by reality factors and defensive behavior concerning the use of time, money, and energy. Furthermore, people cannot revert to the time and psychological situation in which decisions were made. In this sense, an occupational choice is irreversible.

Biological, psychological, and environmental considerations also affect the course of occupational choice; as a result people differ in the timing of occupational decisions. Other factors that affect the occupational choice are reality testing experiences, identification with suitable role models, and the extent to which a person inclines toward work versus pleasure.

A Theory of Personality and Model Environments

John Holland [1959, 1966, 1973] proposed a theory that is only implicitly developmental but it stresses the determinants of occupational choice. The major outlines of Holland's theory, according to Zaccaria [1970], are reflected in the following quotation:

Essentially, the present theory assumes that at the time of vocational choice the person is the product of the interaction of his particular heredity with a variety of cultural and personal forces including peers, parents and significant adults, his social class, American culture, and the physical environment. Out of this experience the person develops a hierarchy of habitual or preferred methods for dealing with environmental tasks. . . . The person making a vocational choice in a sense "searches" for [work] situations which satisfy his hierarchy of adjustive orientations [pp. 42–43].

Through learning, the individual develops habitual preferences in responding to environmental demands, one of which is that each person should make an occupational choice. In making this choice people are affected by their stereotypes and knowledge of the various occupations in the world of work. The depth and accuracy of the self-knowledge and occupational knowledge are critical, both deepening a person's understanding of the range, levels, and adequacy of possible occupational choices.

The Process of Occupational Decision-Making and Adjustment

Tiedeman and O'Hara [1963] offered a unique theory of vocational development in response to a need for a complete characterization of decision-making within the broader framework

of career development. Erikson's theory of general personality development [1950] is used as the foundation. Erikson outlined personality growth in terms of eight psychosocial crises of human life that result in the major components of the healthy personality. Within a framework similar to Havighurst's description of developmental tasks, Erikson portrayed the individual growing and developing while fulfilling biological potentialities within family and community life. At each developmental stage the individual must face a major psychosocial crisis; it is in the resolution of these crises that the person progresses from one stage to another.

Tiedeman and O'Hara defined career development as a process in which the individual resolves a group of general psychosocial crises, occupational aspects of these crises, and a sequence of problems or decisions that lasts throughout life. Each problem-solving task includes a series of decisions. When someone leaves a setting (e.g., school or job), a new decision is necessary. This propels the individual into a new decision-making sequence. Ultimately some form of overall adaptation or integration occurs.

Self-Concept Theory and Career Patterns

Super [1953] synthesized the work of developmental psychologists and added original formulations to construct a comprehensive theory of vocational development. The principal emphasis in Super's theory, however, has continued to be phenomenology or self-concept theory. While the genesis of a developmental framework is evident in Super's early work [1942], Ginzberg's theory stimulated the further research efforts that led to the formulation of Super's theory. Super's theory is perhaps the most comprehensive and generally accepted among contemporary theories of vocational development.

Super's central idea concerns developmental stages through which the individual passes in career development. While everyone goes through the same basic stages, individuals differ in the type, sequence, and duration of work and work-related activities within each stage. These differences are reflected in various types of career patterns.

According to Super, vocational development means developing and implementing a self-concept within the occupational world. This self-concept is defined during the growth and exploratory stages. Through different activities and exploratory behavior people perceive their uniqueness and also their similarity to others. As sensations, perceptions, and experiences become better organized and articulated, early self-perceptions become more abstract and comprehensive until the self-concept itself is formed.

A vocational self-concept is but one aspect of the whole self-concept, which guides the individual into and through career experiences. Preferring the notion of career development to that of occupational choice, Super directed his attention to the processes that occur as people develop, define, and implement their vocational self-concepts. Taken in its entirety, a person's career constitutes a lifelong search for a means of self-expression through work. People work to earn a living, to maintain effective human relations (e.g., to gain recognition as a person, independence, self-expression, status, and so on), and for the satisfactions of work itself. So, Super concluded, working is a way of life, a way of fulfilling needs, and a way of attaining selfhood.

According to Super, when vocational development is full and positive, it is a dynamic synthesis—an interaction of personal needs and resources with the economic and social requirements of society—rather than a compromise as others have suggested. Developmental tasks represent the demands that society imposes on people.

The concepts of career development are essential in vocational counseling with the disabled. It is necessary in rehabilitation counseling to consider the long-range career implications of the client's occupational choice and preparation. Ideally, vocational rehabilitation is a one-time effort resulting in permanent self-sufficiency. Careful vocational counseling with long-range career considerations often fulfills this goal [Dunn, 1974a].

27.2.3. RELEVANCE TO DISABLED PEOPLE

David Hershenson observed in 1974 that relatively little had been written concerning the vocational development of individuals with disabilities. Consequently he suggested a model of vocational behavior that has particular relevance to the handicapped. It utilizes five constructs: (1) the individual's background (physical and psychosocial), (2) work personality (the psy-

chological characteristics such as vocational self-image and motivation that mediate adaptation to work), (3) work competencies (behaviors, skills, and interpersonal relations in the work setting), (4) work choice (appropriateness and completeness of career plans), and (5) work adjustment (satisfaction and effectiveness on a job). Thus, background is one determinant of people's work personalities, work competencies, and work choices. These three in turn affect one another and determine work adjustment. Disabilities most directly affect work competencies, and adjustment to disability relates most directly to work personality. The extent of vocational adjustment to disability depends on the prior nature of these five constructs and their interrelationships, how far into the individual's career development the onset of disability occurs, and its specific impact on each of the elements in this model.

Minnesota Theory of Work Adjustment

To explain the development of the work personality, the Minnesota Studies in Vocational Rehabilitation, under a federal grant for the first Regional Rehabilitation Research Institute, concentrated on how the disabled individual interacts with the environment. According to Lofquist and Dawis [1969], the individual develops many response capabilities through interaction with the environment. The responses utilized most often can be identified as a primitive set of "abilities." At the same time the most frequently identified reinforcers in the environment become a primitive set of "needs." Abilities are thus general but recognizable categories of responses typically utilized by the individual, while needs denote the individual's learned requirements for certain environmental conditions. The primitive set of abilities and the primitive set of needs together make up the individual's salient vocational characteristics.

The sets of abilities and needs become more specific as the individual continues in a particular life style with its own fairly stable set of requirement-reinforcer conditions. When the ability set and the need set are completely formed, successive measurements of ability and need strength will yield essentially the same values. The theory states that work adjustment occurs to the extent that the individual's needs and abilities correspond with the work environment's reinforcers and demands.

In the Minnesota Theory of Work Adjustment, work adjustment is viewed as "the outcome of the interaction between an individual and his work environment," and is defined in terms "satisfactoriness" and "satisfaction." Satisfactoriness is the "evaluation of the individual's work behavior principally in terms of quality and quantity of task performance and/or performance outcomes," and satisfaction is "the individual's evaluation of stimulus conditions in the work environment with reference to their effectiveness in reinforcing his behavior." According to this theory, satisfactoriness "is a function of the correspondence between an individual's set of abilities and the ability requirements of the work environment" and satisfaction "is a function of the correspondence between the reinforcer system of the work environment and the individual's set of needs" [Lofquist, Siess, Dawis, England, & Weiss, 1964, p. 2].

In the Minnesota theory, tenure, which is the amount of time an individual stays in a certain work environment, is the ultimate criterion of work adjustment. Tenure is the most readily observable outcome. The longer a person remains in a given work environment, the more likely it is that an effective adjustment with this environment has been achieved. When a person leaves a given work environment, it may be inferred that the adjustment was not adequate. According to the theory, work adjustment and tenure are predictable if there is knowledge about the correspondence between individual abilities and job requirements as well as knowledge of needs and job reinforcer systems. (There are obvious exceptions, for example, the Civil Service worker who is neither satisfactory nor satisfied, but who stays on the job until retirement.)

For the rehabilitation counselor, the emphasis is on determining how the disability has disrupted work adjustment. Disability is generally considered to result in significant change in the ability set, brought about by physical, mental, and/or emotional trauma, with or without concomitant changes in the need set. Thus disability is seen in terms of its actual consequences for an individual. Information about residual sets of abilities and needs is necessary for counselors, who must identify jobs that have suitable requirement-reinforcer characteristics and that will yield maximum work adjustment.

With respect to the Minnesota theory, successful vocational intervention can be judged in a number of ways. When rehabilitation counseling and disability are considered in terms of the theory of work adjustment, several criteria of the effectiveness of counseling can be used, for example: increases in ability utilization; stabilization (lack of fluctuation) in measured abilities and needs; satisfactory progress in a course of job training; choice of a job, for which work adjustment is predicted; obtaining placement in a job; adjustment (satisfactoriness plus satisfaction) in a job; and tenure on a job.

Other Approaches

Walter Neff [1971a] discussed the work personality as a semiautonomous part of the general personality. He compared his approach to the theory of work to the approach of the Minnesota theory of work adjustment, stating that in contrast to the empirical and psychometric studies of the Lofquist group, his approach is sociological and clinical. There are a number of similarities between the two theories. Like Lloyd Lofquist, Neff utilized the conception of a "work personality," explicitly defined as a semiautonomous segment of the general personality. In contrast, however, Neff was far more interested in work as a type of social behavior and with the relationship between work behavior and the total personality. An important difference is that Neff did not consider the presence or absence of specific work skills, but emphasized the ability of the worker to cope with the social and cultural demands of work. Neff's theory, moreover, stresses those aspects of the work environment—as well as those elements of the work personality—that are likely to lead to problems in adaptation.

In his analysis of the work environment, Neff separated the structural features from the interpersonal requirements and both from the customs and mores that must be learned before the individual is initiated into the work structure. Structurally, Neff pointed out four potential problem areas for the individual with a disability. First, most kinds of work are done away from the home and require travel. Second, work is typically carried on in a public place, so privacy is severely limited. Third, the work situation is not only public, but also quite impersonal.

The final structural characteristic—often related to maladaptive behavior—is the degree to which work is bound by time. These characteristics of work situations comprise major barriers in adapting to work for a considerable number of disabled people.

Each work situation is delineated by customs, rules, and traditions, which stem in part from the culture as a whole and in part from each situation's own particular history and place in society. The work personality evolves in response to the demand of society that people must perform in a productive way. Children are confronted with this demand when they begin their education. The compulsion to work is initially external but becomes internalized. In other words, we learn to become workers. Borrowing largely from the Minnesota theory of work adjustment and Hershenson's pioneering schematization, McMahon [1977] synthesized these conceptualizations into a model of vocational redevelopment for disabled persons whose handicap occurs in midcareer. The model utilizes the ingredients of worker needs and competencies, job reinforcers and demands, and the worker's perceptions of these elements to elucidate such critical aspects of redevelopment as self-assessment, occupational information, impact of disability, and broad categories of vocational redevelopment behaviors. Motivation factors that either facilitate or inhibit vocational redevelopment were also considered by McMahon.

27.3. Self-Understanding

Promoting self-understanding as a principal component in the client's occupational choice is the most challenging task in the vocational counseling process. Shaw [1976] noted that in doing this one helps clients recognize their personality traits, their hopes, their various capabilities, their likes and dislikes, their sense of values. The rehabilitation counselor assists clients to sharpen their perceptions of themselves and increase self-acceptance, to understand their abilities and their limitations, and also to identify their major economic and personal needs.

Early on during rehabilitation, information about the client is collected from interviews, medical reports, school records, social studies, behavior descriptions, autobiographies, home visit reports, personality studies, interest inventories, and aptitude and achievement tests. (The reader is referred to Part III, Assessment, for a further description of these techniques.) Clients require a clear interpretation of this information if they are to increase self-knowledge and make appropriate vocational decisions. But, it is important to recognize that this kind of data can puzzle, mislead, or even alarm people [Dunn, 1974a]; counselor expertise is therefore required for selecting and weighing assessment information as well as in communicating it for client self-understanding.

27.3.1. ASSESSMENT INFORMATION

Information from various sources about interests, aptitudes, and personality improve self-understanding in clients, but it is necessary that clients understand this information about themselves in order to use it properly. This places a responsibility on the counselor to be a knowledge resource for clients that can interpret information from psychological and other evaluations. Assessment information provides a broadened perspective to some clients and suggests promising possibilities that they have not previously considered. For others, further understanding of self serves to narrow down the range of possibilities that deserve serious consideration.

Assembling such a large body of information may seem frighteningly difficult to even the counselor. But despite the very large number of occupations, only relatively few aptitudes and other human potentials account for success or failure after preparation. With all of the intricacies of occupational patterns there remain only a relatively few variables that are critical in occupational choice. Moreover, the round-peg-in-a-square-hole fear is alleviated by the fact that while both people and jobs come in many different shapes their dimensions are flexible. Forcing persons to fit into imprecise job requirements may not be ruinous because they do have the capacity to adapt and grow to accommodate the challenge of demands. The process of choosing a career is not scientifically exact but then neither is the choice of a mate. The making of both of these choices, as projected for a long term, are usually methodologically unsound, emotionally influenced, and based upon inadequate sampling. Remarkably, such intuitive decisions, based as they are on incomplete and biased data, often produce happy outcomes.

The best approach in vocational counseling is to anticipate career difficulty and accommodate a margin for error in the plan. The world of work is constantly changing, with new occupations appearing and old ones vanishing. Trends vary in ways that are difficult to predict. Therefore, counselor and client must guard against occupational obsolescence in career planning. Highly specific job training places one in a highly vulnerable position because specific and narrow skills are not transferable to the requirements of other jobs. Disabled people should seek as much flexibility as possible so as not to compound their physical limitations. When there is a reasonable choice, the client's vocational preparation should be broadly applicable in anticipation of changes in future job requirements.

In many instances, career counseling follows the Parsons model of matching person with job. But in addition to this traditional approach, which helps the client with a specific decision, another vocational counseling method deserves consideration. This alternative approach focuses upon teaching decision-making skills for future vocational choices that the client will encounter. The idea of a single point-in-time career decision—particularly for the disabled person —is an erroneous assumption that will lead to reopened cases every time there is a job

crisis. In rehabilitation the process of choosing an occupational objective can be aimed at both the short-term objective of choosing a job and also the long-range objective of developing the client's capacity for making independent decisions at career choice points in the future.

27.3.2. COMMUNICATING INFORMATION

If rehabilitation is considered a joint effort, it is evident that one counselor responsibility is to determine what kinds of evaluation should be obtained and to communicate the results so that the client can understand them. It is important to bear in mind the kinds of information the person needs. Early on, a fairly clear idea of the individual's needs begins to emerge from interviews. The counselor must develop with the client an evaluation strategy that addresses those needs. Then if evaluation data are to be truly illuminating, and if information that can actually increase self-knowledge is to be provided, the evaluation results must be accurately interpreted (see 24.4.6).

In vocational counseling, a generally useful procedure is to examine all case information with relationship to patterns of interest, potentialities, life-style, and other job-relevant behavior. The client should be encouraged to express reactions and opinions relative to the entire assessment process. The counselor keeps in mind that client evaluations and other case study information are supposed to provide a way of looking at various possible alternatives, not final answers to force the client to make definite choices. Generally, the techniques of self-understanding used in vocational counseling are comparable to those used in other forms of counseling as discussed in the various chapters in Part IV.

27.4. Occupational Information

For clients to make a wise choice of occupations, they must be informed about not only themselves but also about jobs. It is particularly important for disabled people to know the requirements of jobs because their choices are limited by restrictions in activities or environ-

ment. Moreover, the effort to obtain vocational preparation and employment may be complicated by the disability and resultant handicaps.

First of all, handicapped people need to know that there is a wide variety of occupational opportunities suitable to their capabilities and interests. Even physically normal young people, due to their limited experience in the world of work, fail to recognize the many kinds of jobs open to them. The knowledgeable rehabilitation counselor is able to expand the range of choice by providing information about unfamiliar occupations.

The counselor involves the client in this search for occupational information. To learn about the world of work for themselves, clients must know what variables to consider, where to get information, and how to assess it for their own uses. Sources of information extend beyond the counselor's file. The world of work also may be explored directly by clients through observation and through conversation with other people as well as with the knowledgeable vocational counselor.

Too often, however, people choose their occupations on the basis of faulty and biased information or for the wrong reasons. There are a great many considerations over and beyond pay, security, and potential advancement. The more occupations one knows well, the better the basis for an intelligent choice. Through vocational assessment, occupational information, and counseling, clients learn about themselves and are able to match their needs and qualifications to all of the rewards and demands of the various occupations.

A lifetime career choice is implied here because rehabilitation seeks permanent solutions. The process is complicated by the permanent functional limitations of the client, a recurring barrier to employment. Moreover, it is particularly important because without this service the disabled person is less likely to make a satisfactory occupational adjustment. Nonhandicapped people have a broader range of suitable jobs from which to choose. Moreover, they can more readily learn about themselves and different kinds of jobs in their youth by trial and error work experiences before the time comes for making a "permanent" career decision. In practice the use of occupational information is integrated with client assessment (interests, aptitudes, and so on) in vocational counseling to help clients consider vocational alternatives and develop a rehabilitation plan.

Chapter 19, Occupational Information, focused on the collection of such information for purposes of client assessment. The present section is oriented toward using occupational information in the counseling process, but the assessment orientation of the material in the earlier chapter is relevant here.

27.4.1. EFFECTIVE USE

Miller and Obermann [1968] suggested several principles regarding the effective use of occupational information in the counseling interview. First, occupational information will benefit the client most if utilized as an essential element of counseling. That is, a counseling session in which occupational information is the focal point is basically the same as any other type; approaches that are effective in other counseling situations will make the occupational information session successful.

Second, the success of such a session will depend primarily on whether the client is given a reasonable opportunity to respond to the information presented. The presentation of information and passive participation of the client are not sufficient. The client's viewpoints and feelings must be elicited. The client should view the material as a foundation for decision-making.

Third, it is also essential that individuals have an opportunity to look at occupational information as it relates to their concepts of themselves. This implies that clients can utilize occupational data best when they are prepared to assimilate it; when they have gained self-understanding about their own capacities, interests, and limitations; and when they recognize the personal relevance of the material. In other words, occupational information is usually not presented until client assessment has taken place.

Fourth, clients should be involved in weighing the relevance and significance of occupational information. This is necessary for a number of reasons. For one thing, involvement of the client will help the counselor appraise motivation. For another, individuals who have much to do with the planning of their vocational future will invest more in the vocational counseling process. Those who have an active role in the process are more apt to be open to the counselor's viewpoint without feeling threatened. The client's involvement also can help prevent excessive reliance upon the counselor. Finally, being a part of the process can help people who have difficulty making up their minds. Practice in making the easier choices, like where to go first for job information, can increase one's sense of assurance and serve as a step toward making more complicated decisions.

All these principles stress client participation, but there are occasions when it is appropriate for the counselor to carry a major portion of the responsibility. The principles are useful guidelines, but a substantial amount of common sense is also necessary with regard to use of occupational information. Each client is a unique individual and client differences, such as low reading ability and intelligence or inexperience, must be taken into account and reflected in a variety of approaches to the use of occupational material.

Baer and Roeber [1964] reviewed a number of sources in the professional literature and classified the functions or uses of occupational information into three board categories: motivational, informative, and adjustive. Motivational uses include attempts to arouse interest and stimulate activity in vocational planning. The term *informative use* is self-explanatory. The most common adjustive use is to help clients with unrealistically high levels of aspiration test their goals against the realities of actual job demand.

27.4.2. SOURCES

Occupational information is available to the vocational counselor in a wide variety of places, but one can also come across unsound or biased information. It is necessary to estimate the reliability and validity of all available information in order to employ it properly. Like other kinds of information, occupational material is most trustworthy when it comes straight from the source. Material is sometimes unreliable because it has travelled too far from where it originated, has been too condensed through abstraction and summarization, or has been distorted by change in emphasis. Literally, original information about an occupation has to come from engaging in the occupation, but in actuality few have access to knowledge gained in this way. In many instances material that is called "primary" is in fact based on a report by an individual who did not actually participate in collecting the data. Information, then, is often the result of efforts by many persons over a span of time (see 17.2.4).

As the world of work undergoes constant al-

terations, the body of information about it must change as well. Accordingly, it is important to use current information for changing job pictures. The counselor must also be aware that occupational information can be biased or incomplete. The motivations for extensive and glamorous marketing techniques must be scrutinized. The military, volunteer services, and public utilities are examples of organizations that seem to overemphasize desirable aspects of vocational activity (e.g., adventure, travel, and so on) while other, less glorious aspects are ignored (e.g., poor pay, long hours, boredom).

Nationwide Information

Norris, Zeran, Hatch, and Engelkes [1972] discussed fully the various sources of nationwide occupational information, and their compilation is followed here. The federal government is obviously the richest source of information about the world of work in this country. The agencies that have the most to do with this subject are all divisions of the U.S. Department of Labor: Bureau of Labor Statistics, Manpower Administration, and Women's Bureau. These agencies regularly disseminate information pertaining to occupations.

The U.S. Bureau of the Census compiles the most comprehensive data on the country's working force. Census data is gathered periodically for use on federal, state, and local levels. These data reveal conditions and tendencies in the work force according to various categories such as sex, race, income, and so on. Local statistics are compiled in the Census Bureau's *County Business Patterns*. It is published every several years and presents data about workers in all industries according to county.

The Statistical Abstract of the United States, which has been published since 1878, summarizes industrial, social, political, and economic data for the nation at the end of each year. It presents information about the population, the educational system, and the budget along with material about specific industries and many other subjects. The *Catalog of U.S. Census Publications,* prepared four times a year and obtainable from the U.S. Government Printing Office, contains complete information about material published by the Census Bureau.

The Bureau of Labor Statistics, a division of the Department of Labor, issues much valuable information about the national occupational picture. The Occupational Outlook Service, instituted in 1938, examines the present situation and prospects for the future for selected segments of the labor force. Using consultants from many different fields the Service collects, analyzes, and publishes data on the organization, economic situation, technological trends, and other aspects of various occupations and industries. Originally issued in 1949, the *Occupational Outlook Handbook* is revised every other year. The *Handbook* is continually brought up to date by the *Occupational Outlook Quarterly*. With help from the states, the Department of Labor issues total employment figures for all industries in the *Monthly Labor Review* and *Employment and Earnings*. The *Monthly Labor Review* contains very useful material on research and on happenings in labor, industry, and the legislature as well as book reviews. In *Employment and Earnings* one gets in-depth numerical data about directions in employment, weekly economic conditions, and state and area conditions for about 300 industries.

The *Manpower Report of the President* is one of the most important sources of information out of the Manpower Administration. It is issued every year and usually sums up manpower needs, availability, utilization, and preparation.

Many other national sources of material can be used to enhance one's knowledge of current occupational opportunities. General and specialized information comes from a very large number of associations and companies. The Chamber of Commerce, for example, reviews and reports on the overall economy at regular intervals. Labor unions, on the other hand, prepare reports on many specific occupations.

One can find occupational information in many magazines. Sometimes experts participate in the preparation of these articles, but in popular periodicals the truth may be distorted by misplaced emphasis in an effort to attract the reader's attention. Valuable information also comes from professional and trade organizations.

The American Personnel and Guidance Association and its divisions, particularly the National Vocational Guidance Association, publish information on occupational subjects in their journals. Up-to-date information about the work world also can be obtained from annotated bib-liographies and other materials issued by commercial publishers.

The Dictionary of Occupational Titles

A most important occupational information resource for rehabilitation counselors is the *Dictionary of Occupational Titles (D.O.T.)*; it describes most occupations in America and allows for the categorization of these occupations by job components [U.S. DOL, Employment and Training Administration, 1977]. Knowledge of what is in the *D.O.T.* and supplemental publications help one relate needed information to clients. The *D.O.T.* is described extensively in Chapter 19, Occupational Information.

27.4.3. LOCAL INFORMATION

Locating and systematizing local information about available jobs in the community is more important than having extensive knowledge of national occupational information. This problem was dealt with by Tolbert [1974], whose ideas are related here. Tolbert suggested that for a number of reasons most people have only a vague notion of how this information can be obtained. Typically there has been no one channel through which local job information is disseminated. The state Employment Service has the most information about the occupational scene, but its main function is to place people. Even that agency, however, is unable to adequately help disabled people find out about different jobs and go through the process of planning and choosing (see 35.2.3).

Employers

Frequently material about jobs, training, and advancement possibilities is produced by employers, especially those in the larger local companies. This kind of information is also available from large employers with local branches.

Kunze [1967] arranged the spectrum of occupational information gained in order of "directness," that is, how closely the type of information approximates actual work experience. In order of decreasing directness, the spectrum includes: performing the job (working part time or in connection with a training program); trying aspects of the work under guidance; observing workers in a job; working in a simulated occupational setting; participating in work games or role play; talking to people who represent vocations or careers; getting computerized information; reading programmed teaching material; seeing films and other visual presentations; reading material written for a general audience.

Educational and Training Programs

Usually organizations that have training programs outline them in pamphlets, catalogues, and so on. Because these programs, especially in the vocational-technical fields, change frequently, those interested should get new information every year and keep in close contact with the organization. Sometimes local colleges and vocational programs produce films or slides about what they have to offer.

Generally counselors and clients can get the best idea of what local programs are like by visiting the sites. Apprenticeship representatives come to groups to explain apprenticeship programs; after hearing such a presentation, a person will learn more when observing trainees at work (see 36.2.5).

Material on local colleges is the most readily available, but it is not easy to interpret it correctly since the catalogues contain only some of the essential information. There are also regional and national directories for current information about colleges (see 14.4.3).

Facts about local learning opportunities, along with knowledge about various institutions and student populations, are important, as is knowledge of in-school opportunities like work-study (see 14.1). Again, attention must be given to the recruitment nature of materials offered, since educational and training institutions are like any other institution in that each is interested in perpetuating itself.

Community Agencies and Organizations

Public and private services and organizations are valuable information resources. The most useful source of information on a local level is the state Employment Service. Elsewhere in this book a discussion on the U.S. Employment Service summarizes what this service does (see 12.2.9 and 37.2). A visit to the local office is the best way to become familiar with how it operates and to make useful contacts.

Local organizations working together with the town or city government frequently have good information. The Chamber of Commerce is in touch with economic trends and developments. The service clubs—Rotary, Lions, Kiwanis,

and others—often have committees studying the local labor situation. Local executives in these clubs also serve as good employer contacts for job development activity (see 38.1).

Workers and Occupational Groups

Occupational groups may offer very useful information about various kinds of employment opportunities; normally they have material about job preparation and availability in the area. Getting information from people who work in various occupations can be extremely useful. Clients who talk to workers on the job—in the doctor's office, the furniture store, the repair shop—get a much more accurate idea of the work than could be derived in any other way except through personal experience. While the presentation could be slanted if the person being talked to tries to propagandize for the occupation, planning before the visit and follow-up discussion afterward should restore the balance.

Newspaper and Other Local Media

The classified ads give abbreviated descriptions of jobs, and other items in the local newspapers reveal various kinds of information about new companies, training opportunities, and employment agencies. The quality of this material varies from one locality to another, and newspapers may be hard for some persons to read [Gutsch & Logan, 1967].

A considerable amount of material about occupational subjects is presented on radio and television, on the news, in feature stories, and in special announcements. News about summer job opportunities can be very useful, not only for students but for rehabilitants seeking trial work experiences. Interesting announcements about vocational-technical opportunities are made at regular intervals by the National Alliance of Businessmen. Dramatic presentations and non-fictional accounts of occupational subjects, however, often reflect stereotyped notions.

Working with Sources

Decisions about the relative importance of various kinds of data must be made before local information is collected. Two kinds of files are then set up, one for important employers in the area and one for the principal local resource agencies.

Tolbert [1974] suggested the following basic procedures. To build the employer file, one finds out from the state Employment Service office and the Chamber of Commerce the names of the largest employers; consults the telephone book and the state's listing of businesses, if there is one, for additional names; and establishes contact with these companies by mail or phone. The names and numbers of the businesses and contact people are filed, and each one is visited so that more information and knowledge can be obtained and working relationships can be formed. The card file becomes an index to collected materials. There should be cross-references between the *employers* file and an *occupational* file. The list is built up as names of other agencies are obtained. For each one the steps are the same. The established file will contain the names of contact people and information about each organization's purpose. After these two files have been established, other components of the local information system can be established to include resource people, material on former clients' occupations, and local occupational survey data.

27.4.4. INFORMATION PROCESSING

In gathering information it is easy to amass too much that is not relevant and thus collect material that can neither be organized nor used. It is a good idea to evaluate the material as it comes in.

Every piece of occupational information that is to be kept should be identified as to source. The name of the sponsor of the report and the names and credentials of those who prepared it should be recorded. In order to assess the soundness of the work it is important to know what procedures were implemented and how thoroughly the subject was investigated. The date is also important, since occupational patterns may change rapidly. If statistical data is given, it should be current. Finally, materials should be appealing in form and should be intelligible to those who are to use them.

Filing

Material about occupations will be of little use if it is not easy to find, so any organization or office that collects it should have a filing system. All standard systems operate on the principle of classification, but occupational material can be classified in various ways: alphabetically, by tasks, by industry, by product. The files may be organized according to any principle of classification, as long as the system is understood by all who utilize it.

The individuals who will be needing the material should be able to retrieve it easily. In a rehabilitation office, the principal users are members of the counseling staff. Sometimes clients are allowed access to the file, perhaps to find information that will help them make vocational decisions. If clients are sent to the material, they should understand the filing system and how to find what interests them. It is important to remember that this storehouse of knowledge is useless unless it can help clients make vocational plans. Even the problem of disappearing or misfiled information is preferred to the situation in which this material is inaccessible and unused.

The location of the file is important. Its significance will tend to be lost if it is placed along a row of other files, causing congestion in the area; it should therefore be set apart from the mass of routine office paper. Also, other conditions such as lighting and temperature and accessibility for the handicapped should be appropriate.

27.4.5. FACTS ABOUT JOBS

Generally speaking, while clients are willing to learn about themselves through counseling, testing, and other assessment techniques, they do not wish to spend time reading occupational literature. Even university counseling centers find that their elaborate occupational information library is avoided by some students seeking a major field of study or new professional goal. Independent use of occupational materials has not been improved greatly by attempts to package them more attractively.

If clients will not read about occupations on their own, then, it may be necessary for the counselor to assume a teaching role. It is just as important to have a command of occupational knowledge as to have knowledge of client tests and other evaluations, or, for that matter, the knowledge and skills of counseling. The counselor's role is also served by providing information or helping the client find it.

How does one help clients discover what they need to ask and how to find answers? While initial counseling sessions tend to be nondirective, when it comes to gathering occupational information and self-assessment information the circumstances generally require more structure.

Hoppock [1976] devised "A Checklist of Facts about Jobs" that is useful in providing structure for the client's learning. This review of occupational considerations should be done before the client becomes prematurely committed to a vocational objective. In fact, one value of this broad perspective of work dimensions is that it tends to preclude ill-founded judgments about what one wants to do.

Hoppock divided job considerations into various categories: employment prospects, nature of the work, work environment, qualifications, unions, discrimination, preparation, entrance, advancement, earnings, number and distribution of workers, advantages and disadvantages. Under each heading there are various questions that direct attention to concrete details: for example, whether the work setting is clean and safe; whether people work together or alone; what age, sex, aptitude, legal and other requirements exists; what preparation is necessary and at what cost; what weekly earnings are expected; whether the job is seasonal; whether required skills are usable elsewhere.

Reviewing a list of issues in vocational choice should not be a mechanical task, however, but should involve counselor-client discussion about relevant and unresolved considerations. In these sessions the focus is upon client needs and capabilities as they relate to occupations. The factual knowledge of the counselor is naturally brought into these client-focused sessions in an unauthoritative manner.

Unfounded Employer Preferences

At one time employers were allowed to implement unjustified biases against selected applicants by demanding personal characteristics unrelated to the actual requirements of the job. Fair employment practice legislation makes it illegal to discriminate because of disability, age, sex, race, or other personal characteristics that have nothing to do with vocational ability. Employers therefore can no longer refuse to hire or retain a qualified person simply because of a personal bias.

Affirmative action programs aggressively enforced by government have required some employers to rectify past inequalities by special efforts to recruit handicapped workers. These "catch-up" campaigns are improving the quality of employment opportunities in the American labor market for handicapped, women, and nonwhite persons (see 38.4.1).

Legal Qualifications

There are, of course, many other employer preferences that are objectively based and some are required by law. There are legal restrictions governing the employment of certain classes of people; for example, minors are protected from hazardous work or hours, aliens may be prohibited from working in sensitive defense factories.

State licenses (or some sort of certification) are required for employment in certain occupations in order to help protect the public from incompetent practitioners; examples include physicians, electricians, attorneys, and public school teachers. The associations of certain professions and labor unions exert other restrictions on employment that are supposedly designed to protect society. The lack of credentials may, however, constitute barriers to employment to otherwise qualified people who did not investigate the necessary route for entering the occupation.

Medical Qualifications

Each occupation has a unique pattern of demands for medically determined abilities. While most jobs are readily classified as sedentary or light or heavy, a full description of physical requirements is oftentimes more complex. It is often necessary to look beyond the *D.O.T.* for a detailed understanding of the physical requirements of a specific occupation as practiced in a particular setting. Better reference sources may be specific occupational literature; a description of watch repair tasks, for example, will indicate the requirement of finger dexterity. Vocational counselors cannot have an intimate knowledge of the physical demands of all jobs, but they can constantly expand their expertise by turning to the literature, talking with working people, and observing jobs firsthand (see 15.1).

Social Skill Requirements

The general impression of the applicant that the interviewer gets is a subtle but critical criterion for many vocations. Unfortunately, a pleasant physical appearance and manner are often more important than ability, even for jobs that do not involve interpersonal or public relations skills. Realistically, though, many occupations do require a measure of social intelligence or skill. One generally must be able to get along with co-workers, supervisors, and in many jobs, the public. Such requirements need to be understood not only for appropriate occupational selection by clients but also to provide social adjustment training, if indicated, in the rehabilitation plan (see 13.2).

Education

A general or liberal education is a broad academic preparation and does not have a particular occupational objective. In the United States, 12 years of general education is the usually accepted minimum. People with less education may be hired if the available labor supply is low. Interestingly, once in a job, advancement depends more upon practical and explicit learning attainment than general educational credentials such as diplomas.

Educational requirements for many occupations increasingly include a college degree. Specific degree fields and levels are needed for professions. The *D.O.T.* specifies the level of general educational development required as well as levels of "reasoning," "mathematical," and "language development." The feasibility of rapid upward social-vocational mobility through general education development is well demonstrated (see 14.4).

Training and Experience

The term *training* should be differentiated from *education* as defined above. Training is practical instruction for specific skills development rather than general knowledge. Generally in skilled and technical jobs, the specific preparation requirements are referred to as training (see 14.1).

Even unskilled jobs may require orientation training, which lasts only a short time. The *D.O.T.* indicates training times for occupations along with other requirements. The amount and type of training vary greatly with occupations. Training may be on-the-job, in formal apprenticeship, by correspondence, or through courses in technical schools or colleges. After employment, many occupations and employers expect ongoing development through in-service training, conferences, extra college courses, and other forms of continuing development.

In practice it is sometimes difficult to differentiate between training and experience because the product, job skill attainment, is the same. For this reason most jobs are advertised as requiring a specified amount of training or the equivalent in experience. The truly self-taught worker is increasingly rare and it is better to assume that qualifications are more efficiently obtained by preplanned training than through experiential paths.

Duties

Because selection of an occupation requires knowledge of the nature of the actual work involved, the most important information about an occupation is the description of its duties. In fact many jobs are operationally defined by a simple description of their duties. The *D.O.T.* describes ordinary duties in the job definitions.

Any job can be described in detail through analysis of the specific tasks performed by workers. Job tasks, as the elements of what a worker does, can be assessed for the type and level of worker abilities needed. Thus the duties of an occupation can be systematically studied and reported with great accuracy through task analysis. The description may include the tools and materials used in performing the work. More complex occupations may include a description of worker behavior. Particularly appropriate for use in the vocational counseling process is the framework for job analysis developed by Sidney Fine and his associates [Fine & Wiley, 1971].

Working Conditions

The prospective worker should know about the working conditions of the occupation being considered. One's workweek varies as to the amount and pattern of time spent on the job. Some jobs, including self-employment and commission sales, may permit considerable flexibility as to when one works. Other positions, such as that of the rising executive in business, may involve far more work than 40 hours per week without additional compensation. Still other jobs may require long periods away from home (e.g., that of interstate truck driver). Other examples of jobs with unique work weeks include those of firefighters, sailors, and traveling salespersons. While the physical working conditions of one's chosen occupation are of interest to everyone, such information is essential to a person whose disability may preclude adverse environments. The *D.O.T.* lists certain working conditions that are contraindicated for some handicapped persons. Handicapped or not, people should know about hazards and discomforts before becoming committed to a job selection.

Psychological conditions inherent in the occupation are equally important. Included under this consideration are the social climate of the organization, prestige, authority role, interpersonal relationships, clothing, work, and so on.

The location of the employment is another aspect. Jobs are clustered around industrial and densely populated areas. Accessibility by public transportation and freedom from architectural barriers may be important considerations. The Bureau of Census has compiled data of this nature.

Remuneration

The pattern, amount, and security of remuneration vary according to the occupation selected. Monetary return generally increases along with the educational and other requirements of the occupation, although this is not always true. Supply and demand as well as other factors influence the median (typical) salary and wage range of occupations. As a higher percentage of the labor population becomes college-educated, the potential salary incentive for education alone is reduced. Thus it is wise to try to project future income potentials.

Employment Outlook

The future of an occupation over many years to come cannot be predicted with much confidence. It is known whether workers are currently in demand and whether the prospects are likely to go up or down, yet the prediction of future trends is based on many assumptions: worker supply and demand, predictable replacement rate from attrition, stable business and economic conditions, stable technological and industrial conditions, predictable population growth, and absence of war, to name just a few. The number of persons currently employed in an occupation may well be the best single statistical indicator of future employment prospects. Technological advancements provide some clues as to larger shifts in employment patterns. The best hedge against obsolescence of one's job qualifications is the flexibility or transferability of one's skills, without the necessity of extensive retraining.

Availability

Another variable is the steadiness of the availability of work. Some occupations, such as construction work, are dependent upon uncontrollable conditions (e.g., the weather). The advent of a guaranteed annual wage may reduce the disadvantages of irregular and seasonal employment.

Self-employment in one's own business provides for independence from supervision but requires greater self-discipline for assurance of success. While the financial rewards of an established, successful business can exceed those of working for others, there are no guarantees of adequate income and many small business attempts fail before the first year ends (see 39.3).

Finally one should be aware of the fringe benefits of the job—paid vacations and holidays, retirement plan, insurance provisions, profit-sharing, bonuses, and opportunities for outside income.

Other Considerations

While all of the above considerations are important in deciding on a career, there are many others. Some of the critical variables in job satisfaction are subjective and may be peculiar to the individual. Intrinsic benefits—such as self-expression, societal contribution, personal development, fulfillment, independence, responsibility and authority or the lack of it—are difficult to describe and assess. Yet such benefits are particularly associated with certain occupations.

While the advantages of occupations have been cited, one must consider the disadvantages as well. Disadvantage is either a lack of an advantageous circumstance (such as opportunity for future advancement) or a negative circumstance (such as boredom or nervous strain). Consideration must be given to both positive and negative circumstances in view of the person's own needs and capabilities.

27.4.6. COUNSELOR CONSIDERATIONS

Beginners especially will sometimes find the task of providing occupational information staggering; clients will ask endlessly different questions and no one could be expected to know the answers to them all. In discussing this issue, Hoppock [1976] first recommended the frank acknowledgment of ignorance, when appropriate. But, Hoppock stated, the magnitude of the problem does not justify a passive attitude toward the information function; it is not a good idea to stop learning and to rely on the library for every answer. Neither should clients be expected to obtain all information for themselves. First of all, in many instances, what the client needs to know is not recorded in writing. Secondly, a great deal of library material is outdated or incorrect. While the library is probably the best single source of occupational material, clients should not be routinely sent to conduct an independent search.

The Big Three

A good approach for the new rehabilitation counselor is to learn as much as possible, become really knowledgeable about, three occupations. These should be selected according to their importance for rehabilitation in the locale: the largest employer of clients, the largest local employer generally, and the employer in which most clients are presently interested. Time spent becoming thoroughly familiar with these three job choices will be time well spent.

Follow-up

It is essential to keep track of what former clients are doing vocationally. Follow-up investigations should be conducted regularly. There is no better way to evaluate the success of the rehabilitation effort. The continuing contact and information about closed cases also help the counselor to keep informed about the local labor market.

27.4.7. MEDIA

The many types of instructional media that can be used to convey occupational information were discussed by Campbell, Walz, Miller, and Kriger, [1973]. Whether the material is in written, audio, audiovisual, or programmed form, it should be selected in accordance with the client's requirements and capabilities.

Written Materials

While print is more prevalent than any other medium, there are drawbacks to the use of written material. Some people have poor reading skills; others are not enthusiastic about reading. In essence, writing is an extremely effective medium but sometimes fails to engage an audience's attention [Havelock, 1969].

Audio Media

Radio and recordings can reach many people simultaneously, can reach people who cannot or do not want to read, and can capture the listener's interest. These media are especially effective if the individuals at whom they are directed have preexisting knowledge of the subject matter.

Audiovisual Media

Films, television, and slide presentations can follow actions taking place. This may be important as a teaching device, as material that the audience can both hear and see is more readily intelligible than that which involves only one sense. For individuals who know little about jobs, the audiovisual medium is sometimes the most efficient way to present facts about occupations.

27.5. Occupational Decision-Making

Making decisions about a prospective career is a difficult and complex process. Clients may need help in overcoming obstacles to decision-making. Self-understanding and adequate knowledge will not automatically enable people to make a logical choice. On the contrary, in vocational rehabilitation arriving at the decision presents the major difficulty. Occupational choice is the end result of a series of decisions in which the individual processes both self-knowledge and occupational data and then arrives at a choice.

27.5.1. FUNDAMENTAL QUESTIONS

Does a person choose an occupation, a place of work, or a career? Should the perspective be on the choice of an occupation when on the average people may have six or more entirely different occupations during a working life? The development of technology and automation creates new jobs and old ones disappear. Lifelong stability is most likely limited to professional occupations, crafts, or clerical jobs. Would it not be better to choose an organization to affiliate with for life—as many industrial workers do in Japan? Up to 85 percent of American workers are employed by organizations. Perhaps it would be best to prepare and place people for life-time participation and relationships in a selected organization (e.g., a particular type of industry, business, or government service). Realistically, career counseling means helping a person to begin a pattern of occupations or to enter an organization for a succession of jobs.

Since career development is a never-ending process it might be thought that career counseling also continues throughout the client's work life. But the purpose of counseling is to make perpetual assistance unnecessary. The objective rather is to initiate successful decision-making, and by extension, a successful career pattern, in an organization (e.g., Postal Service), employment sequence (e.g., electrical work) or in a permanent occupation (e.g., secretary).

27.5.2. IMPLICATIONS OF CHOOSING

There are many reasons why a wise choice of an occupation by the client is important. While the full impact of the decision may not be known for years, an occupational choice influences one's life in various ways: the amount, stability, and assurance of income; the degree of vocational success experienced; the amount of personal satisfaction derived from work; the extent to which one's life is influenced by the work environment and associates; the contribution one makes through work to society; and the experiencing of fulfillment as to purpose in life.

In choosing the vocational objective, it is important for both the counselor and client to be aware of the career implications of the decision. Most clients will be spending upward of twenty years in the labor force. This step gives them the opportunity to engage in meaningful careers. It is suggested here that the counselor must be prepared to assist the client in examining the long-term career implications of possible alternatives during the decision-making process.

27.5.3. THE PROCESS

The skills that are needed in making an occupational choice are very similar to those needed in obtaining employment. For job interviews people must be familiar with their strengths and liabilities. They must know how to get information before they talk to prospective employers and during the interview itself, or the dialogue will probably not be successful. And, people need to make reasonable determinations as they look for work, building on a foundation of self-understanding and learned information. So, it is logical to prepare rehabilitation clients for making an occupational choice and to help them develop the appropriate skills [Dunn, 1974].

Much of what is written on vocational counseling applies mainly to young people starting their careers. Rehabilitation counselors also deal with older clients whose problems are different in some respects. Whether it is necessary in midlife to change career because of either disablement, technological changes, layoff, or other reasons, there are certain commonalities. Generally the choice of a new career should utilize the transferrable knowledge and skills from one's prior training and experience. It is usually best for middle-aged people to avoid revolutionary changes in work patterns if their previous position was satisfying. Moreover, radical changes in life-style produced by a second career may tax their adaptability. The scope of options is superior for broadly educated and experienced individuals who have mastered a variety of tasks.

27.5.4. PROBLEM-SOLVING SEQUENCE

A significant number of client concerns can be translated into problems to be solved or decisions to be made among two or more alternatives. In the context of this chapter, the primary client concern is the client's decision regarding an occupational choice.

The problem-solving and decision-making sequence described by Brammer [1979] can be used to help a client solve a problem or make a decision. It can also be taught to clients so that they can apply the steps without outside help to solve their future problems. Sequentially it is as follows:

1. The individual's involvement is essential because no final decision can otherwise be made. So, the first step is to attain client ability and willingness to engage in the process of self-understanding and problem-solving.
2. The problem must be defined clearly and the goals pinpointed.
3. Alternatives to the obvious answers or decisions are identified.
4. Pertinent information is collected, either through investigation by the client or through verbal explanations, other instructional devices, and tests.
5. The ramifications of the data and the end results of the various choices are investigated.
6. The individual's values should be examined so that priorities become apparent; likes and dislikes, abilities, family situation, social aims, and practical considerations should be discussed.

7. Before the decision is made it is important to review the previous steps; goals, possible choices, and negative and positive results are analyzed again.
8. A choice is made and an appropriate course of action is devised.
9. The whole sequence should be generalized to other circumstances.
10. The chosen alternative is tried out and evaluated at intervals in case the situation changes or relevant new information is discovered.

While this process generally proceeds sequentially when considering specific alternatives it also may recycle through new alternatives suggested by the client-counselor exchange.

A client's choice of occupational objective is the key to the vocational rehabilitation plan and influences its outcome to a great extent. This choice is the culmination of client assessment, the end result of decision-making based on self-knowledge and occupational data. It is the foundation and start of the client's preparation for occupational adjustment through other services such as restoration and training.

27.5.5. TECHNIQUES

The counselor not only conveys information about the client and jobs, but also interprets its meaning in view of situational variables and client perceptions and acceptance. In other words, the counselor provides the bridge for the client's personal understanding of the information. It is a matter of self-concept change and reformation in the counselee. Certain guidelines, given below, may be helpful. These are not inflexible rules, but it is well to consider them in such counseling.

1. The ultimate responsibility for making decisions about career choices belongs to the client.
2. Counselors strive to minimize their own role and to maximize client participation.

3. Client involvement and assertiveness may need to be developed through counseling since many disabled people have been taught to be dependent and avoid making their own decisions.
4. Evaluation procedures should lead to self-understanding and, therefore, should come first—at least before client self-appraisal is finalized.
5. Timing is critical since the final decision in selecting a vocational objective must be held in abeyance pending adequate assessment and vocational exploration.
6. Client readiness for information is sometimes an issue, as it may be dangerous to give unsolicited information too early.
7. Language and concepts must be expressed in ways readily understandable to the client.
8. Information must be presented objectively and neutrally so that the counselor's values and interests do not intercede in the vocational choice.
9. Even though the counselor guards against advice-giving, it is often necessary to help assure that biased influences from others (including occupational information) are exposed.
10. While the client is engaged in self-appraisal the counselor is also collecting data for the vocational assessment. These are concurrent endeavors and not independent. Confirmation is achieved when both counselor and client arrive at the same conclusion.
11. When the client's choice appears to the counselor to be incorrect, the counselor is obliged to continue the collection of information to allow for better self-appraisal by the client. It is not a matter of dissuading a client from a bad decision. Rather, if the counselor is to be a party to a workable plan, consensus is a reasonable basis for collaboration in implementing the service program.

27.6. The Rehabilitation Plan

Once a vocational objective has been decided upon through rehabilitation counseling, a plan of services is necessary to facilitate the goal. A knowledge of the present abilities and potential capacities of the individual is essential in the

development of a rehabilitation service plan. This information in conjunction with facts about the worker characteristics required for effective performance in the chosen occupation is used to determine what services will be needed to bridge the gap between the client's present level and that which will be required for success in the job.

27.6.1. WRITTEN PROGRAM

The rehabilitation plan (or program) is designed for and with a disabled individual as a service strategy for that client. It is mandated according to the 1973 Rehabilitation Act and its ancillary regulations. The Individualized Written Rehabilitation Program, IWRP as it is called, is initiated at the certification of eligibility for rehabilitation services. It is a separate part of the case record and can be amended by the counselor and client at any time. The IWRP must document:

1. Financial responsibilities for the services to be provided.
2. Counselor and client responsibilities in the rehabilitation process.
3. The long-term vocational goal and intermediate objectives toward that goal.
4. Services to be provided.
5. Criteria and procedures for evaluating progress.
6. Annual review for as long as the case is open.
7. Closure information, such as the reason for closure, employment status, and type of job.
8. Postemployment services, if these are planned at the time of closure.

These components are the essence of an organized, purposeful rehabilitation plan. Its development requires careful planning and considerable time, more so because of the disabled person's involvement in the planning process.

There are three important tasks in rehabilitation plan formation. The first is to determine what obstacles stand in the way of occupational effectiveness and what must be done to decrease or remove these obstacles. In order to do this, knowledge of the client's capabilities and needs and of available resources is necessary. Then the client must learn about these obstacles and the ways in which they can be cleared away. Frequently clients will show opposition to suggested services; this opposition must be handled immediately so that it does not interfere with progress later or cause the client to leave. The third step is setting up a schedule that provides for evaluation of success at definite points; this is for the client's use in adjusting the program as necessary. While the schedule is frequently

overlooked, it is very important. A problem in rehabilitation case service planning is that frequently it is difficult for clients to understand themselves, especially in a long, complex program; this has a serious effect on motivation. By means of carefully designed schedules, clients can tell what will take place and for how long, and they can later evaluate their accomplishments.

27.6.2. GUIDELINES FOR FORMULATION

The formulation of the plan is a process the client must understand and be involved in. It should be agreed that the program adequately meets the requirements of the client, that the chosen means are suitable, that the help of relatives and other resources will be incorporated into the effort. The rehabilitation plan per se is the written description of the particular means by which the client will be helped toward adjustment goals. Several guidelines should be applied in this formulation of a plan of services, as explained by Thomason and Barrett [1959].

Completeness and Comprehensiveness as to Kinds and Number of Services
The comprehensive rehabilitation plan consists of all the measures that will be taken to help the client attain rehabilitation goals, from determining the vocational objective to its attainment. The more immediate activities will obviously be covered most thoroughly. Almost every plan, however complete, must have explanatory material added to it later, but segments of plans, dealing with only small parts of the whole, are not adequate. The formulation should encompass all aspects of the program.

Amount of Detail as to the Execution of the Plan
The formulated program is composed of all services that are indicated for equipping the client for achievement of long-term vocational and life adjustment objectives. A given rehabilitation agency either offers the necessary services or coordinates the provision of these services with other participating facilities. The plan should include any course of action indicated, but, if it does not, the reasons for the omission(s) should be stated.

Justification of Services
The provisions of the plan need to be justified, in terms of the client's requirements and the

agency's guidelines for services. As a separate document for the record, the plan states explicitly that its components will answer to the requirements of the client and will help the individual progress toward the chosen vocational goal; that the plan is in keeping with agency guidelines; and that the program involves a "substantial service" expected to lead to rehabilitation.

If counseling is the only kind of service to be included, the plan should make explicit the kinds of difficulties the client is having, the specific measures that will be taken, and the ways in which they will facilitate resolution of the problem. The rationale behind the choice of each service and activity should be stated. Agency policy will dictate the format of the plan and will determine how particularized each statement of the plan must be.

Any time an important alteration is made, the plan should reflect this through additions or revisions. But, the plan should not be changed solely because of additional information.

Provision of Services

During rehabilitation, clients get the assistance they need in order to proceed satisfactorily through the program. The best service resource for each provision of the plan is chosen. If the client's needs are physical, appropriate professions or facilities are selected in accordance with agency criteria and client wishes. Likewise, services such as training and/or equipment are contracted for with careful attention to appropriateness and client desires.

When a client goes away for training, it is important to keep in close touch with the personnel involved. Practical problems should be worked out with the training facility on a cooperative basis. The same holds true for clients undergoing physical restoration. Close monitoring and additional facilitation enable the objectives of the plan to be carried out; for instance, it may be necessary to provide transportation or equipment that was not initially anticipated. The plan should be revised as new information suggests the need.

In personal interviews with the client, specific developments with relation to service provisions and delivery are discussed and evaluated as appropriate. In this way possible difficulties can be foreseen and their development prevented. Any breakdown of the plan is immediately discernible; remedial steps are then taken promptly to assure achievement of the planned vocational objective.

Chapter 28

Personal Adjustment

It is not within the province of this book to describe psychotherapy, which is a responsibility of other professions (i.e., psychiatry and clinical psychology). However, rehabilitation counselors must deal with a variety of human reactions that often interfere with their client's vocational adjustment. These various reactions and life adjustments are interrelated and may at times be best attended to by the rehabilitation counselor. When there is a deep and disabling emotional problem, however, the rehabilitation agency refers the client to a psychotherapist. Rehabilitation counselors are unprepared to deal with the intensive personality restructuring required in the therapy of emotionally disturbed individuals, but they must recognize such disablement. Moreover, rehabilitation counselors are partners on the mental health team and require professional knowledge of this role.

The function of personal adjustment counseling is traditional in rehabilitation counseling with the physically as well as the emotionally disabled. It predates even the emergence of rehabilitation counseling education (RCE). Despite lack of training in psychology, rehabilitation personnel had to cope with their clients' negative reactions to disability, this being seen as a necessary function to achieve vocational goals. In the 1960s, however, many RCE programs overemphasized counseling for personal-emotional adjustment—the therapeutic role—at the expense of instruction in counseling for vocational objectives. And for a number of years after RCE programs started, students were generally more interested in working with psychiatric cases than with the physically disabled. But, by the 1970s there was better balance of interest, and owing to a matured professional identity, rehabilitation counseling in

personal adjustment matters was in good perspective. Personal adjustment counseling is now generally regarded as an adjunct to rehabilitation professional service.

This chapter provides a description of some of the common client reactions and problems that rehabilitation counselors encounter as well as some of the techniques to use with clients when they show these reactions. Also described are the more severe adjustment problems, the human abnormalities requiring psychotherapy.

28.1. Motivation Problems

Motivation refers to the internal and external factors that account for differences in the nature, intensity, and direction of behavior [Barry & Malinovsky, 1965]. The internal conditions are an individual's capabilities, personal characteristics, knowledge, and the like, as well as sense of values, opinions, and self-image. External factors are barriers (social, physical, financial) that stand in the way of action or inhibit incentive.

28.1.1. CONCEPTUAL FRAMEWORK

The highly complicated nature of motivation is recognized. In working with clients one must be aware that extrinsic and intrinsic forces are interacting in a powerful way to affect clients' behavior. Insufficient motivation in handicapped clients is seen as common and is usually treated as a counseling problem. In many cases, however, what appears to be lack of motivation in reality are barriers to motivation—obstacles that prevent the client from trying.

Motivation as it applies specifically to the rehabilitation client must be considered in its dynamic context. This is to say that to deal with the motivation of the rehabilitation client, one should be concerned with interconnections between personal relationships and the social system the individual comes from. Consequently it is necessary to be sensitive to the meaning of a rehabilitation program for relatives and for other people who influence the client. Awareness of social interactions helps in appraising the dynamics of a client's motivation. When the pressures and barriers of the social systems involved are understood, it is possible to

strengthen the positive elements and decrease the negative influences [U.S. IRS, 1963].

28.1.2. EXPLANATIONS

Observable behavior is frequently taken to reflect motivation; in other words, it may seem that whether or not a client is motivated will be somewhat obvious. Against this traditional view, however, is one that distinguishes between an individual's desire (to work, for instance) and the attempt to obtain a desired goal. For various reasons people may not try to achieve objectives they actually do believe are desirable.

Several points made by Deitchman and McHargue [1973] should be considered in working with clients who seem "unmotivated." First, clients sometimes fail to work toward goals because they are apprehensive or anxious about taking a chance. Anxiety is not unusual in people who are contemplating some untried course of action that involves risk and uncertainty. Clients who have feelings of inadequacy, who lack confidence in their capacity to become self-reliant or to make decisions, will tend to prefer the security of the status quo. They will not usually embark on a course of action they feel will throw them on their own resources with no one else to help. When doing new things or merely contemplating changes such as a new training program or placement, unknown people and places, and the like, such individuals may feel great anxiety.

People can be helped to face risks in a variety of ways. A rehabilitation plan that consists of very slight changes, to be made one at a time, can be devised. The client receives help and encouragement while taking these steps; none of them seems too unsafe but each constitutes progress toward the final objective. At the same time the client can be taught what behaviors are suitable in different circumstances and what can be anticipated in novel situations; this will enhance feelings of adequacy. Role-playing employment interviews, sheltered work, on-the-job evaluation and training, and structured social situations can diminish apprehension. An effective strategy is to focus on the attempting itself rather than the outcome. For instance, the rehabilitation counselor would reward the client for arranging and going through an interview with a prospective employer, regardless of how the interview turns out. The trying behavior may signify real progress; the counselor can stress the idea that one failure is not as significant as the apprehensive client may think.

A second factor that keeps some clients from trying is a sense that their lives are dominated by external forces. In contrast to the belief that people shape their lives through their own industry, energy, self-fulfillment, and accomplishment, there is the notion, which some people have learned, that people's destinies are mainly the product of forces beyond their control. This idea may have its roots in a certain social background, for instance, a family with very authoritarian parents. But however they have come to believe it, clients who feel this way are not likely to exert the effort needed for making major alterations in their lives. They may need to be shown how they actually could change their ability to cope with their life situation. In the rehabilitation plan, provision should be made for equipping such a client with increased personal and vocational skills so that desired achievements can be anticipated.

Another cause of low motivation, one which may overlap with the others, relates to the idea of "payoff." Some people who do not seem to be trying to reach desired goals believe that they are getting a better payoff from their present behavior. The likelihood is that most people will try to change if the prize is valuable enough. Generally people will not work toward change unless they believe that the new behavior will be more positive (e.g., more enjoyable) or less negative (unenjoyable) than their present mode of conduct. This may apply to vocational behaviors. Payoff might be financial but is usually

intangible. Clients who feel that the process will cause too much apprehension, for instance, or who believe that a given rehabilitation goal may endanger their welfare support, may not respond to the opportunity for change.

The right payoff is difficult to determine because its appeal depends upon the person. For this reason it is useful to discuss with clients the incentive considerations in formulating the rehabilitation plan. The counselor, for instance, could do this with a dependent, institutionalized individual who resists rehabilitation because it seems to mean that help and security will be taken away. Planning could provide for a community living environment in a residential facility, which would lessen anxiety and offer the client needed emotional support; at the same time the client could be assured of other available help in the community. Generally, clients must see the payoff in a rehabilitation plan.

28.1.3. SOLUTIONS

The following are some general approaches in the effective management of clients who seem to be unmotivated. They are the result of three regional mental health training conferences sponsored by the Florida Division of Vocational Rehabilitation and were explained by Deitchman and McHargue [1973].

Client Investment

Sometimes the client is asked to make an investment in the rehabilitation plan; this makes undercutting the effort or dropping out more difficult. Active participation of the client is feasible from the beginning, as decisions are made and information is obtained [Kravetz & Thomas, 1978]. The client should select which (approved) physician will do the physical examination and find out what training programs have openings. The individual takes on more responsibility and gets less direction as the program evolves. The amount of work and time invested by clients must relate, obviously, to their physical and mental abilities and maturity.

Services as a Contingency

Some of the problems that arise with extremely dependent or resistant clients can be prevented by a contract that specifies obligations and relationships between the agency and the client (see 29.3.3). This may make it more unlikely that the individual will try to thwart the effort. Instead of the agency's continuing to offer services regardless of what the client does—an unrealistic situation anyway—services become contingent upon the client's actions. The rehabilitationist, however, should be quite assertive in insisting that clients fulfill their contractual obligations; a passive posture by the professional results in premature closure of potentially successful cases.

Setting Subgoals

Many times rehabilitation clients need to improve their understanding and adaptation with respect to job interviews, personal appearance, occupational behaviors, handling of money, social adjustment at work, and the like. While their final objective is to obtain appropriate employment, they must acquire these capabilities first. It may be necessary to select a number of subgoals before expecting a client to handle a job; if job placement is too big a step, success is not likely. The subgoals are selected to fit the client's disability and present capacities, so that each separate achievement will represent success and progress toward the ultimate goal.

Setting Time Limits

In somewhat the same way, time can be analyzed and divided up. Together the rehabilitationist and the client estimate how long the entire program and each of its steps should take, again considering the present level of functioning. Establishing time boundaries is particularly appropriate with clients who have been through several different kinds of programs to no avail and who have been working without such limits. The element of time can be dealt with when the contract is first formulated.

It is important to note that time schedules, like other components of the client's rehabilitation program, must be individualized. A recently or catastrophically disabled applicant may need substantial time and help by the rehabilitation counselor in the personal adjustment phase before arranging for purchased or other services. The agency policy should not dictate the time frame of the individual's plan.

Assessing Assets

Sometimes rehabilitation clients have been through the assessment process more than once. They have been told the nature of their pathology and the severity of their handicap, and sometimes their self-concept has been weak-

ened. It is important to deemphasize the negative aspects of a client's condition and to ascertain what this individual is able to do, perhaps pinpointing the skills that will be needed for coping in a job. It is especially important to remember that one problem some disabled people have results from mistaken notions and invalid judgments about their capacities and limitations as well as from erroneous ideas about the world and ways of dealing with it effectively.

Family cooperation may be essential in the motivational process (see 31.2.1). If relatives are an important part of the client's life, they have the power to further rehabilitation or undermine it. If the family is brought in early, the likelihood of various kinds of later difficulties is diminished.

28.1.4. COUNSELING TECHNIQUES

The First Institute on Rehabilitation Services addressed the concept of motivation in their *Training Guides in Motivation for Vocational Rehabilitation Staff* [U.S. IRS, 1963]. Some of their suggestions to rehabilitation workers are paraphrased below:

Accept the fact that there are no simple formulas either for understanding the concept of motivation or for dealing actively with it in a specific case.

Continually make, test, and evaluate assumptions and inferences.

Identify and then deal with barriers to movement toward goals.

Probe for the real problem of clients as distinguished from the presenting ones.

Develop suitable alternatives with clients and do not lose interest in the case when the client fails to follow through.

Recognize the numerous factors within the rehabilitation agency that affect motivation.

Help clients to understand themselves and to recognize their self-worth and assets.

It was also suggested that in dealing with clients who have a problem in motivation, counselors should ask themselves the following questions.

Have I gone beyond the surface facts and come to know this client in some depth?

Do I know the client's aspirations and problems? Are the problems presented the real ones?

What pressures—positive and negative—are there on the client (wife, mother, lawyer, doctor, and so on)? Is this person entrapped in pressures from another system (e.g., insurance benefits)?

Can I and the services of my agency help this client within a reasonable period or would another agency be of more value in this case?

Have I helped this person to develop and understand suitable alternatives?

Why is it that I am not able to deal with this case effectively and what can I do to correct these reasons?

What is the client really saying? What clues can help me to understand the client better?

Am I working too fast with the client?

What are the barriers to case movement toward the goal of work?

To what types of incentives and values has this person responded in the past?

28.2. *Reluctance Reaction*

Reluctance on the part of clients is met with in every phase of counseling and rehabilitation, and it shows up in many different ways. People sometimes will not talk at all, sometimes they will only nod their heads or shrug their shoulders, in other words, barely respond. Reluctance is also expressed when clients try to outguess the counselor and say only what they think the counselor expects to hear. An extremely eager and pleasant demeanor, the habit of evading important topics, and silliness can manifest reluctance. Other behaviors that can indicate reluctance are defensiveness, unwillingness to talk about oneself, and denial that help is needed [Vriend & Dyer, 1973]. A dynamically different client reaction, hostility, discussed later, has the same repercussions as other forms of uncooperativeness in counseling.

28.2.1. COUNSELING TECHNIQUES

Benner, Burke, and Miller [1976] outlined a four-step method of dealing with reluctance: showing concern, showing awareness, rearrangement, and evaluation. In the first step, one expresses concern by describing the counselor's functions, emphasizing confidentiality, detailing one's role, and explaining what is expected of the client.

The next step is to enhance awareness of the reluctance, to recognize the reaction and accept it. The counselor explains that one purpose of the discussion is to look into the causes of the reluctance and to examine ways of helping the client understand it. The here-and-now technique may be useful in getting at the reasons the client is reluctant and facing them directly. Direct decision methods and various problem-raising and problem-solving tactics are suitable.

Next it is necessary to rearrange the factors that have produced the reluctance by examining the reaction with the client. The reasons for evading a difficult situation and the methods of evasion are dealt with outright.

Another technique is to concentrate on what is reinforcing reluctance, without explicitly mentioning the behavior itself. The question can be raised whether individuals close to the client, in an institutional setting or at home, are strengthening reluctant attitudes. The answer may emerge if the client is asked to talk in detail about daily routines, people, and incidents that might have this effect. These influences then can be examined and the client may see that other individuals and various events play a role in shaping attitudes of avoidance.

The reluctance can be confronted head-on. One explains outright how the client appears to be shying away from difficult situations and what this reluctance consists of. Confronting may include one of the following or a combination of these methods.

1. Naming and explaining the significance of "games" the client is playing. Some common games are maintaining an ambiguous attitude (responding with "I guess," "maybe," and so on); playing stupid (answering with "I don't know"); playing helpless; seeking pity; placing responsibility on other people ("That makes me feel . . ."); being a reactor (responding as though one were the pawn of chance or external happenings).
2. Analyzing techniques that the client is using to impede or distort communication. Some of these are interrupting or switching the subject, speaking for another person, and speaking inaudibly.
3. Pointing out the oppositional style of a client who tends to respond negatively by saying

things like "No, that isn't it" and "Yes, but . . .", or who uses negative body language such as head shakes, tapping of feet, and so on.

As a last resort one may purposely insult and criticize the client. This is a hazardous technique, however, because an individual's reaction cannot be anticipated or regulated. Moreover the relationship may be ruined. Even if the technique stimulates the client to change, the changes may not be desirable.

Finally, appraisal of the intensity of the client's reluctance should always be taking place. If the techniques being used are not lessening the behavior, a return to the concern step or the acknowledgment step may be indicated.

28.2.2. SILENCE

Silence on the part of the counselee can be a difficult thing to deal with. Those working with the individual may feel rejected, opposed, or thwarted by the silence, but it is important to see the silence for what it is and not to respond as if being personally attacked. People may be silent because they resent what they consider to be probing. They may view the counselor as an authority figure to be put down or avoided, or they may simply not be ready to reveal what is on their minds. It should be noted that the client will usually be able to keep silent longer than the professional worker.

Demonstrating acceptance of this resistance may be an effective way of breaking the silence. One might say, "I don't mind the silence, but I feel you are resenting me in some way. I wish you would tell me about it so we can discuss it together." Another suggestion for breaking a silence is to begin talking in a way that does not involve the client, gradually involving the person in nonthreatening questions. The following steps provide an example.

1. Talking about the agency and about what rehabilitation may mean to the client.
2. Asking questions that require only a yes or no answer, or a nod of the head as an answer.

3. When the client responds to the above, beginning to ask more open-ended questions, such as "What kind of job would you like to have?"
4. Remaining patient and not rushing the conversation, as this may only make the client more anxious.

28.2.3. HOSTILITY

A client may be hostile for a number of reasons, such as being referred to the agency in the first place or having a disability. Hostility may be expressed during a counseling session by verbal outbursts, or by nonverbal cues such as grimaces, frowns, and voice quality. People express hostility overtly by failing to show up for appointments, being late for them, dismissing the counselor, and refusing agency services.

Techniques for Handling Hostile Client Reactions

Four steps can be taken in an attempt to initiate a working relationship with a hostile client. First, one acknowledges and reflects the client's hostility by saying, in a matter-of-fact, uncritical manner, something like "Maybe you feel angry about the fact that you are here."

The next step is to express acceptance of the way the client feels, by making a statement such as "I don't like being told what to do either." Third, one takes an open-minded approach to the subject of the client's need for help rather than speaking as though the need were self-evident. The subject can be handled as an open question and the client invited to tell about apparent problems. Finally, when enough information has been revealed, the possible usefulness of counseling can be suggested, in an understated way. It might help to mention another individual with the same kinds of problems who found a satisfactory job after working with rehabilitation personnel.

To resolve hostility a client must be able to admit the hostility, identify its sources, and understand its causes. Only after this is done can the hostility be faced realistically.

28.3. Dependence Reaction

Rehabilitation can often serve as a way of taking clients out of their dependency mode and placing them in a more adaptive position in life. Individuals who have excessive dependency needs are frequently overtly cooperative, but being both dependent and angry, they will often sabotage agency efforts. The dependency seemingly produces either passivity or hostility.

Goldin and Perry [1967] dealt with dependency in detail in their notable monograph, *Dependency and Its Implication for Rehabilitation*. Their discussion, which is related in this section, shows dependency to be a complicated and critical problem in rehabilitation. Overlooking dependent reactions may be interpreted by the client as rejection; on the other hand, merely accepting this behavior may encourage dependency and interfere with the rehabilitation goal of independence.

Regression into dependency is a well-known concomitant of most illnesses and disabilities, and severe disablement often drives a person into unhealthy dependence not only on family and professionals who try to help, but also on the society at large. Therefore, in bringing a disabled individual out of dependency, rehabilitation accomplishes two very important goals. The client is able to attain greater self-sufficiency and thus life enjoyment; and the rehabilitation becomes a method of contributing socially and economically to society as a whole.

Client dependency is an obstacle that must be overcome in vocational rehabilitation as well as independent living rehabilitation. For this reason it is absolutely necessary for those who participate in the rehabilitation of disabled people to learn as much as they can about dependency and the reactions associated with it.

Goldin and Perry analyzed dependency from the standpoint of the social, emotional, financial, institutional, and psychomedical stimuli that apparently induce it. This approach lets rehabilitationists consider manipulating the environment in a therapeutically beneficial way so that they can use counseling to clarify a client's excessive dependency needs within a given social context. As a prime example, rehabilitation workers are better equipped to plan counseling strategies if they understand the manifest differences between the dependency occurring in the institutionalized client and the dependency seen in the welfare recipient living in the community.

28.3.1. SOCIAL DEPENDENCY

Working from the premise that some degree of dependency is necessary for human development, one must ascertain when dependency ceases to be a positive aspect of growth and becomes a hindrance. The threshold is different for different people, as it is linked to the development of personality and functional abilities and also to the circumstances that surround each individual. Dependency as it influences personality positively and negatively is also related to the individual's acceptance of disability: people who accept their disabilities as not devaluating may be more willing to accept needed help from other people. In rehabilitation it is well understood that some clients think any assistance (dependency) is a sign of inferiority. When a person feels this way, counseling must be aimed at helping the individual learn that such reliance upon others is not a weakness.

As a result of opposing feelings about dependency, it is common for people to avoid facing their real needs and to present a self-reliant exterior. Rehabilitation clients will sometimes refuse to admit their dependent feelings, take a distorted view of their functional limitations, and select inappropriate vocational objectives.

Understanding

Social dependency may occur because people feel that they do not belong or because they are apprehensive about handling unfamiliar situations. It may also come from feelings of antagonism or anxiety. A socially dependent person perceives anyone whose position seems to be authoritarian, or anyone associated with an authoritarian organization, with mistrust, so that a professional worker or employee of a state agency might be regarded in the same way as a law enforcement officer.

The mode of the socially dependent individual is a kind of withdrawal from the rest of the world. These people find normal social activity too much to handle, so they are always asking others to help them in these interactions. It is not uncommon for physically or mentally disabled people to become social dependents.

Intervention Techniques

Dealing with the dependent individual can call for extreme tactics. Sometimes such a client must be directed through the first steps of the rehabilitation effort. As the process goes on the individual should be helped to outgrow the need for the intervention of others in interactions with staff members. Typically the client will oppose this effort and make it more arduous, but as independence is gained the opposition will lessen. The strategy should consist of providing some of the needed help while at the same time putting pressure on the client to handle some situations alone. The use of force is not appropriate, however, since it will accentuate the client's feelings of apprehension and may make any change impossible. Instead the client is taught, through the use of rewards and other psychological principles, to increase independent efforts. The change will not be rapid or dramatic, however.

One of the principal difficulties in working with socially dependent individuals is that progress is so gradual. However, if the working relationship is good, progress will be made. It should be remembered that socially dependent people have been injured not in just a few relationships but generally in their whole social life. Progress means their becoming part of the rest of the social world for the first time.

28.3.2. EMOTIONAL DEPENDENCY

Emotional dependency differs from social dependency since it occurs most frequently among family members and usually results from one member's neurotic behavior. In some cases, it is a striving to satisfy unfulfilled needs for affection and nurturance; in other cases it is a conscious or unconscious expression of hostility toward the person who is the target of dependent demands.

Understanding

Emotional dependency can be critical to the rehabilitation plan, since significant members of the family are highly important in motivating the client either positively or negatively. In particular, family attitudes toward a client's dependent strivings can profoundly influence motivation toward self-help. Overprotective relatives, for instance, might intensify the apprehension to the extent that the client is unwilling to do what is necessary for rehabilitation. At the other extreme, relatives who cannot understand that the dependent behavior is not unusual may take a harsh approach and try to force the client into independence.

Identification

Emotionally dependent people continually lean on others for emotional support. Some need it as a more or less steady diet in order to conduct their lives at all effectively; others feel the need only in particular situations, a man might rely on his wife to handle all of the family's monetary affairs.

Intervention Techniques

The task of decreasing emotional dependency in rehabilitation clients is a difficult one because the behavior is strongly influenced by relationships with relatives. Sometimes this kind of dependency, although very difficult to eliminate, can be redirected. If the dependency of a man on his wife is quite intense, for instance, the wife can be taught how to encourage her husband to engage in certain activities without her. The husband's dependent needs will still be satisfied, but he may be able to act on his own with regard to aspects of his rehabilitation.

28.3.3. FINANCIAL DEPENDENCY

Financial dependency is almost always associated with other pathological conditions—illness, disability, and so forth. Sometimes it has a basis in inadequate educational opportunities or other disadvantagement.

Understanding

A high incidence of family stress seems to exist in families that are financially dependent and families in which the provider of support is disabled; it is not understood whether the financial dependency has produced the stress or vice versa. In rehabilitation it is understood that efforts to provide financially dependent clients with opportunity must go hand in hand with an effort to increase their motivation [Goldin, Perry, Margolin, & Stotsky, 1972].

Identification

Various methods of categorizing financially dependent people have been proposed. Traditionally, however, people who have received assistance from one or more welfare organizations for an extended period are categorized as being chronically dependent.

Intervention Techniques

When a rehabilitation client is financially dependent, counseling outcome may be affected adversely. The extraordinary emotional needs of the financially dependent person make the helping relationship difficult to maintain. These clients often make heavy demands on the time of rehabilitation counselors.

28.3.4. INSTITUTIONAL DEPENDENCY

The rehabilitation of disabled people may begin in different kinds of hospitals, residential centers, and various institutions. Institutional dependency complicates the rehabilitation process. (See 5.7.)

Understanding

According to Goffman [1964] institutions have four common elements: (1) life in its totality is carried on in one location under a single authority; (2) all elements of the daily routine of an individual are conducted among a large group of people who all receive the same treatment; (3) there is a strict schedule, everything is done at a fixed time, and the entire routine is determined by the authorities; and (4) the components of daily life have been designed to fit together into a program that will fulfill the mission of the institution.

Many influences of institutional life accentuate people's dependent feelings. They know, for example, that whatever they do, the bare necessities will be provided. Furthermore, the organization of daily life discourages individuality and creativity, and sometimes people who express skepticism about official policies are looked upon as troublemakers.

In addition to the dependency imposed by the social structure of the institution, the residents (inmates or patients) are also prey to feelings of personal inadequacy because they know that they are institutionalized because of some defect or inability to function outside the institution's walls. They know they are deviant, even if temporarily so, from what is considered normal by society.

Intervention Techniques

Rehabilitation work with dependent individuals in institutions can proceed more satisfactorily if the tremendous impact of the institution's social organization on the client is recognized. While the institution itself will remain essentially the same, it is possible to enter into the client's relationship with it and arrange with staff members to encourage more autonomy in the individual. Programs that involve clients in the world outside the institution can prepare them to move into it when the time comes. To provide this sort of preparation the facility should be an integral part of the community and of the system of services within it.

When deinstitutionalization was instituted by state governments in the 1970s, severely disabled residents of large mental hospitals were returned

to (or retained in) their community for care. Special efforts were and are made to find satisfactory, even useful activity in small housing units for mentally ill or retarded people who formerly were sent—often for life—to a big, custodial "hospital" removed from society.

28.3.5. PSYCHOMEDICAL DEPENDENCY

Psychomedical dependent behavior is caused by physical illness or disability; its foundation is in reality when the individual is actually incapable of autonomy. Ill or disabled people are dependent by necessity and they typically regress for a certain length of time. But the extent and duration of the regression usually relate to how self-reliant the individual was before onset and how significant others view the situation. A normal and symptomatic phenomenon, psychomedical dependency should be viewed as an element of the disabled person's condition. At the same time, other people's attitudes and responses to it have an important effect on the individual's recuperation and on the progress of rehabilitation.

Understanding and Identification

Important advances have been made in the past two decades with regard to the management of dependency in disabled people. The most notable contribution may have been the idea that dependency can have positive value. Coburn [1963] suggested that in our society self-reliance has been overemphasized and dependence associated too strongly with failure. As a result people who are dependent because of disability think of themselves as worthless and unwanted. It is perhaps the case instead that independence is of questionable value and often destructive.

Dependency, Havens [1963] maintained, is functional in that everyone participates in a vast system of dependent interrelationships. For clients to be helped, dependency must exist.

Because dependent behavior is associated with many illnesses, those who work with rehabilitation clients must know what dependent reactions accompany various kinds of disability. Severely disabled adults who must rely on others for their physical needs frequently experience a sense of helplessness like that of a child, and this can result in discord. People whose past social adjustment has been good can use their former coping methods to guide them in adapting to new life circumstances. In doing so they associate rehabilitation personnel with the adults—parents, teachers, and so on—who had a significant impact on their early growth. In progressing through each stage they experience a renewed sense of dependency. They must recognize that this feeling is natural in order to progress toward full rehabilitation.

People who have obvious and unattractive disabilities may experience dependency more intensely because their handicap is conspicuous and their self-image is altered (see 5.5.l). As a consequence of this, people sometimes cannot come to terms with dependency; while in other cases the reliant behavior becomes excessive since the reason for it is so evident. Other difficulties arise because such individuals feel that they are set apart socially from nondisabled people. They may try to make up for this by behaving in an extremely dependent or demanding manner.

In severely debilitated individuals dependency may result from their inability to do the things nondisabled people can do (see 5.13). But since their limitation in function may not be obvious they frequently hesitate to rely on someone else; they may be torn between the wish to demonstrate independence and the need to ask for help. The fact that cardiac and other debilitating disabilities are not apparent contributes to the problem of acceptance on the part of the individual and makes the rehabilitation task more challenging.

Rehabilitation of mentally ill persons is particularly difficult, partly because of the strong dependency engendered by a prolonged and sheltered stay at a mental hospital (see 5.7), and partly because of the discrimination that such people experience in the community when independent living is attempted. In addition to these difficulties, it is frequently true that mentally ill individuals had been excessively dependent even before the onset of illness (see 5.8). For all these reasons, dependency in such cases is a very serious problem.

Dependence in the chronically ill is a very important issue in rehabilitation. For some, dependent behavior stands in the way of remunerative work; for others, it even prevents efforts toward independent living. In preparing people to live on their own, rehabilitation is assuming an increasingly important role, both because of its value to the client and also because of its economic advantages.

Dependency in chronically ill people is protracted; this puts caregivers under special pressure and makes the behavior more difficult to deal with. Extremely dependent or domineering behavior is frequently a vehicle for expressing disappointment and frustration, especially in aged people who have chronic impairments.

Intervention Techniques

Rehabilitation for highly dependent handicapped individuals must be tailored not only to their present psychological environment but also to the developmental aspects of their dependency. Counseling is of fundamental importance because rarely does the person know how to cope with the dependent behavior. The helping relationship provides a threat-free psychosocial situation in which the client can prepare to face and cope with feelings and problems that will occur when the stresses of the community at large are confronted.

The chronically ill person's behavioral style —mandated inactivity, physical dependency, decreased responsibility—may become an ingrained feature of life. Goldin and Perry [1967] set forth guidelines for counteracting extreme dependency.

1. Dependency must be viewed as a normal by-product of disability, and clients must be helped to understand that it has its foundation in reality. They can thus begin to accept this behavior, learn to stop blaming themselves for it, and work to reconcile opposing feelings about dependent needs.

2. Those who work with these clients should make clear that they believe dependency can be decreased. Clients will tend to adopt this positive attitude. A realistic sense of what can really be accomplished, however, should be maintained. Usually the dependent person will put up some opposition to the idea of working toward greater self-reliance because it will entail some risk; fundamental emotional needs and security must be provided for. The process of gaining independence does cause some fear because the end results cannot be anticipated, but clients derive support from the helping relationship.

3. When, with the help of others, the client can handle increased apprehension, various aspects of dependency can be explained: for instance, its roots in personal adjustment patterns, social relationships, and so on.

4. The client, with help, decides what course of action will be best in striving toward self-sufficiency. A sheltered workshop, for instance, may provide the best environment for lessening dependency.

The families of disabled individuals should participate in the struggle toward independence; this is essential when relatives are contributing in some way to the dependency. Sometimes relatives foster dependency because they are afraid that the client's physical or mental well-being will be threatened by increased independence. When this is the case, telling the family the facts will often set things straight. Sometimes, however, when family members encourage the individual to remain dependent it is because they have serious emotional difficulties that need to be addressed. (See 31.2.)

Independent living techniques that enable the person to perform the tasks necessary for self-care are, of course, basic to solving such problems of dependency. Counseling is one of the techniques that facilitate a life of independence for the severely disabled population. Other techniques for independent living are described in Chapter 40.

28.4. *Effects of Crises*

A crisis is definable as a turning point in a person's life, resulting from a decision or event, and marked by either sharp improvement or sharp deterioration of great psychological significance. Brammer [1979] expanded on this concept, stating that in a situation of crisis the individual confronts the idea that major life objectives are in jeopardy, or encounters severe disturbances in the passage of life and usual ways of handling stress. The word *crisis* normally refers to the response to the disturbance rather than to the disturbance itself. Periods of crisis typically last no longer than a few weeks.

Various kinds of crises can be distinguished. Having a baby or having children leave home are natural developmental crises. Situational crises occur when one suffers a great loss: the death of someone loved, loss of a job. Existential crises, Brammer said, are the reactions people have when they confront "the significant human issues of purpose, responsibility, freedom, and commitment" [p. 104]. These experiences are natural but they become real crises when they cause people to question their usual assumptions and consider new choices. When these situations do not eventuate in creative action and positive solutions, the emotional cost is great. People can lose their sense of involvement and purpose, lose hope, and break down completely.

A disabled person must cope not only with the crises that are encountered in everyday life but also with those related to the disability. This means that rehabilitation counseling involves helping clients cope with crisis situations. For example, a crisis may occur when a client is trying to adjust to a newly acquired disability, facing the prospect of looking for another job, or planning to enter a workshop. According to Carkhuff [1969], helping in a crisis is the essence of helping. A crisis state can be an opportunity for the client to reach higher levels of personal functioning if it is encountered fully and if resources are used to resolve it.

It is important to distinguish between crises that have disrupted a well-integrated client from those that accompany a chaotic life-style. A client whose crises are a result of a chronically chaotic life can usually not be helped in a short period of time and often requires some form of therapy. Those who work in a rehabilitation setting will more likely have to deal with a crisis in a client who, until recently, had been progressing along well in the rehabilitation process.

Obviously when clients are in a crisis or are depressed or suicidal, they will not be functioning adequately at their jobs or will not be progressing well in the rehabilitation process. It is at these times that it becomes necessary to intervene.

28.4.1. INTERVENTION TECHNIQUES

According to Carkhuff [1969], specific steps can be followed in working with a client experiencing a crisis. These crisis intervention techniques include:

1. Making contact with the client on a feeling

level; identifying the client's feelings and accepting them. Reflecting the feelings can be helpful.

2. Exploring the crisis in the here and now; focusing on the last six weeks of the client's life and identifying events, situations, or persons that may have precipitated the crisis. Open-ended questions at this time will encourage the client to do the talking. Clients should be asked to be concrete and specific in their descriptions.

3. Summarizing the problem to the client so that its definition and main elements can be agreed upon.

4. Focusing on specific areas of the problem that are causing the client immediate difficulties—the areas most likely to give positive results after immediate action.

5. Exploring resources. Clients are asked what they have done so far about the crisis, what they wish to do, what they are afraid to do, what they have done in similar situations, whom they have talked with, and, whom they would like to talk with.

6. Suggesting alternative resources after talking with the client.

7. Planning together some kind of action; specifying what the person can do, what others will do; specifying goals.

Brammer also offered guidelines that may help to alleviate the stress clients feel during periods of crisis. First, one depends primarily on the positive quality of the relationship for supportive reassurance rather than on verbal reassurances. Second, stress can be reduced through verbal encouragement, specifically stating facts and predicting outcomes. That is, words are used to assure clients about the consequences of their actions or feelings, to lessen stress and build confidence. "You are competent," "You will solve your problem," or "You will feel better" are reassuring comments. Eye contact is important in every effort at reassurance; it expresses empathy and understanding. Touching can be very comforting but should be used discreetly because of the wide variety of responses it may elicit. A third guideline relates to the physical tension that usually accompanies stress. A direct method of inducing comfort is to reduce muscle tension through relaxation techniques.

Brammer also discussed the importance of building hope. Hopelessness, despair, and depression, he noted, are common components of crisis, and persons in stress depend heavily on professionals for constructive help under these conditions. Hope gives relief from the tension and frustration of unmet goals. Clients are helped when they can be brought to feel that the future may bring relief from their present pain. Reviewing growth experiences helps people focus on other pleasant or unpleasant experiences that have had a profound positive effect on their growth. This process leads them to re-experience good feelings and heightens their image of themselves as capable persons with the strength to handle stress and crisis.

28.4.2. REFERRAL

Sometimes the people involved with a rehabilitation client will feel that they are unable to offer adequate help in a crisis; in such cases a referral will provide a new opportunity. Referral, Brammer stated, can be considered a skill that is most effectively utilized in accordance with certain principles.

Knowledge of the available resources is the first requisite (see 10.2.1). Then it must be determined whether a referral is right for the client at a given time. The individual may have initiated the idea or, on the other hand, may be frightened by it. People are sometimes alarmed by a referral, taking it to imply that their problems are extremely severe. It is important to explain candidly the reasons behind a recommended referral, with relationship both to the client's conduct and to one's own professional scope. If it appears that a given individual would benefit from working with someone with special training, it is appropriate to say "Let's think about who else might be able to help you here" or to make some other statement that does not suggest that the client's problems are too difficult to cope with.

The prospect of referring someone should be discussed with the referral facility or agency before it becomes immediately necessary. One should also discuss the case with others who have helped the individual in the past. Parents should know of the referral and agree to it if the client is a minor.

Clients should understand what kind of agency they are being referred to and what it can and cannot do. False hopes should not be raised. While sometimes it might be helpful to offer practical assistance like transportation, generally clients should handle their own contacts with the new resource.

No data about the client should be given to any referral agency without the written consent of the client. Finally, the person who has had the principal responsibility for a client should continue the relationship until the client has completely transferred to the other agency and has begun to establish another such relationship.

28.5. Depressed Reaction

In a crisis the emotional reaction is one of fear and confusion to some short-term situation in a person's life. A depressed person, on the other hand, is someone who has resolved some life crisis with self-blame, discouragement, passivity, and loss of interest in external events. In a normal individual depression can be described as a state of despondency characterized by feelings of inadequacy, lowered activity, and pessimism about the future. In pathological episodes of depression, there is an extreme unresponsiveness to stimuli, coupled with self-deprecation, delusions of inadequacy, and hopelessness.

Depression is an affective disorder: emotions and feelings are disrupted, but thinking processes remain logical. The depressed person's emotions are restricted to negative and critical evaluation of the self, and no action is taken to change or clarify the situation. Depressed persons often communicate that they cannot, should not, or are afraid to act, or feel otherwise inhibited from doing what they want to in a decision-making situation.

28.5.1. CAUSES OF DEPRESSION

Although there is almost always a reason for depression, the depressed client may not know the reason or may be confused about it. The reason may be real, or it may stem from a fantasy about something that happened in the past or is expected to happen in the future.

Cammer [1971] discussed depression in terms of three principal variables: intensity, duration, and quality. Depression ranges from mild to moderate to severe; typically, when it is mild, although causing stress, it is fairly easy to combat. In duration depressions are acute, recurrent, or chronic. The acute form arrives rather suddenly, regardless of its causes, and lasts for a few days or a few months. Recurrent depression occurs in the acute form but instead of being overcome reappears at various times; between these episodes "remissions" occur. The chronic type evolves more slowly and continues for any length of time up to two years; eventually normalcy returns.

Depression can be "endogenous"—the result of internal disturbances that prevent the nervous system from operating in the normal way. Examples include senility, drugs, infections, and glandular disorders. On the other hand, depressions can also occur as a reaction to certain external conditions. These so-called reactive forms of depression may be the result of a relationship loss through death or divorce or a situational change such as retirement or displacement.

28.5.2. IDENTIFYING DEPRESSION

Depression is characterized by loss of the capacity to control one's emotional life. A depressed individual cannot govern feelings and attitudes such as sadness, resentment, fear, listlessness, and the like. Primary verbal symptoms of depression are statements of self-blame, guilt, or despair and feelings of inadequacy, and feelings of hopelessness, isolation, or loneliness, all of which may find expression in statements such as "I can't do anything right." Primary nonverbal symptoms of depression include: sadness, sleep difficulties, poor appetite, loss of interest in surroundings and loss of pleasure drive, loss of sexual desire, self-neglect, loss of self-confidence, loss of self-esteem, preoccupation with body function, lack of concentration, memory troubles, inability to make decisions or use will power, poor judgment, agitation, crying and tearfulness, fear of being alone, fear of death, and loss of hope.

28.5.3. COPING TECHNIQUES

The counseling techniques described for use in crisis intervention are also applicable in work with a depressed client. While in a depression, clients are often unable to recall positive feelings about themselves or to feel good about themselves in the present. With help, however, they can learn to identify their feelings, take action, and realize they can have a good future. Antidepressant medications can be prescribed in severe cases.

28.6. Suicidal Reaction

Suicidal persons are in a state of crisis and are at a turning point in the resolution of problems. Overwhelmed by an intolerable situation and with feelings of helplessness, they reach a point of ambivalence between living and dying. Helping a suicidal individual is a very challenging task for a well-qualified professional.

The possibility does exist that rehabilitation counselees may consider suicide as an alternative to facing the many problems that may arise because of their disability. The realization that a disability is permanent or progressive may lead a person to consider suicide. Or a disabled person may not be able to stand the thought of being dependent on others for care and may decide on suicide as a way to end this dependency.

Those who work in helping professions will almost inevitably be faced with the need to evaluate and handle a suicidal client at some time.

28.6.1. SUICIDAL SYMPTOMS

The most common psychological states in which suicidal symptoms are expressed are depression, psychosis, and agitation. While depression is often evidenced, self-annihilistic tendencies are not restricted to persons who are depressed. Evidence of a client's severe depression may be revealed in information about sleep disorders, loss of appetite, loss of weight, social withdrawal, apathy and despondency, severe feelings of hopelessness and helplessness, and feelings of physical and psychological exhaustion. Psychotic states are characterized by delusions, hallucinations, disorientation, loss of contact, or highly unusual ideas and behaviors. Such descriptive information often comes from associates or the family of the client.

Persons in a state of agitation will show tension, anxiety, shame, and poor impulse control; they will exhibit feelings of rage, anger, hostility, and revenge. The anger may be indirectly felt, or expressed as a desire to commit suicide: "I'm going to kill myself; then they'll be sorry."

Suicidal persons always give clues to their impending action. The clues may be overt, clear, and specific, or they may be quietly presented and easily missed. Verbal clues might take the form of statements such as "I can't take that exam, I'm sure to fail it;" or "I just can't take any more, it's not worth it and nobody cares anyway." These comments might be made in a flippant manner with the implication that no one will take them seriously, but when hearing such comments one should analyze them and consider whether or not the person has shown other behavior congruent with a suicidal communication. If one is uncomfortable and feels there may be a possibility of suicide, questioning the person is indicated. And even when other indications have not been noticed, it is appropriate to probe into the possibility by asking, "How bad does it get: Do you sometimes think you'd rather be dead? Have you thought of killing yourself?"

There should be no hesitation in asking a person about suicide if verbal or nonverbal clues have been given, because asking about it will open up the subject for discussion and reduce the potential for suicide. Persons contemplating suicide are usually in the midst of internal crisis, and having people around who are uncomfortable with death and suicide will compound the crisis because avenues for expressing and discussing feelings are cut off. Merely having someone to listen to them will reduce some of the anxiety associated with the crisis and open other alternatives for discussion.

Vague suicide clues often indicate high lethality. Significant nonverbal clues are being left when people suddenly put their affairs in order, make out a will, pack belongings in boxes, or clean up their room. Insignificant gifts might be given to others as if the occasion were a big event in the life of the giver.

28.6.2. INTERVENTION TECHNIQUES

Four basic principles for use in preventing suicide were described by Farberow, Heilig, and Litman [1968]. These are presented as advice to workers in a telephone "hot-line" crisis center. Paraphrased below, these principles may be helpful to the rehabilitationist.

1. The first step is to establish a relationship, keep in contact with, and get information from the caller. A calm, interested, self-confident, optimistic attitude is appropriate. The individual should get the message that it was a good idea to make the contact and that the listener can and wants to help. An initiative in making contact is in itself a plea for assistance, and the individual should be permitted to talk about the problems and concerns that prompted the call without being questioned or criticized. Listening effectively and projecting the appropriate attitude will have an important effect on the suicidal person.

The worker gives identifying information and asks the caller's name and number, as well as those of others such as family members, friends, and the person's doctor. The first objective is to collect information that can help in assessing how strong a possibility suicide is. Asking how the individual plans to carry it out—whether with a gun or pills—and inquiring about other details will elicit this information. Calm discussion will help the person to become less anxious about the feelings that are prompting thoughts of suicide.

2. Next the main problem should be isolated and clarified. Many times the thinking of a person contemplating suicide is extremely chaotic and unfocused. The individual has no clear idea of what the central problem is and is concentrating on many smaller ones. It can be of great help to sort all these thoughts out so that the most crucial concern stands out from the others.

Sometimes the person is aware of the focal problem but feels that all possible solutions are inadequate. In this case someone else may be able to see and suggest new approaches.

3. The next step is to evaluate the person's strong points and inner resources. These are just as material as the pathological elements of the situation. In many cases the individual's negative or destructive responses are somewhat offset by constructive qualities or behaviors. These might be exemplified in the way the person responds to the attempt to clarify; answering the questions and going along with suggestions would signal positive attitudes, as would a change for the better in the person's mood or thought processes.

4. Finally, a strategy is devised and all avail- able assistance is brought into play. The kind of approach will depend on how serious the possibility of suicide is and on the data that has emerged. Usually people who seem most likely to take their lives will need the most help. If it is determined that the probability of suicide is high and there seems to be no way to lessen the dangerousness of the situation, hospitalization is in order; but, these cases appear to constitute only about ten percent of the total. Relatives and friends should be called in to assist and to provide transportation, and they should be told to stay with the person.

Most of the time the chances of suicide are relatively low. Sometimes empathy and intelligent listening, and suggestions given over the phone, are all that is required. More frequently the worker must play a more extensive role, typically by recommending that the individual make use of another local resource. The choice will be determined by the nature of the problem.

It should be remembered that problems seem more serious at night. If someone calls during the nighttime hours, the first objective is to keep the individual going until the next day. It is important to get the data needed to decide whether the situation is critical. Generally, if the worker feels uncertain in any way, the individual should be referred to an appropriate professional or agency to be evaluated thoroughly. A suicidal individual whose difficulties are not imminently severe should go to a mental health center or a family agency, but this is appropriate only if the person can handle the waiting period.

28.6.3. SUICIDE POTENTIAL

Suicide potential refers to the probability that a person will attempt to commit suicide in the immediate or near future, and varies from minimal lethality, in which there is no danger of loss of life, to maximal lethality, in which the possibility of death is great and immediate. Criteria developed at the Los Angeles Suicide Prevention Center (reported in Farberow et al) for evaluating suicide potential are as follows:

1. Age and sex—older male is highest risk, young female is lowest.
2. Suicide plan—gun and jumping are a greater risk than pills or wrist slashing.
3. Preparation—has the person made out a will or note?
4. Nature of stress—loss, success, anxiety?

5. Symptoms—depression, agitation, psychosis?
6. Life-style—has the person attempted suicide before?
7. Communication—has the person severed communication with others?

In general, no single sign need be alarming, with the exception of specific, lethal plans being actively made.

Inevitably some attempts to help suicidal individuals will fail. The person who tried to help will feel sorrow and should deal with it by seeking the support of others and trying to keep on learning. Suicide is in many ways a mystery about which much remains to be discovered.

28.7. Abnormality

The rehabilitation counselor requires a breadth and depth of knowledge of abnormal behavior. This understanding of abnormality requires an organizational framework. Because of medical relationships, the diagnostic system of the American Psychiatric Association is important to rehabilitationists—although there are other ways of conceptualizing abnormal human behavior (see 5.4).

Various conceptual models for abnormality are used. The statistical model asserts that a person who does not deviate much from average in either direction in a particular behavior (i.e., excess or deficiency) is "normal." The psychoanalytic or psychodynamic models and the learning or behaviorism models are described in other chapters as are other views of psychology. The medical or disease model has communication value to rehabilitationists who work with psychiatrists and deal with legal classifications [Nicholi, 1978]. The circular reasoning in the system, however, is a weakness that results in abuses. Labeling does not automatically reveal cause and treatment alternatives. A withdrawn or hallucinating person is diagnosed as schizophrenic; then, when it is asked what is causing the withdrawal and hallucinations, these problems are attributed to the fact that the person has schizophrenia [Davison & Neale, 1978].

Rehabilitation counselors should know the conceptual organization of the *Diagnostic and Statistical Manual of Mental Disorders* (DSM) of the American Psychiatric Association [1980]. It provides the most extensive classification scheme of its kind. Much of the material in this section consists of paraphrased condensations of the categories presented in a prepublication draft of the Manual's third edition (DSM-III) prepared by a task force of the Association. The Association's permission to include this information is especially appreciated because most rehabilitation counselors will not possess a personal copy of their DSM-III.

28.7.1. CLASSIFICATION

The DSM-III is based on a framework consistent with complete psychiatric diagnostic evaluation. Multiple categories representing separate parameters are coded for any individual. Thus every case is coded on each of several of the axes in the classification scheme.

Following the multi-axial classification as recommended, individuals are evaluated on each of the following axes:

1. Clinical psychiatric syndrome (i.e., a pattern of symptoms) and other conditions.
2. Personality disorders (adults) and specific developmental disorders (children and adolescents).
3. Physical disorders.
4. Severity of psychosocial stressors.
5. Highest level of adaptive functioning (past year).

Most of the DSM-III is devoted to the description of mental disorders (to be summarized later).

28.7.2. PSYCHOSOCIAL STRESSORS

The rehabilitationist is particularly interested in the *psychosocial stressors* of a case. This information and the method of rating facilitate communication between the psychiatrist and rehabilitation counselor. Psychosocial stressors are identified as significant contributors to the development or exacerbation (i.e., an increase in severity of symptoms) of the disorder. A stressor may play a formative or precipitating role in a disorder or it may be a consequence of the individual's psychopathology. For example, alcoholism may cause marital problems and divorce, which themselves are stressors, contributing to the development of depression. The impact varies with the individual.

The following psychosocial stressors—listed with examples—are suggested for consideration in psychiatric evaluation:

Conjugal (marital and nonmarital)—engagement, marriage, discord, separation, death of spouse.

Parenting—becoming a parent, friction with child, illness of child.

Other interpersonal (all problems with one's friends, neighbors, associates or nonconjugal family members)—illness of best friend, discordant relationship with boss.

Occupational (includes work, school, homemaking)—being unemployed, retirement, problems at school.

Living circumstances—change in residence, threat to personal safety, immigration.

Financial—inadequate finances, change in financial status.

Legal—being arrested, being in jail, being involved in a lawsuit or trial.

Developmental (the meaning given to phases of the life cycle)—puberty, menopause, "becoming 50."

Physical illness or injury—illness, accident, surgery, abortion.

Other psychosocial stressors—natural or man-made disaster, persecution, unmarried pregnancy, out-of-wedlock birth, rape.

Family factors (for children and adolescents other stressors may be considered)—distant or hostile relationship between parents, physical or mental disturbance in family members, insufficient social or cognitive stimulation, anomalous family situation (single parent or foster family), institutional rearing, or loss of nuclear family members.

More than one stressor may be judged etiologically significant, in which case they are ranked according to importance.

The severity rating of the summed effect of all of the psychosocial stressors that are listed for an individual is based on the clinician's assessment of the stress that an average person with similar sociocultural values and circumstances would experience from the psychosocial stressor(s). Severity ratings (with code numbers) for adults—with examples—are as follows:

0 Unspecified—no information or not applicable.
1 None—no apparent psychosocial stressor.
2 Minimal—minor violation of the law, small bank loan.
3 Mild—argument with neighbor, change in work hours.
4 Moderate—new job, death of close friend, pregnancy.
5 Severe—major illness in self or family, bankruptcy, marital separation, birth of child.
6 Extreme—death of close relative, divorce, jail term.
7 Catastrophic—concentration camp experience, devastating natural disaster.

28.7.3. LEVEL OF FUNCTIONING

For the highest level of adaptive functioning the clinician judges the individual's highest overall level. It is a rating of the best several-month period of the last year.

As conceptualized, adaptive functioning is a composite of three major areas: social relations—all relations with other people, with particular emphasis on family and friends (the breadth and quality of interpersonal relationships); occupational functioning—functioning as a worker, student, or housekeeper (the amount, complexity, and quality of the work accomplished); and use of leisure time—recreational activities or hobbies (the range and depth of involvement). While considered together for the evaluation, social relations may warrant greater weight because of their high prognostic significance. Leisure time significantly affects overall judgment when there is no impairment in social relations and occupational functioning or when occupational opportunities are curtailed because of retirement or a vocational handicap.

Adaptive functioning level is rated and recorded by code. There are six levels, from superior to grossly impaired. A zero code is used for "unspecified," meaning there is no information. The highest level during the past year frequently has prognostic significance.

28.7.4. MENTAL DISORDERS

The American Psychiatric Association, for the third edition of their *Diagnostic and Statistical Manual of Mental Disorders* (DSM-III), broke away from many older concepts and labels presented in books on psychiatry and psychology published before 1980. While subject to further refinement the present classification scheme, presented here, will help the rehabilitationist understand the classifications and descriptions of the whole range of mental disorders.

Organic Mental Disorders

The essential feature of the organic mental disorders is transient or permanent dysfunction of the brain attributed to specific organic factors. Medical laboratory evidence (such as X-ray, brain scan, EEG, spinal tap), physical examination, or a history of the etiological organic factor is necessary before the diagnosis can be made. Differentiation of organic mental disorders as a separate class does not imply that the nonorganic, the so-called functional mental disorders are somehow independent of brain processes. On the contrary, it is assumed that all psychological processes, normal and abnormal, depend on brain function.

Substance Use Disorders

In American society, use of certain substances to modify mood or behavior under certain circumstances is generally regarded as normal. This includes recreational or social drinking of alcohol as well as the use of caffeine as a stimulant in the form of coffee. On the other hand, most behavioral changes due to taking substances that affect the central nervous system are viewed in almost all subcultures as extremely undesirable. Examples of such behavioral changes include impairment in social or occupational functioning as a consequence of substance use, inability to control use of the substance or to stop taking it and the development of serious withdrawal symptoms after cessation of substance use. The substance use disorders are generally subdivided into substance abuse and substance dependence.

Schizophrenic Disorders

The essential features of this group of disorders are: disorganization of a previous level of functioning, characteristic symptoms involving multiple psychological processes; the presence of certain psychotic features during the active phase of the illness; the absence of a full affective syndrome concurrent with or developing prior to the active phase of the illness; a tendency toward chronicity; and the fact that the

disturbance is not explainable by any of the organic mental disorders.

A schizophrenic disorder always involves at least one of the following: delusions, hallucinations, or certain characteristic types of thought disorder. No single clinical feature is unique to this condition or evident in every case or at every phase of the illness. Significant impairment always occurs in areas of routine daily functioning such as work, social relations, and self-care. Family and friends often observe that the person is "no longer himself." Invariably there are characteristic disturbances in several of the following areas: language and communication, content of thought, perception, affect, sense of self, volition, relationship to the external world, and motor behavior. No one of these features, however, is invariably present or seen only in schizophrenia.

Almost any psychiatric symptom can occur as an associated feature. The individual may appear perplexed, disheveled, or eccentrically groomed or dressed. Abnormalities of psychomotor activity are common, either pacing, rocking, or apathetic immobility. Ritualistic or stereotyped behavior that may be associated with "magical" thinking may occur. A dysphoric mood is common; it may take the form of depression, anxiety, anger, or a mixture of these. Feelings of unreality and estrangement from self and environment, as well as thinking that reads personal significance into trivial remarks and misinterpretation of experiences are common, as are hypochondriacal concerns that may or may not be delusional.

Onset is usually during adolescence or early adult life (i.e., before age 30). The diagnosis of schizophrenia requires that continuous signs of the illness have lasted for at least six months of an active phase of psychotic symptoms, with or without a prodromal (i.e., initial or precursory) stage or a residual phase. Prior to the development of the active phase of the illness, there is frequently a clear deterioration in functioning, with such symptoms as social isolation or withdrawal, impairment in role functioning, eccentric or peculiar behavior, impairment in personal hygiene and grooming, blunted or inappropriate affect, disturbances in communication, odd or bizarre ideation, and unusual perceptual experiences. The length of this prodromal phase is extremely variable and its onset may be difficult to date accurately. In those cases in which the prodromal phase is characterized by an insidious downhill course over many years, the prognosis is especially poor.

The onset of the active phase is frequently associated with the occurrence of a psychosocial stressor. During the active phase there are prominent psychotic symptoms, such as delusions, hallucinations, derailment (loosening of associations), incoherence, poverty of speech content, illogicality, and behavior that is grossly disorganized or catatonic.

Usually a residual phase follows the active phase of the illness. The clinical picture of this phase is similar to that seen in the prodromal phase, although affective blunting or flattening and impairment in role functioning tend to be more common. During the residual phase some of the psychotic symptoms, such as delusions or hallucinations, may persist but have lost their affective coloring. A complete return to premorbid functioning is unusual but full remission or recovery is possible. There is a strong tendency, however, for acute exacerbations requiring therapeutic intervention—usually with increasing residual impairment between episodes.

Prodromal or residual symptoms of schizophrenic disorders are: social isolation or withdrawal; marked impairment in role functioning as wage-earner, student, or homemaker; markedly eccentric, odd, or peculiar behavior (e.g., collecting garbage, talking to self in corn field or subway, hoarding food); impairment in personal hygiene and grooming; blunted, flat, or inappropriate affect; speech that is tangential, digressive, vague, overelaborate, circumstantial, or metaphorical; odd or bizarre ideation, or magical thinking (e.g., superstitiousness, clairvoyance, telepathy, "sixth sense," "others can feel my feelings," overvalued ideas, ideas of reference, or suspected delusions); unusual perceptual experiences (e.g., recurrent illusions, sensing the presence of a force or person not actually present, suspected hallucinations).

Several classic types of schizophrenia are described below:

1. Simple. Appears during or after puberty and is characterized by an insidious loss of ambition and deterioration of personality.
2. Hebephrenic. Appears during late adolescence and is marked by thought disorder and

limited social contact. The person appears disheveled and unconcerned about self. Emotional responses may be inappropriate (e.g., silly grins or laughter, unresponsive).
3. Catatonic. Appears in late adolescence or early adulthood and has the feature of abnormal motor activity. Spontaneous activity may be reduced to stupor: muteness, negativism, stereotype, automatic obedience, excitement, outbursts—all may occur. Without drug therapy (tranquilizers) the person may die.
4. Paranoid. Tends to become symptomatic in the late twenties or thirties. Paranoid schizophrenia is characterized by delusions of persecution and of grandeur. This person is tense, suspicious, and guarded (reserved to the point of being vague or mute)—like a catatonic. Intelligence is relatively well preserved and is used freely in areas not affected by pathological ideas.

Paranoid Disorders

The essential feature in paranoid disorders is a clinical picture in which the predominant symptoms are persistent persecutory delusions or delusions of jealousy, not explainable by another mental disorder. The paranoid disorders include paranoia, shared paranoid disorder, and paranoid state. The boundaries of this group of disorders and their differentiation from other disorders, particularly severe paranoid personality disorder and paranoid schizophrenia, are unclear.

The persecutory delusions may be simple or elaborate; they usually involve a single theme or series of connected themes, such as being conspired against, cheated, spied upon, followed, poisoned or drugged, maliciously maligned, harassed, or obstructed in the pursuit of long-term goals. Common associated features include anger and resentment, which may lead to violence. Ideas or delusions of reference are common. Often there is social isolation, seclusiveness, or eccentricity of behavior. Suspiciousness, whether generalized or focused on certain individuals, is common. Writing letters and complaining about personal injustices or instigating legal action often occurs. There is some evidence that immigration, migration, deafness, and other stresses may predispose to the development of a paranoid disorder.

There is rarely impairment in daily functioning. In contrast to schizophrenia, intellectual and occupational functioning are usually relatively well preserved even in chronic forms of paranoid disorder. Social and marital functioning, on the other hand, are often severely impaired. These individuals rarely seek treatment on their own. The age at onset is generally later than that of schizophrenia. Although this disorder is rare in its pure form, the symptoms are common.

Schizoaffective Disorders

There is controversy as to whether this disorder represents a variant of affective disorder or schizophrenia, a third independent entity, or part of a continuum between pure affective disorder and pure schizophrenia. The term *schizoaffective* is still used, however, as a classifiable mental disorder. The essential features are a depressive or manic syndrome of at least one week's duration that precedes or develops concurrently with certain psychotic symptoms thought to be incompatible with a purely affective disorder; this diagnosis is not made if the disturbance is due to any organic mental disorder.

Affective Disorders

The essential feature of this group of disorders is a primary disturbance of mood accompanied by related symptoms. Mood refers to a prolonged emotion that colors the whole psychic life, and generally involves either depression or elation. There are several categorical groups. The first group is termed "episodic affective disorders." The term *episodic* is used to mean a period of illness in which there is a sustained disturbance clearly distinguished from previous functioning. The second group of disorders is referred to as "chronic affective disorders." The term *chronic* is used to indicate a long-standing (at least two years) illness that usually does not have a clear onset. The third group consists of residual categories classified as atypical depressive, manic, and bipolar disorders.

The essential feature of the episodic affective disorders is an episode of illness with a prominent and persistent disturbance in mood with either the full manic or depressive syndrome clearly distinguished from prior functioning.

A manic episode is a distinct period when the predominant mood is either elevated, expansive, or irritable and is associated with other symptoms of the manic syndrome, which may include hyperactivity and excessive involvement in activities without recognition of the high potential for painful consequences. Lability of mood with rapid shifts to anger or depression are associated. The depression, with tearfulness, suicidal threats, and other depressive symptoms, may last moments, hours, or (more rarely) days. Manic episodes typically begin suddenly with a rapid escalation of symptoms over a few days. The episodes usually last from a few days to months, are briefer, and have a more abrupt termination than depressive episodes. Most of these individuals will eventually have depressive episodes and be reclassified as having a bipolar affective disorder. In a bipolar affective disorder the initial episode is usually manic.

A depressive episode is a period of either depressive mood or a pervasive loss of interest or pleasure. These symptoms may include loss of interest or pleasure, sleep disturbance, appetite disturbance, change in weight, psychomotor agitation or retardation, cognitive disturbance, decreased energy, a feeling of worthlessness or guilt, and thoughts of death or suicide. Common associated features include a depressed appearance, tearfulness, feelings of anxiety, irritability, fearfulness, brooding, excessive concern with physical health, panic attacks, and phobias. Paranoid symptoms may be present and range from mild suspiciousness through ideas of reference and more rarely to frank delusions. Common paranoid delusions include the idea that one is being persecuted because of sinfulness or some inadequacy. Major depressive disorders may begin at any age, including in childhood. The onset of depressive episodes is variable, with symptoms usually developing over a period of days to weeks; but, in some cases, it may be sudden (e.g., when associated with a severe psychosocial stressor).

The course is variable for all of the episodic affective disorders, with some individuals having episodes separated by many years of normal functioning, others having clusters of episodes, and yet others having an increased frequency of episodes as they grow older. Usually the level of functioning between episodes returns to the premorbid level. However, in some cases—

when there are frequent recurrent episodes—there is considerable residual impairment.

During manic episodes there is usually considerable handicap in both social and occupational areas. When there is no gross impairment in judgment or ability to hold a meaningful conversation, such episodes are commonly referred to as "hypomanic." When impairment is extreme the individual usually requires protection from the consequences of poor judgment or hyperactivity.

During depressive episodes the degree of handicap varies, but there is always some interference in social and occupational abilities. If the depressive episode is extreme, the individual may be totally unable to function socially, occupationally, or even to feed or clothe himself or herself or maintain minimal personal hygiene.

The most common complications of manic episodes are substance abuse and the consequences of actions resulting from impaired judgment, such as financial losses and illegal activities. The most serious complication of a depressive episode is suicide. The likelihood of a serious suicide attempt increases with the age of the individual.

Psychoses Not Elsewhere Classified

Some disorders with psychotic features are not classified as either an organic mental disorder, or a schizophrenic, paranoid, schizoaffective, or affective disorder. There are several categories: schizophreniform disorder, brief reactive psychosis, and atypical psychosis. The term *psychotic* denotes the existence of any of the following: delusions, hallucinations, incoherence, repeated derailment, marked poverty of content of thought, marked illogicality, and behavior that is grossly disorganized or catatonic. The essential features of schizophreniform disorder are identical to those of schizophrenia with the exception that the duration is less than six months but more than one week. Brief reactive psychosis differs from schizophreniform disorder in that the duration of the disturbance is less than one week (although secondary effects may persist for a longer period); also it always follows an environmental stressor, which frequently is not present prior to the onset of a schizophreniform disorder. In atypical psychosis the symptom picture is consistent with that of psychosis but it does not meet the criteria for any specific mental

disorder (e.g., confusing or unusual clinical features, short duration).

Anxiety Disorders

In other classifications, these disorders are grouped together under the neuroses or neurotic disorders. As classified in the DMS-III, in this group of disorders some form of anxiety is either the most predominant disturbance in the clinical picture, as with panic disorder and generalized anxiety disorder; or anxiety is experienced if the individual tries to resist giving in to the symptoms—avoidance of a dreaded object or situation in a phobic disorder and obsessions or compulsions in an obsessive-compulsive disorder. It is estimated that 2 to 4 percent of the general population has had an anxiety state or a phobia. Perhaps 10 percent of patients in cardiology practices are suffering from an anxiety disorder. (See 29.3.1.)

Factitious Disorders

The term *factitious* means not real, genuine, or natural. Factitious disorders are therefore characterized by physical or psychological symptoms that are produced by the individual and are under voluntary control. They are distinguished from acts of malingering in which the person is also in voluntary control of the symptom production, but the act is for a purpose that is obviously recognizable with a knowledge of the circumstances: for example, claiming to have a physical illness in order to avoid conscription into the military would be classified as malingering. In a factitious disorder there is no apparent goal. Whereas an act of malingering may, under certain circumstances, be considered adaptive, by definition a diagnosis of a factitious disorder always implies psychopathology, most often a severe personality disturbance. In other classifications some of these disorders are subsumed within the category of hysteria.

Somatoform Disorders

In this group of disorders there are physical symptoms suggesting physical disorder (hence *somatoform*) without any demonstrable organic findings to explain the symptoms, and for which there is positive evidence, or a strong presumption, that the symptoms are linked to psychological factors or conflicts. Unlike factitious illness or malingering, the symptom production in somatoform disorders is not under voluntary control (i.e., the individual does not experience the sense of controlling the production or withdrawal of the symptoms).

The disorders in this category are: (1) somatization disorder—elsewhere referred to as hysteria; (2) conversion disorder; and (3) psychalgia—psychologically induced pain not attributable to any other mental or physical disorder.

Dissociative Disorders

The essential feature of the dissociative disorders is a sudden, temporary alteration in the normally integrated functions of consciousness, identity, or motor behavior, so that some part of one or more of these functions is lost. If this alteration occurs in consciousness, important personal events previously registered in memory cannot be recalled. If the alteration occurs in identity, either the individual's customary identity is temporarily forgotten while a new identity is assumed or the customary feeling of one's own reality is lost and replaced by a feeling of unreality. If the alteration occurs in motor behavior, there is also a concurrent disturbance in consciousness or identity.

Personality Disorders

The essential features are deeply ingrained, inflexible, maladaptive patterns of relating to, perceiving, and thinking about the environment and oneself that are of sufficient severity to cause either significant impairment in adaptive functioning or subjective distress. Thus, they are pervasive personality traits and are exhibited in a wide range of important social and personal contexts. The manifestations of personality disorders are generally recognizable by the time of adolescence or earlier and continue throughout most of adult life.

The personality disorders are grouped into three clusters: (1) paranoid, introverted, and schizotypal personality disorders—individuals with these disorders often appear "odd" or eccentric; (2) histrionic, narcissistic, antisocial, and borderline personality disorders—individuals with these disorders appear dramatic, emotional, or erratic; (3) avoidant, dependent, compulsive, and passive-aggressive personality disorders—individuals with these disorders often appear anxious or fearful. Finally,

there is a residual category for other or mixed personality disorders.

Psychosexual Disorders

The psychosexual disorders are divided into four groups: (1) gender identity disorders—characterized by the individual's feelings of discomfort and inappropriateness about his or her anatomical sex and by persistent behaviors generally associated with the other sex; (2) paraphilias—characterized by arousal in response to sexual objects or situations that are not part of normative arousal-activity patterns and by gross impairment in the capacity for affectionate sexual activity between human partners; (3) psychosexual dysfunctions—characterized by inhibitions in the appetitive or psychophysiological changes that characterize the sexual response cycle; and (4) ego-dystonic homosexuality and other psychosexual disorders.

Disorders Usually Arising in Childhood or Adolescence

These disorders usually arise and first manifest themselves in childhood or adolescence. A child or adolescent is given this classification of diagnosis only if no other diagnosis is appropriate.

Reactive Disorders

The essential feature of reactive disorders (not elsewhere classified) is that they do not meet the criteria for any of the specific disorders previously described as a reaction to life events or circumstances. All of the reactive disorders may be prolonged or brief, depending upon the duration of the stressor, the personality characteristics of the individual, and the environmental support systems that are available. These disorders include posttraumatic stress disorder and adjustment disorders.

Disorders of Impulse Control

This is a residual category for disorders of impulse control that are not classified elsewhere (e.g., substance use disorders). A disorder of impulse control is characterized by the following, in order:

1. There is a failure to resist an impulse, drive, or temptation to perform some action that is harmful to the individual or others. There may or may not be a conscious resistance to

the impulse. The act may or may not be premeditated or planned.

2. Prior to committing the act, there is an increasing sense of tension.

3. At the time of committing the act, there is an experience of either pleasure, gratification, or release. Immediately following the act, there may or may not be genuine regret, self-reproach, or guilt.

The classification contains five specific categories: pathological gambling, kleptomania, pyromania, intermittent explosive disorder, and isolated explosive disorder.

Other Disorders

"Unspecified mental disorder" is a residual category used when, following a psychiatric evaluation, there is evidence of a mental disorder but without any features suggesting a psychosis, and not meeting the criteria for any of the nonpsychotic mental disorders; in some cases, with more information, the diagnosis is changed to a specific disorder. Also classified as "other disorders" are "psychological factors affecting physical disorder" and "no mental disorder."

PSYCHOLOGICAL FACTORS AFFECTING PHYSICAL DISORDER. The judgment that psychological factors are affecting the physical disorder requires evidence of a temporal relationship between the environmental stimulus and the meaning given to it, and the initiation or exacerbation of the physical disorder. This category, which has been referred to as either "psychosomatic" or "psychophysiological," is used with any physical disorder in which psychological factors are judged to be contributory. Common examples of physical disorders for which this category may be appropriate include: obesity, headache, migraine, angina pectoris, painful menstruation, sacroiliac pain, neurogastric ulcer, duodenal ulcer, cardiospasm, pylorospasm, nausea and vomiting, regional enteritis, ulcerative colitis, frequency of micturition, and hyperthyroidism.

CONDITIONS NOT ATTRIBUTABLE TO A MENTAL DISORDER. This category includes conditions that have led to contact with the mental health care system, but without sufficient evidence to justify a diagnosis of any of the mental disorders noted previously. An example is malingering, the essential feature of which is the presentation of fake or grossly exaggerated physical or psychiatric illness apparently under voluntary control. It should be noted, however, that the act of malingering may be associated with or be symptomatic of another mental disorder, such as antisocial personality disorder or substance dependence.

The differential diagnosis of malingering begins with the ruling out of a true physical or psychiatric disorder as an adequate explanation for the individual's symptoms. Depending upon the medical sophistication and theatrical talents of the person, this may be difficult, particularly when the malingering takes the form of grossly exaggerated symptoms of true medical illness.

28.7.5. GLOSSARY

Abnormality and psychotherapy are the focus of this glossary. Selected techniques, disorders, and symptoms from an extensive nomenclature are covered. Symptoms are a deviation from normal functioning that indicate a disorder; a syndrome is a group of such symptoms suggesting the diagnostic category of the disorder. Other relevant concepts are described in Chapter 25 and elsewhere in this book.

ACTING OUT. This is the expression of unconscious conflicts or feelings of hostility or other emotion through overt behavior.

AFFECT. A person's emotional feeling becomes an affect when it is expressed in observable behavior. Common examples include euphoria, anger, and sadness. Affect and emotion are often used interchangeably but affect is distinguished from mood. Affect ranges are described as broad (i.e., normal), restricted (i.e., constricted), blunted (i.e., reduced in intensity), or flat (i.e., virtually no emotion is expressed whatever the stimuli). Labile affect is characterized by repeated rapid and abrupt shifts—tearful one moment and combative the next.

AGGRESSION. Forceful hostile action of a physical, verbal, or symbolic nature against people or things is known as aggressive behavior. It is supposed to release tensions or attain something the person desires by establishing fear in those being attacked.

ALIENATION. The lack or the loss of relationships with others is referred to as alienation. An individual who is disabled may feel set apart from the mainstream of society due to a combination of factors. There may be a sense of powerlessness over what is happening and a sense of meaninglessness.

AMBIGUITY. Ambiguity refers to an incompleteness or vagueness and a lack of structure so that the situation does not elicit a clear response. Ambivalence refers to the universal, sometimes extreme, coexistence of contradictory emotions, attitudes, ideas, or desires with respect to a particular person, object, or situation.

AMNESIA. Total or partial loss of memory can be associated with hysteria, an organic brain syndrome, or hypnosis.

ANTISOCIAL PERSONALITY. This diagnosis is applied to individuals who have repeated conflicts with society, are selfish, do not experience guilt, and are incapable of loyalty to others. The terms *sociopath* and *psychopath* have been used for such people.

ANXIETY. A chronic emotional condition in which there is apprehension, tension, dread, and uneasiness, anxiety stems from the anticipation of danger, the sources of which are largely unknown or unrecognized. Anxiety is distinguished from "fear," which is an emotional response to a consciously recognized and external sense of danger. A "phobia" is an obsessive, persistent, and unrealistic fear of an external object or situation.

APATHY. The absence of feeling or emotion, apathy may be a symptom of a pathological condition. It may appear as indifference toward life.

APHASIA. This word means loss or impairment of the ability to use language because of lesions in the brain.

AUTISM. Autism is an absorption in self or fantasy as a means of avoiding communication and escaping objective reality.

CATHARSIS. This is the discharge of emotional tension or anxiety associated with repressed traumatic material by reliving, through speech or emotional reaction, those incidents or events in the past that contribute to the present difficulty.

COMPULSIVITY. The personality characteristic of excessive adherence to rigid standards is seen as compulsive behavior.

CONFABULATION. This refers to filling in gaps in memory caused by brain dysfunction with made-up and often improbable stories that the person accepts as true.

CONVERSION. Repressed ideas or impulses and the psychological defenses against them are converted into somatic symptoms.

DELUSION. This is a false belief firmly held in spite of what almost everyone else believes and in spite of obvious proof to the contrary. Delusions are subdivided according to their content (e.g., persecutory, grandiose, nihilistic, somatic).

DEMENTIA. Dementia is the progressive and marked deterioration of mental functioning.

DEPENDENCY. Applied to the relation of one individual to another or to society, dependency means receiving aid for maintenance. The role of a sick and disabled person often demands passivity and cooperation from others, beginning with acquiescence to the decisions of medical authority. If this becomes extreme, the person may fear being declared well [Goldin & Perry, 1967]. The term *dependency needs* refers to infantile needs for mothering, love, affection, shelter, protection, security, food, and warmth.

DEPRESSION. A morbid sadness, dejection, or melancholy, depression is differentiated from grief, which is realistic and proportionate to what has been lost and which gradually subsides.

DEREISTIC. Mental activity is dereistic when inconsistent with reality, logic, or experience. It is similar to autistic behavior in that it is subjective, directed toward oneself.

DETERIORATION. A progressive disintegration of intellectual or emotional function, deterioration is apparent in persons with psychoses and may or may not be reversible.

DISORIENTATION. This is the loss of awareness of the position of one's self in relation to space, time, or person.

DISSOCIATION. Dissociation occurs when a group of mental processes is split off from the mainstream of consciousness, or behavior loses its relationship with the rest of the personality.

ENDOGENOUS. This refers to conditions attributable to internal causes; exogenous refers to external causes.

ETIOLOGY. This refers to all of the factors that contribute to the development of an illness or disorder.

FLIGHT OF IDEAS. This rapid shift from one subject to another in conversation, with only superficial associative connections, is a symptom of manic psychosis.

FUNCTIONAL PSYCHOSIS. This is a condition in which thought, behavior, and emotion are disturbed without known pathological changes in tissues of the brain.

GENOTYPE. This refers to an individual's unobservable, physiological genetic constitution (i.e., the totality of genes possessed by an individual). Phenotype refers to the totality of a person's observable characteristics.

HALLUCINATION. A hallucination is a sensory image without external stimulation of the relevant sensory organ. The term usually implies a pathological state.

HYPERACTIVITY. Hyperactivity, generally purposeful excessive motor activity, is frequently but not necessarily associated with internal tension.

HYSTERIA. Physical incapacity that makes no anatomical sense is called a hysterical state or hysterical conversion reaction.

IDEAS OF REFERENCE. This refers to delusional thinking that reads personal significance into seemingly trivial remarks and activities of others.

INSECURITY. Feelings of insecurity may lead to restriction in activities, to fearfulness and apprehension, and to failure to participate fully in one's environment.

INSIGHT. Self-understanding is a major goal of counseling and psychotherapy. Insight is understanding of the origin, nature, and mechanisms and of one's own attitudes, abilities, and behavior.

INTERACTION. Behavior that affects two or more persons is called interaction when it assumes mutually dependent activity.

INTROSPECTION. Introspection is self-observation of one's own mental processes.

LABILE. *Labile* means easily moved or changed, quickly shifting from one emotion to another, or easily aroused.

MILIEU THERAPY. This treatment procedure attempts to make the total environment and all personnel and patients of the hospital a "therapeutic community" conducive to psychological improvement.

NEGATIVISM. Negativism is a perverse resistance to influence from others. Suggestions and advice are rejected by people who subjectively feel "pushed around."

OBSESSION. Intrusive and recurring thought that seems irrational and uncontrollable to the person experiencing it is referred to as obsessional.

ORGANIC BRAIN SYNDROME. In this mental disorder the intellectual or emotional functioning, or both, are impaired through a pathology or dysfunction of the brain.

PANIC REACTION. A sudden and inexplicable outburst of acute and overwhelming fear is known as panic reaction.

PERSONALITY DISORDERS. This is a heterogeneous diagnostic category for maladaptive patterns that are considered neither neurotic nor psychotic; some are self-defeating traits and others are social problems, such as alcoholism and unconventional sexual practices.

PHOBIA. An intense irrational fear and avoidance of specific objects and situations is known as a phobia.

PREMORBID ADJUSTMENT. This is the social adjustment of the individual before the onset or diagnosis of symptoms.

PRIMARY GAIN. A term used in connection with neurotic symptoms, primary gain refers to the basic internal psychological gain of an emotional illness. "Secondary gain" refers to the external, additional gains derived from disability.

PROGNOSIS. Prognosis is the prediction of the likely course and outcome of an illness or disorder.

PSYCHOPHYSIOLOGICAL DISORDER. This disorder has physical symptoms involving actual tissue damage produced when the person was under stress; examples are hives and ulcers.

REGRESSION. The partial or symbolic readoption of more infantile ways of gratification is seen as regressive behavior.

SOMA. The totality of an organism's physical makeup is referred to as its soma.

SOMATOGENESIS. Somatogenesis means development from bodily origins as distinguished from psychological origins (psychogenesis).

STRESS. Stress is any stimulus that strains the physiological or psychological capacities of an organism.

THOUGHT DISORDER. A thought disorder is evidenced by problems such as incoherence, loose associations, and concrete reasoning.

TRAUMA. A severe physical injury or wound to the body caused by an external force or a psychological shock that has a lasting effect on mental life is a trauma.

VISCERA. The internal organs of the body located in the great cavity of the trunk proper are the viscera.

Chapter 29

Behavior Techniques

Behavior is anything a person actually does, although the term *behavior* usually refers to observable acts (i.e., explicit behavior). People behave in one way or another because of feelings, habits, available alternatives, need satisfaction, avoidance of unpleasantness, learned responses, and informed choice. As the science of human behavior, psychology is concerned with why people act the way they do and how to influence behavior to make it adjustive.

Behaviorism, as a term of psychological import, was originally coined by J. B. Watson [1930]. Behaviorism, as a psychological theory, employed the concepts of "stimulus," "response," and "reinforcement" in its account of the bases of human behavior. Behavioral techniques that have been developed more recently as a practical approach use a variety of procedures (e.g., modeling, rewards and punishments, and cognitive restructuring) to help a client learn to act in more positive ways.

The behavioral model of rehabilitation posits that psychopathology is largely a set of maladaptive behaviors that are learned in exactly the same way as are adaptive behaviors. Psychopathology refers to psychological as well as behavioral dysfunctions experienced by individuals. Behavioral treatment involves procedures derived from theory and experimentally established principles of learning and related concepts. Thus, maladaptive behavior can be modified or eliminated and more adaptive behavior patterns can be acquired by exposing individuals to appropriate learning strategies.

Behavior modification and social learning theory approaches have been successful in rehabilitation with a wide range of client difficulties (viz. behavioral problems, mental retardation, and emotional disturbances). Most frequently behavior modification utilizes tangible or verbal reinforcement for desired behavior and nonreinforcement (e.g., inattention) for undesired conduct. But influencing behavior through the giving of rewards, tangible or intangible, is not the only effective method of altering behavior.

Modeling, which is derived from social learning theory [Bandura, 1969, 1977], is defined as a process by which one learns as a consequence of having observed another person perform (see 25.3.4). It has been found to be quite effective with a variety of clients and for a variety of problems. Using reinforcement and modeling, separately and together, according to a report of the Regional Rehabilitation Research Institute at the University of Missouri [Bruch, Kunce,

Thelen, & Akamatsu, 1973], holds promise in clients who do not respond to other counseling approaches. Behavioral modification, modeling, and counseling need not be used in isolation but can be effective together in a treatment plan.

All counselors, either consciously or unconsciously, use behavioral principles in interacting with clients. A simple nod of the head may serve to encourage a client's verbalization on a particular topic; personal warmth reinforces the client-counselor relationship and makes it productive. Such courtesies as showing up on time

for appointments model appropriate behavior. Even the development of the individual written rehabilitation program (IWRP) involves a number of behavioral principles and techniques.

This chapter sets forth the behavior modification concepts and techniques that the rehabilitation counselor needs to know in order to provide clients with adequate services. Also included are discussions of behavior change procedures such as relaxation training, assertive training, and contracting, all of which are also important in working with rehabilitation clients.

29.1. Behavior Modification

A great many behavior modification strategies are based on the principles of operant conditioning. "Operant behavior" denotes the complex behavior of voluntary responses, which are the observable activities that affect one's environment. These range from simple gestures such as a smile to an intricate set of responses such as those involved in obtaining a job. Operant behaviors can be decreased or increased by systematically controlling their consequences. This system of altering operant behaviors by modifying their consequences is called "operant conditioning" or "instrumental conditioning."

In the terminology of behavior modification, client behaviors that are undesirable and frequently exhibited are called "behavioral surpluses;" behaviors that are desired but not exhibited are called "behavioral deficits." The rehabilitationist's goal—eliminating undesirable behaviors in the client and increasing desired conduct—becomes a matter of decreasing behavioral surpluses and increasing behavioral deficits. This section explains the procedures by which behavior modification principles are applied, as related by Marr and Krauft [1975], and also by Hosford [1969], Hosford and de Visser [1974], Kanfer and Goldstein [1975], and Thoresen and Hosford [1973].

29.1.1. DEFINITION OF TERMS

Behavior modification involves a number of unique techniques that have been developed to change behavior. Definitions of some of the techniques used by behavioral counselors will be helpful since the terms and concepts are explicit to this approach.

DESENSITIZATION. The technique of desensitization aims at teaching the client to emit a response that is inconsistent with anxiety while in the presence (real or imagined) of the anxiety-producing stimulus. Thus, the therapist attempts to train the client to remain calm and relaxed in situations that formerly produced anxiety.

IMPLOSIVE THERAPY. Like desensitization, the implosive approach regards maladaptive behavior as involving the conditioned avoidance of anxiety-arousing stimuli. The client is asked to imagine and relive aversive scenes associated with anxiety. Rather than trying to banish anxiety from the treatment sessions, the therapist deliberately attempts to elicit a massive flood, or "implosion" of anxiety. With repeated exposure the stimulus loses its power to elicit anxiety and the neurotic avoidance behavior is extinguished.

ASSERTIVE TRAINING. A means of developing more effective coping techniques, training in assertiveness is particularly helpful with individuals who have difficulties in interpersonal situations because of conditioned anxiety responses that prevent them from "speaking up" for what they feel is right.

AVERSION THERAPY. Punishment is used to modify undesirable behavior. The punishment may involve either the removal of positive reinforcement or the use of aversive stimuli (e.g., drugs), but the purpose is to reduce the "temptation value" of stimuli that elicit undesirable behavior.

Other terms that are useful to know have to do

with reinforcement techniques typically used in behavior modification.

RESPONSE SHAPING. Positive reinforcement is used in establishing or shaping a response that is not initially in the individual's behavioral repertoire. Response shaping starts with the reinforcement of very simple initial behaviors and works gradually toward the development of more complex terminal behaviors. Each behavior reinforced in shaping can be viewed as a link in a chain that has a single function: the occurrence of a terminal response.

MODELING. Terminal responses can be acquired more readily if the subject observes a model and is then reinforced for imitating the model's behavior. Modeling involves essentially a process of response acquisition whereby clients are given verbal instructions and/or demonstrations by which to model in order to establish a viable behavioral repertoire. Through verbal and demonstrational modeling procedures the process of learning new behaviors can be considerably shortened, accelerated, and made more effective.

BEHAVIORAL CONTRACTING. A behavioral contract is a written agreement governing the exchange of positive (or negative) reinforcements between clients and their helpers. Such contracts detail the responsibilities of each party and the privileges to be gained by fulfillment of these responsibilities. In some instances the counselor negotiates a contract between other parties, such as between worker and employer.

EXTINCTION. Extinction involves withholding the reinforcement for a conditioned response, which results in a gradual reduction in the rate of the maladaptive response. Because learned behavior patterns tend to weaken and disappear over time if they are not reinforced, the simplest way to eliminate a maladaptive pattern often is to remove the reinforcement that is maintaining that specific behavioral pattern.

TOKEN ECONOMIES. Token economies involve programs in which appropriate behaviors are rewarded with tangible reinforcers in the form of tokens that can later be exchanged for desired objects or privileges. Token economies have been used to establish adaptive behaviors ranging from elementary responses such as eating and making one's bed to performing responsibly on a job. The ultimate goal in all programs of extrinsic reinforcement is not only to achieve desired responses but to bring such responses to a level at which their adaptive consequences will be reinforcing in their own right, thus enabling natural rather than artificial reward contingencies to maintain the desired behavior.

SOCIAL REINFORCEMENT. Social reinforcement refers to the use of attention, praise, and so forth from human beings contingent upon the client's demonstration of a desired, positive behavior.

29.1.2. BEHAVIORAL DEFICITS

The goal when there are behavioral deficits is to increase the desired behavior. Either positive or negative reinforcement may be used.

Positive Reinforcement

Rewarding (e.g., reacting positively to a particular client behavior), will increase the frequency with which clients perform that behavior. Disabled people who show new interest in becoming independent should be given praise, attention, and smiles upon their demonstration of behavior indicative of efforts in this area. This kind of approval could be a reward by itself, or it could be accompanied by some material benefit or privilege. For verbal rewards to become reinforcers, they should be paired with some other comment, object, or event that satisfies a need for the client. Another factor is the client's attitude toward the person as a reinforcer per se in that social approval is often not rewarding unless it comes from someone admired. Desired behavior should be positively reinforced as soon as it occurs; behavior that is not reinforced will probably decrease in frequency. Determining what rewards are effective is a problem because people value things differently.

Negative Reinforcement

To use negative reinforcement, the counselor looks at the client's world to identify unpleasant situations and then works with the individual in an effort to select behaviors that, if increased, will eliminate the unpleasant situations. Better adaptation to society is the general goal. Thus, the termination or withdrawal of an aversive situation (stimulus) is termed "negative reinforcement."

29.1.3. BEHAVIORAL SURPLUSES

As with increasing a behavior, there are two principal methods by which a behavior can be decreased: adding and subtracting. Behavioral surpluses, those kinds of conduct that occur too frequently, are the ones that need to be decreased. Such behavior, when performed often enough, can damage one's general welfare or that of others. Stealing, lying, yelling, fighting, and smoking and drinking excessively are behavior surpluses; these, if they happen at all, might be categorized as surpluses because they detract from an individual's capacity to deal successfully with other people. In all these instances the goal is to decrease the frequency with which this kind of activity is performed so that the client's life is not so disturbed by it.

Two major ways of reducing behavioral surpluses are punishment and time-out. Punishment is added·to the undesirable behavior to decrease its frequency. With the time-out technique, one subtracts a reinforcing element from the person (or removes the person from the reinforcement) in order to reduce the undesired behavior.

Punishment

The technique of punishing to decrease undesirable behavior is far from new. Years of research suggest that this technique does permanently suppress a behavior if the selected punishment is intense enough. But apparently strong punishment tends to lessen desirable behaviors also. For instance, an adolescent who receives strong punishment for lying will probably respond in one of two ways. The individual will stop communicating with the person inflicting the punishment or will stop lying to the punisher but keep lying to other people.

Another punitive measure that can decrease surplus behavior is embarrassment, but this frequently arouses resentment, which in turn leads to other problems. Likewise, reproving someone in public causes resentment; also it does not seem to have a lasting effect on behavior.

Frequently, rehabilitation clients have received a considerable amount of inappropriate punishment; they have been told in various ways that they are inept, incompetent, no good. When client aggressiveness occurs, it frequently has resulted from an effort to avoid punishment; these people have learned that when someone rebukes them, fighting back puts an end to the criticism.

Time-out

Another important method of reducing surplus behavior is time-out. It means taking an individual away from a pleasurable activity or withdrawing the reinforcing agent. Experience shows time-out to be extremely effective in decreasing disruptive behavior.

The client or the reinforcing activity should be removed for only a short period of time: a few minutes usually suffices. It is the removal of the person from the enjoyable situation that makes the difference, not the length of time. Time-out can be used at any time the client is engaged in a liked activity but is demonstrating inappropriate behavior. When using it, one should make clear that time-out is being used because the individual has performed a specific behavior.

During the time-out, the client is usually not required to do anything. The behavioral objective will presumably be achieved by the time-out itself (i.e., withdrawal of the reinforcer). In two variations on time-out, however, performance of certain activities during the period is required.

With the "negative practice" technique, the person is asked to demonstrate repeatedly the inappropriate behavior. Someone who has been verbally aggressive, for instance, is taken to a nearby but somewhat isolated room for the time-out. While there, the person is asked (in a neutral way, not with anger) to repeat whatever the behavior is—swearing, name-calling, shouting, and so on. After having repeated the behavior and stopped, the individual is asked to continue for another two minutes. If throwing something had been the problem, the person is asked to throw some nonbreakable object over and over during the time-out. This technique is effective in decreasing aggressive behavior, but the practitioner must remember to give positive reinforcement contingent upon the demonstration of positive behaviors as well as using negative practice to reduce the frequency of the inappropriate behavior.

Overcorrection

The technique of "overcorrection" requires clients to correct or repair whatever damage to themselves, their environment, or others that may have been caused by their negative behavior. In this process the time-out period is used to improve the situation in which the person was involved. In a rehabilitation setting, the client is required to make the correction immediately after performing the undesired act, spending no less than 3 minutes and no more than 10 minutes on the correction. In explaining why the correction is necessary and guiding the client through it the worker uses a firm, neutral manner—showing anger, displeasure, or amusement is inappropriate. If someone has been putting out cigarettes on the floor and leaving them there, for example, the overcorrection technique would require the individual to pick up the last cigarette immediately and put it in an ashtray. The last step could be to clean up the room, pick up cigarettes, and empty ashtrays in several rooms, or empty and wash nearby ashtrays. Overcorrection has proved successful with severely retarded people, the very intelligent, and the severely disabled.

Extinction, Signaling, Reinforcing Incompatible Behavior

Extinction involves removing the reward for a behavior that shows signs of disappearing altogether if it is not reinforced. When people get no reward for a particular response, they will look for responses that get attention and rewards.

Although weak punishments have no permanent effect on behavior, a signal can sometimes be used to indicate that a behavior is inappropriate. In effect, the signal is a light punishment that expresses disapproval. Saying "No" or "No, that's wrong" can communicate disapprobation of a certain form of conduct and temporarily suppress it so that an appropriate behavior can be substituted and learned. It is important to focus on the behavior rather than the client when signaling, and to avoid condemning the behavior in front of other people, which can cause resentment.

Since acceptable responses are distinctly different from unacceptable responses, increasing a positive behavior through reinforcement will sometimes extinguish the inappropriate behaviors that are its alternatives. Mild punishment can be used to suppress incorrect responses, and then when desired responses occur they can be rewarded. If particular desired behaviors do not occur, they can be suggested.

29.1.4. REINFORCEMENT

A continuous reinforcement schedule involves using reinforcement every time a desired behavior occurs. This is the desired technique when behavior initially is being strengthened. Extinction of the behavior begins when the reinforcement is withdrawn.

Reinforcing the response only occasionally or intermittently will slow the extinction rate and in many cases maintain the behavior level that has been established by a continuous reinforcement schedule. A partial reinforcement plan involves first establishing the behavior and then choosing a less frequent reinforcement schedule while observing whether the behavior is maintained or decreased. The schedule that maintains behavior with the least reinforcement is then chosen for use.

29.1.5. TOKENS FOR REINFORCEMENT

A "token economy" has been used with success in rehabilitation and institutional settings to motivate clients to increase positive behaviors. In effect, a token economy is an extended system for positive reinforcement of appropriate behaviors.

One of the problems in employing traditional methods of positive reinforcement is that the rewards lose their value when used frequently enough to increase behaviors. Approval by smiling or saying "Good," can be used only so many times before it loses its value and becomes boring. To keep its value, approval must be paired with a primary reinforcer (e.g., food, drink, or otherwise strong conditioned reinforcement such as an interesting activity or game). The problem with such strong primary reinforcements is that they usually cannot be given immediately after occurrence of the behavior for which they are the reward, and their value as a reinforcement is diminished in proportion to the time between the act and the reward. In using a token economy, both approval and a token are given for an appropriate behavior. The token can be exchanged for a reward at a later time. The use of tokens helps the client bridge the gap between the time of the correct behavior and the time that the primary reinforcement is obtained.

Other advantages of giving tokens for positive behaviors are also worth mentioning. One is that the client has immediate and continuous possession of the token until the reinforcement is given, whereas the smile or comment of approval lasts only a short time for most clients. Also, clients can accumulate a large number of tokens as reminders of their positive behaviors and future rewards, but they can have only one smile at a time. The number of tokens given for each type of reinforcement, moreover, can be different, or the type of token can be different for each type of reinforcement; in either case, the type and number of tokens will vary with the behaviors and make distinctions between acts that approval might not distinguish as well. Finally, the number of tokens held by a client might be recorded and used as an indication of the frequency with which the client has demonstrated correct behaviors in a day or week; increases in number of tokens reflect an increase in appropriate behaviors.

In summary, the simplest token economy, to be effective, has four basic components: a list of target behaviors for the client to increase; the tokens themselves; a list of reinforcers (rewards) that the client can buy with the tokens; and a record system for charting the client's holding of tokens.

Target Behaviors

Behavior(s) targeted for clients to learn or demonstrate are those desired behaviors that would ordinarily be followed by positive reinforcement. Once selected, they should be specifically described in behavioral terms so that everyone involved can agree on what is to be reinforced.

If behavior in the workshop were to be targeted, for example, specific behaviors must be described. "Working hard" is too vague and imprecise for either the client or the reinforcer. "Completing the task in 10 minutes" is acceptable because it is explicit. Specifying target behaviors explicitly is an economical way of describing the client's problem in a certain area, and a clear statement of a problem is often a large part of solving it. Discussion with the client to identify and describe target behaviors will clarify what responses will be expected and rewarded with tokens and verbal approval.

Uses of Tokens

Many types of tokens can be used: poker chips, punched holes on a card, stars on a chart, points recorded in some manner. Regardless of type of token used, however, it should be paired with a signal of approval, such as a smile, pat on the back, or complimentary comment. Ideally the token should immediately follow the verbal approval, and the client should be told what specific behavior the token is given for. This procedure accomplishes three major goals. First, it increases the probability that the client will repeat the behavior. Second, describing the behavior for which the token was given will help clients articulate for themselves or others the reason they have received reinforcement; subsequently, they will learn how they can acquire more tokens by controlling their behavior. And third, giving the token with verbal approval or immediately afterward will not only strengthen the value of the verbal signal but will also encourage the client to seek verbal approval apart from the tokens.

Back-up Reinforcers

This component of the token economy provides the incentive for clients to demonstrate the desired behaviors. The back-up reinforcers are the activities or things that the clients can purchase with their tokens, hence the consequences that give the tokens reinforcement value. Without strong back-up reinforcers that interest clients, the tokens will be worthless; in most cases the reinforcers will be tailored to the client.

The back-up reinforcers are typically recorded on a card called the reinforcement menu, which contains activities or things a client can purchase and the cost of each. Persons working closely with the client can construct the list from their knowledge of what the client likes. The list can be revised and expanded as needed, with the goal of maintaining a list of fresh, interesting activities or objects that will motivate the client to change behaviors.

Token economies may have reinforcer menus that contain things such as food, drink, and personal items, although such a system can be costly. Token economies seem just as effective when the back-up reinforcers are activities that require supervisory time but little expenditure of money.

Record System

Experience has shown that a record system showing behavior change over a period of time adds much to the motivational power of a token economy. One quite simple way is to graph the frequency of a certain behavior as a function of time. The first part of the graph will show baseline behavior; the second will show improvements (or deterioration) over the succeeding duration. Because it records and displays a behavior very specifically, the graph allows for discussion of behavior and exploration of problems associated with it. Group situations such as a workshop detail may involve having all clients reinforced for the same behavior, in which case it is convenient and helpful to have a master record to keep track of individual behavior.

Clients who are consistently receiving tokens and showing appropriate behaviors for rehabilitation progress are often moved into a second stage of the token economy, one in which they are no longer paid tokens for each behavior but are paid a salary of tokens or points at the end of the week. The points or tokens can be spent or saved as desired. In this stage, the appropriate behaviors are expected of clients, and there is little supervision to check that they are being demonstrated. Appropriate behaviors will likely become habitual in this stage, and the back-up reinforcers might be expanded in variety. Nevertheless, clients should still receive verbal reinforcement for their efforts in this stage.

29.2. *Modeling*

Modeling is the utilization of models, real or symbolic, who perform the behavior the client needs to learn. Nearly everything that can be learned through personal experience can also be learned through observation or vicarious experience. By observing someone else's behavior and its consequences for that person, one can gain much the same knowledge one would gain from actual experience. So, a suitable "model" may expedite social learning. This method is especially appropriate for use with clients who show gross behavior deficits: children, for instance, who do not speak or respond at all to others. By means of modeling procedures, clients can acquire new behaviors, increase or decrease inhibitory responses, and reestablish behaviors acquired previously [Bandura, 1969, 1971, 1977].

Since observational learning has been shown to be an effective procedure for the promotion of many kinds of behavioral change, Hosford [1969] said that helping clients to acquire new ways of behaving can be accelerated through the methodical use of models. Many times all that is needed to promote more adaptive behavior is one social model, presented one or more times. In cases involving particularly complex or anxiety-provoking situations, the models are best presented in graduated sequences, with the client having undergone relaxation training.

Daniel Cook [1976], on the basis of research with modeling, in rehabilitation, concluded that for it to stimulate learning, several specific and interrelated conditions must be met:

First, an observer must attend to the modeled behavior. Merely exposing an observer to a model does not insure that the observer will attend to the model. . . . Second, for the modeled behavior to be retained or learned, the modeled behavior must be effectively cognitively encoded. Observers who transform modeled actions into visual imagery or verbal codes through post-modeling discussion obtain the highest level of response retention. Third, to achieve behavioral reproduction of the cognitively encoded behavioral representations the observers must be physically able to perform the behaviors. . . . Finally, if negative sanctions or unfavorable incentive conditions for the acquired behaviors exist in the observer's behavioral field, it is highly unlikely that the cognitively encoded behavior, which exists in representational form, will be activated into overt performance [p. 33].

In short, for modeling to be effective, the client-observer must attend, must comprehend, must accept, and must eventually act the modeled behaviors. Cook thought that failure to meet any of these conditions can result in ineffective modeling.

29.2.1. ESTABLISHING THE SITUATION

Setting up the modeling situation was discussed by Bertcher, Gordon, Hayes, and Mial, [n.d.]. They dealt with several key issues: specifying of cues, consistency of the model's behavior, client's response to the model, and practicing the behavior.

Specifying the Cues

It is necessary not only to be clear about what the client is to learn, but also to specify what cue the model (the counselor or another who is serving as the model) will be responding to when performing the chosen behavior. The use of this cue must be understood by the client. The term *cue* refers to some element of a situation that elicits a certain response, one which determines that this behavior, instead of some other possible reaction, is the one appropriate to the time and situation.

Consistent Models

Clients will often have difficulty understanding clearly what is to be imitated unless the model performs consistently in response to a particular cue. Models tend to make either one of two mistakes that can result in inconsistency. It is common to respond to a cue differently at different times because of the presence of other cues. If the client has been prepared to watch the model's response to a given cue, it may be confusing when the model reacts to another one. The client may not realize what is going on.

Another kind of inconsistency results when the model instructs the client in how to behave in response to the cue but does something different; people tend to copy things they see others doing rather than behave as they are told. If the model's message seems to be "Do as I say, not as I do," the client may feel resentful, perceiving that there seem to be two sets of rules—one for the client and another for authority figures.

When Clients Will Model Behavior

Clients will follow the model's conduct in a given situation when they feel that their own reaction is not rewarding or suitable, and when they believe that the model's behavior will meet with more reinforcement. They will usually not change their own behavior unless they feel uncertain or displeased about it; when they feel this way, they will be more likely to imitate a model who appears to have some expertise than one who does not. Although people tend to choose methods somewhat like themselves, the element of expertise is more important than that of similarity when people feel that they themselves lack expertise.

Practicing the Behavior

If one element of a model's conduct is supposed to be imitated, getting rid of strong distractions will help ensure that this element stands out clearly. A lot of noise or an unfamiliar setting might be quite distracting, for instance. But, if most potential distractions are eliminated, the client may learn to respond correctly only when there is little interference. The learning process may be quick, but the client may have difficulty performing correctly in another environment that includes many distractions. So, it is probably a good idea to begin by eliminating major sources of interference and then to accustom the client gradually to various situations.

29.2.2. USES IN REHABILITATION

For a number of reasons pointed out by Bruch, Kunce, Thelen, and Akamatsu [1973], modeling procedures are especially useful in rehabilitation. These techniques are compatible with the philosophy of rehabilitation; they are appropriate to the emphasis in rehabilitation on interpersonal relationships; and they facilitate behavioral generalization.

Emphasis on Client Assets

Learning by imitation is consonant with the rehabilitation principle of emphasizing the client's assets. Through modeling the disabled can learn directly and efficiently to take advantage of their strengths in spite of handicapping conditions. Most disabled people have premorbid behaviors, skills, and abilities that counterbalance the handicap resulting from impairment; to emphasize these resources is to facilitate the development of a satisfactory new vocational or social status.

When a disability strikes, an individual's sense of perspective is often temporarily dulled; it is difficult to envision going on in the usual fashion. Observing models whose disabilities are similar, but who have learned to do many things not prohibited by the handicap, may make it more probable that the client will do the same. A client who sees someone else coping with a disability may be able to understand that, despite the handicapping condition, it is possible to learn alternative ways of doing things.

Interpersonal Relationships

Rehabilitation programs make considerable use of dyadic and group relationships as vehicles for behavior change. The implications of modeling for these relationships are many. Modeling techniques are appropriate in staff-client relationships and also among peers as ways of working toward rehabilitation goals.

Behavioral Generalization

A behavior is said to be generalized if, after it is learned, the individual performs it not only in the setting in which it has been learned but in other situations as well. Generalization of acceptable social and vocational behaviors is a perplexing problem, both from one treatment setting within a particular facility to another and from the treatment environment to the community at large. Modeling procedures alone or in combination with reinforcement techniques may be more effective in achieving generalization than the use of direct reinforcement by itself. The advantages of modeling in this area are several.

There are various ways in which modeling can increase internal control of responses. Seeing models express feelings about particular activities in a treatment setting can enhance a client's awareness of the satisfaction that accompanies performing certain tasks, regardless of the social situation. Observing a model behaving the same way in more than one context, and seeing the consequences vary according to the context, may teach an individual what to expect from doing this. In the same way, seeing models different in personal attributes (age, sex, occupation) displaying the same behavior may help an individual generalize responses.

29.2.3. CLIENTS FOLLOWING TRAUMA

Bruch and colleagues described the modeling procedures that are useful in addressing rehabilitation clients' problems. They identified the following stages in the rehabilitation process in terms of the kinds of learning problems faced by the client: onset of disability, extinction of inappropriate behaviors, acquisition of appropriate behaviors, and transition to a nontherapeutic environment.

Onset of Disability

A physical disability that comes on suddenly, such as traumatic spinal cord injury, stroke, and so on, results immediately in noticeable sensory alteration. Impairment of autonomic nervous system functions along with extended confinement to a hospital bed decreases sensory input. This abrupt alteration causes disorder and turmoil at the same time the person is suffering from grief and depression.

Modeling techniques can be particularly helpful in dealing with the sense of inadequacy such an individual feels. The strategy involves exposure to models similar to the client in background and occupation and identical with regard to the disability. The client observes these models involved in social, occupational, and physical activities; in this way, it is hoped, the individual will begin to see more possibilities in the disability situation.

However, models should not seem to demonstrate that the client's condition can be miraculously overcome. In a state of doubt and dejection after the onset of disability, the client will probably have difficulty identifying with models who manage superlatively. What will work better are models who also feel discouraged at the beginning but who gradually show determination to handle disability and proceed to take on more and more challenging tasks. These models can demonstrate specific motor activities for the client to imitate, for example, physical therapy exercises and skills like those required to handle a tool with an artificial arm.

Modeling is useful for the period following onset; first, because during this phase the client is immobilized to some degree and therefore unable to practice behaviors. Learning through observation is feasible, however, unless, of course, cerebral functions have been impaired. Learning from models also helps to accelerate later learning as it heightens motivation to undergo the strenuous process of restoration. Modeling is also appropriate in this early stage for another major reason: because clients in this situation may be very dependent, their capacity to be influenced by the models is especially great. Hence, observational learning can be exceptionally effective.

Extinction of Inappropriate Behaviors

Decreasing or eradicating inappropriate behaviors in the newly disabled individual may involve reduction of fantasies about returning to a particular job or lessening of apprehension about treatment or training. It may be necessary during this phase, especially with socially disadvantaged or emotionally disturbed clients, to decrease undesirable social behaviors and negative opinions about occupational training.

As pointed out earlier, inappropriate behavior can be extinguished in three ways: by not reinforcing it, by punishing the individual, and by rewarding for a form of conduct inconsistent with the undesired behavior. These contingencies, however, can be presented vicariously. That is, having a model perform a behavior and then be reinforced or punished can promote much the same outcome as reinforcing or punishing the client directly. The consequences for various responses of the model and for the observer must be clearly explained. A modeling strategy for the extinction phase might start with the presentation of a model performing unlike behaviors that are followed by unlike consequences. This kind of strategy might be especially helpful for people whose effective social responses need to be increased. A videotape could specifically present undesired behaviors in a work situation, such as interfering with and manipulating others or seeking undue attention from supervisors. The model would suffer consequences like being separated from the others, having no say in the choice of assignments, being ignored by supervisors, or losing the job. This presentation could be followed by one that depicts opposing responses and positive rewards.

People who are extremely apprehensive about training for some reason may be helped by another kind of strategy. Someone who must use a wheelchair, for instance, may wish to avoid trips into the community because of fears of getting hurt or stranded. Such a person could observe a model getting around in a wheelchair without negative results, or the positive rewards for this behavior could be depicted.

Acquisition of Appropriate Behaviors

Modeling is useful in helping the client acquire behaviors necessary for educational, vocational, and social adjustment. It is especially important for the rehabilitation effort to focus on those behaviors that will be required in the target environment. First a careful study of the target environment is conducted to identify the specific behaviors that the client will need to acquire and that can be presented vicariously through modeling. For instance, the client can observe models going through the various steps of the routine in a workshop, with time allowed between steps for the observer to practice these tasks. The client can learn each facet until competent to perform the entire cycle.

Besides acquiring the actual vocational competencies, the client must also develop positive attitudes toward the work. The model can present appropriate attitudes while demonstrating how the vocational tasks are accomplished; observing the model's enthusiasm or interest can

greatly enhance the client's own performance and involvement in the therapy program.

Transition to a Nontherapeutic Environment

At this stage more emphasis is placed on development of the special behaviors that will be needed in environments other than the rehabilitation setting. Now, external management of the client's behavior through approval or other rewards will end, since in the community behavior is not controlled this way. The client must therefore learn self-governance so as not to rely on incentives that come from without.

Modeling can be used to demonstrate responses important for self-control. First, criteria for self-reward must be defined because the community will typically have different standards for performance from those of the institution. In some cases, raising the standards may help a client adjust to more demanding work or more difficult social circumstances. In other cases, adopting looser criteria may help less confident clients perform more competently.

Before moving from the relatively insulated rehabilitation setting to a work site in the community, the client should observe models working in the outside setting, either in actuality or on film. Self-reward criteria, more strict than standards in the workshop, can be modeled. Both the improved work itself—increased production—and the intangible benefits of performing well—the reward of satisfaction—should be demonstrated.

The informal modeling that takes place in a rehabilitation workshop may not be appropriate. For example, clients in a work adjustment setting observe the work habits of fellow clients who may be inappropriate models. On the other hand, the opportunity to watch persons with similar disabilities overcome their handicaps may help a newly disabled person to capitalize on residual abilities.

29.2.4. OTHER MODELING USES

In addition to its usefulness for rehabilitation work generally and for dealing with newly disabled people in particular, modeling is especially suitable at several other points during the rehabilitation process. Bruch, Kunce, Thelen, and Akamatsu [1973] discussed how modeling can facilitate vocational counseling, work adjustment training, and training for job-seeking.

Vocational Counseling

Since a primary objective for vocational rehabilitation clients is to find a job objective suitable to their capabilities, vocational counseling is central to the rehabilitation effort. Modeling can be used in conjunction with vocational exploration during the early stages and also during the decision-making process when the client is selecting a particular training program.

Modeling techniques can be used along with group counseling to mobilize the potential enthusiasm of people working together. Models seen on tape by the group can demonstrate how prevocational endeavors may help people choose a particular training program. Modeling can also be used to generate group discussions on employment objectives.

Demonstration tapes can be made to deal with subjects like getting and using vocational information. Others can dramatize certain behaviors such as responses during vocational counseling. Other kinds of presentations are devised to display the rewards of vocational exploration. After the group is exposed to such tapes, discussion about the conduct of the models and its relevance to the group can take place.

Later on during rehabilitation, modeling may be helpful in teaching clients how to decide upon a vocational objective and rehabilitation preparation plan. First, the decision-making process is divided into separate steps; then peers who can demonstrate the relevant behaviors are selected as models. They can be taped while going through the sequence that culminates in choosing a specific training program. Besides showing these steps, the tape should convey the idea that following this pattern is self-reinforcing. The clients can learn the whole set of procedures by imitation and practice. Once they have mastered the decision-making process, its relevance to the practical matter of selecting a program can be discussed.

Work Adjustment Training

Work adjustment is very much emphasized in rehabilitation. A rehabilitation workshop gives clients the opportunity to do various kinds of jobs and to develop a positive work personality. The objectives of work adjustment training are to develop physical capabilities and social behaviors suitable to the work situation. Modeling procedures are used in helping clients attain these goals.

It is important during rehabilitation for the client to acquire the physical capacities that will be needed in a particular job. Someone who will be doing benchwork or working in an assembly line, for instance, may need to develop increased tolerance for sitting or standing. For this purpose a training schedule should be devised to help the client learn to remain in one posture for longer and longer periods of time. Also the client must learn to work more efficiently and to approach the job more positively. Clients who make these efforts should be reinforced; explaining how this progress improves job qualifications is rewarding to clients who want to work.

Modeling techniques that are aimed at improving physical adaptation can also be beneficial to many rehabilitation clients. Learning to cope with a particular disability frequently necessitates acquiring new skills, such as handling small objects with an artificial arm. Models can show how this is done in a particular work situation, and they could also exhibit the rewards of increasing proficiency with the prosthesis. It is easy to display not only external rewards, in the form of attention from staff or progression to vocational training, but also intrinsic rewards, such as satisfaction expressed by the models.

Work adjustment training includes as a principal goal the acquisition of social behaviors that will help the client operate in different kinds of work environments. Many clients need to develop a set of fundamental behaviors for this purpose, whether they be adolescents with most of their occupational life ahead of them or adults whose disability necessitates retraining. Frequently they must learn what is and what is not acceptable social behavior in a particular work situation. Sometimes a great deal of personal interaction is allowable or even necessary, whereas in other cases a great deal of social contact would impede productivity.

Multiple models are especially suitable for illustration of the desired social behaviors, such as cooperation; they can be observed at the work site itself. As Bandura [1971] pointed out, multiple models work better than a single exemplar in teaching complex behaviors in which the timing, duration, and frequency of responses are important. Multiple models can create the illusion of a real situation and also, because different models react in different ways to a given stimulus with different consequences ensuing, they can illustrate contrasting behaviors effectively.

Finally work adjustment training, in addition to developing physical capacities and furthering social adaptation to the work environment, addresses clients' apprehensions about various aspects of working. It is not only long-term or severely disabled people who need this kind of help in order to transfer successfully from a sheltered setting to an industrial environment; most clients are apprehensive about certain aspects of a new work situation. Sometimes they hesitate to talk about these fears out of embarrassment and as a consequence appear unmotivated or uninterested.

Clients may be excessively fearful of contact with equipment or of certain industrial materials believed to be harmful; they may have other phobias such as fear of heights, confined spaces, and so on. A technique called "contact desensitization" [Ritter, 1969] can reduce excessive fears through a combination of systematic desensitization and modeling tactics [Wolpe, 1958]. A model illustrates appropriate behaviors and draws the client physically into the demonstration. If someone were afraid of handling a particular piece of machinery, for instance, the client's hand can be placed on the model's while the model operates it. In addition to illustrating the desired behavior and helping the client practice it, the model uses rewards that indicate approval, both verbal and nonverbal. The model's instructions diminish gradually as the client performs the behavior more independently. This strategy should be organized so that the least difficult steps are practiced first, with progression to more difficult tasks as the client's fears lessen and proficiency increases.

Some clients, having mastered work skills, are still unable to get a job because their interview behavior is unacceptable. Sometimes they need to learn where to look for work, while in other cases they need more perseverance. Modeling and role-playing are effective in improving clients' interviewing and job-seeking skills and also in teaching suitable ways of dressing, speaking, and the like, as Sarason and Ganzer [1971] and Walker [1968] reported.

Job-seeking

To teach interviewing behaviors, models first demonstrate, to a group of clients, appropriate forms of conduct. Then, after discussing what they have seen, the clients take turns playing the role of the applicant, to be taped and played back. Each client's performance is evaluated, and then everyone continues practicing the effective behaviors until they are established.

This sort of training has been shown to increase the success of clients looking for jobs. Rehabilitation clients prepared in this way have reported that after training they feel less apprehensive about interviews; sometimes their self-esteem is enhanced when they realize that someone else in the group is imitating their role-playing. Possibly, as Bruch and colleagues suggested, the experience of being imitated increases the likelihood of one's repeating a behavior.

29.2.5. CONCLUSIONS

Sometimes, as Hosford [1969] wrote, modeling alone may influence the client to adopt the behavior in question; at other times, the use of modeling along with other strategies may be the best way to achieve the desired goals. For clients who need to increase or maintain already acquired responses, operant conditioning techniques are extremely successful and dependable; but, when it is necessary for people to learn new ways of behaving or complex sets of responses, these techniques may work very slowly. Modeling by itself, or modeling combined with operant procedures, may be a better choice in these cases.

One important advantage of modeling, as Krumboltz and Thoreson [1969] reported, is that it seems to work as well with groups of people as with individuals. Hosford pointed out that modeling may also be useful as a form of prevention. Films and tapes designed to illustrate how to make decisions, handle anxiety, and behave in appropriate ways may reduce or eliminate problems before undesirable behaviors have had time to become ingrained habits.

An excellent review of behavior modification in rehabilitation facilities was published by Robert Couch and Conrad Allen [1973].

29.3. Improving Self-Control

Management (control) of one's behavior to achieve self-selected outcomes is a critical developmental process for every person. Behavioral techniques are frequently useful for clients who exhibit difficulty in self-control. Self-control behaviors, according to Wehman [1975], may be best characterized as "independent decision-making in different conflict situations" [p. 27].

29.3.1. ANXIETY-REDUCTION TRAINING

Haddle [1976] discussed anxiety and methods of dealing with it. He pointed out that in order to function well people actually need to feel some anxiety but that when it is "maladaptive," it becomes a problem. Anxiety is adaptive when it involves openness to the environment as well as strong contact with the real world. It is maladaptive when it results in a closed attitude relative to the environment and poor contact with reality. Haddle discussed how to assess anxiety level, the use of relaxation training and exercises, and cognitive restructuring for anxiety relief.

Assessing Anxiety Level

In order to help people learn to decrease maladaptive anxiety through self-control, it is useful to teach them how to measure their anxiety level. Through practice, people can become adept at determining how intense their anxiety is.

Relaxation Training

Individuals whose anxiety is maladaptive can receive relaxation training either individually or in groups; the training begins after clients have been taught how to assess their anxiety levels. Deep muscle relaxation is frequently used to teach clients how to relax themselves. The physically disabled person should enter into a relaxation training program only if it is certain that the exercises could not be injurious in any way. For some severely disabled clients, a quadriplegic client for example, verbal suggestion techniques are a more appropriate form of training than deep muscle relaxation.

Relaxation Exercises

Relaxation exercises consist of producing tension in one part of the body at a time, noticing the difference between this tension and the relaxed state of the rest of the body, then loosening, and again observing the contrast between tension and relaxation. The individual is told first to get comfortable in a chair, breathe deeply, and rest as completely as possible. Then the instructor gives directions for going through the cycle: "Now while you relax the rest of your body, clench your right fist. Clench it tighter and tighter. Notice the tension. Keep it clenched. In your fist, hand, and forearm, notice the tension. Notice the difference in the tension in your right hand, fist, and forearm in contrast to the relaxation in the rest of your body. Now relax. Allow your right hand to become loose; allow it to completely relax."

The person is told to observe and appreciate how it feels to move from tension to relaxation, to note details ("the nice, warm feeling"), to enjoy relaxing after tightening, for 5 seconds, each part of the body in turn: fists, biceps, triceps, face (eyes, mouth, lips, tongue), neck, shoulders, chest, stomach, lower back, hips, thighs, calves. "Press your toes upward again, toward your face with your heels on the floor. Notice the tension. Now, relax them, and allow the relaxation to spread all over your legs and the rest of your body." After the whole process is complete, the instructor again names all the different body parts while the client relaxes them further and further, letting the relaxation spread over the whole body.

Cognitive Restructuring for Anxiety-Relief Training

Anxiety can be produced by irrational thinking, but through cognitive restructuring people can be taught to recognize illogical thinking and thereby reduce the anxiety. A technique known as "thought-stopping" is a way of helping clients isolate and deal with irrational notions. The client is asked to give a verbal description of the obsessive ideas that are causing the problem. The counselor suddenly yells "Stop!" Then the individual is asked to voice other irrational ideas; as soon as they are mentioned, the counselor yells "Stop!" again. The next step is to have the client do the yelling whenever mentioning these ideas; and finally, after practicing, the client learns to stop the flow of irrational thoughts silently and independently.

29.3.2. ASSERTIVE TRAINING

Another important self-control approach, also discussed by Haddle, is assertive training—also referred to as assertiveness training. This method is extremely effective in teaching people certain social skills and in helping them deal verbally with interpersonal problems. "To assert" is to state or affirm positively and plainly; assertive behavior is behavior that enables people to act in their own best interests, to defend their rights without excessive anxiety, to articulate feelings without discomfort, or to exercise their rights without infringing upon those of others. At the core of assertive training is the idea that all people have fundamental rights, which they can be taught to exercise by means of a set of verbal skills.

It is important not to confuse assertive conduct with two other forms of behavior that do not work effectively: nonassertive and aggressive behavior. The nonassertive individual tends to be inhibited, self-effacing, passive, and dependent, and frequently arouses guilt or anger in others. The aggressive person is overdoing self-assertiveness. This type of individual, often negative and critical, will interfere with the rights of others. Crime is an extreme form of aggression; verbal abuse is a milder form.

Assertive behavior, on the other hand, is a way of solving problems. Assertive people have learned to express themselves effectively, to control their own behavior, and to take responsibility for their conduct. They make their own choices; they have confidence that comes from self-control and from the knowledge that they cannot be manipulated by others. Among the topics Haddle dealt with in his treatment of assertive training were: the teaching of assertive skills to the severely disabled, assertive training groups, collecting data and selecting targets of change, training procedures, and use of homework.

Teaching Assertive Skills to Severely Disabled Clients

There are many ways in which assertive training can help the severely disabled. These people frequently suffer psychologically not only because of their physical problems but also because they are stigmatized in our culture; this can damage self-concept and create a sense of vulnerability. Competing for jobs is often difficult for the severely disabled. Assertive training is useful in helping these individuals prepare for employment interviews, and also appropriate for teaching them how to improve relationships with others and how to carry on an effective conversation.

Assertive Training Groups

For the severely disabled, group training is effective. Clients usually benefit from this approach and develop self-regulation through practicing assertiveness. Groups usually meet once a week for several months and consist of eight to ten members.

Data Collection and Targets of Change

Individuals are interviewed before joining a group to find out what problem areas particularly need attention. An interview schedule or inventory that covers major potential problems is helpful.

Clients should learn as soon as possible to pay attention to their own conduct. They can keep journals recording situations in which they were assertive or failed to respond assertively; this can help them decide what kinds of changes are desirable. After this has been done, they can select specific behaviors to concentrate on, and strategies for each client can be planned.

Training Procedures

The main assertive training procedures for groups are modeling, coaching, behavior rehearsal, and covert rehearsal. Models in person or on tape can demonstrate assertive behavior, instructing clients in a set of basic skills as well as focusing on particular problems. Role-playing can illustrate the contrasts among assertive, nonassertive, and aggressive responses. Dividing the group into pairs gives clients an opportunity to practice different assertive responses.

Coaching is another useful technique. The leader and those members of the group with more background help others by explaining various assertive responses and helping them behave assertively in the group. In behavior rehearsal, clients role-play the behaviors they are trying to develop. Covert rehearsal differs in that clients merely envision how they would react in particular situations instead of role-playing or verbalizing the behaviors. By picturing themselves coping satisfactorily in certain circumstances they practice vicariously the assertive behaviors they need to demonstrate in real-life situations. Covert rehearsal is quite often done before role-playing in the group.

Use of Homework

Clients in groups are assigned problems to practice on between meetings. This homework is important because it emphasizes the element of self-regulation. It also furnishes subject matter for people to bring to the next meeting. In this way they can get the reactions of the others and gain further insight into particular difficulties.

29.3.3. CONTRACTING

Contractual counseling utilizes both behavioral counseling and self-regulation procedures, as explained by Scott and Maxwell [1975]. By means of contracting, the counselor and the client select certain goals and outline in sequence the behaviors needed to attain these goals. The "contract" is the plan they agree on. While it is not a legal document it has a binding influence. When this technique is used, clients understand that they are responsible for their own conduct and that the counselor has had a specific but limited helping role.

Formalized written goals require the client and counselor alike to focus upon the tasks that, as given priority through careful thought, are most important. As Westman [1974] said:

The advantages of this system are many: it objectifies and also helps to eliminate the myths in the process of counseling; it helps all staff relate to the same objectives for individual patients; and it individualizes patient care and makes evaluation easier. It also helps us to tell anyone who has a right to know what we are doing for the people who come to us for help and something about how well we are doing it. It also produces in the staff a very realistic and pragmatic approach to their own work and the nature of their limitations, the limitations imposed from the patient, the treatment methods or other sources [p. 17].

A further advantage concerns the built-in evaluation mechanism inherent in Goal Attainment Scaling.

Basic Concepts

Thomas and Ezell [1972] showed how the underlying concepts of contracting apply to counseling. At a point during counseling when some future course of action can be mapped out, the counselor must determine whether a contract would be suitable. Relevant considerations are the character of the problem itself and the attributes and needs of the client. The kinds of issues most appropriately addressed through contracting are the simpler behavioral problems resulting from poor self-discipline, ineffective thinking, or low motivation.

If contracting seems like a good way to proceed, the system is explained to the client. It is emphasized that the client is free to reject the idea, that the contract will be worked out mutually and will require certain behaviors on the part of the client, that the counselor's role will be to help, and that the only rewards or punishments will be self-imposed. Now the client decides whether to adopt the system or not.

If the contract system is agreed upon, counselor and client prepare to draw up the contract. This involves analysis of many different plans of action, followed by selection of the one that seems most appropriate. The contract becomes a catalogue of behaviors that fit into the chosen plan. At this point a partial contract may have to suffice until more information has been collected; if so, only the beginning is completed and other material is added as the work progresses. The contract can always be altered along the way as new alternatives become apparent or as elements of the selected plan prove to be inappropriate.

This method encourages the client to analyze problems carefully, construct a strategy for dealing with them, and act on it. The counselor's function is to help the client assess progress, work out new directions, and offer information that comes from sources not accessible to the client. But, the client's signature symbolizes responsibility for work toward the goals in the contract. The contract system, by placing this responsibility on the client, encourages mature behavior.

Contracting Guide

DeRisi and Butz [1975] presented these steps as essential in the drawing up of a contract:

1. Select one or two behaviors that you want to work on first.
2. Describe those behaviors so that they may be observed and counted.
3. Identify rewards that will help provide motivation to do well.

4. Locate people who can help you keep track of the behaviors being performed and who can perhaps give out the rewards.
5. Write the contract so that everyone can understand it.
6. Collect data.
7. Troubleshoot the system if the data do not show improvement.
8. Rewrite the contract (whether or not the data show improvement).
9. Continue to monitor, troubleshoot, and rewrite until there is improvement in the behaviors that were troublesome.
10. Select another behavior to work on [p. 7].

Writing the Contract

According to DeRisi and Butz the essential items for the contract are: the dates of the agreement (including beginning, end, and renegotiation dates); behavior(s) targeted for change; amount and kind of reinforcer to be used; schedule of reinforcer's delivery; signatures of all those involved (client, parents, mediator, and the counselor); and, schedule for review of progress. Optional (but strongly suggested) are a bonus clause for sustained or exceptional performance and a statement of the penalties that will be imposed if the specified behavior is not performed.

Advantages of the Contract System

Thomas and Ezell reviewed the advantages of contracting. The contract itself records the client's choices and intentions, and its formal character and use of deadlines frequently provide incentive for people who tend to put things off. Dividing the contract into separate parts and conducting evaluation at different stages enable clients to sense progress being made. Besides placing responsibility on the client, the technique also helps to keep the client coming back regularly for the counselor's evaluation.

Disadvantages of the Contract System

The disadvantages of the system consist of certain limitations. The method works only if an individual really wants to alter behavior or resolve a troublesome situation. The counselor cannot really ensure that someone will abide by the contract; there are no external incentives or punishments that can be used. Defining elements of the contract can be difficult, and living up to the agreement may be more difficult than it

had at first appeared to be; also the novelty of the whole concept may tend to wear off. This system appears not to be appropriate as a way of addressing difficult psychological problems in which the individual's motivation is unclear. Finally, it is possible for a person to satisfy a contract without really gaining new understanding of the behavior it was designed to change or of why the new behavior is preferable.

Goal Attainment Scaling

Goal Attainment Scaling, generally referred to as "GAS," is a procedure for setting and evaluating client progress on short-term goals. The ultimate goal of vocational rehabilitation is employment but there are short-term goals that must be met before this is accomplished. The procedure has been explained in a publication of the Chicago Jewish Vocational Service, Research Utilization Laboratory (JVS-RUL) [1976].

Goal Attainment Scaling is a way of gauging quantitatively how the client is progressing; it provides for putting goals in order so that results are clearly visible and therefore measurable. Virtually any kind of goal can be placed on the scale; results are assigned numbers on the scale from low to high.

An important element of this technique is expectation. A result that can realistically be anticipated is given a middle value; this is the target. Proportionately higher numbers are assigned to more desirable results up to the best outcome that could take place; lower values are given to results worse than anticipated. Each of these results is characterized concretely—the ability to perform a task in a given time, for instance—so that the scoring is not debatable.

The various outcomes are conceived in terms of time so that there are set limits for their attainment. When the deadline arrives, scoring takes place and the goals may be revised if this is appropriate to new circumstances or an altered strategy. If the scale is composed of items that can be objectively validated, scoring can be done by outsiders if necessary.

In order to construct a scale for a particular person, the goal planners select the material—based on the client's problems and concerns—for the scale to cover. This involves setting goals and defining the hurdles that stand in the way of their accomplishment. Any number of items may be chosen, but they must reflect the client's most important or immediate concerns. Next, signs of progress in each area are identified in accordance with the client's characteristic responses. For instance, if the client's failure to speak to fellow workers is reflective of unsatisfactory social relationships, the number and duration of conversations in the workshop could become an indicator on this subject. However, it should be kept in mind that frequently the behavior is not the actual problem but only its outward sign. Those who use the scale should think of the problem itself, asking themselves how they would be able to tell if it were solved or alleviated.

The last step is to enter the anticipated outcomes on the scale, using criteria as concrete as possible. "Rarely speaks in workshop" is vague; "Speaks only to counselor and supervisor" is specific. The outcomes are arranged according to expectation based on knowledge of the client.

As an example, JVS-RUL presented a scale designed to measure an individual's progress in making vocational plans, conducting social relations, concentrating on a task, and handling suicidal depression. Each vertical column represents one of these and is so titled. Under *Vocational Plans* five steps from "most unfavorable outcome thought likely" to "most favorable outcome thought likely" are:

1. No ideas at all for future work. Hasn't thought about it.
2. Has plans, but they are not realistic (wants to be lawyer, college professor, etc.).
3. Has identified what he can't do and doesn't want to do, but still no positive and realistic plans.
4. Plans developed, but no choice made.
5. Chooses a realistic vocational objective.

From the most unfavorable outcome thought likely to the most favorable in the category of *Concentration*, the criteria are:

1. Can do assigned task an average of 15 minutes or less at a time.
2. Can do task an average of 16–30 minutes.
3. Can do task an average of 31–45 minutes.
4. Can do task an average of 46–60 minutes.
5. Can do task average of 61 minutes or more.

Results listed under *Suicidal Depression* are:

1. Attempted suicide once in last month. Threatened 3 times per week or more.

2. No attempts in last month, threatened an average of twice per week.
3. Threatened suicide 5–7 times in last month, no attempts.
4. Threatened suicide 2–4 times in last month, no attempts
5. Threatened once in last month, or less, no attempts.

The two elements of Goal Attainment Scaling that present the most problems are (1) setting concrete and measurable goals that will really reflect the client's attainments, and (2) setting goals realistically. If the objectives are too easy or too difficult to achieve, the score will be a distortion; if they do not relate to the client's general purposes, the score will not be relevant. If these difficulties are surmounted, Goal Attainment Scaling is objective. It also provides a sound basis for discussing with those concerned how the client is doing.

This scaling method is also useful as a way of considering the effectiveness of various service programs or facilities, which all obviously fail somewhere or to some degree when not presenting a solution. Goal Attainment Scaling can reveal important deficiencies and coincidentally helps accelerate progress by forcing concerned individuals or agencies to look more closely at a client's situation and work harder on potential solutions.

The various steps that constitute the entire process of Goal Attainment Scaling were explained by the JVS-RUL for the rehabilitationist or other user. The steps consist basically of identifying objectives and problems; choosing indicators, methodology, and expected levels; filling in and checking the scale; and assessing the client's current status.

The first step is to identify general objectives for the client, pinpointing also the lesser objectives that must be initially achieved. A rehabilitation counselor would probably select employment as the final goal, perhaps with intermediate objectives such as occupational choice, job training, and the like. After goals have been established, problems need to be scaled down to manageable proportions so that work on them can begin. Specific problems such as poor grooming, specific undertakings such as enrolling in school, or more general problems such as low motivation can be isolated.

Now the indicators of progress must be chosen. Whatever the problem is, the indicators must be observable. Sometimes the difficulty itself is not measurable, but the symptoms of it can be easily discerned; someone overly dependent on family may not leave home often or may show other signs of excessive reliance on people that can serve as objective criteria. The information that will be used to trace the client's progress—the observations of personnel, reports from the family, and statements by the client should be decided upon.

Next, the goal planner and the client together select the methodology by which the problems will be approached. (Clients have the right to be informed about the planned treatment and to reject or accept it.) The client's success should be predicted on the basis of what is known about the individual, what indicators have been chosen, and what treatment plans have been developed to help the client change. Almost any methodology can be used, although it is important to remember that the choice may influence the degree of success anticipated. In choosing levels, the user thinks about what can realistically be expected of this client with reference to each problem and what the client believes is possible. Unrealistic goals will produce poor scores and a sense of failure for the client; obviously the opposite danger is wasting the client's time by expecting too little. The scale will, however, reflect excessively unrealistic expectations, which can then be adjusted.

The user specifies the results that are "most favorable" and "most unfavorable." Again a realistic outlook is the key. Keeping in mind the client's history of reinforcement, characteristic fears, and behavioral patterns, the goal planner pinpoints what could be accomplished in each problem category if everything went well, and what the results would be if any negative influences intervened. As the intermediate levels of success are filled in, a graduated sequence of situational outcomes can be produced. The scale should be checked for scorability and consistency, for poor or missing instructions, nonmeasurable criteria, and unrealistic expectations. Finally, the client's present level of progress with respect to the material on the scales is identified and recorded.

Goal Attainment Scales can be scored in various ways, such as a five-point system in which scores range from +2 to −2 for each scale. The choice of the number system is based on the underlying purpose of the scaler who will do the scoring, on what the scores will be used for, and on how quickly feedback is wanted.

29.4. Rehabilitation Counseling

Terms such as *client-centered counseling* or *behavioral counseling* are often misleading. All counseling is client-centered. And there is no such thing as "non-behavioral counseling." The essence of psychology is to influence behavior. As Krumboltz [1965] said, "The central reason for the existence of counseling is based upon the fact that people have problems that they are unable to resolve by themselves" [p. 383]. In other words, people need help in changing their (problem) behavior and this is the purpose of all counseling. Krumboltz and Thoreson [1969] described the application of behavioral principles in decision-making.

29.4.1. MANAGING CHANGE
Weiner [1976] in his book *Clinical Methods in Psychology* categorized intervention types by which clinicians attempt to meet the psychological problems of their clients. The main methods are psychotherapy or counseling with an individual or group, crisis intervention, and behavioral modification. Although the techniques may be quite different, all are used for the purpose of change and all might be used separately or in combination with each other.

The idea of change is the most fundamental concept underlying all counseling practice. Yet, the complexity of changing people is seldom examined in detail by the counseling practitioner. Probably behavioral counselors have attempted more fully than anyone else to examine each aspect of the change process. Indeed, because the term *counseling* is often misleading, behavioral counselors prefer to think of themselves as change agents. Their job is to help clients unlearn maladaptive behaviors or to learn new behaviors that are necessary for the client to acquire in order to achieve desired behavior change.

William Gardner has written extensively about rehabilitation in which behavioral techniques are used. He and his colleagues [Karan and Gardner, 1973] have advocated a rehabilitation counselor role as a "manager of behavior" whose function would be to "bring about desired changes in behavior by systematically arranging and, where necessary, rearranging his client's environment [p. 294]. In the remainder of their paper they intentionally used the terms *counselor* and *manager* interchangeably to convey the notion that behavioral counseling is more than just applied behavioral modification techniques within a face-to-face relationship. They noted that the role of the behavioral counselor is to arrange an environment that maximizes the probability of vocationally desirable behavior. This implies that the counselor should have a very active role in the change process.

29.4.2. REHABILITATION CONSISTENCY

Biggs and Bowman [1973–1974] have similarly discussed the applicability of behavioral approaches to rehabilitation counseling. Because of its limited use in rehabilitation, they elect to defend the use of the technique:

It is commonplace for those not experienced in behavioral methods to characterize these methods and the people who use them as automating, dehumanizing and impersonal as compared to more traditional methods. However, if one studies the situation closely, it seems more accurate to say that these systems are less, not more, dehumanizing. There are a number of bases for this assertion. One is that these procedures are necessarily highly individualized in their design [p. 242].

Indeed, Hosford [1974] noted that behaviorism is the application in counseling of the true principles of humanism.

Several arguments justify the incorporation of behavioral techniques in rehabilitation counseling. All counselors quite naturally, but perhaps unconsciously, practice nonselective reinforcement through verbal responses. This is inevitable in any verbal exchange, so it is important for the counselor to exert purposeful effort to use these reinforcing statements in the best interest of the client. Secondly, it is clear that rehabilitation counselors are especially concerned with the impact of disability and the need to desensitize situations, and more specifically to help clients deal with the anxiety-provoking problems of life as a handicapped person. Behavioral techniques in certain cases are often more efficient in helping clients overcome these common difficulties as measured by the duration and number of treatments when compared to other techniques (e.g., insight therapy). Finally, the relationship of counselor with client is facilitated by behavioral principles. This is attributable not only to the successful outcome of tangible goals in behavioral techniques, but also to the fact all counselors serve as important models and reinforcement sources for their clients.

The fact that behavioral methods are both action-oriented and goal-directed techniques makes them especially appropriate to rehabilitation counseling. The primary use of behavioral techniques in rehabilitation, however, has been in facilities. Counselors in the public rehabilitation program have utilized the principles of behaviorism less than those in facilities in which a controlled environment seems more feasible. For example, the indecisive client is a very difficult counseling problem in all rehabilitative settings. Yet Kravetz and Thomas [1978] noted that behavioral counseling is seldom used in such cases. As they pointed out, "Although vocational rehabilitation counselors have the resources . . . they continue to use the interview as a principle means for facilitating client change" [p. 199]. It is to be hoped that behavioral techniques will become a common tool of all rehabilitation counselors, to be used along with other methods to improve the behavior of the disabled client with adjustment needs.

Chapter 30
Group Counseling

Group techniques are particularly applicable to the social rehabilitation needs of handicapped people. In fact group counseling in a developmental context is aimed at helping people regain or realize their potential for social functioning. Human interaction skills deteriorate over the long period of incapacity, isolation, and overprotection common to physical or mental disablement. Likewise group methods are especially effective with culturally handicapped people who seek (re)integration into the larger society.

In a broader usage, groups are appropriate for many counseling problems with which individual techniques might be applied. When sev-eral clients face similar hurdles in the rehabilitation process, group procedures may be more efficient as well as more effective. Examples include procedures for choosing a vocational objective, the developing of job-seeking skills, imparting information about agency services, and so on. Desmond and Seligman [1977] described groups with vocational goals.

The rehabilitation and health care perspective of group counseling is addressed in a book by Robert Lasky and Arthur Dell Orto [1979]. They have presented group procedures for use with a wide variety of disabilities. David Hershenson in the foreword of that book made this important observation:

Group procedures were introduced into counseling and psychotherapeutic practice with the aim of serving a greater number of clients within available professional time. With use, however, it was discovered that group methods added new and unique elements which could contribute to successful counseling outcomes. Not the least of these elements is the client's awareness of and support by other individuals attempting to cope with similar problems. For the disabled and hospitalized, who are frequently put into isolated or inferior life situations, these considerations can be particularly significant [p.ix].

Therapy through groups originated with the work of Joseph Pratt [1922], an internist who worked with advanced tubercular patients in a Boston sanatorium. In 1905 he arranged regular sessions with a class of 25 patients to discuss their experiences. Tutored by Dr. Pratt, the patients formed group cohesiveness and mutual support that helped them stave off isolation and depression. Pratt, impressed with the role that emotions played in medical treatment, extended his "thought control" or "inspirational class" methods to diabetic and cardiac patients.

Group therapy was subsequently initiated in hospitals and clinics by various psychiatrists. In the early years they, like Pratt, used a didactic approach. However, in the late 1920s group therapists began experimenting with applying psychoanalytic and other psychological concepts. Jacob Moreno [1946], known for his early work in group methods, had come to the United States in 1925 and introduced psychodrama. He is also known for role-playing and sociometry, a method for charting positive and negative affective ties that exist within a group.

Social group work started with culturally handicapped people. Toward the end of the nineteenth century, settlement houses emphasized the educational development and cultural growth of members, frequently under the guidance of a group worker. While group techniques drew knowledge from many professionals—sociologists, church workers, recreationists, educators, psychologists, physicians—the field of social work pioneered in the education and practice of group work as applied to culturally disadvantaged people. So, there are several major tracks of group counseling in terms of disciplines, techniques, agencies, purposes, and clientele. The knowledge base has been greatly enriched by the varied approaches.

Some rehabilitation agencies use group methods extensively for the personal-social adjustments required to get and hold a job (see 35.1.3). The provision of supervised group associations for clients is provided in the adjustment training programs of rehabilitation centers, workshops, and other facilities (see 13.4.6). Group counseling, however, is not typically offered directly by the state rehabilitation agency counselor. In the context of the public service, vocational rehabilitation has been traditionally defined as an "individualized process." One-to-one counseling is still the rule in state rehabilitation offices, although orientation and information (e.g., resources, occupations, job-seeking) may be conveyed in group meetings. Successful results of group counseling of rehabilitation clients are frequently reported in the research literature but such programs are not routinely conducted in public rehabilitation offices.

The terms *counseling* and *psychotherapy* as applied to groups are often used interchangeably [Seligman, 1977]. This causes some confusion when reviewing the literature on the subject. Group counseling and group psychotherapy have much in common in terms of purposes and techniques, but there are differences. For one thing, counselors concern themselves with conscious, less severe problems that do not necessitate drastic changes in the client. Counseling is generally a short-term approach that addresses problems on a situational level, provides support, and aims at improving awareness in the client. Psychotherapy, in contrast, is thought of as a long-term process that deals with deeper maladjustments, involves reconstructive efforts, and emphasizes the unconscious and the neurotic [Hardy & Cull, 1974]. For purposes of this chapter, *counseling* is the preferred term and approach.

The group format for adjustment through counseling has a number of specific advantages for disabled people. In groups, rehabilitation clients have a special opportunity to help and become close to one another, to express and share feelings, and to develop communication skills. Through the group, severely disabled persons receive attention and care from others.

It is not uncommon for the severely physically disabled to become separated from the rest of the world or socially reliant on close relatives. In group housing these isolated people can safely form new social relationships. The group experience enables them to widen their lives through the making of new acquaintances and also gives them a chance to develop and practice social skills. (See 8.5 and 40.5.)

Group members can serve as resources for one another in identifying new behaviors and approaches to problems. They can also provide a safe environment for reality testing in trying out new ideas and behaviors prior to actually putting them into practice. As their horizons expand, they form continuing friendships and social groups.

Salhoot [1974] pointed out that, for people who find it difficult to express their feelings, the group offers a more relaxed atmosphere than does a one-to-one counseling situation. Many times in groups, people who hesitate to speak up find that someone else is voicing their thoughts. This sometimes encourages silent participants to speak eventually, but even those who remain silent can benefit from the meetings; in contrast, the individual counseling session necessitates that the client actively participate.

Group work is more helpful to some people than individual methods. When the problems of the severely handicapped are the same, group members contribute constructive viewpoints and innovative ideas toward the solution of their problems. Many times the disabled feel that those who have not experienced their situation cannot understand it, and these feelings can be a serious impediment to progress. But in a group, Salhoot thought, people who share the experience of disability can deal with this response.

30.1. Establishing a Group

Before establishing a counseling group, those who are responsible must answer a set of questions: Why? Who? What? When? Where? How? This Kipling structure is suggested in the following discussion.

30.1.1. PURPOSE

The element of purpose is of great importance in the establishment of a group. Salhoot [1974] discussed this idea, emphasizing that the needs and concerns of the clients should be the primary consideration.

The establishment of a group should be contemplated when a number of clients have the same sorts of concerns, and when these needs could be dealt with effectively in a group. The purpose for bringing the clients together should be clearly defined and specific rather than general or comprehensive. Purposes such as the improvement of social adaptation, discussion of problems, looking at feelings about disability, discussion of work, and bettering communication are too vague. More specific purposes that could warrant the formation of a group are: preparing for effective job interviews, discussing good work habits, dealing with the pressures on the family in the disability situation, planning for release from a treatment facility, and working on problems arising on the job.

The purpose for forming the group should be developed with clients before and during the initial meeting. After they have specific objectives clearly in mind, the members formulate an agreement or a contract. This should reflect the goals the counselor expects the members to accomplish and also the clients' expectations of the leader. Frequently, as a group progresses, their purpose alters; the members accomplish some goals and new objectives come into view. When this happens, purpose should be brought up for discussion again, and the agreement amended.

30.1.2. OPEN OR CLOSED GROUP

A closed group is one that does not add members once it has begun. It usually meets for a predetermined number of sessions. An open group, which may or may not have a predetermined number of meetings, maintains its size by adding new members as people leave.

Whether a group is open or closed may depend on its purpose. For example, in intensive group therapy in which the relationships among members are of primary importance, a closed group would be appropriate. On the other hand, a predischarge group in a hospital might be open for practical reasons [Yalom, 1975].

30.1.3. SHORT- OR LONG-TERM GROUPS

Duration of groups was discussed by Northen [1969]. Short-term groups (usually meeting 6 to 12 times) are appropriate for certain counseling purposes. They are useful when the content has been limited and when members are relatively well motivated to participate. A short-term group can be used to help prepare members for new roles in the family or society, or when an individual or family needs help in coping with a crisis or learning about the client's disability. Short-term groups can also be useful in such areas as social skills or assertive training and in facilitating vocational choice.

Long-term groups have usually been used when the goal of the group is to help with problems in psychosocial functioning. It is generally agreed that major changes in emotional or social functioning will take longer than a few months of group treatment.

30.1.4. SELECTION OF MEMBERS

Participants should be chosen so that the group is homogeneous enough to draw together and at the same time heterogeneous enough to provide diverse resources for the accomplishment of group objectives. For group unity the most important ingredient is commonality of needs among the members [Salhoot, 1974].

The individuals also need to be similar in relation to the particular purpose of the group. If members are selected because they have in common a specific and significant purpose, the group will function more effectively: the individuals will identify with one another more readily; they will find it easier to talk to one another, disclose their feelings, and reveal themselves [Levine, 1967].

It is also very helpful if potential group members reveal different opinions, feelings, and ways of coping with problems such as those that may be dealt with in the counseling sessions. If they are somewhat different, members will be able to help one another in their areas of strength and will receive help when they have difficulty. Thus, everyone will learn new ideas and useful solutions from the others.

Levine discussed grouping in terms of two categories: the individual's motivation and ability to benefit from this form of counseling, and also the ability to work toward or attain the group's stated goals. In selecting members, it is important to consider ability to communicate: withdrawn clients and very active speakers should be put in separate groups. It may be necessary at times to change the membership after the group has been established. As it func-

tions the group may turn out to have a combination of personalities too heterogeneous for compatibility.

A common concern is whether to put people with different disabilities in the same group, but, again, the composition of the group must relate to purpose. If, for instance, the purpose will be to assess members' effectiveness in the workshop, the differences in their disabilities are not relevant. On the other hand, if the purpose is to work on problems that result from the disability, the degree and nature of handicap would be important considerations.

30.1.5. SIZE AND SESSION LENGTH

Group size is determined by the nature and purpose of the group. In most cases there are 5 to 12 members [Levine, 1967]. Basically, as Salhoot pointed out, those considerations applicable to other counseling groups with respect to size also relate to groups of the disabled. In general, larger groups will be more difficult to manage, and more group time and energy will have to be devoted to group maintenance as opposed to task functions. On the other hand, larger groups will be able to generate more varied ideas and other resources toward accomplishment of group objectives. It is essentially these two factors that must be weighed in deciding on optimal group size.

The duration of each meeting will vary according to the physical tolerances of the members, the number of meetings planned, and the environment from which the members come. Two hours, Levine said, is the most common meeting length; if sessions are held three or more times a week, one hour for each may be ample.

30.1.6. INTAKE

While in some agencies it may not be crucial or even necessary, depending on the nature of the group, an intake procedure is usually helpful in putting a group together. In some instances enough information comes from the referral process so that the counselor knows, for example, that all the potential group members have the same problem objective.

Interviews with each individual who might join a group are the best way to eliminate those who are not suitable. Interviewing also lets the counselor evaluate the adjustment goals and capabilities of each person and give people information about the group. Salhoot also pointed out that some individuals may feel more comfortable about joining a group if they meet the counselor before it begins.

30.2. Stages of Group Development

Groups go through predictable stages of development. Although there are different labels for these stages, the process is about the same. Groups pass through them at different speeds and sometimes regress to previous phases or completely skip one, but the typical sequence can be described. Helen Northen [1969] characterized this progression in her book, *Social Work with Groups*, and the dynamics presented in this section come mainly from her book.

30.2.1. THE FIRST MEETING

The first meeting, Irvin Yalom [1975] said, is always a positive experience. The group members have usually expected the worst, so they are pleasantly surprised. The counselor sometimes starts by explaining briefly the objectives and procedures of the group, sometimes by introducing important working principles like openness and confidentiality. The counselor may initiate introductions among the members or wait for them to do so. Typically one member who will play a dominant role in the early meetings gets the discussion underway. It is at this session that the counselor's shaping influence over the group begins to be felt.

30.2.2. ORIENTATION

During the orientation phase, the members must decide on their basic strategy with relationship to the group's work; they must also begin working out their interrelationships, each member establishing a social position in the group. This is necessary both for the accomplishment of their objectives and also for the satisfaction each individual derives from belonging to the group. The fact that the work and the social element are intertwined makes group membership a very complex experience for people whose social adaptation is deficient.

Members at this stage are likely to feel anxiety about this unknown situation. They are usually uncertain and self-conscious; they bring their own norms and values into the group situation and do not know what to expect from the others. At this time, group norms and expectations have not been developed. There is a tendency for the members to relate to the counselor rather than to one another; they look to the leader for signs of approval and may be quite dependent.

This stage is characterized by a search for meaning, and by definition of goals, roles, norms, and the direction of the group as a whole.

30.2.3. DEVELOPMENT OF RELATIONSHIPS

Gradually psychological bonds develop among group members, who are usually motivated to participate and work on evolving relationships. People tend, however, to be fearful of change, or some may have had negative experiences with groups of people in the past. So, there is a period of cautious testing during which members observe who listens to them, who snubs them, who seems similar, and so on. Feelings among individuals then start to crystallize and patterns of communication begin to develop. The counselor needs to be aware of the meaning of this new experience for the group members in order to help them develop trust and to minimize any anxiety they feel.

30.2.4. EXPLORING AND TESTING

The members explore and test out the situation at this stage. It is a time of unrest, conflict, and tension: there is competition for leadership and a struggle for power and control. But at the same time group cohesion begins to develop; as conflicts are resolved, relationships form and members are able to work together more freely.

30.2.5. INTERPERSONAL RELATIONS

There is a stage during which many issues of relationships arise, between the members and the counselor as well as among the members. Many members during this phase will view the counselor as a sort of authority figure. They will use many devices to test the counselor's role; the testing may be subtle or quite obvious, brief or prolonged. Group members may ask for special favors, or they may exhibit unacceptable behavior as a test of the counselor's acceptance. The form of testing depends on the type of group and the personalities involved.

In some groups, members become very dependent. They may compete for the counselor's attention or make exaggerated efforts to please. They sometimes make unreasonable demands and feel rejected when the demands are not met.

Problems in relationships between counselor and group members are sometimes accentuated by differences between them. A white counselor with black group members or a nonhandicapped counselor with handicapped group members may exemplify this. If the individuals try to deny or avoid facing the difference, feelings of distrust may be aggravated. Open recognition of such diversities, on the other hand, can break down communication barriers.

30.2.6. PATTERNS OF ROLE BEHAVIOR

As interpersonal relationships are formed, many patterns of role behavior develop. For one thing, leadership emerges. Although the group may have positions of formal leadership, informal leaders will constantly change. Members will vary in the amount of influence they exert on the group, which in turn will depend on the group's activities.

Certain kinds of role behavior will further the group's progress toward accomplishing its goals, whatever they may be. Frequently there is someone who asks the right questions at the right time, eliciting necessary information or explanations. An entirely different role belongs to the person who has valuable knowledge or experience or who can pull a variety of ideas together to make helpful generalizations. Someone may know how to articulate feelings in such a way as to encourage others to do so; or this same person may also be adept at asking others how they feel. Someone else may look at things in a particularly imaginative way and so be able to offer creative suggestions. The elaborator sees and explains the various implications of what others say; the coordinator is able to harmonize disparate viewpoints or organize various activities; the critic evaluates people, ideas, and situations and is perhaps the one to see the flaws in a proposal. There are other kinds of behavior: those

of the teacher, the spokesman, the technician, and the recorder.

Other people contribute to the emotional and social functioning of the group. Those who tend to be encouraging and supporting, those who attempt to resolve disagreements, and those who are able to dispel tension, among others, help keep the group experience positive.

Sometimes a role behavior develops that causes an individual member distress or harm. There may be an isolate, one who has few bonds with others, or a scapegoat, one who creates solidarity by channeling group tensions. Aggressions and hostilities can be projected upon one member.

Other dysfunctional roles result in the satisfaction of one person's emotional needs at the expense of the group. The clown disrupts the group's activities by arousing the others' laughter. The monopolizer feels a need to be the center of attention at all times. The aggressor attacks other members or the group as a whole; the gossip and the bully take over other dysfunctional roles.

30.2.7. DEVELOPMENT OF VALUES

Gradually values and norms develop in a group, and there is pressure on members to behave according to these principles. For example, a standard of behavior will be established that dictates how conflict will be expressed, managed, and resolved. The developing standards will depend on cultural factors and on the personalities in the group.

The norms established at this stage will govern such issues as whether discussion should be rational and practical, deeply emotional and introspective, superficial, and so on. They will also relate to questions of who speaks when and how much, the relevance of what is said, and patterns of communication and interaction. Members will often need to adapt to norms quite different from those they adhere to in their lives outside the group. It may be a group norm to express angry feelings, for example, but not a standard that people apply to situations in training or at work.

The Construction of Norms

The group establishes its norms on the basis of the members' wishes and instructions from the counselor and the more dominant members. If the members do not have definite preferences, there is freedom for the counselor to shape a cultural structure that will seem to serve best the needs of the group. Obviously it is the counselor who has the greatest opportunity to guide the group and set its course.

The particular norms that will be most beneficial will depend in part on the objectives of the group. Examples are as follows: (1) rather than relying on the leader, the group should assume much of the responsibility for itself and its functioning; (2) members should be open and willing to reveal information about themselves; (3) members should be sources of help for one another; and (4) members should view the group as important.

There are several ways in which the establishment of norms can begin. Frequently a norm is incorporated into the group's operation by a member who states it and tells the others to accept it. Norms can also be initiated through modeling; members learn to conform to a group norm by watching others conform. Norms may even be imported from other groups. The leader frequently influences norms: for example, the norm of group responsibility for its own functioning may be promoted by the leader who, instead of answering questions, throws them back to the group members. Generally, however, the most effective way of creating group standards is through discussion.

Johnson [1970] presents a set of general guidelines for the establishment of group norms and for ensuring that the members will support them:

1. Norms will work only if the group members know what they are, see that the others adhere to them, and have a sense of their validity.
2. In order for members to follow and internalize norms, they must find these standards useful for the achievement of group objectives. It is therefore a good idea for the members to discuss the relevance of a norm to their work on goals.
3. People will follow and internalize norms when they feel responsibility for them, for instance, when they have participated in selection of the principles.
4. Group members should invoke norms as soon as possible after an unacceptable behavior has occurred. Consistency is important.

5. Models and examples of adherence to the norms should be available, as should opportunities for members to rehearse desired behaviors.
6. The group should make use of general cultural standards that would aid in the pursuit of group objectives.
7. Norms should not be thought of as absolute but should be changed any time this would contribute to the progress of the group.

It should be remembered that norms are established near the beginning of the group's evolution, and that altering them is a laborious and time-consuming process. Because often they can be changed only after the composition of the group has changed drastically, the counselor should remember that the important task of setting up group norms should be undertaken with thought and care.

30.2.8. PROBLEM-SOLVING

According to Northen [1969], during the problem-solving stage two major trends in group life are discernible. First, a unit is formed in which the individuals are no longer separate but depend on one another. Second, they begin to make use of the group as an instrument for problem-solving.

This is a time of cooperative activity, interdependence, and mutual identification. There is a strong sense of group feeling and an ability to work together productively; the members feel that the group is important and worthwhile. (However, while relationships among members are generally positive, there will inevitably be some hostility and conflict.) At this point the members are less concerned with testing, and they begin working intensely on whatever the group is supposed to be about. Whatever the goals may be, members are able to work together on a more meaningful level.

Problem-solving is often the primary focus of the unit as it becomes capable of dealing with the designated tasks. As discussed by Johnson and Johnson [1975], the process begins as the group assesses its problem-solving competency and continues with a consideration of what problem-solving involves. The group is capable of work on problems if there is: (1) consensus about what they are working toward, (2) a way of obtaining the data they need in order to understand their present status with regard to this objective, (3) a plan for devising, selecting, enacting, and assessing various solutions, and (4) the ability to carry out these steps without detriment to the group's effectiveness.

The group should learn that five steps compose successful work on problems: defining the problem, diagnosing its causes and magnitude, drawing up proposals for its resolution, selecting and putting the best plans into action, and evaluating their effectiveness. Of these steps, definition may be the most difficult. It may be a more manageable task if all the members first state what they believe the problem to be. Then, through the process of elimination, the group can select the definition that seems most accurate.

30.2.9. ACHIEVEMENT OF COMPETENCE

Achievement of competence is the stage in which there are many opportunities for group members to learn and practice new behaviors, first in the group and then outside. Rehearsal is useful at this stage, so that people can plan how they will face difficult situations. Role-playing may be used to try out various alternatives as responses to stressful circumstances.

Competence is also developed more informally. As members learn to express their needs, share in decision-making, communicate effectively, and show empathy toward others, these behaviors will carry over into the member's daily life.

30.2.10. CLARIFICATION OF REALITY

Often individuals in groups learn from other members or from the counselor that their social behavior, attitudes, or beliefs are inappropriate or irrelevant to a situation. A member may be thinking irrationally or performing behavior that is self-destructive or detrimental to the group. At this stage in the group process, there will probably be enough mutual support to enable members to cope with criticism of their behavior or thinking. The incentive to change may come directly from the counselor or from the group assisted by the counselor.

30.2.11. THE TERMINATION

This is the final period in the group's life. The termination process differs somewhat according to the type of group. Some groups begin with a time limit, but in others the counselor and clients work together to decide when they are ready to

conclude. In open-ended groups in which members enter and leave at different times, the termination process will be very different from that of closed groups, which end as units. In planned terminations, it is recognized that a member has no more need of the group; an unplanned termination occurs for unanticipated reasons, such as the client's or the counselor's moving away.

As Levine [1967] wrote, when someone who has been involved in the group for a long time leaves, anxiety is caused for the individual and everyone else. The event may serve to remind some members of past separations; many emotions can be stirred up in the client; and they all have the opportunity to rework their ability to separate from others in the group. Time will be needed to prepare the individual for leaving and to help members deal with their reactions.

After a member leaves there will be disequilibrium in a group until the individual's role and function are replaced. Groups will have a variety of reactions to termination. There may be constructive reactions such as decreasing dependence on the group, or less constructive responses may take place. Some individuals may simply deny that the experience is ending and behave as if termination were not going to happen, while others may regress to earlier patterns of behavior. All kinds of negative symptoms may occur: increased conflict among members, sudden inability of members to cope with situations they could handle before.

30.2.12. ANOTHER CATEGORIZATION

Yalom [1975] suggested a somewhat different division of the group development process. He identified the three basic stages as periods of orientation, conflict, and cohesiveness. During orientation members participate hesitantly, depend on the counselor, and search for a meaning for the group. In the conflict stage the question of dominance is salient. As the group develops cohesiveness, the element of conflict recedes and the members concentrate together as a unit on the work at hand.

Knowledge of this basic pattern, Yalom stated, will guide the counselor in helping groups form appropriate norms, and also in recognizing problems and helping the group work past them. Moreover, the counselor who knows what stages most groups go through will have a sense of control rather than the uncertainty that would have a negative effect on the members.

But each group, Yalom explained, differs from every other in its evolution, as all the members' unique personalities reveal themselves and change under the counselor's direc- tion. Because human relationships are invariably complex and because in groups adaptive problems further complicate this interplay, each group will evolve in an unexpected way.

30.3. Techniques

In counseling groups, discussion is the primary medium through which objectives are accomplished. Consequently, the most important techniques are those that facilitate discussion that is productive relative to group objectives. The techniques used in groups, Levine [1967] pointed out, are as varied as the counselor's creativity.

It is important that members communicate with one another and not just with the counselor. The counselor must help members express themselves by showing understanding, helping them feel at ease, or encouraging them to clarify a confusing statement. If group members do not seem to understand what is being said, the counselor may need to help them clarify it for themselves. Often a counselor will need to encourage individuals to respond to one another's communication.

Satir [1972], in her book, *Peoplemaking*, drew attention to the importance of communication skills in a disabled individual's adjustment. To help the disabled learn these necessary skills, one can use games that are entertaining and effective. Through games, group members can become sensitive to the significance of body language and eye contact, and they can also learn about such aspects of communication as presumption of meaning, response to criticism and praise, and the like.

30.3.1. GROUP PROCESS TECHNIQUES

Group counselors are as different in their techniques as individual counselors, but there are similarities within the two approaches that differentiate the group counseling approach from one-to-one counseling. In the individual format the counselor functions solely and directly as the agent of change. The approach is much more indirect in group counseling, since change is primarily mediated not by the counselor but by the members of the group. The counselor's task is to help the group function.

Necessary group functions can be divided into task and maintenance activities. Paraphrasing Johnson and Johnson [1975], these are the various task functions that, when assumed by any member, contribute to the accomplishment of the group's work:

1. Information- and opinion-giver—to help group discussion.
2. Information- and opinion-seeker—to help group discussion.
3. Starter—to initiate action within the group.
4. Direction-giver—to focus attention on the task.
5. Summarizer—to pull together related ideas.
6. Coordinator—to harmonize activities of various subgroups and members.
7. Diagnoser—to figure out sources of difficulties.
8. Energizer—to stimulate work from the group.
9. Reality-tester—to examine the practicality of ideas.
10. Evaluator—to compare group accomplishments with group goals.

In contrast to task functions, which refer to the actual work the group is engaged in, the maintenance activities relate to the way in which members are relating to one another. Maintenance activities are very important, because interpersonal relationships within the group may either facilitate or impede accomplishment of task objectives. Someone who acts in any of the following ways is maintaining or increasing the smoothness of the group's operation (also paraphrased from Johnson and Johnson):

11. Encourager of participation—to demonstrate acceptance to ideas of others.
12. Harmonizer and compromiser—to reconcile disagreements.
13. Tension-reliever—to ease tensions and increase the enjoyment of group members.

14. Communication-helper—to make sure that each group member understands what other members are saying.
15. Evaluator of emotional climate—to ask members to share their feelings.
16. Process-observer—to help examine group effectiveness.
17. Standard-setter—to get acceptance of group norms and procedures.
18. Active listener—to be an interested audience and to be receptive to others' ideas.
19. Trust-builder—to reinforce risk-taking and encourage individuality.
20. Interpersonal problem-solver—to resolve conflicts and increase group togetherness.

A basic difference among counselors who conduct groups is the extent to which they assume primary responsibility for the task and maintenance functions as opposed to delegating that responsibility to group members. All group counselors, however, assume some degree of responsibility in the conduct of the group. The techniques that follow may assist the counselor in carrying out that responsibility.

30.3.2. USE OF THE PRESENT

Focusing on the present or the "here-and-now" is effective because an individual's interpersonal behavior inside the group and elsewhere will be quite similar [Yalom, 1975]. As described by Lassiter [1974], this technique disregards the elements of time and place. It fosters interaction based on feelings and encourages members to give and get one another's honest reactions. The atmosphere and chemistry of the group, rather than any kind of prescription, dictate what will happen next.

30.3.3. USE OF THE PAST

There is disagreement, Yalom pointed out, concerning the use of the past in group sessions. Some believe that focusing on the past can at times aid in the development of group cohesion by helping members understand and accept each other. While emphasis on the past is traditional, some feel that the past is important only as it influences here-and-now relationships.

30.3.4. ACTION ORIENTATION

Action-oriented techniques, often referred to as "nonverbal," are the many group activities be-

sides discussion. They may include arts, crafts, games, trips to the zoo or park, dancing, drama, meal preparation, and so on—essentially anything appropriate to the group. Activities are selected on the basis of how well they will contribute to group cohesiveness, what demands they will make, and what equipment will be required. Such questions as whether an activity will stress competition among members and what ultimate purpose it will serve are considered [Yalom].

30.3.5. INTERPRETATION

In discussing interpretation, Yalom used the term in its broadest sense to denote any kind of statement that makes something clearer or more intelligible. As used in groups, interpretation either illuminates an element of a relationship between one individual and another or it explains some aspect of group interaction as a whole. (See 26.1.5.)

30.3.6. WARM-UP TECHNIQUES

Exercises can be used initially in a session to help participants begin responding to one another on a here-and-now level more quickly. Members may, for instance, be asked to take turns articulating the feelings they have toward the person on their right; then these people might describe their responses. Or all the participants may talk about how they feel toward one person. The leader can organize the discussion further by asking speakers to focus on qualities they have the most difficulty accepting; these instructions will also help members keep in mind the distinction between individuals as people and their traits or habits. Another exercise would be for everyone to point out someone else's likable qualities.

30.3.7. STIMULATING DISCUSSION

There are times in any group when things begin to lag or seem to come to a stand-still. Certain techniques can be used at this point to stimulate discussion; some of the more common ones, as discussed by Glass [1969], are related here.

Summarization

After group members have discussed a topic, a summary of what has been said may be helpful. The technique should be used with definite goals in mind. For example, if a question has been discussed thoroughly and interest in it is starting to wane, a summary can be used to conclude the discussion. Summarization can also be very helpful in preparing the group for the next topic of discussion. (See 26.1.4.)

Pick-Up

A good device, especially when counseling goals have been well outlined, is the pick-up technique. In using this, the counselor takes something that has been said by a group member and uses this statement or question as the introduction to a new phase of discussion.

Comparison

The counselor selects a subject with which all the group members are familiar, and then draws a comparison with the present issue. This can stimulate understanding.

Leading Questions

In leading by a series of questions the counselor continually asks questions until the desired answer is given. This technique can be used for introductory purposes to stimulate the group members' interest in the subject matter to be presented. There are some hazards in the leading technique. In seeking one particular answer, the counselor may be imposing personal values on the group members. If they do not agree with a counselor who they feel has taken a dogmatic stand (as waiting for the "right" answer may seem to indicate), group interaction may decrease. The technique can be used in an entertaining way, playing a "twenty-questions" game, for instance. It may have a novel effect and thereby stimulate the interest of the group. It should be done, however, in a spirit of fun.

It should be noted that Glass used the term *probing*, rather than *leading*. Clinicians usually consider probing to be an in-depth intervention of the subconscious or otherwise defensively guarded material. (See 26.1.2.)

Direct Questioning

The technique used most frequently in groups is the direct question. This method can be particularly helpful when it is important to organize the group in a definite way. When used to the exclusion of other techniques, however, direct questioning tends to cut off or decrease opportunities for interaction among members.

Didactic Technique

The didactic approach is appropriate when information is what is most important. The emphasis is not on discussion; the counselor lectures to the group just as a teacher conveys knowledge to a class. (See 26.1.6.)

Confrontation

In confrontation, which is used less in group counseling than in other types of group work (i.e., group therapy), the group member is confronted directly by the counselor. Unless the counselor is extremely skilled with this technique and has been working with the group for a long time, this is not the technique of choice in a group counseling session. (See 26.1.7.)

Problem-Oriented

Many times groups are organized and their goals planned in relationship to problems. The counselor structures the group on a problem-solving orientation, that is, plans for the members to try to rectify or correct something that is perceived as wrong.

Sentence Completion

Asking someone to complete a sentence is an excellent way of getting at unexpressed thoughts and feelings. A person who seems to be hiding fear, for instance, might be asked to finish the sentence, "People are afraid when . . . ." After completing the thought a few times, the person may become aware of some of the reasons for avoiding or suppressing the fear.

Unfinished Business

Almost always there are unanswered questions or unresolved problems left over from the earlier part of a meeting or from other meetings. It can sometimes be helpful for the group to go back and complete discussion of these matters. Pfeiffer and Pfeiffer [1975] suggested that the leader bring up unfinished business by saying to the group something like, "I often find that after a conversation is over and I've left, I start thinking of the things I wish I'd said. I'd like you to picture yourself on your way home after this session. Are there things you would wish you had said?" This lead often encourages people to mention issues that can then be dealt with further. However, not every issue can be resolved, and some subjects should be explored only so far at one time and then set aside until later.

30.3.8. EXPERIMENTAL TECHNIQUES

Certain experiments in group counseling sessions can generate activity that gives insight into the personality or problems of the clients. The following are among the experiments appropriate for groups, as described by Pfeiffer and Pfeiffer.

Making the Rounds

A relatively simple but very forceful technique is to ask an individual to go from one person to another in the group and say something or interact briefly with each. For instance, someone who continually engages in self-criticism might go up to each group member and say, "I am a worthwhile person because . . . ." The effect of saying something boastful to everyone, as appropriate to the other person, would probably be similar.

Mimicry

Mimicking, unlike many other techniques, can point up what is going on without a distractive effect. If an individual is discussing something that has a great deal of emotional significance and is also expressing tension through body language, such as clutching at the chest, it would probably be distracting for the counselor to present a verbal picture of the behavior: also, the speaker would probably stop the behavior immediately. But if the counselor imitates the behavior, the individual can see the point.

30.3.9. BRAINSTORMING

At some stages of their work on problems the group will need new ideas and fresh viewpoints. "Brainstorming" is a technique that can be used to elicit many divergent views quickly. It is important for everyone to participate in a brainstorming session. While it is going on, no judgments are made and no organization is imposed; everyone throws out all the ideas that come to mind. The purpose is to discover and explore.

There are a number of guidelines for brainstorming. Ideas are presented without critical discussion. "Wild ideas" should emerge if the group is really getting into the free spirit of the session; the discussion should be uninhibited. What is important is the number of ideas

that are suggested, not their validity; the more new ideas, the greater possibility that a really good one will emerge. The members should work together, adding one idea onto another or combining what two people have said. It is important that they concentrate on one relatively simple topic rather than try to cover a number of problems at once or deal with very complex issues. The climate should be friendly and unstrained, and every member of the group, however reticent, should have an opportunity to be heard. Finally, all the ideas that have been produced should be written down.

30.3.10. ROLE-PLAYING

In role-playing, an individual plays the part of an imagined person in order to acquire different or new behaviors and habits of thought. It is an important group counseling technique, an excellent way of making a situation seem real so that it can be felt and discussed. In group counseling sessions in job placement agencies, role-playing works well as preparation for interviews (see 35.4). It is also useful as an approach toward difficulties people have at work in dealing with employers or other employees. A leader can suggest role-playing whenever it seems difficult for others to visualize what someone is talking about. It can also help people who cannot clearly envision themselves in a given set of circumstances.

Role-playing, Ohlsen [1977] explained, gives people a way of expressing how they feel about aspects of their lives that they find difficult to explain or possibly even to face. It gives them an opportunity to try out and rehearse different behaviors, to find out whether they can accomplish some new task, to get the reactions of others, and to view themselves from another perspective. If role-playing helps people talk candidly about difficult situations, learn more effective behaviors, and perform them confidently and easily, then their capacity to articulate their problems is improved.

Uses of Role-Playing

Ohlsen summarized research on the uses of role-playing, stating that most of the literature is positive. The following are the uses of role-playing upon which there is most consensus in the literature.

Role-playing can help an individual who is having difficulty explaining or admitting a problem or perceiving an important relationship clearly. It can enable people to recognize "unfinished business" with other people, choose what to do, and rehearse it, as well as to examine ways of improving significant relationships. Generally, this technique is useful in the determination and definition of a client's counseling goals.

By imitating an imagined person, an individual can present ideas to others and get their reactions. Role-playing can also provide training in asking others to help select and reinforce new forms of conduct.

In groups this technique is effective in enhancing people's perceptions and understanding of experience, and in getting members to work together to help one another. A client can re-enact an experience that revealed resistance, acknowledge it, and ask for the group's help in dealing with it. By acting out new responses with another group member an individual can generalize to other situations, that is, evaluate the potential effectiveness of these responses. Role-playing is a means of developing in people the sense of freedom to feel safely and speak honestly; it serves to heighten group members' concern for one another, gives them the opportunity to experience rather than merely theorize, and increases their awareness of their own and one another's feelings and needs. They can then respond to others more completely and also learn to control their own lives better.

Role-playing enables people to look at themselves more objectively, and it also provides training in decision-making. It is a tool for self-scrutiny, permitting people to isolate important questions about themselves and helping to show them how to look for the answers.

Bertcher, Gordon, Hayes, and Mial [n.d.] discussed role-playing in terms of six purposes. As a diagnostic instrument, role-playing can show how an individual will tend to respond in certain circumstances. The diagnostic purpose of the technique is better served if the role-play is timed to occur close to the actual situation that it is imitating; then the client's responses in the role-play will more closely approximate the real-life behavior.

Second, role-playing can be used for rehearsal, to equip an individual to deal with situations that will arise in the future. Other purposes are problem-solving (to summarize a problem and enact various solutions), modeling (to provide an example behavior), attitude change (to alter someone's negative attitudes toward others), and self-awareness. If through role-playing people can learn how others see them, their self-awareness will be enhanced as well as their capacity to relate effectively to others.

Role-play should have a practical application; people will not have much desire to learn behaviors they do not anticipate using. Therefore, the more similar a role enactment is to the situation to which it refers, the more probable that the learned behavior will actually be practiced.

Introducing Role-Playing

There are various ways of introducing role-playing to the client. Bertcher and colleagues maintained that the client should first learn new behaviors from a model and then try them out initially when no audience is present. They suggested that the pattern for learning role-play should consist of (1) modeling, (2) private or semiprivate practice of the role-play, (3) role-playing in front of the group, and (4) further improvisation. Having the client practice role behaviors first from a model helps to conform the learning of the desired behavior; once the behavior has been learned, the client can be encouraged to improvise variations on the behavior for different situations. The improvisation helps to ensure the client's commitment to the behavior, increasing the probability that it will be practiced voluntarily outside of the learning situation.

These authors contended that moving a client into a group role-playing situation too quickly can inhibit learning and lead to dislike of role-playing in general. They recommended that certain conditions be established before clients role-play in front of a group. The members should have become well acquainted with one another so that there is a climate of friendliness and cooperation. The counselor should stress the fact that role-play permits one to make mistakes with impunity, and that, as may not be true in actuality, a role-player can correct errors. The imagined circumstances should be carefully explained and the basic outlines of the performance indicated. It is important for the counselor to preface criticism of a role-player with positive comments, and other members should do the same. People should be urged to take parts that approximate their roles in daily life, and they should participate in choosing the role. There should usually be no more than ten spectators, in keeping with the idea that the role-play is an exercise, not a performance for an audience.

Ohlsen's [1977] book, *Group Counseling*, deals with the use of role-playing in a group and explains how the technique can be presented to group members. A counselor should talk about role-playing while telling prospective members about the group. Then during a session when someone has trouble talking about a difficult situation, the counselor can state that it might help if everyone had a clearer idea of the problem—what is disturbing the person, what other people have to do with it. Role-play can then be suggested as a way of presenting this information. The speaker probably plays the individual who is making the situation most difficult to handle, and casts the rest of the players. After the initial role enactment, the counselor should recapitulate the uses of the technique, explain it briefly, and indicate when the members of the group might suggest it in the future. Then a group member may propose role-playing anytime it seems useful. If, however, another member is the primary client (the person the play is about), that individual may veto the idea or suggest waiting until a later time.

The Role-Play

Ohlsen explained the functions of various people relative to the performance itself, pointing out its value for the primary client, the other participants, and the audience.

If the primary member does want to do the role-playing as suggested, this individual becomes the director, explaining the subject to the group, setting up the scene, selecting players, and getting the participants ready to take their parts. The counselor assists, but the client should be in charge as much as possible. Typically the primary member distributes roles among those who wish to participate; many times people who have seldom spoken up before will offer to take roles that have meaning for them. If not enough people volunteer, the counselor urges group members to help the director cast the rest. Puppets and dolls should be handy, because there are people who will feel more comfortable speaking through a puppet.

Without taking a managing role like that of the theatrical director, the counselor helps the role-play director, particularly in explaining roles to the players and helping them make up their lines. The counselor's function is to explain, when necessary, aspects of the encounter or of relationships to be portrayed, and to help players trying to express a feeling.

Usually the primary client learns the most from taking two roles in turn. First the individual acts the part of the most important "supporting" character and then, in a re-run, that of the primary character. This client usually gains much insight into the problem and the people involved during the process of getting ready to do the scene, regardless of the distribution of parts. It happens that people staging role-plays find their purposes have been accomplished even before the scene is enacted.

The counselor tries to get across to the actors the idea that this is to be an unrehearsed play. All the players, after discussing their parts, should feel that they can present their characters as they see fit. Even if words and sentences have been more or less set, the players should not worry about adhering literally to a script. Rather their aim should be to portray their characters' thoughts and feelings as well as they can, improvising as seems necessary. It is also suggested that the players use soliloquies as a way of showing that a character's words and actions do not really reflect inner feelings.

As the scene is about to be presented, the counselor ascertains that all the players comprehend their parts, giving everyone a chance to ask questions or seek advice. During the enactment the participants should not hesitate to stop when they run into any difficulty, perhaps because they have nothing more to say or because there is a response they cannot imitate. If the latter happens, the group can take a break and try to provide help. Knowing that there is this element of flexibility enhances the confidence of the players and probably helps them feel more free and relaxed.

When an actor stops the play and has asked for help or explained the interruption, the other participants and then the spectators should get an opportunity to comment, interpret, or ask questions. The director most often interrupts the play in order to make changes or simply to talk about what has been going on. The counselor's function is to direct the clients' attention to how the characters feel and to alternative forms of conduct.

Discussing the role-play gives the primary participant an opportunity to uncover inner reactions to the events in the scene, to talk about any knowledge gained, and to give thought to the advantages of doing the scene again with parts distributed differently. In discussing the scene, the other members can offer their views of the dramatized interrelationships and the primary character's position and behavior, and they can recommend new behaviors.

The other participants in the drama also learn from getting one another's responses, trying on different parts, and attempting to deal with circumstances that present a special challenge (because most often people ask for roles that have particular significance for them, though they do not always realize this). They also get criticism of how they handled themselves in terms of the demands their characters faced. All the actors should have a chance to explain how it felt to imitate the imagined characters and what insight they gained from the exercise. Role-playing can show an individual how to cope with a situation without ever actually experiencing it; more typically, people enacting various parts recognize a relationship between the drama and their own lives and are able then to talk more freely about their problems.

The spectators, although they learn less from the role-play than the performers, do become very wrapped up in the dramatization. They may want to participate if the play is repeated. The value of the exercise for the audience is in their involvement; as Moreno [1946] emphasized, all the group members should be encouraged to enter into the role-playing in some way and all should be viewed as possible participants. The technique should be used with the idea of providing everyone with a chance to look inward and do some rethinking.

Recording of the Role-Play

The taping and audio replaying of role dramatizations enables the participants to "observe" themselves. Unless there is a way of hearing the scene again, the primary member forgets many important details and has only a vague idea of what went on. But listening to a recording of the dramatization, this individual gains a new perspective. Video recordings have the same advantage and their impact is greater. Body language that would otherwise remain unnoticed or be forgotten becomes visible (see 26.1.8).

Usually people who resist the idea of recording will agree if they understand its purposes, which the counselor should make clear: to show people how others see them, to help the counselor make better comments, and to enable clients and supervisors to provide better criticism for the counselor. Another advantage of recording is that it tends to promote greater understanding and sympathy among clients. Individuals who place themselves in another's shoes tend to become more empathetic and doing this also come face to face with themselves [Shaftel & Shaftel, 1967].

Counselor Role-Playing

The counselor may be invited to play certain roles that are inappropriate. Depending on what kind of part the counselor might take (possibly that of a parental figure or someone else in authority), distortions in relationships with various clients might result. While these difficulties might be worked out, they could detract from the beneficial effects of the role-play.

Individual Role-Playing

The guidelines for group role-play can be adapted to role enactment by one person or by one client and the counselor. Bertcher and colleagues showed how this would work. The counselor can use role-play for diagnosis by having the individual pretend to answer a certain question in a job interview. Rehearsal involves getting the client to experiment with another type of answer. Role-play can be used for problem-solving; the counselor explains possible responses to anticipated situations. The counselor can model by role-playing employee or employer behavior in a work situation.

On the one-to-one basis the organization and pacing of the role-playing and the preparation of the client are essentially the same as in a group. For individuals the procedure is less systematized, it is worked into the dialogue that is going on, and the counselor becomes the audience.

The Value of Role-Playing

Role-playing is a valuable adjunct to group counseling. Ohlsen [1977] summed it up as a technique that gives people a chance to experiment with alternative modes of conduct, practice them, learn to express themselves better, get the reactions of others, and look at themselves as though from the outside. It is an appropriate procedure to use along with counseling rather than being in itself a major mechanism for change. It is no longer necessary when individuals through language alone can explain difficulties in their lives and work out ways to resolve them.

30.3.11. ART THERAPY GROUPS

In recent years several rehabilitation professional specialties connected with the arts have been established. Three of the best recognized ones are music therapist, art therapist, and dance therapist — all of whom may work in a group setting and are used in mental health and other facilities. These three specialties have established professional organizations: National Association for Music Therapy headquartered in Lawrence, Kansas; American Art Therapy Association, in Baltimore, Maryland; and American Dance Therapy Association, in Columbia, Maryland. Professional workers interested in psychodrama as an art may affiliate with the American Society of Group Psychotherapy and Psychodrama, New York, New York. All of these professional groups have stipulated preparational standards (e.g., the masters degree). Recreation therapy, described in detail later as an important service in independent living rehabilitation, can also employ group techniques (see 40.7).

In addition to psychodramatists there are new specialties such as drama therapist, poetry therapist, and bibliotherapist. Not all of these approaches from the creative arts are understood and accepted as useful by the established professions. Supervision by others (e.g., occupational therapists) is common. An important new book entitled *The Arts in Therapy* has been written by Robert Fleshman and J.L. Fryrear (in press).

Chapter 31

Family Counseling

The family, traditionally, is the basic unit of the social order. As the most enduring of human institutions the family structure not only provides stability and strength to the larger society but also serves vital human needs. Through families the race is reproduced and offspring are nurtured. Children are not only protected, housed, fed, and educated in their upbringing, but also grow as social beings through natural family ties of affection. The feeling of belonging derives not merely from common ancestry or the physical household but from the related goals and shared convictions (e.g., religion) of kindred learning.

Family patterns and dynamics have changed with cultural systems. Clans and tribes have been replaced by systems of government for protection and education. The intradependency of the large family unit found in early rural communities and in industrial city life has been reduced to "nuclear" families of only the married couple and their children. Modern housekeeping and changes in childrearing responsibilities have given married women occupational and other opportunities within and outside of the home. Whereas the functional family once included grandparents and many relatives, most persons today have smaller, contained or isolated families—first as children born into the family and second as adults and parents in the "conjugal" family established by marriage. A

"new morality"—couples living together without marriage or in communes—may also affect responsibility patterns for minors.

Rehabilitation is concerned with the nature of the family, its developmental role, and its influence on handicapped members. Through family nurturance children build the personality strength needed to adjust to a life complicated by disablement at whatever the age. Understanding the family influence is essential for diagnosis, counseling, and rehabilitation planning. William McPhee in the Utah Rehabilitation Research Institute studies found that family variables greatly contributed to rehabilitation outcomes [Wright & Trotter, 1968]. William Gellman [1961a] at the Chicago Jewish Vocational Service explained the vocational adjustment of handicapped children and the importance of having family chores in developing work habits.

Agricultural life with its "extended" families offered opportunity to contribute through all kinds and levels of work activity. Children all helped, as did impaired and aged kinfolks: there was work for the retarded cousin, the aged grandmother, and the alcoholic uncle. Able members of the family accepted the responsibility for dependent members in the absence of public assistance and institutional facilities. Even very old people remained at home instead of being sent away. Children of that time grew up in a natural communal atmosphere with the aged and those who were "different."

Family life has changed and professional community resources to substitute for personal family care have been devised by the larger society through government and agencies. Professional counseling of families has developed to help meet marital, sexual, and other adjustment problems of people in modern society. Special needs and techniques are associated with family relations and counseling of disabled individuals.

Marriage is often disrupted by disability. The interrelationship between the problems of disability and the marriage may necessitate the professional services of the rehabilitation counselor. The marital relationship of clients has special meaning to the rehabilitationist since family support and involvement are often critical to readjustment—the rehabilitation process involves the whole family.

31.1. Marital Counseling

The term *marital counseling* describes the process whereby a professionally trained person assists couples in preparing themselves for marriage or in resolving problems after marriage. It is conducted by a variety of professionals including psychologists, religious counselors, and, most often, social workers. Specialists in this field, even though from different disciplines, have their own organization, the American Association of Marriage and Family Counseling. Family service and public welfare agencies in communities provide marital counseling and social case work for families. Many people, as in former times, still take their marital problems to their religious leader. The family physician also is often consulted. Now there is a growing number of private practitioners who give counsel on problems of marriage or sex.

Marital, family, and sexual counseling in practice is not readily isolated as to family, marital, or sexual adjustment. Counselors prefer to work with the family unit, which certainly includes both partners of the marriage. Many counselors include the children or other family members because poor functioning in one area affects the entire family unit. Moreover, other members of a family may contribute to marital disharmony. This chapter then has been divided into separate sections on marital, family, and sexual counseling for convenience in discussing each one rather than because of any clear distinctions in counseling methods and purposes.

31.1.1. TECHNIQUES

The purpose of marital counseling is to assist couples in maximizing their strengths and resources to cope with crises and stresses. The problem is identified and goals are set during the initial session with the clients. Agreement between the husband and wife on the purpose of counseling helps to avoid conflict in subsequent sessions. The most frequent presenting problems concern interpersonal communication, financial affairs, personality conflicts, marital dissatisfaction, sexual difficulties, infidelity, the disciplining of children, role concepts, alcoholism, nonsupport, and physical abuse. In rehabilitation, the problems of disability may affect marital relations. The problems that couples request help for may not be the underlying or crucial issues.

All helping relationships, as Carkhuff and Berenson [1977] pointed out, are "for better or for worse." This is most true for the couple in matrimony, but intervention in their lives by the marriage counselor can be either constructive or destructive, depending largely upon the counselor's interpersonal skills. Counselors maintain a neutral position toward the partners in order to focus on their marital relationship. It is difficult to help the marital unit without the participation of both individuals. The perception by each partner of the major problems is sought early.

Marriage counseling usually requires a series of sessions. A single meeting, however, may result in enough insight and improved communication that a couple can carry on without help. Unfortunately, many times the counseling begins too late and is terminated prematurely. Most people do not see a marriage counselor until their problem is so far advanced that saving the marriage is no longer at issue. In fact, in many instances the counseling is directed at helping with the inevitable problem of severing the relationship. Referral to other counseling resources such as legal, financial, psychiatric, or medical is often indicated.

Regardless of the nature of complaints, clients come to the counselor filled with emotion— anger, fear, dejection, or anxiety. Negative feeling should be reduced before attacking the underlying causes of the couple's conflict.

Marital counseling sessions tend to be centered on crisis. It is in this context that the rehabilitation counselor may be drawn into this function with a disabled client. The first task is to help the couple discuss the problem. One solution is to teach communication techniques (e.g., active listening). As in other counseling, also, the client-counseling relationship is important. By the counselor's example—of an accepting relationship and rapport—clients are enabled to try new ways of relating to each other.

Because the emphasis in treatment is on the marital relationship rather than personal pathology, the preference is to work with both husband and wife. The spouses may be seen together, separately, or in varied individual or group sessions. Often marital counseling is conducted in a coordinated plan by a male and a female counselor.

There are many approaches: acceptance of client feeling and actions without censure; recognition and encouragement of positive efforts and improvements; clarification of feelings; interpretation that leads to client insight; suggestions about alternative courses of action; structuring for focus and setting priorities; and, information on factual matters.

As has been discussed elsewhere, in the relationship there is a therapeutic value. Other counseling mechanisms are also applicable in marital adjustment cases. Since interpersonal relationship is often the root problem, the counselor serves as a model to emulate. Audiovisual tapes are used for modeling, or to play back to clients their verbalizations in order for them to get an objective view of themselves. Behavioral techniques can be effective. Bibliotherapy, assigned reading material, is an efficient way of informing clients.

The flow of communication between the clients is improved by modeling the counselor's open communication; reinterpreting what they say to clarify messages; urging the clients to talk to each other rather than about each other through the counselor; and communication in

each other's presence. Compared to working with individuals, family counseling is more active. The passive counselor who seems to be merely listening will find the couple inattentive to professional input. Family counselors exert influence by being quite directive at times. Forceful intervention by the counselor, such as telling one member to be silent, is often needed. Sometimes one member alone is taught to be an expert on family interaction, thus affecting continuing adjustment.

Genetic counseling may be an issue in working with married couples in whom the disability of one or both partners (or of an offspring) may affect reproduction. Estimating the risks of genetically determined disease requires special preparation that is beyond the scope of rehabilitation counselors. But, reproductive risks may be a critical issue with some clients, in which case they should be referred for genetic counseling.

Premarital counseling and the problems of mate selection are also generally outside the realm of rehabilitation counseling. They sometimes arise, however, in special cases: with clients who are considering marriage before completion of their rehabilitation for job preparedness, or with clients who are concerned about their qualifications for marriage and parenthood because of their disability or its effects on family life.

31.1.2. BEHAVIORAL FACTORS

Four factors that describe the nature of marriage, family, and sexual behavior with special significance to rehabilitation have been listed in an unpublished paper by Bruce Thomason [1976]:

1. Marriage is the most emotionally charged of all interpersonal relationships. All emotions come to play in marriage and no other group or two-person relationship is as dynamic or as emotionally satisfying.

2. It is the most absorptive of all our relationships; that is, it is most absorptive of all outside troubles. In the final analysis, all problems are brought to the marriage and family structure for solution. The sexual relationship absorbs outside troubles, creating problems in that relationship. If husband and wife are having in-law problems, these may end up in the marriage as a sex problem. The same may

be true of differences between husband and wife on such matters as discipline of the children, spending the family income, selection of friends, philosophy of life, and differences in religious beliefs.

3. It is the most reflective of all relationships. If sex is a problem, it may reflect itself in husband-wife discord over such matters as

children, friends, philosophy of life, religion, and money matters.

4. The family represents a group relationship. Rehabilitation personnel must always remember that they are not dealing just with a disabled individual but with him, his wife, his children, his relatives, and, very often, his friends.

31.2. Family Adjustment

Counseling with the family of a disabled person is often indicated because chronic illness or disability, whether it is physical or emotional, whether it necessitates hospitalization or not, always creates problems for the family. The tranquility of family life is usually strained and sometimes shattered by the emotions that the disability generates—anxiety, guilt, hostility, unexpressed fears, and displaced feelings [Scherz, 1970]. When these emotions can be expressed and dealt with by family members working together, everyone benefits.

The concept of family rehabilitation thus is based upon the assumption that when disability occurs the whole family is adversely affected. Therefore, rehabilitation services must be designed and delivered so as to meet the needs of the entire family, claimed Nau [1973]. The family, in turn, will frequently have a more "poignant, influential, lasting and significant" effect on the disabled person than all the professionals who work with the individual, observed Buscaglia [1975, p. 119]. Because the family is such a powerful force in the determination of human behavior, it cannot be overlooked in comprehensive rehabilitation.

31.2.1. FAMILY PARTICIPATION
The family has a direct influence on the attitudes and behavior of handicapped persons [Klausner, 1969; Rosenstack & Kutner, 1967]. In fact, family relationships may determine the outcome of rehabilitation [Erba, 1969]. However, rehabilitation counseling usually does not address itself to the family as a whole. While it may be held that the handicapped person should be viewed as a member of larger systems, this perspective is not commonly held. And while some rehabilitation agencies (including the public program) do include work with families, the practice is not general.

Involving relatives in the process is an approach that recognizes that successful rehabilitation rarely takes place without active participation by the family, Lindenberg [1976] emphasized. The family is an important component of the process and must be incorporated into the rehabilitation effort.

It is obvious that some families of disabled individuals need professional help in pursuing the goals of rehabilitation. They may be lacking in the ability, the knowledge, or the desire to work toward these goals by themselves. Families, like individuals, vary in their ability to tolerate frustration and trouble and in their capacity to rise to occasions of crisis. The central goal should be the "interpersonal competence" of the disabled person and the entire family, according to Christopherson [1962].

31.2.2. SITUATIONS OF FAMILY HELP
Family involvement in rehabilitation may be particularly useful in certain situations. When, during the course of treatment, the client's behavior is undergoing a change, participation in the program may help relatives understand this better. The family can also cooperate to try to get the client to change attitudes when necessary. Family participation is indicated when the members are antagonistic to rehabilitation as well as when special understanding and cooperation are needed, for instance during training.

Sometimes relationships within the group are so disturbed that the success of the rehabilitation effort is impeded. In other cases conflict arises from differences between the family's objectives for the client and those of the counselor or the client. The process can also be threatened by relatives who are contributing to the client's difficulty in developing independence and responsibility. In all these instances, active family participation is likely to have a positive effect on the client's progress. If the client is a young person and therefore still an integral part of the family, or if the client's rehabilitation will cause an economic problem for the family, participation of the whole group may also be essential.

31.2.3. FAMILY REACTION TO TRAUMA

Just as the traumatic event usually strikes the person without warning, the family is also poorly prepared for the event and its consequences. The family's reactions are roughly parallel to those of the disabled person. While the person attempts to deny the reality of the disability, relatives also suffer through a period of disturbance in reaction to the trauma.

The disruptive effect of the event is usually multiple on the family. Financial resources are likely to be severely strained, especially if the disabled individual has been the breadwinner, and family objectives may need to be revised. In turn, this may cause alterations in the roles of various members—the housewife turning provider, for instance—and, as a further consequence, situations of adaptive stress for everyone in the group.

In addition to the economic impact of the event, members will feel its effect on all the various activities and relationships that together contribute to the maintenance of the family unit. Former patterns of decision-making are no longer practical if they had depended upon the full-bodied participation of the now incapacitated member. While continuing to answer to the underlying purposes of the family—the bringing up of children, the providing of emotional support for everyone, the maintenance of fulfilling activities—the family must now accommodate itself as a group to the incapacity [Shellhase & Shellhase, 1972].

According to Christopherson [1962], whose ideas are related here, the incapacitation may be considered in terms of four distinct stages that sharpen one's perception of clients in their important relationships. While individual histories vary, many will include: (1) the acute stage, (2) the reconstruction stage, (3) the plateau stage, and (4) the deteriorative stage. These phases are conceived as rough categories and are not mutually exclusive. Nor are they universal; every individual will not go through all of them, and everyone will not experience them in the same way.

The Acute Stage

The acute period begins when a member of the family is suddenly and, it seems, inexplicably stricken with a disability. There is frequently a sense of panic in the family as the members begin to realize what is happening and to consider the long-range implications. At this point the family may turn in alarm to those with easy answers or even fall prey to exploiters; normally rational people may risk financial disaster in attempting to alter what is medically inevitable.

At this stage the family probably needs counseling in order to mobilize all of its resources most effectively. In practice many families receive only medical advice when financial and emotional problems also need to be addressed. During this phase the establishment of a practical and orderly routine is most desirable, for routines provide people with a sense of meaning and direction. The rehabilitation team should begin its work as soon as the person is physically capable of participating.

Usually a crisis of this kind brings members of a family closer together initially, as they unite to meet the challenge ahead. Emotional relationships between the disabled person and other family members are usually good at this stage; these responses are resources that should be carefully and conservatively utilized for the next stage.

The Reconstruction Stage

The term *reconstruction stage* may be useful as a designation for the period when the disabled person, having been through the acute stage, is now attempting through surgery, therapy, and other types of treatment to recover as much physical status as possible. Its duration, short or long, is an entirely individual matter, but it is usually a very crucial time for everyone. Frequently it is during this period that people begin to understand the full implications of the disability, perhaps realizing intuitively that the chances for recovery are minimal. Perhaps the details of life in the future become clear: confinement, limited physical capacity, and social isolation. It is common for the rehabilitation client and other family members to differ in the realism of their perception.

Frequently the severely disabled person feels a "peripheral status" with regard to the family and society in general, and the rehabilitation team should address this question of perceptual adjustment. A sense of change in status may stem from physical alteration or changes in occupational, social, or sex roles. The professional workers should help the client achieve a realistic sense of place within the family and larger reference groups. It is not desirable for a disabled person to withdraw from the occupational world and society, but neither should unrealistic goals be set. Part of the rehabilitative process should consist of helping the individual and other family members strike a realistic balance, from which point integration can take place.

During the reconstruction phase it is crucial that the entire family get all the motivational help necessary to recover as much as possible of what has been lost. Many barriers will have to be overcome. The afflicted individual may feel bitter and may have to contend with pain and boredom as well as the financial burdens of practical concern to the whole family.

The Plateau Stage

When all possible reconstructive measures have been taken, the disabled person enters the plateau stage. The goals now are the maintenance of progress already made and the development of skills to compensate for those that have been lost. Because there can be little hope for further medical improvement and yet a long period of care looms ahead, and also because economic and emotional resources have dwindled, the plateau stage may be the most difficult for the whole family.

If the disabled person is confined to the home and family members must provide care for a long period of time, relationships that had been good before can drastically deteriorate. Caregivers in the family may sacrifice their own mental and physical health if they do not pay enough attention to their own lives, pursue their own interests, and spend time outside the home. Another undesirable result of long confinement is the development of a "locked relationship" between the disabled individual and the family care-giver. The interaction of the two parties becomes stereotyped and a tension cycle develops

that neither is able to interrupt. When this happens, the rehabilitation worker can sometimes suggest practical changes that may break the pattern. In any case, because the postreconstruction period is relatively long, it is usually a strain on relationships.

Even though the term *plateau* signifies the end of medical reconstruction, it need not denote the end of all progress. The rehabilitation counselor might do well to help the client and family look back and see reconstruction as part of a larger process, and also help them to perceive compensatory alternatives and encourage working toward realistic objectives. The family's interest and cooperation can help the person continue to grow. Relatives should encourage client plans to develop or adapt vocational and avocational competencies and interests, to find ways to overcome limitations of energy and mobility, and in general to increase independent and productive life.

The Deteriorative Stage

The disabled individual may go through another, final period, which can be called the deteriorative stage. It may be associated with a terminal attack or the person may simply give way to the process of attrition.

It is important to examine the kind of power structure that is likely to develop in the family that includes a severely disabled individual. Some clients may unconsciously dominate the household by unnecessary dependency or exploitation of their "helplessness"; the family may even unknowingly encourage this, but more commonly the reverse is true and it is the disabled one who is dominated.

The client's role in conserving the family is very nearly as important as the reciprocal role of the family toward the disabled person. Clients should plan ahead and pace requests for service, avoid overwhelming the care-giver with complicated requests, and take the practical needs of the other family members into consideration. If clients plan intelligently so as to avoid imposing on the rest of the family, much antagonism can be avoided. On the other hand, families can promote harmony if they recognize how important it is to respect the disabled member's most critical needs.

The above model best fits the chronically ill but it illustrates stages of the adventitiously disabled whose functioning does not so deteriorate. Family involvement in various stages is comparable.

31.2.4. COUNSELING APPROACHES

Usually in work with families of the disabled, dealing with pathological processes is less important than helping the family recognize the realities of the disabling condition. Members must adapt to life with the disability, mobilizing emotional and practical resources in order to preserve the family unit. They must also cooperate in rehabilitative efforts so that the person can make the best progress possible toward functioning as a member of the family and society.

Continuance of the family during such a crisis is of the utmost importance. A severe disability constitutes a very serious threat to family cohesiveness, especially if the stricken person had been integral to the functioning of the group. Sometimes the situation results in the disintegration of the family, either in a gradual way, such as dispatching children to the homes of relatives, or as a sudden breakdown, with members renouncing their obligations to one another. To prevent this, Shellhase and Shellhase [1972] advised, the family must gather itself together and use all the resources at its command.

There are a number of ways in which the participation of relatives can be promoted: contact with families of new clients—for joint goal and program determination—as a program begins; orientation groups; progress reviews; family therapy to help family members make role adjustments when necessary [Lindenberg, 1977]. The family should contribute to the rehabilitation process, and one family can help another within community service agencies.

Client Participation

The disabled person can be taught how to help relatives adjust to the disability situation. This is an eminently desirable and even necessary strategy because counseling contacts with the family directly may not be feasible. Clients can use some of the counseling techniques about emotional problems and changing behavior they themselves have learned.

The person with a disability can learn how to understand what other members of the family feel. It is up to the disabled individual to put other people at their ease and allay their anxieties, to help the nondisabled cope with their guilt feelings. This is true for two reasons: first, because there is no other way in which the disabled can change their human environments, and second, because the disabled are better qualified to help others adjust to disability than anyone else. The handicapped person constantly has the opportunity to practice on others, as Dishart [1964] put it, "to try out the perceiving of and accepting of their feelings. If he goofs with several, and doesn't perceive their feelings correctly, during the course of a day he will meet many other nondisabled people on whom to practice . . . " [p. 43]. The relatives and friends of the disabled individual, however, have only one person to practice on, so their opportunity to learn is much more limited.

The counselor, then, can teach rehabilitation clients to help those around them, in the family and beyond. "If a client wishes to include his friends, or his community, or even the whole world among those persons he would like to put at ease and accept—then that is his family," said Dishart [p. 43].

Other Approaches

The inevitable and multiple needs of the disabled and their families must be met in a variety of ways. In most rehabilitation centers, the service procedure includes assessment of family resources for accommodating the continuing limitations of one of its members. The focus is on the client's needs and the capacity of the family to meet these needs as the program goes on. Relatives are informed about the client's special requirements, about the measures they can take in order to prevent "pressure sores" from developing, and about medication, signs of adverse reaction, and the like. The rehabilitationist must first evaluate the group for its strengths and weaknesses and then help the members utilize and maintain all the resources they have.

The functioning of the family as a unit is the pivotal concern as the needs of all those involved are considered in balance. The client needs support in order to adjust to the problems of disability; the other members of the family need support if they are to adapt to the situation and learn to function adequately in the face of it. The professional discriminates between the two sets of needs in an effort to help reconcile them. If a family shows lack of consideration, the rehabilitationist may work with them to increase their understanding. Or, if a client has become inconsiderate of the rights of other people in the family, there is need for intervention. All this comes after everyone involved has had time to accept the disability situation and it no longer has an immobilizing effect upon the family as a whole.

This work with the family should begin early in the rehabilitative process. People are helped to become more sensitive and more perceptive about their relationships. The extra stress disability places on a family may well cause it to function less satisfactorily; the members may need help in evaluating themselves, their goals, their success or failure as a group. In these situations, family counseling is indicated.

The goal of family counseling is the return of the disabled person to full membership in the family group. Preventive attention to the entire family throughout the rehabilitation effort may keep the disabled member from becoming separated from the others. "In this way the trip home is never a long one," said Shellhase and Shellhase [1972, p. 550].

31.2.5. COUNSELING NEEDS

The rehabilitationist performs a very active function when working with clients and families. The interaction is a facilitative one in coping with needs. Goolsby [1976], in discussing this topic, recognized that handicapped people and their families have basic needs that must be acted upon if services are to be effective. She said that the most critical of these needs are:

Education. This is obvious and should not need to be stressed, but, unfortunately, it does. People need to know, have the right to know, as much about their problem as they can: factual information, definition of terms, clarification of what is known and not known, what to expect.

Emotional support. This does not mean pity, but it does mean providing a climate where feelings can be expressed and support provided. For most professionals, this is the most difficult thing they have to do . . . .

Identification of realistic alternatives. Along with special knowledge about the problem, the professional brings perspective. We all know how emotional involvement obscures logic. A forum, where ideas can be tested and feedback given on probable consequences of a specific course, can be of real help.

Needed services. We know that chronic problems require the provision of ongoing services, intense at times (e.g., at points of potential crisis such as upon diagnosis) but always with an ongoing supportive base. The model service system will be designed to make possible a flexible response to the client's changing needs [p. 333].

31.3. Sexual Adjustment

The client's sexual adjustment is an important part of rehabilitation. Counselors need to gain greater awareness and understanding of sexuality in order to help the disabled as total human beings. They can no longer ignore psychosexual problems, avoid discussion of sex with their clients, and plead incompetence to give information on sexual issues. These are legitimate aspects of human functioning and counselors must be willing to face the problems.

In 1970 *Human Sexual Inadequacy,* the basic text on treatment of sexual problems from laboratory experimentation and clinical experience, was published by William Masters and Virginia Johnson. Their therapeutic concepts and format provided the foundation for professional respectability and for treatment of sexual problems through counseling.

Most health science professionals now agree that sexuality should be regarded as part of the whole person. Until recently, however, sexuality has been a neglected element of medical education, and this is certainly true in the field of rehabilitation. Even though professionals in rehabilitation have been affected by the tendency in our culture to consider the physically disabled as nonsexual beings, they are not sufficiently aware of this influence. Out of a sense of inadequacy, they have suppressed their clients' need to talk about sexual concerns [Berkman, 1975].

False ideas abound about the sexuality of the physically disabled. This is comprehensible in view of the negative connotations that surround words like *crippled, paralyzed, maimed,* and *deformed,* as well as the durability of myths about sexuality in general. Many people believe that a partially paralyzed person is unable to engage in sexual acts; a smaller number even believe that the disabled have no need for or interest in sex. "In addition, the conspicuously disabled person," Anderson and Cole [1975] observed, "is often stereotyped as also being mentally retarded" [p. 117].

Rehabilitationists now recognize that sexuality is a vital concern of the disabled. Berkman [1975] reported that the effectiveness of the rehabilitation effort can be greatly increased when professionals combine the concepts of rehabilitation and sex counseling.

31.3.1. SEX COUNSELING APPROACHES

Acceptance and understanding may not be of much help when a client brings up sexual concerns, nor is exploration of the client's feelings likely to suffice. Specific behavioral methods have been developed by which such problems as impotence, premature ejaculation, inability to reach orgasm, and pain during intercourse can be alleviated, and the counselor should be familiar with these methods. The professional, according to Kelly [1976], should be able to explain dysfunctions to clients and also inform them of the various ways in which these conditions can be treated. If the rehabilitation counselor's expertise is not appropriate, referral to other professionals or to a sex therapy clinic is in order.

So that they can help clients choose among alternative treatments for sexual problems, counselors should be familiar with the various therapeutic approaches that have been developed. "Misunderstanding and misdirected advice in dealing with the sexual problems of the disabled is often the result of ignorance of human sexuality plus judgments based on personal experience alone," according to Berkman [1975, p. 15]. Counselors therefore need to be aware of their limitations and recognize the necessity for referral.

Therapeutic Approaches

The World Health Organization [1975] reported on a number of applied therapy techniques that are used at present to treat sexual dysfunctions: somatic therapy, behavioral therapy, psycho-analysis, hypnosis, couple therapy, and group psychotherapy. According to the report there are certain general trends in therapy going on.

Somatic therapy deals exclusively with the body. Although few sexual dysfunctions are organic in origin, it is essential that treatment begin with a physical and, when appropriate, an endocrinological examination. Physical, pharmacological, and surgical therapies have been developed for a number of sexual dysfunctions.

Modern behavioral therapy begins with systematic definition of the goal of treatment. Because certain sets of attitudes can hinder the whole process of sexual functioning, practitioners insist on the changing of attitudes rather than immediate behavioral changes. The orientation is flexible and rational so that needs of patients can be met on an individual basis.

Psychoanalysis is appropriate as a means of determining the significance of particular symptoms in relationship to the whole personality. It is useful as an approach to the quality of sexual functioning and also addresses the place of fantasy and imagination in sexuality.

Although it is not fully understood, hypnosis can aid the process of desensitization and can induce relaxation. Subjects can be helped, for example, by visualizing the sex act while under hypnosis; hypnosis can induce positive sensations, such as a feeling of heat at the base of the abdomen, to facilitate achievement of sexual pleasure.

Couple therapy is based on the Masters and Johnson model, focusing on the partnership and its pathological aspects. The couple works intensively and continuously for two weeks; expression of feelings is insisted upon. With this approach, the goal of therapy is not merely the relief of symptoms but also the enhancement of the sexual relationship. Richer fantasy, greater sensitivity, and more positive attitudes toward sexuality are positive results of this goal.

Group psychotherapy encourages the sharing of experiences in an atmosphere in which sexual attitudes can undergo change. In addition to this method and the other major types of applied therapy, other less well known approaches have been developed. Unusual and original in methodology, they include, for instance, psychotherapy with a psychodynamic orientation and techniques aimed at increasing physical sensitivity.

Despite the divergent trends in therapy, there is general consensus on a number of points. One is that practitioners are tending increasingly to consider human sexuality in terms of relationships, treating couples rather than individuals. When both partners participate in therapy, better communication becomes an important goal. Another point on which experts agree is that therapy is still in the development stage and that experience is still being gained. There are no universal answers to the question of what types of therapy are most effective; rather, therapists must choose the method best suited to a specific problem, to the patient as an individual, and to their own skills. There is general agreement that therapists are continually learning more about the causes of sexual dysfunction and the value of sex education. Finally, experts feel that, generally, there is decreased emphasis on the medical model that has been commonly used for the diagnosis and cure of sexual dysfunction.

Many kinds of institutions have programs for sex counseling and therapy. There are comprehensive programs that involve many people and many approaches to sex counseling, sex therapy, and family therapy; and there are small programs in which relatively few people participate. The training therapists receive varies in intensiveness, but preceptor models and extensive group discussion are commonly used in this training.

Referring

Before making a referral, the counselor should check on the credentials and competence of the individual or institution of referral. It is a mistake to assume that representatives of certain disciplines, such as psychiatry, are necessarily qualified to handle sexual dysfunction. On the other hand, people without the usual professional training for treatment of sexual problems may have special qualifications that enable them to deal with these problems.

The counselor should bear in mind that referral for the treatment of a sexual problem may be somewhat delicate. It may be necessary to prepare the client and especially to provide emotional support so that the revelation of intimate sexual concerns will be easier. The counselor should help make contact with the referral source so that careful definition of the problem and aim of treatment is formulated. Following up is also important.

Many clinics specializing in sex therapy are now operating across the country, in the larger cities primarily in association with hospitals or medical centers. A number of private resources are also available. In making any referral to a sex therapy clinic, the counselor should try to become acquainted with the staff, according to Maddock and Chilgren [1976].

Explicit instructions for sexual expression for paraplegic and quadriplegic men and women has been published in films and in a book by Thomas Mooney, Theodore Cole, and Richard Chilgren [1975] of the University of Minnesota, Minneapolis, Medical School. As they say: "The disabled are people, and people are sexual. Much of one's sense of personhood comes from our ability to play a sexual role" [p. vii]. Mooney and his colleagues went on to say this:

Virtually nobody is too disabled to derive some satisfaction and personal reinforcement from sex—with a partner if possible, alone if necessary. When a disabled person is unable to enjoy sex, the greatest obstacle to enjoyment usually isn't the difficulty or impossibility of making particular movements, but the social convention that sex consists of putting the penis in the vagina and that all the rest of the rich range of human and mammalian sexual responses—oral, manual, and skin stimulation—are abnormal. Human sex is widely versatile and not limited to the genitalia [p. viii].

Financial support for this book came from the federal rehabilitation agency, Lutheran and Methodist church organizations, the Playboy Foundation, and other groups.

31.3.2. SEXUAL PROBLEMS

The sexual concerns of disabled clients have not traditionally received much attention during the rehabilitation process. One reason for this is the difficulty people have in sharing problems that are so deep and emotional. Rehabilitation counselors, too, have generally been trained to concentrate on the goal of returning a disabled person to work. Moreover, sexual counseling has not been viewed by state rehabilitation agencies as one of the regular responsibilities of the counselor or the agency. Now, however, as Diamond [1974] said, "The professional, more than anyone, must realize that meeting an individual's sexual concerns can go a long way in reestablishing or establishing a general feeling of self-worth conducive to general rehabilitation [pp. 35–36]."

Clues to Sexual Problems

People cope in various ways with anxiety about sex. While most individuals do not want to talk about the subject per se, the disabled frequently do discuss concerns about their physical condition. Anxiety about sexuality can take the form of concern about purely physical matters: the ability to function in the sexual role, or bowel and bladder functioning.

In the early stages people tend to react to disability with depression and denial. These two reactions are probably less difficult for the rehabilitationist to deal with than the client's later responses to the sexual implications of disability. In proceeding through the rehabilitation process and envisioning a return to the community, the person is likely to form new attitudes toward sex [Berkman, 1975].

Effects of Disability on Sexual Function

The counselor should know how various physical disabilities affect sexual function. Some disabilities impair functioning in the sexual areas of masturbation, coitus, and fertility; some are related to an individual's sexuality less directly in that their conspicuousness affects the person socially. Conspicuous disabilities seem to force people to examine their images of themselves and to face the question of their sexual adequacy.

Many disabilities acquired at birth or early in life (for example, brain injury, spinal cord disease or injury, skeletal amputations and deformities, blindness, deafness) are conspicuous but not progressive. Progressive prepubertal disabilities like cystic fibrosis, the juvenile form of diabetes mellitus, and muscular dystrophy, like most progressive disabilities, are also conspicuous. The individual with a highly obvious disability is treated differently from nondisabled people. Children and adolescents who are treated differently from their peers are robbed of normal experiences in daily life and as a consequence may have problems with human relationships. When they cannot use the body language and other forms of nonverbal expression available to the nondisabled, another gap is created. "The net effect of societal forces on the disabled developing child," noted Anderson and Cole [1975], "has often been to arrest or deflect the normal maturational processes" [p. 120]. The end product is an adult who may lack some of the basic components of the adult personality.

Although not all the disabilities acquired at an early age limit sexual function, some disabilities have genetic implications that may place another kind of strain on the disabled person. Sometimes young people with these conditions feel that they should not have children and consequently do not have the right to complete sexual fulfillment.

Among physical disabilities acquired after puberty, the following are nonprogressive: brain and spinal cord injury, skeletal amputations and deformities, genital injuries, disfiguring burns and injuries, blindness, and deafness. Most of these are conspicuous, unless they can be concealed by clothing. Heart disease, stroke, diabetes mellitus, multiple sclerosis, and the last stage of renal disease may be progressive. The latter disabilities have a special effect on sexual relationships; either partner may be afraid that sexual activity will harm the disabled person [Anderson & Cole].

Various disabilities and their treatments create other miscellaneous sexual problems. Spinal cord injury, diabetes, and treatment of kidney disease may cause impotence; medication, especially the drugs used to treat high blood pressure and psychiatric disorders, can lead to sexual dysfunction, and some medications are sexual depressants. Sometimes the patient with cardiac disease is advised by a doctor to modify sexual habits; frequently people suffering from stroke, polio, spasticity, amputations, and arthritis must learn new sexual patterns. Berkman [1975] reported that not until recently has there been a systematic review of the influence of illness and medication on sexual function.

Knowledge about sex and the spinal cord-injured person is needed by rehabilitationists. These people can participate in sexual activities. Women have no loss of physical sexual function and some spinal cord-injured men can ejaculate and experience orgasm. All can experience sexual pleasure, Coleman [1974] advised, through reflexogenic responses, genital relationships, and other caressing of erogenous zones. Marital counseling is indicated, however, because of the need for adjustment in sexual styles and also because of difficulty the spouse may have in maintaining interest when responsible for bowel care, feeding, and other such nursing duties.

Disability typically affects the sexuality of men much more drastically than that of women.

Disabled women are usually able to engage in sexual intercourse, and their fertility is hardly ever affected by physical disability; but, in men certain disabilities frequently result in infertility or impotence. A young man with diabetes may be able to have a relatively normal sex life, but frequently he becomes impotent as an adult. Disabled individuals must deal with their own special feelings and differences and with the attitudes of others, all of which has a bearing on sexual relationships. Many do have active sex lives within the limits of their condition. (Anderson and Cole have described these matters in detail.)

Relationship of Self-Esteem and Work

The self-esteem of disabled individuals appears to be related to their ability to develop alternative coping mechanisms with which to become involved with the world. When disabled adults participate in activities that enhance self-esteem, they have fewer medical complaints and are more independent; their lives are more satisfying. Sexuality may be important in an individual's adaptation to an acquired disability.

Rehabilitation emphasizes, and society underwrites, efforts to return the disabled to work. It is possible that counseling to help clients accept and adjust to their sexuality may also enable them to adjust better to the condition of disability. It may be that if everyone has only a given amount of energy to tap, the disabled individual must conserve and expend that energy more carefully than the nondisabled. If physically handicapped individuals can save psychic resources by realistic adjustment to their sexual limitations, they may be able to channel more energy into self-actualization.

31.3.3. PROFESSIONAL QUALIFICATIONS

Indications are that it may be possible to identify groups of professionals most likely to be interested in sex counseling with the disabled. Sex therapists might appropriately move into this role, but at present sex therapy seems to be only for the nondisabled; people whose sexual functioning has been impaired because of illness or disability have been systematically excluded. The professionals who will do this kind of work with the disabled will need training not only in human sexuality but also in rehabilitation practice, according to Berkman [1975].

Most rehabilitation workers know very little about the sexuality of the disabled; neither their academic background nor their field work has provided adequate training. They do not expect, and are not prepared, to deal with their clients' sexual problems. Sometimes the policy of an agency contributes to this gap in practice by limiting the scope of the professional's participation. Thus, an agency's orientation toward the vocational aspects of the disability situation may result in minimized attention to clients' personal problems. In such an agency workers tend to refer clients with these problems elsewhere, or, worse, stop working with them until the personal difficulties are resolved.

There are a number of ways in which sex counseling can be integrated into the rehabilitation process. The agency can provide an organizational structure that encourages workers to deal with clients' sexual problems. Rehabilitationists who work in comprehensive medical settings can turn to their colleagues, either for consultation or referral. The person's physician is probably the first professional to be consulted, especially when the client has a spinal cord lesion. The doctor can help the person gain at least an intellectual comprehension of how a disability affects sexual function. Of course, once this understanding is reached, it is important that the client go on to the next step, emotional acceptance.

When the physician feels that the client has adequate knowledge, referral to a rehabilitation worker is in order. The worker with whom the patient has the best relationship is the obvious choice. Although the orientation of the agency, the self-confidence of the worker, and the feelings of the client are factors, there is no intrinsic reason why any rehabilitationist cannot help a client face sexual problems. Official titles and responsibilities should have no relevance to the question of who handles these problems.

When the rehabilitation worker is the only professional in the agency, approaching the sexual concerns of clients is more difficult. This is also true when the worker does not have good contact with other members of the traditional team. For instance, if a client who is in psychotherapy comes to the agency worker and pours out sexual problems that are being worked on with the psychotherapist, the worker may wonder how best to help. Trying to find out why the client is bringing the problems to the agency worker might be the best idea. Frankel [1967] suggests the questions, "Is he using the worker as a friend? Is he using him as an antagonist to the psychotherapist? Is it in the client's best interest to declare this topic off-limits? The latter might be the most productive type of support that the rehabilitation worker can offer . . . ." [p. 20]. The worker must talk with the psychotherapist, certainly, before attempting to give any therapeutic support.

Coping with clients' sexual problems might also be difficult in a facility where the clients are mentally retarded adolescents. When such individuals begin to act sexually, parents are upset and the situation looks explosive. The best tactic is for the professional to look at each individual's deviant conduct separately.

The need for rehabilitation counselor expertise in normative sexual behavior has been explained by Robert Flynn and Ami Sha'ked [1977]. They described the principle of normalization as applied to the sexual behavior of the disabled and the role of rehabilitation agencies and personnel.

31.3.4. COUNSELING TECHNIQUES

Physical, emotional, or cognitive impairment will generally affect an individual's sexual behavior. Using the broad principles of sex counseling as a base, workers can develop appropriate techniques for extending their rehabilitation efforts to include the sexual aspects of their clients' lives.

Developing Effective Attitudes

The counselor's own acceptance of sexuality, knowledge, and willingness to deal with clients' sexual problems must underlie effective counseling. Most importantly, counselors must accept and feel at ease with their own sexuality. A counselor's unresolved sexual problems may inhibit discussion if the counselor is embarrassed over what a client says about sex or the language used. In order to help others cope with these problems, professionals should take time to examine their own feelings about and attitudes toward sex.

There will be those who find that sex counseling is simply not for them. An individual may not be able to overlook personal biases, may not be able to distinguish personal needs from those of the client, or may not feel comfortable talking about sex. When for any reason the professional does not want to do sex coun-

seling, admitting this to the client is the only fair thing to do. The counselor should help the client find another professional who can help with sexual concerns.

It is of the utmost importance that a person who does choose to do sex counseling have sound knowledge. As with any other subject on which a client needs information the counselor should become familiar with the subject of sexuality—read about it, attend conferences, and see informative films. If the counselor has done research and is well prepared to explore the topic with the client, discussion of this delicate subject will probably be more open and relaxed. It is important for the client to know that the professional is ready to deal with any and all subjects.

There should be no promises about the progress a client can make in regaining sexual function. Especially in the early stages of disability, time is a very important factor. Statistics cannot be relied upon to predict the future sexual capabilities of a given individual, and no client should be arbitrarily categorized according to generalizations. The counselor must always view the client as a person with a unique set of problems and attitudes.

Finally, any professional who works with clients on sexual problems will at times need to say, "I don't know." This is highly preferable to dodging the question, which may give the client the impression that certain topics are off-limits or suggest that the counselor is unwilling to talk about more than a few subjects. Boyle [1976], in writing about this, points up the dependency of the client when there is no other source of professional help.

31.3.5. SEX EDUCATION

Sex education in itself can help the disabled and their partners understand sexual interaction and be more comfortable sexually. It involves three dimensions: information, attitudes, and communication skills [Berkman, 1975]. Information encompasses the facts about sexual function, sexual development and behavior, male and female sexual response, and related topics. But the teaching of facts is not sufficient; sex education should include attitude training. People taught to change their attitudes toward sex are much more at ease with sexuality and more tolerant of the varying sexual behaviors of others. Communication comprises the third dimension of sex education; in this area, then, counselors who wish to deal with the subject of sex will use skills they already possess. A common mistake is speaking in unfamiliar language. Sex education in counseling can be successful if the professional is forthright, nonjudgmental, relaxed, and sensitive to individual needs, and uses terms the client can understand.

After the disabled have become convinced that their sex drives are normal and important, they can take the next step: making the adjustments necessary to fulfill those drives. When a disability makes intercourse difficult or impossible, couples should explore other means of achieving sexual satisfaction. Petting, manual stimulation, and the use of artificial devices to enhance sexual excitation may provide an answer in such a case; the goal should be for each couple to find the most suitable and satisfying means of sexual expression. It is essential that sexually active disabled individuals receive information on contraception.

It is also very important, Schneider [1976] pointed out, for handicapped men and women to participate in mixed group activities. The social interaction contributes to general as well as sexual adjustment.

Precautions

There is no right way to convey sexual information to a client. A cross-cultural and cross-disciplinary approach stimulates both counselor and client to look in new ways at reasons for the client's sexual problems, Calderone [1976] reported. In addition to dealing with each case on its own terms, the counselor should always exercise caution. A nondogmatic attitude about the nature of a sexual problem as well as the way to approach it will prevent new problems from being created.

Because clients may be disturbed by talk about sex or may feel that the subject is "dirty," counselors must be especially sensitive to these feelings. A calm, polite manner and scientific use of the appropriate language can ease the tension of the situation and help to break the language barrier the client may have. Eventually the client recognizes that worthwhile communication uses sex-related words, including the less euphemistic ones.

Overteaching or underteaching are pitfalls. In underteaching the counselor fails to use all the information and resources at hand. Conversely, stretching the facts to reach some conceptually satisfying conclusion or to round out the picture is overteaching. Clients are usually most concerned with a specific problem or want the answer to a particular question; seldom are they seeking an education on the subject as a whole. It is important to avoid asking academic questions and to keep the dialogue relevant to the client's special concerns.

Through overconfidence in their knowledge of sexuality, counselors can complicate the problems with which clients confront them. A false sense of expertise can lead a counselor to underestimate the variability in human sexual behavior, mistakenly attribute sexual inadequacies to psychological factors, or overemphasize the role of sex in a problem.

Counselors should remain aware of their own ethical codes and should not attempt to impose their moral notions on clients. Calderone [1976] further warned that, "Some counselors have a pet theory or method that has worked in the past for some clients but may actually tend to close doors for other clients with whom it is inapplicable" [p. 350].

Physical and Psychological Dysfunction

Since sexual dysfunction may be either physical or psychological, particular emphasis on psychological factors in sex-related problems could obscure the possibility that real physical problems are involved. Also, the counselor should be aware that there are individuals who, because of disability, age, or other factors, experience a decline in sexual drive and are happy anyway. There is no reason to impose other values on these clients. Naturally, clients should not be forced to talk about sexuality when other subjects seem more important to them.

A journal on the subject of sex and the disabled was introduced in the spring of 1978, *Sexuality and Disability* [1978]. It is edited by a rehabilitation counseling psychologist, Ami Sha'ked. The aim of this journal is to promote a more humanistic, normalized approach in dealing with the sociosexual aspects of the disabled person.

Isabel Robinault [1978], of the New York ICD Rehabilitation and Research Center, has written a valuable book for professional rehabilitationists entitled *Sex, Society, and the Disabled.*

Dr. Robinault has listed many relevant resources and sources of further information on the topic.

31.3.6. THE COUNSELOR AND SEX

All counselors have a special obligation to maintain their professional commitment and roles. In the process they establish a helping relationship with their clients. But the psychological mechanisms of relating and helping can go beyond professional ethical and moral bounds. This is particularly dangerous in personal-sexual adjustment counseling. The most unfair and potentially dangerous thing one can do is to abuse the counseling trust by allowing any sort of sexual act during, or as a result of, one's professional work.

Chapter 32

Written Communication

Providing written communication about cases is an essential responsibility of all professionals who work directly with clients. Operationally defined, case communications is the succinct and prompt report-writing or recording of the important information about a particular client by the professional worker. The broader term *client records* refers to the collection of all materials from all sources that communicates information concerning a client. There are three categories of client records: (1) objective data checklists and printed forms filled out by the counselor for automated processing of data for computer storage; (2) case folder files, for holding important documents (medical, psychological, and educational reports; the individualized written rehabilitation program (IWRP) or case plan; and agency forms, agreements, and other papers pertaining to the client); and (3) case notebooks for written entries by the counselor immediately after each contact with or regarding the client and summarizing everything important that transpired.

32.1. Case-Recording

In case-recording, the counselor enters various subjects: (1) counseling and other communications with the client; (2) contacts—personal, telephone, and correspondence—with others (e.g., family, colleagues, collaborating agencies, employers); (3) abstracts of vocational assessment and other reports; (4) notes on case-planning and decisions (including the IWRP); and (5) a summary written periodically or at points in the rehabilitation process (e.g., eligibility determination, plan implementation, closure). This chapter focuses upon case-recording as a professional function. This so-called paperwork is disdained by many rehabilitationists. As a consequence their recording is unwisely postponed or done in haste without thoughtful or complete coverage, without key facts, and without clear composition or even legibility.

Neglect of this recording responsibility may be due to the counselor's natural interest in working with people and concern that time spent with records is at the expense of more client contact. Some counselors lack adequate skills in written communication, while others simply fail to understand how case records are critical to professional performance as well as program administration. Counselors who shun case-recording need to understand why it is important and how to improve their proficiency. (Incidentally, there are some professional workers who conversely spend disproportionately large amounts of time on paperwork in order to avoid the more challenging professional functions, perhaps out of feelings of incompetency.)

Good case-recording is probably highly correlated with good casework. To be good the recording must provide the reader with a full and accurate description of the casework, the revelation of which constitutes a motivation for the rehabilitation counselor. Counselors are naturally influenced by the necessity of disclosing their performance with each client: they must reveal what they consider to be the most important facts of the case, their interpretation of those facts and rehabilitation planning implications, their understanding of and interactions with the counselee, their utilization of outside resources, and their construction and implementation of a vocational rehabilitation plan. The quality of the counselor's work is laid bare since the case record shows not only the wisdom but also the vigor of the counselor throughout the rehabilitation process. The record even gives quantifiable information about the number of contacts and the time required for each phase. While such documentation is threatening if acceptable professional judgment or performance is lacking, the well-qualified counselor takes pride in the record as a documentation of skill and devotion.

Recent "disclosure" legislation prevents assurance that the counselor's case recording will not be revealed. Antisecrecy provisions permit clients to request seeing their records, or having the material interpreted by an authorized representative who is qualified. This potential violation of the ethics of professional confidentiality (see 2.2.2) unfortunately inhibits adequate recording practice.

32.1.1. PURPOSES

In addition to the motivation to demonstrate a good job, good case-recording actually helps the counselor perform case duties better. The act of faithful recording forces the professional to pause and reflect upon information received after each critical incident. Thus the important facts are screened and their implications considered as they are written for the record. Obvi-

ously this structures the counselor's understanding and planning functions. In fact, case-recording is an integral part of casework and contributes to client success. Moreover, in complex and long-term cases and with larger case loads (i.e., many active clients), the counselor needs these notes as a memory jog and as an aid in planning counseling sessions and providing services.

Agencies collect records for various reasons and in the case of government agencies this is mandated by law (see 7.1.3). Private agencies may also be legally required to keep auditable client records under terms of government contracts for services rendered. In any event, documentation provides a safeguard against charges of malfeasance or misfeasance by the agency staff. To state it positively, the record proves the effectiveness of the work of the agency for all interested parties (e.g., agency directors, funding organizations, regulatory bodies). (Naturally, safeguards for client confidentiality must be assured in all uses of case records.) Thus case records can protect both the agency and the employee by providing data to correct unfair or erroneous interpretations of how a case in question was handled.

The case record is the client's permanent record at the agency and should be accurately kept and in a useful format because it will be consulted not only by the worker in charge, but also by colleagues and by successors if the case is ever reopened or transferred (see 10.2). Moreover, under certain circumstances the record may be inspected by representatives of other agencies, and possibly by courts, employers, and other individuals obtaining the right to access—including the client. The case record, then, is seen as a fundamental and continuing mode of communication about the client for use within and among agencies and other authorized people.

Case study, the subject of Chapter 24, provides the information base for client assessment. In constructing the case study the counselor interprets selected data from materials in the case record (the client's application for service, school transcripts, medical examination forms, employment history, psychological test results, work evaluation reports, counselor interview notes, and other recordings). The counselor's case study, therefore, depends upon gathering case record information from many sources, in various formats, and on innumerable facets of client and environmental considerations relevant to rehabilitation planning.

Professional people are always keenly interested in learning how they can improve their effectiveness in helping clients. An ongoing review of one's case records is a splendid way to see what one is doing well, what procedures work, and how to do better. Insights are obtained by rereading the history of the case, which through chronological notes gives a clear indication of case movement and the dynamics of the process. The value of the feedback for purposes of self-assessment—as well as individual case-planning—warrants frequent case reviews by the counselor.

A review of case folders is probably best when done with a training supervisor in the course of an organized program of professional development. This training can be either individualized, with a critical appraisal of a counselor's casework by the supervisor (see 7.1.6), or in student groups that study sample cases (perhaps composite or hypothetical) in formal preservice or in-service training.

Finally, the case record is a primary source of data for purposes of evaluation. At the personal level the file yields information about the counselor to be used by the supervisor in personnel decisions such as retention, pay increases, transfer, task or client assignments, and promotions. The case file is also used for program evaluation data—an administrative activity federally required of all state rehabilitation agencies. Case reviews, when using comprehensive information, provide for an appraisal of the effectiveness of the rehabilitation process and the quality of the rehabilitation effort; this is far better than basing the judgment simply on the total number of case closures. Moreover, case records facilitate program evaluation and other research that correlates client characteristics and rehabilitation process variables with desired client outcomes; this provides information needed by administrators and counselors to improve service delivery. (See 7.4.)

32.1.2. USES

Ten critical uses of case-recording are summarized below:

1. As a professional tool, forcing the counselor to utilize a period of reflection after each client contact in order to crystallize emerging understanding about the case and the diagnostic implications.
2. As a case review for the counselor's future use as a memory aid for purposes of case study and planning and before key contacts.
3. As documentation of evidence of action taken, in the case of program and fiscal audit.
4. As intra-agency communication to others on the professional team working with the case or to another counselor in the event the case is transferred or reopened.
5. As interagency communication for purposes of client referral or cooperation (including exchange of information) with another community service agency.
6. To aid in the professional development of the counselor by means of joint review of the counselor's casework practices under the tutelage of the immediate supervisor or staff trainer.
7. To be used in supervisory assessment of the counselor through case folder review of professional performance and productivity by an administrative supervisor for personnel action data.
8. To aid in training by means of the detailed presentation of a well-recorded case experience (either successful or unsuccessful) to rehabilitation staff or students.
9. As a methods study, through examination of a sample of agency cases for discovering better professional techniques (e.g., the study of the relationship of successful case outcome to client or process variables).
10. As evaluative research through case study to assess the program effectiveness of the agency in accordance with its goals.

These are ten commanding reasons for the professional worker to write complete but concise notes as each client progresses through the rehabilitation process.

32.1.3. PROBLEMS

Effective case-recording is hampered perhaps more by the writer's attitude toward the task than by the lack of writing skill. Lack of appreciation for the value of a good report, or the agency's misuse or release of case records, may make staff members reluctant to prepare thorough records. Rehabilitation counselors, for example, may feel that the files could be used against them by the administration and that they should therefore present only the positive aspects of cases, omitting information about mistakes, delays, and so forth. An atmosphere of openness requires a realistic attitude on the part of the administration, a clear-cut division of labor among the staff, and agreement among personnel about the agency's objectives.

Hamilton [1946] suggested that the ability to select and organize material is critical and that case-recording will take shape without difficulty if the practitioner can think clearly about the client's needs, the client's circumstances, and the flow of the rehabilitation plan.

Hartley, Wolfe, and Clark [U.S. IRS, 1963a] prepared the following list of reasons why case-recording often breaks down:

1. Lack of an organized approach to the rehabilitation process. Some rehabilitationists experience difficulty in following a systematic approach such as "study-diagnose-plan-follow-up," and this will be reflected by disorganization and breakdown in case-recording.
2. Lack of clear agency standards for casework. When the rehabilitationist is not provided with clear guidelines for agency policy and procedure, omissions and vague generalizations in case-recording can result.
3. Poor case load management techniques. The rehabilitation worker may be too busy completing other activities to get around to recording.
4. Inability of the rehabilitationist to make decisions. Sometimes the case does not contain recording at critical points because the professional worker does not want to "go on record" or is indecisive when faced with a critical decision.
5. The lack of written case-recording guides. Without a predetermined structure, the rehabilitationist may fail to record essential material.
6. Lack of training. Some rehabilitation professionals have never received training in case-recording techniques.
7. Very high case loads. Abnormally high case loads make it difficult to find time for proper case-recording.
8. Aversion to use of recording equipment. Evidence indicates that some professional workers are not comfortable with dictating

equipment and procrastinate with recording for this reason.

32.1.4. STYLES

The preferred style of recording is determined both by the purposes of the record and agency practice. Several common styles are presented below, with suggestions about their use. Many of the descriptions of recording styles used in this section are adapted from the proceedings of the First Institute on Rehabilitation Services [U.S. IRS, 1963a] which were edited by Robert McDonald.

Established Forms

Printed forms that must only be filled in, such as fact sheets or social history or work history forms, are useful when the amount and type of information to be gathered is small and when the data from all cases must be gathered in a uniform manner and format.

With the advent of high-speed computers and automatic data processing hardware, machine-readable forms that are completed serially by the worker provide empirical, comprehensive, and immediate data on the performance of entire programs. (This facilitates regular computerized reporting, printouts on case flow progress for each counselor, for more effective case load management.)

Summary Recording

This is a condensed account of transactions between the counselor, the client, and the agency. It may summarize what happened in a particular session or series of contacts and may contain notations about important characteristics of the client or of the events during the contacts. The summary recording may also describe ongoing progress toward an established objective. This style of recording, however, does not tell a story of client progress, as the narrative style of case-recording would do.

Summary recording works best after rehabilitation objectives have been clearly spelled out and case-recording can focus on progress or retrogression with regard to the objective. Changes in the client's situation or in program objectives during the time span covered by the summary can also be noted.

Narrative Recording

This standard format of case-recording essentially presents a sequential story about the client, circumstances, and services. The narrative contains factual data about the background of the client's problems, actions, and motivations. It describes the client's full situation and gives a clear picture of the relationships between the client and significant people (family, friends, associates, authority figures, counselors, and so on). Dates are recorded for each step and inferences are provided.

The narrative form lends itself to a variety of lengths, from brief shorthand descriptions to longer journal-style entries; it may even sometimes approach the style of the novel. The narrative style may be descriptive, analytical, or both. It is extremely important, however, for the record to clearly differentiate between observed fact and conclusions drawn from interpretations and implications of fact. In any case, the recorder strives for a dynamic picture of what is happening to the client.

Process- and/or Verbatim-Recording

Process-recording is a highly detailed description of the series of incidents and feelings that occurred during a session with a client. Hamilton used the analogy of a slow-motion picture to describe the way in which process recordings enable the reader to "see" the details of the personal interaction unfolding. The process record will be familiar to anyone who has ever attempted to write a detailed description analysis of the feeling tones, attitudes, and behavior of a client in a counseling session. Process-recording focuses on the counseling and about what is happening during counseling. It is more useful in training than in practice.

Verbatim-recording is a complete transcription of remarks and behavior, and it is used when such a detailed record is essential, such as in clinical evaluation. Process and verbatim records are not often used because they are time-consuming to prepare, impractical to keep, and difficult to read for ordinary purposes.

Topical Headings (Captions)

Case record notes can be organized under topical headings or captions to facilitate use of the information. "Structured caption-recording" results when the agency dictates which topics must be covered in a record, such as disability, financial determination, justification for acceptance, and so forth. Such areas usually represent the minimal standards for a brief record-

ing. "Unstructured captions" may be inserted to draw attention to an event in the case, or to label the content of a section of the record.

Caption-recording saves time, when it is necessary to review previous case entries, by making it easy to find the subject matter of interest. The headings serve as a subject index. Captions also help the writer to organize thoughts while recording. Mentally categorizing material into categories such as "impressions" or "case evaluation" prevents rambling and helps to define perceptions of the client's rehabilitation problems. Time is saved because it forces organization of the information before the labor of writing. Moreover, this structuring of thought about the case helps to eliminate gaps in information and planning. For those who dictate the case record to a stenographer or a machine, it is essential to prepare an outline listing key points to cover.

32.1.5. PRINCIPLES

Case-recording is not only for agency files; effective professional communication also helps clients. It demands understanding and facilitates planning, no matter what style the rehabilitationist chooses for describing the process. Recording reflects and thus becomes an integral part of the procedure through which a client plan is developed and implemented by the rehabilitation worker.

Set forth here are nine principles of rehabilitation case-recording that appear to be representative of guidelines found in the literature. The guidelines that follow were suggested by Kagan [1962].

1. Case records should present meaningful case data and should present it accurately. Biases will be difficult to avoid unless a conscientious effort to be objective is made.
2. Case records should reflect casework practice, the working diagnosis, how well the client is doing, and what the treatment plan is accomplishing.
3. The record should contain a judicious selection of case material. The length of a record does not determine its usefulness or accuracy. Skill in appropriate selection is learned through practice. Relevant material for the record is selected from rough notes jotted down during or right after counseling sessions.

4. Facts, client perceptions, and the counselor's perceptions should be clearly distinguished in the case record. Since case records are an account of communication and human interaction, they cannot be devoid of judgment. What must be avoided, however, is the intermingling of verifiable fact with judgments that are stated but not attributed to a source. Case records have two basic types of verbalizations: descriptive (factual) and interpretive (inferential or predictive). As the case progresses, the rehabilitationist marshals the facts, assesses their implications, draws interpretations from them, finally acting on them, and then checking interpretations and perhaps reinterpreting as new data may indicate.

5. Case record data should be presented in the simplest and most economical form. The recorder tries to avoid unnecessary complications, trivia, and redundancy in the presentation of case record information or duplication of information in other records. Handwritten notes must be legible, of course, for permanent records. Routine reports may sometimes be filled in by clerical or paraprofessional staff.

6. Proper grammatical construction is required.

Good organization, specificity, sequence, and clarity of case information makes the record more useful.

7. Technical terminology and professional jargon must be used carefully. Any professional or technical field of practice has its own unique materials, concepts, and processes and usually possesses a small but important vocabulary of terms to describe phenomena in the field. New words are often created, and new meanings are given to old words in order to produce terms that are economical to use and capable of imparting minute and specific shades of meaning. This technical nomenclature is valuable, but only if the reader is familiar with the terminology and when simple terms cannot convey the precise meaning intended.

8. Case records must be kept up to date to be fully used. Case-recording that occurs too late to be used as a professional tool in a case becomes a tiresome administrative chore.

9. Case records should be formulated according to the needs of the agency. They serve as documentation of agency function and provide supervisors and administrators with the means to measure worker performance and monitor agency activity.

32.2. Records

Recording is a professional function, but there are ethical and legal considerations regarding the resultant records (see 2.2.2). Rehabilitation workers are bound professionally to respect the rights of clients and to cause them no harm. Appropriate confidentiality of information about and from clients is an ethical responsibility as well as an agency requirement. Consequently, case records are written on the premise that they will be held in confidence or, at least, not misused. It is also generally assumed that the information is gathered for the purpose of helping a client to achieve rehabilitation. There is always the possibility, however, that case records will be unintentionally misused. Some of the potential uses and misuses of records are discussed below to help the practitioner know how case records can be handled.

32.2.1. CONFIDENTIALITY

Professional codes as well as the client's permission and agency guidelines dictate how, when, and where a record is to be used appropriately. Use of client information for extra-agency purposes may require not only consent but also a signed legal release.

Client material should be altered in some cases to protect the client's identity, such as when records are used for personnel training (i.e., client names and identifying information are omitted) [Lindsay, 1952]. A case record is a legal document and is thus subject to legal sanction that may take it out of the professional worker's control. In the field of medicine, for example, a patient's medical chart is a legal record that might be required as evidence in malpractice suits. The legal and ethical guidelines on confidentiality are provided by legal statutes, agencies, and professional associations. These mandates are not always consistent and consequently become issues in rehabilitation.

32.2.2. CAUTIONS

Past records label people. An outstanding illustration of this is the untold numbers of mentally competent citizens who were once diagnosed "schizophrenic" through a hasty psychiatric judgment and were forever falsely so known. This misuse of permanent files grossly ignores the fact that diagnostic errors are common and that people change and are always developing. At best the labeling entry represents a client at one point in time. Worse yet, the description is biased by the writer's perceptions, emphasis, and distortions of fact. Consequently, records that would permanently label former clients with derogatory or even erroneous descriptions should be destroyed when their specific purposes have been served.

Nothing that has been said here about the possible inaccuracy of case records should deter the rehabilitation worker from perusal of all available records for greater understanding of the client. The professional worker, forewarned of the occurrence of errors in both description and interpretation in case records obtained from various sources, is in a position to assess the validity of such outside information and obtain verification when indicated. Sometimes naive students are disturbed by the possibility that their reaction toward a client will be biased by negative implications in the client's history. Carrying this notion to the extreme, such students actually avoid explanatory information that could help in counseling and planning. Rehabilitationists must be able to accept clients for their personal worth without regard to negative characteristics. The true professional can handle all the facts with objectivity. Moreover, the capable professional can screen out of the case history unfounded assumptions and invalid reports.

A static view of the person may be propagated by the worker's own descriptions and assessments and may even become actualized in those disabled clients who unconsciously assume the behavior that they believe is expected of them [Riscalla, 1974]. This consideration, along with the possibility that records may in fact contain misrepresentations resulting from bias or judgmental error, makes it doubly important that when professionals read or write case records, they try to see how the contents match the current behavior of the client. If it is not possible to place complete confidence in the full accuracy of client information, collaboration from another source is mandated.

Case records occasionally deliberately misrepresent the client's situation for a purpose. For example, clients might be called functionally mentally retarded in the record when what they actually have is minimal brain dysfunction or a learning disability. Such a misrepresentation might be done in order to obtain services not available under the real diagnosis. The consequence, though perhaps not apparent at the time, is that the practitioner has actually created and will perpetuate an additional handicap.

When previous records are requested, the client being asked to release the information often does not know the nature or the accuracy of the previous records and does not know the impact that past records may have on the present case. Many are therefore understandably hesitant about releasing past information. Yet, such clients are often considered uncooperative. They find themselves obliged to release the information for fear that the agency staff will think they are trying to conceal something if they voice their reservations. It is important, therefore, for workers to determine how the client feels in such situations and to alleviate fears by proper explanation.

After reviewing the literature, Riscalla suggested that more intensive involvement by clients in decision-making and case-reviewing would help alleviate some of the problems and abuses of case-recording. Professional organizations and the courts have also taken measures to prevent abuses of personal recording and personal records. In its standards for development and use of educational and psychological tests, the American Psychological Association [1974] recommended that obsolete test information be eliminated from a person's file, that descriptive labels be avoided, and that access to information be given to the person in question.

32.2.3. LEGAL ISSUES

Legal precedents have been set that apply to a broad range of helping disciplines. In the case of Corrubut vs. San Diego Unified School District, for example, punitive damages were sought for diagnostic mislabeling [Vergason, 1973]. According to Riscalla, a New Jersey Supreme Court ruled that a patient or a patient's representative possesses the right to subpoena a psychiatric evaluation report and to contest the findings.

Riscalla believes that consumer activity and legal measures should not be considered policing procedures aimed at professional people; that rather these efforts should be viewed as a means of helping professionals to help others and an attempt to provide clients with some control over the information and decisions that are used to govern the course of their lives.

Client rehabilitation file information is subpoenaed by the courts in certain cases. More often, confidentialities are leaked inadvertently. Loose talk about clients, even in the office, is an abuse of client trust and certainly cases should never be discussed in public places even when names are not attached. The potential loss of records makes the contents of the case folder a hazardous possession. Client files should always be housed properly and then destroyed or closed in accordance with agency regulations. The clerical as well as the professional staff must be sensitive to this issue of confidentiality, and only authorized employees should have access to client information.

Tape-recording of counseling sessions must have the advance consent of clients, of course, and with their full knowledge of how it is to be used. Information that is potentially damaging to the client should not be recorded by any method that might result in its loss by the professional worker.

Selectivity in what is recorded has become a keen issue ever since clients were granted the legal rights to examine their own files. Clearly, information that would harm the clients and their self-concepts and relationships should not be freely circulated. In actual practice clients rarely demand to search their files, but it remains a serious issue. Particularly explosive information or conclusions may need to be withheld from the rehabilitation record.

32.3. Reports

The writing of reports is an extremely important part of the rehabilitation process, because the report is a form of communication among the members of the rehabilitation team. Reports make known to those involved with the case the facts that serve as the basis for decision-making about the client. If a report does not fulfill this purpose, it wastes the time of both the writer and the readers for whom it is intended. But the client, of course, is the person who loses the most when written communication fails. Therefore the responsibility of the writer to prepare effective reports is very great.

Since rehabilitation agencies and services differ markedly from one another, there is no set of guidelines that can fit the purposes of all. The report writer and the reader both benefit, however, if there is some uniformity in report organization and content. Formats are tailored to the requirements and activities of particular agencies. A very useful principle in the constructing of formats is to ask those who will be reading reports how they can be made most useful [Esser, 1974].

Reports in clear, accurate, concrete language can contribute substantially to any human services endeavor [Huber, 1961]. A written report becomes a kind of contract that divides up the responsibilities in a case; it sets forth the problems, states who will perform each task, and indicates procedures and deadlines. Plans, activities, conclusions, and the interpretations and logic underlying a particular case are set down for everyone to see, ensuring that the program makes sense and that follow-through is consistent [Coffey, 1970].

The written report is above all a document that integrates information from the variety of sources utilized during the progress of a case [Jacobs and Hay, 1961]. It synthesizes this data so that all the members of the rehabilitation team can understand the client's unfolding situation. Unsupported generalizations should not be used.

32.3.1. TYPES OF REPORTS

Although there are many different kinds of reports prepared during the rehabilitation process—intake reports, work evaluation reports, medical examination reports, psychological test reports, training reports, progress reports, status reports, social service reports, counseling reports, incident reports, behavior observation reports, placement reports, termination reports, follow-up reports, among others—they usually follow one of three principal types of formats: the narrative report, the basic checklist, and the narrative checklist. The discussion here is adapted from that of Esser.

The Narrative Report

Reports are more frequently written in narrative form than in any other form by rehabilitation workers, even though they are more time-consuming. In order to be effective the narrative report must first of all be well organized. Usually a topical outline is used, and the writer, while relating events chronologically, arranges the material under subject headings.

Relevancy is the other important principle. About each of the subjects in the outline the writer selects the essential information. The temptation to write long reports that contain a great deal of information, however interesting, should be resisted. Narrative reports are generally quite comprehensive, but the writer has selected, from the wealth of material available, what is significant and relevant in terms of the purpose of the report. As an example, the fact that a client's father was a watch repairer may or may not be relevant. If the father died when the client was young and his occupation had no impact on the client's life, the data is probably not relevant. If, on the other hand, the client learned how to fix watches from the father, the topic may have a great deal of bearing on some phase of rehabilitation. It is the writer's job to weigh information for relevance so that the reader will not have to sift out, and possibly miss, what is essential.

Even when a subject outline is used, there is no simple formula by which a narrative report can be made useful. The principles that underlie good writing in general will make the difference. It is to be hoped that those with superior writing skills do not use them to misrepresent aspects of the case, by making inadequate services appear better than they really are.

Those who question the value of the narrative report do so on the grounds that it makes heavy demands on the time of both writer and reader. A logical organization goes a long way toward solving this problem. And if a writer tests all the available information for relevance, striking a balance between completeness and utility, the report will probably be a suitable length.

The Basic Checklist

On the basic checklist, a rating scale is used to indicate whether the client has a particular skill, attribute, or behavior, or whether the characteristic is acceptable in relation to work. Checklists are used mainly to facilitate report-writing rather than as sources of comprehensive information. Unless used in conjunction with other material, therefore, the checklist is not an adequate form of communication.

The Narrative Checklist

In the narrative checklist, the most important data about the client is recorded in narrative form, and factual details such as test scores, work sample results, production data, and information about work behaviors are recorded on a checklist. While the end result is a comprehensive report, the narrative checklist—utilizing the advantages of both other forms—is efficient in terms of the writer's energy. The advantages of this combined form are that it takes less time to write than the narrative report, results in an easy-to-read document, tends to foster uniformity in report content, encourages the writer to be objective, and standardizes information.

32.3.2. COMMON PROBLEMS

Following is a list of the most typical problems in reports, all of which seriously detract from the value of a report.

1. Failure to answer the questions that prospective readers have asked or to provide the information they need.
2. Excessive length—more material than is necessary.
3. Repetition of information that the readers already possess.
4. Failure to use all the information that has been obtained.
5. Presence of conflicting material.
6. Failure to express realistic negative opinions or present negative information.
7. Failure to support recommendations with evidence and reasoning.
8. Failure to interpret facts and findings.
9. Presentation of plans and suggestions that are unrealistic.

10. Failure to consider or propose alternatives.
11. Lack of summary material.
12. Excessive brevity, resulting in lack of information.

32.3.3. EFFECTIVE WRITING

Amazingly little emphasis is placed on the development of writing skills in graduate training programs in rehabilitation, and seldom is the gap filled during in-service training or when a new staff member joins a rehabilitation agency. Rehabilitation professionals are usually initiated into report-writing when the time comes to write the first report on the first client, and the task can seem quite intimidating.

These principles for effective report-writing can help inexperienced writers.

1. The main purpose of the report is to provide information.
2. The report should meet the reader's requirements, basically by answering the questions that have been asked.
3. Accuracy and objectivity can be achieved to the extent that the information in the report is verifiable.
4. Neither facts nor generalizations are sufficient by themselves; facts must be brought together and generalizations, deductions, or conclusions drawn from them.
5. A clear organization will save the writer's as well as the reader's time.

32.3.4. WRITING STYLE

The writing done by rehabilitation professionals is similar to business and technical writing. It is not done for its own sake but for practical purposes, and therefore the style is important not in itself but as a vehicle by which information and understanding can be conveyed. The report writer, then, should not be concerned about evolving a style. Instead the aim is to give readers the information they need in the most efficient, direct way possible. The following rules about words and sentences will guide the writer in this direction.

1. Unnecessary words should be avoided. Seldom is there any excuse for using ten words when two or three will do as well.
2. In general, simple and familiar words are preferable to polysyllables; the big word is not justified when a shorter one will convey the same meaning. Excessive use of jargon is the most obvious and common violation of this rule. If "The client does not want to work" is what is meant, to say so is far more preferable than to say, "The client's motivation in terms of employment-oriented activity is low."
3. Active verbs are more direct and forceful than passive verbs. Thus, "Mr. Harbage was seen on Feb. 24" is less direct and clear than "I saw Mr. Harbage . . . ."
4. Concrete language and descriptive detail should be used to make more general ideas meaningful. "Mrs. Greene seemed extremely nervous" is a general statement; "She jiggled her leg continuously" provides detail, making the broader statement clear.
5. Prepositional phrases and other connective devices make the relationship between one idea and another understandable. *Although, because of, in keeping with, therefore, in addition to,* and dozens of other such terms, are selected by the writer so that the reader will not have to work out these relationships.
6. Short sentences are preferable to long ones; each sentence should express one thought or two that are closely related.
7. Variety in length of sentences will help keep the writing from becoming monotonous.

If the writer keeps in mind the purposes of the report—to help the client and help others to do so, there will be less of a tendency to become absorbed with style or even with following these rules. When the writer's attitude is positive and helpful, this will be communicated through the report to the readers, for the ultimate benefit of the client.

All those who prepare written communications so that decisions about rehabilitation clients can be made must be responsible for improving their own writing skills. With effort and practice, and through experience, this can be accomplished; the writer may well be able to think more clearly and to communicate more effectively in other ways, and the client will eventually benefit.

32.3.5. REPORT CONTENT

Obviously it is crucially important for the writer to make careful decisions about what will go into the report. In the narrative report, the topical outline dictates the overall organization, but the writer decides what will be covered under each heading.

While no ideal model exists, it is generally accepted that certain types of information should be included in any report: the specific pieces of identifying information, summary material, and recommendations that are almost always needed were discussed by Esser [1974] and Korn [1976b].

At the beginning of every report a certain amount of identifying information should be recorded: the client's full name, date the report is written, period covered by the report, agency case number, date of birth, name of report writer.

Summary material and recommendations compose the core of the report. The summary includes a composite picture of the client, identifies goals and objectives, and mentions the alternatives that can be considered. Recommendations should be specific. This section especially should be written in a clear and economical manner.

Part V

Placement

Chapter 33

Essentials

Job placement is a fundamental rehabilitation service for people who are vocationally handicapped by disability or other disadvantage. In fact it was one of the several original provisions of the public rehabilitation program in America. Ever since 1920, placement has been regarded as the culminating service, the goal of the entire vocational rehabilitation process. Moreover, it continues to be provided directly by the state rehabilitation agency staff while other services, such as training and physical restoration, are usually purchased for the client.

Placement refers to the professional activities involved in assisting handicapped individuals to seek and obtain employment. These activities may include guidance in vocational decision-making, training in job-seeking skills, supportive counseling, finding job leads, negotiating with employers, participating in the hiring procedure, educating supervisors and co-workers, and providing follow-up or post-employment services. The extent of placement assistance depends upon the vocational maturity of the client, the nature of the handicap, and many other factors.

An effective rehabilitation placement program consists of client preparation services, professional staff trained in placement techniques, and other resources to support the agency program. Depending upon the nature of the agency and the community served, there is a wide range of available placement services that will benefit the clientele. Among these are vocational assessment and counseling, vocational and adjustment training programs, public information campaigns, sheltered employment, selective placement services, tax incentives for employers, mediation between handicapped worker and employer, job development and job bank listings, and affirmative action implementation.

The goal of vocational rehabilitation is placement of rehabilitants at their highest level of employment potential. Most of Part V consequently focuses on the objective of remunerative work. But since this may not be feasible for some severely disabled persons, public rehabilitation services are authorized for nonvocational objectives. Thus a legitimate objective in lieu of job placement is independent living, the topic of Chapter 40.

33.1. Principles

Job placement of disabled persons is a well-developed technology that is an integral part of total rehabilitation. It is an explicit responsibility of rehabilitation counselors but the placement and job development functions are often conducted by a specialist because of the unique knowledge and skills needed. All rehabilitationists should find that placement success is a source of personal satisfaction because of their own first-hand involvement. Also, it is a continuing source of professional growth by means of direct feedback about people and occupations gained during the placement process. Expertise in placement techniques, however, is essential for success with difficult cases [Bowman & Graves, 1976].

33.1.1. PLACEMENT FUNCTION

Some rehabilitation agencies have a placement specialist who relieves the regular counselor of work in this final phase of rehabilitation (see 2.4.4). This specialist may be a former staff rehabilitation counselor who proved particularly proficient in placement. In any case, the rehabilitationist assigned to placement should have no less professional preparation than other counselors (see 3.4.8). In fact, all of the counseling functions (e.g., assessment, support, understanding) remain challenging and critical throughout client placement and follow-up procedures. Patricia Livingston [1978] of New York University has stated convincing reasons for requiring the masters degree in rehabilitation counseling for the function of job placement.

Successful placement is based upon a depth of professional knowledge about a client in the complicated process of matching the requirements and rewards of a job. The complexity of this process is comparable to that of the sales engineer who has, along with theoretical engineering education, a detailed knowledge of the product (e.g., a highly complex machine) and also of its unique uses and potential users or customers. When it is a human being to be put to work the rehabilitationist has a first responsibility to the client as a "sales product" that is far more precious and complicated than any machine. Yet both machinery and work force are selected carefully by business from competing sources. Consequently both need effective sales representation.

Although placement is a traditional function of rehabilitation counselors and an integral part of rehabilitation counselor education there is a movement to spin off this function and assign it separate disciplinary status [Usdane, 1976]. Such boundary disputes are irrelevant for the purposes of the present discussion but the term *placement specialist* as used here means a rehabilitation counselor who is especially prepared for the job placement function. Such a person has a professional masters degree in rehabilitation counseling and is not to be confused with the subprofessional agency employee who is called upon to help with job placement.

33.1.2. COUNSELOR INVOLVEMENT

The amount of direct counselor involvement in job placement varies substantially. Some clients after physical restoration or training are fully able to get their own jobs or return to former employment. A group of clients will have access to better resources for job-finding, such as their college placement service, and there are a number who use other placement or employment agencies to find jobs. Many clients need only minimal help—for example, ideas for locating vacant positions, practice in interviewing—but do not need the direct assistance of the rehabilitationist in employer negotiations. Finally, there are an increasing number of severely handicapped and unsophisticated rehabilitants who must have a great deal of help in identifying jobs suitable to their limited ability, in locating employment opportunities, in communicating to employers their suitability and the reasons for hiring, and/or, in becoming oriented and adjusted to the job.

Agency intervention is often great in vocational rehabilitation for blind people. Placement service for blind workers in industrial jobs may use agency specialists who are themselves blind in order to demonstrate to the employer how blind people can operate a machine (perhaps with modifications) or can function on specific jobs. The placement specialist for blind rehabilitants may participate in the hiring and orientation training of clients who are blind and may stay with them in the plant until they are securely settled and accepted.

33.1.3. THE NEED

Counselor involvement in placement should not exceed what is required to help a client secure appropriate employment. Minimal intervention by the rehabilitationist reduces client dependency and also prevents employers from forming misconceptions that would damage their image of the disabled applicant. Nevertheless, situations calling for substantial client assistance are important to recognize.

Intervention is dictated by placement problems that relate to many client variables, including: the type and the extent of functional limitations; sophistication in job-finding, preparation, and other occupational qualifications; personality, work record, and recommendations; and affiliations and employer connections. Other personal characteristics that may influence the difficulty of placement include age, race, and sex, although there are statutes prohibiting employment discimination due to disability or other characteristics that do not reduce performance potential.

Still other circumstances that indicate a need for extra help in job placement include: (1) poor labor market conditions in the locality for the kinds of occupations for which the client is suitable; (2) resistance or misinformation of the target employer with regard to hiring this applicant or handicapped people in general; and (3) inadequate qualifications of the client for the work due to improper selection of vocational objective, incomplete rehabilitation restoration, inadequate vocational training, or insufficient personal adjustments and job readiness—in other words, inadequate rehabilitation procedures.

Research shows that (all other things being equal) the ease and success of job placement are positively correlated with the amount of counselor time and agency funds invested in the rehabilitation effort preparatory to placement [Reagles, Wright, & Butler, 1970]. In actual practice, placement difficulty and employment sustention problems are too often the result of imperfect planning and inadequate service. Successful job placement of handicapped people requires occupational enablement through prior provision of needed client services.

After clients are readied for employment, success may depend upon locating, through local job surveys, industrial and other jobs appropriate for the disabled. Ironically, rehabilitation workshops in the community, in their aggressive efforts to subcontract work suitable for their own production, may have reduced the number of simple, light assembly job stations in area factories that could have been filled by clients. An effective approach to employment of the disabled population in the competitive labor market is to earmark suitable jobs, designated by agreement with business and other employers, to be filled by available and qualified disabled personnel.

33.1.4. REASONS FOR DIFFICULTY

Where suitable jobs are nonexistent the best of rehabilitation efforts are destined to fail. Rehabilitationists, having no authority over the free labor market, cannot be held responsible for rehabilitation client failures due to lack of job opportunity. This is not an uncommon problem; a study of state agency closures for example, revealed that one-third of severely handicapped cases, even after adequate rehabilitation services, could not be found suitable work [Sha'ked, Bruyere, & Wright, 1975].

Many of the very severely handicapped group never have a chance to get a competitive job because employers who are in a competitive business cannot afford to have substandard producers. Governments need to subsidize the pay of these marginal workers or otherwise to provide employer incentives and earmark suitable positions for severely handicapped workers. Moreover, governments should provide adequate subsidies to community sheltered workshops for the permanent employment of the noncompetitive disabled population. Otherwise, there will be a substantial group of people who never have an opportunity to work and are permanently dependent financially. Experience and research indicate that governments must intervene for people who are not quite fit or competitive for regular employment but who could be partially productive if given a subsidized or protected work setting.

Community employer practices in hiring disabled workers influence the ease of job placement and the need for intervention by the rehabilitation agency. Notwithstanding national or statewide fair employment legislation, local practices vary.

Attitudes of employers toward hiring handicapped workers, while a potential barrier, are subject to improvement. Publicity campaigns are conducted by the President's Committee for Employment of the Handicapped as well as associated Governor's Committees in the 50 states. Additional public relations efforts are made by the state rehabilitation and Employment Service agencies as well as private health groups and rehabilitation facilities. The media of press and air collaborate in these general public education efforts to increase factual knowledge and reduce unfounded fears about disability.

Professional workers individually in personal contact with potential employers are the best agents for inculcating constructive attitudes toward disablement. Still the most successful way to overcome resistance of employers is through placement of disabled persons who turn out to be good workers.

Placement is a process that may superficially seem to reflect just the actions of the rehabilitationist and the client. Actually there are many forces working either to impede or facilitate the employment of rehabilitants.

The paramount factor over which the rehabilitationist has no control is the labor market in the area—its character (e.g., number of sedentary jobs in local factories) and fluctuations (e.g.,

instability due to sensitivity to depressions in the national economy or due to seasonal production). It is said that the handicapped population is the last to be employed in an expanding economy and the first to be laid off as times worsen. Difficult economic conditions require proportionately greater rehabilitation effort.

In large measure, employment opportunity for the disabled depends upon the job pattern of local industry: communities with a concentration of heavy industry or mining offer relatively few jobs suitable for those disabled people who require sedentary work. And the unavailability of suitable jobs may even be compounded by local industrial conditions as, for example, when there is a high prevalence of disability due to industrial disease from the predominant business in the area (e.g., unemployed coal miners with black lung disease who cannot return to the mines).

33.1.5. PLANNING

Placement is mistakenly regarded by some as a discrete activity performed at the end of the vocational rehabilitation program. Experienced placement specialists, however, recognize that placement planning should be an integral part of the entire rehabilitation plan. Placement is the ultimate purpose of each service provided to a client. It is this explicit goal-directed structure of vocational rehabilitation that makes the whole process dynamic.

Program integration at the beginning of the rehabilitation process requires counselor consultation with placement specialists if available. Even when paraprofessionals serve as placement specialists or when other agencies perform the placement function, the rehabilitation counselor seeks their advice in client training programs and vocational choice. Their frequent contact with community businesses places them in a unique position from which to predict feasible employment alternatives.

The rehabilitation literature emphasizes the need to integrate placement, the final phase of the process, with the initial phase of planning [e.g., Decker, 1972; Dunn, 1974a]. Indeed, with some clients, continuing employment may require periodic placement assistance interspersed with other rehabilitation services. Clearly, the service model of placement as a discrete activity occurring at the end of the rehabilitation process does not hold in practice for most rehabilitants.

In some situations, however, placement may be the only service vital to a client's sociopsychological recovery. In other cases, it may not be needed at all, as many rehabilitants eventually obtain their own employment without professional assistance.

33.2. Definitions

The many technical terms that are relevant to job placement come from various fields—personnel and industrial psychology, industrial sociology, personnel management, and organized labor, as well as educational guidance and personnel work, vocational assessment, and rehabilitation counseling. Much of the nomenclature that is important in the realms of job placement and job development for the disabled population has been presented previously in other chapter discussions and in lists of definitions (e.g., see 17.2 and 27.1). In particular, many relevant terms are defined in Part III, Assessment.

33.2.1. JOB PLACEMENT

A number of terms that are useful in describing job placement, development, adjustment, and follow-up of rehabilitation clients that have not been described before are given here.

PLACEMENT. This term refers to obtaining a job for a client. Rehabilitation placement differs significantly from employee selection, in which the personnel worker seeks qualified job applicants for available openings. In placement work with disabled people, the counselor or rehabilitation placement specialist begins with the client and tries to find a job consistent with the vocational assets and limitations of the client. A rehabilitation placement is not completed until follow-up for a reasonable period of time determines that all needed services were provided, that the job is suitable, that the client is satisfied, that the employer is satisfied, and that the client will have some permanency on the job.

SELECTIVE PLACEMENT. The special process of matching the requirements of a specified job with the relevant characteristics of the client to achieve compatibility is known as selective placement.

WORK TOLERANCE. This is the ability to sustain a work effort for a prolonged period of time, to maintain a steady flow of production at an acceptable pace and level of quality, and to handle work pressure—all without acting in an unsatisfactory manner or quitting.

WORK OR JOB READINESS. Preparation of physical, mental, emotional, and other vocational resources for entry into competitive employment is termed the person's readiness for work and a potential job.

EMPLOYMENT INTERVIEW. This is a means of obtaining from applicants the facts about their experience and qualifications on which selection and placement are based. It serves, also, to give the applicant a picture of the position, the firm, and the disadvantages and demands as well as the opportunities of the job.

JOB ORIENTATION. Job orientation enables a disabled person to become familiar with aspects of a particular job, including the job site, tasks, rules, supervision, and co-workers.

JOB-SEEKING SKILLS. Job-seeking skills enable a person independently to find job vacancies and apply for them successfully. It includes knowledge of where to find information about job openings, how to fill out application forms, how to take employment tests, how to handle job interviews, and other skills that are effective in getting employment.

JOB RETENTION. The retention of a job after it is obtained prevents loss of client self-confidence, dissatisfaction on the part of the employer, and difficulty in obtaining another job. Jobs are mainly lost because of absenteeism, tardiness, poor work performance (quality or quantity), and problems with co-workers or supervisors. "Postemployment" services by state agencies are available to help rehabilitants to keep their employment after case closure. Ongoing support is provided by the rehabilitation counselor's follow-up visits and through other techniques (e.g, the "buddy system," in which a "job buddy" (fellow employee) provides help to a newly placed rehabilitant; and "social or alumni clubs" composed of graduates of job-finding clubs who continue to meet in order to help one another succeed in the world of work).

JOB (FINDING) CLUB. A number of job-ready clients may be brought together as a group (a so-called job club) to help in the job-finding attempt.

JOB MODIFICATION. Charting revisions for a position suitable for a rehabilitant is called "job modifying." The strategy is to get employers to make changes in the job or work structure (or hiring practices) to make existing work suitable or available to the disabled. Job restructuring is one approach, it involves examining the relationships among a number of the employer's jobs and rearranging tasks performed to create a position that is suitable. Job modification alters a workplace or specific job function to match an applicant's capabilities by eliminating tasks that the person's functional limitations preclude.

JOB-SHARING. A single job can be held by two (or more) persons who may share its responsibilities. This accommodates clients who do not have the stamina to work full days or who can perform only certain tasks. Other clients work the rest of the day or perform the other tasks.

JOB TRYOUT. This is the use of on-the-job work experiences, within the rehabilitation facility or in conjunction with outside establishments, to help handicapped individuals acquire knowledge and develop skills or assess their readiness for job placement when they must meet expectations or standards set for nonhandicapped workers. It is actually a "placement" used as an evaluation tool with the understanding that the client may not succeed and will be assisted further through the additional information.

FOLLOW-ALONG SERVICES. These are extended services provided after job placement to assist the handicapped individual maintain employment. All research demonstrates the particular importance of continuing follow-through with the very severely handicapped rehabilitant.

FOLLOW-UP SERVICES. This is the term for sup-portive assistance during the initial stage of job placement to evaluate the adequacy of rehabilitation services, to ascertain the client's need for further services, to determine whether the job placement is satisfactory, to decide when the case can be closed, and to provide closure data.

JOB BANK. The model job bank is the computerized system, developed by the U.S. Department of Labor, that maintains an up-to-date listing of job vacancies available through the state Employment Services.

SELF-EMPLOYMENT. Self-employment is any work for one's self, as a small business enterprise or service, for which one directly receives the profit from sales or fees for service. Self-employment is contrasted with work for others on a wage or salary basis.

GAINFUL EMPLOYMENT. This includes employment in the competitive labor market, practice in a profession, self-employment, homemaking, farm or family work (including that for which payment is in kind), sheltered employment, and home industries or other gainful homebound work.

JOB DEVELOPMENT. Developing job opportunities for hard-to-place rehabilitants is a comprehensive professional service and not simply the solicitation of jobs. Continuing and mutually beneficial relationships with community employers are established through agency services (e.g., selective placement, job modification, adjustment counseling). Job development activities should provide disabled workers with a chance for a career in cooperating firms as opposed to temporary or otherwise substandard employment.

AFFIRMATIVE ACTION REGULATIONS. This consists of government mandated efforts by employers to actively seek women, the disabled, the aged, and minority persons as employees, and to treat such employees without discrimination in all employment practices (i.e., advancement, rate of pay, and selection for training). It involves a written plan outlining specific active steps, timetables, and complaint and enforcement procedures to assure such equal opportunities.

33.2.2. THE STUDY OF JOBS

Techniques for the study of jobs are fundamental to the entire process of client placement. Consequently, the following terms are basic to Part V, Placement.

Many of the concepts related to work were formulated in the nineteenth century by Frederick W. Taylor [1911] in his development of "scientific management." In the beginning, "Taylorism" involved simply the study of methods and movements of workers to increase output and reduce costs by introducing changes in jobs. Human betterment applications came later.

JOB ANALYSIS. Job analysis provides systematic and detailed information about a job: what the worker does in relation to data, people and things; the methodology and techniques employed; the machines, tools, equipment, and work aids used; the materials, products, subject matter, or services that result; and the traits required of the worker. The process of observation, interview, and study identifies job duties, responsibilities, purpose, qualifications for employment, relation to other jobs, equipment and material used, and training and physical demands.

METHODS STUDY. The systematic recording and critical examination of existing and proposed ways of doing work, as a means of developing and applying easier and more effective methods and reducing costs, is known as methods study.

TIME STUDY. Time study is a work measurement technique for recording the times and rates of performance for the elements of a specified job. Carried out under specified conditions, it shows the time necessary for carrying out the job at a defined level of performance.

MOTION STUDY. This is the study of repetitive movement in order to eliminate unnecessary motions and to determine the most efficient and least fatiguing movement or combination of movements.

TASK ANALYSIS. Task analysis is breakdown of a particular job into its component parts. Information gained from task analysis can be used to prepare or select qualified workers for the required task performance.

JOB CLUSTERS. Jobs are grouped together on the basis of similar job requirements (e.g., specific duties of the job, materials worked with, equipment used, necessary skill and knowledge, and worker characteristics). Such clusterings reveal "job families."

EMPLOYMENT PHYSICAL DEMAND FACTORS. Physical activities required of a worker in a job include: lifting, carrying, pushing and/or pulling (strength); climbing and/or balancing; stooping, kneeling, crouching and/or crawling; reaching, handling, fingering and/or feeling; talking and/or hearing; and seeing.

PHYSICAL DEMANDS ANALYSIS. This is a component of job analysis by which the physical activities and working conditions involved in jobs are determined. Physical demands are those physical capacities required of a worker in a job and are of primary interest in determining the suitability of a job for a physically handicapped worker. There are three subfactors: physical activities, working conditions, and hazards.

PHYSICAL CAPACITIES APPRAISAL. This is a medical procedure whereby a determination is made of the physical activities a person is capable of performing and the working conditions under which the person can safely be employed.

WORKING CONDITIONS. Working conditions are the physical surroundings of workers in a specific job: inside, outside, or both; extremes of cold plus temperature changes; extremes of heat plus temperature changes; wetness and humidity; noise and vibrations; hazards; fumes, odors, toxic conditions, dust and vapor, and poor ventilation. They also include environmental conditions over which the workers have no control and that affect their mental or physical well-being or comfort. Those situations make specific demands upon a worker's capacity.

WORK ENVIRONMENT. Surroundings in which, and conditions under which, workers perform their occupational duties—including lighting, equipment, state of cleanliness, and type of supervision—are referred to as the work environment.

WORK STATION. A work or job station is the physical site where a production operation is performed.

JOB BREAKDOWN. This is the division of a complex job, one requiring extensive training for mastery, into a number of work units, any one of which can be mastered by less skilled workers.

ADAPTATION OF JOBS. Sometimes referred to as "job reengineering," this is defined as the means of improving employment opportunities for disabled workers by means of simple adjustment, adaptation, or redesign of tools, machines, and workplaces. In this way, stresses and strains of work can be reduced or eliminated, thus opening up a much wider field of employment possibilities for rehabilitants.

INDUSTRY. An industry is a group of independent but similar establishments where business is conducted, or where services or productive operations are performed. It includes stores, factories, farms, mills, and mines, in which similar services or industrial operations are performed or business is carried on.

INDUSTRIAL CLASSIFICATION. This system is used in assigning code numbers to employers and establishments, based on the nature of their activities, so that data reported by them can be grouped into industries for purposes of analysis.

INDUSTRIAL STANDARDS. These are actual worker requirements in a given industry based on the expectations of employers in terms of quality, quantity, and worker traits.

STANDARD PERFORMANCE. This is the rate of output that qualified workers will naturally achieve without overexertion as an average over the working day, provided they know and adhere to the specified method and provided they are motivated to apply themselves to their work.

33.2.3. LABOR TERMINOLOGY

Labor, as a word of many meaings, is important in this book meaning the "expenditure of physical or mental effort," as a "trade or industrial union organization," and as the "group comprising the workers of the nation." The following terms particularly address the last definition.

LABOR FORCE. This usually refers to the total number of persons over a certain age (e.g., 14 years old) who have a job (the employed) or are looking for a job (the unemployed). Not considered a part of the labor force are people under a certain age (14 years), housewives, full-time students, people in institutions, and retired people neither working nor seeking work.

MANPOWER. The term was formerly used to describe military strength, but, since the 1960s, it has been used to describe the nation's total production strength in terms of all available workers.

MANPOWER PROGRAMS. These programs were originally developed for administration by the U.S. Department of Labor (DOL) to retrain workers who would lose their jobs because of automation. When technology proved less threatening than anticipated, the DOL Manpower Administration switched its concentration to the "hard-to-employ." There was a proliferation of programs (e.g., Job Corps, Work Incentive Program, Neighborhood Youth Corps, JOBS).

MANPOWER DEVELOPMENT. This is a collective effort to assure the availability of an adequate supply of qualified workers.

OCCUPATIONAL STRUCTURE. This is a standardized classification of occupations according to the kinds of work involved.

OCCUPATIONAL MOBILITY. This means shifting from one occupation to another. When the movement is between occupational status levels, it is called vertical occupational mobility. When it involves a change to another occupation at the same occupational status level, it is called horizontal occupational mobility. Horizontal mobility does not necessarily involve economic or social changes in status or geographic mobility.

LABOR MOBILITY. The concept of labor mobility refers to the ease with which workers can move from one place to another or from one occupation to another. It is also used for the rate of movement into and out of an industry.

LABOR TURNOVER. Labor turnover is the ratio of the number leaving (or newly employed) to the average number on the payroll for a specified period of time (e.g., one year).

MIGRATORY LABOR. These are workers who periodically change their residence in order to obtain seasonal or temporary employment.

33.2.4. PERSONNEL TERMINOLOGY

The term *personnel work* has a broad meaning covering a wide range of functions in industrial, educational, governmental, and agency establishments. It embraces the whole policy of management toward employees: methods of remuneration, human services, union relations, and promotion or transfer, as well as hiring and discharge.

It is important for the rehabilitationist to know about personnel work in order to make use of this knowledge in assessment, vocational planning, and placement of clients. In working with industrial personnel and employment offices the rehabilitation worker should know that these are usually "staff" as opposed to "line" offices. Line structure involves the division of an organization according to authority from top to bottom; staff organization is division according to functions performed. Most organizations have both line and staff offices and employees. Traditionally only line employees (e.g., administrators, supervisors) give commands, while staff personnel are concerned with consultation, coordination, fiscal affairs, and the like. In other words, the "employment officer" of a firm may be unable to make final decisions, as the authority to hire a handicapped applicant may belong to the "line" production superintendent or foreman.

The following terms are useful to rehabilitationists in dealing with personnel workers.

WAGE STRUCTURE. The system or pattern of wage rates existing in a given establishment, industry, or occupation, or prevailing in a community, is known as its wage structure.

WAGES. Recompense given on a time basis to workers (often those engaged in manual or mechanical occupations) is known as the hourly wage. Additional pay is customarily given for "overtime" work.

SALARY. Salary is a stipulated recompense paid at regular intervals to an employed person for services rendered. The term generally applies to professional, administrative, or supervisory personnel and often does not include additional pay for overtime service.

OCCUPATIONAL DISEASE. In general terms, this is a pathological condition brought about by the work done, or by the circumstances in which such work is done.

OCCUPATIONAL ACCIDENT. This is an occurrence in a work setting or work-related activity that involves injury and may result in disablement. Work accidents may have many causes: lifting, handling, falling, falling objects, hand tools, machinery in motion, dangerous substances, and so on.

EMPLOYMENT INJURY BENEFITS. These are benefits provided by industrialized nations in one of two ways: through a government social insurance system, with a central public fund, or through various private arrangements that are required by law and referred to as workers compensation. Benefits often differentiate between temporary incapacity and permanent disability, total or partial.

OCCUPATIONAL ABILITY. The person's ability to perform all of the essential requirements and demands of an occupation in its normal environment and according to normal standards without hazard to self or jeopardy to the safety of others and without aggravating medical conditions, is called occupational ability. This refers to whether a person can do the job—not whether the individual will be employed.

PLACEABILITY. This is the condition of the client following completion of the rehabilitation process and prior to employment on a job, indicating the probable success of the placement effort by personnel of the rehabilitation agency in helping the client to obtain employment.

EMPLOYABILITY. This refers to the likelihood that one will be employed and retained. It is different from the ability to work, although it is sometimes used in this connection.

WORK HISTORY. Important in vocational rehabilitation and personnel work, a person's work history consists of: periods and places of employment and unemployment, kinds of positions held, work proficiency, pay received, duties and responsibilities, the reasons for leaving, and so forth.

33.3. Disabled Workers

Employment of disabled people occurs within the context of the norms and expectations of society—a complex fabric of prejudices and good will, misconceptions and enlightened action. It is within this social framework that rehabilitationists seek to place their clients. This requires not only making the rehabilitant a capable worker and locating a suitable job but also developing employer willingness to hire the person.

Confidence in the occupational potential of disabled populations is necessary for rehabilitationists to convince employers. The rehabilitationist's best source of enthusiasm is personal experience with the many clients who succeed in the face of overwhelming odds.

Much is written about the work performance of the disabled population, including subjective case-experience reports published by employers. These employer opinions have a great influence on other employers and may well have more to do with overcoming employers' misconceptions and bias than valid scientific data. However, the student of rehabilitation does need the evidence from the research literature on the subject, which extensively documents the job abilities of disabled people [Wright & Trotter, 1968]. The literature covers: the full range of disabilities; considerations pertaining to various types of occupations and employers (e.g., manufacturing, transportation, government); production considerations (e.g., work performance, rates of production, quality, wastage); personnel considerations (e.g., absenteeism, labor turnover, accident rates, insurance coverage); special arrangements to change the job or change the person (e.g., job modification or job training); employment adjustment techniques; and employer and employee attitudes.

The first research of this type dates back to 1929 when J.W. Dietz conducted a longitudinal study of 652 disabled employees of the Western Electric Company matched with 652 control (nondisabled) subjects [Dietz, 1931]. The disabled employees compared favorably with the nondisabled on variables that included rate of production, absenteeism, accident rate, and turnover. Such early studies led to the conclusion that almost all handicapped people can work at some kind of productive labor. In fact the U.S. Federal Security Agency, Office of Vocational Rehabilitation, concluded in 1946 that practically any job can be performed by some disabled person.

33.3.1. EMPLOYMENT POLICY

A statement of employment policy that would provide full opportunities for disabled persons and preclude discrimination in employment because of physical or mental disability was approved by the 1976 meeting of the Council of World Organizations Interested in the Handicapped (CWOIH) in Geneva, Switzerland. This policy was recommended for adoption by all nongovernmental organizations:

Each candidate for employment shall be evaluated and employed on the basis of his or her qualifications to perform the functions of available positions regardless of the presence of physical or mental disability.

Disabled employees shall receive the same pay, benefits and employment security as other employees doing equal work and shall be entitled to promotion on the same basis as all other employees.

Whenever possible, all places of work and related facilities such as rest rooms, toilets, lunch rooms and others shall be fully accessible to persons whose mobility is limited by disability. When complete accessibility is not yet accomplished, special arrangements will be made to meet the needs of disabled employees in a manner fully respecting their rights and dignity and protecting their safety and that of their co-workers.

Technical aids and adaptations of office machines and equipment, tools, furniture and other items required for the safe performance of tasks for which a disabled employee is otherwise eligible shall be provided by the employer unless they are available from other sources.

The employer should consider reorganization of the tasks being performed by all employees with the objective of identifying clusters of functions that will result in positions more readily performed by disabled employees.

When the employer provides transportation, or assists in making transportation to and from the places of work available for employees in general, suitable and accessible transportation shall be made available for disabled employees.

All possible assistance shall be given for the provision of the education and training needed by potential employees who are too disabled to qualify for suitable positions, by disabled employees to qualify for advancement and by employees requiring retraining after accidents or illness.

Activities planned for the orientation and training of all personnel shall include information about the problems of disabled persons and measures to assist in the solution of such problems, particularly those associated with social integration. Special training shall be given to employees assigned to supervise or work in close association with disabled individuals.

Recreational programs planned for employees shall be designed to encourage and facilitate the maximum possible participation by disabled employees.

The above statement represents a thoughtful analysis of the problem and an informed employment policy to assure equal opportunity for workers who have a disability.

33.3.2. FOCUS ON ABILITIES

Not more than one percent of all workers is physically fit for all work, according to Bert Hanman [1951]. This means that the great mass of the working population is physically limited to some degree. Whether the physician finds an impairment or not, the truth is that the so-called disabled and the so-called physically fit are both handicapped. Both groups are physically limited for numerous occupations and activities in life, since practically every human being is physically limited in one way or another for some occupations. Then in addition to the physical demands, every job has other necessary requirements—education, intelligence, emotional, and skill factors. Physically fit or not, no one possesses all of the other abilities needed to perform all jobs.

While this discussion addresses the placement services and techniques for so-called handicapped people, the fact is that all workers need selective placement services. The principles of placement focus upon the individual's capacities and abilities. The individual abilities of all applicants require matching with work demands. As a consequence, rather than thinking in terms of disability and handicap, it is best to consider abilities instead. Jobs are performed—and obtained—on the basis of abilities. This is not merely a plea for positive thinking. The fact is that negative concepts and terms are of little value and may be counterproductive in job placement considerations for all people.

33.3.3. DISABILITY NOT HANDICAP

Misunderstanding of the terms *disability* and *handicap* has contributed greatly to confusion. Employers as well as the rest of society fail to distinguish between these two quite different conditions.

The term *physical disability* refers to causes of limitations in function(s), whether the disability stems from disease, injury, or birth condition. A physical (or emotional) disability may be either temporary, the individual recovering with no marked residual defects, or permanent, in which case, after all medical, surgical, and natural measures have been taken, the damage continues to be limiting in one or more functions. Also the disability may be rated in terms of severity of the functional limitation. The difference between disability and functional limitations was discussed in previous chapters (see 4.1.1).

The term *occupational handicap* refers to the lack of ability to fill all of the requirements of a specific job, including the knowledge, skill, intelligence, interest, personality, physical, and emotional requirements. As pointed out before, one is occupationally handicapped for any job for which one cannot meet the requirements. Most people can fill all of the requirements for a comparatively small number of jobs, as Hanman pointed out. In the large remainder people are occupationally handicapped, not always because they cannot meet the physical demands but rather because they cannot fulfill the skill and knowledge requirements. This is repeated because it is important that those working with the disabled use these two terms, *disability* and *handicap*, with proper discrimination. It is especially important that rehabilitationists do not use the word *handicap* without stating how, that is, "Handicapped for what?"

33.3.4. THE ULTIMATE GOAL

"Work, in American culture," Chapple [1972] thought, "is too often considered the ultimate value. . . . If a job with some kind of remuneration is not being aimed at as a consequence of our efforts, we have a tendency to feel that our basic goals are being perverted." [p. 11]

Employment, and more specifically competitive employment, is not always the proper objective for many disabled people. It is necessary to examine the context of each client's value system, functional abilities, and needs in order to determine how important that goal is. This is not to discount the significance of productive activity for most people in most societies. Generally speaking, a vocational objective at the highest level of the client's potential is clearly preferred in the rehabilitation program.

Most clients going through a rehabilitation program want to become contributing members of society. They would prefer to work for pay than receive pension benefits [Towne, 1972a]. Homebound clients involved in a job program, it is noteworthy, will generally speak with great pride about their work and have especially friendly manners; noninvolved patients, on the other hand, will often be passive and withdrawn and suffer feelings of worthlessness, according to Springer [1961]. Whether handicapped, disabled, disadvantaged, or not, people who are unemployed for long periods of time generally experience sociopsychological difficulty of some sort.

Not all work is therapeutic, however. In some instances employment may actually be harmful to a client, according to Esser [1975a]. Occasionally an overambitious client will rashly attempt a former level of productivity before redeveloping the necessary work tolerance. Jobs must be consistent with physical and environmental capacities. Moreover a client who becomes disabled at an advancing age may suffer so much humiliation because of job downgrading that it might be better for the person to retire than work at a job considered inferior [Olshansky, 1974].

33.3.5. THE CHANGING WORLD

Behind every new technological development and social experience is new potential for rehabilitation services. The existence of electronic, computer, and telecommunication systems, in addition to the efforts of rehabilitationists, is enabling severely handicapped individuals, once considered incapable of competitive employment, to attain increasingly higher levels of self-actualization and production. An example was given by Overby [1973]:

Frequently one reads or hears about the mobility problems of handicapped people and of the efforts being made to ease their transportation problems. It is important that such efforts continue for this minority segment of our society. Another dimension of the problem, however, should perhaps be given equal attention—namely, taking employment to the immobile.

Present and not distant future technological developments in the computer-telecommunication area suggest that much can be done in the "here and now" about taking information handling jobs to persons rather than transporting persons to such jobs [p. 18].

Of course, technology cannot solve every problem. The implications of whatever changes technology effects, however, are worth consideration. The feasibility of a disabled client's seeking rehabilitation services and obtaining employment is not a static situation.

As social values change, many persons previously denied access to employment may hope for social and economic fulfillment. Though stereotypes and prejudices are difficult to change, public attitudes toward the capabilities and contributions of the disabled population also are continually improving. The disabled themselves are improving their public image: a retarded person invents a device to improve assembly line production; a person with epilepsy achieves popularity as a major league hockey player; and a person who suffers from a debilitating neurological disorder, while confined to a wheelchair, becomes a leading physicist.

33.4. *Alternative Models*

This section surveys selected program models for job placement of handicapped individuals. Different approaches have been studied in rehabilitation research and demonstration projects. A number of alternative placement models have been described by White, Goldston, Leeder, and Soloff [1976], and, since 1978, in various issues of a research utilization publication, *Rehab Brief,* prepared by John Muthard of the Florida Rehabilitation Research Institute for the federal rehabilitation agency.

Some kinds of improvements would require

major revision of the employment structure in the country. Other innovations suggest substantial changes in the human services delivery systems. Certainly new methods are needed to provide employment opportunity for all of the disabled population who can and want to work. Rehabilitationists still have difficulty in creating occupational opportunities for many disabled clients because of the backdrop of employer hiring practices aimed at increasing profits. A comprehensive adjustment of resources, whether by adequate tax incentives for businesses that hire disabled workers who are handicapped, greater authority for rehabilitationists to require job redesign in industry, or other arrangements for employment of those with serious placement handicaps, may be necessary to alleviate the problem of high unemployment among the disabled population.

33.4.1. PLACE AND TRAIN APPROACH

The "place and train" approach has been tried in many ways. For some clients who come to rehabilitation agencies, immediate placement is feasible if a suitable job is available, even though the individual will still need training or other help. Others have been successfully placed on part-time jobs that serve as a "transition" into full-time employment after rehabilitation services are completed. The purpose in both approaches is to enable the individual to benefit from the therapeutic aspects of combining a real work situation with the rehabilitation program [Kaufman, 1975].

The 1978 Amendments to the Rehabilitation Act authorized funds to sponsor projects for the training and employment of disabled people (see 33.4.14). While this approach incorporates the element of subsidized employment—which is another model—it retains the rehabilitation goal of preparation for competitive employment (at the conclusion of the project).

Dunn [1974a] noted that the rehabilitation process has attempted to develop some "alternative service delivery approaches" that promise to be more effective than the usual linear sequence of referral, evaluation, services, and placement. He cited Taylor's [1970] analysis to explain the reasoning behind these alternative models. While the conventional model of rehabilitation service delivery is effective for those disabled people who have middle class values, he thought that it would not work as well for the disadvantaged population, because the latter see

their problem as merely "joblessness" and are often unwilling to embark on long-term rehabilitation programs to prepare for an eventual job.

The culturally disadvantaged client needs a more rapid delivery of meaningful services. When the client is involved in meaningful activity at an earlier stage, much of what is attributed to lack of motivation is overcome. The client receives some of the rewards of the system at an earlier point in the process than in the traditional rehabilitation agency.

Dunn's emphasis throughout is on early contact, immediate placement, ongoing service while the client is working, and assistance for advancement from "low-level, dead-end jobs." He further suggested that reciprocal contracts be drawn up, according to which employers would provide a given number of positions and the rehabilitation agency would provide the manpower. Stress is placed upon the reciprocal nature of the contract: if sufficient numbers of clients are unavailable for positions, or if an individual is unsatisfactory in a position, the rehabilitation agency still has the obligation to fill contracted job slots at all times—even if the professional staff has to perform those jobs.

The development of job-sites for the place-and-train approach is more feasible in metropolitan areas than in rural areas, which favor traditional on-the-job training. Where clients and opportunities are few, more specific and lengthy arrangements are required. Even so, job-site development for transitional employment takes time and it is a continuing task. An employer will sometimes hire an individual in a training slot to that same position as a permanent employee. It is better to accept the loss of a training site than antagonize the employer.

33.4.2. EXTENDED WORK EXPERIENCE

The extended work experience program is used for severely disabled persons whose functional limitations are such that they may have difficulty learning how to do a job or handling job interviews. Employers in large businesses agree to allow the agency to do screening without the prerequisite of an employment interview, thereby enabling placement of individuals who would normally be excluded from employment by the job application process. A guaranteed probationary period of up to six months allows the agency to complete adjustment services and training as necessary, and to substantiate the individual's productive capability to the employer.

Another approach with employers is that of Fountain House in New York City, called "transitional job placement." Here the staff person works alongside the clients on jobs guaranteed to Fountain House by the employer in return for reliable coverage of the jobs and supervision and training of the work group.

33.4.3. EMPLOYER ACCOUNT SYSTEM

The employer account system used in metropolitan areas consists of a systematic and concerted effort to develop ties with large businesses. Individual counselors are assigned to coordinate agency contacts with particular businesses to ensure that quality service is provided and to nurture the "prime contact" relationship. Typical services to the employer include: affirmative action assistance; workers compensation assistance; aid in establishing companybased programs for troubled employees; direct employee services; awareness training for supervisory and general personnel; and manpower assistance in the form of job analysis, screening of rehabilitants for job referral, and intensive follow-up.

Account systems with large corporations provide wider access to a variety of jobs. Successful placements have been made at all levels of employment including skilled and semiskilled, clerical, managerial, and professional. Another advantage of the account system is that beginning salaries are typically higher because the participating companies are large corporations.

The account system requires extensive inservice staff preparation. Considerable staff time and experience are needed for job development activities. Agency supervisory personnel are utilized in both training and account development activities. It may take many months just to establish an employer account with a major corporation.

33.4.4. THE MONTHLY BULLETIN

Though not widely used, the monthly bulletin is one of the most effective ways of maintaining contact with employers. According to Wuenschel and Brady [1959], this list of available workers should be mailed monthly to employers who have formerly used the placement service. The bulletin lists clients by their qualifications, experience, special assets or problems; employers interested in clients on this list then call to arrange an interview with the placement counselor. The counselor then learns details about the job and the employer gets fuller information about the client. Then, if the employer feels that client and job will be compatible, an interview can be set up with the client. Properly handled with adequate follow-up, the monthly bulletin is a most useful aid in placing disabled clients [Echols, 1967].

33.4.5. THE LODGE PROGRAM

The "Lodge Program," used successfully in Alaska, consists of the organization and training of a group of disabled people to operate a joint business venture. The original project began with the selection of 20 men and women residents of a mental hospital who had shown little or no improvement under traditional treatment programs.

The step-by-step plan began with training the group to operate independently. The program emphasized treatment that fostered patient responsibility in problem-solving and decisionmaking. Using this approach, vocational rehabilitation managed, in a little over a year, to move patients into a lodge where they alone bore responsibility for their treatment. Not only did they become the "expert" mental health workers who had to deal with other members' problems, but they ceased treating mental illness as a disease and dealt with it instead as a deviation from social norms. In establishing their own society, the patients set their own norms, chose their own leaders, settled their own problems, and used the staff not as problem-solvers but as information-givers.

Daggett, James, and Singley [1975] reported that training in the institution was conducted for approximately one year before the group moved into a house in the community. A housecleaning business of proved local need was chosen to provide a basis for independent support. One nonresident staff person worked with the group for several months after the move to help with adjustment problems and to serve as liaison to local business.

Reporters on the lodge program cited several reasons for its effectiveness. First of all, it provides a community situation in which a patient may still be psychotic but can also be self-supporting. Second, the society of the lodge sets its own norms; its acceptable behaviors differ from those of normal society, but its members are also much less judgmental. The patient also has companionship, an important factor for mental patients who have undergone long hospitalization with its accompanying physical and psychological isolation. Most important, perhaps, is the fact that the program takes the treatment one step beyond the ordinary. It insists that the patient act responsibly and provides a setting for responsibility to flourish in.

Considerable problems of hostility and resentment are often encountered from neighbors of residential situations like this (e.g., halfway houses). Neighbors fear a drop in property values or perceive some imagined threat from the nonconformity of the deinstitutionalized residents. Public education campaigns and careful selection of the residential site minimize such hostile reactions.

33.4.6. SHELTERED BUSINESS

In spite of effective job development and placement efforts, many of the severely disabled people will not succeed in competitive employment. Kaufman [1975] noted this growing recognition of an "awesome, but sobering" problem in vocational rehabilitation: the "largest bulk" of clients do not reach successful placement at all, while of those successfully placed, a significant percentage fail to hold their jobs beyond a few months. But these same disabled workers in sheltered workshops, job stations in industry, client-operated businesses, and other employment programs of rehabilitation facilities behave adequately and produce good products (see 8.3.5).

Kaufman said that "the answer lies in supervision of clients employed, and not only in the clients themselves. Between the low level 'Chronic' client who requires traditional sheltered workshops and the client successful in competitive employment, is this larger group—the group that needs tolerant, but firm supervision, and who requires more understanding than that usually found in industry" [p. 17].

Horizon House Industries, which Kaufman described, is organized as a "sheltered-competitive" business employing psychiatrically disabled clients who perform complex production tasks. It competes with light manufacturing industries in work quality and is financially self-sufficient. The essential differences between this type of business and profit-making companies are that its staff is trained to work with the handicapped worker-clients and that personnel of the rehabilitation agency that owns the business can make decisions freely with the clients more consciously in mind.

33.4.7. UNION-MANAGEMENT PROGRAMS

Rehabilitationists trained without much contact with business may be largely unaware of the considerable resources within management and labor to help return disabled employees to work. Large unions have their own counseling staff, and large businesses often have job-engineering, safety, or personnel staff who can redesign job characteristics in order to reintegrate employees who have become disabled. These business people may not be capable of handling the most severely disabled individuals without outside consultation, but their experience and expertise is often extensive [U.S. IRI, 1975].

A noteworthy effort was a New York City project in which retired union members were hired to contact unions and solicit opportunities for disabled members. The retirees were trained in basic methods of rehabilitation, then sent to union meetings. The combination of union affiliation and rehabilitation knowledge led to immediate rapport and subsequent help with placement [New York City Central Labor Council AFL-CIO, 1970].

33.4.8. REINSTATEMENT OF EMPLOYEES

Another type of placement program is operated by industry for rehiring or reinstating (former) employees who, because of a disablement, are unable to return to their former position. This would include workers compensation cases as well as others. The National Industrial Conference Board [1957] developed guidelines for companies to use. Most firms attempt to "make a place for" handicapped people who have a good record or whose disability was incurred on the job.

One way to promote regular rehabilitation placement services with businesses is to offer the consulting services of the professional staff to help with the business' own disabled employees. Counselors can meet on a preventive basis with managers, disabled employees, and individuals who have potential problems. At the same time, these visits enable the counselor to learn about job openings for other disabled clients.

33.4.9. BUSINESS ASSOCIATIONS

There are many advantages to the utilization of associations of employers such as the National Alliance of Businessmen (NAB). People in private business are more likely to be successful in convincing other business people to pledge meaningful jobs. Moreover they have a better working knowledge of both current job locations and potential locations. This type of cooperation saves job-searching time that can be used by the rehabilitation agency in other job development tasks. To strengthen relations with personnel and business leaders, the job development specialist should participate in meetings of their associations. Membership in the local personnel club is particularly important.

33.4.10. EXCEPTED APPOINTMENTS

The U.S. Civil Service Commission has an "excepted" appointment procedure that can be applied to disabled people to facilitate their employment if they meet certain requirements. There are several certification requirements of this procedure. The Commission requires that a rehabilitation counselor must certify that the client can perform the duties of the position, can physically do the work without undue hazard to self or others, and is socially competent in the work environment. Several thousand severely disabled individuals have found federal jobs through this *noncompetitive* channel.

33.4.11. WORK EXPERIENCE PROGRAMS

The federal government sponsors short-term programs for handicapped people. One such program provides federally funded training positions for up to one year in local government agencies. The positions are tailored to the capabilities of mentally retarded individuals with the expectation that upon completion of one year in training, the local government will continue a position under its own funding arrangements. State Employment Service personnel coordinate the job-site development and placement aspects of the operation. CETA and other federally sponsored programs are discussed elsewhere in this book (see 12.2.4 and 37.1).

33.4.12. JOB DEVELOPMENT LABORATORY

Many seemingly unsuitable jobs can be adapted for the severely disabled worker through the use of social and mechanical engineering. Electronic communications equipment, for example, can allow some kinds of full-time competitive work to be performed at home (called satellite work stations). (In developing work for homebound clients the idealized image of commuting to the place of work must be overcome.) Work hours can be varied using "flex-time" scheduling. In another solution, groups of variously handicapped individuals can be organized to handle complementary work components of a particular job or business.

A "job development laboratory," utilizing the job placement model, can enhance productivity and place many severely physically handicapped persons who would otherwise be considered as infeasible by vocational rehabilitation agencies.

33.4.13. PROJECTS WITH INDUSTRY

Projects with Industry—or PWI, as it is called—is not really a set model, but it is a very effective means of helping people who are disabled into paid employment. The program was authorized by the 1968 Amendments to the Vocational Rehabilitation Act and is based in the federal offices of the public rehabilitation agency. Corporations and other participating organizations make contracts directly with the federal Commissioner. The intention is to involve the private sector in the rehabilitation process, especially in relationship to unemployment [Hadley, 1979].

The project contract provisions vary but they offer opportunity to employ, train, and furnish needed services. PWI plans differ, with a wide range of activities and approaches. There are three major models for PWI programs:

1. Job placement. Seeks immediate employment on a full-time and permanent basis for the client. This model is characterized by client selection (to assure job readiness) and supportive services or job coaching by staff.
2. Work adjustment. Provides a time-limited work experience to help clients improve work attitudes and behavior. An outstanding aspect of this model is the relationship established with employers.
3. Skills training. Teaches work-ready rehabilitants the technical skills needed to be competitive for jobs. This model recruits clients at a relatively high level of functioning and provides group instruction.

33.4.14. FEDERAL SERVICE PROJECTS

In 1978 the U.S. Congress amended the Rehabilitation Act to authorize "community service employment pilot programs for handicapped individuals." This provision was made to promote useful opportunities in community service activities for those people who have poor employment prospects. Administered by the U.S. Department of Labor (DOL), the DOL Secretary may make agreements with either public or non-profit organizations for pilot projects for the employment of state rehabilitation clients in work that "will contribute to the general welfare of the community."

Community service programs include those providing social, health, recreational, educational, or other human service or assistance as well as projects for the conservation of natural resources, for the betterment or beautification of the community or its economic development. These federally sponsored projects must pay the handicapped worker at the prevailing rate for the work. The projects must also pay for the employee's work related expenses (e.g., transportation, attendant care, interpreter, reader services). Moreover, necessary training for the job (and subsistence) is provided. Finally, these projects are to provide appropriate placement services to employees to assist them in locating unsubsidized employment when the federal assistance for the project terminates. (See 37.2.3.)

Chapter 34

Methods

Job selection is an important activity for the able-bodied as well as for the disabled person. To be precise the process consists of a comprehensive assessment of the requirements of a particular job and the capabilities of the individual. Matching the person and job, known as "selective placement," assures that the rehabilitant is able to deal with job tasks and that the job is, in turn, appropriate to the needs of that person. Advantages of selective placement over less precise methods are increased production and worker satisfaction, and greater employer cooperation in placement activity.

Precision in job selection then requires an understanding of the job, which is discussed in the following section, Job Analysis. The final section of this chapter deals with job modifications and client adaptations sometimes needed for appropriate match of job and worker. The highly formalized methods discussed in this chapter are most frequently modified in actual job placement practice, but, even when informally used, the approaches are effective.

34.1 Job Selection

Matching a worker's capabilities with the requirements of a particular job is the objective of the job—or the employee—selection process. As Mallik [1975] noted, from first job to last, workers should be productive without exceeding their physical and emotional abilities or causing harm to themselves, to others, or to property. Proper rehabilitation planning, therefore, must consider the client's entire work-life span, including preparation, placement, and continued adaptation.

Hanman [1951] clarified what is meant by successful adaptation to a job by saying that a worker is suited to a job when the individual's own health is not impaired, disease is not spread to other workers, and the person neither becomes injured through accident nor causes accidents to others. Almost everyone has some functional limitation; thus, the same job placement (or employee selection) principles apply to those ordinarily labeled "physically fit."

34.1.1. INTUITIVE METHOD

The intuitive method of worker selection, as characterized by McFarland [n.d.], is "still the most widely used of all employment methods" [p. 18]. The method is completely informal, involves very little paperwork, if any, and relies upon trial and error. The guessing may be done by the potential employer, the personnel worker, the physician, or various combinations of these three as they try to decide whether or not a worker will fail or succeed at a given job. While small business especially uses the intuitive method, McFarland feels it is a poor one since it relies on chance and intuitive flashes and not on systematic analyses of jobs and workers.

Whether disabled or not, workers also use this intuitive, uninformed method for selecting employment. This is a good example of the fact that methods of job selection by workers and for employee selection by employers are counterpart approaches. It is in the best interest of both employer and worker that precise selection methods are used.

34.1.2. DISABILITY LIST METHOD

The "disability list method" is a placement approach based on the notion that jobs can be listed according to the various disabilities that each can accommodate. At one time it was common to compile lists of jobs suitable for one-armed or one-eyed or one-legged persons or even for "elderly" people. The thought was that people could be placed on any of the jobs listed as being suitable for a person with their specific disability. This approach, however, ignored all other considerations. Moreover, it was based on subjective and frequently changing concepts of average disability tolerances, and it ignored the highly individual nature of both workers and jobs. It was centered on the idea that an "average" one-armed person, for example, was capable of performing only certain kinds of jobs; it thus excluded the individual from consideration for any jobs not on the list. The approach limited and stigmatized people by stressing their handicaps rather than pointing up their capabilities, the latter of which may be used on a much greater variety of jobs.

34.1.3. RATING METHOD

This widely used approach to job selection relies upon comprehensive rating scales that are applied to both job and worker variables. For example, a rating of the amount of lifting a job requires is compared to a rating of an applicant's lifting strength. Unfortunately, subjective judgments reduce the usefulness of rating scales, by making their application imprecise. (See 21.2.)

34.1.4. INDIVIDUALIZED METHOD

The individualized method of job selection consists of matching only those capabilities of an individual that pertain to the specific requirements of a particular job. Capabilities and requirements are compared on the basis of their frequency and intensity during the course of a typical week on the job, making it possible to assess the person's capacity to cope with the range of fluctuating conditions and sustained effort that would be required. More potential jobs are open to the applicant with this procedure than with the rating or disability methods because the field of choice is not narrowed by "average characteristics" that are not applicable to individual cases. Furthermore, the confusion caused by generalized categories of physical demand rating scales is eliminated by specification of the tasks, frequency of movement, and strength required in the particular job. Thus, inappropriate placements resulting from misunderstanding among supervisors, plant physicians, and rehabilitationists can be virtually eliminated [U.S. GTP, 1955b]. The rest of this chapter will deal with the individualized approach of matching the person to an appropriate job.

34.1.5. DEMANDS AND CAPACITIES

Individualized placement involves having two kinds of information: requirements (demands) of the job and qualifications (capacities) of the applicant. Rehabilitationists gather information on job requirements by means of on-site job analysis and interviews with job supervisors and workers. Simulated job tryouts, medical examinations, and work capacity evaluations are used to identify qualifications of the applicant. Samuelson [1967] noted that successful placement of people with medical limitations requires particular attention to the physical requirements of jobs and the physical capacities of workers.

This concentration on physical capacities of workers and physical demands of jobs is coordinated in the following way. A physical demands analysis, one part of the full job analysis, gives information about the physical requirements of the job itself, while a physical capacities appraisal, conducted by a physician, gives information about worker capacity. The two analyses are presented in the same terminology and compared by the placement or employment professional in an attempt to match the worker with a job.

This matching procedure has a number of advantages: it emphasizes positive qualities in the workers; it is both individualized and specific; it is nonsexist and nondiscriminatory; it provides a common terminology for all participants in the placement process; it allows medical diagnoses to remain confidential; and, it can be used both in placement and transfer of workers. When an analysis stresses what a worker can do rather than listing limitations, the need for "pass" or "fail" standards is removed and replaced with the idea that all workers have varying physical capacities for work. Classifications like "physically fit" and "disabled" are no longer applicable.

The matching approach is intrinsically individualized; it overcomes the disadvantage of job lists that group disabilities, people, and jobs. Moreover, the .individualized matching of job and worker avoids classifying workers as able to do *heavy work* or *light work*—terms that tell very little about actual physical capacity.

A common or shared terminology is used by the examining physician, the job analyst, the employment interviewer, and the rehabilitationist—thus translation of the terms of one profession to another is unnecessary. Furthermore, the match technique is equally applicable whether a worker is seeking a first job or must transfer from one job to another because of injury or disability.

34.1.6. PROFILING

In the job selection process, rehabilitationists and personnel workers use forms as a tool to compare client and job characteristics. Forms may be developed by the rehabilitation agency or obtained from another source. Basic to the forms in use is the *Profiles of Physical Demands and Abilities,* which was originated in 1951 by Hanman. The state Employment Services and many agencies and companies use the Physical Capacities Report found in *Placing Handicapped Applicants: An Employment Service Handbook* [U.S. DOL, 1976]. The U.S. Civil Service Commission (e.g., 1947, 1975) has also developed guidelines. Job descriptions, such as those obtained from employers or found in occupational handbooks, provide information on classes of jobs but they are not always applicable to individual positions (see 19.3).

One of these aids, the *Dictionary of Occupational Titles (D.O.T.),* describes jobs and general characteristics required for performance (see 19.2). However, the physical demands estimated for the average job relate only to ablebodied persons. The *D.O.T.* approach assumes that the worker has physical capacities at least equal to the physical demands of the job; this, by definition, eliminates those who, despite handicaps, could perform with the aid of rehabilitation engineering or orthotic devices. Furthermore, the *D.O.T.* classification system is not foolproof; in actual work settings a job can be a combination of two or more jobs in the *D.O.T.,* and tasks listed under the same job title can vary greatly. Since one cannot depend on the *D.O.T.* in every instance, a site analysis may be needed for an understanding of the tasks and possible environmental barriers of a particular job [Mallik & Sablowsky, 1975].

The profile of the job and its demands is most adequately provided in a formal job analysis as described in the next section. The worker characteristics profile is obtained by medical, psychological, and other evaluations in the case study. The term *worker characteristic* refers to any quality that is required of the worker for the performance of a job.

34.2. *Job Analysis*

Since the individualized method of job selection requires a simultaneous knowledge of specific clients and job characteristics, placement of some clients will necessitate a job analysis. Usually, general information on jobs may be obtained from analysts in the public employment service or the staff of large businesses. Motion and time studies, lists of job tasks, physical demands ratings, fatigue and monotony studies, wage ratings, and safety evaluations are sometimes available for specific positions. Nevertheless, placement of severely disabled individuals, or placement into small businesses, may require that the rehabilitationist gain a first-hand awareness of the activities and surroundings of the work (see 19.3.7).

A valid determination of jobs feasible for some clients can be made only through personal observation of all facets of a particular job. Verbal descriptions of a position may be unsatisfactory since only the counselor is fully aware of the client's assets and liabilities. An employer's verbal description may gloss over minute but relevant details that might well rule out a particular client's adaptability to the job.

These descriptions of job analysis techniques are, in part, summarizations from federally sponsored Guidance, Training and Placement Workshops that were edited by Bruce Thomason and Albert Barrett [1960].

34.2.1. METHOD

Any worker has both physical and mental involvement in the work situation. Physically the worker may transport materials, cut, bend, grind, put together, make ready, set up, tear down, insert, regulate, clean, finish, or otherwise change the position, shape, or condition of the work by the expenditure of physical effort. Mentally, the worker may plan, compute, judge, direct, or otherwise govern the expenditure of his own or others' physical efforts by a corresponding exercise of mental effort. A worker may expend any combination of physical and mental effort in doing a job. To determine what the worker does, the analyst must therefore consider all of the physical and mental activities involved.

Job Tasks

Most jobs are composed of more than one task, each of which may involve different physical and mental activities. The job analyst must discover those tasks and describe them in clear, direct language; the tasks may be grouped chronologically or categorically, depending on whichever is more descriptive. Considerations of what the worker does include:

What tasks have been observed in the job?
Are there additional tasks that have not been observed?
Are these additional tasks customary for all workers on the job?
Are the tasks included for this job performed by all workers designated by the job title?
What is the frequency with which the tasks are performed?
What is the relative difficulty of each task as compared with the rest of the tasks of the job?

Have the data obtained by observation been verified by the proper authority?

Job Methods

How the work is done concerns the methods used by workers to accomplish their tasks. Physically, this involves the use of machinery and tools, measuring instruments and devices, and other equipment; the following of procedures and routines; and the movements of the worker. Mentally, the methods lie chiefly in the "know-how" that must be applied to the task. This may involve the use of calculation and formulae, the application of judgment or decision, or the selection and transmittal of thought. Workers may use a single method in the accomplishment of a task or they may have at their command several alternate methods, any of which may be used with equal success. Considerations of how the work is done include:

What tools, materials, and equipment have been used to accomplish all the tasks of the job?
Are there other tools, materials, or equipment that have not been observed and if so, how do they work?
What methods or processes have been used to accomplish the tasks of the job?
Are there other methods or processes in the plant by which this same work can be done and, if so, what are they?

Job Purpose

What a worker performs on a job is the purpose of the job itself and is indicative of the relationships among the tasks that compose the total job. The purpose may be the conversion of material from one form to another, the maintenance of conditions under which other jobs can be performed, the catching or preventing of errors, the development of new methods or the improvement of existing methods, and so forth. The purpose of the job must be ascertained before the analysis can be made. Considerations of why a job is done include:

What is its overall purpose?
Why is each task done and what is the purpose of each?
What is the relationship of each task to other tasks and to the total job?

Interrelationships

The "how, what, and why" of a job are held together by an interior logic: the "why" of a job sets the stage for "what" and "how." The job analyst begins by stating the purpose of the job clearly and by clarifying relationships of component tasks to the job as a whole.

34.2.2. OTHER JOB FACTORS

The job analyst must also consider various other aspects of the job. Each factor must be first identified according to descriptive consideration, after which they must be measured in meaningful terms.

Supervisory Responsibilities

Supervisory responsibility refers to directing the work of others or assisting and instructing them in their work. It is identified by the number of workers supervised and type of work supervised. It is measured by the nature and extent of supervision given. Considerations of supervisory responsibility include:

What is the nature of supervisory responsibility?
How closely are subordinates supervised?
How many workers are supervised and what are their duties?
Is the supervision direct or indirect?
What supervision is received by the worker?
What is the nature of nonsupervisory responsibility?
What tools, equipment, materials, or products could be lost by work failure?
What would be the value lost?
What time loss would be caused and what would be its value?
What is the likelihood of loss and what can the worker do to prevent it?
What injury can occur as a result of work failure?
If others can be injured, what can they do to protect themselves? Or are they entirely dependent on this worker?
What safety devices or checks exist?
How and to what extent is the worker required to cooperate with other workers?
In what manner, if any, is the worker responsible for contacts that include outsiders?

Job Knowledge Requirements

Job knowledge means the practical knowledge of equipment, materials, working procedures, techniques, and processes that the worker must have to do the job successfully. Job knowledge is identified by the amount and complexity of the worker's practical knowledge gained by actual on-the-job experience, prior training, or both; it is measured by the kind of job instructions and the degree of supervision received. Considerations of job knowledge include:

Does the job require the reading of blueprints?
Is the worker required to follow written instructions?
Does the job require knowledge of machine operation, machine setup, or repair?
Does the job require make-ready or other preparations for performance?
Does the job require mathematics, and if so, what kind (i.e., shop, bookkeeping, actuarial, engineering)?
Does the job require use of formulae?
What tools, gauges, or instruments are used?
What materials are used and what must the worker know about materials?
Does one worker sharpen tools and what must be known to do this?
Does one worker inspect or check and what must be known to do this?
Must the worker know preceding (or subsequent) processing operations?

Mental Application

Mental application means the mental alertness demanded by the job because of diversity of work or variety of problems, that is, by the complexity of tasks and skills required, importance and frequency of problems, and the planning and decision-making needed for their solution. Criteria for its measurements include the repetitiveness of tasks, degree of supervision received, and speed of reaction necessary to meet changing work situations.

Subfactors involved are: initiative—the taking of independent action; adaptability—the versatility required of the worker to handle quick changes in assignment, process, or personnel; judgment—the independent decision-making exercised by the worker; mental alertness—the concentrated attention of the worker to avoid work failures. Considerations include:

Does the worker plan the operative sequences and if so, how?
Does the worker assign work to others, and how?
Does the worker decide the method by which the work is done?
Must the worker make decisions regarding other persons' jobs? What decisions?
Does the worker make routine, emergency, or unusual decisions?
Does knowledge of preceding or subsequent operations guide the worker in decisions?
Does the job require the analysis and correction of problems?
Is the job repetitive or routine?
Must the worker be constantly alert to prevent errors or work failure, or is the job one that requires only casual attention?

Does the worker originate designs, create original models, or devise new procedures and techniques? Must the worker improvise expedients in the course of the work?

Dexterity and Accuracy Requirements

Dexterity and accuracy refer to the manipulative ability needed to perform the work accurately and precisely. Dexterity means the quickness, of coordination of sight and other senses with the muscles, required to perform the tasks of the job; accuracy means the precision necessary to handle products or materials, equipment, and tools. These are identified by difficulty of maintaining accuracy, number and type of movements, repetitiveness of job, and required precision of movement. They are measured by the allowable error or tolerance and the required speed of manipulation. Considerations of worker manipulative abilities include:

To what tolerance is work done?
Does work require the coordination of sight or other senses with physical movements?
Does the job require rapid physical movement?
Does the worker use small parts or devices that are difficult to manipulate?

Required Experience

Experience comes from any related job, either equivalent or less skilled, in which a worker acquires the physical and mental abilities necessary for a job. Entry jobs require no previous experience but may require a large amount of previous training. Experience is identified by the type of experience or the occupational field in which experience is required and is measured by the time required to acquire satisfactory proficiency in the work. Considerations of experience include:

What is considered to be acceptable experience for placement on this job?
How much additional training is required for the worker to reach full competency and of what must this training consist?
Is there any type of training that can supplant the acceptable experience?
Is there more than one source of acceptable experience?

Required Training

Training may be considered as the means whereby physical and mental skills are developed by the worker. Training differs from expe-

rience but is similar because it indicates that the worker has the proper skills for a job. "Required training" refers to the minimum acceptable for job placement; "desirable training" refers to additional skill development above the minimum requirement. Training is identified by the kind required and the time spent in acquiring it, and is measured by the job skills acquired during its course. Considerations of a training nature include:

What kind of training will assist the worker in acquiring the ability to satisfy the performance requirements of the job?
What specific courses of training contribute to the acquisition of required job knowledge and dexterity and accuracy?
What training is not provided and how can it be supplied on the job?
Is there training that can be considered as an alternate to an experience requirement?
Are the experience or training factors logical in light of the skill involved in the job?
Are these requirements consistent with available sources of labor?

Physical Demands of the Job

"Physical demands" refer to the demands placed on the worker by the physical characteristics of the job. These demands are key issues in determining the suitability of a job for the physically handicapped client. When physical demands are extreme, they also limit the suitability of workers normally not considered as physically limited. Physical demands discussed in subsequent subsections are: physical activities, working conditions, and hazards.

34.2.3. PHYSICAL ACTIVITY

The physical activity required by a job must be considered in selective placement of the handicapped person, and when requirements are extreme or severe, the matching process becomes even more critical. Physical activities are identified by specific requirements of a job and measured by the intensity of the required activity. Considerations include whether and how much of the following are required: walking, jumping, running, balancing, climbing, crawling, standing, turning, stooping, crouching, kneeling, sitting, reaching, lifting, carrying, throwing, pushing, pulling, handling, fingering, feeling, talking, hearing, seeing, color vision, depth perception, and working speed. The measurement of intensity asks how much, how often, how long, and so forth.

34.2.4. WORKING CONDITIONS

Working conditions are environmental circumstances over which workers have no control and that affect their mental or physical well-being. The incompatibility of working conditions with the medical characteristics of the rehabilitant may preclude selection of the person for a job. Working conditions are identified by the nature of the job's surroundings and measured by the effect of those surroundings on the worker. Considerations of the conditions of work include: is it inside, outside, hot, cold, humid, dry, wet, dusty, dirty, noisy; are there sudden temperature changes, adequate lighting, adequate ventilation, vibrations, odors, mechanical hazards, moving objects, cramped quarters, high

places, exposure to burns, electrical hazards, explosives, radiant energy, toxic conditions; does person work with or around others, work alone.

34.2.5. HAZARDS

Hazards are the possible deleterious effects of either physical activity or working conditions upon the worker. They include both injuries and occupational diseases; they are identified by the nature of possible injury or occupational disease and measured by the potential severity of injury or disease and the likelihood of its occurrence. Considerations of the hazardous nature of the work include the possibilities of: cuts, bruises, burns, sprains, hernia, fractures, loss of parts, impairment of sight, impairment of hearing, occupational diseases, collapse, electric shock, sudden death, and other problems.

34.3. Modifications

Many functional limitations can be counteracted by changing aspects of either the client or the job, thus making it possible for the client to secure employment that would otherwise be unsuitable. Client change or adaptation involves physical restoration (surgery, medication, therapy) as well as the use of rehabilitation engineering, adaptive techniques, and artificial devices. Job adaptation or modification includes barrier removal, job task modification, and job restructuring. Large companies often have their own staff to provide the necessary industrial engineering work; smaller companies are reliant upon outside resources for this service.

The rehabilitation counselor's responsibility is to organize the talents and resources available in the locality, focusing attention on the most significant mobility problems, job barriers, and client adaptations. Advice and information regarding useful modifications are frequently obtained from rehabilitation workshops and other facilities, industries employing disabled people, architectural firms, and device manufacturers. The personnel of these organizations provide a useful source of consultive services. The advice of such consultants is helpful in persuading business executives to make necessary modifications of structures and job characteristics. In many cases, employers will expect the rehabili-

tation agency or the government to finance the required modifications, while in other cases, the rehabilitationist may be able to get business or local service groups to donate materials and labor. Telephone companies and other public utilities often have a policy of providing free analysis and installation of equipment designed particularly for disabled people.

The rehabilitation counselor can make employers aware of tax credits that are available as an incentive for their assistance and can inform the local media services of their efforts in order to assure that public recognition is given to the businesses. In this manner, continued assistance and a mutually rewarding relationship can be encouraged.

34.3.1. CLIENT ADAPTATIONS

Some functional limitations can be overcome by redesigning the job tasks and fitting the client or the work environment with mechanical and electronic devices. The useful provision of such devices is limited by the staff expertise and financial resources of the rehabilitation agency. Most rehabilitation agencies cannot provide technical assistance to help the employer. Fortunately, however, many large companies have engineers who can assist the rehabilitation counselor in analyzing and adapting the work environment.

Adaptive Techniques

The following material is summarized, in part, from a staff manual, written by A. G. Garris and K. D. Koonce [1970] for the California state rehabilitation agency. An adaptive technique is used as a method of adjusting to an environment. It creates a better person-environment fit by modification and connotes pliability or readiness. Adaptive techniques are primarily concerned with physical limitations, but they also include attitudinal acceptance and willingness to change. They increase productivity and may make possible self-care and job tasks formerly considered to be impossible.

A technique, to be maximally useful, must be socially acceptable. It cannot differ too radically from the way that normal persons perform a task. For instance, a man with a double leg amputation may crawl to the bathroom in the night, not wanting to go through the difficulties of installing his prosthesis. This adaptive technique, however, will be restricted to moments of privacy or some emergency situation such as a fire in the home.

Adaptive techniques are devised to meet identified needs, which may include conserving energy, and are often met by performing in habitual patterns. For example, a person may use a stick or cane to open doors, reach for objects, or steady something. Though the individual may be physically capable of doing these things, the stick is used to save the energy expended in bending over, climbing, or walking. The conservation of one's energy is an important consideration.

Assistive Devices

Mechanical assistive devices are tools that may be used while performing adaptive techniques. Devices increase in complexity as the degree of functional limitation increases. Inventiveness and creativity vary from person to person. Learning the use of pertinent personal tools is sometimes a formal process within a rehabilitation center; here the client is fitted with braces, splints, or specially designed and constructed devices. Here, too, the person learns basic adaptive techniques of self-care; training in adaptive techniques often enables one to function better in areas other than self-care. Rehabilitation center training is especially valuable because people can learn from others and observe how they do things. Without exposure to such training, people usually do not use the adaptive tools and techniques that could make life easier.

Observing and asking the right questions will reveal problem areas. Existing devices and aids may solve the problem only if properly selected and fitted, and mistakes in this area are easily spotted. For example, a cane or crutch or walker may be too long or too short. The cane user's arm should have a bend of 15 to 20 degrees. This is important as a shock absorber and permits quick adaptation to irregular terrain.

Newly disabled persons may have difficulty in utilizing adaptive techniques if their use requires a change in lifelong habits. A common adaptive technique is early arrival for appointments, especially if the patient walks slowly or has long distances to travel. (Doing this often requires asking for prior information on facilities, such as parking lots, steps, and architectural barriers.) For the chronic latecomer, such drastic changes in behavior can be annoying or painful.

Planning ahead is an adaptive technique to avoid problems and is probably the most important. Such planning includes second-guessing probable happenings. For example, weakness and incoordination of the lower extremities make falls a probability. The accepted adaptive technique is to learn how to fall and how to get up again. Properly prepared, a person can avoid entanglement, can roll with the fall, and can prevent serious injuries.

Employer acceptance can often be gained with use of proper devices and adaptive techniques. Instability of gait has caused rejection of many disabled individuals for jobs they might well have performed. Many handicapped persons who reject assistive devices and stumble around would be much more employable in a wheelchair, partly because the employer does not have to be afraid the employee will fall.

Rehabilitation Engineering Aids

There is a real advantage if a device can be suggested for use by other workers as well as the disabled job applicant. In one case a counselor studied a task in which employees had to pick up and feed small bearings into a machine. The client had both visual and manual limitations, but he could do the total job, though the pace was slower and clumsier than that of co-workers. The counselor, cooperating with the supervisor, designed and developed a chute that fed bearings directly from stock into the machine. This chute was so efficient that it not only saved the client's job but was duplicated on all machines and improved production in the department.

Other devices have become so common that they are more standard than special: brailled micrometers for the visually handicapped, light instead of sound signals for the deaf. The rehabilitationist need not hesitate to suggest performance aids that make industry as a whole more efficient.

Right controls in place of left controls and leg controls in place of arm controls, which aid only one handicapped worker, must be considered "special" devices; they should be recommended only when absolutely necessary. Before making such recommendations, the counselor is advised to know the employer, the job, and the client thoroughly and to get information about the source, installation, and cost of the device according to the Tenth Annual Workshop on Guidance, Training and Placement [U.S. GTP, 1957a].

Orthotic Devices

Orthotic devices are mechanical assistive devices fitted to the body with precision. They have three basic functions: to support body weight, to control joint motion, and to change the shape of body tissues. Examples of the body weight support are such devices as the arch support or the weight-bearing long leg brace. Examples of devices used to control joint motion include long leg braces that serve to lock the knee, short leg braces that control ankle movement to prevent drop foot, and the stop in drop-foot braces that limit motion by acting against a spring or tight joint. Orthotic devices that change the shape of body tissues include corsets, shoe inserts that bend or twist bone structures or correct positions when weight is applied, and braces that stretch tight heel cords. (Note that prosthetic devices, by contrast, replace body parts.)

The purposes of orthotic devices, prescribed by a doctor, are to prevent additional deformity and to improve function. Although interested in improved function, the person may be more directly concerned with conserving energy, appearance, and reliability. The purposes of these devices should be carefully explained, since people who understand the purposes of orthotic devices are more likely to wear them.

Rehabilitationists need to develop observational skills in order to see when an orthotic device might be helpful. The client's gait, for example, is often revealing. A limp may signal legs of different lengths, a bad back, a dislocated hip, a tipped pelvis, or a bent knee. Studies show that aberrations from normal gait greatly increase energy use. For instance, a four-inch difference in leg length in someone weighing a hundred pounds means the loss of hundreds of foot pounds of energy in a single day. Limitations or lack of control in joint movement, and problems with shoulders, elbows, fingers, wrists, and thumbs can be visually checked.

It should be remembered that even though a client has had excellent medical treatment, maximal physical potential may not have been achieved, and that orthotic devices can save energy and improve work abilities. Moreover, intelligent use of orthotic devices frequently precedes reconstruction through surgery. For instance, an "opponens" splint, which positions the thumb opposite the index finger in order to grasp and pick up objects, can sometimes be duplicated by a transplant. Similarly, a splint-stabilized wrist can be surgically fused. Such improvements sometimes have dramatic effects for the client; an improvement of as little as 5 percent can make the difference between employability and idleness. (Other aspects of this subject are discussed in Chapters 5, Functional Limitations, and 40, Independent Living.)

34.3.2. JOB MODIFICATIONS

During the process of job analysis, the rehabilitationist can consider how a particular set of job tasks and equipment could be modified to enable disabled persons to do the job. Many times, the rearrangement of job tasks, the provision of adaptive mechanical devices, or the redesign of equipment will enable clients who would otherwise have been unacceptable to perform at the required level of production in jobs. The placement counselor needs to become familiar with the basis of production engineering, the adaptive devices available, and the margin of flexibility in a given plant. These, in turn, will define the limits in which job modification activities will take place. Some employers will be receptive to change, others will not, often depending on the rehabilitationist's consultation skills and expertise, but sometimes depending on the employer's willingness to take the risks involved in making a modification.

Reengineering Jobs

An important selling point in the placement of vocational rehabilitation clients is that many can compete for jobs, without special favor. Consequently, any request for a major reengineering of a job or ways of doing it may be seen as contradictory. But, if the counselor sees that the client could benefit from minor modifications such as realignment or placement of work materials, such a recommendation should be made. Because job engineering requires money and, sometimes, special working conditions, the counselor consequently diminishes chances for placing disabled persons if either cost or special conditions are so obvious that they attract special attention.

There are instances in which reengineering of jobs for clients has resulted in the use of production improvement devices useful throughout the plant. The nonhandicapped workers often find such energy-saving devices attractive. For example, many ablebodied people prefer to use gradual ramps (constructed for wheelchairs) rather than climb steep stairs.

Job Task Modification

Sometimes work can be made more suitable for severely disabled persons by rearranging the job schedule. "Flex-time" scheduling, for instance, can be used with clients who do not have sufficient strength to function at a job for a regular "eight-hour day." Several individuals could share a portion of the time of a single job with part-time pay. Another alternative is for workers to divide assigned job tasks. At times, the activities of several persons having different disabilities may be organized to compensate for one another's functional limitations in a particular job, or it may be convenient to have an "ablebodied" worker exchange tasks with a disabled person.

For the most part, the rehabilitationist will find job task modification difficult to implement because of the inconvenience and production risks to the employer and co-workers. It is only

when such risks can be balanced or surpassed by other incentives (e.g., tax credit, increased production or safety, subsidized training) that the approach should be considered.

Job Restructuring

This is a specific technique useful in any type of job development or job creation activity. It involves examining the relationships among a number of jobs within a production system and, through the application of job analysis, rearranging the contents or tasks performed in these jobs to achieve desired purposes. There are usually two purposes for job restructuring: first, the development of new employment opportunities for inexperienced or presently unskilled workers by creating entry-level jobs, and second, the development of meaningful promotional opportunities [U.S. DOL, Manpower Administration, 1970a]. The promotional opportunities are usually stated in the form of career ladders that allow for employment of unskilled recruits and their promotion to higher level jobs as new skills and competencies are acquired.

Job restructuring is facilitated by job analysis—especially the accurate identification of levels of worker functioning and task complexity [Wilson, 1974]. The job analysis technique developed by the U.S. Department of Labor is the most widely used; it has the advantages of a well-written manual, *Handbook for Analyzing Jobs* [U.S. DOL, Manpower Administration, 1972], and clear-cut applications to job restructuring.

Most of the reported research and demonstration projects on job restructuring have been in the area of human service and public service employment [Dunn, 1974a]. These projects tend to remove routine tasks from the professional's workload and create new entry-level positions assigned to "aides," or paraprofessionals. This redistribution seems sensible, but the actual practice has been somewhat less than successful.

Ferman [1969] said that job restructuring is accomplished by means of segmentalizing, enlarging, or simplifying the required tasks. Segmentalizing the job means breaking it into simpler tasks to fit the talents of handicapped workers. Job enlargement is the combining of a series of simple tasks to produce a more interesting and mobile job unit. Job simplification is done by modifying the preparation required to hold the job (e.g., education or training completed) so that the preparation period is shortened, modified, or eliminated in favor of on-the-job training. The restructuring of jobs requires a technical knowledge and should not be attempted by untrained staff members of a job development unit.

Ferman continued by observing that "knowing how" is not enough. Employers need to know how job restructuring will affect the firm's cost-profit structure. A number of vested interests militate against easy persuasion. Since union-management contracts outline the content of jobs, unions may see job restructuring as a threat to the job rights of union members. Such changes often lead to long negotiations and revisions of the union contract. Furthermore, those who do cost-accounting will be concerned about increased labor and supervisory costs when a job is broken down into a series of jobs. Added to this is the national resistance to change in any entrenched network of work relationships in which adjustments will be required (for example, new workloads, lowered status). Smaller firms, especially those without on-site experts to examine job structures, are more likely to find job restructuring attractive than are larger firms with their complex fabrics of vested interest.

Job restructuring, Ferman warned, "poses the danger that the resultant jobs may be so simple in structure that they are 'dead end' rather than 'stepping stones.' The goal of job restructuring should be to create jobs that have mobility potential and are meaningful rather than dead-end jobs in the company for the hard-to-employ" [p. 13].

Major problems have been encountered in restructuring human and public service jobs. Job analysis has been naively applied to restructuring existing jobs with a failure to recognize the interrelationships of tasks. In rehabilitation, for example, a common temptation has been to separate routine clerical and recording tasks from counseling and to assign these to an aide. However, recording cannot be delegated, simply because the professional is the only one who possesses the information to be recorded. Another problem is that the new positions created offer no opportunity for advancement because of the educational and credentialing requirements of professional organizations.

Competency-based credentialing and certification would seem to relieve this barrier, but the more fundamental issue is preparation for competency. Certain necessary educational requirements are not readily or quickly available. Still another problem is the reluctance of organizations to create new entry-level or career-ladder positions.

Dunn noted, however, that though job restructuring has not worked well in public service, it has had better success in private business and industry. Much of this private experience was summarized in *Work in America* [W. E. Upjohn Institute for Employment Research, 1973], whose authors saw job restructuring techniques as the "keystone" in a program that would not only create meaningful jobs for the unemployed and underemployed but also improve the quality of life for the employed.

Obviously, job restructuring has economic advantages because it does create new jobs and tends to increase productivity. Dunn, however, issued warnings. He felt that job restructuring must be joined with an active program of worker improvement and a system of upward mobility. Unless workers are provided with the necessary opportunities for skill and competency development that will enable them to progress up the newly established career ladders, or to enter existing ladders, the approach is doomed to fail. The expense involved in implementing the technique is a major problem to rehabilitation agencies with inadequate financial resources. Skilled job analysts must be added to the staff. Analyzing and restructuring jobs within production systems is a time-consuming and costly process.

34.3.3. REMOVAL OF BARRIERS

Sometimes job modification has to be extended beyond the workplace and specific tasks to include the entire work situation. As Lorenz [1974] said, it does no good to modify a job only to find that the job setting itself is inappropriate because of architectural barriers. Consequently, the removal of these barriers through the provision of ramps and other necessary structural changes must be an integral part of the job modification program. This can be a costly operation on old buildings. Yet, as Dunn [1974a] pointed out, the architectural barrier legislation passed in most states generally applies only to new construction and leaves unresolved the problem of renovating existing structures, including places of employment.

Architectural Resources

To assist the rehabilitationist, several handbooks are available that describe the essential modifications for making job sites, transportation modes, and dwellings accessible to the disabled population. These include *Removing Architectural Barriers* [State of New Mexico Department of Education, Division of Vocational Rehabilitation, 1975], *Into the Mainstream —A Syllabus for a Barrier-Free Environment* [Kliment, 1975], and *Barrier-Free Design* [Rehabilitation International, 1975]. These handbooks and other materials available on barrier-free design are useful to the rehabilitationist in assessing the need for modifications and in documenting that need to employers. They contain illustrated designs and specifications for the following: bathrooms, entrances, corridors, drinking fountains, emergency and danger signals, curbs, elevators, ramps, identifications for the blind, showers, parking, and transportation.

Since potential employment opportunities may come from businesses under construction, it is appropriate for the rehabilitation representatives to contact builders and architects to assure that design considerations have been made for the disabled. Modifications done during construction of the original building are much less costly than those installed at a later time.

Imposing flights of stairs impossible for the person in a wheelchair or with a heart condition, restrooms with facilities too narrow for wheelchairs, hazardous doorways with no sense-of-touch markings for the blind, drinking fountains out of reach of the handicapped: these are some of the architectural features that unfortunately bar many handicapped men and women from industrial buildings all over America. As Williams [1965] concluded, "If they can't even enter, they can't possibly hold a job there."

Architectural barriers affect many people. It is estimated that one out of every nine persons in the United States would benefit by removal of architectural barriers.

The American Standards Association drafted and released a landmark set of standard specifications to make buildings fully accessible to the handicapped. Among many other items, their specifications are the following notable examples cited by Williams:

1. Ground for new buildings should be graded so that at least one entrance would be at ground level.
2. Special parking should be set aside for the handicapped.
3. If entrance-way ramps are needed, the slope should rise not more than one foot in 12 feet.
4. At least one stall in each rest room should be made to accommodate a wheelchair.
5. Doors leading to danger areas should be identifiable by touch for the blind.
6. Telephones should be installed within reach of those in wheelchairs; some should be adapted for the hard-of-hearing.

Transportation to Work

Because transportation is a major problem of many disabled persons, representatives of disabled people and rehabilitation programs seek to develop resources for coping with this problem. The rehabilitation counselor's role may consist of making arrangements for a car pool with fellow employees when the worker is too shy or lacks the social awareness to do so independently. Volunteers may be organized as drivers and agency funds used for vehicles and insurance. Knowledge of community resources in addition to the potential assistance of former clients places the counselor in an advantageous position for providing service.

Through organized efforts, special transportation systems for mobility limited people have been installed to supplement public conveyances that these people cannot use (see 5.1). Availability of suitable transportation is important not only for work but for deinstitutionalization, social integration, recreation, medical care, and many critical areas of normal living. Chapter 40, Independent Living, covers the subject of accessibility, including housing and transportation.

34.3.4. JOB CREATION

Ferman [1969] has also described "job creation," which means the creation of subprofessional or nonprofessional employment opportunities in the public sector and the creation of completely new occupations in the service sector. This definition refers to such subprofessional jobs as teachers' aide, medical aide, counselor aide, and social worker aide. Job creation requires as much expertise as job restructuring. Counselors need to know the professional field, its decision-makers, and the needs of the profession before constructing training programs for subprofessionals. Such jobs must be created before training begins. One common failing in job creation is to train subprofessionals first and later find that the conditions of the profession preclude their employment. As is the case with job restructuring, the new jobs should represent career advancement opportunities rather than dead-end employment.

Where the job creation method has been tried, Ferman noted problems. Professionals tend to resist segmenting of jobs, assuming that costs would naturally increase; they also tend to defend the routine or repetitive elements of the professional role on grounds of traditional practice. Professionals also may object to definitions of their roles from the outside and may resist the creation of truly subprofessional jobs. Moreover, developing subprofessional career jobs proves difficult because of civil service regulations: usually the regulations contain no legal definition for such work, no clear job description, and no wage scale. Despite the formidable obstacles, however, Ferman calls job restructuring and job creation "two hopeful avenues" to new jobs for persons who have a functional limitation.

Chapter 35

Client Preparation

In a very competitive job market it is often not sufficient to send a disabled individual, armed with vocational skills, off to an interview with a prospective employer. There is a body of knowledge and skills that should be taught to disabled job applicants regarding the process of *obtaining* employment. This includes where to find job openings, whom to contact, how to fill out an application, what to wear to an interview, how to act, and, of great importance, how to deal with interview questions about the disability. These "job-seeking skills," as they are called, are presented individually to applicants or as part of an organized curriculum to a group of disabled job-seekers. Job-seeking skills training goes hand-in-hand with work adjustment training: in the former, behaviors are learned that will enable people to find and secure suitable jobs; in the latter, behaviors are learned that

will enable them to act appropriately within a job situation after they are hired (see 13.3).

As in the case with other kinds of training, there are commercially marketed materials for teaching job-seeking skills. Workbooks, programmed learning packages, curriculums, and videotapes typify the resources available. The video tape recorder has become an essential tool in job-seeking skills training. It is used not only to play sample interviews and other instructional material, but also to record trial job interviews by job-seekers within the classroom situation itself.

Job-seeking skills training is found primarily in rehabilitation facilities, preferably under the auspices of a counselor specialized in job placement. Other organizations sponsoring job-seeking skills training include mental health facilities, correctional institutions, schools, the state Employment Service, and other agencies with rehabilitation programs.

Many clients, though capable of obtaining jobs on their own, lack the job-seeking skills essential for success. As a result, rehabilitation agencies have programs to assist clients in the development of these skills. The goal of an agency program that provides assistance to job-seekers is to maximize each individual's capability of functioning in the labor market. Regardless of the employment procedure used in a given society, the agency attempts to accomplish the following: (1) increase individual self-confidence about obtaining work with a minimum of assistance from a social agency; (2) instruct individuals in the skills, behaviors, and attitudes required to survive the employer's selection process; (3) maintain job listings and employer contacts to provide applicants with a range of employment opportunities; and (4) provide timely emotional support and guidance.

Job-seeking skills training helps job applicants become as independent as possible by teaching them the basics of competitive employment, including what to do and say in a job interview situation. One study conducted by Anderson, Hutchins and Walker [1968] at the Minneapolis Rehabilitation Center and also published by the Multi Resource Centers [1971] showed that clients had three types of adjustment problems: lack of appropriate job goals, problems in job retention, and poor job-seeking skills. Further analysis of the third area revealed that 80 percent of the clients did not look for work frequently enough, 85 percent could not explain skills to their employers, 40 percent had poor personal appearance or inappropriate mannerisms, and 90 percent could not explain their handicapping problems.

The ability of clients, even those who are severely disabled, to find their own employment is well documented. In fact, about half of the clients whose cases are closed by the public rehabilitation program as rehabilitated find their own employment without the need for direct placement services by the counselor. From their experiences, from leads and suggestions supplied by the counselor as well as their friends and relatives, from their own knowledge, interests, and preferences, these clients are able to find suitable work. Nevertheless, experience and research both indicate that the job-seeking activities of most clients, and indeed in the population at large, are inefficient and often inappropriate [Akabas, Medevene, & Victor, 1979].

McClure [1972] noted that many clients, even though they have marketable skills, fail to get jobs because they mismanage the initial interview, do not know how to present themselves, or do not understand job-procurement procedures.

Employers and other hiring personnel have attested loudly that most of the applicants who appear before them just do not know how to apply for work. Worse yet, clients will often settle for inappropriate jobs because of their fear of unemployment. The resulting frustration, failure, and aggravation of the disability continue to plague the individual, negating the satisfaction that derives from self-placement. The agency attempts to overcome these difficulties by training clients in appropriate job-seeking skills and by providing guidance in job-selection and decision-making.

Placeability refers to the amount of assistance a client needs to find employment, and while placeability can be thought of as one aspect of job readiness, the term can also apply to those who have marketable skills yet have trouble finding a job. The level of placeability may be determined by the use of placement readiness scales in the form of psychological tests or observed behaviors, or by a clinical assessment of the individual's performance. Self-reliant clients will determine on their own when they feel confident to seek work. Clients needing substantial counselor involvement, however, usually require intermittent appraisal of their readiness level.

Obtaining a job is not a "once-or-twice" phenomenon but is repeated surprisingly often. Long-range independence therefore becomes important for sustained employment. The labor market is a very unstable place with a tremendous flow of workers in and out of jobs. The average duration of employment is around three years. Considering that the average rehabilitant is about 30 years old and has a labor force life expectancy of another 30 years or more, it can be projected that the average rehabilitant will change jobs 10 times. As Dunn [1974a] pointed out, "normal" vocational behavior is characterized by short job tenure so that a "normal" worker independently searches for and obtains a new job at frequent intervals. Consequently, the goal of normal vocational behavior requires the development of placeability competencies as an integral aspect of the rehabilitation program.

Group training and counseling programs are not efficient unless all of the participants have been adequately prepared (see 30.1.4). Among the criteria frequently stipulated for entrance into client-training courses are the following: (1) desire to obtain employment; (2) determination of an appropriate job objective; (3) completion of skill training and work adjustment to adequate levels; (4) ability to explain the functional aspects of the disability as related to vocational goals and situations; (5) completion of independent living skills training; and (6) medical clearance indicating that an adequate adaptation has been made to the disability. These criteria

assure that the client is prepared physically and psychologically to work as soon as an opportunity is arranged [Minneapolis Rehabilitation Center, 1971].

A well-organized agency program of assistance to job-seekers saves both time and effort. Group work can help to avoid the duplication of counselor efforts with individual clients while increasing the opportunities available to individuals from the combined resources of the group. Videotapes, instruction manuals, and audiovisual materials substantially increase the efficiency of counselor involvement as well as the skill level achieved by the clients. Skillful case management reduces recidivism and increases the mutual enjoyment of counselor and client in this rehabilitation phase.

35.1. Placement Counseling

Counseling during the placement phase focuses on the emotional stresses experienced by the client and the decision-making that must be done to acquire employment. A positive self-concept during the placement process is an essential ingredient of getting a job, but this is difficult to develop for many clients who have been confronted by repeated rejection and prejudice in the job market. Many agencies have full-time placement counselors to help the client in this final phase of rehabilitation adjustment. The application and interview process itself is usually an emotionally charged situation. Furthermore, as most jobs offered to clients will not immediately fulfill all of their needs and desires, counselor assistance may be solicited in decision-making (see 27.5).

35.1.1 GUIDANCE IN DECISION-MAKING

During the placement phase of the process, the rehabilitant may be concerned about accepting a particular job. While some clients feel comfortable in making decisions without counselor involvement, others desire assistance from someone who has a broader knowledge of the labor market. Since the client's economic security and emotional well-being are of primary importance, the risks and disadvantages of a particular job should be weighed against the likelihood of obtaining a more suitable position. Counselors may

assist their clients in examining the suitability of the job to the disability, interest in the job tasks, the status and security of the position, opportunity for promotion, fringe benefits, working conditions, co-worker and supervisor personalities, adaptability to changing disability limitations, safety, and plant location.

Since disabled individuals are frequently offered positions that are below their capacity or that pay less than a job held before onset of the disability, serious feelings of inadequacy, hostility, or depression may result if the job is accepted. On the other hand, a tight labor market and competitive hiring practices often leave the individual with little choice. The negative emotional reactions caused by working at a marginal job may, in turn, result in perpetuation of a failure syndrome on the part of the client. The counselor's role is to attempt to resolve unfortunate situations by encouraging the clients to achieve their potential employment growth. Regardless of the need for an income, clients should not be abandoned at entry-level positions when there are resources to enable them to progress to more suitable positions. The opportunity for growth must not be overlooked in client placement. Employers generally expect new employees to prove their worth to the organization before they are allowed to obtain better-paying jobs, and in some situations, counselors may obtain a commitment from the employer to promote the worker at the end of the probationary period.

A major concern regarding job acceptance by people collecting disability insurance benefits is the result it will have on their total income and health care costs. Occasionally, the sum of insurance benefits and savings from free medical treatment surpasses the income that a disabled person would have from competitive employment. Furthermore, disability benefits are tax-free and may be assured for life, while income from a job is taxed and tenure on the job uncertain. Many unfortunate conflicts arise from this dilemma. Social pressure and security tend to reinforce unemployment, while mental health may suffer from inactivity. After careful examination of the situation, the counselor may encourage some form of productive but volunteer activity in order to sustain the client's level of functioning.

Throughout the counseling process, the counselor should guide clients to be responsible for their own decision-making and to bear the consequences. As always, dependency is discouraged whenever possible, since it is recognized that clients ideally should function without counselor assistance, if possible, and that they will usually perform more adequately when they feel responsible for their own destiny.

35.1.2 DEPENDENCY OR SELF-RELIANCE

Among rehabilitation clients, feelings of dependency and inadequacy constitute a major obstacle to obtaining and sustaining employment. Dependency is a concomitant of disability, and handicapped people frequently become used to having others—including the counselor—do things for them. Not only do many clients expect the rehabilitationist to find them employment without actively participating themselves, but this attitude is reinforced by misconceptions regarding the role of the agency (the agency's title or reputation may suggest that it is a place where jobs are obtained), or even by governmental policy (such policy may place responsibility for placement on the agency). Whatever the cause of dependency, effective placement is seldom achieved until the individual develops a sense of responsibility and self-reliance. Jobs obtained by a counselor for a client are less highly regarded and more readily abandoned than those a client obtains independently.

Goldhammer and James [1976] noted that clients must become aware of their own self-concepts and of attitudes exhibited by friends, relatives, and spouses. Unfortunately those closest to clients may also be the biggest roadblocks to a career. Doctors, parents, siblings, schools, friends, and acquaintances often create the very dependency that the rehabilitation counselor on occasion describes as "lack of motivation." This is sometimes the rehabilitant's greatest barrier to success.

Dependency is often characterized by feelings of weakness and helplessness. Dependency also creates in people fear of failure, actual failure, and resulting unhappiness, and a vicious cycle sets in: lessened ability to make decisions followed by loss of self-respect. Since nondependent people characteristically feel right, strong, and self-sufficient, it follows that strong self-concepts help people satisfy needs and wants (see 28.3).

As Goldhammer and James pointed out, the healthy, assertive personality has the best chance to succeed at self-directed placement. Characteristically, however, the disabled have been rewarded for being obedient and quiet. In them, assertiveness may unfortunately be viewed as aggressive.

Disabled persons who feel confident and worthy of rehabilitation can be expected to perform well throughout all phases of rehabilitation. Levels of anxiety are lowered by an infectious air of confidence that accompanies feelings of worth.

35.1.3. GROUP COUNSELING

Small group counseling, which provides an effective and efficient way of assisting job-seekers, also results in a substantial savings in time to counselors, greater self-reliance on the part of clients, reduced time in obtaining employment, and higher-paying jobs (see 13.4.6). The rehabilitationist is in a unique position to identify the job-seeking skill needs of clients. Videotaping of mock interviews, discussions with employers, and reporting of individual job-seeking efforts provide a basis for sharing information. In the stress-filled situation of job-hunting, group support helps to combat depression, anxiety, frustration, lowered self-esteem, and self-deception. Often, clients are more willing to take advice from those in a similar situation than they are from counselors. And the emotional dependency usually placed upon individual counselors is appreciably diminished.

Anderson, Hutchins, and Walker [1968], of the Minneapolis Rehabilitation Center, described a job-seeking skills group that changed client behavior in a relatively short time. "All client problems are described in behavior terms—which the client can understand, which specifically state what it is that the client will need to change, and which allows for measurement to determine whether our methods of correcting a problem are effective."

These researchers noted that group participation produced surprising behavior changes. "Before" and "after" interviews on videotape showed a transformation from fearful individuals to people who were confident and comfortable because they had successfully interviewed for a job. Frequently client motivation also increased through group participation. Counselors worked with individuals who had a job goal but were not really committed to the idea of working. With help in job-seeking skills, motivation for seeking work increased and they became employed. Furthermore, a contagious "we want to get

hired" attitude set in, inspiring some apathetic individuals.

35.1.4. JOB-FINDING CLUB

The so-called job-finding club addresses a number of complex skills assumed to be best learned in a structured and continuing learning situation. The program provides help with transportation, peer assistance, job-seeking, family support, interview skills, job leads, scheduling of time, resumé preparation, and professional advice.

Regular attendance at daily meetings is stressed, since there is a high correlation between attendance and securing employment. At counseling sessions of one to two hours, discussions are held on topics such as the buddy system, car pooling to employers, manner of telephone inquiry, review of resumés, sharing job leads, and mutual encouragement by a peer group.

The club encourages clients to view job research not as incidental but as a full-time activity requiring daily counseling sessions, phoning, being interviewed, writing letters, and contacting friends and relatives.

35.2. *Job-Finding Assistance*

Clients are frequently encouraged to use traditionally formal job finding methods, to watch the newspaper want ads and submit applications to many employers. But as Dunn pointed out, evidence suggests that while these are common methods they are also the least effective and often result in fruitless searches for jobs. Certainly disabled persons (or their families) should use available social contacts to secure employment, but for those who lack such contacts, or who may lose their contacts because of a lengthy rehabilitation program, the development or maintenance of social contacts with employed persons should be an integral part of vocational programming. "Social rehabilitation" is often thought of as extraneous or ancillary to a vocational rehabilitation program; research suggests, however, that disabled persons who have active contacts with employed people have increased chances of getting jobs themselves.

Moreover, Dunn said, rehabilitation counselors can be better sources of job leads if they

have contacts in informal job information networks and can obtain early information about job openings. Effective rehabilitation counselors have usually developed and cultivated informal networks of job informants.

One of the best sources of information on job-finding assistance is Dennis Dunn [1974a], of the University of Wisconsin–Stout, whose ideas are incorporated into this and other chapters on job placement and client assessment.

35.2.1. JOB-INFORMATION SOURCES

The agency's role in developing employment opportunities consists of a series of ongoing activities. These include solicitation of jobs from employers; maintenance of contacts with key workers, employers, vendors, service professions, and former clients; operating or initiating small businesses; and the use of media in developing community relations contacts. As former clients begin to work their way into the employment structure, they are able to keep the rehabilitationist informed of changes in production, promotions, transfers, and so on that result in potential job openings. Assistance from former clients, of course, requires long-term maintenance of a relationship between them and the agency personnel. Other staff members of an agency are a valuable source of potential job leads, as long as incentives are present for sharing information. A failure on the part of supervisory staff to encourage cooperation may result in missed opportunities for placement [Zadny & James, 1976].

Civic and Religious Organizations

Good relationships with various organizations within the community can be of help in aiding rehabilitation clients. Counselors should sustain contacts with civic and service clubs willing to sponsor a project that will contribute to the rehabilitation of a handicapped person. Churches, either through their administrative structures or their organizations, will help in the rehabilitation of their members. Service clubs, veterans' organizations, health associations, and welfare services often respond to special appeals for help with difficult placements.

Radio and Television Stations and Newspapers

Since radio and television stations are required to allot time to public service programs, job opportunities may be solicited by spot announcements. These announcements should provide details on the qualifications of the client, and permission from the client for release of case data should be obtained. The station program director should be asked for cooperation, for advice on type of materials that might be acceptable, and for help in preparing the script. (See 10.4.1.)

The press, especially in the smaller communities, will often cooperate in stimulating job opportunities for qualified handicapped workers. Editors are always looking for "human interest" stories. Information should be submitted in a clear, concise, factual style. Again, it is important that permission of the client be obtained prior to release of case data.

Client Advisory Committee

The client advisory committee is a committee of community members selected by the counselor to advise and assist in planning and carrying out a placement program for a particular client. Members are selected for their interest in re-

habilitation of the client and their willingness to devote time to the work.

A committee is particularly appropriate when a very special job or self-employment opportunity is required (for example, if the client's disability is unusual or severe and placement seems unlikely without considerable community assistance); when the counselor and client have been unable to work out a satisfactory placement plan and recognize the need for a committee; and when the client has a good reputation and is well known in the community.

Although the counselor selects the committee members, the list of nominees should be reviewed with the client. Citizens of stature and civic leadership are likely to be familiar with community resources and thus be able to contribute best to the resolution of the client's placement problem.

A committee of five to nine people who represent a cross-section of interests is desirable. A spiritual advisor to the client, an important public officer such as the mayor, a judge, a city council member, a school principal or superintendent would be suitable for the committee. Remaining members may be selected from the service clubs, business, or professional groups. While members may be chosen from the state Employment Service or a social welfare agency, this should be principally a "lay" committee.

JOB (Just One Break) Committees

With difficult placements, a counselor may choose to organize a JOB committee composed of leaders in business and labor in one or more communities. A JOB committee is similar in form and function to the client advisory committee. The JOB committee differs in that it continues to operate as long as there are clients who need help, while the client advisory committee is ad hoc and works with one client only.

Various medical facilities, trade and vocational schools, and industrial and labor organizations provide job training and employment opportunities. Coordination or rehabilitation agencies with these various private and public employment services is the responsibility of the labor-management team. Under the JOB concept, such coordination can be performed in a relatively easy fashion. JOB should make full use of existing rehabilitation services and their many offerings in training, evaluation, and treatment. A seriously interested, committed group of business and labor leaders should constitute the board, which devotes time to finances, policy decisions, and the everyday problems that such boards customarily handle. The board seeks to set up a continuing program of community and public relations and to open areas of employment for the disabled citizens referred to JOB.

The board conducts its business by mail, and individuals are called upon for their special areas of expertise. For example, an advisory board member may be asked to contact someone in upper management of an industry and the chain of communication can then spread to supervisors and foremen.

It is important that the JOB committee be chosen from industry in order to work with a full knowledge of industrial and labor problems; hence the members operate as if they were the personnel department of a large company or a private employment agency operating for profit. A JOB committee should operate within the association of private employment agencies as well as with the public employment and social welfare agencies; this network then provides the community with a coordinated service in the employment field.

The JOB committee should have research and education as a goal, to orchestrate the isolated efforts of job placement in the community; to provide a clearinghouse for various companies and their forms, policies, and problems; to confront the problems of casualty liability, labor contracts, transportation, health and welfare and pension programs; and to provide an existing laboratory from which management, labor, and the community can seek assistance.

35.2.2. DEVELOPING CLIENT RESOURCES

One of the difficult tasks of the rehabilitation counselor is helping clients become aware of their own potential employment resources. Although relatives, friends, acquaintances, and former employers are the source of most successful job leads, clients are sometimes reluctant to contact them after the onset of a disability. In fact, there is a tendency for those out of work to drift away from their successfully employed peers, thus losing a valuable source of information about openings.

Family and Friends

When clients hesitate to discuss their employment situation with family and friends, it may be necessary for the counselor to encourage these people to take advantage of their contacts with potential employers and friends who can provide job leads. Once an initial contact for a job has been established through a friend or family member, it is important for the client to indicate sincere interest in the position in order to overcome the negative effect that is associated with favoritism.

The individual who uses a variety of job-search methods stands a better chance of finding a job, but—depending on the type of job—some job-seeking methods are more effective than others. The use of friends and relatives is the most effective means of obtaining a job among blue-collar workers although they do not recognize this fact. It is an even more effective means among job-seeking white-collar workers. There is an informal job-information network in which persons with early knowledge of job openings (employers and employed persons) selectively and privately pass this rewarding information on to their unemployed acquaintances, who are then likely to reward the job informants in social ways [Jones & Azrin, 1973]. This employment process is an active exchange of inside tips and personal favors. The result of these relationships is reflected in family businesses and trade union membership, in nepotism, and in hiring discrimination against minorities. A major barrier to the employment of the disabled and disadvantaged, Dunn [1974a] concluded, is their lack of social contacts within the essentially private and informal job availability information network.

Former Employers

Zadny and James [1976] pointed out that former employers are excellent potential sources of jobs and that they serve as contacts for openings in related industries. The worker who returns to a former employer, even if to work at a different job, has a higher rate of satisfactory adjustment and usually receives more pay and promotions. Former employers have hiring authority and often are more concerned for the client's well-being—particularly if the person received an injury while working there. The system of disability claim insurance may even provide a monetary incentive for rehiring.

Volunteer Position

Volunteer work by clients can be used as a way of finding job leads in an area of interest. The client gains experience, makes contacts, and is usually the first to be considered for a full-time position when an opening occurs. Many jobs result from unique situations that lead to a chance encounter between an employer and job-seeker. The person sensitive to the situation will get the job. The person who takes time to develop contacts has a better chance of finding work than the person who stays at home, despondent over being unemployed.

35.2.3. COMMUNITY JOB INFORMATION

The counselor's role in helping clients utilize community sources of job information is mainly one of keeping aware of the most reliable sources and encouraging clients to use them (see 27.4.3). These may include public and private employment services, trade schools, unions, civil service, construction sites, and the media. Material for the following originated in a federal rehabilitation agency publication [U.S. GTP, 1957a] but has been updated.

Public Employment Service

The state Employment Service is the major source of information on local job vacancies. For the most part, the agency's services are geared toward meeting the needs of employers for production, sales, and service personnel. The requirements of each job are matched against the skills of the applicant. Many of the jobs posted with the Employment Service are part-time, limited-term, or high-turnover positions.

The state Employment Service agencies also provide special testing, counseling, and placement services for the handicapped job applicant. Cooperation between the state rehabilitation agency and the state employment agency is mandated federally. The mutual assistance of staff from both agencies provides additional opportunities for disabled clients. This mandated cooperation between the two agencies, however, is not as important as local, direct-level working relationships among professionals who care about their joint clients. To make full use of placement facilities of the Employment Service, the rehabilitation counselor must maintain good relationships, work cooperatively with Employment Service counterparts, and provide full exchange of information (see 12.2.9 and 37.2.2).

Training Agencies

The training agencies—the colleges and universities, technical trade and vocational schools,

workshops and other rehabilitation facilities—have their own employee contact and placement programs and can supply leads to employment openings for state rehabilitation client-trainees.

Business Reports

Considerable information on business and industrial relocations, expansions of existing business concerns, industrial changes, and trends indicating the probability of future job opportunities is to be found in industrial report manuals and chamber of commerce surveys.

Construction of new plants and factories, stores, gas stations, and building renovations are indications of potential job openings. Employers should be contacted about possible jobs before construction is completed.

Civil Service

Whether clients are looking for white- or blue-collar work, they should consider government employment at the federal, state, county, or local level as a possibility. Handicapped people are considered a "protected class" by affirmative action standards and are mandated by federal law to be hired into civil service positions. Civil service policy states that employment may not be denied an applicant for public employment because of disablement if the person is qualified (see 38.4.1).

Unions

Officers, agents, stewards, and other union personnel generally keep informed of events that will affect the employment of the members, although direct job referrals are of course reserved for union members. Nonunion clients may consider joining if this would improve employment prospects. Union officials are particularly helpful to members or former members who become disabled and who, following rehabilitation, seek reemployment (see 12.1.13 and 38.3).

Help-Wanted Advertisements

Local newspaper want-ads are not a very good source for most employment opportunities, but they should not be disregarded. If immediately pursued, they can put a client in direct contact with an employer who has an expressed need for a worker. Counselors need to assist clients in learning how to interpret personnel ads to determine misleading content.

Private Employment Agencies

Private firms, their profits derived from commissions paid by employers or workers (based on a percentage of wages), offer employment services. Counselors should help clients evaluate such an agency and determine legal obligations of any written agreements. These firms canvass potential employers in the community to compile their job list, but the client pays for this service; on the other hand, the state agency has the jobs listed and available without charge (see 37.2.4).

Salomone and Rubin [1979] compiled strategies for rehabilitation counselors and their clients to secure job leads. They advocated the development of new job leads that are not yet available to the general public.

35.3. Information Presentation

The job resumé as described by Morgan [n.d.] is basic to any job search. Its one or two typewritten pages conveniently list a person's background, skills, and former jobs, arranged so that potential employers can quickly ascertain salable assets. The counselor will usually help the client with the resumé, checking to see that it is clear and that it presents a complete description of the client's qualifications. The resumé gives the client a chance to apply for many jobs and saves time otherwise lost in filling out long application forms. Finally, it structures the interview. Many job-seekers are frustrated by interviews that never bring their best qualities to light. A good resumé prevents this because it individualizes the client and focuses on his or her unique combination of attitudes, skills, experiences, personality, and ambition.

35.3.1. THE RESUMÉ

The key to an effective and useful resumé is its sensitivity to the information needs of the prospective employer. A creative resumé written in short lines of dynamic narration stands out and calls attention to the applicant. One advantage of many handicapped individuals is that eliminating the dates and chronology of the standard resumé format reduces the emphasis on embarrassing blank periods in the employment record. It is possible to thus emphasize the individual's accomplishments.

References may or may not be included. While some employment interviewers prefer to see them in the resumé, others assume that references will be filed with a placement office where they will be readily available. Many will expect to contact former employers personally. References related to work experience are preferred to those of social acquaintances.

Usually a job list will begin with the last job held. Listings appear in reverse order, ending with the earliest. If the client has ever held successively more responsible jobs, the resumé should emphasize that growing responsibility, since demonstrated progress impresses an employer. While the resumé should describe the client's strengths, no mention should be made of physical or mental limitations that might cause the person to be screened out without consideration.

35.3.2. COVER LETTER

A cover letter should accompany the resumé and should contain a statement of background, skills, and the job being applied for. It may be helpful for the applicant to suggest arranging an interview appointment for the job, since this makes the applicant seem confident of eligibility. The introductory letter should be typed neatly, on a good grade of letter-sized white bond paper, and addressed, if possible, to the person responsible for hiring. Care in sentence structure, spelling, and punctuation should be used. The rehabilitationist can show the client several sample letters for use as a guide, review the format and grammar, and arrange for typing assistance if necessary.

35.3.3. THE APPLICATION FORM

Employers routinely require applicants to fill out an application blank before an interview, in order to structure the discussion. A good indicator of literacy, for example, is the client's ability to fill out the blank without assistance. A well-prepared job applicant should therefore be able to deal with the questions on an application blank unassisted. This ability usually develops quickly because the information requested is predictable. A sample application should contain complete information, names, and dates that may be needed for reference in order to fill out an application in the employer's office. Clients with limited reading and writing skills will need assistance in filling out the application. This is where the placement specialist can be of help. Clients must realize that the application makes an important first impression and will often determine whether an interview is offered; neatness is essential.

35.3.4. APPLICATION QUESTIONS

Some clients have difficulty answering certain questions on the application form. These are items that may reveal personal problems such as physical limitation, diseases, periods of emotional illness, workers' compensation claims, arrest or imprisonment, military status, marital status, education, and employment history. Even though some of the questions are illegal and should not be on the form, a client should know how to respond without fear of recrimination.

Employment interviewers usually base their questions on the information given in the application. It is necessary, therefore, that the applicant state the answers carefully. The counselor can assist the client to prepare for these initial questions and for related questions that may follow.

35.3.5. COMPLETING AN APPLICATION

Anderson, Hutchins, and Walker [1968] provided the following guidelines for completing an application form and answering problem questions. First, the client must give accurate information indicating those skills necessary to do a particular job and evidence showing potential to be a good employee. The counselor's role is to help make the client aware of the information that is necessary and show how to present it in a favorable way. Second, past problems should be considered only if they might affect the ability to perform on the job. Third, while important facts should be given to the employer, insignificant or irrelevant ones should not be mentioned. And fourth, the client should be helped to select information that is useful to the prospective employer and encouraged to concentrate on skills and abilities rather than problems.

35.3.6. DISCLOSURE

Most application forms ask the applicant to specify any special medical or personal conditions that need to be considered in placement. Personnel managers and employers expect the applicant to be honest in disclosing the nature of any disability that might affect job performance or personal safety. If it seems best to tell an employer that a problem exists, it should be described in functional rather than medical or psychiatric terms. Disability labels, for instance, usually cause the employer confusion, elicit a prejudicial reaction, or result in rejection. It is easier for employers to ignore applications that mention unfamiliar defects than to risk finding out what they mean. Some employers will automatically reject applications that specify a disability, even though it is illegal to do so.

There is another alternative. Since the space in the application form is often insufficient to explain adequately a mental illness or prison record, the counselor may suggest to the client that these spaces be left blank or marked "N/A." (This procedure is unnecessary in situations in which the counselor has a working relationship with the personnel manager or when the company has a reputation for giving fair consideration to disabled applicants who are forthright about their disability.) Once a decision has been made to postpone answering a question until a job interview is obtained, the counselor should be certain that the client is capable of answering the question appropriately in the interview situation. This will provide an opportunity to offer a more thorough description of the problem. In this way, the client's abilities will be maximized and the disabilities minimized [Goldhammer & James, 1976]. It should be remembered, however, that honest disclosure is required in direct counselor-employer contact. There must be no question of agency candor and forthrightness in such relationships.

35.3.7. ADDITIONAL INFORMATION

Additional information about the job application form needs to be discussed with clients. If clients are asked what position they would like to have ten years from now, their answers should be directly related to the kind of job for which they are now applying. Minimum salary desires may be expressed after considering what the job in question usually pays, or they may be said to be "open." If the question deals with what led the applicant to consider becoming an employee of this company, "Good company to work for," "Good working conditions," or "I've heard good things about this company" are appropriate answers. If clients are asked to state outstanding debts, it is acceptable for them to list major items such as a house or a car, but they need not mention the amount of each debt. If asked why they left the last job, they should answer "laid off," "to take a better job," "moved," or the like. If asked how many days of school or work were missed in the last year, they should specify the number of days if it is six or less; otherwise they should leave it blank and explain. To questions that do not apply, the client should simply write "nonapplicable" in the blank.

References are often important. Besides the names of former employers, clients can also use the names of local businesses or professional people who know them. Former instructors, vocational counselors, and ministers are equally good references. If the client is new in town and cannot offer local referrals, as usually requested, this should be stated while offering those references available. Physicians, psychiatrists, or social workers are not advisable references. And if clients use a counselor's name they should be prepared to explain why they have sought the agency's services. In some cases, the client may need to prepare a "prompt card" with a list of references to be copied onto the application [Anderson, Hutchins, & Walker, 1968].

35.3.8. THE JOB CAMPAIGN

Placement counselors generally agree that searching for a job should be a well-organized, full-time activity. Like any other such activity, it needs to be learned. People who have not sought work before (or for a long time) thus are not good at job-hunting. Motivation may be a problem with persons collecting unemployment benefits, for they may not seriously look for work until their benefits are exhausted—then panic sets in.

The job search should follow regular working hours and be regarded as a job in itself by the client. A minimum number of applications should be made daily, in person if possible, and follow-up contacts scheduled to ascertain the results. The majority of employers note that their primary source of personnel consists of job-seekers who apply in person, by which they indicate a sincere interest in the company. On the other hand, many unemployed people wait for openings to be advertised, and this often does not happen. Some employers will not hire individuals until they have returned several times to reapply or check on job openings. Often, employers will hire the best person who is available whenever an opening happens to occur. Blanket mailing of resumés may be useful in uncovering job openings outside of the local community, although the positive response rate is low [Irish, 1973].

35.4. Employer Screening

While finding job vacancies is an important first step, it is obvious that in order to get the job the disabled person must manage to be chosen in the selection process. The process and formality of the selection procedure vary with employers and with the level of the position. Large firms generally have personnel managers, sophisticated programs and staff, including job analysts, employment interviewers, and industrial physicians who facilitate the employee selection process. In small firms applicants may be selected by the manager or line supervisor with the necessary paperwork done by a clerk. Medical examina- tion, contact with former employers, and other references—even the completion of a written application form—may be waived for temporary and low-level jobs, or by a very small organization. Union shops also have less complicated procedures of selection if stipulated in the labor contract. The particular method of selection used to make hiring decisions is affected by a number of factors, including size of company, kind of activity, community attitudes and expectations, and labor market demand. The problem is complicated by the stringency of some of the criteria. Many companies screen prospective workers according to multiple criteria, only some of which are directly related to an applicant's ability to perform the tasks involved. For example, criteria may include a high school diploma or a superior test score even though the job does not require such attainments.

Hamilton and Roessner [1972] found, in a survey of hiring qualifications and disqualifications used in a national sample of employers, that over half of them would disqualify applicants with "health problems." Persons with medically based problems (health, drug use, alcoholism, and overweight) seem to be even more likely to be disqualified for employment than those with socially based problems (prison record, arrest record, garnishment, and language problems).

Stereotyping disabilities and inferred labeling may be more important than covert attitudes and outright discrimination. Dunn [1974a] observed that while employers may use a variety of screening methods, hiring standards, and criteria, the relationship between these and the actual requirements of jobs is often scant. The difference between meeting the requirements of the job and meeting the hiring criteria of the employer is often considerable; those who make hiring decisions are less concerned about what the disabled can do than they are about the possible health and accident problems of the disabled person and the concomitant costs to the company in increased worker compensation insurance premiums. In spite of ample evidence that insurance costs do not rise as a result of employing disabled workers, the wide belief in this myth continues to affect hiring practices negatively. Another myth, a cruel stereotype, may be operative: that a disabled person is an unhealthy person. Because physical fitness and health are closely allied and are highly valued in our society, disability, by inference, implies ill health in the minds of employers.

Affirmative action regulations of the 1973 Rehabilitation Act on employment of people who have a disability are helping to change employer rejection practices. These regulations, which require federal contractors and subcontractors to take affirmative action to employ and promote qualified disabled persons, are especially effective with larger firms and organizations (see 38.4).

35.4.1. TRAINING FOR INTERVIEWS

Most employment interviewers usually decide whether or not to hire an individual in the first 5 minutes of an average 10- to 15-minute interview. If a negative impression is gained in these first several minutes, this impression remains 90 percent of the time and the applicant is not hired; if the first impression is positive, the applicant is hired 75 percent of the time [Anderson, Hutchins, & Walker, 1968]. Applicants must immediately appear self-confident and must present positive information (focused primarily on skills and abilities) in the first part of the interview. Personal problems such as an apparent disability should be mentioned casually by the applicant early in the interview so that the employer will not form a negative impression before the information is given.

Good preparation for job interviews can eliminate problems. Clients thoroughly familiar with their assets and prepared for problem questions can answer quickly and properly if they have sound information and some practice prior to the interview. It is crucial that they not have to stop and think for the correct answer.

Typically, for interview training, four to eight clients have two days of instruction. The clients learn to identify their assets and describe them advantageously to potential employers. The rehabilitation worker prompts and clients rehearse ready answers to questions about possible problems or deficiencies (e.g., poor work record) so that responses show self-confidence. In the same way, clients are rehearsed to focus on their abilities rather than their problems. Help also is given on where to look for job leads and how to inquire about a job and get an interview. Practice applications are completed by clients and criticized by staff to pinpoint problems and refine answers.

Practical experience in interviewing with a staff member who takes the employer's role is very helpful. These exercises teach the client the importance of a firm handshake and a friendly greeting, ways of speaking about competency or experience in the desired job, and techniques for showing confidence and enthusiasm for the job during the interview. The applicant then learns how to leave by asking for permission to call back to check the outcome.

Videotaping practice interviews gives clients an opportunity to see what they are doing right and wrong during these role-playing sessions with the rehabilitation staff. The replay draws attention to annoying mannerisms or to a demeanor that detracts from a good impression. Instruction on eye contact and other behavior, attire, grooming, and hygiene are offered as necessary. Viewing role-played interviews, recorded both at the beginning and the end of training, show clients their progress and boost confidence for attempting real job interviews.

More elaborate courses may last for weeks. They may involve tours of local companies; lectures by Employment Service representatives; discussions led by personnel managers, a charm school instructor, or public health nurse; and continued participation by graduates of the course (viz., rehabilitants who have been successful in obtaining suitable employment). Instruction in large cities may be needed on how to use the public transportation facilities. Near the conclusion of training, the clients may be allowed to try out their new talents, under tutelage, by developing a list of prospects and telephoning them. By this practice remaining flaws can be rapidly detected and corrected.

McClure [1972], from a study with rehabilitants, reported that those trained in job-seeking skills obtained jobs at about twice the rate of other clients—in about half the time and with less counselor assistance.

35.4.2. APPEARANCE AND MANNERISMS

Appropriate appearance and mannerisms often require an extended period to develop; for some clients this improvement will involve a rehabilitation facility program. Consequently, they should be dealt with long before interview training and the job search begin.

Appropriate Appearance

Though counselors differ in their opinions regarding the type of dress a client should wear to a job interview, they generally agree that the attire should be consistent with the interviewer's expectations and standards. Applicants should wear clothing similar to, or perhaps just slightly better than, that of the people working at the job for which they are applying. If applying for a job as a machinist, for instance, the client should dress like other machinists working for the company so the interviewer will have no difficulty visualizing this person working at that job.

Regardless of the position applied for, neatness and cleanliness are always essential. When necessary, counselors encourage clients to be aware of the positive responses possible when they are appropriately groomed. Employers regard the overall appearance of all applicants as an indication of their competency.

Use of Polaroid Pictures to Improve Appearance

Another technique that has also produced excellent results, according to Anderson, Hutchins, and Walker [1968], is the use of polaroid pictures. Clients with an appearance problem are first photographed, then given information about personal appearance matters, usually through a checklist of attributes. They are then asked to compare their photograph with standards on the checklist. Through use of the photograph the situation is somewhat depersonalized and the clients can be more objective about their appearance and how they must change. Often, such clients maintain their new standard of grooming because it is usually reinforced throughout the day by the people they meet. If the person's grooming should deteriorate, the process is repeated to show that good grooming is a daily effort.

Use of Monitor to Improve Appearance

Appeal to a client's vanity has produced excellent results with clients who have grooming problems. When they learn ahead of time that they are going to be on television they make a special effort to appear well-groomed. (The monitor that is used with various audiovisual equipment is similar to a television set.) The members of the group subsequently reinforce the positive change of behavior, which is maintained for the employment interview.

Nervousness

If the client is particularly nervous, the counselor might say it is normal for many people to be nervous, especially during an interview. Experienced interviewers pay little attention to a certain degree of nervousness. Nevertheless, clients should keep their hands still and listen attentively to the interviewer. Usually nervousness will decrease substantially as interviewing skills improve and clients become aware of the nonthreatening behavior of most interviewers.

Self-confidence and Positive Attitudes

A friendly, confident, sincere attitude is one the prospective employer is most likely to appreciate. The composed applicant, secure in presenting skills and fielding difficult questions, will no doubt have an effective job interview. Enthusiasm as reflected in the applicant's voice and expression—and firm handshake—is also important.

There are corresponding negative attitudes, however, that should be avoided. Inability to relate to others is the most frequent cause of dismissal. Generally employers try to screen out "troublemakers" and individuals whom they consider insubordinate. Such individuals, they feel, cause supervisors difficulty and their lack of sociability creates morale problems among fellow workers. Group counseling sessions provide the means to help the client develop positive attitudes. Positive reinforcement hastens learning and retention.

35.4.3. THE MODEL INTERVIEW

The model interview is a role-playing technique in which an audio- or videotape is used to improve a client's verbal responses in job interview situations. It can be used in either group or individual counseling sessions. Lasting about 10 minutes, it illustrates every important interview behavior (see 13.4.7).

The model interview shows clients the standard that is the goal. In actual practice, if they see the model interview before participating in a mock interview, they will have a better idea of the sorts of answers needed. They begin to see that there is a definite way to answer questions and to present information in an interview. Were they asked, on the other hand, to participate in a mock interview before seeing the model, they might feel that the counselor is unjustly critical.

Many clients, in addition to some physical disability, have a poor vocational history and no relevant work experience. Problems similar to this will be discussed on the model tape. Usually client attention during the showing of the model interview is strong and nods of agreement showing identification are frequent. In the group discussion following the model interview, the counselor can ask questions about the applicant's appearance, enthusiasm, and general poise. Eventually as the whole group begins to participate in the discussion, the term *inter-viewing* begins to lose its frightening connotation. The participating clients are now prepared to do their own mock interview.

35.4.4. THE MOCK INTERVIEW

Lasting about 5 minutes, the first mock interview is based upon an application form previously filled out by the client. For maximum effect, the interview should focus on issues covered on that application. Since the clients usually have little experience explaining their problems in an interview, they will answer questions inadequately or indecisively. The counselor should show a visual negative response such as raised eyebrows or a pause after the client gives such an answer. Usually the client will expand this answer during a pause. This technique not only makes the client aware that the original answer was unacceptable, but it also makes the group aware of ineffectively presented information.

Anderson, Hutchins, and Walker [1968] suggested that the mock interviewer assume a businesslike approach and ask pointed questions unhesitatingly. Their list of fundamental questions that may be used is paraphrased as follows: What job are you applying for? How did you hear about it? Will you tell me about yourself? Why did you leave your last job? Have you ever been unemployed for over two months? If so, why were you not working? Do you have any physical or emotional problems? How do they affect you? How did you do in school? What makes you think you can do this job? Have you ever been in trouble with the law? How often have you been absent from work or school? Have you ever had trouble with other people on the job? How much money do you expect to make on this job? Can you work an evening shift? Why should I hire you?

Questions that can be answered with a simple Yes or No should not be asked. Professional interviewers use open-end questions such as "Tell me a little bit about yourself." The client will need to respond to such questions by personnel interviewers. (See 26.2.)

Through mock interviews clients become aware of the problems that they would have in an employment interview. They are uncomfortable with the feeling of ineptness resulting from their mistakes in the mock interview. Starting with "explaining skills" at this point is advantageous because this provides an opportunity for clients to learn positive things about themselves. They begin to build confidence in themselves and to feel they have marketable attributes. After they know their skills, they can convince an employer to hire them.

Clients need to be told that explaining their skills is their most important task in an employment interview. Past work experience, related experience, training, aptitudes, and hobbies are areas of information developed for the client's skills presentation. All of the person's vocational assets should be listed.

After this asset information has been gathered, the client's skills statements should be written out and the client should learn to state them as they will be expressed in an interview. Several different asset statements should be used to support a job choice. In describing work skills the names of machines and technical terms should be used. Clients must be able to answer the question, "Why should we hire you?" by referring to their assets and skills relevant to the job. This information must be supplied within the first few minutes of the interview.

The counselor helps the client remember a skill by saying, "That is a skill you should mention to an employer; now let me hear you say it in sentence form as if I were the employer," as each asset stated is identified and the statement is recorded. To help clients remember their asset lists and rehearse their statements the counselor can role-play a partial interview with them, asking only about their skills. Practice in reporting these skills aloud in front of the group makes the presentation more natural.

Asking Questions

An applicant who does not ask any questions during an interview indicates little interest in the job. Toward the end of an interview employers usually ask if the applicant has any questions. Clients should listen carefully throughout the interview so as not to ask questions the interviewer has already answered. Even if the interviewer does not ask for questions, the client should show interest in further information about some aspect of the job or business. The exception is an instance when the interviewer's coverage is so complete that there is nothing left to ask about. In this case the client should say: "I had questions to ask in the beginning of this interview, but I think you have gone over them completely" [Anderson, Hutchins, & Walker, 1968].

Counselor Role-Play Deficiency

In comparison with the group training method, there are disadvantages when counselors role-play interviews with a single client. Zadny and James [1976] pointed out, "It is doubtful that a counselor will take the time to cover all aspects of the training; his presumptions about what to omit could be erroneous. He knows the client too well and may no longer notice things that might put off an employer. Preparation for interviewing is likely to be deficient because it will not be anxiety-provoking enough if the counselor, whom the client has learned to trust, takes the employer's role. The point of the role-play is to isolate not only those difficulties that appear in the relative safety of an agency office, but also those likely to surface for the first time in the employer's office" [p. 23]. (See 30.3.10.)

35.5. Problem Areas

Most vocationally handicapped people have some problems in their personal or work histories that need to be explained to the employer in a job interview. In fact, the major reason that these individuals require vocational rehabilitation services stems from these problems that have caused employers to be skeptical of their ability. Anderson, Hutchins, and Walker [1968] have identified problem areas and described how to help individuals cope with their employ-

ment handicap. Their ideas are used in this section.

Employers cannot be expected to hire an individual who has problems that would interfere with the job applied for. The job objective, therefore, must be carefully selected so that it is certain that such problems are minimized. The completion of a standard application form helps to identify problems the person will need to explain in an interview. Problem questions include those on physical limitations, diseases or mental illness, workers compensation, arrests or imprisonment, gaps in employment history, and level of education.

An additional type of problem that the individual will need to explain relates to personal characteristics that are noticeable to an interviewer. These include not only apparent physical disabilities but also outward mannerisms, peculiarities, and unpleasant negative personality attributes such as hostility or withdrawal (see 5.5).

35.5.1. PREPARING ANSWERS

Helping individuals develop answers to problem questions simply means determining what positive statements the client can make on the subject. Framing such a statement is the key consideration. A review of the examples offered shows that positive answers are formed by: stating that the problem the person once had no longer exists; focusing on residual abilities (rather than limitations), thereby showing suitability for this particular job; and turning the problem into an asset.

The answer should be developed so that it counteracts the employer's expected reaction to the problem. Typical employer reactions to a physical disability, for example, might be that the individual would be a slow worker or a shop hazard or might have a high rate of absenteeism or tardiness. Answers should, therefore, be structured to put the employer at ease about these concerns; for example, "I know that most people with a condition like mine might be slow workers, but I turn out as much work as the average assembler because I can work at a steady pace all day. I usually finish more than the people who take a lot of breaks."

A job applicant's answers to questions about disability, job history, institutionalization, and other problem areas should be brief and should be stated in such a way as to relieve the employer's concern. For example, a demonstration of abilities or an explanatory statement about the disability may be all that is necessary to refute an employer's bias about disability. As Twomey [U.S. IRI, 1975b] said, when problem areas are brought up in an interview, the applicant should present pertinent information at once and in a positive way. This results in a far better impression than is created when the interviewer has to ferret out negative information on a piecemeal basis.

The disabled person should routinely cover potential issues even though the interviewer might not have thought of them until later. It is important to say, for instance, that transportation arrangements are adequate and that the disability will not be the cause of excessive illness or absence from work.

Obvious Disability

As was stated before, if the disability is obvious it should be mentioned early by the interviewee whether or not the employer asks about it. Even though employers are hesitant to ask about physical problems, they may harbor reservations about hiring the individual. Consequently, if they do not learn more about the individual's limitations, the person may not be hired. For the client to mention any apparent disability in the interview clears misconceptions and offers the applicant an opportunity to explain how the limitation will not interfere with job performance. When the individual has a device such as a prosthetic hook, it is advisable not only to provide information about it but also to demonstrate its function.

The interviewee should be aware of the employer's possible reaction to the disability and should make a reassuring statement. For example, if the individual is in a wheelchair or on crutches, the employer is likely to suspect that the person will be frequently tardy or absent from the job. The applicant can say, "Most people think that my condition would prevent me from getting to work every day but I have transportation that will get me here even in a blizzard."

Occurrence

There are various suggestions for explaining the occurrence of the condition. For example, the individual with a congenital problem might say, "I have had this all my life, and I've learned to do most things that other people can do." If it's an old injury, the person should mention the time it has existed and how the effects are overcome. In case of a recent injury, it is best to say something about completion of medical care, the doctor's permission to work, and the fact that no further difficulty is expected. With a contagious disease, it is important to explain to the employer that the person is not a disease carrier. A physician's statement that there is no possibility this person could give the disease to anyone else is indicated for an individual who recently recovered from a contagious disease.

Limits and Abilities

Clients should be supplied with information about their abilities as found through the assessment process. For example, a client can say "I am all thumbs when it comes to working with real small pieces, but I can handle larger objects like the kind of things you have here without any difficulty." In another case the person says, "I wouldn't have any trouble with my back on a job like this since I can lift up to 20 pounds, and I can sit for three hours at a time before I take a break." Still another client explains, "It is true that I cannot see, but I have had special training in learning to get around, so I wouldn't have any difficulty finding things here once someone shows me where they are." A client with a speech defect says, "I have a little difficulty with my speech, especially when I'm a little nervous like now, but if I talk more slowly so people can understand me, I never have difficulty being understood."

It is good to draw the interviewer's attention to any special devices that the client uses to become a better worker. If the condition is stable or improving, the person should mention this. On the other hand, if the condition is commonly known to be progressive (such as muscular dystrophy) the person should say how long it has been stable and what the doctor says about the future.

35.5.2. OTHER COMMON PROBLEMS

There are many other problem areas that require explanations such as those formulated by Anderson, Hutchins, and Walker [1968], below.

Age

People who are younger than most people applying for the job can say "I know that I am young but that means I can learn the job quickly, and I'm interested in getting a steady job that I could keep for several years." This explanation presents youth as an asset that means the applicant can learn quickly; it anticipates the possibility that the employer expects a young person will not stay on the job long.

Older people explain, "I know that I am older than most people applying, but I feel just as good as I did when I was 30. I have worked all my life, and I know what employers expect of a worker. This will be a steady job for me as I do not plan to do like the young people who will leave a job just as soon as they can find something else." This presents age as an asset that means the applicant knows what is expected of a worker. It also presents an image of reliability and steadiness. Such explanations should be volunteered by the applicant before the employer mentions the problem area.

Hospitalized for Emotional Problems

These clients simply say "Yes, I did have some treatment for my nerves. I became uncomfortable sitting around home after my injury and my doctor and I decided that I could use some help so I went into the hospital for a while. I am really glad that I did because they helped me a lot. I am fine now and ready to go to work." This message presents a problem in a way that dispels the employer's possible concern about hiring someone with serious mental illness. Clients explain their former mental illness in terms of a precipitating external situation that no longer exists. They avoid using psychological terms to describe the problem.

Prison Record

A prison record must be explained. The public offender can say "Yes, I spent some time in prison. I did some dumb things that I really regret now. I was young and foolish but I have really learned my lesson by spending some time in prison and I haven't had any problems since coming out." If the employer asks for further explanation of the offense, it is best, if accurate, to provide information that indicates that the offense was in no way connected with work or with the former employer. The fact that the offense was committed because the individual was influenced by undesirable—*former*—friends, or happened following a drinking party (if the person no longer has such problems) makes the offense appear less serious to the employer.

As mentioned earlier, a poor job history is in itself a problem. Several explanations for a poor record are described below.

Poor Work References

A bad reference can be explained by saying "If you call my last employer they will probably tell you that I was not a good worker. Actually, I found out that the kind of work I was doing there didn't suit me very well. If you call some of my other employers I am sure they will give me a good reference." This prepares the interviewer for a bad reference from a past employer so that it will not be a surprise. The applicant provides information about what went wrong on the job, thereby making clear that the individual accepts the blame in a mature way.

Too Many Short-Term Jobs

"Job hopping" must be explained: "It's true that I have worked at a number of different jobs in the past. I've been searching around for steady work—something that I would like, and on one or two of the jobs I had there were layoffs. I'm sure now that this is the job I want, and if I get it, I expect to still be here when they hand out the Social Security checks." This tells the employer that there has been a search for steady work and that some of the jobs had layoffs (which no new worker can avoid). It concludes with a statement that shows that the applicant really wants this particular job.

Gaps in Employment History

Answers depend on the individual's circumstances, such as what it was that caused the person to be unemployed. Sample explanations are "I was self-employed during that time," or "It took some time for me to recover from my injury, but I'm fine now and ready to go to work," and "I had a number of part-time and seasonal jobs during that time that I didn't bother to put down."

For women, there are a number of good explanations, involving such things as "I was needed by my parents," or "I was raising my family," or "I was helping care for a relative." Everyone who has been unemployed has been engaged in something, so the counselor should find out what it is and put the best construction on it for the interview. The idea is to tell the truth but to use the most acceptable reason out of the several that the client may have. The impression to convey is that the individual was occupied with some meaningful activity, even though it was not paid employment.

If the person has not worked recently, it is important to avoid the impression that attempts to find work for a number of months have been unsuccessful. No employer wants to hire someone whom all others have rejected.

Has Never Worked

If the individual has just left school or is a housewife just entering the labor market, the fact of never having worked is readily understandable. The counselor must determine what the individual was actually doing during the period of unemployment and expand acceptable reasons. Examples are "taking a correspondence course" or "helping on the family farm or business"—anything that suggests constructive activity.

Change of Job Area

People who have spent most of their lives in a particular type of occupation and are now trying to get into another field for which extensive training is not required, will naturally cause the employer to wonder about the decision to change occupational areas. If there is an obvious physical problem that has occurred to prevent such a person from returning to a former occupation, and which the individual is going to explain in the interview, the problem is already clarified. If possible, however, the individual should convey the idea that the disability does not preclude return to the former type of job but only that the change is preferred.

Not Returning to Former Employer

If the client was previously employed in the same type of job but by another company, the employer will wonder why the person is not returning to that company. Usually the individual will need to indicate this former job on the application blank as verification of job skills, so the employer will be aware that the person did similar work before.

When the other company is in another city, or another part of the city, one says "I wanted to be closer to my work." Otherwise, it may be necessary to explain "I was not happy with that job because of the working conditions (or pay, or some other factor), but I heard a lot about your company, and I'm sure I would enjoy working here."

Have Received Workers Compensation

In this case it is best to admit "Yes, I received workers compensation for my back injury, but my doctor has told me that I can do this kind of work without any further problems. (I have a medical statement here for you to see.) I am also covered under the Second Injury Law, and this means that if I should have any trouble with my back while I'm working here, the expenses could come out of a special fund so there wouldn't be any liability on your part." It is helpful for the individual to carry a copy of the state Second Injury Law, which defines the protection for the employer, because many employers who are not familiar with this protection hesitate to hire anyone who has had a previous injury.

Educational and intellectual problems are another category for which Anderson, Hutchins, and Walker suggested explanations by the disabled job seeker.

Learns Very Slowly

The slow learner can say "It takes me a little longer than most people to learn a job, but once I know what to do I don't forget."

These individuals are telling the employer that they may not be able to learn academic subjects quickly, but that their performance will be consistent once they know what to do.

Memory Problem

It is rare that a memory problem would be so severe that it would be apparent in the interview. However, an individual with such a difficulty might say, "I do have a little difficulty remembering things, but I carry a notepad with me and write down instructions." This tells the employer that the person has learned to cope with the memory problem.

Little Education

People with this deficiency should explain, "As you know I haven't graduated from high school, but I have kept up with my reading and math in everyday life. I read the newspaper, and I had to use fractions on my last job. I was tested recently and I read at the seventh grade level and my math is at the sixth grade level. My counselor tells me that a lot of high school graduates don't get scores better than that." This tells the employer that this person does have fair basic skills, even without formal education.

Too Much Education for the Job

Some individuals, especially those who have emotional problems, may be unable to perform at the level for which they were educated or trained. The application blank could be completed so that advanced education, inappropriate to their current job goal, is not indicated. If indicated, the individual will need to offer an explanation: "I did have college training, but I found out that I did not like the kind of work that this prepared me for. I would much prefer to do this type of job instead." Or the person might explain, "I'd like to work here for a few years at least before I decide whether or not I want to go back to college, and then I would probably take evening courses." In this way the client is expressing real interest in this kind of job, despite educational or training background. This counters the employer's fear that the individual will work for a few months and leave to go to school or to a higher level job.

School Dropout

The young person who has dropped out of school can say, "I was having a little difficulty in school and decided it would be better to quit and get a job. I know now that I made a mistake by not finishing my education, but I'm going to get my GED."

The older or culturally disadvantaged person who did not finish school can explain, "Times were pretty hard for my folks so I quit school to get a job and help out. I wish now that I'd had a chance to finish. I do keep up with my reading and math, and the tests I've taken show that I am intelligent and well-informed."

Cannot Read or Write

People with literacy problems should carry a completed application to copy from or to give to the prospective employer.

They can say "I cannot read or write very well, but I feel that I can do these things well enough to be a good worker on this job. I've looked into the requirements for the job, and I understand that there is not much reading or writing required." This statement tells the employer that the applicant understands what is required on the job and feels able to do the kind of work required. Bringing a completed application form indicates that the person is aware of the difficulty and can compensate for it in situations in which reading and writing are required.

35.5.3. PREPARATION

Preparing for an interview includes keeping a schedule of place and time of the interview and getting the full name of both the company and the interviewer correct. If necessary, clients should have a dossier or portfolio that will demonstrate as well as substantiate expressed skills and achievements. When appropriate, they should have medical documents and releases available should the employer want information regarding physical status.

A Research of Companies

Clients will benefit from acquiring information about the companies they are applying to before the interview. Information may include: how old the company is, how many branches it has, what its line of products or services is, what its growth has been, and how its future looks. This will give the client something to talk about during the interview and give the interviewer an opportunity to go beyond the basic application information.

Information about a company may be obtained from its employees, local libraries, chambers of commerce, and business organizations. It helps to know the kinds and number of jobs available in a particular company, the physical requirements of various jobs, the turnover rate in regard to certain company jobs, salary levels, fringe benefits, the labor unions involved, working conditions, the person with final authority on hiring, the company's affirmative action plan for disabled workers, and its financial situation. Only a knowledgeable applicant can convey to the employer an interest in and enthusiasm for the job.

35.5.4. THE UNSUCCESSFUL INTERVIEW

If the client has had an unsuccessful employment interview, counselors may call the employer to learn the reason(s) why. If personality factors caused the rejection, the agency may suggest further counseling or work adjustment. If lack of skills was the cause, more training is considered or the appropriateness of the job choice is evaluated. In this way employers may offer indirect help to enable the client to become more employable. Occasionally, clients are rejected because company policy defers the hiring of applicants until they return a second or third time to ask for the job. In other cases a prejudice or fear may be involved that the counselor can address.

Negative Factors Related to Rejection

A survey of 153 companies by Northwestern University, designed to discover the particular negative factors that frequently led to an applicant's rejection, was reported by the New York Life Insurance Company [n.d.]. Selected reasons are paraphrased as follows: poor personal appearance; overbearing (overaggressive, conceited); inability to express self clearly (poor voice, diction, grammar); lack of planning for career (no purpose and goals); lack of interest and enthusiasm (passive or indifferent); lack of confidence and poise (nervousness or ill-at-ease); failure to participate in activities; overemphasis on money; poor scholastic record; unwilling to start at the bottom (expects too much too soon); makes excuses (evasiveness, hedges on unfavorable factors in record); lack of tact; lack of maturity; lack of courtesy or ill-mannered; condemnation of past employers; lack of social understanding; marked dislike for school work; lack of vitality; failure to look interviewer in the eye; limp hand-shake; indecision; loafs during vacations; unhappy married life; friction with parents; sloppy application blank; merely shopping around; wants job only for short time; little sense of humor; lack of knowledge of field of specialization; parents make decisions for him; no interest in company or in industry; dependence on sponsor; unwillingness to go where assigned; cynical; low moral standards; lazy; intolerant (strong prejudices); narrow interests; spends much time at movies; poor handling of personal finances; no interest in community activities; inability to take criticism; lack of appreciation of the value of experience; radical ideas; late to interview without good reason; never heard of company; failure to express appreciation for interviewer's time; asks no questions about the job; high pressure type; and indefinite response to questions. It is noteworthy that these objectionable factors may be applicable to any person, whether or not that person is disabled. Moreover these reasons for being rejected for employment are correctable.

Chapter 36

Securing Employment

Securing employment as described in this chapter refers to arranging a placement and making the job secure for the client. Generally, placement activity follows the completion of services of career planning, training, work adjustment, and job development; then it proceeds concurrently with the job selection process and solicitation of employment opportunities. As with every other rehabilitation counselor service, it is an alternative used only to the extent required after careful analysis of the individual situation. Its several components, which are fashioned to suit the individual situation, include the following:

1. Serving as an intermediary between personnel manager, supervisor, and client.
2. Examining the need for modifications of the job or the client (see 34.3).
3. Arranging for on-the-job training.
4. Orienting the client to the job.

5. Helping co-workers and supervisors adjust to the new employee and providing other follow-up services as needed.

The primary sources used in writing this chapter include: *Job Opportunities for Handicapped Workers* [National Association of Manufacturers, 1964]; *Placement Services in the Vocational Rehabilitation Program* [Dunn, 1974a]; *Physical Capacities and Job Placement* [Hanman, 1951]; *An Introduction to the Vocational Rehabilitation Process* [McGowan & Porter, 1967]; *The Placement Process in Vocational Rehabilitation Counseling* by Thomason and Barrett [1960]; and several reports from federally sponsored rehabilitation institutes.

An especially valuable source of information is the material published by the Portland State University Regional Rehabilitation Research Institute from its series of "Studies in Placement and Job Development for the Handicapped";

but, as Zadny and James [1976] pointed out in their first monograph, "The placement literature has grown mainly in bulk instead of depth by the addition of variations to basic principles set forth 30 years ago by Bridges" [p.1]. In this book, *Job Placement of the Physically Handicapped*,

Clark D. Bridges [1946] proposed a steady concentration on job placement throughout the rehabilitation process aimed at selectively matching requirements of a job to the talents and needs of a competitively prepared client.

36.1. Direct Placement

Some clients—even after other vocational rehabilitation services are successfully completed—are unable to secure work on their own. In many such cases, however, the rehabilitation counselor can provide the services required to obtain employment. These may include appraising the job site and employer, meeting with employers and personnel managers, orienting the client to the job, and working out problems with co-workers. The techniques used by the counselor often determine whether or not a job is obtained. *Direct placement*, as the term is used in this section, means that the rehabilitation agency counselor or placement specialist provides appropriate client assistance without the necessity for outside intervention or other service strategy.

Arrangements for individual client placement are appropriate only after the individual has achieved a status of "employment readiness." The completion of an appropriate rehabilitation training and adjustment program and the attainment of a sufficient level of job skills and social functioning to sustain employment indicate that the person is ready for work. An appraisal of the level of employment readiness also may be obtained from counselor observation, vocational assessment, or monitoring at a rehabilitation facility.

36.1.1. INTERMEDIARY SERVICE

Due to the severity of the disability or an inadequacy in social functioning, certain clients—even after they have reached their maximum readiness for work—will need a counselor's personal participation in securing employment. The intermediary service provided by the rehabilitationist may consist of the following:

Appraising the client's need for assistance.
Determining appropriate alternatives to the usual situation between an applicant and potential employer.

Guiding the visually impaired or otherwise providing physical assistance.
Acting as an interpreter for the hearing- or speech-impaired.
Assisting those who have difficulties in writing a job application.
Providing support for the emotionally disturbed, retarded, or shy clients who cannot cope with interviews alone.
Soliciting employment opportunities.
Documenting the client's suitability for a particular job.

When judiciously applied, this service complements client job-seeking efforts while saving employers from the inconvenience of inappropriate applications and awkward interviews.

The counselor's presence, however, is not always regarded positively by prospective employers. Some view agency involvement with mistrust, doubting the applicant's ability to do the job and to get along with co-workers, and questioning the agency's motivation as well [Zadny & James, 1976]. Others regard the counselor's presence at client interviews as a sign of excessive dependency or lack of counselor trust or as an appeal to the employer's charitable obligations. When employers have such negative impressions about the agency's involvement, or when the counselor fails to perform in a skillful, professional manner, the client's chances of getting a job are severely diminished. In the long run, however, attention to the proven techniques of rehabilitation and their consistent practice improve the professional's skill as well as the agency's reputation in the business community.

36.1.2. PLANNING

Precontact planning for the placement of individual clients is essential for efficient case management and the effective use of the interview situation. It includes an analysis of the needs, problems, and management practices of those local businesses in which appropriate jobs are available. It also includes a final, comprehensive appraisal of the client's suitability for the particular job. As a final component, the rehabilitationist should ascertain the experience of prior contact with the business in order to determine the agency's reputation and the employer's level of awareness of the agency services that are available.

The counselor's approach determines the success or failure of the employer interview. McGowan and Porter [1967] stressed the importance of planning for the interview because the counselor's and employer's time are valuable. They also emphasized that the counselor should explain the purpose of the visit clearly and concisely, not with an overrehearsed "pitch," but rather with a carefully planned and sequential presentation devised to raise informed questions and comments from the employer.

To secure the best job placement for a client, it is essential for the counselor to have a sincere belief in the client's ability. The counselor must be able to convince an employer that the client can do the job, and that there are substantial reasons for hiring the rehabilitated person rather than another applicant. Experienced counselors, according to McGowan and Porter, warn against appealing to the employer's "humanitarian interests" or "concern as a taxpayer with the problems of the handicapped" (p. 132). They did recommend that the counselor approach the employer in a businesslike fashion and explain the merits of the proposition (i.e., that the employer should hire the client because it would be in the best business interests of the employer). Finally the counselor should show a willingness to accept the employer's decision based strictly on those considerations.

Knowledge of the Business

Although a thoroughgoing examination of the nature of each prospective employer's business should precede the job solicitation interview, this often is not possible when case loads are large and time is short. In many agencies, the essential background details of local businesses will be examined and recorded as part of a job development program, or they may be obtained from the chamber of commerce, business acquaintances, a management association, and state departments of industry or labor. Twomey reported for the Second Institute on Rehabilitation Issues [U.S. IRI, 1975b] that this information may include: kinds of products or services, seasonal business trends, number of employees at various skill levels, hiring practices, turnover rate, presence of unions, key personnel with hiring authority, entrance requirements, and the company's future outlook.

From this precontact information, the counselor can develop an interview procedure that recognizes the employer's needs and anticipates possible objections to hiring disabled people. Twomey cited problems relating to turnover and affirmative action requirements as especially promising areas in which rehabilitationists can assist employers. If the counselor is armed with specific information before the interview, the interview discussions will be focused and relevant.

Information regarding the management structure, the nature of interstate commerce participation, company growth record, and community reputation may also be useful. When possible, mutual friends, business associates, and employees may offer clues regarding the employer's personality, likes, dislikes, problems, and prejudices that will assist in guiding interpersonal communication. At the very least, the rehabilitationist should become familiar with the general kinds of problems faced by local businesses and the characteristics and terminology of the jobs under consideration. Even more importantly the counselor must know all that is relevant about the client and be able to convey this information clearly in terms the employer can appreciate. This knowledge provides the basis, in both mutual understanding and vocabulary, for discussing the client's suitability for the job (see 17.2 and 33.2).

Preparation of Client Information

The job solicitation and employment interview will require complete preparation of information on the client's job-relevant background. This procedure assures that the rehabilitationist is familiar with the client's current level of functioning and can communicate to the employer specific examples of the individual's proven ability for handling job requirements. The employer will be primarily concerned with the client's ability to perform the job tasks safely and adequately; the rehabilitationist, therefore, prepares the substantiating information in advance for presentation during the interview. Occasionally the preparing of a dossier, resumé, or portfolio—including transcripts of scholastic performance, letters of recommendation from former employers and samples of work—will help portray the client's assets. Knowledge of the functional limitations of the disability as well as evidence of the individual's personality characteristics will also be of concern to the employer. A physician's statement indicating the client's ability to handle certain job tasks safely or a release of medical information may be required by the employer's industrial physician. With these materials at hand, the rehabilitationist offers a professional service that is comprehensive and reliable. Such service will increase an employer's faith in the wisdom of the placement recommendations.

Avoiding the Use of Slogans and Labels

Rehabilitationists should avoid sweeping generalizations about the capabilities of individuals who have a disability. They should also avoid using slogans, professional terminology (jargon), and labels that might confuse or embarrass people in business. While it may be true that the work characteristics of disabled people are better than average, the employer knows that some individuals will be worse than average. The employer, consequently, is concerned not with national averages but with the record and potential of the individual applicant in question. Moreover, the employer is likely to be impressed by the specific accomplishments of the rehabilitant, the experience of similarly disabled people in other jobs in the community, and the results of workers placed at competitors' businesses [Ortale, n.d.].

Avoiding such terms as *retarded*, *epileptic*, or *mentally ill,* which serve to evoke a fear or prejudice in the ill-informed businessperson, counselors describe the client's limitations in specific functional terms, emphasizing that the limitations will not interfere with the performance of a particular job. By so doing, they seek to defuse the emotionality attached to such labels and encourage practical, relevant conversation.

Previous Contact

Soliciting employment opportunities from employers unfamiliar with the rehabilitation agency can lead to an anxiety-provoking situation for the employer as well as the counselor. Consequently, the agency's job development program should be presented as an "employer awareness" program effort to inform the employer of the services offered and to create a receptive mood for any job solicitation contacts that may follow. Another advantage of having the agency's job development program precede the actual job soliciting development program is its provision of background information on the company. This will save counselors the chore of repeating research already done by their coworkers.

When previous contact has not been made, however, the initial job solicitation also becomes the initial job development contact. Not only will there be more concerns and uncertainties on the employer's part that will require detailed explanation of the agency's services to help employers, there will be greater consequences resulting from the performance of the first client recommended for placement. Most agencies will, in this case, select a "model" client for the initial placement and refrain from referring high-risk cases until a viable relationship has been established with the employer. After several new workers have performed adequately, most employers are likely to be more tolerant of subsequent placements that may require special attention and agency adjustment services.

Team Interviewing

Usually the rehabilitationist will meet with employers on a one-to-one basis. In some instances, however, it is useful for professionals to team up in pairs for interviewing, especially if one of them belongs to an agency more experienced with the employers in businesses that will be contacted. When the expertise of counselors from both rehabilitation and job service agencies is combined, employer questions are answered more thoroughly and job solicitation is facilitated. At the very least, teamwork enables professionals to share the valuable potential of personal business contacts that agencies or individuals within that agency have developed independently.

36.1.3. PRESENTING THE CLIENT

In hiring and paying for the services of a worker, employers have one thought in mind: they want the best available person for the job. They may or may not use the term, but they are certainly going to apply some of the principles and techniques of *selective placement*, that is, the optimum matching of job requirements with the worker's qualifications. If they can be convinced that the rehabilitation client is the best available applicant, the client will be hired. It is the counselor's job to help the employer to understand that this client is the right person for the job. The following material is largely from McGowan and Porter [1967].

Presenting Client Qualifications

Rehabilitation counselors might begin by stating that they are not just looking for *a* job for their client, but for *the* job, one that is right for the client and for which the client is right. They can then explain the client's qualifications in these terms:

1. Vocational assessment. An interpretation of medical data, psychological testing reports, work evaluation results, training and work experience reports, personal and other history.
2. Rehabilitation services provided. An explanation of the physical restoration, training, and other services furnished.
3. Client's readiness for employment. An explanation to the employer of the client's readiness for employment with emphasis upon qualifications.

Revealing Client Information

How much is the employer told? The counselor's first responsibility is to the client, and confidential information cannot be disclosed without permission. On the other hand, the counselor must be fair with the employer. For example, psychological test data may be used, with the client's knowledge, to the extent that this will assist in the placement; medical information is interpreted in terms of the client's abilities to perform the functions of the job sought. Pertinent emotional components of disability should be explained to the employer, but counselors should be certain that they are correct in their evaluation of these factors. A vocational history indicating the kinds of jobs a client has had, their rates of pay, and reasons for leaving previous jobs is also relevant. The employer is entitled to know the facts that directly relate to the job in order to make a decision in the matter. One employer may want to know only about the client's qualifications as a worker; another may want to know these and also more about the client as a person. Pertinence of the information is the rule; discretion governs the practice of releasing information about the client.

Explaining Selective Placement

Selective placement, the matching of worker qualifications and job requirements, can be described as an employment technique applicable to the hiring and assigning of ablebodied workers. It is equally applicable in the employment of the vocationally handicapped person. The counselor can explain how, through the preparatory rehabilitation services, considerations of selective placement have been observed; in other words, that the employment objective has been determined feasible in terms of the client's physical and other capacities, interests, skills and knowledge, and potentials, and that there is every reasonable assurance that in the job category of the vocational objective this person will prove to be a competent and satisfactory worker.

In the course of explanation, the counselor can note other selective placement principles. Few, if any, jobs require all of the mental, physical, and other capacities and potentials of the workers employed. Theoretically, then, any given job can be suitably performed by a specially selected disabled person. Performance duties vary widely in jobs of the same title from place to place and even within the same factory or organization. Good placement requires more than a matching of the applicant's mechanical and physical capacities to the requirements of a job; consideration must be given to the degree of responsibility that must be assumed; the amount of initiative, adaptability, judgment, and mental alertness that must be exercised; environmental working conditions; individual temperament; and an individual's social and economic background and needs.

36.1.4. EMPLOYEE SELECTION PROCEDURES

For the most part, counselor assistance in selective placement will involve some form of job solicitation or consulting before a client's employment interview. At this stage counselors can obtain for a client an opportunity for an employment interview by overcoming interviewer prejudices or fear of hiring disabled workers. Then they will interpret the functional capabilities and limitations of the client based upon the particular job under consideration. The standard employee selection procedures are often modified if a rehabilitation facility has developed an ongoing program of supplying workers in service occupations or if counselors have a particularly notable reputation with a local businessperson.

Selection Interview

The selection interview should concentrate on job interests and skills, the applicants' future, and jobs that best serve their interest. If there is no suitable vacancy, the applicant may be willing to wait if assured of first consideration when a vacancy occurs, or may agree to a lower-grade job if assured of eventual transfer. However, if decisions are based on job vacancy alone and people are placed at too low a level of skill or interest, they may quit.

Selection interviews not only involve decisions made by interviewers; they involve decisions by applicants as to what is best for them [Hanman, 1951].

Interview with Supervisors

The employment interviewer for the firm has the responsibility for properly involving the applicant's prospective supervisors in the hiring of a rehabilitation client. No matter how astute, the interviewer may still wonder if the new worker will like the job, get along with supervisors and co-workers, and work well in team situations.

The wisdom of an informal preemployment interview with the supervisor, in which the applicant can be shown the job and be introduced to co-workers, has been demonstrated. In preparation, the interviewer makes an appointment with the supervisor, recognizing that the applicant's first impressions of the supervisor and the job will be critical. If supervisor and applicant reject each other, it is better to know this early. Since the final decision rests with supervisors and not with the personnel department, supervisors may need assistance in dealing with applicants.

36.1.5. COUNSELOR INTERVIEW ASSISTANCE

Counselor assistance in the client's employment interview is advisable only when a preliminary study has indicated its need. Since employers will usually regard the counselor's performance as an indication of the client's capability, conversational guidelines are followed to better the standing of the client as much as possible. Accompanying the client, the counselor is introduced to the employer by the client and acts as an interpreter only when consulted for explanations. Indeed, when the client and employer are conversing, the counselor refrains from interruption, knowing that this could be regarded either as interference or as an admission of the client's inadequacy.

The employer who sees a client come to a job interview with a counselor will question whether the person can function on a job if unable even to apply independently. Alternatives to obvious help are worth considering. For example, as one counselor—a woman who serves blind adults —pointed out, even though she may locate the job, sit by as the client telephones for an interview, and drive the client to the appointment, she coaches the client to be able to go to the employment office unassisted. By delaying her entrance until after the client and employer have exchanged greetings, she notes an improvement in the latter's assessment of competence and finds that discussion focuses on the particulars of the job at issue rather than on irrelevant aspects of the disability [Zadny & James, 1976].

36.2. On-the-Job Training

When an employer hesitates to hire a disabled individual and is uncertain of the applicant's ability to handle a job, the rehabilitationist might arrange for trial work experience (see 22.1.2). While small businesses are often receptive to a counselor's request for on-the-job training or trial-work experience, larger companies may be hesitant because of more stringent organizational, union, or legal requirements. Nevertheless, opportunities may be developed in large businesses by arranging for guaranteed job stations that can be used as transitional employment for a number of clients. In this way the effects of cost efficiency, compensation laws, management policy, and insurance regulations may be overcome. As with other employer-client services, one of the responsibilities of the professional is to study their legal and practical implications for training clients on the job before soliciting opportunities within the business community. (See also 14.1.6.)

36.2.1. PLANNING

In setting up on-the-job training (OJT is a common abbreviation), the counselor identifies the operations to be learned and the sequence in which they are studied. This is done through job analysis, by conference with the employer and the supervisor, and by discussion with qualified workers in the selected vocational setting who are employed where the client is to be trained. The time allocations for each unit and for the program as a whole may vary from extended to very short periods, depending upon the nature of the operations in each phase to be mastered. Agreement is then reached with the employer on what person(s) will supervise and instruct the client. Since the function of training is delegated to the employer-trainer, provisions or performance of such responsibilities should be unmistakably clear.

Similar to OJT are workshops, set up within major industries, that serve as evaluation and training programs. They can demonstrate whether unskilled or "problem" persons can adjust to the normal work demands of that industry. They use actual machinery and production items from the factory but they are located apart from the main assembly line at a place—referred to as a "vestibule"—where different speeds and quality variations can be tolerated. Disabled persons can develop specific skills and directly demonstrate to management their ability before they are accepted as regular employees. These shops usually represent more specific skills training than shops located in rehabilitation facilities, the latter offering more opportunity for personal adjustment training and task exploration. (See 23.5.)

36.2.2. FINANCING

Financing on-the-job training can range from "tuition" paid by the state vocational rehabilitation agency to the employer-trainer, or funds from a subsidized employment project, to full and regular wages, comparable to those paid a regular worker. Large factories or plants tend to

be more willing to take the client as a trainee for the position at full wages. If they have already established training programs and trainee positions, they may train the client on the same basis as other trainee-applicants.

Sometimes the counselor may have to agree on behalf of the state agency to pay tuition to the trainer (the employer) for providing on-the-job training to the client. A rather common arrangement is the progressive trainee wage scale. For example, the average experienced gas station attendant's wage is so many dollars per week for an experienced worker. The counselor talks with the owner about training a client as an attendant. The employer is not willing to pay the trainee that much a week because an experienced worker in the community can be hired for the same wage. In such a situation, the counselor might set up a progressive wage and tuition scale with gradually decreasing tuition and gradually increasing wage payments adjusted as the client acquires the knowledge that makes the rehabilitant a more useful worker.

The counselor seeks assurance that the client is neither exploited nor used as "cheap labor" and that the client actually receives full training and wage increments as provided in the training program. The client's own awareness and self-responsibility are the primary safeguard of employment rights and benefits. The counselor should also inform the trainer as to minimum wage laws, some of which grant exemptions as a way of encouraging employment and training of handicapped people. Procedures are carefully prescribed by law and must be observed judiciously.

36.2.3. SUPERVISING

The on-the-job training program outline will show the job operations to be learned, the time allocations for studying the separate operations, the person(s) who will provide the instruction, and the trainee wage scale, if any, to be paid. Copies are prepared for all parties so that each one involved will have a precise understanding of the arrangement.

Careful and close supervision by the counselor is even more important in on-the-job than in other kinds of training. The employer or designated trainer may have had no instruction in teaching principles and procedures; clients may become impatient and feel that they are not being moved ahead as rapidly as they should be or according to the training plan—perhaps without realizing that their training must be fitted into a regular work schedule. The counselor must be ready with help, advice, and explanations—and be alert for danger signals. If, for example, on one call at the station, the client is manning the pumps while the employer is greasing a car, that observation would not mean much; but, if the counselor repeatedly finds the same situation, it would indicate that the trainee is not being taught the salient skills of the job and the matter needs attention. Another part of the counselor's supervision is the periodic check on reports on training units covered, the quality of teaching and learning in these units, and the satisfaction of the trainer and client with the training arrangement.

36.2.4. ADVANTAGES

The advantages of an on-the-job training program for the client include: learning a job through practical experience, possibly receiving wages during training, and having a good chance for employment at the training place when the training program is over.

On-the-job training programs have advantages for the employer as well. The client can be taught job operations as the employer wants them done. The financial arrangements for the training are an incentive to many employers; moreover, the employer can come to know the client from trainee to employee status and gain a better idea of how effective the client will be as a regular employee.

On-the-job programs may also be used as a trial work experience. A client who has had vocational training or experience in a related field but has had no actual work experience in the selected vocational objective, may nevertheless feel well qualified to perform the particular duties of a job. The counselor may also be convinced that the client can perform those duties, but the employer may have doubts about hiring the client as a regular employee without an "on-the-job" demonstration of ability. The counselor should proceed here (as with a training program) by listing the job operations with time allocations, specifying the person(s) to rate the client's performance in each component, and negotiating a progressive wage scale completing an on-the-job demonstration or trial work program.

36.2.5. APPRENTICESHIP

An apprentice is defined as "a worker who learns, according to a written agreement, a recognized skilled trade requiring two or more years of work experience on the job through employment, supplemented by appropriate related trade instruction." Approximately ninety general trade classifications contain one or more apprenticeable occupations (e.g., airplane mechanic, bricklayer, carpenter, cook, electrician, furrier, millwright, painter, etc.).

Criteria for Apprenticeable Occupations

An apprenticeable occupation is generally understood to mean one that meets the following criteria:

1. Has been learned customarily in a practical way through training and work experience on the job.
2. Is clearly identified and commonly recognized throughout an industry.
3. Requires several years (4,000 or more hours) of work experience to learn.
4. Requires related instruction to supplement the work experience (144 hours of such instruction during each year of the apprenticeship is usually considered the minimum).
5. Does not fall into any of the following categories: selling, retailing or other distributive occupations; managerial occupations; clerical occupations; professional and semiprofessional occupations; agricultural occupations.

Standards of Apprenticeship

Standard apprenticeship programs contain provisions for the following:

1. Apprentice must be a minimum of 16 years of age.
2. A schedule of work process or operations in which experience is to be given on the job.
3. A progressively increasing schedule of wages to be paid the apprentice, which, as a minimum, should average over the period of the apprenticeship at least 50 percent of the rate paid journeymen during that period.
4. Related classroom instruction.
5. Adequate supervision of the apprentice and keeping of appropriate records of progress.
6. Joint establishment of the apprenticeship program by the employer and the employees.
7. Indication that the number of apprentices to

be employed conforms to the need in the community.

8. Review and registration of the written apprenticeship program by an apprenticeship agency of government.
9. Registration of the apprentice with the recognized apprenticeship agency.

Conditions Controlling Placement of Clients as Apprentices

During normal times, apprentices are usually selected from those in the 17 to 22 age group. The number of apprentices who can be trained at one time in one place is controlled; this is usually done under a plan that allows one apprentice to a shop and additional apprentices according to a prescribed ratio to the number of journeymen employed—perhaps one to six. For example, a plumbing shop with three journeymen plumbers could have one apprentice; but, under the one to six ratio, it could not take on a second apprentice for concurrent training with the first until at least seven journeymen plumbers were employed.

Advantages in Apprenticeship Training

Some workers do become fully qualified in occupations designated as apprenticeable without serving a regular apprenticeship. In fact, the re-

habilitation counselor may discover that establishing an on-the-job training program for the client is easier than having the client registered and trained as an apprentice. Of course, apprenticeship training and placement has its advantages: written apprenticeship training outlines have been developed and organized to produce qualified all-around skilled workers; records are kept so that apprentice and future employer can be sure of the training received; and the apprentice, upon completion of the course, receives a Certificate of Completion of Apprenticeship as evidence of proper qualifications for journeyman employment and pay.

Steps in Placing Apprentices

The counselor should take several planning steps. It is well to have a list of apprenticeable general trade classifications and occupations. (The list, with sample schedules of work experience and training required in different occupations, and a roster of the state apprenticeship agencies may be obtained from the U.S. Department of Labor, Bureau of Apprenticeship, in Washington, D.C.) The counselor should also be certain that the client is qualified and eligible for acceptance as an apprentice and for licensing. Finally the client must be registered as an apprentice. (See also 14.1.4.)

36.3. *Employee Orientation*

Counselor involvement with clients during their orientation to a new job situation will vary. Often the move into a new and uncertain work setting will provoke in a client feelings of bewilderment and anxiety, which may force return to the sheltered, protective environment of the rehabilitation facility. During the orientation process there are several ways for a counselor to ease the client's transition to the job site.

During the training and adjustment period the counselor can, first of all, build in the client a desire to work in an independent situation as well as bolster feelings of competence and self-esteem. The counselor can familiarize the client with the job site itself, using introductions to prospective supervisors and co-workers as a way of showing that they are willing to cooperate. Personnel policy, company rules, and the physical layout of the plant can also be ex-

plained, although the client should rely on the company's orientation program as much as possible. Throughout the orientation period, the counselor should be available if difficulties arise over attendance, production, co-workers, or a desire to terminate employment.

There are special considerations. If, in some cases, a client is distressed by the probation period or if initial placement is below the client's level of capability, the counselor can relate the procedures for advancement to the client. If, in other cases, a client feels suddenly abandoned, follow-up contact can be reduced gradually until the client is well integrated into the job setting. Finally, if a client fails to maintain employment, the counselor can carefully analyze the difficulties and try again.

Generally, the degree of counselor involvement will have been decided on jointly by the counselor, work supervisor, and client. Occasionally, however, the supervisor will feel equal to the task single-handed and will need no special assistance. Occasionally supervisors even resent the counselor's presence in the work area. And some company personnel officers will not give the rehabilitation counselor permission to have direct contact with a line supervisor. In any event, to make the transition from rehabilitation to competitive employment as smooth as possible, counselor should learn the biases and limitations of the employee orientation situation. Until the client feels at ease with the situation and the counselor has verified this with verbal and behavioral cues, the orientation phase is incomplete.

36.3.1. CONSIDERATIONS FOR SUPERVISORS

Supervisors should try to take special note of the extent of the handicapped worker's adjustment to physical limitations. If workers have not completely adjusted to their own physical limitations, they may be: unusually concerned about acceptance by co-workers and bosses; uneasy about special attention or provision made for their disablement; worried that handicaps will block consideration for promotion; concerned (if on incentive pay) that their functional limitations will affect the earnings of the entire group; or fearful that the handicap(s) will act as deterrents to regular consideration for seniority or transfers to other kinds of work. In other words, if workers have adjusted to their disablement, their concerns are no different from those of any other new employee: they have questions about ability to do the work, kinds of work preparation to be expected, chances for promotion, and acceptance by co-workers and supervisors [National Association of Manufacturers, 1964].

The National Association of Manufacturers (N.A.M.) has provided supervisory guidelines, which follow. "In addition to the usual preparation made for all employees, the supervisor expecting a handicapped worker to report for work may also ascertain:

1. The nature of his handicap and pertinent facts about his case history.
2. His ability to perform assigned duties (by matching the physical requirements of the job against his capacities).
3. What other jobs in the department fit his qualifications in the event a future need arises.

4. How the first conversation may be planned to put him at ease, thereby relieving any self-conscious feeling he may have.
5. How job leaders and fellow employees may be coached to receive a handicapped person without making him feel conspicuous [p. 12].

N.A.M. went on to advise that ". . . the supervisor is the key man in welcoming and accepting the new employee. It is his task to acquaint the newcomer with his assignment, help break him in and develop in him the feeling that he has something to contribute which the company needs" [p. 10].

36.3.2. INTRODUCING THE EMPLOYEE

When a new employee arrives, the supervisor should provide information about the kind of work done in the plant and the department, especially about work related to the job to which the new employee is assigned. The supervisor should also explain relationships with other employees as well as regulations concerning pay, attendance, hours of work, rest periods, lunch breaks; rules regarding clothing requirements, smoking, and so on; and any special services such as lockers, first aid, rest rooms, and cafeteria or lunch rooms.

The new employee should be introduced to other supervisors and workers. A tour of the department with an explanation of its work and its relation to the new employee's job, is a good practice. The person should be shown the work site, the desk or work bench, equipment or tools. Good supervisors would conduct such orientation to put newcomers at ease, even if they were not handicapped.

Hanman [1951] suggested that after supervisor and employee have had a conversation and a tour the supervisor then introduce the new employee to a regular worker who performs a similar job for informal demonstration and discussion. Before the new employee leaves, the job and its functional relationship to the operation of the department should be clear. As with all other workers, supervisors should keep disabled workers informed of new developments, be a sounding board for questions about rules, policies, or job routines, and should let the worker know how work is progressing.

Plant Orientation

There are good reasons for showing new workers around the plant. A practical one is to indicate where everything is located. Another is to clarify the relation of the new worker's job to other work in the plant and to emphasize again the significance of this specific job so that the worker understands that significance. But the main idea is to give the worker a genuine feeling of belonging. Many companies are extremely successful in this; workers feel a sincere loyalty to the company from the very first and it becomes almost a family.

As new workers tour the plant, they should be introduced to persons of importance along the way. A welcoming word from a plant manager or president can mean a great deal. Small firms may consider plant orientation for each new worker, while those with larger volume may have a policy of conducting tours on a periodic basis.

Orientation Class

Some hiring procedures and plants are sufficiently complex that a worker cannot grasp in a day the company aims and services. While some firms rely upon a descriptive booklet, progressive firms find that an orientation class for new workers is valuable. The class may easily fill a day, especially when combined with a plant tour and a movie or slide presentation on the industry and products involved.

Orientation classes, sometimes using various kinds of visuals, should explain the functions of the personnel and medical departments as well as the handling of safety, training, and social welfare. From this class, the new employee learns about safety and health measures. The employee should leave the class convinced that the firm can give expert help with any problem that might arise.

Job Instruction

A four-step method of job instruction has proved to be effective in getting the disabled worker into production very quickly. The steps are preparing the worker, presenting the operation one step at a time, having the worker try out on the operation in order to learn by doing (thus making the employee independent), and following up until the employee has demonstrated mastery of the job.

Safety Instruction

The worker who has certain limitations in function may also need careful instruction in job safety, including instruction on: specific safety factors applying to the job, safety equipment, the responsibility of the disabled worker for personal safety and that of fellow workers, medical and accident procedures, housekeeping, regulations (regarding fire, smoking, and hazards), and other information (e.g., availability of exits, fire escapes, and the use of elevators).

36.3.3. ROLE OF PLANT PHYSICIAN

The plant physician is charged with seeing that the work environment provides for the well-being of the workers. When applicants have severe limitations, the physician is advised, when necessary, to establish guidelines for the conduct of the applicant when employed and to set restrictions on activities within the plant.

The physician might deem it necessary in unusual circumstances to confer with the employment interviewer and supervisor, and then to recommend special considerations—such as special lunch hours, parking privileges, or conveyance to help the applicant get in and out of the plant under heavy traffic conditions—to make the placement successful.

Physicians must conduct ongoing and frequent follow-up when the worker has a progressive disability. Periodic medical examinations may well reveal the need for adaptations at the work site or changes in job duties over a period of time.

36.3.4. CO-WORKER ATTITUDES

"The question of acceptance of the handicapped by fellow employees," William Twomey reported, "is often raised by the employer. It is usually the case that within a period of several weeks, fellow employees will get to know the handicapped employee as an individual, frequently overlooking the disability. Counselor reassurance to employers along these lines is usually sufficient to overcome this objection" [U.S. IRI, 1975b, p. 4]. In any event, attitudes of employees at the job are an issue worthy of the counselor's consideration as it bears directly on job tenure.

There are no simple methods for handling problems of co-worker attitudes. Some suspicion and hostility are natural at first but usually these problems will work themselves out as the former client and co-workers become familiar with one another. The counselor, however, can hasten the resolution of these problems by being available for consultation and training to overcome the misinformation and fear that surround all kinds of deviance.

Dunn [1974a] pointed out that stereotyped expectancies about the performance of the disabled person on the part of supervisors, co-workers, or both, could adversely affect that individual: "Consider that if co-workers communicate (either overtly or covertly) that they expect the disabled person to perform at a lower level than an able-bodied person, the result is a reduction in the perceived self competence of the person. This can then be reflected in reduced work performance" [p. 87]. A gradual erosion of perceived competence, self-esteem, and performance can eventually lead to resignation or termination.

36.4. Follow-up

Most rehabilitation agencies maintain contact for a period of time with former clients who have been placed. This is to provide further adjustment services, immediate intervention should mistakes surface, employment maintenance, employer assistance, or verification of the results of the placement for program evaluation and accountability. Although rehabilitation is often a "one-time expense," the provision of postplacement service is sometimes needed to alleviate unforeseen problems resulting from poor work adjustment, underemployment, job loss, or other eventualities. By providing rather minor services, the counselor may be able to neutralize difficulties that could lead to job loss if left unattended. The result of the service is to assure that clients are suitably adjusted to their jobs and that employers are satisfied with their employees and the agency service. Adequate follow-up, consequently, reduces failures and aids in job development. In the case of severely handicapped rehabilitants, some kinds of periodic or maintenance services may be required on a lifelong basis to assure that the benefits of rehabilitation are sustained.

Federal rehabilitation rules require that state agency cases not be closed for *at least* 60 days after the rehabilitant is employed on a job. Even after closure, however, a rehabilitant can be provided "post-employment services," status 32 (see 7.2.2), without reopening the case if they do not entail a complex or comprehensive rehabilitation effort unrelated to the original plan for the client. In some cases the counselor recognizes at the time of closure that a client will need post-employment services; in other cases, an unexpected situation arises that requires further service. The post-employment services are provided to prevent future loss of gains made through rehabilitation or to upgrade the rehabilitant's employment potential. Some rehabilitation authorities have pointed out that post-employment services in fact are essential in order to "close the wasteful 'revolving door' through which clients continuously return" but that such services are not being adequately provided by the state rehabilitation agencies [Sands & Radin, 1979, p. 24].

Job sustention is more difficult for the disabled than for the nondisabled working population due to the added problems of functional limitations, degeneration and relapse, prejudice and stigma, inappropriate behavior, incompatible environment, lack of acceptance by co-workers, lack of job seniority, lack of flexibility, and the kinds of socioeconomic fluctuations in the nationwide economy that exacerbate these conditions. For example, in one study it was found that 27 percent of a group of disabled persons placed into competitive employment had been "fired" at least once during a one-year period [Dunn, 1974a]. Similarly, a follow-up of severely disabled rehabilitants in Wisconsin found that 35 percent were unemployed one year after closure [Sha'ked, Bruyere, & Wright, 1975].

These studies indicate the severity of the employment problems of former clients who are capable of functioning at a competitive level, yet have been denied employment as a result of their own behavior or circumstances beyond their control. Many, though not all, of these employment "failures" could be averted by the provision of postplacement services, while others require a modification in socioeconomic systems that are not now sensitive to the needs and abilities of disadvantaged citizens. Yet many agencies will have neither the resources nor the program guidelines to identify and serve those persons who will need long-term attention.

Since new clients are always coming to agencies for assistance, there is constant pressure to terminate involvement with individuals once they are placed and to concentrate attention on the current demand of new clients. But for some clients, agency severance is a definite disservice, because they are not able to "make it" on their own; they will either deteriorate in a marginal job or develop a cyclical lifestyle of failure-rehabilitation-placement-failure that only serve to drain the agency's resources and reputation in the eyes of the business world [Longfellow, n.d.]. Ferman [1969] suggested that a regular proportion of staff time should be allotted to follow-up activities, and that this service should be stressed for its information-gathering and support functions.

Kenneth Reagles [1979], professor at Syracuse University and director of that university's Rehabilitation Counselor Education Program, has written the *Handbook for Follow-up Studies in the Human Services*, the definitive work in this area. The book's focus is rehabilitation agency program evaluation. Reagles defines "follow-up studies" as "attempts to determine the nature and circumstances of former clients at various points in time after case services have been stopped. [Follow-up studies] are to be distinguished from 'follow-along,' 'follow-through,' or 'post-employment services' which are active interventions intended to assist recently-served clients with problems which threaten their new-found statuses of independences" [p. vii].

36.4.1. PLANNING CONTACTS

The nature of postplacement contact depends on the program limitations of the agency, the needs of each individual client, and operational restrictions made by employers. The counselor can begin planning for follow-up contact by examining the client's attitudes, level of preparation for employment and residual limitations. Follow-up contacts are most essential among high-risk situations and disability groups: the first disabled person hired by an employer, cases having a poor work history, individuals with very severe or multiple limitations. Some clients who need postplacement service will refuse to cooperate while others will cling to the dependency cycle.

It is well to examine the capabilities and restrictions of the business where the placement is made. Some employers regard follow-up as uncalled-for interference and resent the counselor's contacts. In some situations, the business and union will have access to their own counseling, medical, and job engineering staff, in which case the counselor's attempts to assist in a client's adjustment may only serve to disrupt the activities of the business.

The appropriate method of contact will vary. Most rehabilitationists have found the job-site visit most useful for determining a worker's level of adjustment and satisfaction and for maintaining a professional relationship with an employer that will guarantee personal assistance if any difficulty arises. The telephone, however, is the most efficient means for checking on the client and is satisfactory after personal visitation has been conducted for a few weeks and familiarity with the employer is established.

In some instances, the counselor may know that a representative of the state Employment Service, social worker of the welfare department, officer of the parole board, or other professional, has made or will make a follow-up call. If the report of that visit is available to the counselor and it is adequate, the employer and worker should be saved the inconvenience of a duplicate visit.

Flexibility is a primary consideration in an agency follow-up plan. Client needs may include job coaching, counseling, reengineering, or reevaluation. Continuing follow-up to assure job adjustment should be available to the client during the entire probationary period. The disabled employee is most vulnerable to discharge during this time.

Employers will generally take note of a thoroughly professional follow-up and of continuing counselor interest in the client beyond placement. During follow-up, employers can gradually become allies if the counselor talks with them about rehabilitation as a service. Thus, follow-up is also a public relations tool: it protects the placement and often leads to others.

36.4.2. ROLES

Postplacement services are not necessarily confined to the work place. The disabled person, adjusting to work and a new job, also becomes a worker within the community. Attention should therefore be paid to use of wages, budgeting, and leisure time, for example, since problems with any of these may affect the quality of job adjustment. Consequently, the scope of postplacement services must be larger than that of other rehabilitation services. While the rehabilitation counselor typically works with the disabled person and other professionals to provide rehabilitation services, postplacement services often broaden the relationship to include the employer, supervisor, co-workers, family members, friends, and others in the community [Dunn, 1974a].

Follow-up activities with clients can make use of "indigenous workers," whose performance in follow-up work has been shown to surpass that of professionals. "The familiarity with low-income neighborhoods and the ability to establish psychological and cultural rapport," according to Ferman [1969], "gives the indigenous workers a decided advantage in seeking and establishing contact with ex-clients" [p. 83]. The use of indigenous workers, Ferman thought, provides more accurate information about the client's adjustment to the job.

The family is an important factor in the adjustment of the vocationally disabled client. Younger clients, especially, sustain successful placement when the parent is positive and supportive of the counselor's planning with the client. Overprotective or meddling parents who interfere with placement make job adjustment difficult. The attitude of the marital partner is likewise crucial in the adjustment of the married client. (See 31.2.1.) A profoundly emotionally disturbed client, especially one who is leaving the hospital to try to adjust to daily life, is particularly in need of supportive family members or supportive people besides the counselor.

36.4.3. AVOIDING DEPENDENCY
Client dependency is a problem, regardless of the stage in the rehabilitation process. Counselors walk a fine line. They must encourage an appropriate level of independence, yet, as Zadny and James [1976] pointed out, they must do so "without falling into the trap of making a fetish of independence in a world in which everyone is interdependent" [p. 65]. As they said, "One can agree with the necessity for weaning from dependency, and with the necessity for assisting the client with his initial adjustment to his job, without getting into the thicket of the client's overall adjustment to life and the world in which he lives. There is a difference between assisting the client with initial orientation and adaptation to the job, both important to job retention, and a misdirected effort to assure that the client reaches his highest possible level on Maslow's Hierarchy" [p. 65]. There is a point at which the individual is capable of independent growth, and counselor intervention is no longer required. (See 28.3.)

36.5. Postplacement Services

Altogether too many rehabilitants fail to maintain what they have gained from their rehabilitation services. This is primarily due to unexpected job difficulties after the case has been closed and the rehabilitation agency no longer has contact with the client. Such failures are bad for the client, disillusioning to the employer, and expensive to the agency, which must reopen the case and begin again after the setback. It is much better to be assured of the placement before closure, or to provide postplacement services immediately as needed after the client is on the job. Postplacement follow-through services are especially important for the severely disabled. (In the public rehabilitation program this further stage is formalized as "post-employment service," case status 32.)

36.5.1. FREQUENCY AND DURATION
During the first phase of employment counseling services may be essential to the worker's psychological adjustment. The frequency and duration of the counselor's contact with employer or worker will vary, but most contacts in this orientation phase should be made during the first days of employment and no later than two weeks, thus giving the client time to adjust to the job and the employer time to observe the client. All contacts, whether initial or subsequent follow-up, should be planned and scheduled, with special attention paid to use of the employer's time.

Samuelson [1967] also recommended early initial contact but for a different reason: to verify that the job to which the client was referred is actually the job being performed. In large companies, although the personnel staff may understand the client's capacities perfectly well, the supervisor may mistakenly assign the client to unsuitable work.

The counselor must make the determination as to how much support either the client or employer needs; sometimes a call to the employer on the first day of the client's work is helpful, providing assurances of follow-up. Follow-up contacts with the client at the place of work should always have the employer's approval or should be done over the lunch hour.

A logical question inevitably comes up: How long should a rehabilitation counselor continue to oversee employed disabled persons? Dunn [1974a] suggested that some of the probationary periods, both formal and informal, already established in various kinds of work be made to correspond with the follow-up period. For example, union shops customarily use the requisite waiting period for union membership as the probationary period and so tend to discharge unsatisfactory workers before the 30, 60, or 90-day waiting period expires. (Once a worker is a union member, dismissal without substantial cause is difficult.) Typically, public Civil Service has a probationary period of six months; here too, dismissal usually takes place within the probationary period because permanent government workers are not easily discharged. Technical, professional, and management positions often classify new workers as "trainees" for a one-year probationary period, while educational employment and teaching often require three to six years before workers are granted tenure.

The problem of appropriate length of postplacement service has yet another ramification: how best to handle disabled workers in "place and train" situations. Theoretically these workers can be designated as permanently employed but they may need more rehabilitation service before they are truly effective on the job. Dunn notes that such workers may not have contact with the rehabilitation agency for extended periods and that the customary administrative approach is to close their cases as successful rehabilitations only to reopen them later on when services appear to be necessary again. It is a costly approach, both in terms of the repeated case "start-up costs" incurred and the eventual failure in some cases to recover previous levels of self-sufficiency.

While the foregoing discussion seems weighted heavily in favor of longer rather than shorter postplacement service, there are sometimes excellent reasons for limiting both frequency and duration of follow-ups. For example, one study found that the most secure clients are those who feel they are largely responsible for their own successes, that the agency and counselor played minor roles, although they were not indispensable. The clients would probably feel uncomfortable, if not insulted, with the idea of a rehabilitation counselor "waiting in the wings" for a year or more to meet any of their problems. In short, they want to be as independent as possible, as soon as possible, just like other self-supporting people [Zadny & James, 1976].

In another study, reported by Olshansky and Beach [1974], community workshops made it a policy to limit follow-up contacts to three. The policy arises out of the philosophical tenet of "normalization," which holds that workers should be treated as if they are capable of more normal behavior. While employers and workers are told that the counselor will be available if necessary, the main impetus is toward short follow-up as a way of increasing the client's maturity and feeling of autonomy.

36.5.2. JOB ADJUSTMENT

The rehabilitation counselor meets periodically with the employee to see if job adjustment is satisfactory. The counselor should consider the client's job satisfactoriness, satisfaction with the job, and levels of physical and emotional stress. These meetings may reveal latent anxieties about the job that were not communicated to supervisors. The counselor might ask the following questions to make an assessment: How do you feel physically? Are you unduly tired after work? Do you have increased symptoms or pains? Do you feel you are trying to do too much? Are you working at too fast a pace? How are you getting along with your co-workers and your supervisor? Do you feel your work is up to standard, qualitatively and quantitatively? Do you need more moral support or encouragement? Was your training adequate? Do you need more training? Are there other services that the agency could provide? Are you having any difficulties in connection with your job? How could these problems be resolved? Are you receiving full pay regularly? If the interviewer listens carefully and phrases questions thoughtfully, the interview should provide the counselor with insight into any problems endangering retention of the job. As Samuelson [1967] noted, the counselor needs to know if the client pushes or is being pushed too hard physically.

Guidelines are helpful in setting approximate measures of expectation when clients are on the job. Walker [1966] outlines such measures as a bench mark for client behavior, reliability, and work production:

Tardiness—lateness is permitted occasionally (perhaps once a month, not oftener); habitual lateness threatens job retention.

Absenteeism—absence of 6–12 days per year is usually permitted without threatening the job.

Relationships with co-workers—job retention is difficult if co-workers show overt rejection or hostility.

Relationship with supervisors—good relationship with supervisors is essential to job retention; inability to accept criticism or take orders threatens job retention.

Work production—failure to persist at work, wildly variant swings in output, and average daily output below the norm threatens job retention.

Quality of work—lack of concern for quality work or quality standards (even though the client may have the requisite skills) threatens job retention.

36.5.3. THE JOB COACH

A "job coach" is described as one whose principal responsibility is to provide supportive services to clients on the job. This person may perform a number of duties, including "counseling" the new employee, acting as liaison between the employee and supervisors, advising the line supervisor, or handling any number of job-related problems that might arise. The job coach does not police the employee but may have to intervene if the worker is constantly tardy or absent or indulges in behavior requiring disciplinary action.

Ferman [1969], in pinpointing key areas for attention in job-coaching, noted that first of all, arrangements should be made well in advance of worker placement. To make job-coaching effective, management has to know why it is done,

and further, must agree to give the job coach access to the worker and supervisors if circumstances require this. However, the job coach should avoid becoming a "truant officer" who disciplines the worker for the employer.

Second, the most effective job coaches are indigenous workers who have a real understanding of the client's life situation; these coaches are frequently recruited from neighborhoods where the hard-to-employ reside and thus can empathize with the worker's problems away from the job as well as on the job.

Third, the job coach is a connecting link between worker, agency, employer, and community services. The coach may need to explain the worker's behavior to upper management, refer the worker back to the agency, provide psychological support or access to other resources: in brief, the coach smooths the transition into the world of work.

36.5.4. EMPLOYER CONTACT

Besides checking with an employer to see if the applicant has been placed on a job after referral, the counselor may be able to suggest adaptations to assist the worker's adjustment on the job. For instance, the employer of a lip-reading worker may appreciate information on how to face the light when speaking. Suggesting a better placement of work materials or adjusting the height of the work bench may considerably assist orthopedic cases in proper job adjustment.

In interviewing the employer, the counselor can use the following questions as guidelines: Is the client acceptable as a person and as a worker? If not, why? Can existing difficulties be resolved, or should the client be removed from the job? What is the employer's reaction to the rehabilitation services program in terms of this client? What are the employer's suggestions for improvement of services? What other jobs are available? What are the requirements? Will the employer accept additional clients? Will the employer recruit through the counselor? Can the employer suggest other placement leads? Supportive services for the employer should be more than mere moral support and should help the employer "normalize" work for rehabilitants.

Chapter 37

Placement Resources

Placement resources as described here include all of the special efforts made by agencies of the community to find and maintain suitable employment for disabled people. This involves not only making people able and matching them with jobs but also their training in job-seeking skills and the education of business as to the vocational potential of disabled workers. It also includes special help in locating available work and financial support pending readjustment. This constitutes a system composed of various agencies and specialists.

The distinct responsibilities of the placement phase of rehabilitation were listed by Sieder [1966]:

1. To obtain information about the types and numbers of work opportunities in the community which are suitable for handicapped people;
2. To convince individual employers that many disabled people are excellent workers and that by giving them a chance at jobs they are equipped to fill, the employer is not making a charitable gesture, but is performing a profitable act for the company;
3. To work closely with the industrial engineers, personnel workers, and job analysts of business and industrial firms to discover what jobs are best suited to the skills of handicapped people;

4. To select workers and refer them to jobs which have been judged suitable to their skills;
5. To follow through, after handicapped workers have been placed in a job, in order to help them in the orientation process, advise them when unexpected problems come up, and evaluate their progress from time to time;
6. To enlist the interest and assistance of plant or office supervisors and other management personnel for rehabilitation; and
7. To give constant encouragement to the handicapped workers as they try to advance in their chosen vocations.

Community resources that provide placement services for people with disabilities include: the state Employment Service, the CETA programs and projects, the state rehabilitation agency (and the state rehabilitation agency for the blind), veterans' services (public and private), the community rehabilitation facilities (e.g., workshops and service centers), and various other organizations. Other community resources are an integral part of the system of agencies participating in the job placement phase of the rehabilitation process; for example, insurance programs for income and other services help the handicapped person in the job placement process.

There are many resources and influences in a community that affect the outcome of placement efforts. An informed public, understanding employers, and vigorous affirmative action programs make a more favorable climate for handicapped job-seekers. People in America's communities are beginning to realize that unless more of the disabled and aged persons in the population continue to be employed, the tax burden for their care will grow larger; and these taxes are falling on a smaller segment of the population. Communities are becoming more articulate and realistic not only about tax loads, but also about the humanitarian values associated with the rehabilitation and employment of handicapped people.

Government, insurance, health groups, and community agencies stimulate the employment of handicapped people. Among the most outstanding of these groups are the Governors' Committees on Employment of the Handicapped, which enlist the cooperation of community employers in a year-round program. The committees encourage local employers to "hire the handicapped." The Governors' Committees, like the President's National Committee, are organized on a statewide basis.

Insurance firms also exert an influence on a community. They appreciate the advantages of rehabilitation and reemployment of disabled people as an alternative to insurance benefit payments. Another source of community pressure is found in the voluntary health organizations that are concerned with the effects of disabilities.

The most direct pressure on employers to employ people who are disabled derives from the affirmative action provisions of the 1973 Rehabilitation Act. But, many employers, even without these outside pressures, had begun to develop a sense of responsibility. In particular, there is a sense of obligation toward their own employees who become disabled.

Finally, communities are realizing that rehabilitation agencies and facilities are producing employable persons who are well qualified and highly motivated to return to a productive and independent life.

37.1. CETA

CETA, a "manpower" program, reflects the programs associated with the federal Comprehensive Employment and Training Act (and its Amendments). *Manpower,* a term that back in the 1940s generally meant military strength became popular in the 1960s as a characterization of the nation's total strength in available workers. The fear of rising unemployment due to technology spurred Congress to pass laws to provide training for those who would lose their jobs to machines. This fear, however, proved less threatening than anticipated and job training under the Department of Labor's Manpower Administration subsequently focused on the hard-to-employ who were the first to lose their jobs in a slow economy.

A number of programs were initiated on both the national and local levels. Federal programs such as Job Corps, Neighborhood Youth Corps, Mainstream, Concentrated Employment Program, and New Careers were basically "categorical" in nature in that they were designed to serve specific segments of the population in a prescribed manner. Some worked well in some areas and not well in others. Complicating matters were the myriad local programs that were run by state governments, city governments, community agencies, and business enterprises. Many of these programs were funded by a variety of federal agencies, thereby creating severe coordination problems.

In order to make manpower resources more responsive to the diversity of local needs and to integrate more effectively the manpower resources of the Department of Labor, the Congress passed the Comprehensive Employment and Training Act of 1973 (PL 93-203).

37.1.1. GOALS

In CETA terms: "The purpose of this Act is to provide job training and employment opportunities for economically disadvantaged, unemployed, and underemployed persons, and to assure that training and other services lead to maximum employment opportunities and enhance self-sufficiency by establishing a flexible and decentralized system of Federal, State, and local programs." One of the primary concepts behind the passage of CETA was that of bringing the responsibility for solving manpower problems down to the local level in the belief that these problems can be most effectively dealt with there. CETA attempted to do this through a community manpower system that provides training, job-related services, and job placement. Basically, it shifted the burden of responsibility from the federal government to the states, cities, and counties, which administer their own programs, but still using federal funds.

In the hope of achieving efficiency and coordination of manpower programming, Congress authorized CETA to provide for decentralization of decision-making, maximum local flexibility, and coordination or categorization, or both, of local programming. Although coordination and efficiency at the local level are two primary goals of CETA, one of the major criticisms of the program is that CETA just does not achieve them. More specifically, CETA has been criticized as not adequately structured to prevent overlapping at the local level. Overlapping weakens programming, and lack of definition of programming leads to criticism of local administrators as "uncooperative." Whatever the case,

there are many conflicting views as to the efficacy of CETA programming and services.

Generally, the ultimate goal of CETA is the individual's attainment of self-sufficient, unsubsidized employment. In this sense, vocational rehabilitation and CETA share a common purpose: both help their clients prepare for, secure, and retain gainful employment. The common target group of public vocational rehabilitation and CETA is the handicapped population in accordance with the rehabilitation agency's definition, and the unemployed, underemployed, or economically disadvantaged as defined by CETA regulations. "Potential to achieve economic self-sufficiency" might also be added as a criterion, in light of the basic CETA purpose.

37.1.2. CONGRESSIONAL AUTHORIZATIONS

Administered by the U.S. Department of Labor (DOL), CETA's activities are authorized under the following titles.

Comprehensive Manpower Services

Title I emphasizes the provision of training manpower and supportive services leading to unsubsidized employment. Grants are made to states and localities serving as prime sponsors of comprehensive employment and training programs that offer various services: recruiting, testing, and placement; classroom and on-the-job training; work experience; transitional public service employment; and supporting services to prepare clientele for participation. Eligible people include the unemployed, underemployed, and economically disadvantaged.

Public Employment Programs

Title II creates public employment programs in areas where unemployment is high; these are transitional subsidized positions in the public sector that will lead to permanent unsubsidized employment for those who participate. Grants are made to Title I prime sponsors and Indian tribes in areas with 6.5 percent or higher unemployment for three straight months. Participants must have been underemployed or unemployed for at least 30 days.

Special Federal Programs and Responsibilities

Title III programs are administered directly by the Department of Labor, whereas programs under the other Titles are administered under grants to chief elected officials. Title III programs deal with special target groups, special manpower problems, and special geographic areas to provide manpower training and related assistance. Title III is divided into three parts. Part A is for special target groups such as Native Americans, migrant and seasonal farmworkers, other national emphasis groups such as offenders, older workers, persons of limited English-speaking ability, and (through the summer program) economically disadvantaged youth. Part B is for research and development, technical assistance and training, and labor market information. Part C is for youth programs.

Job Corps

Title IV is a residential program of intensive education, training, and counseling for disadvantaged young men and women, ages 16 through 21, that operates at 60 centers across the country.

National Commission for Manpower Policy

Title V established the National Commission for Manpower Policy, appointed by the President, to identify the nation's manpower needs, do research, and evaluate the effectiveness of federal programs.

Emergency Jobs Program

Title VI was passed in 1974 as an amendment to CETA. It establishes public employment programs for unemployed individuals; it was passed as an emergency measure to lessen the impact of high national unemployment. Jobs subsidized under Title VI need not lead to unsubsidized employment. Grants under this Title are for emergency programs to augment the number of subsidized jobs available under Title II during periods of severe unemployment. Requirements such as transitional jobs and previous unemployment of 30 days are modified somewhat because the program is an emergency one.

General Provisions

Title VII states administrative requirements: the general provisions applicable to all titles such as definitions, conditions of work and training, and prohibitions against discrimination and political activities.

Young Adult Conservation Corps

Title VIII provides jobs and training for disadvantaged youth, ages 16 through 23, from all economic backgrounds. Through an interagency agreement with DOL, it is operated by the Departments of Agriculture and Interior in both residential and nonresidential settings, offering work on conservation, wildlife, and recreation projects for 22,000 young people [U.S. DOL, Employment and Training Administration, 1977].

37.1.3. ADMINISTRATION

CETA is administered by the DOL Employment and Training Administration. Cities and counties with populations of 100,000 or more are eligible to apply for CETA funding. States may also apply for those areas that do not meet population requirements. The state program is referred to as the "Balance-of-State" program. The Prime Sponsor—either the city, county, or state program—is responsible for program design and administration. The Department of Labor reported 445 state and local governments as CETA prime sponsors in the 1977–1978 fiscal year. In effect, CETA became the first full-scale special revenue-sharing experiment by placing program design and control in the hands of the chief elected officials, who take on the responsibility as Prime Sponsors of the local CETA programming. As previously stated, this decentralization of responsibilities leads to one of the most important aspects of the CETA program because it facilitates local differences. The flexibility in determining which CETA programs are appropriate is thought to be necessary in order to deal with the specific needs in various geographic areas. Differences have been demonstrated by the ways in which local prime sponsors have designed new programs, combining traditional employment and training efforts with more experimental and innovative approaches. For example, special programming under Title III has been developed for target groups such as Native Americans, migrant workers, summer programs for youth, the School-to-Work Transition Program, older workers, and offenders.

37.1.4. SERVICES

Three general types of services are supplied by CETA: manpower services, supportive services, and other activities. Manpower services basically recruit people for CETA programs; make assessments of employability, interests, and capabilities; and develop plans for attainment of specific goals. Some typical manpower services are outreach/recruitment, assessment, counseling, classroom training, on-the-job training, temporary subsidized employment, transitional employment, job development, and job placement.

Supportive services essentially assist the individual in overcoming other personal or environmental handicaps. They help the individual to make whatever arrangements are needed to take advantage of employment opportunities, for example, transportation, health care and medical services, child care, residential support, family planning services, and legal services.

The third type of service rendered is a catch-all entitled "other activities." These may include the removal of artificial barriers to employment (e.g., discrimination, rigid attitudes of supervisors), job restructuring, revision or establishment of a merit system, or development and implementation of affirmative action plans.

37.1.5. PROGRAMS

Public service employment under CETA is designed to provide an individual with a consistent work history in a particular occupation and/or on-the-job training, and/or access to a public sector unsubsidized position. Most public service employment jobs are located in public or private nonprofit organizations. CETA normally reimburses the organizations for wages and benefits paid to CETA participants.

Another aspect of manpower services provided by CETA is exemplified by the Job Corps. The Job Corps, initially instituted under the Economic Opportunity Act of 1964, was later brought under CETA. The Corps is concerned with both basic education and vocational skills training. The unique aspect of the Corps is the concept of residential living. Job Corps is an attempt to assist disadvantaged youth to become more responsible, employable, and productive citizens. Eligible are young people, ages 16 to 20, who are out of work, out of school, and in need of education, training, counseling, and other services to help them obtain employment,

return to school, qualify for other training programs, or enlist in the Armed Forces.

Two basic concepts underlie Job Corps: first, that a change in environment is needed for the youth, and second, that the young person needs a variety of services in order to benefit from training. The Corps client is sent to a residential center that offers a variety of services to help discover and develop job potential. Job Corps is the only national manpower program that has its separate identity under CETA.

37.1.6. AGENCY COLLABORATION

Under the various titles of CETA many resources and activities are available to benefit the clients of a rehabilitation counselor. Since many potential clients for rehabilitation would also be potential clients for CETA, and a duplication of some types of services as authorized by the federal government exists, local professionals in these agencies must cooperate for the benefit of their clients.

As in public rehabilitation, services by CETA are comprehensive and flexible. One of the major differences, however, is that CETA focuses on finding the right individual for the job, while public vocational rehabilitation services are centered primarily on finding the right job for the individual. This approach is more feasible for rehabilitation because its assessment procedures are much more extensive.

Both CETA and rehabilitation finalize assessment through the use of an individual plan: for CETA the Employability Development Plan (EDP) and for public rehabilitation the Individual Written Rehabilitation Program (IWRP). Though the EDP is not compulsory, as is the IWRP, it is in general usage. It has been suggested that rehabilitation and CETA work out a joint IWRP/EDP for those clients whom they both serve. State rehabilitation counselors are required to seek the collaboration of other agencies to provide services called for in the IWRP; such available resources are called "similar services."

37.2. Employment Services

The 1978 Amendments to the 1973 Rehabilitation Act authorized "Community Service Employment Pilot Projects for Handicapped Individuals" as a U.S. Department of Labor program. This program placed DOL and its affiliates in administration of rehabilitation projects with considerable potential for the hard-to-place disabled people. These projects to create employment opportunities for the handicapped population are described elsewhere (see 33.4.14 and 37.2.3).

The primary resource discussed here is the state Employment Service (ES), although others will be mentioned. With the 1978 legislation, it is especially important for rehabilitation counselors—wherever they are employed—to be aware of the services and practices of the public employment agency.

37.2.1. HISTORY

The public ES is a federal-state system of public employment offices located in over 2,500 sites across the country. In some states the agency is now referred to as the "Job Service," although it is officially called the "Employment Service." The state ES agencies are linked to the federal government through the Employment and Training Administration (formerly the Manpower Administration) under the U.S. Department of Labor.

Background

The United States Employment Service was created in 1918 in response to the extensive manpower needs associated with World War I. The Service continued to be useful during the postwar period by assisting the reentry of veterans into the civilian labor force. After this period, however, it was continued only as a clearinghouse until the employment situation of the depression necessitated reestablishment of services. Federal legislation was then enacted to mandate a permanent bureau. The Wagner-Peyser Act of 1933 (PL 73-30) stated that, "In order to promote the establishment and maintenance of a national system of public employment offices, there is hereby created in the Department of Labor a bureau to be known as the United States Employment Service (USES)."

The history of the USES has been one of change, reflecting the current economic and social climate by adapting its programs and priorities. The main objectives of the Service are: (1) to help people become successfully employed; (2) to help employers meet their manpower needs; and (3) to help communities develop their manpower resources. The emphasis on each objective and the techniques used to pursue them are what vary with the times. One of the major conflicts within the Service concerns the priorities placed on objectives 1 and 2—worker services versus employer services. The USES was first conceived in response to the needs of employers. It was and still is a division of the Department of Labor, which suggests a focus on large-scale manpower needs rather than the needs of the individual worker. In fact, up until 1962 the USES stressed finding the best worker to fill employer needs. During the 1960s the Employment Service became much more involved in services to the disadvantaged—assisting the individual poor, unskilled, or minority worker into the labor force. Coincident with this was a marked decrease in the number of job placements. Because of this and the changing political climate, in 1973 emphasis once again moved toward satisfying employer needs.

The primary focus of the public employment agency is still job placement. Their experience and studies over the years have provided a specific body of knowledge of how successful placements can best be accomplished. Because job placement is also part of the rehabilitation process, it is important to utilize and to adapt the USES placement resources and techniques in the vocational rehabilitation of disabled people. Although the rehabilitation purpose is clearly and rightfully to respond to the needs of the disabled individual, greater attention to employers' needs is a practical approach to more and better job opportunities for clients.

37.2.2. STATE EMPLOYMENT SERVICE

The programs and services of the state employment agency as placement resources for rehabilitation are described below.

Clientele

The state ES is available to all workers who are legally qualified to work. There are no restrictions except the federal and state laws defining the types of jobs and hours of work permissible for youths under 18. Placement assistance can also be given to foreign nationals. (They may enter the United States when the Employment and Training Administration certifies to the Immigration and Naturalization Service that a shortage in the labor supply exists for a specific occupation, or for certain hiring specifications.) The ES cannot extend preference in referral to any applicant or group of applicants except in accordance with legal requirements. The Service does have a legal obligation to give priority in selection and referral to qualified veterans and to give disabled veterans priority over other veterans [Haber & Kruger, 1964].

Programs

The range of people served by the state ES network is great. They are veterans who are assisted in obtaining civilian jobs through counseling and testing, who are helped with arrangements for needed job training and other services, and who are accorded priority in referral to suitable employment. They are older workers, served by staff familiar with the special problems senior citizens encounter in finding work, and they are members of minority groups. They are youths who get needed guidance in choosing a career and preparing for it, and they are women seeking to reenter the labor force. They are people with mental or physical handicaps who only need to find suitable employment. They are poor people with limited education and few job skills, and workers with none of the special characteristics noted who may need counseling or testing or who may wish to change jobs or know what the job market is like. They are professionals who use the professional placement service [U.S. DOL, Employment Standards Administration, 1974].

The ES likewise serves all employers whose jobs to be performed or terms and conditions of employment are not contrary to federal, state, or local law. It serves large employers whose manpower needs require continuous access to the widest possible supply of labor. It serves small employers with limited personnel for recruiting and evaluating worker qualifications. It serves employers engaged in seasonal or intermittent production who, at the beginning of each work period, must recruit their entire work force. It serves those who need workers not readily available through their normal channels of hiring. For the most part, these employers are in manufacturing, retail and wholesale trade, and service industries.

Services Provided

The main services provided by the ES can be described as follows: to place people in jobs; to provide employment counseling; to assist employers in locating applicants; to render special employment services to groups such as vet-

erans, youth, the handicapped, and rural workers; to conduct labor market studies and other research related to employment; to work with other agencies involved in the employment process; and to administer or otherwise assist the Unemployment Insurance Program and special job programs such as CETA. The emphasis placed on each of these functions may vary from time to time due to legislative changes, federal guidelines, economic conditions, and local needs.

In regard to the handicapped, the ES may provide or refer handicapped job applicants to other agencies for the following services:

1. Evaluation of the handicapped job-seeker's interests, abilities, education, and work experience; and occupational testing, to help in determining a suitable vocational goal.
2. Evaluation of the handicapped person's physical and mental capacities to be sure that the chosen occupation will not aggravate the person's physical condition or jeopardize anyone's safety.
3. Referral to institutional, on-the-job, or remedial education training to prepare the handicapped person for competitive employment.
4. Referral to other agencies for supportive services, such as health and rehabilitation.
5. Analysis of jobs for the purpose of determining their physical and mental demands, or for restructuring or modifying them so they can be performed by handicapped workers.
6. Providing a wide range of high-priority services to veterans, especially disabled veterans, including preferential treatment in job placement [Committee for the Handicapped, 1974].

The term *handicapped applicant* is used to identify applicants whose handicaps meet certain definitions. The ES has established a range of handicaps with code numbers that specify the nature of the handicap (i.e., upper extremity, lower extremity, cardiovascular, and so on). State ES interviewers spend time obtaining and recording information about physical capacities of handicapped applicants so that this information can be matched with the physical demands of a job. Two methods have been used by ES offices to assess physical capacities of applicants: a physical capacities appraisal completed by the Service or a physical capacities report filled out by a physician.

Labor Market Information

Another service of interest to the rehabilitationist is the labor market information and occupational research performed by the ES. This includes data obtained not only from the community, but also from the day-to-day operations of the local ES offices in their job applicant records, occupational analysis information, and hiring specifications as indicated on employer orders for workers. The local offices collect information on the trends and levels of employment and employment opportunities in various industries and occupations; the activities that are expanding and those that are declining; the number and characteristics of unemployed workers; and the practices in the community with respect to employment of women, new workers, youth, older workers, and minority groups [Haber & Kruger, 1964].

Information on current employment, by sex and skill, is obtained from area employers along with estimates of future labor requirements for two to five years. Limited information on the age distribution of current employees is usually collected to help in developing estimates of the number of workers needed for replacements because of deaths and retirements. To give an indication of future labor requirements by occupation, the surveys cover current training programs, including apprentice programs.

Labor market information has various uses. In vocational counseling, it is necessary in assisting the counselee to choose a sound vocational objective—what openings he or she is qualified for, how stable the potential job is, and the advantages of moving or staying in the locality. Employers use labor market information for planning personnel activities, such as scheduling of operations. They use it in the making of decisions with respect to location or relocation of facilities. Various organizations interested in manpower problems, economic development, affirmative action, training, and social welfare as well as rehabilitation require such information [Haber & Kruger, 1964].

Job Placement

A critical summary of the placement program of the public employment agency is required here. There have been improvements in the 1970s through program changes in the U.S. Employment Services that now provides a "job bank book," a computer printout of job openings in area labor markets, and various management changes. Still, ES offices are not very effective in developing or otherwise locating employment opportunities for hard-to-place rehabilitation clients. Only half of all applicants are placed through this agency's efforts. Moreover, only a little more than a third of job vacancies in business and industry are filled through ES referrals. The preponderance of their job listings are in the lower to middle occupational echelon, which tend to be less desirable.

37.2.3. EMPLOYMENT PROGRAMS

In November 1978 the federal Rehabilitation Act of 1973 was amended to establish the Employment Opportunities for Handicapped Individuals Act. The first part of this legislation authorized federal subsidy for "Community Service Employment Pilot Projects for Handicapped Individuals." It was enacted to "promote useful opportunities in community service activities for handicapped individuals who have poor employment prospects." Administered by the U.S. DOL, it authorized exactly what its name said, a community service employment pilot program for handicapped individuals. Eligible persons may work in public or nonprofit projects that contribute to the general welfare of the community. The purpose is to increase employment opportunities for the disabled without displacing currently employed workers. Authorized services include training and work-related expenses, transportation, and attendant care incurred by people employed in these projects. The prevailing rate of pay is specified for project employees who also are entitled to placement services for locating unsubsidized employment when the project terminates.

Federal matching funds of 90 percent are authorized for these projects with the federal appropriation allocated to the states on a per capita basis. Preference in awards for projects is given organizations of proven ability in providing employment services to handicapped individuals.

In another part of this federal legislation, further provision was made for projects in industry for handicapped individuals. The federal rehabilitation agency was authorized to enter into agreements with individual employers and other organizations to establish jointly financed projects providing clients with training and employment in realistic work settings to prepare them for competitive employment. The law provides for modification of jobs to accommodate the clients' special needs, distribution of special aids, appliances, adapted equipment, and modification of facilities or equipment, as well as appropriate placement services. Minimum wage or better is required along with equal employment benefits. Payments to such projects cannot exceed 80 percent of the project's cost.

Also in this part of the legislation, the federal rehabilitation agency (in consultation with the Secretaries of Labor and Commerce) was authorized to make grants to or contracts with handicapped individuals to enable them to establish or operate commercial or other enterprises to develop or market their products or services.

37.2.4. PRIVATE AGENCIES

There are approximately 9,000 private employment organizations in the United States. Fees are charged to the employer or job-seeker, but only when and if the individual is hired. (About 2 or 3 million of their clients are hired each year.) Usually a percentage of the job-seeker's salary (e.g., half of one month's salary) is charged. Guidelines for ethical practice for these firms are suggested by the National Employment Association, with headquarters in Washington, D.C.

Clientele

Many private employment agencies specialize in executive, skilled, or white-collar jobs that are appropriate for only a few selected clients. Because most of these agencies operate a volume business, requiring a rapid turnover of highly marketable job-seekers, they may have little patience with problem cases. An exception to this is found when the employer is actively cooperating in affirmative action efforts. The public rehabilitation agency even then may be compromising its role if it becomes a partner in the profit-making work of a private employment firm.

Services Provided

Despite various shortcomings, the private employment agency can help the job-seeker gain access to companies and organizations that are not available through other channels [Angel, 1969]. Such firms often serve as a negotiator between the employer and job-seeker. The number and reliability of these companies vary among the states according to local labor composition and state legislation. In some countries in which public employment service is poor private firms dominate the market.

37.2.5. OTHER AGENCIES

Many government agencies and private organizations consider job placement one of their most important services and problems. Handicapped workers and their counselors should not overlook the possibility of seeking help from these sources. Sometimes they are in a unique position to help because of their contacts or procedures. Furthermore these placement channels do not carry the stigma of disablement that prospective employers may associate with a rehabilitation agency. This list, suggested by Angel, includes a few of the many available sources of help in placement: labor unions' hiring halls, religious groups and charities, Civil Service (federal, state, and local), college and university employment bureaus, nurses' registries, political patronage sources, professional societies, sales and service organizations, and so on.

37.3. State ES Guidelines

This section, which is an overview of the guidelines provided in the in-service training of their professional employees, provides an operational description of the state Employment Service (ES) agencies. It was prepared with assistance by Marilyn Groves [1978], who utilized much of the literature search for her masters thesis. Materials and information were provided by state and federal employment service personnel. It does not necessarily represent preferred methods for practitioners [e.g., McGowan & Porter, 1964; Ehrle, 1966].

In reading this material, one should remember that the basic purpose of the state ES is twofold: to find people to fill job openings and to find employment for job-seekers. It is fundamentally a manpower program designed to meet the needs of American business, but in doing this it operates as a human service agency. Agency operations reflect these dual purposes and resulting role conflicts. The ES interviewer tries to serve not only the unemployed of the community but also business, industry, and other employers.

37.3.1. APPLICATION-TAKING

When individuals come to a state ES for assistance in finding work, they complete an application that is then reviewed with an interviewer. This application contains much of the same information that would be found on an employer's application. This is a good opportunity for an applicant to develop a written record of job-related qualifications. The thoroughness with which the application is completed will then influence the quality of the selection and referral process. If all pertinent information is readily available and presented in a meaningful way on the application, then it is easier to refer the individual to suitable jobs.

Staff training stresses that it is the ES interviewer's responsibility to be sure that the application is complete, clear, and clean prior to the conclusion of the initial interview. This means that the interviewer makes certain that all questions are answered with current relevant information, that nothing is ambiguous, and that the form is legible. The application should stand on its own. When discussing an applicant with an employer, the interviewer must be familiar with necessary facts just from looking at the application.

The employment history section of the application contains the data most often used for assigning an applicant a *Dictionary of Occupational Titles (D.O.T.)* code. Because coding requires information concerning occupational capabilities about the client that is important for job placement, the process of *D.O.T.* coding develops valuable insights concerning an applicant's actual abilities. The job orders received by the agency are also described in functional terms, facilitating matching of applicants with jobs.

The application also requests job-relevant supplementary information (e.g., union status, type of work preferred, educational level, willingness to relocate, driver's license, and disabilities). Disabilities are always noted for statistical purposes even if the applicant requires no special service. In describing a disability on the application the interviewer provides information that is clear and meaningful; this means giving the functional limitation rather than medical diagnostic information. Limitations on activity are expressed specifically, showing intensity, duration, and frequency of limits. To state that a person has a cardiac impairment as a result of rheumatic fever does not provide adequate guidance. If this is all that is given a prospective employer, it will probably increase reluctance to hire the individual since the employer may misunderstand and exaggerate what the medical disability label means in terms of what the applicant can do. Much more helpful is specific functional activities information: "No damp, cold, wet environment or sudden change in temperature; no continuous lifting, carrying, pushing of objects over 50 pounds; continuous activities for under 50 pounds all right." The greater the lack of knowledge about a disability, the more important it is to state the difficulty in functional terms. Thoroughly understanding the situation, the employer will be more comfortable with it.

There is a section on the state ES application on which the interviewer writes comments. The intention here is to supply personal information that will assist further in the appropriate selection and referral of the applicant. The types of comments that are constructive and those that are inappropriate are suggested in unpublished Employment Service personnel training materials digested below.

37.3.2. COMMENTS ON APPLICATION

The "interviewer comments" section on an application offers the opportunity to describe an applicant further. Recording pertinent characteristics helps to identify an individual and is of assistance in determining job suitability and the applicant's acceptability. Consequently, personal comments by the interviewer are encouraged, but the following ground rules are set forth.

1. Avoid the discriminatory—anything that would disqualify or harm an applicant because of race, color, creed, sex, age, national origin, or handicap.
2. Avoid the derogatory—any comment that would not be suitable for the applicant to see.
3. Emphasize the positive—if an applicant makes an excellent first impression, is job-ready, has attractive manner and appearance, communicates well, and so on, it is appropri-

ate to say as much in the comment section. The comment section also offers an opportunity for positive emphasis by amplification of an applicant's training, experience, or work history or by inclusion of volunteer activity that has helped prepare an applicant for a job.

4. Avoid psychological theorizing or editorializing—these remarks should be confined to a counseling folder or not said at all. Examples are: "May be a drunk, but I'm not sure" or "Very low frustration tolerance."

5. Include relevant information on the applicant's situation or condition. Examples are: "Has large family; anxious to get off welfare and into a job" or "Recently suffered serious illness. Sufficiently recovered to return to part-time work."

ES interviewers are told that case notes provide valuable information for increasing the understanding of a client's situation. It is stressed, however, that the worker must be careful not to write notes that are discriminatory, judgmental, or speculative. These comments should be suitable for the client to see upon request.

37.3.3. INTERVIEW TECHNIQUES

Each ES applicant talks with an interviewer immediately after completing the application to be sure that all the necessary information is obtained. Agency guidelines are recounted here. To initiate the interview and encourage the applicant to talk, one must establish rapport: a friendly greeting and a relaxed manner of speaking are appropriate, as are establishing good eye contact, smiling, and sitting in a relaxed position. The interviewer starts with nonthreatening general questions. Questions phrased indirectly will assist in getting maximum information; questions that are broad and non-leading, allowing the applicant to determine what is important to share, can accomplish this. An example would be, "Tell me about your last job" as opposed to "Did you like your last job?" If the applicant should ask for clarification by asking "What do you want to know about the job?", the interviewer may respond, "Tell me whatever you think might be important." This type of questioning is likely to provide more information and information of better quality and accuracy. The question "Did you like your last

job?" can be answered with one word and may lead into the answer that the applicant feels the interviewer wants to hear. One should avoid expressing approval or criticism as this may also cause the applicant to slant answers to gain interviewer approval. The best attitude is one that is understanding and interested but not judgmental.

As the interview progresses it is helpful if the interviewer occasionally, briefly, summarizes what the applicant has said. Repeating a critical sentence controls the content of the interview and helps the applicant stay on the point. When the applicant is on a topic that merits further discussion, additional details are elicited by asking "how" or "why" questions. Taking care not to appear threatening or challenging is helpful. Example questions are, "How did that happen?" or "Why did it work that way?" Another interviewing technique is to allow pauses. A pause in the conversation gives the applicant a chance to think out the answer and also encourages conversation to fill the silence. These techniques all stimulate the applicant to talk about those topics that are relevant to the interview.

Interviews are terminated after the application and notes are completed. To signal the conclusion the interviewer can: (1) ask the applicant to summarize the discussion, (2) suggest the finish by asking if there are questions, or (3) show the conclusion by putting away papers and finalizing the discussion.

From a counselor's point of view, these agency guidelines may be professionally lacking.

37.3.4. JOB ORDER-TAKING

The process by which the ES gains information from employers about their job openings is called "order-taking." The person receiving the order obtains all relevant information and records and classifies it. The order is then filed on microfiche copy in a "Job Bank" for statewide referrals to this opening. The information on the order must be as thorough as that given on a good application.

The best approach for job order-takers, according to agency instructions, is to use the information volunteered by an employer and then ask selected questions to guide and expand the employer's job description. Questions are avoided that might lead an employer to state arbitrary hiring requirements. For example, asking about willingness to employ the physically handicapped may cause employers to describe the job as more physically demanding than it actually is. The best technique is to get the employer to elaborate on established requirements rather than suggesting additional requirements through questioning. It may be noted here that it is illegal for an employer to ask for "able-bodied" people only or otherwise to discriminate against a specific group. Placement through ES is a question of finding a qualified applicant whose capabilities match the demands of a job, not of finding out whether an employer has a willingness or reluctance to hire the handicapped or other special group. When order-takers are sure that all the necessary information has been gathered, they close the conversation by reviewing the information and action to be taken.

A complete state ES order contains the employer's requirements for performance, hiring, and acceptance, as well as address and contact person. The work performance requirements should answer these questions: What function(s) is the worker to perform? What is being used to perform the function or who receives the services? What is the technique or method? What is the product or service? This job description provides the basis for the *D.O.T.* coding of the job order. The comments in the application section pertaining to an individual's description of previous employment apply equally here. The more functionally specific the information is, the more successful the matching process between applicant and position will be. This is particularly important when a physical requirement is given. Saying "some lifting" is not sufficient, but "must lift 50 pounds every 30 minutes for 6 hours" gives important information. The order-taker should try to get performance requirements in terms of frequency, intensity, and duration of activity. Whereas performance requirements describe the job, hiring requirements represent the specific abilities and background the employer feels will be necessary for an individual to succeed. This will include amount of education, training, and/or experience. Employers may also request more subjective abilities such as, "the ability to communicate effectively verbally and in writing" or "initiative and drive." The applicant acceptance requirements are those items the employer is offering the applicant. They include information on wages, bonuses, incentives, overtime, promotional op-portunities, hours, benefits, and other working conditions that contribute to an applicant's acceptance or rejection of the job.

During this conversation with employers, the order-taker also provides information. The general characteristics of available workers are discussed using applicant files (arranged according to *D.O.T.* codes). Employers are informed of any potential problems involved in filling the order, such as unrealistic hiring requirements. Employers are also told of the services they will receive in the effort to fill the order.

37.3.5. SELECTION

"Selection" in the ES state agency is the process of choosing suitably qualified applicants for referral to job openings. The interviewer's goal is to best match the qualifications and interests of an applicant with the requirements of a job order. The recorded information gathered on applications and job orders according to agency instructions assists in this process.

The first step is to be sure the job order is fully understood, that is, to determine the performance requirements, then to establish which ones are essential and how important the others are. The interviewer also evaluates an applicant's qualifications and employment preferences in terms of the requirements of the specific job. The degree to which qualifications can be matched with job requirements is influenced by the amount of time available for the search and the number of applicants available for selection. The interviewer should refer only those who meet requirements essential for satisfactory placement. However, when applicants or time are limited, less essential requirements may be waived. The interviewer is comparing the three requirements described in relation to order-taking: work performance, employer-hiring, and applicant acceptance requirements. If necessary, the interviewer may consult the employer again to obtain further clarification of requirements or possible modification of them in light of the availability of qualified applicants. The interviewer continually strives to meet the manpower needs of the employer while at the same time assisting the applicant to find suitable employment.

37.3.6. REFERRAL

Following selection of a qualified applicant for a job order, the ES interviewer initiates the referral process: the interviewer contacts the employer to determine that the job is still open, to obtain any final instructions concerning the interview (place, time, interviewer), and to review the selected applicant's qualifications. This affords an opportunity for the interviewer to help the applicant. The interviewer discusses the applicant's abilities in light of the requirements of the job, suggests to the employer why this individual was selected for the job, and explains why this applicant is likely to be successful in that position. If the person is handicapped, this is the time when the interviewer may mention the handicap. If a handicap is readily evident or potentially related to the job it should be discussed with the employer. An invisible or minor handicap that is not job-related is not usually mentioned. When discussing an applicant's handicap, the ES interviewer is advised to present the applicant's performance ability first and then make an objective statement of the handicap. An example is, "Mr. Smith has recently performed your same kind of work quite successfully, despite a hearing loss that requires that he be given written instructions." As discussed under application-taking, a functional description of a disability will be most useful to the employer. An employer does not need diagnostic labels such as "schizophrenia" or "mental retardation" but should have information such as: this woman prefers routine work and has difficulty adapting to sudden changes in her work requirements, or this man cannot lift more than 20 pounds.

To complete the referral process the interviewer prepares applicants for the employer's interview. One gives the applicant the requisite data about the interview: time, address, whom to ask for, and so on. The better prepared the applicants are, the more successful are referrals. Applicants need to know the specific job requirements so that they may emphasize their most relevant qualifications. Knowledge about the employer's organization will help them ask pertinent questions. From the interviewer's contact with the employer they may have a good idea of questions the employer is likely to ask. Handicapped people should be prepared to discuss the handicap but also instructed to concentrate on their abilities and present themselves most positively. When it appears necessary, ES offices offer more extensive instruction in job-seeking skills.

37.3.7. JOB SOLICITATION

The primary focus of state ES' public relations efforts with employers is to promote the overall placement service and obtain more job orders. More job orders means more opportunities for applicants. However, when there are no suitable job orders on file for particular applicants, a special effort can be made to assist them. Either ES counselors or interviewers engage in what that agency refers to as "job development" (i.e., contacting employers on behalf of the specific individual to arrange an interview); the procedure as described here is actually "job solicitation."

Agency personnel are told that every applicant must have a specific job goal and the qualifications to support that goal. "Selling" an employer on an individual who cannot perform the job will only serve to alienate the employer against future contact with the referring agency. For the same reason, the job solicitation contact must be well planned. To prepare for the contact one must know all of the applicant's qualifications (experience, training, aptitudes, hobbies, motivation) and restrictions (general health, handicaps, wages, hours, location, transportation). Knowledge about employers (type of business, jobs, hiring practices, possibility of staff expansion or reduction) helps ensure productive contacts. The job solicitor should also know all possible employer objections and be prepared to answer them.

There are several agency steps in soliciting jobs. First, one establishes contact with the person who has responsibility and authority for hiring. This contact may be in person, by phone, or through a letter of introduction. Then, with a carefully planned statement, one arouses the employer's interest by introducing an applicant in terms of skills that the employer values. Interest is developed by further description of the applicant's qualifications. The job solicitor must be prepared to meet employer objections with a short positive statement. If the employer responds positively, it is time to promptly "close the sale." Since the aim is to get an interview for the applicant, this is the time to set a specific appointment and politely close the conversation.

It is reiterated here that the material in this section is from various in-service staff training guides of the U.S. Employment Service and state ES agencies. It was included to show the operations of the public employment service and its orientation.

37.4. Workers Compensation Programs

Workers compensation programs are the oldest form of social insurance in the United States. They were first enacted by state governments around the time of World War I to overcome injustices to occupationally injured or diseased workers and their families. A fixed schedule of benefits and simple claims procedures was designed to replace the uncertainties of litigation at common law or under employers' liability laws. The cost of industrial injury and disease was seen as part of the production process and was held to be a proper charge against the expense of business.

The cost to an employer for workers compensation insurance coverage varies with the risk involved (type of business and experience). It has been thought that employers would minimize work accidents if they bore the resulting cost. In the 1970s, the average cost to American employers was a little over one percent of the payroll. (Individual employer cost, however, varies widely.)

Bibliographic material on workers compensation relevant to vocational rehabilitation includes: Conley and Noble [1978], Ross [1976a], and Jaffe [1960], as well as the proceedings of a U.S. Department of Health, Education, and Welfare national training institute on the industrially injured that took place in 1976 and included papers by D.E. Galvin, L. Smedley and G.P. Sawyer.

37.4.1. HISTORY

The ancient concept of justice, that one who is injured due to the fault of another may recover payment for damages from the aggressor, was an element of English common law. Under this law the worker hurt on the job could sue the employer for damages. In actual fact, however, this was not a generous stipulation. To bring the employer to court was often too expensive for the injured worker. Furthermore, because the employers could afford the best legal help and because they were influential, "justice" was often less than even-handed. The injured employee even often had difficulty finding fellow workers who would be courageous enough to testify in their favor and against their employer. (This

historical material is from C.E. Obermann's 1965 book, *A History of Vocational Rehabilitation in America*.)

According to common law, plaintiffs in these cases had to prove that their injuries resulted from a lack of due care on the part of the employer in protecting the worker from injury. Three kinds of defenses evolved, and were accepted by the courts, that could prevent the plaintiff from recovering damages. Workers could not recover if it could be demonstrated that they took the job recognizing that there were risks involved—they were assumed to have accepted those risks. They could not recover if it could be shown that another worker contributed to the accident and injury. They could not recover if it were established that they themselves were negligent and thus contributed to the injury.

These defenses deprived many workers of payments they might justly have obtained from their employers, payments they needed in order to live and to rehabilitate themselves. However, social consciousness was increasing at the close of the last century: there was movement to improve the situation of the injured workmen. It certainly was not best for the community to have larger and larger numbers of workers become dependent because of injury.

The problem was partially alleviated in some of the American states in the early 1900s by laws that amended some of the common law defenses employers could use. The assumption-of-risk rule, the fellow-servant rule, and the contributory negligence rule were invalidated and could no longer be used against the worker. However, the necessity of going to court, the lack of uniformity and uncertainty in the awarding of payment, and the long waiting periods for decisions by the courts were still problems. It was obviously necessary to devise a better system of protecting workers and compensating them for injury.

Although the common law was accepted throughout most of the colonies, and later the states, this was never so on the European continent where a more liberal tradition for protecting workers had evolved. The concepts underlying workers compensation laws in the United States were imported from Germany and Austria, which by 1884 and 1887, respectively, had specific legislative plans for compensating injured industrial workers.

In 1908 the United States government placed into effect a law that provided for "workmen's compensation" for federal employees. Following this action and influenced by European examples, some of the states passed similar laws. It was a long time, however, before all the states had workers compensation laws. These state programs vary greatly and are generally inadequate as to vocational rehabilitation provisions.

The early rehabilitation literature stressed the intent of the rehabilitation program in relation to injured industrial workers. The original Rehabilitation Act, Public Law 236, 66th Congress, June 2, 1920, began: "That in order to provide for the promotion of vocational rehabilitation of persons disabled in industry or in any legitimate occupation . . . ." Although Section 2 of the Act provided "That for the purpose of this Act the term 'persons disabled' shall be construed to mean any person, who, by reason of a physical defect or infirmity, whether congenital or acquired by accident, injury, or disease . . . ," the early emphasis in many states was on industrially injured persons.

Vocational rehabilitation was thought of as the third step in the process of protecting and salvaging industrial workers, the first being accident prevention and the second compensation for people injured in accidents. The third step was to treat and prepare people so that they could return to some kind of work.

Those who led the movement for workers compensation contended that the program could not be completely effective unless a well-administered vocational rehabilitation endeavor was part of it. They also maintained that it was necessary to provide injured workers with all the medical treatment they needed, financial help during a retraining period, and a second-injury fund to facilitate reemployment when the time came to return to work.

Unfortunately, litigation still stands in the way of vocational rehabilitation. The motivation of a disabled worker to go back to work while awaiting settlement of a workers compensation claim is usually poor. The compensation laws were intended to reduce legalistic complexities and expedite settlements in industrial diseases and injury cases. However, the procedures have become very complicated in most states; litigation continues to delay compensation settlements and the application of effective rehabilitation procedures.

37.4.2. STATE OPERATIONS

Because of great variations in provisions of different state laws as to type, coverage, amounts of benefits paid, insurance requirements, and administrative procedures, it is not feasible to give detailed descriptions of state worker compensation provisions. However, the broad purposes of these laws—to provide medical aid and financial compensation to workers for disability sustained as a result of accident or disease in the course of their work—are important rehabilitation resources for job placement.

Not all workers are covered by workers compensation. According to particular state laws, some areas of employment (e.g., agriculture, domestic, religious, or charitable work) are exempted from coverage; too, the compensation law may not apply unless the employer has a designated minimum number of employees. About 10 percent of American workers are not covered.

Compensation insurance, again according to the state law, may be carried under a "State Fund" insurance plan, with a private insurance company, or under a self-insurance plan if the employer can qualify. Under all workers compensation laws, medical aid must be furnished to injured employees; in some cases, however, there are specified limitations on the period of time and the cost of medical aid that must be provided.

The amount of compensation that disabled workers receive for their injuries or diseases is usually computed on a percentage of their weekly wage rate (in most instances it is two-thirds of former pay). However, because of requirements or lapsed waiting periods before payments begin and maximum dollar restrictions on the amount payable, a temporarily disabled worker may actually be paid as little as one-third of actual pay loss.

Money payments to the injured worker for certain disabilities such as loss (or loss of use) of hearing, speech, and vision or of a member, including finger, hand, arm, toe, foot, and leg are usually made according to a "schedule" determined by the state (i.e., a designated payment on a weekly or monthly basis for a specified length of time). "Weeks of compensation" means that in a given state every covered worker so disabled will receive a specified number of weeks of compensation for the loss. Some idea of the disparity in the provisions of workers compensation laws is obtained by comparison of scheduled benefits among the states. For example, 100 weeks of compensation for the loss of the use of an eye are paid under the schedules of several states, while in another state, provision is made for payments up to 275 weeks for the same disability.

Disabilities resulting from head and back injuries, heart conditions, and others are recompensed on a "nonscheduled" basis. Except as maximums may apply as to total dollar payment or length of payment period, compensation benefits are adjusted to individual circumstances.

37.4.3. CLAIM PROCESSES

It is generally required that workers must give prompt notice of any injury, accident, event, or symptom that might establish their eligibility for coverage under workers compensation laws. They may forfeit their right to benefits if they fail to do so. However, under certain conditions, claims may be filed one year and even several years after the date of the attributed cause. Applicants for rehabilitation services who are disabled by injury or disease sustained in the course of, or in causal relation to, former work—particularly when there has been a delay in the onset or manifestation of disability or when they have been separated from the liable employer—may not realize that they have a legal claim for medical and compensation benefits.

There has been a liberalization in interpretation of liability under workers compensation regulations; for example, cardiac conditions that in earlier years were rarely compensable are commonly accepted under many jurisdictions when the claimant is disabled immediately after unusual physical and other trauma. In some instances, claims are being accepted even when the "attack" is delayed. This same kind of liberalization is being applied with respect to a variety of disabilities resulting from accident and disease.

Compensation payments for disability are generally spread out over a period of time to protect workers and their families against economic disaster. Experience has shown that lump-sum settlements are generally not advantageous to the long-term welfare of the disabled worker. However, many compensation boards will consider lump-sum financial settlements of the worker's claim for disability on recommendation of a qualified person or agency, including the state rehabilitation agency. It is necessary to show that the money will be invested or utilized to rehabilitate the worker.

37.4.4. TECHNICAL EXPLANATIONS

Although there are substantial variations from state to state, there are six major classifications of workers compensation benefits. These are defined below, along with an indication of their implementation.

TEMPORARY TOTAL DISABILITY PAY. This is a weekly income replacement benefit that is payable after a brief waiting period, usually three to seven days. If the disability continues for a longer period of time, typically two to four weeks, benefits may be paid retroactive to the date of injury.

TEMPORARY PARTIAL DISABILITY BENEFITS. These are provided during the convalescent period if the injured employee works part-time and is earning less than full pay.

PERMANENT PARTIAL DISABILITY AWARDS. These are lump-sum payments, according to a fixed schedule, for loss of an eye, hand, finger, foot, toe, and so forth. In most states the amount payable is a specific number of weeks of benefits (based on the body member lost or impaired) multiplied by the worker's weekly disability pay entitlement.

PERMANENT TOTAL DISABILITY AWARDS. When a total disability is considered to be permanent, the time limit for benefit payments is extended to life in most states. However, more restrictive limits (time or dollars) still exist in a number of states.

MEDICAL CARE BENEFITS AND REHABILITATION. Nearly all of the states now provide for full medical care and physical rehabilitation service without limitations on time or dollars.

SURVIVOR'S BENEFITS. All states provide for a burial allowance. Weekly payments for widows and dependent children are specified also, but with state variations in weekly and lifetime maximum allowance.

Thirty-six states have compulsory laws requiring employers to accept state provisions and to provide the benefits specified. The remaining states have elective laws that permit an employer to reject the state's law and to defend the company against worker suits, but without the protection of common-law defenses (assumption of risk, contributory negligence, and negligence of fellow workers). On the other hand, if an employee rejects the state law and sues an employer who has accepted it, the employer usually retains the right to use the three common-law defenses, which are listed here.

ASSUMPTION OF RISK DOCTRINE. It is presumed that the worker who is injured was aware of the hazards and accepted the risk along with the employment.

CONTRIBUTORY NEGLIGENCE DOCTRINE. Employers are not liable if an accident results from the employee's own negligence.

FELLOW-SERVANT RULE. If an employee is injured through the negligence of a fellow worker, the employer is not responsible.

37.4.5. SPECIAL PLACEMENT PROBLEMS

The most frequently heard excuse for not hiring a handicapped worker is that workers compensation insurance costs would be increased. A federal report [U.S. GTP, 1956a] made this rebuttal:

It is true that a poor accident experience—that is, a relatively high number or cost of claims over a period of time—will cause an increase in an employer's compensation insurance rates. It is equally true that if a disabled worker would be more apt to have accidents and consequently suffer greater disability, as some people once believed, then an employer's insurance costs might eventually go up. But, and this should not be forgotten, research studies . . . have shown that when placed at the proper jobs the handicapped have an accident experience that is as good as their able-bodied fellow workers—and is often superior. So then, this possibility for an increase in an employer's compensation insurance costs is nullified [p. 48].

It must be remembered, too, that workers compensation insurance is a lucrative business for the several private companies that write this type of policy. They are unlikely to interfere with such an important social issue as the employment of disabled people by penalizing employers who do so.

37.4.6. SECOND-INJURY PROTECTION

To protect the individual employer against excessive claims for permanent total disability when an occupational injury is superimposed upon a preexisting disablement of an employee, most states have included second-injury provisions in their state compensation laws. World War II provided the stimulus to increased enactment of these laws because of the wartime need to utilize handicapped persons, and because of a desire to ease the employment problems of returning disabled veterans.

Provisions of these laws differ in the various states, but their main objective is to avoid penalizing either the worker or the employer should the former be injured again and, as a result, be totally disabled. The worker is protected in this contingency by receiving compensation for total disability, but the employer is assessed only with costs of the second injury. The assessment for total disability is spread among all employers by charging it to a second-injury (sometimes called subsequent-injury) fund. The interpretation of eligibility differs widely among the states, but ideally it is designed to spread the cost of second injuries among all employers rather than to charge the individual employer with the entire cost.

Methods of financing the second-injury fund (some states use a combination of two methods) include: special appropriations by state legislatures; assessment against insurance carriers (or self-insurers) proportionate to total compensation paid by all such carriers; assessment of employers or their carrier with specific charges when a worker has been killed and leaves no dependents; and payment of flat amounts in cases of permanent partial disability.

Most cooperating companies believe the idea behind second-injury laws is good, but they criticize such laws as being too limited in scope and too vague in defining their coverage. For example, the law may be effective only when the worker who is missing an arm, leg, hand, foot, or eye suffers the loss of another such member.

Liberal interpretation of compensation laws sometimes results in awards for aggravation of diseases, even without evidence that work duties of the claimant did affect or could affect the disease. Since few second-injury laws cover this type of case, the employer may become liable for the full claim [National Industrial Conference Board, 1957].

"Waiver of compensation" is another legal issue. The establishment of the second-injury fund helps to prevent pressure on employees already handicapped to waive their right to compensation in the event of subsequent injury. Such waivers are now restricted or prohibited in most jurisdictions. There are still a few states, however, where employees handicapped by an existing disability such as blindness, epilepsy, or loss of a member, may by special contract waive their right to compensation in the event of a subsequent injury, subject to approval by the compensation agency. Where such a practice exists, the scope of the compensation law is narrowed and workers and their dependents may personally suffer losses [U.S. GTP, 1956a].

37.4.7. DEFICIENCIES

Serious deficiencies exist in the present state workers compensation system: inequity, inefficiency, and incomplete coverage, as summarized from a two-year federal study. A 1977 federal Interdepartmental Workers' Compensation Task Force reported on the need for reform of state workers compensation. The report was signed by officials representing the U.S. Departments of Labor, Health, Education and Welfare, Commerce, and Housing and Urban Development, as well as the Office of Management and Budget. While they did not go so far as to recommend federalization of the system "at this time," they did state the need to "monitor" activity and to "assist" the states with their workers compensation programs.

The problem lies with permanently disabled persons rather than the "medical only" or temporary disability claimants. Based upon their research and investigations, the Task Force stated:

Our overall assessment of the system today is mixed. We believe that the medical only and temporary disability claimants are handled well. These cases represent about 95 percent of those in the system.

However, we are deeply concerned about the permanent disability, work-related death, and occupational disease cases. Although the permanent disability and death cases constitute only about five percent of workers' compensation claims, they are responsible for about 50 percent of the benefit payments. With respect to these cases, we find excessive litigation, long delays in payment, high subsequent rates of persons without employment, and little relationship between the benefits awarded and the actual wage loss.

Most of the problem comes from a settlement system focused on ending the liability of carriers and employers, either by compromise and release, or by a lump sum or "weeks of benefit" arrangement that attempts to foretell the amount of wage loss that will be sustained by a person with a specific type and degree of impairment. Studies for the Task Force indicated that such estimates are subject to large error.

Compensation for wage loss should be separated from other benefits provided under workers compensation. These wage-replacement benefits should be paid as wage loss accrues. Under present state workers compensation procedures, the start of payments is unduly delayed after onset of disability, and there are arbitrary limits in the amount and duration of benefits. Future income needs are often unmet because of this, and also because of inaccurate estimates of losses. The latter is compounded by legal compromises on the amount of the employer's liability and by lump sum settlements through which the injured worker relinquishes further recompense.

Workers compensation as an insurance for those persons who become vocationally handicapped should focus on wage replacement or rehabilitation and reemployment, or both. (Prompt and adequate medical care is essential in all cases of industrial accident and disease whether or not a handicap results.) It is necessary to separate income protection from the issue of indemnity (i.e., a sum of money given in settlement for personal damage suffered). The latter, for example, compensation for the loss of an ear, is permanent but may be only partial in that the worker returns to the same job without wage loss other than for a short period after the accident.

Since the World War I period when state workers compensation began, there have been many advances in the human service systems. Workers compensation should be integrated into other public programming for income maintenance, health care, vocational rehabilitation, and also programs for the prevention of industrial diseases and accidents. The 1970 federal Occupational Safety and Health Act (PL 91-596)—OSHA—established the "National Commission on State Worker's Compensation Laws." This has led to many analytical reports covering various subjects (e.g., litigation, data systems, program interrelationships, and experience ratings). It is clear that the administration of state workers compensation does not fully utilize modern components of the human services delivery system.

Litigation is costly and time-consuming and often results in unfair settlements—particularly in the instance of occupational disease. It is difficult to understand how profit-oriented systems can be fair to workers who are impaired in industry due to probable exposure to hazardous substances that may result in long-latency diseases. As presently constituted, it is an adversary system that expends too much of the premium dollar in the "friction" costs accruing to the workers compensation insurance carrier and other costs for purposes alien to the reparation of the injured worker. Only slightly more than half of the premium dollar goes to the claimant as benefits. A great deal of money is spent in the adjudication of claims in the absence of a "no-fault" doctrine.

The lack of program interrelationships and data systems is another sign of program obsolescence. This means that workers who are entitled to compensation are uninformed about their rights—particularly those who suffer from industrial diseases. Moreover, claimants are not well informed about rehabilitation and other services. There is also a lack of coordination with social security insurance provisions for retirement and disability insurance and medical care.

Companies should be compelled to pay higher premiums if they fail to provide a safe environment for their workers or fail to rehire those who are disabled. But, the present system does not properly set premium rates for workers compensation insurance coverage. Government should have input into rate-setting for high-risk companies. And the state rehabilitation and Employment Service agency experience with employers who hire handicapped workers is neither reported nor considered in setting insurance rates on the basis of the company's (re)employment experience.

There is no public insurance provision for product liability (i.e., compensation to consumers for injury from a faulty or dangerous industrial product). Although this issue is closely allied to workers compensation, no provision for this problem is made by the states.

Finally, as suggested earlier, there are substantial exclusions and gaps in coverage by the state workers compensation laws. Those who do receive benefits have often fought long-term and expensive legal battles, and even then the settlements vary greatly from state to state and do not pay a reasonable portion of the total wages lost. There are not even adjustments for inflation in most of the states.

37.5. Unemployment Insurance

The 1935 federal Social Security Act (PL 74-271) set up a state-federal system of unemployment insurance financed by employer payroll taxes. Subsequently the federal government has offered financial backing for the state systems and in recession periods has provided extended benefits. Both benefits and contributions are determined by the states, but federal law sets minimum standards and financial arrangements that structure the program. Still there are substantial variations among the states in the amount and duration of benefits.

37.5.1. THE NATURE OF UNEMPLOYMENT

Fluctuations in the labor force result not only from changes in supply of workers but also from changes in economic conditions. Recession stages in the business cycle cause higher unemployment. These recessions affect some workers more than others. People in the "primary" labor market have relatively stable employment as well as good pay and working conditions. The "secondary" labor market employs the residual labor supply; this disadvantaged category includes a disproportionate number of minority, undereducated, unskilled, and disabled or handicapped persons as well as youths and women who have not been working. This group is most drastically affected by periods and places of high unemployment.

The federal government defines the rate of unemployment primarily in terms of the activity of looking for work on the part of persons who did not work during a survey week. This criteria of job-seeking excludes many people who are in fact unemployed (e.g., temporarily laid-off employees awaiting callback, persons waiting to start a new job, temporarily ill people, and individuals who have been rebuffed for so long that they have become demoralized and have given up looking for work). Likewise, statistical provisions are not made for the subemployed: (1) labor market "dropouts," (2) part-time workers who want full-time employment, (3) people working at substandard wages in full-time jobs, and (4) self-employed people with inadequate income.

It is customary to classify unemployment as cyclical, seasonal, between jobs, and so on. All forms of unemployment other than that attributable to the business cycle are referred to as "frictional unemployment." "Structural unemployment" refers to shifts in techniques and equipment or labor market structure. Automation and other changes not only cause unemployment but also change the training requirements needed. There has been a long-term market shift in the United States from manufacturing to service and other occupations with less demand for unskilled people.

37.5.2. INSURANCE PROVISIONS

While the federal government determines the major characteristics of unemployment insurance, there are variations among the states. Inadequacies in some of the states' provisions led the federal government in 1970 to extend benefits for an additional 13 weeks after 26 weeks of regular benefits. In 1974 the maximum was extended to 65 weeks. The $25 billion disbursed to the unemployed during 1974 to 1975 moderated the impact of the economic recession of that period.

Federal employees, ex-servicemen, and railroad workers are covered in separate federal systems. Special federal benefits may also go to workers temporarily unemployed because of national disaster or increased foreign imports.

Unemployment insurance protects workers only against *involuntary* unemployment. To qualify, they must have been laid off recently from covered jobs; those who quit or were fired for misconduct are denied benefits for part or all the time they are unemployed. To apply for payments, jobless workers must file a claim and register for work at the nearest state Employment Service (or unemployment insurance) office. While drawing benefits, they must be available for work.

Unemployment benefits are a right, not based on need. Hence income unrelated to former jobs does not affect benefits. Since the program is designed to compensate workers for their wage loss, however, the receiving of payments related to wages—such as severance pay, workers compensation, and pension benefits—are considered disqualifying in some states.

State laws determine the amount workers receive and the length of time they are paid. In general the weekly benefit amount is based on a person's employment and earnings during a recent one-year period and is limited by state maximums. In most states, the number of weeks a worker can draw benefits is related to earnings or length of employment [U.S. DOL, Employment Standards Administration, 1974].

Chapter 38

Job Development

The primary goal of a job development program is to assist employers in developing an environment conducive to employing disabled people. Relationships with businesses are established that lead to the provision of services for the mutual benefit of employers and clients. Job development, in the perspective of a long-term agency program, is not viewed primarily as the activity of soliciting employment opportunities. Rather, it is regarded as a comprehensive professional service that seeks to involve employers in the process of creating viable career patterns for their personnel. In this context, job opportunities come about as a result of the successful consequences of selective placement, agency training services, adjustment counseling, and job modification.

Acknowledgment for ideas and information used in this chapter is due to Louis Ferman of the University of Michigan. Ferman's 1969 book, *Job Development for the Hard-to-Employ,* is available from the publications office of the Institute of Labor and Industrial Relations, Ann Arbor, Michigan.

38.1. Principles

The strategy in job development is to work with the employer in evolving a logic of operation rather than trying to place a particular client. Employers are asked to go beyond the mere hiring of disabled applicants by making changes and modifications in their occupational and work structure and creating suitable "new jobs." These modifications are undertaken as improvements in operation rather than rationalized as a social cost. As this approach is implemented and the efforts for job development gain acceptance with employers, increased involvement of rehabilitation services and more job opportunities for clients can be expected. Job development needs to be more intensive at the beginning of a project, requiring a substantial initial investment of resources. After a foundation of satisfactory employer relations is laid, a steady flow of job openings can be expected to follow.

38.1.1. PLANNING

Job development, as Ferman [1969] emphasized, does not begin with a random solicitation of employers for jobs suitable for the disabled. Before any firm is approached, it is wise to know the dynamics of the local labor market, the power structure of the community, and the internal workings of local companies. Technical expertise is required to chart these influence patterns and to analyze circumstances of community manpower utilization and underutilization. It is also necessary to inventory the work skills that are currently in demand by employers and the characteristics of the local labor force. Attention is given to personnel employment practices. Knowledge of these community business patterns enables the staff of the job development unit to influence decisions about the creation and structure of jobs, selection criteria, and other planning strategies.

Job Solicitation

Multi-agency job development efforts may overemphasize the solicitation of jobs from employers to place individuals or to form a job-pool in the agency. Finding job openings is important, but the whole program may fail without the broad perspective and planning necessary to convince the business community of the need for reassessing old employment practices and assumptions. The job solicitation campaign should be conducted primarily as a means of producing job pledges or openings.

Telephoning employers who place classified ads in newspapers or pursuing leads in the yellow pages of the phone book may result in placements but such methods offer two dangers. First, the object of job development is to produce meaningful job opportunities that are consistent with the client's expectations and needs—not unsuitable and dead-end jobs. Second, the jobs solicited may be temporary (e.g., seasonal work) and may not solve the client's long-range job problems. As Ferman said, contacts between agency and employer should develop on an "order-placing" rather than "job-begging" basis.

The oversolicitation of jobs by competing agencies often leads to complaints by employers. Federal funds for "job development programs for the handicapped" are disbursed through a proliferation of authorities and overlapping programs. Without providing clear guidelines, federal (and state) officials charge local practitioners with the responsibility for interagency cooperation. And the professional is evaluated on the basis of placements. The resulting competition and duplication of effort are time-consuming and confusing to local employers. Anyway, constant solicitation alone is seldom fruitful when it is not an intrinsic part of a coordinated and persuasive approach to job

development as a well-grounded, comprehensive service program.

Employer Involvement

"It is axiomatic," Ferman [1969] said, "that the first step in effective job development is to involve the management community in the goals, practices, and activities of the job development unit [p. 54]." In organizing a program of job development, the expertise of management executives should be actively recruited. It is a sound strategy to ask for committed support from participating management at the very beginning. Too frequently, however, involvement by management is simply a verbal commitment to pledge jobs, which evaporates without effective follow-up.

Survey Information

The information accumulated about the employment community includes the nature of the business—products, services, location, number of employees, and suppliers; the composition of the labor force—types of jobs performed, number of males or females, turnover, and seasonality; hiring practices—personnel, procedures, preferences, medical and intelligence requirements, testing, training, wage scale, fringe benefits, interview content; job characteristics—required level of flexibility, lines of promotion and transfer, union participation, shifts, hours, safety experience, supervisory relationships, and co-worker attitudes; and the local system—union influence, state Employment Service effectiveness, involvement of other groups and human service agencies, local climate for affirmative action programs. Records are made on each contact, noting receptivity to the agency program, names and functions of contact people, union-management issues, influence and decision-making processes and people, interests and activities of management personnel [Forde, 1963].

A comprehensive survey can be conducted to obtain information, train the agency staff in business characteristics, and introduce agency services to employers. Approaching employers for information in this way makes the initial contact nonthreatening; it allows them to express their interests and needs, thereby facilitating future cooperation. When coordinated with the agency's job development program, the survey may be conducted by re-habilitation students, paraprofessionals, or new counselors, but, with high standards of preparation, organization, and performance because the agency's job development reputation depends upon their behavior [Zadny & James, 1976].

Community Business Information

Daniel Sinick [1962], a noted authority on placement issues in rehabilitation, has pointed out the importance of being well-informed. Since the establishment of relationships with business leaders can be a delicate and long-term process, a current base of information enables counselors to identify potentially desirable contacts and to coordinate their efforts. Employers expect the rehabilitationist to be aware of their company needs and goals and to collaborate within a framework of a mutually beneficial joint policy. Recording information and summarizing the activities of each employer are essential in job development programs in order to enable the counselor to review pertinent information before each contact. Sources of general information include employer associations, chambers of commerce, state Employment Service agencies, affirmative action offices, service clubs, fraternal organizations, civic and religious organizations, trade journals, newspapers, labor unions, former clients, safety engineers, and school placement counselors, as well as business surveys.

Labor Market Information

Inadequate information about the labor market can be a serious drawback in planning job development efforts. Nationally, the best labor market information is developed and filed by the state Employment Service offices. The U.S. Department of Labor compiles and analyzes this data on job market trends. Various forms of these studies are issued through the U.S. Government Printing Office and are available periodically. State and local Employment Service offices also make reports available.

These data can be used to construct profiles of labor market trends. Unfilled openings studies are probably the best single source of job vacancies, although they will not give a portrait of the opportunities in particular companies. Moreover, the unfilled job orders at the state Employment Service office are more likely to reflect shortages of technical or skilled workers than entry-level job opportunities for the hard-to-employ.

Community Patterns of Influence

Job development must operate in a community context. Knowledge of community attitudes, resources, and influence patterns has obvious implications for the development of job opportunities for the handicapped. It is crucial to build an understanding about the subtleties of influence and decision-making and to accumulate knowledge about the resources of the community.

Job development units can effectively utilize the services of retired business leaders in the community as well as loaned or volunteer executives from local companies to give the unit consulting and training expertise on local corporate structures. Understanding can be gained also by appointing local business leaders to an agency advisory board. These leaders may also act as intermediaries between staff and their companies. In this way, the agency gets the information required to plan an approach to management and a strategy to induce change in job policy.

Familiarity with Business Practice

Communicating with people in business requires some familiarity with management practices. Although the counselor is not expected to be a specialist in business law, personnel administration, labor relations, industrial engineering, and marketing, basic sensitivities need to be acquired by the rehabilitationist in order to convey an appreciation for the employer's position. This requires some awareness of the pressures of the competitive marketplace, the struggles of new businesses to survive, the concern over reputation, deadlines for production, and the responsibilities for the employment and safety of employees. Employers appreciate placement workers who are perceptive of their problems and point of view.

Developing a sensitivity to the employer's situation and needs encourages a willingness on the part of employers to discuss these problems with rehabilitationists, thereby providing information useful to the job development program. The rehabilitation staff can consult on problems of a personnel-related nature (e.g., worker behavior, production, absenteeism, or turnover).

Particularly with handicap-related difficulties, the rehabilitationist is in a position to suggest agency services that might help alleviate the difficulty [U.S. IRI, 1975b].

Preparing for the Initial Contact

The weakest link in the development of an agency-employer relationship, according to Ferman, has been the lack of preparation preceding the initial contact. Cold solicitation either in person or by telephone is not effective in selling job development to the employer as a viable concept. Five basic steps should precede the initial contact.

1. A thorough study is made of the structure of the industry, including manpower and technological trends, growth patterns, status of handicap employment, and previous experience with employment of the handicapped. It is important to identify job areas suitable either in their present form or through restructuring.
2. The target firm should be analyzed for its traditional sources of manpower, competitive position, growth/decline picture in earnings, technological development, and production plans. More important than current job vacancies is data on the potential of the company to create jobs and to restructure other jobs.
3. The power structure of the firm should be outlined, with emphasis on assumptions about employment and decision-making patterns. For example, the front office personnel worker may not set job standards or qualifications but merely acts to fill a prescribed job order. The actual decision as to what goes into the job order may be made by the department head or a company job analyst, so any change must be negotiated at their level.
4. Previous experiences with inducing change in the company should be analyzed to identify the strategies that led to success.
5. Finally, it is necessary to determine how the individual may be reached (i.e., to select a proper setting and strategy of persuasion).

Public Relations

A component of planning is to develop a receptive attitude on the part of employers and to in-

form them of agency services. There are various techniques, such as having counselors speak before fraternal organizations, public service groups, personnel management and business associations, and other groups that provide an informal setting for making contacts. Feature articles, awards for public service, and new promotional campaigns are brought to the attention of the radio and television networks and newspapers as a means of encouraging general public awareness and the consequent influencing of public-minded employers. Various nonprofit groups and public committees on the employment of the handicapped can also provide assistance in introducing the agency program to employers. (See 10-4.)

Small Businesses

It is best to contact small businesses (under 25 employees) on an informal basis. Since most of these business managers are intimately involved in the day-to-day operation of the business, they can be visited during periods of reduced activity and without making advance appointments. Personnel procedures in the small business are generally less restrictive and more flexible than those of larger businesses, making it easier to arrange on-the-job training or trial employment for clients. The rehabilitant must be versatile, however, because the small business employee must usually work at several different jobs as production demands vary or absences require temporary replacement at another job station. As the survival of these businesses is closely associated with community relations, they will tend to be responsive to agency services that have public support, are used by competitors, are approved by bankers, or are discussed in local media and associations. As many small businesses are on shaky financial ground, however, philanthropic interests tend to follow practical concerns in the matter of hiring workers [Mallas, 1965].

Medium-Size Businesses

The medium-size business (employing 25 to 100 persons) may be the most viable size for job development purposes. It is large enough to provide a constant potential for job openings, while financially it is usually secure enough to make long-term planning and arrangements for client occupational growth possible. As the personnel staff is likely to be small, agency services such as client evaluation, selective placement, and training are likely to be appealing, especially in regard to jobs showing a high turnover problem. In addition, the employer, having achieved a higher financial status in the community, is more influenced by public opinion, bankers, and the attitudes of the affluent social set, all of this generally creating interest in the social-service orientation of agency programs. The need for appointments for interviews is more common in this group than among small businesses [Mallas].

Big Business

Big business is most vulnerable to regulations of the 1973 Rehabilitation Act requiring affirmative action in the employment of disabled employees by companies with federal contracts. Moreover, they provide the largest variety of jobs and consequently the best situation for applying the techniques of selective placement. Sophistication in their hiring practices and personnel policies, however, has made it difficult to get disabled clients past the screening procedures. Many large companies, it should be realized, have a good record of retaining employees who become disabled on the job. Personnel managers and supervisors are often far removed from the administrative branch of the business, with the result that favorable hiring policies toward the disabled may not be implemented at the operations level. While approval of the company president of large multi-city corporations is a prerequisite for a job development program, time and effort must also be invested to get the assistance of local management. As the company president will usually have time and interest for meeting with agency representatives, on an appointment basis, there exists the opportunity of getting administrative support and the assistance of medical, engineering, marketing, and legal staff as well.

At this level, business executives generally can afford greater altruistic interests and can be receptive to an approach that emphasizes the social service orientation of the agency program and the goal of achieving self-sufficiency. Familiarity with business practices, the nature of the business being visited, employment laws, and insurance for disabled workers is essential in this situation, as the employer and staff are used to operating at a high level of sophistication and

efficiency. Visitation by two representatives may be effective in providing the breadth of expertise that may be expected by the company head [Mallas].

38.1.2. PRESENTING THE SERVICE

Employment of disabled workers is based on the same principles that result in the effective use of able-bodied workers—matching individuals to jobs for which they are suited by virtue of education, aptitude, skill, experience, interest, and physical abilities. Those employers who use hit-or-miss methods of selection, depending upon subjective impressions of the applicant's physique, personality, and qualifications, often do a disservice to themselves and those they hire. While many employees selected on the basis of such criteria do work out satisfactorily, misfits, poor producers, and disgruntled employees also result from this subjective method. The rehabilitation agency helps employers to avoid these problems through its job development and placement services.

Techniques

The presentation of the agency service package as a professional activity is not to be confused with the "hard sell" tactics sometimes used in retail merchandising. The presentation does not take place in a pressure atmosphere, there is no false advertising or misleading persuasion, and the goal is not to take advantage of a gullible employer. The rehabilitationist's function is to provide a professional service that results in satisfaction for both the employer and the client. Nevertheless, ethical sales techniques can be incorporated into the presentation of the agency service. The employer's curiosity and interest are stimulated by an explanation of the advantages of the service. Evidence of the value of the service is set forth in the form of client performance statistics, examples of successful cases, portfolios of client work samples, and commentary on the participation of competitors in the program. The staff of the agency are pledged to assess and refer only qualified applicants and then to provide the follow-up adjustment services necessary to assure optimal results from individual placements. Job openings are solicited from employers, but not in the context of slogans, their social obligations, or their guilt. Rather, job solicitation is viewed in the context of the employer's overall, long-term participation in job development programs that are available when needed by the employer. Persuasion of the employer to participate is based upon the agency's ability to demonstrate the value of its services.

Professional Behavior

The rehabilitationist's success in communicating with employers is largely dependent upon appropriate professional behavior in the employer interview situation. The rehabilitationist prepares information on the business in advance, dresses appropriately, and comes prepared to answer employer concerns regarding disabled people. Employers appreciate the depth and dependability of professional knowledge about clients as potential employees. The rehabilitationist presents the service package concisely, gives evidence of its successful use, expresses an interest in the employer's business concerns, is attentive to the employer's comments, expresses enthusiasm, and shows appreciation for the time being spent. Descriptive explanations are given without using professional terminology (jargon) that might confuse the employer. The rehabilitation worker brings the interview to a close at its appointed time, or when the employer wishes, and then follows up by a letter with thanks, summaries, and promised information on job-ready clients.

Advantages of the Service

The major focus of the job development interview is an explanation of the advantages of the agency service including employee evaluation, training, provision of skill bank, selective placement, job modification, and follow-up. The goals of the program are to: increase quality and quantity of worker productivity, reduce production costs, decrease labor turnover, lower accident rates, reduce sickness and absenteeism, and improve worker morale and job satisfaction. While these goals may be clear, employers usually focus their attention on the first five, which appear to affect production directly. Actually, the morale and job satisfaction of workers, as Hanman said in 1951, are "the master factors which influence not only production costs but the whole production process" [p. 12]. While in the past, industry often stressed the importance of machines, viewing the worker as subordinate, modern thought holds that the opposite is true.

Worker satisfaction is now a featured goal of job development and placement programs.

Especially in small businesses, the employer may not have the time and professional expertise for learning about applicants. The counselor's service in assessing clients for job suitability becomes a valued resource to employers [Forde, 1963].

Employer Responses

When employers have had previous experience with disabled workers in the plant, their immediate reaction is influenced by this experience—even though it may be based on only one or two cases. If this experience was good, the employer is usually receptive and is ready to talk about possible jobs, either for the present or the future. The placement counselor, however, must be ready to counter the impact of negative experiences. By simple questioning, one can show in an unobtrusive way either that the failure was not attributable to the disability or that the person was not put on the right job. Often the problem of clarifying the identity of the rehabilitation agency arises because the employer has confused referral sources.

When employers have not had previous experience with disabled workers or have done so only without realizing it, their first reaction may take several forms: operations are at too fast a pace, all jobs require standing, there are no light jobs, and other reasons for the nonacceptance of any person who has a disability. This shows misunderstanding of the variations of handicapping and of the wide range of jobs suitable for various disabled individuals. Stereotyped images of "handicapped people" are not uncommon, but they can be corrected quickly by specific examples of the range of disabilities that rehabilitants have and of the types of jobs they do well. It is well to emphasize that disabled people represent a cross-section of the population in age, intelligence, education, sex, experience, and skills. An employer who has disclaimed having any disabled workers, after a clarification of what a disablement is, may then recognize that various (successful) current employees are disabled in one or another way.

Some employers hesitate to show too much receptivity because they fear that if they do they will be overwhelmed with handicapped applicants. Consequently, the rehabilitationist emphasizes that clients are well screened before referral and that the agency might have only two or three prospects for a specific job opening; moreover, it is pointed out that the counselor will always call before referring a client and (with client permission) will submit records of the person's work, education, and medical background to allow the employer to decide whether to see the specific client.

An employer may hesitate to hire rehabilitants because if they do not work out well, it is not pleasant to be obliged to release them. Again, it is stressed that the employer is expected to apply the same criteria to the disabled worker as to all other employees, and that the rehabilitation client will be counseled so that no special consideration is expected. Moreover, the counselor accepts responsibility for telling any client who is unsatisfactory and must be discharged.

Job development is concerned with the long-range opportunities for placement, so it is unimportant if the employer says there are no current openings. This gives the rehabilitationist opportunity to plan for future services. After discussing the above points it is good to be shown through the plant, observe the jobs, and be able to ask questions. What is learned about the jobs and operations and the vocabulary of the industry is used in subsequent visits to this and similar concerns [Hart, 1962].

Employer View of Job Development

Employers should see job development as a manpower service concerned with the solution of a personnel problem. In this context, job development is perceived as a means of increasing company efficiency and reducing costs. Viewed as a resource, the job development unit of the rehabilitation agency is given access to key decision-makers within the company and to company personnel information.

While the job development program is properly perceived as a resource for the company's personnel operation, this does not mean that the problems of hard-to-place clients should not be frankly and openly discussed with prospective employers. Even more important than the number of jobs pledged for the hard-to-employ is the employer's conviction that the jobs provided must be meaningful employment opportunities. Employers must not come to view job development for rehabilitants as a convenient device to fill dead-end jobs. They must perceive the problem as one involving human values and as a so-

cial issue demanding their attention. But whether the employer's motive is self-interest or a social consciousness, or both, there must be a commitment to reexamine the company's assumptions and practices about employment. It may take considerable initiative and imagination on the part of the job development unit to persuade the employer of this.

Principles for convincing the employer follow: (1) Efforts are first directed toward officials in the highest ranks of the company. (2) After the top executives agree, lower echelon (operational) people must be informed and convinced. (3) It should be recognized that personnel workers and production supervisors may have anxieties in these situations, and particular attention should be paid to their concerns about worker performance, quality control, and productivity. (If possible, assurance should be obtained from top echelons in the company that there will be some relaxation of traditional standards in evaluating the performance of work departments in which hard-to-place workers are employed.) (4) Business association groups and business leaders can be influential. (5) Combining the appeals of two or more job development, civil rights, and employment opportunity agencies induces employer acquiescence to job development as a coordinated program.

Obtaining Supervisory Cooperation

Supervisory personnel are a vital link in any employment program. Important to the successful employment of disabled people is teamwork on the part of the employment manager, the safety officer, the industrial physician, and the direct supervisor. From a practical standpoint, it would be difficult for any company to continue to hire disabled persons if the department heads and supervisors objected. After a policy has been established, the authority for its implementation is delegated to line subordinates (department heads and supervisory staff). This level of management, however, will not be an obstacle to placing rehabilitated people if the company administration makes proper preparation for nondiscrimination practices.

Reasons for Lack of Supervisory Cooperation

When a firm lacks the cooperation of its supervisors in its program to employ disabled persons, the fault is usually at the management level. A company's management may express interest in employing rehabilitants but may do nothing to communicate this spirit to the supervisors and other company personnel. And if supervisors do not understand the important reasons for employing disabled persons, they may resent the interference in their departments and fear their production rates will suffer.

Conversely, supervisors may be so soft-hearted that they shelter disabled persons in their departments and keep them from performing any worthwhile duties. As a result, such supervisors are unwittingly keeping disabled workers from being placed in jobs they are able to perform. This usually stems from the supervisor's lack of knowledge about disabilities and about how a job development and employment program operates.

Plan for Putting Policy into Practice

Top management needs to put into writing its policy regarding the employment of disabled people and to make someone responsible for implementation of the decision. To put a policy into practice, adequate lines of communication must be established, usually by a company official charged with affirmative action and equal employment opportunity (EEO) affairs.

Direct supervisors of disabled individuals may be resentful if they are not given specific information about those persons assigned to their department. With management approval, the supervisors can receive consultation from the rehabilitation staff as to how to cope with functional limitations (e.g., communication) of the worker who is handicapped. The supervisor may also need outside assistance in the employee orientation procedures. Continuing follow-up helps the supervisor cope with special problems and appreciate the team effort on the job program.

Cooperation of Other Employees

Companies are wise to make a special effort to persuade rank-and-file workers of the importance of employing disabled people. It is advisable to include stories about the contributions that disabled persons make to a company in circulated company newsletters. In some cases, announcements provide helpful medical information about how to deal with certain types of disabilities—what to do, for example, when a person with epilepsy has a seizure.

It is natural that the pattern of understanding and cooperation shown by the plant work force becomes a reflection of the attitudes of supervisors. It helps if everyone in the work area understands the importance of treating the impaired person in the same matter-of-fact way that any other employee would be treated. Again the supervisors play an important role. Through their actions they can demonstrate to all personnel within a department a positive attitude toward people who have a disability. If they are well-prepared for a unique situation, for instance, that of the first paraplegic worker being wheeled into the department, a positive reception by fellow workers can be assumed [National Industrial Conference Board, Inc., 1957].

38.1.3. RURAL AREAS

Most discussions on job development apply mainly to urban areas. Although many of the same principles apply in rural areas, Ferman [1969] said that the job development activities may be different. There are several reasons for the difference. First, rural areas, particularly depressed rural areas, lack the agency resources to assure job opportunities and support programs for the hard-to-place worker. Special counseling, corporate planning, and management education services may need to be brought in on a part-time consulting basis. Second, a surplus labor market often characterizes these areas and employers tend to keep job qualifications high. Persuading management to revise standards for the hard-to-employ is less difficult in urban labor markets with marked shortages of workers. Third, the handicapped population remaining in rural localities generally have less employment potential since there is continued out-migration of most workers to other areas of employment, even when those workers have only marginal skills. Another reason is that the geographic area is large and the population so dispersed that it puts considerable strain on a small staff. The lack of job opportunities coupled with declining industrial economics, as in Appalachia, requires an intensified job development effort: job creation through economic development and expansion, geographical mobility to seats of employment, and technical assistance to employers in the area.

Economic Development and Expansion

The most effective approach in a depressed rural area is to create jobs through economic expansion. In planning economic development, the primary problem for job programs is to maintain open channels with the business community at the policy-making and grant-making levels. Economic expansion must be linked with labor needs and resources.

In addition to public announcements and contacts with people in the management community who are privy to expansion plans, the following contacts can provide rural job development programs with advance information of impending economic developments: industrial sales representatives, local contracting firms, public officials who must grant licenses for various forms of expansion, local public and private employment agencies, county extension agents, and the chamber of commerce. Financial institutions with loan applications from local businesses will be aware of their expansion plans. Thus, financial leaders can provide current information about firms that will be hiring new workers. Not only banks and local lending agencies but also the Small Business Administration (SBA) can help. They can understand that job development is an important collateral service in their own economic development activities.

The strategy is to build job development into the fabric of economic expansion. Most communities have economic development programs that provide information and other services to attract prospective manufacturing and other new firms.

38.2. *Employer Concerns*

Management may think that hiring disabled workers involves greater risks than hiring the "able-bodied." They may think that there will be additional expenses due to costs of training, redesigning plant facilities, absenteeism, and production problems. Worker flexibility, co-worker attitudes, motivation, social skills, and adjustment to the job become additional concerns to the employer.

These concerns are eased when they learn that through the evaluation, training, and selective placement process, the risk is smaller than it is when hiring nondisabled people who have not been screened for the job. Moreover, the agency's follow-up and job adjustment services provide assurance to the employer that agency assistance will be available throughout the probationary period and that the agency will take responsibility for termination of employment should that become necessary. The rehabilitationist must be prepared to answer all employer concerns honestly but convincingly.

A U.S. Department of Labor survey found that the record of physically disabled workers was comparable to that of nonimpaired workers on similar jobs [U.S. GTP, 1956a]. In a general way, the counselor can cite this and other research that shows that when rehabilitants are given the chance to do work for which they are suited, they achieve work records that average a little better than those of nondisabled workers.

38.2.1. SAFETY AND INSURANCE

Two associated problems that most often make employers reluctant to hire the disabled applicant are safety and the fear of increased worker compensation insurance premiums due to accident. Behind the fear is the notion that some people are "accident-prone." This is a needless fear because disabled people do not have a psychological need, conscious or unconscious, to be reinjured. Employers may also assume that the disabled are less capable of avoiding injury: for example, if there is a fire, can the person hear a warning or escape without help? Safety precautions should be part of the job development package.

Safety

Many studies show that properly placed disabled workers have safety records equal to or better than those of other employees. For minor injuries, the safety record of disabled people is substantially the same as that of unimpaired workers. For disabling injuries, workers who were already disabled in some way have a significantly better safety record than unimpaired workers.

An employer takes a risk in hiring any employee, whether able-bodied or not. As Williams [1965] said, the degree (of risk) depends on two factors: (1) proper placement of the worker in a safe job, and (2) effectiveness of the company's safety program.

Insurance

The question of insurance premiums increasing as a result of hiring disabled people is a serious concern of management. In most cases, the concern, while unfounded, arises from lack of experience or misunderstanding of the statutes. In a few cases, however, there is good basis for concern, and it rests with the placement person to know the state's laws in order to explain the situation to potential employers. Some veteran rehabilitationists believe that the insurance problem is the most difficult obstacle to placement efforts. (Enactment of national health care with worker insurance coverage could render the whole concern in this matter irrelevant.)

Workers compensation insurance rates are determined by two factors: the relative hazards in a company's work and its accident experience. The formulae for determining the premium rates include no consideration of the kind of personnel hired. The insurance contract says nothing, by implication or directly, about the physical condition of the workers the insured firm may hire. As said before, however, a poor accident experience (i.e., a relatively high number of accidents or cost of claims over a period of time) will cause an increase in an employer's compensation insurance rates. The fact remains that if a disabled worker would be more apt to have accidents and consequently suffer greater disability, as some people once believed, then an employer's insurance costs might eventually go up. (See 37.4.6.)

L. N. Loban [1972] queried 15 insurance companies about their group coverage limitations on hiring policy. He asked the companies to comment on the statement, "I can't hire the handicapped because my insurance company won't let me." In all 14 replies, the letters stated clearly that insurance companies do not tell employers whom they may hire. Not one of the 14 insurance carriers suggested any kind of dictation of hiring policy to employers. It is also noteworthy that businesses primarily employing disabled people—such as Epi-Hab in Los Angeles—have been given (workers compensation insurance) premium *reductions* for their better than average safety record. Epi-Hab U.S.A., Inc. is a chain of industrial workshops founded by Frank Risch for people with epilepsy.

Job Site Modifications

Another major concern on the part of management is the potential expense involved in modifying the work site so that it is safe and accessible. The rehabilitationist should be available to assist the employer in making modifications. The modifications for a particular severely disabled individual may be extensive. Most disabled employees, however, require no special work arrangements at all [Wolfe, 1973].

38.2.2. JOB PERFORMANCE

Some employers fear that an individual's disability will result in poor work performance. Surveys usually indicate, however, that the performance of disabled individuals is equal to or better than the average—again with the proviso that proper placement has been achieved.

Again, survey research shows that on the average disabled workers are: adaptable—they adjust quickly and satisfactorily to the conditions of the job; productive—they often surpass the production records of other employees; careful—their safety records are substantially the same as for unimpaired workers; regular— job attendance records of disabled employees equal those of other workers doing the same type of job; reliable—disabled workers do not job-hop; and capable—they have the same wide range of skills, abilities, and interests as the rest of the population.

Inflexibility of the Work Force

Another productivity concern of employers is that there may be a limit on the number of disabled individuals they can employ due to the nature of their businesses. Some of these potential difficulties can be anticipated at the time of the initial placement.

Changing jobs or changing the requirements of the position, for example, may result in displacement of an individual because of physical inability to perform the new operation. If no other suitable job is open, the company has no choice but to lay off that person. Even the most enthusiastic employer realizes that the functional limitations of employees must be considered when a change in production requirements entails changing operations and shifting employees among jobs. At this stage, a company may find itself hampered by a work force that is not flexible. Consequently some companies, depending on their type of operation, feel obliged to restrict the number of disabled persons employed. In this case, if it is possible that a plant may radically change its operation, perhaps the employer should *not* hire a substantial number of people with the same functional limitation. This could be an argument for having a variety of disabilities—conversely stated, abilities—on the work force of a company.

An individual's inflexibility also restricts opportunities. When workers are employed in only one or two jobs in the company, their lack of opportunity to learn the entire operation reduces their potential value. In order to advance in many companies, employees must rotate through several jobs and acquire a broad knowledge of varied company operations. This situation must be explained to disabled persons when they are hired, in order to avoid later disappointment. Nevertheless, some disabled workers become discontented over remaining stagnant in a job.

This problem of inflexibility is in part resolved through the application of job development techniques, rehabilitation client service, and selective placement. The principle of compensation for disability also applies: for instance, blind persons usually develop more perceptive hearing, there is residual muscular development in persons who lose limbs, and so forth.

Rigid union rules regarding seniority traditionally kept employers from achieving satisfactory placement of disabled people, both newly hired employees and those already on the payroll. Some union contracts have required all new "hires" to be assigned to the least desirable work, such as jobs involving heavy lifting or unpleasant environments. Disabled applicants unable to tolerate these entry-level jobs were not allowed to be placed in suitable positions. Seniority rules also have permitted "bumping" handicapped workers from the only job they can perform when there is a reduction in plant work force. The 1973 Rehabilitation Act and its Amendments speak to this problem in such a way that it should be resolved.

38.2.3. ATTITUDES

Attitudes toward and of disabled people are discussed in other chapters. In general, differences in expressed feelings related to disablement interfer with the employment and retention of workers who have a disability.

Attitude of the Disabled Worker

The attitude of the disabled worker is of considerable concern to the prospective employer. Any disruption of the human work environment by the attitudes of clients toward their disabilities or toward co-workers means decreased production and lost money for the employer.

Physical disablement does not automatically preclude the person from having the disagreeable personality characteristics common to many individuals, and in fact some do develop negative attitudes. While that is understandable, it is not excusable. The solution is in preemployment rehabilitation services such as personal adjustment training and counseling (see 13.1 and 28.1).

Favoritism

Another concern voiced by employers is that considerable time may be required in adjusting disabled individuals to their job and to co-workers. In the case of certain disabilities, this is definitely true. However, the time lost and inconvenience caused often appear as greater obstacles than they in fact turn out to be. Co-workers who originally resent clients who get privileges will often come to accept the situation, especially if the disability is highly visible. Nevertheless, the counselor can offer to help adjust the client to co-workers and the job.

While it is true that certain disabilities are upsetting at first, experience has shown that initial negative reactions do not last. In fact, most supervisors report that employees who have an obvious disability seem to have a positive rather than a negative effect upon morale.

Many supervisors take the position that they do not have the time to "pamper a handicapped person" or that they feel obligated to show "favoritism" on the job [Williams, 1965]. But, as a rule, disabled people want to be treated like everyone else, and when placed properly no extra supervision is needed.

Reactions to Specific Disabilities

While most employers are willing to "hire the handicapped," many of them make reservations with regard to certain disabilities. Employers' fear of the epileptic employee, for example, is tremendous: they are concerned with the danger of an industrial accident, although with selective placement on nonhazardous jobs, people having convulsive seizures are not a significant safety risk. Although clients with epilepsy, emotional problems, and some other disabilities meet with resistance, usually orthopedic disabilities are acceptable. Perhaps this is because it is easy to see and understand the orthopedic disability—the exception is low-back pain from previous (often worker-compensated) injury, and this really frightens most would-be employers. Many companies that claim a nondiscrimination employment policy actually screen out severely disabled applicants. It should be pointed out, however, that although they may hire few people who were previously disabled, they often make adjustments within the company for their own employees who develop epilepsy, heart trouble, emotional conditions, and other disabilities during the course of their employment.

Social Relations

Rehabilitationists would like to see their clients considered for work purely on the basis of their ability to meet the requirements of the job. However, prospective employers and co-workers may also consider prospective employees in terms of how they fit into the personal-social life of the group. In after-hour activities, will the client contribute to the recreational interests of co-workers or constitute a burden for them? Such concerns should be discussed during planning for a job development project in a plant.

38.3. Organized Labor

The commitment of organized labor to rehabilitation is evident at the national and local level (see 12.1.13). Nationally, organized labor has contributed to the studies and proposals of the President's Committee on Employment of the Handicapped. And unions have produced pamphlets and films that describe the mutual role of union and management in restoring handicapped workers to a productive life. It is the stated policy of the American labor movement that "every practical means shall be used to insure equal opportunity in employment for all qualified handicapped workers" [American Federation of Labor and Congress of Industrial Organizations, 1973, p. 10].

Rehabilitationists find union leaders very cooperative in discussing the problems that arise in placement. Their knowledge of the area and the labor market and their experience with local employers help in setting up and operating a job development unit. In a tight labor market, however, unionists may caution against trade training for disabled people because of the likelihood of frequent lay-offs and the inability of the individual to build up sufficient seniority to provide for job security. Since the union has ultimate responsibility for all its members, it will share in the burdens and frustrations that result when training is provided for jobs that are not available.

When employers cite union regulations as a cause for not considering a prospective disabled employee, the rehabilitationist may suggest a joint meeting of labor and management to examine alternative ways of resolving the difficulty. Both sides usually cooperate if the rehabilitationist shows understanding and sensitivity to the issues at hand. In some cases the employer may be using the union as an excuse to conceal prejudice about hiring disabled people.

38.3.1. UNION POLICY

Labor unions, along with management, are exerting an increasing influence on the placement of disabled workers in employment (see 33.4.7). Counselors should be familiar with the positions and programs of unions, particularly those concerned with employment in the major trades and industries. An example is the United Mine Workers of America, which (through its Welfare and Retirement Fund) has provided for many years an excellent program for the physical restoration of their disabled members and is concerned also with their vocational rehabilitation.

A comprehensive policy was adopted in 1960 by the Executive Council of the American Federation of Labor and Congress of Industrial Organizations (AFL-CIO). It said in part:

Organized labor, as spokesman for the working force and as representative of citizens concerned with individual, community and national well being, has a vital role in the development and improvement of rehabilitation services. Labor's already well-expressed concern for the placement of handicapped persons in the right job prompts an even more compelling concern to work for the greatest possible reduction of individual handicapping conditions.

For these reasons, the Advisory Council of the AFL-CIO Community Services Committee recommends that the AFL-CIO support a program for comprehensive rehabilitation services (i.e., a Labor Program for Rehabilitation).

The primary role of organized labor in rehabilitation is that of knowledgeable and dedicated stimulator of, and participant in, organized action in support of better rehabilitation services.

A more specific policy statement on the employment of handicapped persons, adopted subsequently, established an "AFL-CIO Program for Union Management Action to Provide Employment for Handicapped Workers." That statement is, in part, as follows:

The trade union movement from the earliest days has recognized the right of the worker, disabled by accident on or off the job, to an opportunity to earn a living. The labor movement has taken the lead in securing the enactment of workmen's compensation legislation and second injury funds to protect the worker who suffers injury in employment. The AFL-CIO has fostered and supported legislation to promote the return of injured workers to suitable employment. The reemployment of persons handicapped by industrial injury or disease has always been high on the trade union program. The return to employment of veterans disabled in the service of their country is likewise labor's major concern.

38.3.2. UNION ORGANIZATION

One of the most serious barriers to working with unions in job development is that few people in rehabilitation placement and job development are familiar with the nature of unionism in the United States. There has been a failure to understand the organization and internal operations of labor unions and management, the services that unions attempt to give members, and the status of a union as a legal entity within the employer establishment. Louis Ferman [1969] has provided much of the information used in the following overview.

Labor organizations, unlike business firms, have elected officials who are accountable to their membership and constituencies. Arbitrary decision-making power is limited by union constitutions, by-laws, and even legislation. Membership privileges, leadership responsibilities, and authority spheres are explicitly defined to ensure a measure of democratic control over the officers by the mass membership. Since unions are not generally incorporated, the officers exercise only the control that is delegated to them by the governing instruments of the organization (constitution, by-laws, approval actions of the members or delegates representing the members). Thus, officers of unions may often lead and influence the thinking of the membership, but there is a feeling of constraint as well as actual restriction on the flexibility permitted to them. The democratic process may be no more viable in unions than in other political, quasi-political, or voluntary organizations, but it does set limits, and leaders who ignore these limits would be seriously challenged.

Another consideration is that most local unions are joined to regional bodies that in turn are part of international unions. While many local unions have extensive autonomy, decision-making power also resides in regional and national bodies. In some unions, winning approval of the local union for job development may mean little if the decision-making process of the regional organization has been bypassed.

American labor unions cover a variety of working groups in a wide range of organizational types. Most of them attempt to rigorously define the dimensions of the bargaining unit (that is, what workers fall under the union jurisdiction for bargaining purposes) to: set a pay scale; establish criteria for promotion and training; protect seniority and pension rights; establish dispute-handling procedures; and set forth work relationships between supervisor and worker.

Industrial Unions

These unions are large in size and are primarily designed to cover workers engaged in mass production, manufacturing work in which training and skills are minimal. The prerogatives for hiring new workers are often completely in the hands of the employer, although this situation may be modified if the labor contract specifies recall rights of laid-off workers as a basis for filling vacant job slots. There is strong emphasis on the expansion of union membership, a goal favorable to the hiring of disabled persons. A separate local union represents the members in the bargaining unit in a particular plant.

Service unions and the retail trade unions have similar structures, although they tend to merge members from many physically scattered units into a single local. Thus, all nursing aides from 10 or 12 nursing homes may form one local, and all the clerks in a chain of grocery stores may form another local.

Job development programs are usually easier to arrange with industrial union shops than craft-type unions.

Craft Unions

Largely in the building and printing trades, the members of craft unions have a well-defined career line, with members beginning as apprentices, moving to journeymen, and finally achieving master craftsman status. Entry to the occupations represented by these unions requires entrance to the apprenticeship system, a combination of formal and informal training on the job. These unions rigorously define the hiring practices and criteria for employment in these trades. Their objectives are twofold: control of the labor supply into the trades and maintenance of skill standards. They negotiate ratios of apprentices to journeymen, and these become the guidelines for admission into the apprentice system. These unions tend to be smaller, more closely knit, and more conservative than industrial unions. They have a long historical tradition, tracing their origins back to the guild system of medieval Europe. In the past, it was not unusual for membership to be passed down along family lines.

White-collar and Professional Unions

So-called white-collar unions represent clerical and technical personnel who are engaged in various occupational specialties that may or may not require extensive formal preparation for nonmanual and noncraft work. Jobs may range from office clerk to draftsman. These unions have many of the same concerns as industrial unions, but their major focus is on the preservation of status prerogatives such as relationships with supervisors. White-collar union members traditionally were drawn from the broad middle class with homogeneous political and social attitudes.

The so-called professional unions include members who have obtained some measure of formal preparation in institutional instruction and who are hired for their professional skills and values. This kind of union has as its major concern the promotion of good working conditions and benefits for its membership.

38.3.3. UNION RELATIONSHIPS

Union participation in job development programs is governed by informal reactions of union members and by the labor contract provisions. The labor union contract regulates the relationships between the union and its members and management. The contract defines the bargaining unit, describes the entry-level jobs and seniority rules, and specifies transfer and promotional systems. Since manpower assignment within the establishment is prescribed in the labor contract or by established practice, these rules must be understood by the job development staff. Suggestions for client placement that violate contract provisions are seriously resisted by both union and management.

Newly employed workers under a union contract begin at the bottom. Fundamental to the thinking of union members is the fact that a job is a property right, and that as new jobs appear, the property values shift. In an expanding employment situation, the workers who are already employed may "bid" on a new job as a more valuable property to which they have a right because of their seniority. The inverse is also true in a job situation that is contracted, so that "bumping" causes the newer workers to be laid off first. This bidding system for new jobs is well structured in most union contracts. Disrupting this bidding system by unplanned job development efforts can be extremely upsetting to employees who believe that their rights are being abrogated.

There are various provisions for the placement of disabled workers made through advance agreement of all parties to the job development proposal. Exceptions to seniority rules take several forms. In most cases these provisions are of assistance principally to the employee who becomes disabled. They may give greater protection to the worker who has an occupationally incurred injury or disease than to the one whose disability is from other origins. But they can and should be expanded to provide equal employment opportunity to all disabled people who can work in appropriate jobs. Labor and management may agree to reserve certain positions in jobs that are sedentary in nature and do not require a fast pace. Another special provision may allow reassignment of a disabled worker by waiver of seniority rules or by automatic (e.g., five extra years) seniority advancement.

The nature of contracts between management

and labor varies greatly; however, the rehabilitationist must be aware of those clauses affecting employment of disabled people and must seek the participation of management and labor in removal of barriers. A constructive attitude and sound knowledge help in the establishment of a reputation and provide consequent leverage in using labor and management to assist in placement efforts.

Unions should be involved in job development because the union is part of the industrial relations system in any firm and its collaboration is needed in both planning and implementing the continuing program. Another sound reason for getting union involvement is that the union is a prime influence on worker attitudes and close involvement may result in a more favorable co-worker climate for the handicapped person. Sometimes, of course, unions may have nothing to say about hiring, and their involvement would be only symbolic.

Union leadership is usually well informed and generally has a natural compassion for the disadvantaged person. Throughout the history of the labor movement, these organizations have supported economic progress for all people, social reforms, and aid to the dependent population. Still, protection of membership sometimes places unions in the position of seeming to exclude nonmembers (viz., the medically disabled and also the culturally disadvantaged who wish to enter the work force).

The potential for jobs for disabled workers in unionized firms is generally overstated. Only about one American worker in every four is working as a union member, and the vast majority of jobs are nonunion. It must be concluded that in some respects nonunionized companies face fewer problems in employing handicapped persons than do firms with a union contract. A lack of understanding among rank-and-file union members and local officers of the importance of employing disabled or disadvantaged people suggests the need for a continuing public relations effort by rehabilitation programs (see 10.4.1).

38.4. Affirmative Action

Affirmative action statutes—the "bill of rights" for disabled Americans—have been hailed by rehabilitationists as a major advance in the cause of the disabled population. They followed in the wake of the successful civil rights movement that brought equal rights in employment to people who had been discriminated against on the basis of race, color, sex, religion, and national origin. These rights were secured by passage of the Civil Rights Act of 1964 and were strengthened by establishment of the federal Equal Employment Opportunity Commission in 1972. Federal protection of the employment rights of disabled people came into being with the passage of the Rehabilitation Act (PL 93-112) of 1973 and its subsequent Amendments. The result of this legislation has been to encourage the growth of affirmative action programs in commerce and industry and in nonprofit and governmental organizations, and to expand the role of the rehabilitation counselor as a consultant in job modification, placement, and job development.

38.4.1. LEGISLATION

The primary intent of affirmative action legislation as specified in the Rehabilitation Act of 1973, Sections 501, 503, and 504, is to delineate those employment practices of employers that are discriminatory or that must be undertaken to overcome the ill effects of past discrimination. The law further covers accessibility to programs, services, and employment opportunities of all employers and programs receiving funds from the federal government.

Section 501 stipulates affirmative action policies to be followed in the internal employment structure of the federal government. Departments and agencies of the executive branch are directed to prepare an action plan indicating how the needs of disabled employees are to be met. This includes the specification of adequate hiring, placement, and advancement opportunities for disabled people as well as designation of staff to perform the special personnel functions. The plans are updated annually and reviewed by the federal Civil Service Commission. Each agency of the government appoints a selective placement coordinator to manage the program and to negotiate with the Civil Service Commission when complaints are filed. The coordinators can be a valuable source of training positions, employment opportunities, and selected placement for rehabilitation clients when an ongoing liaison is established by the rehabilitation agency.

Section 503 of the Act requires affirmative action of all public and private employers who are contractors of the federal government, when the amount of the contract is in excess of $2500. (Subcontractors are also required to observe the provisions of the law.) The law covers all "qualified handicapped individuals," defined in the act as persons who have a physical or mental impairment that substantially limits one or more major life activity, or who have a record of such impairment, or who are regarded by others as being handicapped.

The law requires a clause in the contract indicating that the contractor or subcontractor will not discriminate against a qualified employee or applicant and that affirmative action will be taken to employ and advance in employment such individuals without discrimination. Hiring, upgrading, demotion or transfer, recruitment, lay-off or termination, rates of pay, compensation, and selection for training are all covered by the statute.

Contractors and subcontractors having contracts of $50,000 or more and 50 or more employees are required to specify and follow an affirmative action program. The program requires written policy statements and procedures to be followed, including enumeration of employees who qualify for protection under the act, confidentiality of information, grievance procedure, recording of pertinent information, and methods of placement coordination and outreach with agencies serving disabled job applicants. Enforcement of the law is handled by the Office of Federal Contract Compliance Programs (OFCCP) of the U.S. Department of Labor. Complaints regarding this section of the Act must be made to the OFCCP within 180 days of the alleged violation. The Office may then seek informal conciliation, require a formal hearing or corrective action, or in extreme situations, terminate the contract and declare a contractor ineligible for future contracts. The annual review of affirmative action plans and the strict measures that can be imposed for failure to observe the law provide powerful incentives for employers to seek qualified employees who have a disability and to obtain the assistance of a rehabilitation counselor in selective placement.

Regulations issued in 1976 by the DOL, OFCCP pursuant to Section 503 specify actions to be taken by employers as part of their affirmative action plan. Contractors are encouraged to enlist the assistance of state employment and vocational rehabilitation agencies, sheltered workshops, college placement officers, education agencies, labor organizations, and other groups to develop meaningful employment opportunities. Furthermore, rehabilitation agencies and facilities are regarded as sources of technical assistance in placement, recruiting, training, and accommodations for employment. Contractors are also required to make reasonable accommodations, including job modification, job restructuring, modified work schedules, and removal of in-plant architectural barriers. They must review personnel procedures related to the physical and mental demands of jobs to assure that qualifications are indeed necessary for the task performed. Positive recruitment and outreach are mandated when substantial discriminatory practices of the past have denied employment opportunities to qualified handicapped individuals.

Section 504 of the 1973 Rehabilitation Act extended a similar protection of equal rights for disabled people, to cover all programs and activities of organizations receiving federal financial assistance or grants, including education, social services, housing, and transportation programs. Besides prohibiting all discriminatory practices in employment, the law extends to other areas. Most guidelines and regulations under this section of the Act follow those issued in 1977 by the U.S. Department of Health, Education, and Welfare (HEW). Employers are prevented from practicing segregation or classification of handicapped workers in a way that would adversely affect their employment status or opportunity, or from participating in a relationship with other organizations, such as unions or subcontractors, that would have the same effect.

Recipients of grants from the federal government are expected to make reasonable accommodation to the physical and mental limitation of applicants and employees unless it can be shown that to do so would constitute an undue hardship on the program. Reasonable accommodations include, but are not limited to, providing accessibility to buildings as well as restrooms and program facilities, providing translators for those who have sensory impairments, restructuring schedules or relocating program components, and modifying equipment. Preemployment tests that do not relate to specific job tasks involved are not allowed and are prohibited when there is a failure to allow for the handicap when administering the test. Employers cannot require a preemployment physical examination or disclosure of information regarding a handicap as a condition of employment. However, they may request information or an examination of an applicant if it is part of voluntary participation in an ongoing affirmative action program. Medical exams are otherwise allowable only if all applicants take the same exam and if there is a direct correspondence between the exam and job-task performance. Medical information must be kept confidential except for those specific aspects that relate directly to the job to be performed, and then information may be given only to appropriate company officials.

Employers of over 15 persons are expected to designate a coordinator for the affirmative action program, which is usually the equal employment opportunity (EEO) officer, and to maintain records of the program. Grievance procedures for handling complaints of employees are specified, and notification must be given to applicants, unions, and subcontractors regarding the non-discrimination policy.

The U.S. HEW Office for Civil Rights was charged with enforcement of the provisions of Section 504. (Most of these civil rights enforcement functions were transferred in 1980 to the new U.S. Department of Education although some of them remain in the reorganized U.S. Department of Health and Human Services.) Complaints are made to branch offices within 180 days of the alleged violation. The Office may require remedial action to be taken, require a formal hearing, or refer the matter to the U.S. Department of Justice for court action. In extreme cases, federal assistance to the employer may be terminated or suspended. Direct lawsuits may also be undertaken by individual complainants.

Other federal statutes offer protection of equal rights for the handicapped population in employment. The Civil Rights Act of 1971, for example, has been successfully used as a basis for redress against county and local government units that benefit from federal revenue-sharing. Grievance is first filed with the Secretary of the

Treasury and subject to conciliation before being referred to the United States Attorney General if a satisfactory settlement is not achieved. Another federal statute affecting employment opportunity for disabled individuals is the Vietnam Era Veteran's Readjustment Act (PL 93-508) of 1974. Contractors and subcontractors with contracts of $10,000 or more are required to take affirmative action in hiring qualified veterans whose disability is rated at 30 percent or more.

The affirmative action requirements of recent legislation may affect union practices that have tended to exclude handicapped individuals. Union contracts often require new employees to start on entry-level jobs, which tend to be the heaviest and dirtiest, thereby excluding those disabled workers who could handle the tasks of intermediate level positions. After employees have been on the job for a period of time, they can bid for "easier" jobs. This practice makes it more difficult to place some clients, particularly those with severe handicaps.

State government activities in the area of civil rights for the handicapped population began in the 1970s but the pattern varies. Many states have adopted statutory provisions, often as amendments to fair employment practices legislation to prohibit discrimination in employment based solely upon a person's physical or mental disability where that disability is not a detrimental factor for performance of a particular job.

The equal opportunity commission or human rights commission in a state, for example, may have authority under the state's statute to investigate complaints, arrange conciliatory agreements, require formal hearings, and make settlements to compensate for violations. Statutes of limitation may be less than the 180 days allowed under Sections 503 and 504, requiring the complainant to make timely notice of the grievance. Job applicants who are denied employment because of an employer's concern about insurance rates under a self-insured workers compensation program may have recourse under state statute. In some states the self-insured status can be revoked if an employer refuses employment unreasonably on the basis of a disability. Other statutes require construction and building modification after a certain date to bring physical plants into conformity with accessibility standards. Following that date or new construction, employers may no longer deny employment on the basis of inaccessibility.

38.4.2. ROLE OF THE COUNSELOR

In addition to providing employment opportunities for disabled people, a major consequence of Sections 501, 503, and 504 of the 1973 Rehabilitation Act is the encouragement of closer bonds of cooperation between employers and rehabilitation counselors [Akabas, 1976]. By and large, most employers are anxious to support the goals of affirmative action and do recognize the vital role that disabled people can play in their businesses. Many industries and business concerns are, on their own initiative, developing outreach and aggressive employment programs for the handicapped [Jeffers, 1974]. However, many others lack expertise in working with disabled people and in implementing the technological improvements that can enable these individuals to function at their highest level of ability in the company. The rehabilitation counselor can play a vital role in selective placement, in educational training of supervisory staff, in job modification, reengineering, referral of applicants, and counseling. Many businesses encounter emotional disorders, substance abuse, and other disability-related problems with their own work force and welcome the opportunity for rehabilitation counselors to offer new program alternatives to help solve these problems. Planning conferences can serve as a springboard in job development and affirmative action programs by bringing employers and rehabilitationists together in a common forum to discuss the resources and expertise that can be shared to move them toward the common goal of equal opportunity for qualified handicapped workers [Maloney, 1976].

Employers need assistance in developing affirmative action plans that are acceptable to the federal government. They also need a reliable source of job applicants to fill the new positions that are opened up in order to bring disabled people into the work force. Coordination of job banks with the employment service and with other agencies serving disabled job applicants becomes a primary concern on the part of employers. Job analysis and face-to-face contact with supervisors, personnel managers, and designated Equal Employment Opportunity (EEO) officers become expanding activities for the re-

habilitation worker, requiring a greater investment of time but yielding more accurate placements. It is through such personal visits that the rehabilitationist is able to perceive the potential for nontraditional adaptations of jobs and to encourage modifications that would enable individual clients to find suitable places in competitive employment.

Since most employers voluntarily practice affirmative action, deliberate discrimination in hiring practice is not often encountered by the rehabilitationist. However, there may be more subtle forms of discrimination, built in by years of traditional company operating procedures, that are hard to identify. Differential treatment in the form of wages, fringe benefits, and advancement may be given to different groups, following a pattern based on sex, race, or disability criteria that may not be related at all to ability to perform a job. The employer may not be aware of the effect of the traditional practice until a worker's complaint brings the discrimination to light.

Another type of company policy that may have a discriminatory effect is the use of screening procedures, employment tests, or the requirement of certain levels of qualifications that are applied equally to all persons, yet selectively eliminate certain groups of people. If the tests of qualifications are not directly related to performance criteria on the job, their effect may be discriminatory (see 20.5.2). Since most discriminatory acts are unintentional, they usually will be resolved, through conciliation proceedings, in a manner favorable to both the employee and employer. Occasionally, however, the rehabilitationist will encounter situations of outright discrimination on the part of an employer who has misunderstood the intent of state and federal law.

Some employers have decided that they already have their "share" of disabled workers so feel they are justified in automatically excluding any new disabled job applicants. For those businesses covered by the statutes, however, each individual must be evaluated only on the basis of the ability to do the job, not whether or not a disability is present. Other employers make the, mistaken, assumption that people with certain disabilities, such as those who are blind or who have epilepsy, are not safe, refusing to hire them for any position. However, the law specifically requires the employer to make reasonable accommodations and to consider that selective placement might entirely eliminate either safety concerns or handicap as a reason for refusing employment.

It is to be hoped that, by observing the concerns expressed by employers, the kinds of jobs being offered, the questions asked in job interviews, and the hiring patterns and experiences of other applicants, rehabilitationists will be able to identify intentional and unintentional discrimination and take the steps necessary to resolve the situation. Furthermore, individual clients can be informed of their rights under the statutes and encouraged to seek assistance or to file a complaint when they believe that their rights have been violated.

Although rehabilitation counselors are encouraged to inform clients of their rights under the statutes, it is usually not advisable for them to participate in the proceedings in a way that might compromise their role as an advisor to the employer in job development. Clients who need advice, guidance, or assistance can be given whatever help is necessary to file complaints or to seek redress of grievances as individuals, and the counselor might play the role of conciliator in the situation. In some situations, a complaint may be filed anonymously or by a group in favor of an unnamed individual if there is some fear of reprisal, although the statutes prohibit retaliatory action by employers and prescribe harsh sanctions to discourage it from happening. Clients should not be disheartened by long waits for action to be taken; sometimes settlements can be made within a few months or other jobs become available. In large metropolitan areas, advocacy groups for disabled people may also have access to independent legal aid that can bring rapid action in civil court.

Counselors and clients should be aware, however, that in spite of settlements in behalf of the client, unsatisfactory working relationships may result that would render remaining at the company unsatisfactory. Further caution is advisable when clients file groundless claims to cover up for their own inadequacies or out of resentment of company personnel who do not let them have their own way. In such cases, rapid follow-up counseling, not litigation, is in order.

Although most employers will accept the involvement of the rehabilitationist as a blessing, others will react with suspicion and uncertainty in the face of yet another example of government interference in private enterprise. The rehabilitationist can attempt to overcome this concern by serving in the role of consultant-educator and by encouraging distrustful employers to consult the agency record with colleagues in other businesses. Affirmative action statutes have given needed impetus for employers to become more involved with job development and other rehabilitation programs. This puts a responsibility on vocational rehabilitation personnel to be prepared to provide the information, assistance, and referrals necessary to help employers conform to the law.

Of particular value to the counselor is a legal understanding of the employment rights of people who have a disability. A handbook on the subject was prepared by the George Washington University Regional Rehabilitation Research Institute [Hermann & Walker, 1978]. Publications of the National Center for Law and the Handicapped at South Bend, Indiana and its Director of Legal Services, Kent Hall, contain authoritative information on the legal rights of disabled people.

Chapter 39

Small Business Enterprise

Public rehabilitation programs have traditionally provided special services that help eligible clients establish and operate small business enterprises (SBE). These SBE plans may be for either a product or a service to be provided in a business venture owned and operated by the rehabilitant. Product businesses include both sales of manufactured articles and the manufacturing, assembly, or preparation of products for either wholesale or retail distribution. Services include such businesses as bookkeeping, typing, and telephone answering services.

A small business enterprise, then, is defined as an independently owned and operated venture that involves such activities as the manufacturing of products; processing of raw materials; assembly of components; provision of services; and marketing, sales, and other activities by the operator. In the vocational rehabilitation context, the venture must constitute substantial gainful employment as opposed to marginal employment or avocational activity. In other words, since SBE programs generally entail a great deal of counselor attention as well as "seed money," the income or income security is expected to exceed that which would have been possible if the individual had been trained to work as an employee for someone else. Moreover, the state rehabilitation agency cost should not be excessive when compared with the anticipated profit. Generally speaking, "homecraft" clients are not considered a part of the SBE program (see *homebound training* in the Vocational Preparation section of Chapter 14, Educational Services).

39.1. Introduction

The small business enterprise is an option for individuals who have the capacity and desire to acquire independent business skills. Implementing a small business plan is a difficult and demanding activity, both physically and psychologically, and the consequences to the client if the enterprise fails can be serious. Irreparable loss may be incurred by the client as the result of premature insurance settlements, investment of personal funds, bad business debts, unfulfilled community expectations, strain on family support, and personal anxiety. In some instances the stakes and risks will both be high, less so in other instances. Nevertheless, the SBE option is not viable for individuals who show a pattern of failure in the rehabilitation process or who do not possess the basic personal characteristics that make an independent business possible.

The fact that approximately 10 percent of all placements in the public rehabilitation program during recent years have been in the area of self-employment—mostly in small business operations—shows that handicapped individuals do have an opportunity in such operations. Well over half of the severely disabled persons operating small business enterprises with the help of the state rehabilitation agencies remain in business. This is remarkable in the light of the overwhelming number of small business failures in general after less than a year. This record is made possible by rigorous assessment, supervision, and training of clients in the SBE program.

The material for this chapter is based primarily on information provided by William Georgiles who, since completion of his professional preparation in rehabilitation counseling, has specialized successfully in helping state rehabilitation clients establish small businesses. Georgiles [1973], the author of an unpublished manual on the subject, is responsible for many of the original ideas recorded here. Additional information sources are miscellaneous federally sponsored training materials [e.g., U.S. GTP, IRS, IRI], including *Small Business Enterprises for the Severely Handicapped* [U.S. HEW, Office of Vocational Rehabilitation, 1955].

39.1.1. ESTABLISHING A NEW BUSINESS

For a successful business operation a number of elements must be combined. The most important of all of these is the individual who is to run the business. The responsibility of running a business is quite different from that of working for someone else. The smallest retail store or service shop requires sound managerial judgment; decisions must be made many times every day; action must be taken. Some people are more adept at this task than others. Equally important, no business person, despite technical training and management judgment, can succeed without liking and getting along with people— every successful business is based upon good customer relations.

But no matter how personable or good a manager a person is, the business cannot earn a profit without a market, that is, people who need and will buy the product or service offered for sale. In a proposed business, careful thought must be given to competition, sources of supply, location, necessary financial backing, and the length of time it will take to get the business on a self-supporting basis.

Every prospective operator must be acquainted with those laws and regulations of the federal, state, county, and municipal governments that apply to the prospective type of business. Any question or doubt should be clearly resolved by a consulting authority before the venture is undertaken. Also, every prospective entrepreneur should keep up to date in business practice. This means joining appropriate trade associations, reading trade bulletins, and subscribing to and carefully reading trade papers.

39.1.2. AGENCY PROGRAM

As is the case with all placement options, success in implementing small business plans depends largely upon the appropriateness of agency programs and staff training. The kinds of assistance that agencies can provide include assessment of the client's capabilities and the feasibility of the enterprise; provision of funds, materials, and information; and intercession with other agencies involved in the management of small businesses. In some situations, the agency will maintain a variety of buildings, equipment, and sales outlets under direct management and supervision. In other cases the agency may provide long-term assistance to business operators—including managerial and supervisory consultation—and centralized purchasing and distribution [McCavitt, 1967]. This practice makes possible independent business operation by severely disabled people who require occasional assistance. The ultimate intent of an SBE program, however, is to nurture client businesses that will become self-sufficient.

39.1.3. SMALL BUSINESS ADMINISTRATION

To assist Americans who desire to establish independent small businesses there exists an agency of the federal government called the Small Business Administration (SBA). This agency provides training sessions in management and marketing techniques, publishes extensive materials on business practices, and maintains a staff of local business people to counsel those in need of advice. In addition to these services, the SBA can assist individuals in obtaining bank loans by guaranteeing payment by the federal government should default occur. One qualifies for such assistance after an accountant examines the business plan and analyzes the profit, loss, and operating costs projected for several years.

39.1.4. PUBLIC REHABILITATION POLICY

The state rehabilitation agency is authorized to provide various services to help clients establish their small business. Many state rehabilitation agencies have SBE specialists, but all rehabilitation counselors need to be able to provide consultation services. The client usually needs help developing and assessing the feasibility of a small business plan. This requires a prediction of the problems and knowledge of consulting and other resources.

The state rehabilitation agency can purchase the equipment, initial stocks, and supplies necessary to establish the business. They can also provide training and consulting services needed by the client to get started. Most important in many cases is staff consultation, counseling, and advocacy.

The 1936 federal Randolph-Sheppard Act (PL 74-732) and similar state laws in many states provided for rent-free use by blind people of selected concession space in public buildings. As arranged by the state rehabilitation agency, the client is not only set up in a counter to sell snacks or sundries but also is trained in business practices, sales techniques, facility upkeep, and inventory control. When the operator retires or otherwise abandons the stand, the state agency, as the contractural or licensing authority with the building management, finds another disabled operator. Vending machines are likewise purchased (or rented) for the use of blind vendors who are taught to maintain them for the profits from product sales. These operations usually receive closer counselor supervision than independently established small businesses.

The Wagner-O'Day Act (PL 75-739) of 1938 stipulated that blind and, as amended by Public Law 92-28 (by Javits, *et al*) of 1971, other disabled people, have first priority in supplying products and services under federal contracts. Usually the government purchases have been ashtrays, mattresses, flags, and other such items manufactured by rehabilitation workshops (see 8.3.5).

The 1978 Amendments to the 1973 Rehabilitation Act authorized a new program of "business opportunities for handicapped individuals." In this unique provision the federal (not the state) rehabilitation agency can *directly* provide funds to handicapped individuals to enable them to establish or operate commercial or other enterprises and to develop or market their products or services.

39.2. Assessment of Potential

Assessment of client potential for SBE success consists of examining a number of variables, not all of which are equally important for determining client success in business. Research, for instance, to discover what characteristics separate the successful from the unsuccessful business entrepreneur indicates that managerial and personality factors count for more than the disability condition in predicting success in business.

Managerial ability is difficult to evaluate. The counselor looks for cues such as how the client is handling personal affairs, has the person been successful in making decisions involving significant amounts of money, and other indicators that the client knows how to capitalize on opportunities. Managerial ability is also marked by an appropriateness in timing and the ability to organize and maintain complex activities.

39.2.1. PERSONAL VARIABLES

Personality and other characteristics are related to SBE success. Those listed below are worth considering when trying to predict success.

Self-confidence

Self-confidence is a very important factor, especially since other desirable traits flow from it, such as initiative, aggressiveness, and sociability. Here again, careful observation of the client's behavior is essential. Another way of measuring self-confidence is to require the client to contribute substantially toward the effort. This contribution should consist of client financial resources (e.g., workers compensation settlement), if available, as well as the work required for planning and preparation prior to any cash outlay in establishing the business. Overconfidence without a sound foundation in managerial ability is characterized by an abundance of boasting and a lack of past accomplishment.

Steadiness

Steadiness (self-control) is also needed, since a client who cannot cope with frustration is unlikely to carry on to success. An SBE plan is not for the emotionally unstable, those given to depression, and the easily discouraged. Ample cues to this type of stability are provided by observation of how the client handles the various obstacles that occur in SBE planning phases.

Reputation

A good reputation, or at least the absence of a bad one, is essential when starting a business. This is required for access to lines of credit and to outlets for services or product sales. In the community it is vaguely referred to as "a good name, reliable, dependable, honest, and well liked," but reputation has tangible value for the business person. The counselor must therefore consider the risks of an SBE objective for a client who is on probation or who has a history of bad checks, bankruptcy, and the like. It is important to find out, for example, if this person can secure a small but quick bank loan. A credit check is considered standard procedure. A client who is stigmatized in a town because of a prison record or other non-business-related reason may be able to get established in another community.

Age

The client's age must be considered. Young people with other alternatives may be tempted to give up too easily. Are they lacking in the mature judgment obtained through general life experiences and, as a consequence, likely to make too many basic errors such as indiscreet purchasing, flip decisions, abuse of credit, imprudent expenditures or agreements? On the other hand, old clients may not be able to put in the very long hours a business demands or may not be motivated for the future and prepared to make the personal sacrifices required. Middle-aged clients are often successful because they usually have established a good reputation, have some capital they can invest, and have family support that can help get things going.

39.2.2. VOCATIONAL CONSIDERATIONS

Another group of variables that may be used to predict SBE success has to do with performance of tasks.

Knowledge and Previous Experience

Relevant knowledge and previous experience of the SBE client, rather than formal education, are the critical issues. The counselor will rarely have the intimate knowledge for evaluating a client's job knowledge and business capacity and the client may overestimate it. The opinion of a person knowledgeable in the proposed line of work should be sought. For such an evaluation a lay person may be better qualified, because of personal experience, than psychometrists or work evaluators. For example, a successful restaurant operator can determine if a prospective restauranteur is qualified. On the other hand, the successful business person may not know the impact of disability and other considerations. The physical aspects of the work required should be carefully assessed by the rehabilitationist as soon as the question of job knowledge has been answered. A very simple and effective way of measuring the physical aspects is to ask the client to provide an on-site demonstration. Sometimes workshops can help with this issue.

Family Support

Family members can be an asset. Does the client's wife or husband have the requisite knowledge or characteristics to help the client? Is the family (including offspring) interested and able to work in this type of business? Many banks consider this in deciding whether or not a loan should be approved. Furthermore, family members may cover for a client who must be hospitalized or is for another reason not available. Other friends and connections of both client and family are important in business. Other assets are good relationships with the mayor, bank manager, business people, and others in the community.

Client Contribution and Effort

The ability of clients to contribute toward their own cause is important. It has been found that the small business enterprise plans with the highest rate of failure are those with no financial participation by the client. The reason is not so much the client's failure to contribute financially in the SBE, as the person's ineptitude in accumulating money for investment. It follows that the greater the personal investment of the client the better the chances of success.

Disability

Type of disability may not be a critical issue in determining the feasibility of an SBE plan. The relationship between success in a small business and the disability of the operator is not high. There are exceptions, of course; for example, quadriplegic clients often have physical difficulty, and the problems of business operation by emotionally disturbed or alcoholic clients are obvious.

Public Assistance

Persons who have been on long-term public assistance or come from a home background of long-term reliance on such assistance are usually poor risks for this type of plan. The main reasons are a lack of available capital, absence of a good community reputation, and a past life-style that has not resulted in the person's learning independent managerial skills.

39.2.3. CLIENT CHARACTERISTICS

Tseng and Parker in 1976 compared successful and unsuccessful rehabilitation clients placed in self-employment projects. Significant attributes for success were: a positive perception of success and attitude toward work, self-acceptance, never married but receiving family backing, seeing value attached to being one's own boss, need for autonomy, self-controlled, conservative, having a desire for profit, and a positive attitude toward self-sufficiency.

39.3. Suitability of Business

Determining the suitability of a proposed SBE involves consideration of the demand for the product or service, the current state of competition, the business location, and the expected level of income. The determination of suitability is a joint activity of the counselor and the client since each will have access to different sources of information.

Counselors specializing in SBE programs for an extended period of time develop an ongoing awareness of current marketing opportunities in their areas. Former clients and business contacts keep them informed of fluctuations in the availability and demand for goods and services. Consequently, clients have an advantage at the outset when working with specialized SBE counselors. The role of the counselor is to get the client started by showing how to establish a business rather than doing all the work for the client. This approach assures that the client has a stake in the program and can successfully deal with situations that arise in the counselor's absence.

39.3.1. MARKET ANALYSIS

The client's market analysis begins with the designation of an enterprise line and the delineation of the geographic territory in which sales are likely to occur. Determination of a need for the particular SBE line begins with an assessment of the number of establishments the area could potentially support. A rough estimation of the market size can then be made by listing the size of the particular establishments already in existence. Further refinements in the analysis require a survey of competitors and consumers, information on business and population trends from business advisors, and examination of the business setting.

Competition

While the number and size of competitors' businesses are important in determining the market size, their reputation and management quality are even more important. A new enterprise may find it difficult to pull steady customers away from existing businesses, but a well-managed concern can thrive in the midst of abundant mismanaged competition. In some lines of business, however, the presence of highly regarded competition gives rise to a reputation in the community that increases the sales for all concerned. Employees, other businessmen, consumers, chambers of commerce, and better business bureaus are sources of information.

Consumers

A market analysis of consumer attitudes and behavior usually means interviewing a fair sample of competitors' customers and area residents. They are asked questions regarding what they need, where they shop, and how satisfied they are with the existing establishments. Usually the pattern that develops in the overall results of such a survey will indicate if there is support for a new business. There is no real substitute for talking directly to the prospective consumer.

39.3.2. BUSINESS ADVISORS

Part of the market analysis consists of contacting the business advisors of the rehabilitation agency or the Small Business Administration, the chamber of commerce, bankers and other lenders, business research institutes in universities, trade organizations, and U.S. Commerce Department branch offices. Wholesalers and suppliers of commercial equipment are often in an excellent position to offer advice due to their relationship with retailers across a large area. These people and agencies are aware of the financial condition of existing businesses as well as the demand for their products. Their advice is also important for a determination of the appropriate formal structure in line with local business practice, codes, and taxation.

Credibility of Information Sources

In order to determine if there is a market for the proposed product or service, the rehabilitation counselor resorts to knowledgeable sources who will give valuable data. For various reasons even good consultants will be overly optimistic. Sometimes the comments of a public official or family friend will be influenced by a desire to see the disabled person get even a slight chance—if the state takes the financial risks. One way to offset this sort of thing is to request written opinions. Another problem is that even what should be a solid source of information (e.g., the

Small Business Administration), may often refer to national trends, which may not even apply to the proposed locale, as a basis for judgment.

39.3.3. COMMUNITY SETTING

The commercial characteristics of every community are different, depending, for example, on whether it is primarily a mining town, an agricultural community, an industrial city, or a residential area. The nature of the community determines the type of people attracted to it and the kind of businesses needed to serve the residents.

The business character of any area is determined in part, too, by its proximity to population concentrations. For example, in a suburb of a larger city, business places serve the immediate needs of the suburban residents. If, on the other hand, the community is quite close to a city shopping area, the tendency is for consumers to drive there for goods and services.

Consumer values, spending patterns, and the physical layout of the business areas will also affect the viability of the SBE plan. Certain kinds of businesses usually occur in clusters, giving complimentary services to the consumer. The specific location can be critical, and the nature of other establishments in the area is a clue to the patterns of success. Some businesses traditionally do well in ethnic districts, small towns, or rural areas. Usually a small business does not have the advertising and capital resources necessary to sway consumer behavior toward favoring a new line of goods.

Retail and service businesses fall into classes with common characteristics. For example, retail stores are sometimes broken down into three classes: convenience, shopping, and specialty. A convenience store must be located so customers need not go out of their way to buy cigarettes, food products, hardware, drugs, and other types of small items it sells.

A shopping store primarily carries items in which style plays an important part. Women in America typically buy much of this type of merchandise and they are willing to go further to shop and compare and finally buy a hat, a dress, shoes, or furniture. In order to accommodate comparison shopping, competing stores must be located near each other in a fairly large shopping district. Department stores are the best example; they are often grouped together and surrounded by apparel shops.

The specialty store, on the other hand, carries well-known brand and trademarked items, often of considerable value, such as automobiles or appliances. Customers know these products by brand and will go fairly far out of their way to find the brand they think they want to buy. Such stores are often located on side streets or on secondary shopping streets or centers.

39.3.4. EXPECTED INCOME

Any projection of expected income depends upon a summary of all of the above appraisals of business potential and client suitability. The business must at least meet the client's financial needs to make living expenses, retire debts, and replace obsolete equipment, as well as meet other business expenses. If heavy state rehabilitation agency expenditures or investment are involved, there is an obvious official reason to look very closely at the projected income factor. If a commercial loan is anticipated, expected income is one of the main considerations for approval. The rehabilitation counselor's concern for correctly predicting the profitability of an SBE is equally great when the client is the principal underwriter of the expense. For example, a house or farm used as collateral for a loan might be lost if the business fails.

The services of a public accountant are advisable in estimating the profit potential of a proposed business. If it is an existing business for sale, an accountant should examine the owner's books in order to form an opinion. Banks also offer this type of consultation.

39.4. *Implementing the Plan*

The rehabilitationist's role in the SBE program usually involves client assessment, guidance in selection of the enterprise, and assistance in implementation of the SBE plan. This role requires a familiarity with business practices and the development of a team of consultants. When judgments concerning marketing, business trends, management, funding, accounting, and business law are beyond the expertise of the counselor, specialists may be able to provide the counselor and client with information on the consequences of and alternatives to a plan of action. Some agencies will have a formally designated consulting unit consisting of a lawyer, an accountant, a business management technician, and a financial advisor. In other cases, the rehabilitationist may be able to cultivate personal friendships in the business community for advice or use agency funds for purchasing occasional consultation services. At times, information and consultation on business matters can be provided by other public agencies.

39.4.1. THE SBE PLAN

The SBE plan, like the individualized written rehabilitation program, serves as a statement of goals, stipulates the responsibilities of client and counselor, and schedules steps to be taken. The SBE plan is more complex, however, because it requires the finite stipulation of funding mechanisms, market analysis, and contractual obligations of suppliers. Clear statements of the legally binding obligations of all parties involved are necessary, as well as the title to equipment purchased by agency funds, schedules for repayment of loans, consequences of default, and criteria for termination of affiliation. The plan should describe the client's functional limitations and the methods by which they will be overcome or the reasons why they will not interfere with the individual's ability to carry out the plan. It indicates the rationale behind the business line, expected income level, operational expense figures, and the reasons why a successful outcome is expected. Partial agency investment requires justification for the goods and services purchased, consultation fees, and client expenses, as well as an explanation of why the client is unable to afford the entire cost without assistance. The plan constitutes the primary document to be used in negotiating bank loans and settling disagreements that may arise between the client and the counselor. Like other behavioral contracts, it should be mutually understood by the client and counselor and have the signatures of both.

Client Involvement

Obtaining client participation in the development and implementation of an SBE plan often presents many difficulties that require the counselor's attention. While it is essential for clients to be responsible for implementing the plan, most individuals are not experienced enough to perform many of the tasks involved. The counselor's role becomes one of appraising clients' capabilities, involving them gradually in the process, advising them when appropriate, and referring them to training programs for business skills. An inaccurate estimate of the client's preparedness for a responsibility can result in frustration and can undermine the plan.

As clients usually respect the counselor's knowledge of the business world, there may be a tendency to misjudge the counselor's capability and time available for the individual project. Each client needs to be informed of the counselor's limitations in expertise and time and of program problems (such as lags in approval of vouchers and the need for accurate specifications for preparing purchase orders). Clients need to be encouraged to participate in the plan implementation by contributing their own funds to cover incidental expenditures, seeking their own business consultants, attending management seminars and trade conventions, and subscribing to trade journals. Their increasing knowledge and skill shows their commitment to the enterprise plan, a good indication of the SBE's likelihood of success.

Initial Capital Investment

The initial investment of capital necessary to establish the enterprise usually comes from a variety of sources. These include the client's personal savings, insurance settlements, loans from relatives, sponsorship from the state rehabilitation agency, donations from private groups, and business loans from banks and other sources. Some clients will have personal property that can be converted into cash or used as collateral for a note. In other cases, branches of national organizations for disabled people, churches, unions, civic clubs, and newspapers will make contributions to the establishment of the business or assist efforts to raise funds. An alternative available in some states is the use of disability insurance by arranging an immediate lump sum settlement to be invested in a gainful business in lieu of the regular payments that serve as subsistence and compensation.

Agency Investment

There are several reasons for using agency funds to support a feasible business plan. A substantial agency investment may be essential to acquire the initial operating equipment and/or supplies necessary to begin an enterprise that lacks capital but is otherwise a sound undertaking. The agency's tangible backing in turn will help to make available the financial resources of banks and other agencies, since these organizations will regard the investment as a sign of the potential success of the business. Furthermore, the agency's investment can serve as a motivating force to encourage client efforts.

Since the purpose of the SBE plan is to earn the client a return on the initial investment, it is possible in some types of enterprises to finance later stages of business growth out of early profit. Nevertheless, since there is always a risk of temporary reversal in business fortune resulting from seasonal market fluctuations, the climate, and so on, it is necessary in any enterprise to guard against precipitous business failure by maintaining credit or cash reserves that may be drawn upon as the need arises. Consultation with an accounting firm or a financial advisor is one way to maintain control over levels of investment capital needed for successive stages of plan implementation and the size of cash reserves necessary to cover future purchases, salaries, tax obligations, and other contingencies.

The SBE plan may call for incremented investment on the part of the rehabilitation agency at successive stages. For example, there may be an agreement with the client to provide backing for business expansion once the reputation of the business has been established and the market potential has grown.

39.4.2. DECISIONS

A number of decisions are required in implementing the SBE plan. Some of these matters have legal implications.

Equipment Rental

Whether to purchase or rent equipment must be decided. Business sites and equipment can be leased or rented. Such an approach is often a solution when sufficient funds for outright purchase cannot be mobilized. It is also an excellent approach when the counselor has doubts about either the client or the merits of the business proposition. It creates less pressure and responsibility on the agency and the mechanics are easier to execute. More important, such an approach does not entail a great risk for the client and permits a trial period. Lease-purchase agreements can be made. But in all leases and rentals the parties concerned are informed in writing in a very specific fashion as to the extent of commitment and responsibility.

Partnership

Partnership arrangements may be a suitable business option for some clients. Clients with complementary skills or resources may be able to compensate for each other's limitations and make a viable business team if their goals and personalities are suitable. Such might be the case in a joint venture by an individual who is capable at production with someone else who is talented at marketing. The key to successful exploitation of such arrangements lies in the clients' mutual needs for the relationship. Partnerships require a good deal of extra research into the motivation, resources, and experience of the parties involved. Clients are counseled to be prepared for eventual termination of the business relationship should the viability of the partnership deteriorate. Evaluation of the suitability of relatives in partnerships should be based on personality and family history factors as well as incentives for cooperation. Generally partnerships with relatives are beneficial, although sometimes they are disastrous.

Business Purchase or Franchise

Vacant businesses, closing businesses, and franchises provide a variety of tempting but risky alternatives to the small business entrepreneur. Pursuing any of these options requires a thorough-going investigation of the business line and the owner's motivation for selling. Building, equipment, and stock should be appraised to ascertain their real worth and a check made to determine whether the existing business conforms to zoning and health ordinances. Also, the growth and volume of business, margin of profit, adequacy of suppliers, and community reputation must be determined. This information needs to be substantiated by financial advisors after an audit has been conducted to ascertain profit of the business. Also to be considered is the risk of inheriting the bad debts or other legal obligations of a former owner. The situation calls for an attorney and tax accountant to examine the legal documents (e.g., lease, contracts) and financial records of the business. Building inspectors,

electricians, and plumbers may be required to examine the condition of premises that are desired for the business. If equipment is included in the sale price, an appraisal by a dealer is worthwhile.

Legal Requirements

The establishment of an SBE may require attention to state and local licensing regulations, building permits, insurance coverage, labor laws, zoning ordinances, mortgages, incorporation, and leasing. Incorporation is a method of protecting the business venture from the client's personal creditors. Liability and fire insurance are standard considerations.

Purchase of Equipment and Stock

The SBE plan includes a listing of equipment and stock necessary for operation of the business. The listing indicates the level of priority: materials essential for starting operation, equipment that would improve production, materials essential for later stages of operations, and items that are nonessential but desirable. The listing is further classified by specifying which items are to be purchased by the agency or the client. Second-hand equipment may be specified to reduce initial costs—although with some kinds of equipment maintenance costs outweigh this advantage. A consultant should examine expensive second-hand equipment before it is purchased.

The client's funds should be used to purchase equipment that is personal in nature or to pay for improvements to the client's own property. Other kinds of expenditures that the client should cover are those that may prove embarrassing to the agency or awkward to its funding authority.

Residual Title

The state rehabilitation agency policy of retaining ownership of equipment, property, and buildings purchased at public expense is to protect the agency's investment. In case of business failure, death, or a client's abandonment of the SBE, tangible assets can be reclaimed for use with other clients. Procedural guidelines for retaining "residual title" require the agency to maintain possession of title documents and contracts that indicate that, ultimately, items purchased with agency funds are to be returned. In many cases, the client will be able to acquire ownership of the business property by reimbursing the agency for its investment. The loss accrued to the agency by depreciation of its investment and the likelihood that the client can eventually purchase the material at a depreciated value serve as incentive and reward for maintaining good business practice. Some agency investments are granted outright after a successful business record has been achieved.

Closure and Follow-up

The counselor's goal in the SBE program is to make the client increasingly more independent and self-reliant. Termination of the counselor's involvement occurs when one of three conditions is met: (1) the client is capable of successfully operating independently; (2) the counselor has tried all practicable approaches with a client without achieving substantial progress; or (3) the client's enterprise is suffering because of business factors that are beyond the counselor's power to change.

Some clients will benefit from continuing contact for an extended period of time, especially if assistance is required in adjusting to debilitation. Status 32 allows for brief intervention to keep the business from failing or to overcome unexpected medical setbacks after the plan has been completed (see 36.5). In other cases, local business people may volunteer to assist the client from time to time as situations require the expertise of someone who is more experienced.

39.4.3. BOOKKEEPING

Adequate bookkeeping is a primary requirement for operating a business. It is the means by which records are kept of purchase orders, inventory, wages, sales and other income, loan repayments, and profits. Accurate information enables the owner to take advantage of pur-

chasing opportunities as well as to plan for varying work schedules to conform to fluctuations in sales and work demand.

Bookkeeping skills may be learned in vocational school, but the services of a public accountant may also be required. At times, clients will doubt the need for recordkeeping and will be skeptical of this advice. An accountant or business advisor who is experienced in the kind of enterprise being considered may be quite valuable in informing clients of the skills to be acquired and the pitfalls to avoid. Among the errors most likely to be committed by the inexperienced persons are the following: (1) failure to take advantage of legitimate tax reductions for depreciation and obsolescence of equipment; (2) failure to keep an exact record of expenses or to distinguish between "gross profit" and "net profit"; (3) failure to set aside funds for quarterly tax payments and replacement of worn equipment or depleted inventory; (4) failure to plan for the effect of interest charges or principal repayment on loans; and (5) failure to anticipate seasonal fluctuations in earnings that require prorating of payments over lean months.

A primary concern in bookkeeping is that personal and household funds must be kept separate from business income and expenses. All expenditures above a few dollars should be in the form of business checks, and all income should involve a register receipt or written sales slip.

Counselors should expect monthly income-expense reports from their clients as a way of learning of the suitability of accounting methods and the need for assistance. Occasionally, clients will be mistrustful of the counselor because of their personal pride in being independent, or because of fear that the counselor's knowledge of success might jeopardize assistance or result in taxes on unreported income.

39.5. Causes of Failure

Chances of failure can be minimized by close adherence to careful selection and matching of clients and business objectives; provision of whatever is necessary to offset client deficiencies in terms of knowledge and experience; provision of sufficient resources including capital, thorough planning, active supervision of the plan; and adequate follow-up over whatever period of time proves to be necessary. Failure

does at times occur, however, and can usually be related to the following causes.

39.5.1. FINANCIAL MANAGEMENT

Perhaps the major reason for SBE failure is inadequate financing or poor financial management. Some of the more frequent problems are discussed here.

Insufficient Capital

There should be proper equipment and adequate stock, and at least sufficient cash for one month's operational expenses, presuming that the client's domestic expenses are not an issue. Just having sufficient cash for one month's operating expenses is cutting things rather fine, however, especially in a business in which collections are delayed. The client might make arrangements with the bank whereby, for a fee, the bank allows credit but collects later. Most businesses suffer from periodic setbacks and can survive only when there is a reserve of funds or the ability to borrow.

Mismanaging Credit

The management of credit is a question not only of the rehabilitant's borrowing money, but also of extending credit. The latter can involve expertise, expenditure, and a capital outlay that the client cannot afford. On the other hand, volume of business can be hurt if the business cannot offer, say, a 30-day grace period.

Faulty Use of Capital

The faulty use of capital includes such errors as the purchase of inappropriate or superfluous equipment with a resulting lack of capital for needs that should have taken priority, such as payroll and other operational expenses.

Drawing Too Much Out of the Business

Drawing too much out of the business is not so much a business error as a matter of a lack of self-discipline. However, any counselor can see how a client is likely to give way under the pressures of previous personal debts and deprivation just as the business is getting under way with encouraging results. The best way to avert this kind of problem is to have the client approach all creditors just before getting started in the business and let them know of the situation and to work out an agreement for a reasonable repayment schedule.

39.5.2. OTHER PROBLEMS

Miscellaneous other causes of SBE failures are briefly described below.

Inexperience

The owner-manager of a small business must be a sort of jack-of-all-trades as opposed to executives in larger businesses who can depend on departmentalization. Very often the SBE case lacks experience in one area or another. Gaps in knowledge can be overcome in time while outside consultation is made available as the client gains experience.

Bad Location

That this type of error figures prominently among the causes for failure will not startle anyone. What is startling is that it should be committed so frequently by entrepreneurs ranging from the most sophisticated managements of giant companies that open subsidiaries and later have to close them down, to bootblacks who choose the wrong hotels. A good guideline is to choose the location solely on the basis of market search, and not be influenced by any motive other than profit.

Dependency on Limited Outlets and Suppliers

Perhaps the easiest way to describe this cause of failure would be to refer to the old expression of "putting all your eggs in one basket." The danger of having only one big customer is self-evident. The more suppliers that are accessible to the business, the more likely it is to get such things as free advertising and technical assistance. Dependence upon a single source of vital supplies places the business in a vulnerable position.

Business Neglect

Relatively recently established business owners, after having achieved success following a lot of hard work, sometimes make the mistake of delegating certain responsibilities or the operation of the business to others. A poor selection of managers and a lack of close personal supervision by the SBE owner often lead to rapid failure. Lack of motivation, a related cause of failure, refers to the owner's reluctance to work long and industriously. The desire to succeed is very necessary and thus very important.

Disappearance of Demand

The use of outdated methods and procedures are prominent among the reasons for business failures. The main problem is a decrease in the demand for the SBE goods or services. People are phased out of a job because of, say, automation and they have done nothing to prepare for such an occurrence.

Relatively new business ideas that appear to

have an encouraging and sure market are really untried and may not survive the test of time. New products and services that can be badly affected by new government regulations also can cause the business entrepreneur problems.

Inferior Products and Services

No amount of media advertising or other customer appeal substitutes for good products and services. Reliability, quality, standards, public relations, reputable dealings, fair pricing: these are the hallmarks of continuing business success. Satisfied customers return regularly and bring others to the small business enterprise. Because meeting all deadlines is an important business practice, good judgment is required when promising delivery dates.

Statistical Mortality

Counselors may encounter problems due to the differential assessment of business success by public agencies. A person who builds up a successful enterprise and sells out at a profit may be considered a business failure in the eyes of the SBA. Other examples of "statistical" failure are those who move their business to a new location, change business names, or are hired to more lucrative positions. A business that does not show a gain in profit over time may be considered a failure statistically—even though the owner receives a steady salary and is successful from a rehabilitation standpoint. Such varying perspectives as to what constitutes business success can cause difficulties in getting SBA assistance for SBE programs.

Chapter 40

Independent Living

A legitimate objective of public rehabilitation is independent living (IL) as set forth in the 1978 Amendments of the federal Rehabilitation Act. While an increased level of self-care has significant economic benefits, the humanitarian implications are more important. This emphasis on human values is implied by the definition of *total rehabilitation* as the fullest possible restoration of the individual in all of life's areas. Through IL rehabilitation the client achieves an enhanced place in life of greater value to both self and others. Independent living was defined in a federally sponsored project as "Control over one's life based on the choice of acceptable options that minimize reliance on others in per-

forming everyday activities. This includes managing one's affairs, participating in day-to-day life in the community, fulfilling a range of social roles, and making decisions that lead to self-determination and the minimization of physical or psychological dependence upon others" [Frieden, 1979, p. 6].

Independent living services should be conceptualized as a three-tiered operation:

1. *Prevention of Dependency.* Rehabilitation service needs may be reduced, postponed, or avoided altogether by early intervention that lessens or stops the course of a handicapping condition (i.e., physical, mental, emotional,

or environmental condition) that would, if unattended, adversely affect independency.

2. *Rehabilitation for Independency*. The (re)instatement of ability (e.g., training in daily living skills) to become independent of other people is the change (improvement) process properly called rehabilitation. It is at this level that the traditional vocational rehabilitation service operation and that of independent living are essentially alike.

3. *Maintenance of Independence*. Once rehabilitation is completed it is often necessary to continue selected services (e.g., attendant care) in order to avoid relapse. Thus some independent living services may be needed by a rehabilitant for life.

Prevention, rehabilitation, and *maintenance* for independency are three separate operations occurring at successive time phases and requiring different kinds of services. The public rehabilitation agency structure has been charged by the federal Congress with all three operations for independent living. Pre-service prevention of rehabilitative need and post-service maintenance of rehabilitation gain are new program dimensions for the public rehabilitation agency. The compatibility of these three separate service operations remains to be demonstrated. Clearly one must differentiate between IL service for the maintenance of independence and IL rehabilitation service to achieve independence. This book and rehabilitation counselors focus on rehabilitative mechanisms.

The role of the rehabilitation counselor in the processes of IL rehabilitation corresponds with that for vocational rehabilitation. Counseling and planning based upon client assessment and the selected utilization of community resources to meet client needs: these functions are required whether the rehabilitation objective is independence or remuneration. This expansion of rehabilitation in no way alters the professional strategies for client change. Rehabilitation technology is clearly applicable to the IL client group despite its difference in service needs and objectives. However, in the application of traditional rehabilitation techniques, the counselor requires special information about the additional needs of these most severely handicapped people and the appropriate resources available.

Much of the body of knowledge relevant to independent living rehabilitation has been incorporated in preceding chapters (e.g., chapters on functional limitations, community facilities, case study, advocacy, personal adjustment). Still there are other topics particularly applicable to the objective of self-care and independence (e.g., transportation, attendant care). Sometimes application of this knowledge about overcoming the barriers to independence facilitates placement in remunerative employment.

Rehabilitation counselors gained valuable experience in the IL needs of their clients when the 1973 Rehabilitation Act called for giving priority to severely handicapped applicants. As Pflueger [1977] pointed out, these counselors are finding that "independent living need not be a parallel and separate system, but can complement vocational rehabilitation objectives" [p. 3]. The 1978 extension of public rehabilitation to include independent living was long seen as desirable by many leaders and came close to implementation through congressional debate in 1959 and the early 1960s. (See 6.7 for a legislative history of public rehabilitation.) The delivery system for IL services includes private agencies as well as the public rehabilitation program.

A special note is needed regarding the potential client population for IL rehabilitation. The IL movement has been sparked by young, physically disabled (often spinal cord-injured) people. These vocal young people demanded and obtained government action for themselves and others (e.g., mentally and emotionally disabled). But as yet this constituency of the IL movement does not include the elderly; these people, too, need and would benefit from IL services—and they are a much larger group numerically. While the federal IL rehabilitation program does not exclude people because of age, provisions have not been made (either financially or programmatically) for the services needed to forestall admission to nursing homes by the infirmed elderly. Ultimately organizations for retired persons may be able to rectify this inadequacy in IL program implementation.

This chapter incorporates two previously isolated bodies of literature on the subject of independent living: one covers techniques used with people with severe physical disabilities as treated in rehabilitation medicine centers, while the other literature addresses deinstitutionalization of mentally ill or retarded people. Also included here are techniques relevant to independent living for a third type of clientele, the elderly—those with degenerative impairments —who all too often and too early are placed in nursing homes. A broad perspective of independent living includes all these client groups and the use of all rehabilitation services toward the objective of total rehabilitation.

Bibliographic materials on independent living rehabilitation were published in 1978 by the following: the Center for the Family American Home Economics Association; B. C. Smith at the University of Wisconsin–Stout; and the U.S. HEW, Office of the Secretary.

40.1. Introduction

The concept of *independence* is an integrating influence in the total rehabilitation process— medical, social, educational, occupational, recreational, and living skills rehabilitation. Bilotto and Washam [1979] saw the construct of independent living as inseparable from the concept of growth and maturity: the unassisted disabled person is reduced to "a condition of virtual infancy" with IL rehabilitation the "prerequisite for what we call adult life in this culture" [p. 22].

Independency means freedom from unwanted and unnecessary dependence upon other people (and things) in all areas of life. Vocational rehabilitation is aimed at overcoming financial dependency while rehabilitation for IL focuses on self-care or self-determination. *Self-care* refers to physical self-sufficiency, while *self-determination* means making one's own decisions and having authority over one's own destiny. In part, *physical dependency* is imposed upon functionally limited people because of environmental handicaps (e.g., steps) constructed for so-called "normal" people [Bowe, 1978]. Society also imposes upon disabled individuals a *psycho-social dependency* which deters self-determination. Disabled people properly fight against such unnecessary restrictions to their independence.

Despite all of the positive implications of physical and psychosocial *independence,* however, *dependency* must not be viewed automatically as a totally negative circumstance—or as one to be avoided at whatever the cost to human resources and other goals. In fact, civilization is based upon interpersonal dependency for the fulfillment of both physical and psychosocial needs. Love, a basic need, is exhibited by persons comfortably depending upon one another. Clearly psycho-social dependency can be a treasured relationship, but what about physical reliance upon others? By definition disability

means that certain areas of functioning are limited, and, if they cannot properly be conducted alone, assistance of some kind is indicated. But physical or other functional inadequacy and the need for help does not make a person inferior. When this is not understood by the functionally limited person, the resulting feelings of inferiority unfortunately lead to denial of the disability and of its functional consequences (the need for physical assistance); as a direct consequence of unfounded inferiority feelings, the disabled person may overcompensate and unrealistically reject help from other people (and assistive devices or programs). Conversely, there are overly dependent people who succumb to their disablement and do not fully utilize their potential ability (or rehabilitative opportunities). Ironically, succumbing behavior (too dependent), and denial, which leads to overcompensating behavior (too independent), are both due to basic feelings of inferiority. The point is that the behavioral manifestation of either *dependency* or *independency* can be either *excessive* or *deficient.* (See 4.5, 5.4 and 28.7.)

40.1.1. JUSTIFICATION

A substantial portion of the population need and would benefit from IL rehabilitation services. Survey research by the federal Social Security Administration indicates that about 15 percent of noninstitutionalized Americans between the ages of 20 and 64 are handicapped vocationally, and about half of this group are characterized as "severely disabled" (see 4.5.3). Reviewed before was the "Comprehensive Needs Study" conducted by the Urban Institute [1975a], which established the need and feasibility documentation requested by Congress before passage of the 1978 Independent Living Rehabilitation legislation (see 4.5.1). The substantial size of the dependent population was also estimated from data on vocational rehabilitation applicants declared infeasible for service, recipients of social security disability insurance and supplemental security income, and residents in various institutions and other sources. The State of New Jersey Rehabilitation Commission [1967] pioneered in the early 1960s in the development and demonstration of an IL rehabilitation program administered by the state vocational rehabilitation agency.

Economic benefits of IL rehabilitation have been estimated from demonstrations and other projects. The cost of 24-hour institutional care is staggering—greater than even partially successful IL effort, including the expense of home adaptations, attendant care, and other services that increase independence. The average cost of home care has been estimated at 25 percent (or even less) the cost of institutional care. Extensive personal and household help, of course, drive up the expense of living outside of a group setting.

40.1.2. DEINSTITUTIONALIZATION

Deinstitutionalization as described by Shoenfeld [1975] is an "attitude" that places great emphasis on freedom, independence, individuality, mobility, personalized life experiences, and a high degree of interaction in a free society. The concept encompasses both prevention of admission to institutions and return to the community from them. It should also mean the development of appropriate community residences and IL rehabilitation programs. (IL rehabilitation service is indicated for a substantial percentage of the deinstitutionalized clientele, but it is also appropriate for less severely handicapped people.)

The locational aspects of care have both financial and humanitarian implications. The latter has appealed to socially minded professionals and to reformers: at issue are human rights—self-determination and independence. On the other hand, taxation-conscious politicians saw the financial savings reaped by emptying state institutions for mentally ill and retarded people. (The term *deinstitutionalization* was coined to express President Richard Nixon's goal for the retarded population.)

In the early 1970s deinstitutionalization signified the goal of reducing the census of state "MR" institutions by one-third. Later its meaning widened to denote the process by which disabled people are kept in the community. It now also denotes the actual deinsti-

tutionalizing of an institution, in which those facets of institutional life that foster dependency are reduced or eliminated. Each resident is considered to have potential for community placement, hence programs are created to meet that one's total developmental needs whether the person is capable of leaving the institution or not.

A number of court cases since 1971 have supported the principle of a resident's legal right to receive treatment and programming in the "least restrictive environment." In essence the courts declared that a residential facility shall be used only as a last resort and only if the individual's needs are met. The case of *Wyatt vs. Stickney*, 344 F. Supp. 387 (M.D. Ala., 1972) was precedent-setting in this connection. It declared specifically that the constitutional rights of the retarded to habilitation were being violated in an Alabama public school. More importantly, however, in reaching this decision, it defined the minimum treatment standards required of the state school. These standards, noted below, take into consideration both the boundaries of institutional care and the future direction of deinstitutionalization.

1. No borderline or mildly retarded person shall be a resident of the institution.
2. No person shall be admitted to the institution unless a prior determination shall have been made that residence in the institution is the least restrictive setting.
3. Residents shall have a right to the least restrictive conditions necessary to achieve the purposes of habilitation. To this end, the institution shall make every attempt to move residents from: more to less structured living; larger to smaller facilities; larger to smaller living units; group to individual residence; living segregated from the community to living integrated in the community; dependent to independent living.

Implementation of the states' deinstitutionalization policy for mentally ill and retarded people revealed the need for a government-supported IL program. Previous attempts to expand public rehabilitation to include IL were primarily aimed at those with severe physical disabilities. In fact, IL methods such as teaching daily living skills and fitting assistive devices were developed for the orthopedically or other physically limited population, not for emotionally disturbed or retarded people. Still the philosophy of total rehabilitation and many IL techniques are applicable to mentally disabled people. Another client population needing IL services is the aged, who must otherwise be cared for in nursing homes; geriatric cases constitute a great challenge for deinstitutionalization through IL rehabilitation.

The objective of the deinstitutionalization movement is to provide the least restrictive circumstance that is suitable for each individual who has a severe disability. There are a variety of housing alternatives (see 8.5 and 40.5). While the goal is normalization there will still be residential institutions for those who must have intensive nursing, protective services, or other special accommodations, and also residents who do not wish to live outside of the institution.

40.1.3. PROGRAMMING

The early notion of IL services was the provision of such things as wheelchairs, special equipment and devices, or modifications of quarters, the objective being to permit severely disabled people to care for some of their own *survival* needs. This concept has developed with the growth of rehabilitation. *Total* rehabilitation is now the goal, with vocational and other kinds of life adjustment viewed as integral objectives of the process.

The rehabilitation components of IL programming are comparable to those of vocational rehabilitation in the state-federal system. The rehabilitation plan must be individualized, developed with the client, written out, and agreed to by both parties (see 27.6). Moreover, the choice or scope of services should be as broad as needed to accomplish all objectives. In several respects, however, IL programs do differ from vocational rehabilitation. While vocational rehabilitation may be a one-time expense with only a short-term follow-up, IL may require certain services (e.g., attendant care, meals on wheels) throughout the person's life. Moreover, IL services are not restricted to the work age group. Also, these programs generally make greater use of consumer participation (e.g., peer "counseling").

The public agency services for comprehensive IL rehabilitation involves an even broader range of resources and types of intervention than required in vocational services. Examples include the provision of attendants, maintenance of health, and modification or arrangement of appropriate housing. Other services have long been used for vocational rehabilitation but less often: purchase and training in the use of prosthetic and assistive devices and adapted vehicles; arrangement for the modification of equipment and barrier removal; personal adjustment training or counseling; and physical or mental restoration. (See 7.5.2.)

Service delivery variables are notable in different IL project and private program models as examined by Lex Frieden [1978]: (1) service setting—varies from strictly residential to nonresidential; (2) clientele—ranges from people with a single type of disability to people with any handicap, including aging; (3) delivery methods—either direct service by staff or referral to other agencies may be provided; (4) quality of staff—the pattern ranges from professionals to personnel with various levels of qualification, including lay volunteers; (5) goal emphasis—the vocational objective may be only incidental while other objectives are primary or vice versa; (6) program duration—transitional programs help people move from a level of dependence to independence and then terminate, while maintenance programs provide ongoing service to support a maximal level of independence. Program patterns for public IL rehabilitation are far from crystallized.

40.1.4. CLIENT ASSESSMENT

A guide published by the National Association of Sheltered Workshops and Homebound Programs [1961] stated, "The decision as to whether independent living is the goal for the patient must be made by qualified personnel of the rehabilitation team" [p. 79]. While experience has shown that independent living may not be an alternative for everyone, Frieden [1977] said that "given an adequately supportive environment and certain adaptive skills, most severely disabled individuals who wish to live independently will certainly be able to do so" [p. 55]. Independence, of course, is a relative state with many facets; everyone is dependent upon others to some extent for psychological and physical needs. At the extreme are those people who fear or cannot cope with independence and consequently prefer to live in an institution where life is structured and supervised [Bartels, 1978].

The determination of functional limitations and capacities is the basic evaluation. In IL rehabilitation this has followed the medical model codified within the field of occupational therapy.

While this is appropriate for some physical measurements (e.g., strength, range of motion), it has not covered the comprehensive array of handicapping factors described in Chapter 5, Functional Limitations. Evaluative information should be closely related to assessment goals: the interpretation of living skills as they relate to present task performance ability; the determination of required client services (e.g., adjustment training, recreation therapy, assistive devices); and the provision of environmental modification or equipment redesign.

Situational evaluations for IL is like that for occupational choice: both are based upon an analysis of the tasks involved in the work or activities objective. Activities required for personal independence provide the IL evaluative structure.

Eleven self-care activities can be rated as a measure of independence, based upon the amount of physical assistance required by another person: eating; dressing and undressing; grooming (washing and combing hair, bathing and washing, caring for nails, brushing teeth, and shaving); bed activities (moving about in bed, getting legs in and out, and maintaining balance); transferring to and from wheelchair, bed, toilet, and tub or shower; wheelchair propulsion (being mobile in the wheelchair); ambulation (walking); stair-climbing (going up or down more than one step in succession); food preparation (planning, preparing, and serving a meal); housekeeping (cleaning, caring for floors, dusting, washing dishes, shopping, and so on); and utilizing fine motor skills (turning door knobs, using lock and key, manipulating light switches, turning faucets on and off, tuning radio, operating telephone, writing name). The rating is not influenced by the use of equipment.

In a global assessment of ability (or potential) for personal care the individual may be hierarchically rated:

1. Independent outside the home.
2. Requires limited assistance outside the home.
3. Completely independent at home.
4. Requires assistance at home.
5. Requires the shelter or services of a halfway house.
6. Requires institutional care.

Promotion to the highest achievable level is based upon the assessment and other techniques discussed throughout this book. Client assessment is a rehabilitation counselor *planning*

function to determine service needs and potentials; it should not be confused with eligibility determination, which is an administrative decision.

40.1.5. ELIGIBILITY

The issue of case selection, the determination of eligibility and feasibility, poses a problem when there is no clear criterion for rehabilitation success such as "employed following completion of services." IL cases may require follow-along and other assistance that prevents the termination of services and case closure. Moreover, even the most severely handicapped persons may benefit from independent living services; the quality of their lives is improved by increases in their ability to assume greater responsibilities for themselves, thereby reducing their dependency and improving their self-concept. Partial independence is meaningful even for those who may never live outside of an institution. In addition, increased independence of the client confined at home may improve economic circumstances by permitting a family member to work outside the home.

The public rehabilitation agency's client eligibility criteria for IL and vocational rehabilitation were described earlier (see 15.4). Eligibility provisions for the two program areas are similar but IL is not restricted by the applicant's age (either old or young); vocational services have work-age implications. Client eligibility for public IL rehabilitation services, however, was not defined clearly in the 1978 federal legislation; the Congress did not completely break with the traditional vocational goal for the public program. Moreover, the wording of the law was vague. According to federal regulations, public IL rehabilitation client eligibility determination (briefly stated) is based upon: 1. a severe physical or mental disability, 2. a severe limitation in ability to function independently in family or community, and 3. the expectation that services will assist significantly in improving or maintaining independence (e.g., self-care, activities of daily living, driving, using public transportation, shopping, housekeeping, communicating, or living more independently). Priority is given to very severely handicapped groups.

Various other criteria for eligibility have been considered for IL projects and private agency programs: (1) severe disability (physical, mental and/or emotional), interfering with or preventing self-care for daily needs, must be present; (2) potential for favorable change in vital functions such as mobility, motivity, and communication must exist; (3) physical, emotional, and intellectual capacity or potential must be sufficient to carry out the demands involved in activities of daily living and the rehabilitation program; (4) deteriorative aspects of the disability should not be more rapid than the rehabilitative process; and (5) the IL goal must be the informed choice of the applicant.

As indicated earlier, assessment for IL rehabilitation may be more difficult than for vocational services. It is often necessary to explore for feasibility by the provision of service. Experience indicates, however, that some people have more chance for success than others (viz., those who are under 50 or 60 years of age, are financially independent, are adjusted socially and to their condition, have a strong drive for independence, have relatives available to help, and are referred to rehabilitation soon after onset of disability).

40.1.6. INDEPENDENT LIVING CENTERS

These service centers have the important purpose of enhancing the will and the way to self-care and self-determination by severely disabled persons and providing or securing supplemental services to help them gain and maintain life-support methods. Center programs reduce the time needed to achieve rehabilitation and are often successful when fragmented service provision fails. They have demonstrated the effectiveness of comprehensive services—particularly in the transitional stage after a person leaves a medical rehabilitation facility (see 8.4).

Various models for IL centers and service delivery systems exist. A number of state rehabilitation agencies had programs in operation even before the 1978 congressional authorization in their Amendment to the 1973 Rehabilitation Act. Many state rehabilitation agencies gained valuable experience over the years in a liberal interpretation of the provision of service to severely handicapped cases through "extended evaluation." Other states learned through research and demonstration projects [Wright, 1978a].

In 1947 Timothy J. Nugent at the University of Illinois started the first major program in higher education and by 1962 he had developed a community living program for students with severe physical disabilities in modified housing near campus. This self-help effort and affirmative action program at the Champaign-Urbana campus developed and was copied by many other universities—with grant support by the federal rehabilitation agency—long before the advent of IL legislation and IL Centers founded by consumers or other groups. The Center for Independent Living in Berkeley, California was established as a consumer self-help, outreach program in 1972. The Boston Center for Independent Living, founded in 1974, was established as a residential program, a consumer operated, self-help community of severely disabled people in transitional living facilities. The Boston Center is contrasted with the Berkeley Center which is not a residential program. These IL centers and others serve as models that can be visited and consulted by other communities organizing such programs.

Federal funds were authorized by the 1978 Amendments to the Rehabilitation Act not only for state agency services, but, also, for the establishment and operation of IL Centers. These centers "offer services which enable severely disabled individuals to live more independently in family and community, or to secure and maintain employment." An IL "center" does not necessarily have all services on the premises, but it is the "locus" through which a combination of services required by severely disabled persons are made available. Federal grants for these centers may be made to a private organization or another public agency if the state rehabilitation agency fails to apply.

The IL centers may provide a wide range of programs and services to promote independence, productivity, and quality of life: (1) professional counseling, (2) "peer counseling," (3) help with attendant care, (4) advocacy for legal and economic rights and benefits, (5) teaching IL skills, (6) help with housing and transportation, (7) arrangements for group living, (8) social and recreational activities, (9) health maintenance, and (10) other needed assistance. A long-term service goal may be maintaining a person in a living status which would deteriorate in the absence of supportive services (e.g., homemaker or attendant service). A client's individualized written rehabilitation program (IWRP) for transitional services (e.g., training in independent living skills) must include a plan for IL maintenance (needed supportive services).

40.1.7. DEFINITIONS

The definition of independent living and its related terms have changed over time and have varied according to disciplines. Following are definitions based upon recent notions.

INDEPENDENT LIVING. This term refers to one's ability in the activities of self-care and the processes of self-determination, despite severely limiting disability, in the least restrictive circumstances and setting of choice.

INDEPENDENT LIVING SKILLS. These are the skills needed to minimize dependence on others (e.g., skills for coping, self-help, assertiveness).

ACTIVITIES OF DAILY LIVING (ADL). ADL refer to all the activities arising from the individual's daily living needs (e.g., mobility, personal hygiene, dressing, and eating) and, also, community living. They occur in social, educational, occupational, and recreational pursuits.

ATTENDANT. A personal assistant or so-called attendant is one who facilitates physical or social independency by doing chores required by the disabled person.

AFFIRMATIVE ACTION. Instigated for legal or moral purposes, employers make a special effort to recruit, employ, and promote qualified handicapped persons.

ADVOCACY. This refers to actions by individuals or groups on behalf of one or more disabled persons to insure their rights and interests. (See Chapter 16, Protection and Advocacy.)

ACCESSIBILITY. This term refers to the availability for use by disabled persons of a program, activity, or building. It includes redesigning equipment, reassigning meetings to accessible places, providing transportation, and making aides available.

ADAPTIVE EQUIPMENT. This means any device or mechanical equipment that enables a person to minimize the handicapping effect of a functional limitation.

ARCHITECTURAL BARRIERS. These are constructions designed in such ways as to limit the free movement of a person with a functional limitation (e.g., mobility limitation). Examples include curbs, narrow doorways, inaccessible equipment.

DEINSTITUTIONALIZATION. A program intended to prevent the unnecessary admission to a public institution or facilitate the return to the community of persons who can function outside of an institution. The program requires developing, finding, and using community methods of IL rehabilitation.

REHABILITATION FACILITIES. These community-based facilities have been described in Chapter 8, but there are variations in the nomenclature to be mentioned: activity center —a facility providing social, developmental, and recreational programs for the severely disabled population, without regard to their productivity; adult development center—a facility that teaches severely disabled adults the skills needed for daily living.

CENTER FOR INDEPENDENT LIVING (CIL). A CIL is usually a coordinating office where professional, lay, and volunteer staff and needed resources enable severely disabled persons to live independently. Services typically include advocacy, attendant coordination, housing referral, counseling, and so forth.

TRANSITIONAL LIVING. In a transitional living program a housing facility is provided for a group of people exiting from an acute hospital.

CLUSTERED LIVING. This refers to a small group of persons living in a group setting in the community.

NORMALIZATION. Normalization is the process of effecting a person's exposure and adaptation to the patterns and conditions of daily life that are consistent with the norms of the mainstream of society.

ENVIRONMENTAL MODIFICATIONS. Modifications can be made of many obstacles that impede the functional abilities of the physically or mentally disabled person. Examples include modifications of architectural barriers that prevent wheelchair-bound individuals from gaining adequate access to buildings, substitution of lever handles for knobs, and providing curb cuts with textured material at street level.

40.2. Activities of Daily Living

Activities of daily living (ADL) require a fund of skills that may need to be learned by a disabled person to achieve independence. The ADL program is an essential component of IL rehabilitation. Originally the emphasis was upon self-care by people severely disabled physically. The concept has broadened to include all severely handicapped people and any kind of life activity. The ADL approach as it is related here and in the occupational therapy literature has been associated primarily with physical medicine and rehabilitation patients with orthopedic disabilities. This can be traced back to the early 1940s when the Institute for the Crippled and Disabled, in New York City, developed a scale for rating orthopedic cases in the "physical demands of daily life." Psychosocial aspects of ADL are addressed in the current literature of occupational therapy, however.

The concept of ADL can and will be expanded to address not only functional limitations associated with physical impairments such as paralysis but also limitations in functions caused by other disablements. The narrower focus, however, is reflected in most of the following descriptions of ADL techniques. The potential for future ADL development and application is implied in Chapter 5, which describes many functional limitations.

40.2.1. PROGRAM

Rehabilitation for IL consists of two identifiable procedures to minimize dependence on other people: (1) training the disabled person in the functional abilities required for daily living (ADL), including community living skills; and (2) altering the source of functional limitations by modification of the environment and by providing facilitative devices. The procedures are interrelated, of course, but they involve separate orientations. Training and other professional functions to do with ADL are the focus of this discussion.

The central professional in an ADL program is the occupational therapist, although other members of the rehabilitation team may contribute [Zimmerman, 1971]. Components of the ADL program are: (1) testing and training in daily living activities; (2) testing, providing (or

fabricating), and training in the use of, equipment; and (3) homemaking and housing evaluation and training. The full IL-ADL team may include a physiatrist, physical therapist, rehabilitation teacher, mobility instructor, home economist, prosthetist, orthotist, speech and hearing therapist, nurse, psychiatrist or clinical psychologist, rehabilitation engineer, social worker, rehabilitation counselor and others (see 2.4 and 8.4.3).

40.2.2. EVALUATION OF ACTIVITIES

ADL "tests" are primarily structured lists of activities or tasks performed by the disabled person under the observation of the therapist. These instruments generally do not reflect rigorous psychometric methods but do resemble some of the situational techniques used in work evaluation. Measurement criterion issues—such as validity, reliability, standardization in administration, and norms—are not fully recognized in ADL evaluative devices. As a consequence there is a problem in communicating results to other members of the IL rehabilitation team.

Performance measures of ADL can reflect a variety of factors, including: time, speed, quality, endurance, improvement with practice, effect of personal variables (e.g., incentives), effect of environmental variables (e.g., assistive devices). The primary questions in ADL evaluation are: What degree of independence has been reached? What help (training, equipment, or attendant care) is required? What is the person's overall performance in self-care at home and traveling? ADL activities in the work setting may be neglected in the ADL evaluation, although prevocational evaluation is frequently included.

Major activities and explicit tasks involved are listed on "ADL test forms." Each activity (and/or associated tasks) is rated by the occupational therapist or other evaluator on one or more scoring criteria (e.g., minimal assistance required). ADL items are listed below, along with selected example tasks (in parentheses): bed activities (moving in bed, roll to left and right, sit up); wheelchair activities (propelling, bed to wheelchair and vice versa, wheelchair to chair or to toilet); travel (wheelchair to car on curb—or no curb—and vice versa, place wheelchair in car); hygiene activities (comb hair, brush teeth, shave, put on makeup, turn faucet, wash and dry face or hands, take bath or shower, use urinal or bedpan); eating activities (eat with spoon or fork, cut meat, handle straw or cup); dressing activities (underwear, slipover garments, shirt or blouse, slacks or dress, tying tie or bow, socks or stockings, shoes, coat, braces, or prosthesis); hand activities (write name and address, manage telephone receiver and dial, handle wallet or purse with paper money and coins, turn pages in book or newspaper, use handkerchief); walking activities (open and go through door, walking while carrying); standing up or sitting down (from wheelchair, from bed, from easy chair, from toilet, into car, from the floor); traveling activities (climbing up or down stairs without railing, getting in and out of car or bus, walking one block, crossing street with curbs).

40.2.3. HOME EVALUATION

Planning the ADL program to achieve optimum adjustment is facilitated by a survey of the disabled person's regular dwelling. This investigation, as described by Zimmerman [1971], also provides information about needed adaptations. Checklists are available covering information such as the following: door sills, door widths, sink height, floor coverings, stairs (inside and outside), ramps, elevators, lights, location with reference to transportation and target destinations (e.g., shopping, recreational facilities, church, work).

Alterations advised are as follows: ramp incline five degrees (one to 12 inches) with rails all the way; door sills eliminated or minimized; doorways 30 to 32 inches or more wide; floors without carpeting or slick covering or coatings; wall switches 36 inches (or less) high; electric outlets at least 24 inches high; grab bars for bathtub and toilet. The kitchen area of the disabled homemaker is examined for accessibility of storage, equipment, and work space. It is well to sketch a floor plan with an equipment layout showing barriers and needed alterations for ease, enjoyment, and safety in utilization. Also useful is a list of special utensils and appliances (with supply sources and prices).

40.2.4. SKILLS TRAINING

Training the client in ADL skills is of course the basic function of the professional. To do this it is first necessary to analyze the motions for each particular activity; motions in putting on shoes, for example, are bending, reaching, grasping, pulling, and so on. Other activities may require motions such as standing, walking, or moving in the sitting position. The motions are (re)learned through practice, but going through the motions is not the same as carrying out the activity—the activity must be learned in its entirety and in the various environments in which it will be performed.

A general principle in ADL planning is that of energy conservation. Methods for this have been developed through research in industrial psychology and personnel management. Studies have revealed the following work simplification techniques:

1. Use both hands in opposite and symmetrical, smooth-flowing motions.
2. Arrange work areas within normal reach.
3. Slide objects (do not lift or carry them).
4. Arrange work areas and tools for different tasks, such as preparation and clean-up areas, mixing and baking center.
5. Eliminate unnecessary motions or processes.
6. Avoid holding (use clamps, stationary equipment).
7. Use assistance of gravity whenever possible.
8. Preposition tools for easy grasp or pickup.
9. Locate switches and controls within easy reach.
10. Sit whenever possible (do not stand).
11. Use proper work heights according to the job and the individual.
12. Work under good conditions (proper light and ventilation, pleasing colors, comfortable clothing).

Basic ideas in work simplification are suitable for both IL and vocational placement. The principles are: fewer trips save both time and energy, proper work heights are less fatiguing, sufficient lighting increases productivity, and the organization of work is essential to effective effort [Zimmerman].

Orthopedic disability (see 5.14, Motivity Limitations), such as absence or debilitation of a hand may be resolved with various ADL techniques; examples of adjustments of tasks or equipment in such a case are as follows:

1. Stabilization of tools and appliances.

2. Selection of tools that require only one hand for operation.
3. Selection of tools or utensils for type of handle easiest to grasp.
4. Consideration of type of motion used to operate equipment (whether up and down, push and pull, rotary).
5. Use of electrical equipment to eliminate manual operation.
6. Selection of utensils according to weight, shape, durability, ease of care.
7. Selection of containers (jars, packages) for ease of opening.
8. Use of special, adapted equipment [Zimmerman].

Gloria Hale [1979] has compiled a well-illustrated guide of invaluable practical information to help physically disabled persons live independently; *The Source Book for The Disabled* describes and illustrates specific and tangible steps for coping with the impact of disability.

40.2.5. COUNSELING

Daily living is much more than self-care—it incorporates the larger principle of the right to self-determination and to be a part of the community. True independence is the right of all humans. This right is denied until the barriers to independence are removed; the removing of these barriers to independent living may be considered as "total rehabilitation service" in its broadest context.

Some of the barriers to IL derive from the individual's physical, mental, or emotional condition. The above discussion focused on the physical aspects of ADL. Many of the *personal* adjustment problems, however, respond to counseling or other rehabilitative intervention (see Chapters 13 and 28, Adjustment Training and Personal Adjustment, respectively). Other barriers are of an external nature and are covered elsewhere in discussions on negative social attitudes, protection and advocacy, architectural and transportation barriers, and so

on. The two sets of barriers are interconnected; for example, financial difficulty in paying the rent on one's own apartment or in paying the salary of an attendant may stem from lack of knowledge about available financial assistance resources in the community (see Chapter 12, Agency Structures).

Counseling in IL rehabilitation is so critical to success that professional preparation is needed—preferably in specialization beyond the masters degree in rehabilitation counseling psychology. It is also very important to utilize (as most IL programs do) the personal support and information of "peer counselors" (i.e., lay people who are experienced by their own, similar disablement).

Rehabilitation counseling is targeted at resolving the problems of community living; how to achieve daily living objectives—finding and getting financial and other public assistance, asserting one's self for desired rights, getting along with others, feeling good about one's self, making one's own choices and enforcing these decisions. As in all professional counseling the goal is to put the client into complete control of his or her own life—to become independent. Adaptive information is important to convey in IL counseling. It includes dealing with the following areas: sexuality, social participation, consumer and employment orientation, supervision of attendants, and (perhaps most importantly), the utilization of the human service establishment.

Developmentally disabled persons and others who have been institutionalized or sheltered may not have had the opportunity to participate in ordinary life experiences. To become independent many must learn "community living skills," such as budgeting, personal hygiene and attire, shopping, socializing, and relating to other people. These social ADL training objectives are particularly important for mentally and emotionally disabled persons, but they are also needed to supplement the physical ADL objective for many long-term, severe, physically disabled people who have been overprotected or isolated [U.S. IRI, 1978a].

40.3. *Adaptive Devices*

Adaptive or assistive devices include a variety of technical aids, special equipment, and environmental adjustments designed to overcome the

many forms of functional limitations resulting from disabilities. The initial concept of assistive devices in rehabilitation, particularly within the field of occupational therapy, has expanded, with the application of sophisticated technology, to the ADL problems of disabled people. This expanded concept includes the use of prosthetic and orthotic devices, adaptive driving mechanisms, and rehabilitation engineering technical contributions. At one time special apparatus was used only when deemed essential for treatment. Therapeutic uses are still important, but the newer goal of self-help devices reflected here is to provide independence in daily activities despite functional limitation. This is a supplement to the use of orthoses and other methods in rehabilitative medicine that are prescribed to correct or prevent deformities by proper positioning, support weakened segments, control or stabilize joints, reduce stress on a joint, or prevent undesirable substitution.

40.3.1. PRINCIPLES

Every attempt should be made to improve function without use of an artificial device or to minimize the need for such devices [Zimmerman, 1971]. Often, however, they are necessary to provide greater independence or to increase bodily effectiveness or safety. When the use of a device is deemed necessary, it must be selected with the individual in mind. Because the device becomes an integral part of the person's activities, the relationship between the body and the mechanical construction must be studied.

Evaluation of a device prescribed for a person is based upon at least three criteria: the person's physical performance in the target activities; the person's psychological reactions to use of the device; and the effectiveness of the device itself. Design engineers should be aware of individual needs beforehand; the needs appraisal considers all of the person's functional limitations (e.g., mental and emotional conditions and fatigue, as well as mobility or motivity) and also the desired activities to be performed. Individualization is a principle because what works well with one person may not serve another, even though the two have the same type and severity of disability.

Modifications of standard equipment, according to Bilotto and Washam [1979], should be avoided unless the disabled person is unable to learn how to manipulate the standard version. Adaptation is often unnecessary when the disabled person employs ingenuity and imagination. When modification of equipment is needed it should retain the quality of usability for nonhandicapped persons; often it is found that the redesign is appreciated by everyone—for example, many people would prefer the easy incline of a wheelchair ramp to steep steps. Moreover, devices should be as aesthetically pleasing as they are easy to use. Long-term durability and reliability are also important—too many are constructed so that they do not stand up with the intensive or heavy use demanded for vocational or other activities of daily living.

40.3.2. INFORMATION SOURCES

Everyone is familiar with such commonly used appliances as spectacles, hearing aids, and canes, but there are many uncommon conditions for which standard, mass-produced equipment does not suffice. Severely or multiply handicapped people with unusual body measurements or impairments can also be equipped to cope with their condition and environment. Fortunately there are many unique, even fantastic, functional aids designed for unusual types or sets of limitations. They can be built to help the severely disabled rehabilitation client in many daily activities such as: personal care (hygiene, dressing, eating), mobility (walking, traveling), communication, learning, and so on. An increasing number of such devices are commercially available. Unfortunately, however, these ingeniously engineered designs or mechanical instruments are not well known and may be difficult to locate.

Isabel Robinault [1973], under the auspices of the United Cerebral Palsy Associations of America, prepared a comprehensive resource book of functional aids and equipment for the multiply handicapped. A number of similar reference works have been published over the years, covering not only commercially available devices but also custom-built ones. The American Rehabilitation Foundation [Rosenberg, 1968] has published designs of devices that can be made in a home workshop from simple materials to aid people with paralysis, amputation, cardiac, and other impairments.

The National Academy of Sciences [1975] has a computerized system for information on assistive devices for the physically handicapped. The Academy, which catalogues relevant professional literature, covers the following subjects:

1. Musculoskeletal prostheses for lost, missing, diseased, or injured portions (external or internal).

2. Musculoskeletal orthoses (i.e., assistive devices, aids, and supports fitted to the body) for weakened, painful, or paralyzed portions.
3. Technical aids that are not fitted directly to the body (e.g., powered wheelchairs, buttonhooks).
4. Rehabilitation engineering, which means the design, development, fitting, and evaluation of all of the above.

Recognizing the need for universal coordination and information exchange, Rehabilitation International in 1965 created the International Committee on Technical Aids, Housing and Transportation (ICTA) chaired by Karl Montan [1969], director of the Swedish Institute for the Handicapped, which houses the ICTA Information Center. Through this active affiliate, Rehabilitation International has developed a worldwide clearinghouse of technical aids and related adjustment information.

By its development of new systems and devices rehabilitation engineering strives to make life's needs and pleasures more obtainable or accessible to handicapped people. For example, there is a hand-size "communicator" on the market that prints messages on paper tape (10 characters a second) for people who are mute or deaf. Research on "sensory substitution" opens new vistas for people who are deaf or blind, or both; "biofeedback" research is applicable to various disabilities to restore function and overcome barriers. The U.S. Congress has provided liberal funding for biomedical and other rehabilitation engineering research. This topic was discussed in the Sixth Institute on Rehabilitation Issues [U.S. IRI, 1979].

Information about IL rehabilitation literature is available from the National Clearing House of Rehabilitation Materials at Oklahoma State University in Stillwater as well as the National Rehabilitation Information Center at Catholic University in Washington, D.C. The Rehabilitation Services Administration publishes the bimonthly journal *American Rehabilitation* (formerly entitled *Rehabilitation Record*). The President's Committee on Employment of the Handicapped publishes *Disabled USA*. The *Pathfinder*, a guide to information resources and technology in rehabilitation, has been printed six times a year since May–June, 1979 by the National Rehabilitation Information Center at the Catholic University of America in Washington, D.C. The federal Office for Handicapped Individuals also provides consumer information. Many national health organizations (see 12.1) publish material relevant to independent living rehabilitation (e.g., *Crusader* by United Cerebral Palsy Associations). The Campbell Soup Company and New York University, Institute of Rehabilitation Medicine, prepared a mealtime manual, giving, along with menus, adaptive techniques (or devices) and their sources [Klinger, 1978]. Several consumer magazines are noteworthy: *Rehabilitation Gazette* from St. Louis, Missouri. *Accent on Living* from Bloomington, Illinois. *Accent on Living Buyer's Guide*, published by Raymond Cheever, is a convenient booklet that lists (in the 1980–81 edition) over 450 products for disabled people and gives the company names and addresses.

40.4. Support Services

Support systems must be available to the disabled person for IL. The service system for IL rehabilitation is broader than that for traditional vocational rehabilitation, incorporating various home service programs. In addition to vocationally handicapped clients, these programs serve the acutely and chronically ill, the elderly, and others who are discouraged and overwhelmed, to maintain themselves and their families in their own homes and to enhance the quality of their daily living. Program participants may include nurses, home economists, rehabilitation engineers, physical and occupational therapists, recreational therapists, inhalation specialists, communication specialists, social workers, rehabilitation counselors, chaplains, nutritionists, physicians, dentists, rehabilitation teachers, homemakers, home health aides, attendants, volunteers, peer "counselors," and other helpers. Unfortunately, comprehensive home service programs are not available throughout the United States, are underfunded and understaffed, and are mostly designed for temporary health or family emergencies rather than the permanent needs of the disabled population.

Gini Laurie [1977] has published an excellent book on this subject, *Housing and Home Services for the Disabled: Guidelines and Experiences in Independent Living*. Information is supplemented periodically in *Rehabilitation Gazette*, a magazine founded (in 1958) and edited by Mrs. Laurie.

40.4.1. HOME SERVICES

Home help services in the United States are inadequate and have been for many decades. In an earlier time large family households provided for several generations, including their elderly, sick, or disabled members. With the advent of urbanization and a smaller family circle in America, the government sponsored institutions for those without family help and unable fully to care for themselves. (Western European nations conversely enacted early and comprehensive social security provisions for home help programs.) Deinstitutionalization as an American movement in the 1970s came about because of the overwhelming cost of state hospitalization for mental and emotional patients. Meanwhile private nursing homes continued to be built from patient fees, often paid from public welfare funds. (State penal and correctional institutions likewise expanded in the 1970s for lack of vocational and community rehabilitation aimed at the public offender population.) Adequate funding to enable provision of support services in the home is essential for implementation of IL programming for the partially dependent population. This will require recognition of the economy of home services along with third-party reimbursement to assure their availability.

Nursing and other health professional home care services may be obtained from an expanding variety of resources. These include the Visiting Nurses Association (a nationwide, nonprofit agency), city or county public health nurses, and several other reputable home health agencies.

Homemaker and home health aide services may include housekeeping, meal preparation, personal care, laundry, light cleaning, and shopping on a limited basis. Such services have limited public or voluntary financial sponsorship as they are usually operated by family service or health or welfare agencies. These local agencies are responsible for training and supervising the aides sent into the home. A membership organization, the National Council for Homemaker-Home Health Aide Services, established in 1962, is headquartered in New York City.

Supplementary services as provided by volunteers or nonprofessionals under the aegis of a human service agency may or may not be available in the community. Sustention of IL success often depends on the availability of various kinds of nonprofessional help in addition to health and homemaker services: meals on wheels, friendly visitors, telephone reassurance, shopping, transportation, escort, household repair, and chores. Chore service includes periodic heavy cleaning, lawn care, snow removal for disabled or frail people.

Self-help groups have developed perhaps in part because of lack of government services and general community organization. They consist of individuals (and their families) who have experienced a particular disease or disability (e.g., muscular dystrophy, multiple sclerosis, cancer, sickle-cell anemia). Self-help groups help their members cope with the problems associated with the condition.

40.4.2. ATTENDANTS

Attendant (personal) care is an indispensable service for many disabled or infirmed people. An attendant—*personal assistant* would be a preferable title—is a paid employee who provides regular, in-home, personal care on a full- or part-time basis and is classified for legal and tax purposes as a domestic worker. An attendant is often the most important person in the life of a disabled individual. Attendant care reduces the burden on families of continuing emotional and physical demands; it also reduces the necessity of institutionalizing disabled people.

The needed amount of attendant care varies. Some disabled people need a live-in attendant, in which case it may be cheaper to offer someone room and board as a part of the remuneration. Other people need help only with intermittent personal care for a while in the morning and evening, relying on themselves and families at other times. Then there are those who require an attendant on a periodic basis, such as twice a week for shopping or bathing. In any case disabled people do achieve a measure of independence by taking care of themselves through other people's hands [McGwinn, 1977].

The greatest barrier to IL rehabilitation may

be the lack of available, qualified attendants. This work is often seen as unprestigious, emotionally trying, physically confining, and monetarily unrewarding. Much depends upon the compatibility of the attendant and attendee and their employer-employee relationship. Some disabled people regard their attendants as personal friends or family members; in other instances the relationship is uneasy, at best formal. In most cases there is a high turnover rate.

Disabled people may need outside assistance in the recruitment, screening, and training of attendants. One of the problems in this area derives from the lack of systematic agency programming for this need. Another difficulty is the lack of public funding to help disabled people pay a reasonable salary to their attendants. It is important for disabled persons to employ and supervise their attendants, but the reduced income and other costs of disablement often make this impossible in the absence of government subsidy or tax rebate.

As a personnel problem the morale and qualifications of attendants can be improved through training provisions. The occupation can be professionalized by preparation and certification procedures dignifying the role, improving worker attitudes, and also insuring quality care. Training conducted in a health or IL center should cover a number of skills (e.g., lifting and transfers, wheelchair maintenance, personal care tasks, driving a van, home safety). Attendants should also learn about programs for the disabled, how to work with other members of the IL team, how to relate to the disabled person who is the employer. They need to explore their own attitudes toward disability and their own values. Assertiveness training can help both the attendants and their attendees. During orientation training, unfit candidates can be discouraged from taking this work.

However, providing training and increasing the professionalism of attendants as semi-skilled employment will create an appropriate demand for greater pay in an already underfunded resource. A responsible agency can recruit and train attendants, provide an employment registry, help match the personalities and needs of the people involved, provide orienting consultation, and arbitrate disputes. Recruitment sources of attendant labor include public assistance agencies, senior citizens groups, churches, rehabilitation agencies, and various kinds of schools. More research is needed on selection criteria for attendants as are more demonstration projects on their employment. On their own, many disabled people have hired disabled attendants; the capacities of the one person can make up for the limitations of the other—for example, an ablebodied retarded person can provide the help needed by a quadriplegic employer who can issue intelligent instructions. Recruitment of social security recipients and others, however, is too often blocked by disincentives resulting from entitlement regulations.

In almost every case, IL centers and programs, although assisting in coordination of attendants, do not assume responsibility for selecting, hiring, or terminating attendants. (Legally and in reality, the disabled person is the employer.) Not only must clients receive information regarding payments for employee Social Security and other benefits, but many disabled persons have not had the opportunity to learn the behaviors necessary for this supervisory role. Workshops for learning these skills are an important service to achieve successful IL.

Whether the home care is provided by paid attendants or by family members, they have an occasional need for rest. Respite-care agencies provide relief for vacation time for these caregivers. For all employees, there should also be provision for time-off for holidays or sickness and for other fringe benefits.

In addition to the materials by Donna McGwinn a federally funded study of the attendant issue has been reported by Thornock, Hutchins, Meyer, Kenyon, & Williams [1978].

40.5. Housing

Suitable housing within the community is an essential component of deinstitutionalization and the IL rehabilitation process, facilitating the severely disabled individual's maximal level of community adjustment and personal growth. Many rehabilitation plans require a successive use of different kinds of housing facilities to support the changing level of an individual's capabilities and the contingent factors that emerge during the rehabilitation process. There may be need at times for greater or lesser supervision, medical assistance, psychotherapy, and social participation. The accessibility of housing to health services, social and recreational activities, and employment opportunities will influence the eventual success of the IL rehabilitation effort.

A section of Chapter 8, Rehabilitation Facilities, describes residences for persons with various kinds and degrees of disability (e.g., halfway houses, group homes). Information about such residences is not repeated here.

40.5.1. ALTERNATIVES

The desired living situation of most disabled people is a place in the community where they can live independently in their own housing. Many obstacles besides the disability often make this impossible to achieve. Private housing is costly—often far beyond the means of people who have extra-large medical bills to add to the usual living expenses and frequently an inadequate work record to establish sufficient credit. Housing design places further restrictions on selection, as many homes and apartments contain architectural barriers that make them unsuitable for people with certain functional limitations. Location, transportation, and social barriers add to the limitations; for example, housing that is too far from potential places of employment is inappropriate regardless of how accessible it might be. Lack of housing information and problems in getting around to evaluate available units are other difficulties, as is outright discrimination at times. Professional personnel spend a great deal of time and effort attempting to solve the housing problems that disabled people face in a community designed for a nondisabled population [Columbus & Fogel, 1971].

One solution to the dilemma facing the disabled in their search for adequate and accessible independent housing is in publicly financed apartment complexes. In facilities referred to as integrated housing, provision is made for semi-independent living spaces with a minimum of supervision and supportive services. In this arrangement, because disabled people are given the same kind of housing and right to tenancy as everyone else, they are not isolated from the rest of society. Because many disabled individuals cannot simply move into any apartment or house, required adaptation and assistance must be arranged. There are numerous options in this relative to the degree of independence and integration suited to the handicapped individual. The objective is to provide only as much supervision and assistance as needed for independent living and involvement in normal community activity [Fritz, Wolfensberger, & Knowlton, 1971].

The primary housing alternative for people who are capable of independent living but who do not desire to live in public housing is the formation of a cooperative or self-help housing group. The Center for Independent Living, in Berkeley, California, provides an organizational framework that can effectively support group-owned and operated residences. It bridges the gap for people who want to join others in obtaining housing but are unaware both of others with the same interest and of the community and government resources that can make group living possible. By coming together with other people who have common interests and complimentary needs and capabilities, disabled people are able to pool their resources, sharing the costs of attendant care and maintenance and providing for each other many of the services that would otherwise need to be purchased. Costs are thereby minimized and the experiences of self-reliance and mutual interdependence is fostered. Organizations based on this model enable groups to qualify for federal housing development grants and low-interest loans under the federal Housing and Community Development Act of 1974 (PL 93-383) and other programs administered by the U.S. Department of Housing and Urban Development.

The integrated human services facilitated by organizations modeled after the Berkeley Center include: guidance in the use of the social service system; assistance in obtaining counseling, attendant, interpreter, and respite-care services; development of ADL skills; advocacy; health maintenance; evaluation of housing facilities; and, establishing contact between people who can viably live together and share their resources. Operation of the organization depends upon consumer participation and active community support from the volunteer sector. There are many homes and apartments now in operation that are based upon the principle of mutual assistance. Services that residents are not able to provide for each other and that cannot be publicly financed are purchased by a group, so that the cost to individual residents is reduced.

40.5.2. DIFFICULTIES

One major difficulty faced by community-based, independent housing groups, and often by publicly operated residential homes as well, is an unfavorable response from prospective neighbors. Long-term residents of a neighborhood may feel threatened by the unknown consequences to their personal property value, lifestyle, and sense of territoriality. Their anxiety is especially heightened when the group that is entering the neighborhood consists of persons who have mental impairments or are from a correctional institution. An additional difficulty in establishing a cooperative home in a residential area may be restrictive zoning ordinances. When community officials have been unwilling to consider variances to zoning regulations, the ordinances have often been successfully overcome by legal procedures. Because people who have been severely disabled for a long time were not often seen outside of institutional settings it takes time to arrange their transition into the community and their acceptance by the people who will be their neighbors. Overcoming social barriers such as these requires tactful persuasion and public education.

Another difficulty faced by many disabled people in their desire to be integrated into the community is the presence of architectural and transportation barriers that restrict their movement in their environment and the range of options available to build a productive, enjoyable way of life (see 5.1.6). The concept of communitywide barrier-free design recognizes that ending isolation from common activities and developing a healthy life style for the severely disabled population requires a comprehensive view of the circumstances that integrate people in a community. In Europe the concept has been applied to the development of entire communities. Het Dorp is a village in Holland that has been designed around the housing and transportation needs of handicapped people. It is a community with the primary function of meeting the range of human service needs within a context of normalcy with supportive services rather than custodial care, emphasizing the dignity of independent living. It serves as one of several model projects in Europe in which the community attempts to achieve maximal rehabilitation of all citizens and is prepared to

commit the financial resources required to achieve that goal.

40.5.3. COUNSELOR RESPONSIBILITIES

Although housing resources are largely a consequence of political priorities, the rehabilitationist can play the role of advocate by surveying the need for various kinds of housing, encouraging the organization of consumer groups, and assisting designers during the planning of new buildings. In this way, the general public can be made aware of the needs and wants of the disabled population, and new construction can be designed in accordance with the requirements of accessibility. More typical activities of the rehabilitationist include the compiling of a housing resource directory, weighing housing options to determine which ones are appropriate for individual clients, and making arrangements for referral and financial support.

For the individual who was previously housed in an institution, the rehabilitation counselor can serve as an evaluator, catalyst, and guide to the outside world. Progressively more and more independent settings may be necessary to facilitate the individual's transition, in an incremental fashion, as the person shows an ability to handle the tasks of living in the community. The rehabilitationist stabilizes the transition as much as possible by coordinating living arrangements, and more importantly, by serving as the overall integrator of programs, giving coherence to the myriad social agencies and the ego-threatening experiences that could otherwise overwhelm the individual. Eventually most people may do well on their own, but perhaps only after considerable investment in counseling and case management services. The move from an institution that was once the source of identity, security, and life pattern can involve a great deal of stress as the person adjusts to new expectations and new behaviors. A smooth transition will sustain the individual in the community as coping skills are improved. An uncoordinated move may result in so much uncertainty and stress that the individual's attempt to develop an identity outside of the institution is defeated. By identifying those persons who are severely limited in coping skills and who lack the friendship and emotional support systems that will enable them to survive the adjustment phase, rehabilitation counselors can often intervene in the cyclical recidivism that is characteristic of those who once were institutionalized (see 5.7).

40.6. Accessibility

Housing is not merely a house or an apartment or a flat: "Housing is the total environment—the people who share the housing, the neighbors, the neighborhood, the shops, the recreation, the employment, and the transportation. Housing is the focus of the human need for security and shelter, for privacy and independence" [Laurie, 1977, p. 1]. A person lives not just in a house, disabled or not, everyone lives in a community. All parts of this community must be accessible for true independence. As Hillard [1978] pointed out, barrier freedom means more than curb cuts, wide doors, and other design features of selected sites and buildings; it means accessibility to the entire community for all people regardless of age or physical condition. (See 5.1.)

40.6.1. BARRIER-FREE DESIGN

Barrier-free design aims at the "autonomous functioning" of individuals in the environment —a maximal support for independent living and human dignity. It attempts to equalize access to goods and services, to living and work spaces, to entertainment and education [Kliment, 1975]. For many years, the isolation of disabled people coupled with a lack of public awareness of the mobility problems that they faced resulted in a lack of public interest in or action on architectural barrier removal. Public officials expressed the opinion that problems did not exist because there was no organized expression of need. [U.S. HEW, Rehabilitation Services Administration, 1967]. To overcome this problem of apathy, the Congress and consumer groups began an intense period of public education in the 1960s [McGaughey, 1976]. Action in 1961 by the President's Committee on Employment of the Handicapped, the National Society for Crippled Children and Adults, and the American National Standards Institute resulted in the adoption of uniform specifications for making buildings and facilities accessible to and usable by people who are physically limited. In 1965, Congress established the National Commission on Architectural Barriers (PL 89-333) to provide a nationwide public and professional education program. Studies sponsored by the U.S. Department of Transportation and U.S. Department of Health, Education, and Welfare followed, indicating the need for the removal of barriers to transportation and the barriers to employment that were present in existing systems [U.S. HEW, Social and Rehabilitation Services, 1969]. The recommendation was that successive stages of barrier removal be identified and conducted on an incremental basis, enabling communities to begin the gradual improvements that their limited budgets could afford.

With the emphasis placed upon equal accessibility of programs and services as a result of the Architectural Barriers Act of 1968 (PL 90-480) and the Rehabilitation Act of 1973, transportation resources and mobility in the environment have been increasing. The Rehabilitation Act established the Architectural and Transportation Barriers Compliance Board, which is empowered to encourage compliance with standards by means of investigations, public hearings, and direct order; the Rehabilitation Act as amended specifically requires that recipients of federal contracts make their services and programs accessible to handicapped persons. In addition, guidelines and policy statements have been issued by the Task Force on Barrier-Free Design of the American Institute of Architecture, the National Center for a Barrier-Free Environment, and the United Nations.

According to the 1974 United Nations Expert Group Meeting in Barrier-Free Design [Rehabilitation International, 1975], environmental barriers are elements in the design of buildings and surroundings that cause no difficulty for the unencumbered, able-bodied adult, but that can effectively exclude entrance into or use of the facility by a wide range of people, including the aged, children, pregnant women, mothers with children, and people who have weak heart or lung capacity, as well as those who have obvious physical impairments. Barriers in the approach to buildings may include inadequate space for parking within easy access to the entrance, insufficient space for maneuverability between parked cars, meters placed out of reach, curbs, irregular or slippery surfaces, steep entrance ramps (over a 1 to 20-inch gradient), stairways that are the only means of entrance, steps higher than 7 inches or with projecting lips, handrails that are out of reach, projecting thresholds, revolving doors, doors that are hard to open, and narrow entranceways. The frustrations that such barriers cause to those who have a mobility handicap reflect the difficulty they encounter in their attempt to lead a normal life [Kliment, 1975].

Within buildings, the characteristics of interior design may cause problems as well. These include: areas that are difficult to negotiate when there are crowds of people, especially people moving about in a hurry; door handles that are difficult to turn; drinking fountains, telephone booths, light switches, and countertops that are out of reach; kitchen equipment that is out of reach or difficult to manipulate; bathroom facilities that restrict wheelchair movement, are unclean, or have fixtures that are out of reach; and elevator controls that are difficult to reach or lack braille markings. Safety markings, warning signals, and access to emergency exits are further considerations.

Important in barrier-free design is an awareness of the interdependency of systems, that is, pathways between accessible units of an environment need to be barrier-free as well. Movement-related difficulties include long walking distances between modes of transportation or from transit stop to destination, inadequate waiting facilities or means to signal transit, the effect of crowd movement in boarding and unloading areas, inadequate means for carrying extra objects, timing pressures when there are automatic doors or pedestrian crossing signals, maintaining equilibrium in transit vehicles, handling of transit fare and signaling operators [Brown, 1975].

Suggested building modifications may include: ramps at entranceways; wider entrances; lever door handles instead of knobs; changes in floor or ground surface texture; modification of bathroom, kitchen, and other kinds of facilities; elevators with braille markings; and emergency signals for those who have sensory impairments. To improve accessibility parking spaces should be reserved where there is room to maneuver wheelchairs. At times program activities can be rescheduled to more accessible locations.

Community organizations can make the environment more hospitable to people who have a disability. Public meetings should have available an interpreter for individuals who are deaf and should accommodate those who come in wheelchairs. A wheelchair guide is needed in all communities to identify accessible places (e.g.,

stores, restaurants, theaters, medical facilities, public buildings).

The international symbol of access, the blue and white profile of a person in a wheelchair, has been commonly adopted to indicate facilities that are designed to accommodate those who are disabled. While it is recognized that designing buildings, vehicles, and environments to accommodate the disabled adds approximately one-half to one percent to construction costs, the cost of modification subsequent to construction is very high, as much as five percent or more.

40.6.2. TRANSPORTATION

The availability of transportation is a significant factor in the level of successful, productive, and independent living that a disabled individual can achieve. Employment opportunities may be superfluous if they are not within easy access of public transportation or if the distance and complexity of travel arrangements are beyond the physical or mental capacity of the individual. Private ownership of vehicles may be discouraged by discriminatory laws and by the difficulty of obtaining insurance, even though adequate bioengineering adaptations are provided. Hence, the vital need to get about in the community may be severely restricted beyond any difficulties caused by functional limitations. Isolation and dependency on others are the consequences when disabled people find the environment difficult to use. The rehabilitationist, therefore, seeks to maximize mobility by encouraging the development of transportation resources and by training clients in the effective use of existing means of transportation.

Guidelines for effective design modification to minimize the barriers and difficulties encountered in the use of buildings and transportation facilities can be found in the following books.

Barrier-Free Design [United Nations, 1975]

Barrier-Free Site Design [American Society of Landscape Architects Foundation, 1975]

Freedom of Choice [U.S. HEW, Architectural and Transportation Barriers Compliance Board, 1975]

Barrier-Free Communities [U.S. Department of Housing and Urban Development, 1978]

Rehabilitation International's International Commission on Technical Aids, Housing, and

Transportation is another source of information on adaptation and modification of the physical environment. These and other references assist the rehabilitationist in evaluating the accessibility of work settings, training programs, supportive services, housing, and transportation.

People who have sensory or cognitive impairments often benefit from a rehabilitation program that includes special training in the use of transportation systems. Travel instruction for the blind client includes development of generalized mobility skills in the use of transportation as well as a guided orientation to the particular environment where they work and live. Training enables people to use public facilities in personal comfort, safety, and independence. Travel orientation and mobility training for the cognitively impaired follows a pattern similar to that used successfully with blind rehabilitants. Instructors with specialized training in mobility skills work individually with the learners on specific routes in real settings (see 2.4.8 and 5.1.7). Entrance into the program is based upon evaluation of emotional stability and willingness to learn the tasks of a more independent lifestyle. The transition is difficult for people who most of their life have been reliant upon others, but many persons with severe retardation have mastered the skills of independent use of public transportation systems [Laus, 1977]. The consequences to the rehabilitation effort are substantial; reduction in cost of special transportation vehicles, increased social mixing in the community, increased learning in other areas, and greater feelings of adequacy and self-worth. Blasch and Welsh [1980] have described such training in their useful book on mobility published by the American Foundation for the Blind.

In the United States, disabled people have a preference for private automobile ownership and operation because it is usually the most convenient form of transportation and because of its connotation of "normalcy." In some situations, the most viable rehabilitation approach, both from the standpoint of the individual's personal sense of well-being and independence and from the standpoint of vocational success, will include training in the use of a specially adapted automobile. Many disabled people are able to overcome their functional limitations sufficiently with the aid of rehabilitation engineering adaptations to be able to drive their own vehicles. A considerable array of devices is available to modify the standard van or automobile, including hand-control of accelerator and brake operations, hydraulic lifts and ramps to enable wheelchair entry for a driver, and special communications and guidance systems for people who have sensory impairments. The substantial costs of installation and driver training necessary for safe vehicle operation are usually provided by the state rehabilitation agency, since the resulting mobility is often essential to achievement of a fully productive, independent life. For some physically disabled individuals, ability to use an auto may be an advantage in getting a job due to the effect it can have on an employer's perception of self-reliance.

The potential ability of a disabled person to operate an automobile can be evaluated by rehabilitation engineers, state driver education and licensing departments, and, occasionally, commercial driver education schools. Following evaluation, training, and provision of a specially equipped vehicle, the individual must pass a rigorous examination by the state licensing authority. Most states have adopted a "Uniform Vehicle Code" that does not restrict persons with physical disabilities from driving as long as they can operate a vehicle safely [Finesilver, 1970]. A notable exception has been in the cases of persons who have epilepsy, even if they do not have seizures. Restrictive licensing procedures have forced many individuals to ignore the law when driving was a necessity to hold down a job. All states should adopt licensing procedures to make it possible for all people who can safely drive to obtain a license, regardless of their disability.

In spite of the fact that disabled drivers rank equal to or above the national average in safety, insurance coverage is sometimes difficult to obtain. Some companies, when they are in doubt, will give a new customer a high-risk policy for a period of time and reduce the premium rate if no accidents occur during the trial period.

A primary transportation alternative to private automobile ownership is the volunteer sector (see 9.3). Churches and volunteer service organizations are often willing to offer assistance. The disabled worker who encounters difficulty in using public transit after securing employment may be able to arrange to get a ride with a co-worker; many companies assist in the organization of riding pools as a service to all personnel.

Most communities have responded favorably to federal guidelines by upgrading existing transit facilities and vehicles for the handicapped. The federal government has further encouraged the growth of barrier-free public transit systems by providing funding for local purchase of specially designed buses to accommodate wheelchairs and by providing special considerations for those who have sensory impairments. In order to supplement public transit, specially adapted buses and vans are provided in many communities.

Few severely handicapped people can afford the expense of private taxicab transportation, although it is a frequent necessity for them. Health insurance can sometimes pay the cost if the trip is part of a treatment program. At times the state rehabilitation agency may arrange for a client to be paid for cab service until more favorable alternatives can be found. The monetary difficulty in using private cabs is not the only one, however; many cab companies are forced to restrict the amount of assistance that drivers can offer to handicapped riders because of insurance and liability concerns. Without arranging for someone who is able-bodied to meet the cab at both ends of a journey, it may be

hazardous for some individuals to use this travel alternative.

Intercity travel by air, rail, and bus service has been difficult for some disabled individuals, largely due to problems of accessibility. Modernization of facilities and special assistance for disabled travelers are helping to alleviate burdens that were experienced in the past. The Amtrak system is adding to their routes more accessible rail cars with special accommodations. A major national bus company assists travelers by allowing a needed attendant to accompany the disabled person at no cost. The problem in air travel is often the procedural difficulty encountered in transferring between independent carriers. Although the Federal Aviation Agency sets guidelines regarding accessibility for the disabled, the operational relationship between separate airlines is difficult to supervise. Travel gets easier as the employees of the intercity transit systems become more accustomed to disabled passengers. Disabled persons who are considering long-distance travel are encouraged to contact the carrier in order to become aware of any special service that is available and to clear any arrangements that may be required [Benningfield, Reiser, & Richards, 1975].

40.7. Rehabilitative Recreation

The goal of living for the disabled person, quite as much as for the nondisabled, is individual fulfillment. This comes from using the many capacities with which all are endowed—exercising as it were the intellectual, emotional, and physical talents and the personality resulting from these, that everyone possesses in greater or lesser degree. Individuals who have a disability are, with few exceptions, more normal than abnormal; however great the disability, they have a body, an intellect, a personality, a range of emotions, and a need to utilize whatever resources they possess over and above any limitations. But they may be limited in what they do, how they spend their time.

Leisure is the time people have after they complete their work (or school) as well as eating, sleeping, and other essential tasks. Most people can use this free time as they please;

however, this is not always possible for disabled people even though they may have an excess of idle hours. Leisure is a time for pleasure, for pursuits that broaden life, pursuits engaged in not from necessity but by choice. The opposite of leisure as something positive to do is *idle time*, which is boring and not useful. *Recreation* can be defined as leisure-time activities—particularly those that call for physical or mental participation such as playing handball or bridge. Passive, non-participatory uses of leisure-time such as watching a movie or a ball game are more aptly called *amusement*. Broadly speaking, all activities (mental and physical) that give pleasure and help to renew the mind or body are recreative. Recreative pursuits help the individual to discover new personal talents and interest and to form additional social relationships as an expanded dimension of life.

Recreation is *re-creation;* that is to say, refreshment of the body or spirit from toil, ennui, or frustration. Recreation is by definition rehabilitative. It is a weapon of great potential in the armamentarium of the rehabilitation counselor and an essential element in a comprehensive plan for independent living.

Recreational pursuits offer the individual a diversion from daily routine. With disabled individuals, the feelings of being confined by routine are often even stronger than with the able-bodied person. Yet, opportunities for the disabled population are often limited both in residential and institutional situations and in the community. A need for diversion can be very strong as free time becomes wasted time due to lack of direction or lack of facilitation. This may bring frustration. Disabled persons involved in IL rehabilitation can gain much from personal recreation as they learn to compensate for limitations of function. Recreation allows the client to share common interests and thus to integrate more easily with the community.

Virtually any human experience can be recreative. An experience becomes recreative when it satisfies some need: companionship for the lonely, rest from fatigue, remunerative work after enforced idleness. Pursuits such as arts and crafts, hiking, nature study, field trips, dramatics, games, camping, hobbies, and physical fitness activities can selectively be made part of everyone's daily living. The particular art form, aspect of nature study, or sport must fit the individual's residual potential. Techniques exist through which severely disabled persons, with adapted facilities and training, can participate in many traditional recreations.

In considering the leisure of disabled persons, the rehabilitationist should realize that they have a great amount of "free" time. Because of this one might be led to the erroneous conclusion that leisure is not a problem for them. But to see how little leisure time they really have, it is necessary to become aware of: (1) possible psychological barriers that can be created by the sense of handicap, which in turn may inhibit involvement with strangers; (2) physical, perceptual, or temporal limitations of the individual; and (3) limited choices as to forms of leisure experiences available (e.g., enjoyment of music due to personal background, living environment, or community resources). Because of such factors, the disabled may be channeled into repetitive activities that become boring to anyone.

The unencumbered time of the recreationally handicapped person may be quite different from the leisure time of others. True leisure is an awareness of the freedom to use disposable time as one pleases. For most people leisure is freedom from obligation for a limited period. Too often a disability brings undesired and sometimes unending freedom from obligations and, further, may restrict the scope of behaviors in the time that is free. Leisure for anyone occurs only when there is genuine freedom of choice. One thus needs a diversity of recreative options from which to choose.

The ability to use leisure is not something innate; it must be learned, and the ability to choose wisely is essential. Many disabled persons are even not aware of what possibilities exist for relaxing or what recreative activities are available to them. For example, in some communities there are avocational activity centers for people who are very severely disabled (see 8.3.7).

Leisure counseling is a service that is needed by most people—particularly those who are disabled [Epperson, Witt, & Hitzhusen, 1972]. The objective is to help individuals understand their interests and abilities and to identify and choose from the various leisure-time alternatives available. The process professionally parallels that of counseling for vocational objectives and includes assessment, planning, recreational resources information and referral, and arrangements with preparation programs (e.g., craft classes). The choice options (i.e., recreational objectives) are innumerable: sports, hobbies, do-it-yourself projects, gardening, adult education, volunteer work, tours, games, collecting, picnicking, camping, thinking, reading, writing. Recreational facilities include: theaters, zoos, museums, gymnasiums, auditoriums, libraries, parks, holiday resorts, golf courses, tennis courts, beaches and swimming pools. Unfortunately leisure counselors are generally not specialized in work with physically and mentally disabled people. Consequently, the rehabilitation counselor must share responsibility with other members of the rehabilitation team in educating their clients in the constructive and satisfying use of their leisure.

Persons involved in recreation with disabled people may include: recreation therapist, music and art therapist, occupational therapist, community recreation staff personnel, volunteers, family, and friends. The recreational therapist is most often found in hospitals, nursing homes, rehabilitation facilities, and public service organizations, and is the professional person most informed about the disabled person's needs and the available recreational resources in the community. Recreational therapists base their treatment programs on individual needs. While a one-to-one relationship might be desirable, it is seldom possible with the usual patient-therapist ratio. As a result these therapists bring people of similar need and potential together in groups. The 1978 Amendments to the 1973 Rehabilitation Act authorized therapeutic recreation as a restoration service of the public rehabilitation program.

Some of the important contributions to the literature on recreation include *Recreation for the Physically Handicapped* [Pomeroy, 1964], *Recreation in Total Rehabilitation* [Rathbone & Lucas, 1970], *Why People Play* [Ellis, 1973], *Avocational Activities for the Handicapped* [Overs, O'Connor, & DeMarco, 1974], *Therapeutic Recreation: A Helping Profession* [O'Morrow, 1976], *Helping the Mentally Retarded Acquire Play Skills* [Wehman, 1977].

The *Therapeutic Recreation Journal* is published quarterly by the National Recreation and Park Association of Arlington, Virginia.

40.7.1. TECHNIQUES

Until recently, recreation was not given much attention, even in the lives of ordinary Americans, but it is beginning to become an important adjunct to rehabilitation programs of all kinds. Personal counseling based on an understanding of the individual is the first requisite. Of next importance is the need for a wide range of opportunities for all disabled individuals to grow and function at their highest level of independence and self-sufficiency. Within the rehabilitation process for IL—as distinguished from the community recreation program—this endeavor is called "therapeutic recreation service." A further requisite, the integration of recreation with other services in the medical setting, is of great importance; the treatment situation connects therapeutic recreation daily with occupational therapy, physical therapy, and social services. The need for integrating these services in an individual's complete IL rehabilitation plan is obvious.

The success of recreation service depends upon the effort the rehabilitation staff makes in helping a person to develop a realistic leisure plan. This planning includes these evaluations: leisure needs and personal interests along with previous leisure experiences and knowledge; attitudes toward various recreative experiences and their place in the total life pattern; potential abilities within functional limitations; and available leisure resources.

40.7.2. ADAPTATIONS

Rehabilitative recreation therapists can coordinate community programs and services to enhance client opportunities. This requires interaction with a variety of recreation agency personnel to interpret the needs, interests, abilities, and limitations of disabled persons who might use a given resource. Facilities, equipment, and programs for recreation need to be appraised for suitability. A primary responsibility of the rehabilitationist in coordination and consultation is giving information concerning modifications and adaptations of experiences and facilities to disabled persons, their families, and to professional personnel providing community recreation service.

Generally it is best to avoid elaborate changes, making only those adjustments that prove to be most efficient. The rehabilitation recreation therapist will:

1. Analyze the proposed recreation activity to determine the required intellectual demands, possible emotional hazards, physical movement, strength, endurance, sense perception, and more.
2. Determine the essence of the activity as to what makes it satisfying.
3. Interpret medical information to understand relevant functional limitations and abilities.
4. Determine adaptations for each participant without changing the values of the activity.

The focus of a recreation program is upon the abilities of the individual. Inadequacies become less important to the disabled person as long as remaining functional capacities provide a successful avenue for self-expression and achievement. The tailoring of individualized recreational programs begins with an evaluation of the functional capacities of the individual and of the physical and mental demands of recreational activities. Within this context, the components of an activity can often be adapted to conform to the individual's level of development or recovery. Sense of balance, coordination, limitation of movement, dexterity, ability to communicate, intellectual capacity, ability to reason, fatigue level, and other factors will determine those activity options that are considered and the adaptations that may be appropriate. The techniques of task analysis in the adaptation of sports, games, and hobbies is an established art in the practice of rehabilitation recreation therapy [Overs, O'Connor, & DeMarco, 1974].

Adaptations may be suggested in these areas: the individual's means of moving around, the facilities involved, and the rules surrounding the activity. The game of spot billiards for people with cerebral palsy illustrates an adaptation of rules and equipment. The game can be modified to meet the abilities of the group by using shorter cue sticks with rubber tips, spotting balls near the pockets to eliminate the break, or assisting those severely handicapped people in shooting [Frye & Peters, 1972].

Although medical evaluations may specify or restrict certain activities on the basis of exposure to stress, fatigue, or environmental factors, the therapist is in a position to encourage individuals to discover their own limitations from practical experience and to build capabilities that may go beyond what was thought to be medically possible. For example, many physicians have discouraged swimming for persons who have cerebral palsy, due to the shock effect of cold water, but swimming programs are possible if a tolerance for the temperature change is built up gradually and if the individual really wants to swim. Persons who have epilepsy have been discouraged by some physicians from participating in physically demanding sports because of the possibility of seizures, but many have participated without ill effect.

In some cases adjustments can be made so that the disabled person can participate and compete in physical activities, games, and sports on an equal basis with able-bodied persons. This is particularly true when individual adjustments are made for the disabled participant (e.g., allowing use of a prosthesis or modifying the manipulation of structure of equipment used). A person sitting in a wheelchair, however, can successfully compete with able-bodied persons in archery. There are, however, a number of physical activities, particularly some team sports, which must be organized for participation by disabled people only. For instance, paraplegics cannot play standard basketball with able-bodied players, but wheelchair basketball is a popular sport for all [Frye & Peters, 1972]. *Sports 'N Spokes*, a bimonthly national magazine "for wheelchair sports and recreation," published in Phoenix, Arizona by Nancy Crase, features a calendar of sports events for disabled participants as well as related articles.

40.7.3. THERAPEUTIC APPROACH

Motivation in ADL can be a particular problem with individuals who have been prevented from taking risks in self-expression due to their dependency on other people. In this type of situation a recreational therapist must show a versatility in approach, sometimes being supportive, sometimes directive, and often indirect and subtle. Peer pressure and the awareness of the satisfactory experiences of others are strong incentives for those who are apprehensive, until they too have a chance to experience the enjoyment and self-fulfillment that the activity can provide. But recreational activities are not always enjoyable; for some there may be moments of frustration, anger, and hostility. The therapist helps to alleviate the pain of the emotional crisis if this causes withdrawal, or to facilitate its expression if it can be viewed as an asset to personal growth. The therapist realizes that emotional pain, physical strain, and occasional failure can be important learning experiences in the context of a positive, accepting social environment. Counseling may be indicated with individuals who have serious emotional problems or perhaps moral restraints that interfere with their recreational interests.

The primary concern of the recreationist is not with the teaching of activities, per se, but with the activity as a means of self-expression for the individual. A therapeutic value is evident when the person uses games, hobbies, and recreational opportunities to make contact with other people, to broaden awareness or skills in new areas of life, and to increase physical capacity (strength and endurance) and tolerance for pain as a way of achieving personal goals. If, on the other hand, the activities serve as a way to avoid making contact with others, to avoid meeting the expectations of others, or to avoid encountering unfamiliar situations, the therapeutic value is diminished. Mere involvement in an activity program then is not regarded as therapeutic recreation.

The usefulness of recreation in rehabilitation programs is multi-dimensional. For the individual, it is primarily encouraged as a means of self-expression. It is useful in physical therapy as a way to make appropriate body movement programs enjoyable and in psychological evaluation as a means to observe skills in interpersonal interaction. From a medical perspective, recreation counteracts the effects of physical and mental atrophy that may result from extended periods of inactivity. And from the viewpoint of the rehabilitation counselor, recreation can provide an effective means of reinforcing self-esteem and willingness to take risks that are essential to facilitate personal independence. The need for rebuilding feelings of adequacy and a positive self-image is particularly strong in individuals who have been separated from their families or regular associates as a result of an illness or injury and for those who require long periods of hospitalization. For the most severely disabled persons, leisure activities can help avoid depression and withdrawal, a self-reinforcing syndrome that results from lack of meaningful involvement with other people over long periods of time (see 28.5).

To the extent that recreational therapy can lead to the improvement of a person's self-image and self-reliance, its contribution to rehabilitation will lie in thus bettering relationships with others and producing a greater likelihood of success in vocational areas as well. The goal of recreation therapy in the context of rehabilitation is an involvement of the individual in the affairs of the community and the community's involvement in the rehabilitation of the individual.

Normalization of recreation offerings seeks to minimize the inconvenience caused to both the disabled and the nondisabled populations in seeking a common level for interaction. Programs that demand too many modifications at the expense of nondisabled participants only discourage their involvement. Furthermore, programs that exclude the disabled population or overemphasize modification may reinforce negative attitudes regarding the ability of handicapped people. Volunteers especially are encouraged not to be overly helpful or solicitous since excessive assistance may encourage dependency.

40.7.4. RECREATIONAL RESOURCES

Most disabled individuals experience little difficulty in using standard recreational resources. For those whose disability has resulted in a handicap in their recreational pursuits, how-

ever, modifications of equipment and procedures are becoming more prevalent. Improvements in travel facilities, adaptations of games and sports, and the parallel services of physical therapy, recreational counseling, and rehabilitation engineering make a broad array of alternatives available. Travel opportunities have increased both from the standpoint of facilities and the accessibility of recreation areas. Major air, rail, and bus carriers offer special assistance for persons who have a disability—in some cases this even includes lower fares. Guidebooks indicating accessible points of interest, as well as manuals on how to handle the contingencies of travel, assist the disabled individual in vacation planning.

National parks have developed trails and nature exhibits for the physically disabled, with Braille markings and guide ropes, hardened paths for wheelchairs, and the like. Federal and state conservation and recreation funds assist in developing accessible recreation areas. Ramps and ropes are used at some beaches and swimming pools to enable the physically disabled person to safely enter and leave the water. Promontories have been constructed on trout streams, thus making them accessible to everyone. An increasing number of museums, libraries, bowling alleys, ski resorts, riding stables, and boating resorts have adapted equipment and programs to enable use and participation by all of the people.

The Joseph P. Kennedy, Jr. Foundation is the primary sponsor of Special Olympics programs for mentally retarded youths and adults. The competition, which requires local community co-sponsorship, not only provides a challenging recreational opportunity for the disabled participants but also results in increased social contact and involvement with other community residents.

Hobbies, arts, and crafts provide a rewarding avenue for personal expression to many. A particular hobby can become a source of satisfaction and meaning to the individual: by mastering the skills and knowledge involved, the person develops a channel for interaction and communication that far transcends any limitations the disability may impose. A person skilled in an art or hobby is accorded respect from those who have not developed the talent and from colleagues who share an interest in the same subject. Membership in clubs that focus on the particular hobby or craft becomes a means of forming friendships and gaining status from personal accomplishments and contributions. In some cases, the friendships formed or the crafts produced become the basis for an independent business or for a job offer. Feelings of adequacy, self-esteem, and accomplishment are bound to promote better mental health and to influence performance in vocational areas as well. (See 30.3.11.)

Music, art, drama, and dance are particularly desirable activities for those having sensory or intellectual impairment, as they provide a means of compensating for a deficit in one method of expression by increased involvement in another. Developing an interest in an art form, for example, can lead to broadening experiences such as museum visits, art fairs, and the (possible) display or sale of the individual's work. (See 14.1.9.)

The disabled person as a member of the community is entitled to the same privileges as other taxpayers. City parks, schools, libraries, and public recreation programs are for the use of all community residents. Local chambers of commerce, information centers, city newspapers, and public libraries are good sources of information to the public on current happenings and facilities. The rehabilitation worker should find these sources helpful in learning where the disabled person can participate in leisure time activities. Some agencies have free services from which books, games, and recreation supplies can be borrowed. Often city recreation depart-

ments lend game kits (sometimes for a small fee) to groups planning recreative activities. The American Red Cross has in each of its area offices one or more recreation consultants who give professional assistance to recreation workers throughout the area. Group work agencies such as the Young Men's Christian Association, the Young Women's Christian Association, the Boy Scouts of America, the Girl Scouts of America, and the Salvation Army sponsor selected activities exclusively for people who are disabled. Most communities have a health and welfare council that may be a source of information about camps and other programs designed specifically for disabled people.

One of the greatest benefits of extended service as conducted cooperatively by public and private recreation programs is that while fulfilling the recreational needs of the disabled population they can simultaneously work toward the integration of all of the people in the community. Scheduling activities in typical facilities with the regular recreation leadership staff does not isolate disabled people or set them apart nearly so much as when special facilities are designed for their use. Meeting in facilities also used by the general public creates opportunities for disabled users to be included with others, which is one of the most desirable methods of integration. Special programs are sometimes needed, but whenever possible, persons who have a disability should take part in established programs.

References

Adams, A. S. Disabled should be key shapers of own programs. *Rehabilitation World*, 1976–1977, *2*(4), 25.

Adams, G. S. *Measurement and evaluation.* New York: Holt, Rinehart and Winston, 1965.

Akabas, S. H. Affirmative action—A tool for linking rehabilitation and the business community. *Journal of Rehabilitation*, 1976, *42*(3), 20–23.

Akabas, S. H., Medevene, L., & Victor, J. Pounding pavements: A study of the job hunt of disabled people. *American Rehabilitation*, 1979, *4*(4), 9–15.

Albrecht, G. L. (Ed.). *The sociology of physical disability and rehabilitation.* Pittsburgh, PA: University Press, 1976.

Allan, W. S. *Rehabilitation: A community challenge.* New York: John Wiley, 1958.

Allport, G. W., Vernon, P. E., & Lindzey, G. *Study of values* (3rd ed.). Boston: Houghton Mifflin, 1960.

American Federation of Labor and Congress of Industrial Organizations. *Working together: The key to jobs for the handicapped.* Washington, D.C.: Author, 1973.

American Medical Association, Committee on Medical Rating of Physical Impairment. Guides to the evaluation of permanent impairment. *Journal of the American Medical Association*, March 5, 1960, *172*(10), 1049–1060.

American Personnel and Guidance Association. APGA policy statement: Responsibilities of users of standardized tests. *Guidepost*, October 5, 1978, 5–8.

American Psychiatric Association. *A psychiatric glossary* (4th ed.). Washington, D.C.: Author, 1975.

American Psychiatric Association. *Diagnostic and statistical manual of mental disorders* (3rd ed.). Washington, D.C.: Author, 1980.

American Psychological Association. *Standards for educational and psychological tests and manuals.* Washington, D.C.: Author, 1974.

American Public Health Association and the Health Resources Administration. *Consumer health education: A directory, 1975.* Washington, D.C.: U.S. Department of Health, Education, and Welfare, Public Health Services, Health Resources Administration, 1975.

American Rehabilitation Counseling Association. The professional preparation of rehabilitation counselors. *Rehabilitation Counseling Bulletin*, 1968, *12*(1), 29–35.

American Rehabilitation Counseling Association. *A statement of policy on the professional preparation of rehabilitation counselors.* October 1974.

American Society of Landscape Architects Foundation. *Barrier free site design.* Washington, D.C.: U. S. Government Printing Office, 1975.

Anastasi, A. *Psychological testing* (4th ed.). New York: Macmillan, 1976.

Anderson, A. Real work. *Vocational Evaluation and Work Adjustment Bulletin*, 1968, *1*(2), 2–5.

Anderson, J., Hutchins, R., & Walker, R. A. *Job seeking skills project.* Minneapolis: Rehabilitation Center, February 1968.

Anderson, T. P., & Cole, T. M. Sexual counseling of the physically disabled. *Postgraduate Medicine*, 1975, *58*(1), 117–123.

Andrew, J. D., & Dickerson, L. R. (Eds.). *Vocational evaluation: A resource manual.* Menomonie: University of Wisconsin-Stout, Department of Rehabilitation and Manpower Services, n.d.

Angel, J. L. *Employment opportunities for the handicapped.* New York: World Trade Academy Press (distributed by Simon & Schuster), 1969.

Anthony, W. A., Slowkowski, P., & Bendix, L. Developing the specific skills and knowledge of the rehabilitation counselor. In B. Bolton & M. E. Jaques (Eds.), *Rehabilitation counseling: Theory and practice.* Baltimore: University Park Press, 1978.

Arbuckle, D. S. *Counseling: Philosophy, theory and practice.* Boston: Allyn and Bacon, 1965.

Arkansas Rehabilitation Research & Training Center. *Orientation institute: Evaluation for vocational potential.* Hot Springs, AR: Author, 1966.

Ayer, M. J., Wright, G. N., & Butler, A. J. *Counselor orientation: Relationship with responsibilities and performance.* Madison: University of Wisconsin, Regional Rehabilitation Research Institute, 1968.

Ayers, G. E. White racist attitudes and rehabilitation. *Rehabilitation Counseling Bulletin*, 1969, *13*(1), 52–60.

Ayers, G. E. Counseling in work adjustment programs. *Journal of Rehabilitation*, 1971, *37*(4), 31–33.

Baer, M. F., & Roeber, E. C. *Occupational information* (3rd ed.). Chicago: Science Research Associates, 1964.

Baker, B. Determining the goals and techniques of adjustment services. *Rehabilitation Counseling Bulletin*, 1972, *16*(1), 29–40.

Balthazar, E. F. *Legal, human and economic aspects of developmental disabilities.* Madison, WI: Central Colony and Training School Research Department, November 1975.

Bandura, A. *Principles of behavior modification.* New York: Holt, Rinehart and Winston, 1969.

Bandura, A. *Social learning theory.* New York: General Learning Press, 1971.

Bandura, A. *Social learning theory.* Englewood Cliffs, NJ: Prentice-Hall, 1977.

Barker, R. G. The somatopsychologic problem. *Psychosomatic Medicine*, 1947, *9*(5), 192–196.

Barker, R. G. The social psychology of physical disability. *Journal of Social Issues*, 1948, *4*(4), 28–38.

Barker, R. G., Wright, B. A., & Gonick, M. R. *Adjustment to physical handicap and illness: A survey of the social psychology of physique and disability.* New York: Social Science Research Council, 1946.

Barker, R. G., Wright, B. A., Myerson, L., & Gonick, M. R. *Adjustment to physical handicap and illness: A survey of the social psychology of physique and disability* (2nd ed.). New York: Social Science Research Council, 1953.

Barry, J. R., & Malinovsky, M. R. *Client motivation for rehabilitation: A review.* Gainesville: University of Florida, Regional Rehabilitation Research Institute, 1965.

Bartels, E. C. IL: In Massachusetts. *American Rehabilitation*, 1978, *3*(6), 22.

Bass, R. Group counseling in vocational adjustment. *Journal of Rehabilitation*, 1969, *35*(1), 25–28.

Bauman, M. K., & Yoder, N. M. *Adjustment to blindness—Reviewed.* Springfield, IL: Charles C Thomas, 1966.

Baumheier, E. C., & Welch, H. H. *Interagency linkages in vocational rehabilitation: A preliminary comment on the state of the art.* Denver: University of Denver, Regional Rehabilitation Research Institute, 1976.

Bellamy, G. T., Inman, D. P., & Horner, R. H. *Design of vocational rehabilitation services for the severely retarded: The specialized training model.* Eugene: University of Oregon, Center on Human Development, 1977.

Bellamy, G. T., & Snyder, S. *The trainee performance sample: Toward the prediction of habilitation costs for severely handicapped adults.* Eugene: University of Oregon, 1976.

Bender, M. Special education. In R. B. Johnston & P. R. Magrab (Eds.), *Developmental disorders: Assessment, treatment, education.* Baltimore: University Park Press, 1976.

Benjamin, A. *The helping interview.* Boston: Houghton Mifflin, 1969.

Benner, H. J., Burke, M. J., & Miller, H. R. *The reluctant client: Major response modes.* Paper presented at the American Personnel and Guidance Association Convention, Chicago, 1976.

Benningfield, K., Reiser, K. P., & Richards, S. K. *Rights handbook for Ohio's physically handicapped.* Columbus: Ohio Easter Seal Society for Crippled Children and Adults, October 1975.

Berenson, B. G., & Carkhuff, R. R. *Sources of gain in counseling and psychotherapy.* New York: Holt, Rinehart and Winston, 1967.

Bergman, A. *A guide to establishing an activity center for mentally retarded persons.* Washington, D.C.: President's Committee on Employment of the Handicapped, 1977.

Berkman, A. H. Sexuality: A human condition. *Journal of Rehabilitation*, 1975, *41*(1); 13–15, 37.

Bertcher, H., Gordon, J. E., Hayes, M. E., & Mial, H. *Role modeling, role playing: A manual for vocational development and employment agencies.* Washington, D.C.: Manpower Science Services, n.d.

Berven, N. L. Privileged communication and the rehabilitation counselor. *Journal of Rehabilitation*, 1968, *34*(6), 10–12.

Berven, N. L., & Wright, G. N. An evaluation model for accreditation. *Counselor Education and Supervision*, March 1978, *17*(3), 188–194.

Biggs, S., & Bowman, J. T. Applicability and efficacy of a behavioral approach to rehabilitation counseling. *Journal of Applied Rehabilitation Counseling*, 1973–1974, *4*(4), 239–245.

Bilotto, G., & Washam, V. *A rationale for the integration of independent living with vocational rehabilitation.* Albertson, NY: Human Resources Center, 1979.

Bingham, W. V. *Aptitudes and aptitude testing.* New York: Harper, 1937.

Bingham, W. V., & Moore, B. V. *How to interview* (4th rev. ed.). New York: Harper & Row, 1959.

Bitter, J. A. *Introduction to rehabilitation.* St. Louis: C. V. Mosby, 1979.

Blasch, B. B., & Welsh, R. L. Training for persons with functional mobility limitations. In R. L. Welsh & B. B. Blasch (Eds.), *Foundations of orientation and mobility.* New York: American Foundation for the Blind, 1980.

Blauch, L. E. *Vocational rehabilitation of the physically disabled* (prepared for the Advisory Committee on Education; Staff Study Number 9). Washington, D.C.: U.S. Government Printing Office, 1938.

Blocher, D. H. *Developmental counseling.* New York: Ronald Press, 1966.

Bodine, T. *Utilization of community resources.* Paper presented to the Council of Rehabilitation Counselor Educators, Albany, NY, May 1976.

Bolton, B. (Ed.). *Handbook of measurement and evaluation in rehabilitation.* Baltimore: University Park Press, 1976.

Bolton, B. *Rehabilitation counseling research.* Baltimore: University Park Press, 1979.

Bolton, B., & Jaques, M. E. (Eds.). *Rehabilitation*

counseling: Theory and practice. Baltimore: University Park Press, 1978.

Bolton, B., & Jaques, M. E. (Eds.). *The rehabilitation client.* Baltimore: University Park Press, 1979.

Bolton, B., Lawlis, G. F., & Brown, R. H. Scores and norms. In B. Bolton (Ed.), *Handbook of measurement and evaluation in rehabilitation.* Baltimore: University Park Press, 1976.

Botterbusch, K. F., & Sax, A. B. *A comparison of seven vocational evaluation systems.* Menomonie: University of Wisconsin-Stout, Vocational Rehabilitation Institute, February 1976.

Boudreaux, R. E., Pool, P. A., Henke, R. D., & McCollum, P. S. Rehabilitation—An emerging allied health profession. *Journal of Allied Health,* 1978, *7*(2), 133–139.

Bowman, J. T., & Graves, W. H. (Eds.). *Placement services and techniques.* Champaign, IL: Stipes, 1976.

Bowe, F. *Handicapping America.* New York: Harper and Row, Publisher, 1978.

Boyle, P. S. Totally rehabilitating the physically disabled client: Recognizing the sexuality of the physically disabled individual. *Journal of Applied Rehabilitation Counseling,* 1976, *7*(3), 176–181.

Brammer, L. M. *The helping relationship: Process and skills* (2nd ed.). Englewood Cliffs, NJ: Prentice-Hall, 1979.

Brattgard, S.-O. *Varieties of living for the severely disabled: A life for living.* Paper presented at the 13th World Congress of Rehabilitation International, Tel Aviv, Israel, June 1976.

Bridges, C. D. *Job placement of the physically handicapped.* New York: McGraw-Hill, 1946.

Brill, A. A. *Basic principles of psychoanalysis.* Garden City, NY: Doubleday, 1949.

Brolin, D. E. *Vocational preparation of retarded citizens.* Columbus, OH: Charles E. Merrill, 1976.

Brown, D., & Parks, J. C. Interpreting nonverbal behavior, a key to more effective counseling: Review of literature. *Rehabilitation Counseling Bulletin,* 1972, *15*(3), 176–184.

Brown, E. B. Independent mobility and the disabled. In K. Mallik, S. Yuspeh, & J. Mueller (Eds.), *Comprehensive vocational rehabilitation for severely disabled persons.* Washington, D.C.: George Washington University Medical Center, Job Development Laboratory, 1975.

Browning, P. L. (Ed.). *Mental retardation: Rehabilitation and counseling.* Springfield, IL: Charles C Thomas, 1974.

Bruch, M. A., Kunce, J. T., Thelen, M. H., & Akamatsu, T. J. *Modeling, behavior change, and rehabilitation.* Columbia: University of Missouri, Regional Rehabilitation Research Institute, 1973.

Bryson, S., Graff, R., & Bardo, H. Rehabilitation counselors' biases in referral recommendations. *Rehabilitation Counseling Bulletin,* 1974, *17*(3), 166–170.

Buros, O. K. (Ed.). *Mental Measurements Yearbook* (Vols. I & II). Lincoln: University of Nebraska Press, 1978.

Buscaglia, L. *The disabled and their parents: A counseling challenge.* Thorofare, NJ: Charles B. Slack, 1975.

Butler, A. J., & Wright, G. N. *Research utilization by visiting program consultants.* Madison: University of Wisconsin, Regional Rehabilitation Research Institute, 1975.

Calderone, M. S. Introduction: The issues at hand. *Personnel and Guidance Journal,* 1976, *54*(7), 350–351.

Calli, A. P., & Smith, M. L. Extended employment. In R. E. Hardy & J. G. Cull (Eds.), *Services of the rehabilitation facility.* Springfield, IL: Charles C Thomas, 1975.

Cammer, L. *Up from depression.* New York: Pocket Books, 1971.

Campbell, J. L., & O'Toole, R. *Work adjustment: A dynamic rehabilitation process.* Cleveland, OH: Vocational Guidance and Rehabilitation Services, 1970.

Campbell, R. E., Walz, G. R., Miller, J. V., & Kriger, S. F. *Career guidance: A handbook of methods.* Columbus, OH: Charles E. Merrill, 1973.

Canadian Department of Manpower & Immigration. *Canadian classification and dictionary of occupations* (Vols. I & II). Ottawa: Author, 1972.

Caplan, G. *Principles of preventive psychiatry.* New York: Basic Books, 1964.

CARF, *see* Commission on Accreditation of Rehabilitation Facilities.

Carkhuff, R. R. *Helping and human relations.* New York: Holt, Rinehart and Winston, 1969.

Carkhuff, R. R., & Berenson, B. G. *Beyond counseling and therapy* (2nd ed.). New York: Holt, Rinehart and Winston, 1977.

Center for the Family American Home Economics Association. *Rehabilitation for independent living: A selected bibliography.* Washington, D.C.: President's Committee on Employment of the Handicapped, Women's Committee, 1978.

Chalupsky, A., & Kopf, T. *Job performance aids and their impact on manpower utilization.* Palo Alto, CA: Philco-Ford Corporation, 1967.

Chan, A., Brophy, M. C., Garland, P., Linnane, P., & Screven, R. *Developmental disabilities advocacy project.* Milwaukee: University of Wisconsin-Milwaukee, 1976.

Chapple, E. D. Work or productive participation. *Rehabilitation Record,* January-February 1972, *13*(1), 10–14.

Cherry, C. *On human communication: A review, a survey, and criticism.* Cambridge: M.I.T. Press, 1966.

Chicago Jewish Vocational Service, *see* Jewish Vocational Service—Chicago.

Chigier, E. (Ed.). *New dimensions in rehabilitation* (based on the XIII Congress of Rehabilitation International, Tel Aviv, June 13–18, 1976). Tel Aviv: Gomeh Scientific Publications & Ben-Noon Press, 1978.

Chope, R. C., & McMahon, B. *A classification system for rehabilitation program evaluation technology and literature.* Madison: University of Wisconsin, Regional Rehabilitation Research Institute, 1975.

Christopherson, V. A. The patient and the family. *Rehabilitation Literature*, 1962, *23*(2), 34–41.

Cobb, A. B. *Medical and psychological aspects of disability.* Springfield, IL: Charles C Thomas, 1973.

Coburn, H. H. Dependency—cause and effect. *Journal of Rehabilitation*, 1963, *29*(5), 19.

Coddington, O. L. *Medical considerations in selected vocational handicapping disabilities.* Unpublished manuscript, Columbus, OH, n.d.

Coffey, D. Report writing in work evaluation. In W. Pruitt (Ed.), *Readings in work adjustment—I.* Menomonie: University of Wisconsin-Stout, Materials Development Center, 1970.

Cohen, M., Cote, R., Galloway, F., Hedgeman, B., & Schmones, T. *The role and function of the counselor.* A paper of a committee of the Northeast Rehabilitation Counseling Association, September 1971.

Cohen, S. *Special people.* Englewood Cliffs, NJ: Prentice-Hall, 1977.

Coleman, N. J. Sexual information in the rehabilitation process. *Journal of Applied Rehabilitation Counseling*, 1974, *5*(4), 201–206.

Columbus, D., & Fogel, M. L. Survey of disabled persons reveals housing choices. *Journal of Rehabilitation*, 1971, *37*(2), 26–28.

Colvin, C. R. The utilization of the dictionary of occupational titles in work evaluation. In R. E. Hardy & J. G. Cull (Eds.), *Vocational evaluation for rehabilitation services.* Springfield, IL: Charles C Thomas, 1973.

Commission on Accreditation of Rehabilitation Facilities. *Standards manual for rehabilitation facilities.* Chicago: Author, 1976.

Commission on Accreditation of Rehabilitation Facilities. *Standards manual for rehabilitation facilities.* Chicago: Author, 1978.

Commission on Rehabilitation Counselor Certification. *Application for certification.* Chicago: Author, n.d.

Committee for the Handicapped/People to people

program. *Directory of organizations interested in the handicapped.* Washington, D.C.: Author, 1974.

Conley, R. W. *The economics of vocational rehabilitation.* Baltimore: Johns Hopkins Press, 1965.

Conley, R., & Noble, J., Jr. Workers' compensation reform: Challenge for the 80s. *American Rehabilitation*, January-February 1978, *3*(3), 19–26.

Cook, D. W. Social learning theory and behavior change. *Psychosocial Rehabilitation Journal*, 1976, *1*(1), 32–36.

Cooper, P. G., & Harper, J. N. Issues in the development of a case weighting system. *Journal of Applied Rehabilitation Counseling*, 1979, *10*(1), 7–11.

Cottingham, H. F., & Swanson, C. D. Recent licensure developments: Implications for counselor education. *Counselor Education and Supervision*, 1976, *16*(2), 84–97.

Couch, R. H. The Vocational Evaluation and Work Adjustment Association looks to the future. In R. E. Hardy & J. G. Cull (Eds.), *Vocational evaluation for rehabilitation services.* Springfield, IL: Charles C Thomas, 1973.

Couch, R. H., & Allen, C. M. Behavior modification in rehabilitation facilities: A review. *Journal of Applied Rehabilitation Counseling*, 1973, *4*(2), 88–95.

Council for Exceptional Children, National Education Association. *Careers in special education.* Washington, D.C.: Author, 1969.

Council of World Organizations Interested in the Handicapped, *see* CWOIH.

Criswell, J. H., & Beard, J. H. Community residential facilities for the handicapped. In R. E. Hardy & J. G. Cull (Eds.), *Services of the rehabilitation facility.* Springfield, IL: Charles C Thomas, 1975.

Crites, J. *Vocational psychology.* New York: McGraw-Hill, 1969.

Cronbach, L. J. *Essentials of psychological testing* (3rd ed.). New York: Harper & Row, 1970.

Cronbach, L. J., & Gleser, G. C. *Psychological tests and personnel decisions* (2nd ed.). Urbana: University of Illinois Press, 1965.

Crow, S. H. The role of evaluation in the rehabilitation process. In R. E. Hardy & J. G. Cull (Eds.), *Vocational evaluation for rehabilitation services.* Springfield, IL: Charles C Thomas, 1973.

Cruickshank, W. M. (Ed.). *Psychology of exceptional children and youth.* Englewood Cliffs, NJ: Prentice-Hall, 1955.

Crumpton, A. D. What's it all about—Divisions and NRA. *Journal of Rehabilitation*, 1978, *44*(2); 3; 38.

Crystal, R. M. *A survey of the current status and*

program evaluation needs in the state-federal rehabilitation program. Ann Arbor: University of Michigan, Rehabilitation Research Institute, 1978.

Cubelli, G. E. *Community organization and planning for rehabilitation services.* Washington, D.C.: American Hearing Society, 1965.

Cubelli, G. E. Longitudinal rehabilitation: Implications for rehabilitation counseling. *Professional Bulletin, National Rehabilitation Counseling Association,* 1967, *7*(6), 1–5.

Cull, J. G., & Hardy, R. E. (Eds.). *Vocational rehabilitation: Profession and process.* Springfield, IL: Charles C Thomas, 1972.

Cull, J. G., & Hardy, R. E. (Eds.). *Considerations in rehabilitation facility development.* Springfield, IL: Charles C Thomas, 1977.

Cundiff, G., Henderson, S., & Little, N. (Eds.). *Training guides in evaluation of vocational potential for vocational rehabilitation staff.* Washington, D.C.: U.S. Department of Health, Education, and Welfare, 1965.

CWOIH. CWOIH approves statement on employment policy. *International Rehabilitation Review,* May-June, 1976, 4.

Dabelstein, D. H. Counseling in the rehabilitation service. *Journal of Clinical Psychology,* 1946, *2*(2), 116–122.

Daggett, S. R., James, L. F., & Singley, W. A. *A placement program utilizing the Lodge model: A review and follow-up.* Portland, OR: Portland State University, Regional Rehabilitation Research Institute, 1975.

Dailey, C. A. *Assessment of lives.* San Francisco: Jossey-Bass, 1971.

Davison, G. C., & Neale, J. M. *Abnormal psychology.* New York: John Wiley, 1978.

Dawis, R. V. The Minnesota theory of work adjustment. In B. Bolton (Ed.), *Handbook of measurement and evaluation in rehabilitation.* Baltimore: University Park Press, 1976.

Dawis, R. V., England, G. W., & Lofquist, L. H. *A theory of work adjustment.* Minneapolis: University of Minnesota, Regional Rehabilitation Research Institute, 1964.

Deacon, J. J. *Tongue-tied: Fifty years of friendship in a subnormality hospital.* London: National Society for Mentally Handicapped Children, 1974.

Dean, R. J. N. *New life for millions.* New York: Hastings House, 1972.

Decker, R. S. Holes in the soles of your shoes or: Practical placement techniques. *Job Placement Digest,* June 1972.

Deitchman, P. S., & McHargue, J. *The counselor and client motivation, apathy and dependency.* Tallahassee, FL: Department of Health and Re-

habilitative Services, Division of Vocational Rehabilitation, July 1973.

Dembo, T., Leviton, G. L., & Wright, B. A. Adjustment to misfortune—A problem of social psychological rehabilitation. *Artificial Limbs,* 1956, *3*(2), 4–62.

Demone, H., & Harschbarger, D. *The planning and administration of human services.* New York: Behavioral Publications, 1973.

DeRisi, W. J., & Butz, G. *Writing behavioral contracts: A case simulation practice manual.* Champaign, IL: Research Press, 1975.

DeRoo, W. M., & Haralson, H. L. Increasing workshop production through self-visualization on videotape. *Mental Retardation,* 1971, *9*(4), 22–25.

De Simone, A. S. VR: Viable and reliable. *American Rehabilitation,* 1979, *4*(3), 6–7.

Desmond, R., & Seligman, M. Groups with occupational/vocational goals. In M. Seligman (Ed.), *Group counseling and group psychotherapy with rehabilitation clients.* Springfield, IL: Charles C Thomas, 1977.

Diamond, M. Sexuality and the handicapped. *Rehabilitation Literature,* 1974, *35*(2), 34–40.

Dietz, J. W. An experiment with vocationally handicapped workers. *Personnel Journal,* 1931, *10*(5), 365–370.

DiMichael, S. G. New directions and expectations in rehabilitation counseling. *Journal of Rehabilitation,* 1967, *33*(1), 38–39.

DiMichael, S. G. The current scene. In D. Malikin & H. Rusalem (Eds.), *Vocational rehabilitation of the disabled: An overview.* New York: University Press, 1969.

Dishart, M. Family adjustment to the rehabilitation plan. *Journal of Rehabilitation,* 1964, *30*(1), 42–43.

DOL, *see* U.S. Department of Labor.

Dollard, J., & Miller, M. E. *Personality and psychotherapy.* New York: McGraw-Hill, 1950.

Donlon, E., & Burton, L. *The severely and profoundly handicapped: A practical approach to teaching.* New York: Grune & Stratton, 1976.

Downie, N. M. *Fundamentals of measurement.* London: Oxford University Press, 1967.

Drever, J. *A dictionary of psychology* (revised by H. Wallerstein). Baltimore: Penguin Books, 1968.

Dunn, D. J. Work and behavior change. *Journal of Rehabilitation,* 1971, *37*(4), 22–25.

Dunn, D. J. Work adjustment, work evaluation and employability. *Vocational Evaluation and Work Adjustment Bulletin,* 1971a, *4*(2), 11–16.

Dunn, D. J. *Guide to the use of data, people, and things concepts in work evaluation.* Menomonie: University of Wisconsin-Stout, Institute for Vocational Rehabilitation, 1971b.

Dunn, D. J. Recording observations. *Consumer Brief,* 1973, *1*(1), 1–3.

Dunn, D. J. *Situational assessment: Models for the future.* Menomonie: University of Wisconsin-Stout, Department of Rehabilitation and Manpower Services, Research and Training Center in Vocational Rehabilitation, 1973a.

Dunn, D. J. *Adjustment services: Individualized program planning, delivery, and monitoring.* Menomonie: University of Wisconsin-Stout, Research and Training Center, June 1974.

Dunn, D. J. *Placement services in the vocational rehabilitation program.* Menomonie: University of Wisconsin-Stout, Department of Rehabilitation and Manpower Services, Research and Training Center, December 1974a.

Dunn, D. J. *Process and content orientations in vocational evaluation programs.* Menomonie: University of Wisconsin-Stout, Research and Training Center, December 1975.

Dunn, D. J., Korn, T. A., & Andrew, J. (Eds.). *Critical issues in vocational evaluation.* Menomonie: University of Wisconsin-Stout, Research and Training Center, October 1976.

Dunn, D. J., Korn, T. A., & Schneck, G. R. *What's it mean? Occupational terms in vocational rehabilitation.* Menomonie: University of Wisconsin-Stout, Research and Training Center, August 1976.

Echols, F. H. *Work, Inc.* Tallahassee, FL: Division of Vocational Rehabilitation, December 1967.

Edinburg, G. M., Zinberg, N. E., & Kelman, W. *Clinical interviewing and counseling: Principles and techniques.* New York: Appleton-Century-Crofts, 1975.

Educational Facilities Laboratories. *One out of ten: School planning for the handicapped.* New York: Author, 1974.

Egan, G. *The skilled helper.* Monterey, CA: Brooks-Cole, 1975.

Ehrle, R. A. (Ed.). *Counseling in the public employment service.* Washington, D.C.: Leviathan, 1966.

Ehrle, R. A. An alternative to words in the behavior modification of disadvantaged youth. *Vocational Guidance,* 1968, *17*(11), 41–46.

Ellis, A. *Reason and emotion in psychotherapy.* New York: Lyle Stuart, 1962.

Ellis, M. J. *Why people play.* Englewood Cliffs, NJ: Prentice-Hall, 1973.

Emener, W. G. Clinical supervision in rehabilitation settings. *Journal of Rehabilitation Administration,* May 1978, pp. 44–53.

English, R. W. Recommendations: Alternative strategies for rehabilitating the disadvantaged-disabled. In J. H. Harris & R. W. English (Eds.), *Rehabilitating the disadvantaged-disabled.* Syracuse, NY: Peerless Press, 1972.

Epperson, A., Witt, P., & Hitzhusen, G. (Eds.). *Leisure counseling: An aspect of leisure education.* Springfield, IL: Charles C Thomas, 1972.

Erba, G. Rehabilitation considerations in end stage renal disease. *Journal of Applied Rehabilitation Counseling,* 1969, *5*(6).

Erikson, E. H. *Childhood and society.* New York: Norton, 1950.

Esser, T. J. *Effective report writing in vocational evaluation and work adjustment programs.* Menomonie: University of Wisconsin-Stout, Materials Development Center, 1974.

Esser, T. J. *Client rating instruments for use in vocational rehabilitation agencies.* Menomonie: University of Wisconsin-Stout, Materials Development Center, 1975.

Esser, T. J. The workshop environment: Some essential considerations. *Vocational Evaluation and Work Adjustment Bulletin,* 1975a, *8*(1), 31–35.

Esser, T. J. *A structured guide for selecting training materials in adjustment services.* Menomonie: University of Wisconsin-Stout, Vocational Rehabilitation Institute, 1977.

Esser, T. J., & Botterbusch, K. F. (Eds.). *Token economies in rehabilitation: A book of readings.* Menomonie: University of Wisconsin-Stout, Materials Development Center, 1975.

Experimental Manpower Laboratory, Mobilization for Youth, Inc. *The work sample: Reality-based assessment of vocational potential.* New York: Author, 1970.

Fallows, C. *A complete dictionary of synonyms and antonyms.* London: Fleming H. Revell, 1883.

Farberow, N. L., Heilig, S. M., & Litman, R. E. *Techniques in crisis intervention: A training manual.* Los Angeles: Suicide Prevention Center, 1968.

Farley, R. C. *Basic principles for determining client eligibility.* Fayetteville: University of Arkansas, Rehabilitation Research and Training Center, 1975.

Fasteau, S. Development of a community college program for physically handicapped students. *Rehabilitation Literature,* 1972, *33*(9), 267–270.

Feinberg, L. B. Employment of the certified rehabilitation counselor. *Journal of Rehabilitation,* 1977, *43*(5), 42–44.

Feinberg, L. B., Sundblad, L. M., & Glick, L. J. *Education for the rehabilitation services: Planning undergraduate curricula.* Syracuse, NY: Syracuse University, School of Education, 1974.

Feingold, S. N. (Ed.). *The vocational expert in the social security disability program: A guide for the practitioner.* Springfield, IL: Charles C Thomas, 1969.

Feingold, S. N. Fundamental philosophy of the counseling profession. *Counselor's Information Service,* May 1977, *32*(2), 1–15.

Fenton, J. Rehabilitation programs in the United States. In American Association on Mental Deficiency, *International Research Seminar on Vocational Rehabilitation of the Mentally Retarded.* Washington, D.C.: Author, 1972.

Ferman, L. A. *Job development for the hard-to-employ.* Ann Arbor: University of Michigan, Institute of Labor and Industrial Relations, January 1969.

Fine, S. A., & Wiley, W. W. *An introduction to functional analysis.* Kalamazoo, MI: Upjohn Institute, 1971.

Finesilver, S. G. *A study of driving records, licensing requirements and insurability of physically impaired drivers.* Denver: University of Denver College of Law, Law Center, October 1970.

Fink, S. L. Crisis and motivation: A theoretical model. *Archives of Physical Medicine and Rehabilitation*, 1967, *48*, 592–597.

Fisher, S., & Cleveland, S. E. *Body image and personality.* New York: Dover, 1968.

Flanagan, J. The critical incident technique. *Psychological Bulletin*, 1954, *51*, 327–358.

Fleshman, R. E., & Fryrear, J. L. *The arts in therapy.* Chicago: Nelson-Hall Publishers (In Press).

Flynn, R. J., & Sha'ked, A. Normative sex behavior and the person with a disability. *Journal of Rehabilitation*, 1977, *43*(5), 34–38.

Flynn, W. J. Advocacy programs aid handicapped citizens. *Research Review*, 1975, *2*(2), 1–3.

Forde, W. A. *A special study of on-the-job training prospects for handicapped people in the Phoenix area.* Phoenix: State of Arizona, Division of Vocational Rehabilitation, 1963.

Forster, J. R. What shall we do about credentialing? *Personnel and Guidance Journal*, 1977, *55*(10), 573–576.

Frankel, A. Sexual problems in rehabilitation. *Journal of Rehabilitation*, 1967, *33*(5), 19–21.

Fraser, R. T., & Wright, G. N. Improving rehabilitation personnel management. *Journal of Rehabilitation*, 1977, *43*(3), 22–24.

Freud, S. *The standard edition of the complete psychological works of Sigmund Freud.* London: Hogarth Press & The Institute of Psycho-Analysis, 1952–1974.

Frieden, L. Perspective on Houston: The budding of a seed. In S. S. Pflueger (Ed.), *Independent living.* Washington, D.C.: Institute for Research Utilization, 1977.

Frieden, L. IL: Movement and programs. *American Rehabilitation*, 1978, *3*(6), 6–9.

Frieden, L. Independent living—Consumers and government join hands. *Informer*, 1979, *8*(2), 5–7.

Friedlander, W. A., & Apte, R. Z. *Introduction to social welfare* (4th ed.). Englewood Cliffs, NJ: Prentice-Hall, 1974.

Fritz, M., Wolfensberger, W., & Knowlton, M. *An apartment living plan to promote integration and normalization of mentally retarded adults.* Downsview, Ontario: Canadian Association for the Mentally Retarded, York University, 1971.

Frye, V., & Peters, M. *Therapeutic recreation: Its theory, philosophy, and practice.* Harrisburg, PA: Stackpole Books, 1972.

Galazan, M. M. Evaluation's goal: Prediction or elimination? *Rehabilitation Record*, 1961, *2*(4), 16–18.

Galazan, M. M. Fiscal relationships between state vocational rehabilitation agencies and private rehabilitation facilities. In S. J. Smits (Ed.), *The National Institute on the Interdependence of Rehabilitation Facilities, Workshops and State Agencies.* Washington, D.C.: Association of Rehabilitation Center, 1968.

Galvin, D. E. Problem solving: Vocational rehabilitation for workmen's compensation recipients. In U.S. Department of Health, Education, and Welfare, Rehabilitation Services Administration, Office of Human Development, *Proceedings of National Training Institute: The industrially injured.* Washington, D.C.: U.S. Department of Health, Education, and Welfare, Rehabilitation Services Administration, October 1976.

Garrett, A. *Interviewing: Its principles and methods* (2nd rev. ed.). New York: Family Services Association of America, 1972.

Garrett, J. F. (Ed.). *Psychological aspects of physical disability.* Washington, D.C.: U.S. Government Printing Office, Office of Vocational Rehabilitation, 1952.

Garrett, J. F., & Levine, E. S. (Eds.). *Psychological practices with the physically disabled.* New York: Columbia University Press, 1962.

Garrett, J. F., & Levine, E. S. (Eds.). *Rehabilitation practices with the physically disabled.* New York: Columbia University Press, 1973.

Garris, A. G., & Koonce, K. D. *Technical consultant services to innovate more adequate rehabilitation services to clients with catastrophic disabilities.* Sacramento: California State Department of Rehabilitation, 1970.

Gay, D. A., Reagles, K. W., & Wright, G. N. *Rehabilitation client sustention: A longitudinal study.* Madison: University of Wisconsin, Regional Rehabilitation Research Institute, 1971.

Gazda, G. M., Asbury, F., Balzer, F., Childers, W. C., & Walters, R. *Human relations development.* Boston: Allyn and Bacon, 1977.

Geist, G. O. Internships for rehabilitation counselors: On the way to a professional career. *Journal of Rehabilitation*, 1977, *43*(2), 40.

Geist, G. O., Hershenson, D. B., & Hafer, M. Rehabilitation counselor training: A program evaluation. *Rehabilitation Counseling Bulletin*, 1975, *19*(11), 305–314.

Gellman, W. The vocational adjustment shop. *Personnel and Guidance Journal*, 1961, *39*(8), 630–633.

Gellman, W. Achieving productivity for the cerebral palsied. *Journal of Rehabilitation*, 1961a, *27*(3), 10–12.

Gellman, W. The principles of vocational evaluation. *Rehabilitation Literature*, 1968, *28*(4), 98–102.

Gellman, W. Fundamentals of rehabilitation. In J. F. Garrett & E. S. Levine (Eds.), *Rehabilitation practices with the physically disabled*. New York: Columbia University Press, 1973.

Gellman, W., & Friedman, S. B. The workshop as a clinical rehabilitation tool. *Rehabilitation Literature*, 1965, *26*(2), 34–38.

Gellman, W., Gendel, H., Glaser, N. M., Friedman, S. B., & Neff, W. S. *Adjusting people to work* (2nd ed.). Chicago: Jewish Vocational Service, 1957.

Gellman, W., & Soloff, A. Vocational evaluation. In Brian Bolton (Ed.), *Handbook of measurement and evaluation in rehabilitation*. Baltimore: University Park Press, 1976.

Genskow, J. K. Evaluation: A multi-purpose proposition. *Journal of Rehabilitation*, 1973, *39*(3), 22–25.

Genskow, J. K. The evaluator as the synthesizer. In S. H. Crow (Ed.), *Positions on the practice of vocational evaluation*. Washington, D.C.: Vocational Evaluation and Work Adjustment Association, 1975.

Georgiles, W. *Guidelines to small business*. Madison: State of Wisconsin, Division of Vocational Rehabilitation, August 1973.

Gettings, R. M. *93rd Congress: Federal laws and regulations affecting the handicapped*. Arlington, VA: National Association of Coordinators of State Programs for the Mentally Retarded, 1975.

Gettle, C., & Matthews, S. Ga. Tie-line makes help accessible. *Social and Rehabilitation Record*, 1975, *2*(6), 14.

Gianforte, G. Certification: A challenge and a choice. *Journal of Rehabilitation*, 1976, *42*(5); 15–17, 39.

Ginzberg, E., Ginzberg, S. W., Axelrod, S., & Herma, J. L. *Occupational choice: An approach to a general theory*. New York: Columbia University Press, 1951.

Glass, S. D. *The practical handbook of group counseling*. Baltimore: BCS Publishing, 1969.

Glasser, W. *Reality therapy*. New York: Harper & Row, 1965.

Glasser, W. *The identity society*. New York: Harper & Row, 1972.

Goffman, E. *Stigma: Notes on the management of spoiled identity*. Englewood Cliffs, NJ: Prentice-Hall, 1963.

Goffman, E. The characteristics of total institutions. In A. Etzioni (Ed.), *Complex organizations*. New York: Holt, Rinehart and Winston, 1964.

Gold, M. W. Vocational training. In J. Wortis (Ed.), *Mental retardation and developmental disabilities: An annual review* (Vol. 7). New York: Brunner Mazel, 1975.

Goldenson, R. M. (Ed.). *Disability and rehabilitation handbook*. New York: McGraw-Hill, 1978.

Goldfried, M. R. Behavioral assessment. In I. B. Weiner (Ed.), *Clinical methods in psychology*. New York: John Wiley, 1976.

Goldhammer, M. N., & James, L. F. *Self-determined placement: A guide for vocational rehabilitation counselors and disabled persons*. Portland, OR: Portland State University, School of Social Work, 1976.

Goldin, G. J., & Perry, S. L. *Dependency and its implication for rehabilitation*. Boston: Northeastern University, New England Rehabilitation Research Institute, 1967.

Goldin, G. J., & Perry, S. L., Margolin, R. J., & Stotsky, B. A. *Dependency and its implications for rehabilitation* (rev. ed.). Lexington, MA: Lexington Book, D. C. Heath, 1972.

Goldman, L. *Using tests in counseling*. New York: Appleton-Century-Crofts, 1961.

Goldman, L. The process of vocational assessment. In H. Borow (Ed.), *Man in a world at work*. Boston: Houghton Mifflin, 1964.

Goldman, L. *Using tests in counseling* (2nd ed.). New York: Appleton-Century-Crofts, 1971.

Goodwill Industries of America. *Developing effective work place systems for vocational rehabilitation: A handbook*. Washington, D.C.: Goodwill Industries of America, n.d.

Goodwill Industries of America (J. Hutchison, Ed.). *Goodwill Industries of America rehabilitation manual*. Washington, D.C.: Author, 1975.

Goolsby, E. L. Facilitation of family-professional interaction. *Rehabilitation Literature*, 1976, *37*(11–12), 332–334.

Gordon, T. *Group-centered leadership*. Boston: Houghton Mifflin, 1955.

Graham, E. C., & Mullen, M. M. *Rehabilitation literature 1950–1955*. New York: McGraw-Hill, 1956.

Great Britain, Department of Employment. *Classification of occupations and directory of occupational titles* (in 3 volumes). London: Her Majesty's Stationery Office, 1972.

Greenleigh Associates, Inc. *The role of the sheltered workshops in the rehabilitation of the severely handicapped*. New York: Author, November 1975.

Greenleigh Associates, Inc. *The role of the sheltered workshops in the rehabilitation of the severely handicapped: Vol. 1—Executive summary.* New York: Author, July 1975a.

Groves, M. P. *Wisconsin job service guidelines for professional placement practice: An analysis for vocational rehabilitation.* Unpublished master's thesis, University of Wisconsin-Madison, 1978.

Gutsch, K. U., & Logan, R. H., III. Newspapers as a means of disseminating occupational information. *Vocational Guidance Quarterly*, 1967, *15*(3), 186–190.

Haber, L. D. Disabling effects of chronic disease and impairment. *Journal of Chronic Diseases*, 1971, *24*, 469–487.

Haber, L. D. Disabling effects of chronic disease and impairment. II. Functional capacity limitations. *Journal of Chronic Diseases*, 1973, *26*, 127–151.

Haber, W., & Kruger, D. H. *The role of the United States employment service in a changing economy.* Kalamazoo, MI: Upjohn Institute for Employment Research, February 1964.

Hackney, H., & Cormier, L. S. *Counseling strategies and objectives* (2nd ed.). Englewood Cliffs, NJ: Prentice-Hall, 1979.

Haddle, H. W., Jr. Behavior change through self-control: A training model for helping the severely disabled children. In W. M. Jenkins, R. M. Anderson, & W. L. Dietrich (Comps. and eds.), *Rehabilitation of the severely disabled.* Dubuque, IA: Kendall-Hunt, 1976.

Hadley, F. P. Projects with industry: A marketing approach. *American Rehabilitation*, 1979, *4*(4), 3–5.

Hale, G. (Ed.). *The source book for the disabled.* New York: Paddington Press Ltd., 1979.

Hall, J. H., & Warren, S. L. (Eds.). *Rehabilitation counselor preparation.* Washington, D.C.: National Rehabilitation Association and National Vocational Guidance Association, 1956.

Hamilton, G. *Theory and practice of social case work* (1st ed.). New York: Columbia University Press, 1940.

Hamilton, G. *Principles of social case recording.* New York: Columbia University Press, 1946.

Hamilton, G. *Theory and practice of social case work* (2nd rev. ed.). New York: Columbia University Press, 1951.

Hamilton, G., & Roessner, J. How employers screen disadvantaged job applicants. *Monthly Labor Review*, 1972, *95*(9), 14–21.

Hamilton, K. W. *Counseling the handicapped in the rehabilitation process.* New York: Ronald Press, 1950.

Hanman, B. *Physical capacities and job placement.* Stockholm: Nordisk Rotogravyr, 1951.

Hansen, C. E. Work adjustment in the sheltered workshop. *Vocational Evaluation and Work Adjustment Bulletin*, 1972, *5*(3), 12–19.

Hansen, C. E. Rehabilitation training. *Journal of Applied Rehabilitation Counseling*, 1973, *4*(4), 208–223.

Hansen, C. E. The question of rehabilitation counselor certification. *Journal of Rehabilitation*, 1977, *43*(2), 2.

Hardy, R. E., & Cull, J. G. Standards in evaluation. *Vocational Evaluation and Work Adjustment Bulletin*, 1969, *11*(1), 11–13.

Hardy, R. E., & Cull, J. G. Group counseling with public offenders. In R. E. Hardy & J. G. Cull (Eds.), *Group counseling and therapy techniques in special settings.* Springfield, IL: Charles C Thomas, 1974.

Hardy, R. E., & Cull, J. G. (Eds.). *Severe disabilities: Social and rehabilitation approaches.* Springfield, IL: Charles C Thomas, 1974a.

Hardy, R. E., & Cull, J. G. (Eds.). *Services of the rehabilitation facility.* Springfield, IL: Charles C Thomas, 1975.

Harris, G. *The redemption of the disabled.* New York: Appleton, 1919.

Harrower, M. (Ed.). *Medical and psychological teamwork in the case of the chronically ill.* Springfield, IL: Charles C Thomas, 1955.

Hart, W. R. Effective approaches to employers. *Rehabilitation Record*, 1962, *3*(2), 34–37.

Havelock, R. G. *Planning for innovation through dissemination and utilization of knowledge.* Ann Arbor: University of Michigan, Center for Research on Utilization of Scientific Knowledge, 1969.

Havens, L. L. Dependence: Definition and strategies. In R. J. Margolin & F. L. Hurwitz (Eds.), *Report of a dependency and motivation workshop.* Boston: Northeastern University, 1963.

Havighurst, R. J. *Developmental tasks and education.* New York: Longmans, Green, 1950.

Havighurst, R. J. *Human development and education.* New York: Longmans, Green, 1953.

Heber, R. *Manual on terminology and classification in mental retardation.* Monograph supplement to *American Journal of Mental Deficiency.* American Association on Mental Deficiency, 1959.

Helsel, E. D. Putting it together in Ohio: Parameters, definitions, and alternatives for protective services. In C. K. Sigelman (Ed.), *Protective services and citizen advocacy.* Lubbock: Texas Tech University, 1974.

Henke, R. O., Connolly, S. G., & Cox, J. G. Caseload management: The key to effectiveness. *Journal of Applied Rehabilitation Counseling*, 1975, *6*, 217–227.

Hermann, A. M. C., & Walker, L. A. *Handbook of employment rights of the handicapped: Sections*

503 and 504 of the Rehabilitation Act of 1973. Washington, D.C.: George Washington University, Regional Rehabilitation Research Institute on Attitudinal, Legal, and Leisure Barriers, 1978.

Hershenson, D. B. Vocational guidance and the handicapped. In E. Herr (Ed.), *Vocational guidance and human development.* Boston: Houghton Mifflin, 1974.

HEW, *see* U.S. Department of Health, Education, and Welfare.

HEW, RSA, *see* U. S. Department of Health, Education, and Welfare, Rehabilitation Services Administration.

Hillard, C. Barrier-free communities. *American Rehabilitation*, 1978, *3*(6), 10–15.

Hilliard, T. R. *Rehabilitation counselor personal characteristic type relationship to counselor performance ratings.* Unpublished doctoral dissertation, University of Florida, 1972.

Hills, W. G. *Evaluating vocational rehabilitation programs.* Norman: University of Oklahoma, Regional Rehabilitation Research Institute, March 1973.

Hoffman, P. R. Some comments on vocational evaluation as activity counseling. *Vocational Evaluation and Work Adjustment Bulletin*, 1972, *5*(1), 22–25.

Hoffman, P. R. Work evaluation: An overview. In R. E. Hardy & J. G. Cull (Eds.), *Vocational evaluation for rehabilitation services.* Springfield, IL: Charles C Thomas, 1973.

Holland, J. L. A theory of vocational choice. *Journal of Counseling Psychology*, 1959, *6*, 35–45.

Holland, J. L. *The psychology of vocational choice.* Waltham, MA: Blaisdell, 1966.

Holland, J. L. *Making vocational choices.* Englewood Cliffs, NJ: Prentice-Hall, 1973.

Holvey, D. N. (Ed.). *The Merck manual of diagnosis and therapy.* Rahway, NJ: Merck and Company, 1977.

Hopke, W. (Ed.). *Dictionary of personnel and guidance terms.* Chicago: J. G. Ferguson, 1968.

Hoppock, R. *Occupational information* (4th ed.). New York: McGraw-Hill, 1976.

Horwitz, J. J. Dimensions of rehabilitation teamwork. *Rehabilitation Record*, March-April 1969, pp. 36–40.

Hosford, R. E. Behavioral counseling: A contemporary overview. *Counseling Psychologist*, 1969, *1*(4), 1–32.

Hosford, R. E. Behavorism is humanism. In G. F. Farwell, N. Gamsky, & P. Mathew-Coughlan (Eds.), *The Counselor's Handbook.* New York: Intext, 1974.

Hosford, R. E., & de Visser, L. A. *Behavioral approaches to counseling: An introduction.* Washington, D.C.: American Personnel and Guidance Association Press, 1974.

Huber, J. T. *Report writing in psychology and psychiatry.* New York: Harper & Row, 1961.

Hutchison, J., & Cogan, F. Rehabilitation manpower specialist: A job description of placement personnel. *Journal of Rehabilitation*, 1974, *40*(2), 31–33.

Hylbert, K. W. Experiment at Penn State: Bachelor of rehabilitation. *Journal of Rehabilitation*, 1963, *29*(2), 23–24.

Hylbert, K. W. *Medical information for human service workers* (2nd rev. ed.). State College, PA: Counselor Education Press, 1979.

Ince, L. P. *The rehabilitation medicine services.* Springfield, IL: Charles C Thomas, 1974.

Ince, L. P. *Behavior modification in rehabilitation medicine.* Springfield, IL: Charles C Thomas, 1976.

Indices, Inc. *Functional limitations: A state of the art review.* Falls Church, VA: Author, 1979.

International Labour Office. *Glossary—Vocational rehabilitation and employment of the disabled.* Geneva: Author, n.d.

International Labour Office. *International standard classification of occupations* (rev. ed.). Geneva: Author, 1968.

International Labour Office. *Basic principles of vocational rehabilitation of the disabled* (2nd ed.). Geneva: Author, 1973.

Irish, R. K. *Go hire yourself an employer.* Garden City, NY: Anchor-Doubleday, 1973.

Jacobs, A. E., & Hay, J. Vocational reporting in the vocational rehabilitation process. *Personnel and Guidance Journal*, 1961, *40*, 368–372.

Jacobs, A. E., Jordaan, J. P., & DiMichael, S. G. (Eds.). *Counseling in the rehabilitation process.* New York: Columbia University Teachers College, 1961.

Jaffe, A. J. (Ed.). *Research conference on workmen's compensation and vocational rehabilitation.* Research presented at Columbia University, New York, November 29–December 2, 1960.

Jaques, M. E. *Critical counseling behavior in rehabilitation settings.* Iowa City: State University of Iowa, Vocational Rehabilitation Administration Study, 1959.

Jaques, M. E. *Rehabilitation counseling: Scope and services.* Boston: Houghton Mifflin, 1970.

Jarrell, G. R. Selective training. In J. G. Cull & R. E. Hardy (Eds.), *Vocational rehabilitation: Profession and process.* Springfield, IL: Charles C Thomas, 1972.

Jeffers, J. S. Disabled employment opportunities: Past, present, and future. *Social and Rehabilitation Record*, 1974, *1*(9), 14–19.

Jeffrey, D. Case studies involving medical and vocational information. In Arkansas Rehabilitation Research and Training Center, *Orientation institute—Evaluation for vocational potential.* Hot Springs, AR: Author, 1966.

Jenkins, W. M., Anderson, R. M., & Dietrich, W. L. (Eds.). *Rehabilitation of the severely disabled.* Dubuque, IA: Kendall-Hunt, 1976.

Jewish Vocational Service—Chicago, Research Utilization Laboratory. *RUL #5: Goal attainment scaling manual.* Chicago: Author, 1976.

Johnson, D. W. *The social psychology of education.* New York: Holt, Rinehart and Winston, 1970.

Johnson, D. W., & Johnson, F. P. *Joining together: Group theory and group skills.* Englewood Cliffs, NJ: Prentice-Hall, 1975.

Jones, R., & Azrin, N. An experimental application of a social reinforcement approach to the problem of job finding. *Journal of Applied Behavioral Analysis*, 1973, *6*, 345–353.

Kagan, M. How to improve case records. *Rehabilitation Record*, 1962, *3*(6), 23–27.

Kanfer, F. H., & Goldstein, A. P. *Helping people change: A textbook of methods.* New York: Pergamon Press, 1975.

Karan, O. C. Contemporary views on vocational evaluation practices with the mentally retarded. *Vocational Evaluation and Work Adjustment Bulletin*, 1976, *9*(1), 7–13.

Karan, O. C., & Gardner, W. I. Vocational rehabilitation practices: A behavioral analysis. *Rehabilitation Literature*, 1973, *34*(10), 290–298.

Katz, M. *Decisions and values: A rationale for secondary school guidance.* New York: College Entrance Examination Board, 1963.

Katz, S., Reagles, K. W., & Wright, G. N. A study of counselor time utilization for medically disabled and culturally disadvantaged clients. *Journal of Applied Rehabilitation Counseling*, 1973, *4*(4), 224–233.

Katz, S., Wright, G. N., & Reagles, K. W. *The impact of an expanded vocational rehabilitation program upon intra-agency processes and procedures.* Madison: University of Wisconsin, Regional Rehabilitation Research Institute, 1971.

Kaufman, A. G. *The process of job placement for the psychiatrically disabled: Current focus, emerging trends, and implications.* Philadelphia, PA: Unpublished manuscript, 1975.

Keller, O. J., & Alper, B. S. *Halfway houses: Community-centered correction and treatment.* Lexington, MA: D. C. Heath, 1970.

Kelly, E. L. *Assessment of human characteristics.* Belmont, CA: Brooks-Cole, 1967.

Kelly, G. F. Sex education for counselors. *Personnel and Guidance Journal*, 1976, *54*(7), 354–357.

Kelly, L. J., & Vergason, G. A. *Dictionary of special education and rehabilitation.* Denver: Love, 1978.

Kelso, R. R. Evaluation in the rehabilitation process. *Regional Exchange*, February 1974.

Kessler, H. H. *The crippled and the disabled: Rehabilitation of the physically handicapped in the United States.* New York: Columbia University Press, 1935.

Kessler, H. H. *Rehabilitation of the physically handicapped.* New York: Columbia University Press, 1947.

Kessler, H. H. *The knife is not enough.* New York: Norton, 1968.

Kessler, H. H. *Disability—Determination and evaluation.* Philadelphia: Lea & Febiger, 1970.

Kiresuk, T., Salasin, S., and Garwick, G. *The program evaluation project: Overview.* Minneapolis: Program Evaluation Project, 1972.

Klausner, S. J. *Disabled families: A study of a link between the social contribution of the disabled and the retardation of their rehabilitation in the family context.* Washington, D.C.: U.S. Department of Health, Education, and Welfare, 1969.

Kliment, S. A. *Into the mainstream: A syllabus for a barrier-free environment.* Washington, D.C.: U.S. HEW, Rehabilitation Services Administration, and the American Institute of Architects, June 1975.

Klinger, J. L. (with the New York University Medical Center, Institute of Rehabilitation Medicine; and Campbell Soup Company). *Mealtime manual for people with disabilities and the aging* (2nd ed.). Camden, NJ: Campbell Soup Company, 1978.

Klopfer, W. G. *The psychological report.* New York: Grune & Stratton, 1960.

Knowles, M. S. Adult education. In R. Morris (Ed.), *Encyclopedia of social work.* New York: National Association of Social Workers, 1971.

Kojima, Y. Discrimination of the disabled and seeking ways out. *Japan Christian Quarterly*, 1976, *42*(3), 162–168.

Kojima, Y. Disabled individuals in Japanese society. *Rehabilitation World*, 1977, *3*(2), 18–25.

Kojima, Y. *A history of social work education: A social response to social realities; the historical development and the realities of Schools of Social Work.* Tokyo: Japan Women's University, Department of Social Welfare (Journal "Social Welfare"), 1977a.

Korn, T. A. *Vocational evaluation planning: A model.* Menomonie: University of Wisconsin-Stout, Research and Training Center, August 1976.

Korn, T. A. (Ed.). *A work sample style guide.* Menomonie: University of Wisconsin-Stout, Research and Training Center, October 1976a.

Korn, T. A. *A content based vocational evaluation report.* Menomonie: University of Wisconsin-Stout, Research and Training Center, August 1976b.

Korn, T. A., Ranney, W. C., Schneck, G. R., &

Schober, D. K. *Behavior identification and analysis in rehabilitation facility services.* Menomonie: University of Wisconsin-Stout, Vocational Rehabilitation Institute, August 1976.

Kravetz, S. P. *Rehabilitation need and status: Substance, structure and process.* Unpublished doctoral dissertation, University of Wisconsin-Madison, 1973.

Kravetz, S. P., & Thomas, K. R. A learning theory approach to counseling indecisive clients. In B. Bolton & M. E. Jaques (Eds.), *Rehabilitation counseling: Theory and practice.* Baltimore: University Park Press, 1978.

Krumboltz, J. D. Behavioral counseling: Rationale and research. *Personnel and Guidance Journal,* 1965, *44*(4), 383–387.

Krumboltz, J. D., & Thoresen, C. E. (Eds.). *Behavioral counseling: Cases and techniques.* New York: Holt, Rinehart and Winston, 1969.

Krusen, F. H., Kottke, F. J., & Ellwood, P. M. (Eds.). *Handbook of physical medicine and rehabilitation* (2nd ed.). Philadelphia: W. B. Saunders, 1971.

Kunitz, E. *Community action for comprehensive rehabilitation services and the establishment of a pilot evaluation-referral center.* Martinez, CA: Contra Costa Rehabilitation Council, May 1964.

Kunze, K. R. Industry resources available to counselors. *Vocational Guidance Quarterly,* 1967, *16*(2), 137–142.

Lamb, H. R., & Mackota, C. Vocational rehabilitation counseling: A "second class" profession? *Journal of Rehabilitation,* 1975, *41*(3), 21–24.

Lasky, R. G., & Dell Orto, A. E. *Group counseling and physical disability: A rehabilitation and health care perspective.* North Scituate, MA: Duxbury, 1979.

Lassiter, R. A. *Vocational rehabilitation in North Carolina (1920–1968).* Chapel Hill: University of North Carolina, Rehabilitation Counseling Program, 1970.

Lassiter, R. A. The use of group counseling in achieving adjustment to work. In R. E. Hardy & J. G. Cull (Eds.), *Group counseling and therapy techniques in special settings.* Springfield, IL: Charles C Thomas, 1974.

Laurie, G. (Ed.). *Housing and home services for the disabled: Guidelines and experiences in independent living.* Hagerstown, MD: Harper & Row, 1977.

Laus, M. D. *Travel instruction for the handicapped.* Springfield, IL: Charles C Thomas, 1977.

LaVor, M. L., & Duncan, J. G. Vocational rehabilitation: The new law and its implications for the future. *Journal of Rehabilitation,* 1976, *42*(4); 20–28, 39.

Lee, J. J. The role of the university in the counselor education program. *Journal of Rehabilitation,* 1955, *21*(5); 4–5, 14.

Leshner, S. S., & Snyderman, G. S. Occupational aspects of work adjustment. *Rehabilitation Record,* 1962, *3*(2), 8–11.

Leung, P. The changing work value and the rehabilitation counselor. *Rehabilitation Counseling Bulletin,* 1972, *15*(4), 228–232.

Levin, S. *Volunteers in rehabilitation* (a set of 12 handbooks). Washington, D. C.: Goodwill Industries of America, National Auxiliary to Goodwill Industries, 1973.

Levine, B. *Fundamentals of group treatment.* Northbrook, IL: Whitehall, 1967.

Levine, E. S. *The psychology of deafness: Techniques of appraisal for rehabilitation.* New York: Columbia University Press, 1960.

Levine, L. S., & Pence, J. W. A training program for rehabilitation counselors. *Journal of Rehabilitation,* 1953, *19*(1); 16–17, 20.

Levine, S., White, P. E., & Paul, B. D. Community interorganizational problems in providing medical care and social services. *American Journal of Public Health,* 1963, *53*, 1183–1195.

Lewis, J. A., & Lewis, M. D. *Community counseling: A human services approach.* New York: John Wiley, 1977.

Lindenberg, R. E. *Perspectives on work with families in rehabilitation.* Paper presented at the American Personnel and Guidance Association Convention, Chicago, April 1976.

Lindenberg, R. E. Work with families in rehabilitation. *Rehabilitation Counseling Bulletin,* 1977, *21*(1), 67–76.

Lindsay, A. *Group work recording.* New York: American Book-Stratford Press, 1952.

Lindsley, O. Direct measurement and prosthesis of retarded behavior. *Journal of Education,* 1964, *147*, 62–81.

Linkowski, D. C. A scale to measure acceptance of disability. *Rehabilitation Counseling Bulletin,* 1971, *14*, 236–244.

Linkowski, D. C., & Dunn, M. A. Self-concept and acceptance of disability. *Rehabilitation Counseling Bulletin,* 1974, *18*, 28–32.

Linnane, P. D. *Ombudsman for nursing homes: Structure & process.* Washington, D.C.: U.S. Department of Health, Education, and Welfare, Administration on Aging, 1974.

Livingston, P. J. Professional education for the placement counselor. *Job Placement Division Digest Professional Supplement,* August 1978, pp. 7–12.

Loban, L. N. Group insurance and the handicapped. *Governor's Committee on Employment of the Handicapped,* Santa Barbara, CA: Author, August 3–4, 1972.

Lofquist, L. H. *Vocational counseling with the physically handicapped.* New York: Appleton-Century-Crofts, 1957.

Lofquist, L. H. (Ed.). *Psychological research and*

rehabilitation. Washington, D.C.: American Psychological Association, 1960.

Lofquist, L. H., & Dawis, R. V. *Adjustment to work: A psychological view of man's problems in a work-oriented society*. New York: Appleton-Century-Crofts, 1969.

Lofquist, L. H., & Dawis, R. V. Vocational needs, work reinforcers, and job satisfaction. *Vocational Guidance Quarterly*, 1975, *24*(2), 132–139.

Lofquist, L. H., Siess, T. F., Dawis, R. V., England, G. W., & Weiss, D. J. *Disability and work*. Minneapolis: University of Minnesota, Industrial Relations Center, 1964.

Long, N., Anderson, J., Burd, R., Mathis, M. E., & Todd, S. P. *Information and referral centers: A functional analysis* (3rd ed.). Washington, D.C.: U.S. Department of Health, Education, and Welfare, Office of Human Development, Administration on Aging, November 1974.

Long, N., Reiner, S., & Zimmerman, S. *Information and referral services: The resource file*. Washington, D.C.: U.S. Department of Health, Education, and Welfare, Office of Human Development, Administration on Aging, 1973.

Longfellow, R. E. *Placement—A disservice to the handicapped*. Stillwater: Oklahoma State University, Rehabilitation Counseling Training, The Clearing House, n.d.

Lorenz, J. R. Rehabilitation services: Public versus the private sector. *Rehabilitation Literature*, 1973, *34*(9); 258–266, 274.

Lorenz, J. R. *Job modification for the handicapped*. Carbondale, IL: Unpublished manuscript, Southern Illinois University, 1974.

Lustig, P. Differential use of the work situation in the sheltered workshop. *Rehabilitation Literature*, 1970, *31*; 39–42, 49.

Lynch, K., & Barr, J. *Community assessment training program*. Ann Arbor: University of Michigan, Institute for the Study of Mental Retardation and Related Disabilities, n.d.

Maddock, J. W., & Chilgren, R. A. The emergence of sex therapy. *Personnel and Guidance Journal*, 1976, *54*(7), 371–374.

Mager, R. F. Preparing instructional objectives. In L. R. Dickerson & J. D. Andrew (Eds.), *Work adjustment: A resource manual*. Menomonie: University of Wisconsin-Stout, Research and Training Center, n.d.

Maki, D. R., McCracken, N., Pape, D. A., & Scofield, M. E. The theoretical model of vocational rehabilitation. *Journal of Rehabilitation*, 1978, *44*(4), 26–28.

Malikin, D. *Social disability: Alcoholism, drug addiction, crime and social disadvantage*. New York: New York University Press, 1973.

Malikin, D., & Rusalem, H. (Eds.). *Vocational rehabilitation of the disabled: An overview*. New York: New York University Press, 1969.

Mallas, A. A. *What all persons concerned with rehabilitation should know in making business contacts*. Paper presented in the Placement Workshop at Oklahoma State University, Stillwater, June 1965.

Mallik, K. Books: Homebound employment. *Paraplegia News*, May 1975.

Mallik, K., & Sablowsky, R. Model for placement—Job laboratory approach. *Journal of Rehabilitation*. November-December 1975, pp. 14–20, 41.

Mallik, K., Yuspeh, S., & Mueller, J. (Eds.). *Comprehensive vocational rehabilitation for severely disabled persons*. Washington, D.C.: George Washington University Medical Center, Job Development Laboratory, 1975.

Maloney, S. Section 503 conference—A new day for handicapped people. *Journal of Rehabilitation*, 1976, *42*(3), 14–15.

Margolin, R. J. Rationale for teamwork. *Rehabilitation Record*, March-April 1969, pp. 32–35.

Marinelli, R. P., & Dell Orto, A. E. (Eds.). *The psychological and social impact of physical disability*. New York: Springer, 1977.

Marr, J. N., & Krauft, C. C. *Training package for practitioners in rehabilitation settings: Behavior modification—principles, procedures, and token economies*. Fayetteville: Arkansas Rehabilitation Research and Training Center, 1975.

Maslow, A. H. *Motivation and personality*. New York: Harper, 1954.

Massie, W. A. Partners in improving rehabilitation practices. *Social and Rehabilitation Record*, 1974, *1*(7), 6–8.

Masters, W. H., & Johnson, V. E. *Human sexual inadequacy*. Boston: Little, Brown, 1970.

May, R. *Love and will*. New York: Norton, 1969.

McCauley, W. A. Power, practice and problems in rehabilitation counseling. *NRCA Professional Bulletin*, 1967, *7*(3), 1–3.

McCavitt, M. E. *A demonstration employment training and placement project for small business enterprises in Concourse Village, Bronx*. New York: United Cerebral Palsy of New York City, 1967.

McCavitt, M. E. International cooperation in rehabilitation research. *American Rehabilitation*, 1977, *2*(5), 6–12.

McClure, D. P. Placement through improvement of client's job-seeking skills. *Journal of Applied Rehabilitation Counseling*, 1972, *3*(1), 188–196.

McComb, G. C., & Rice, D. M. *Tomorrow's trends in higher education for the severely handicapped*. Presentation given at the 1976 annual convention of the American Personnel and Guidance Association, Chicago, April 1976.

McCroskey, B. J., Wattenbarger, W., Field, T. F., & Sink, J. M. *The vocational diagnosis and assessment of residual employability handbook*.

Athens, GA: University of Georgia, Department of Counseling and Human Development Services, 1977.

McDaniel, J. W. *Physical disability and human behavior* (2nd ed.). New York: Pergamon Press, 1976.

McFarland, R. A. *Placement methods match a handicap with a job*. Menomonie: University of Wisconsin-Stout, Materials Development Center, n.d.

McGaughey, R. From problem to solution: The new focus in fighting environmental barriers for the handicapped. *Rehabilitation Literature*, 1976, *37*(1), 10–12.

McGowan, J. F. (Ed.). *An introduction to the vocational rehabilitation process: A manual for orientation and in-service training*. Washington, D.C.: U.S. Department of Health, Education, and Welfare, Office of Vocational Rehabilitation, 1960.

McGowan, J. F., & Porter, T. L. *An introduction to employment service counseling*. Columbia: University of Missouri, August 1964.

McGowan, J. F., & Porter, T. L. *An introduction to the vocational rehabilitation process*. Washington, D.C.: U.S. Department of Health, Education, and Welfare, Vocational Rehabilitation Administration, 1967.

McGwinn, D. Attendant care. In G. Laurie (Ed.), *Housing and home services for the disabled: Guidelines and experiences in independent living*. Hagerstown, MD: Harper & Row, 1977.

McMahon, B. T. *A model of vocational development for the midcareer disabled*. Unpublished doctoral dissertation, University of Wisconsin-Madison, 1977.

McMahon, B. T., & Fraser, R. T. The future of subprofessionals: A time for evaluation. *Rehabilitation Counseling Bulletin*, 1978, *22*(1), 30–37.

Mehrens, W. A., & Lehmann, I. J. *Standardized tests in education*. New York: Holt, Rinehart and Winston, 1969.

Mehrens, W. A., & Lehmann, I. J. *Measurement and evaluation in education and psychology*. New York: Holt, Rinehart and Winston, 1973.

Meister, R. K. Diagnostic assessment in rehabilitation. In B. Bolton (Ed.), *Handbook of measurement and evaluation in rehabilitation*. Baltimore: University Park Press, 1976.

Miller, L. A., & Obermann, C. E. *Inservice training program*. Menomonie, WI: Stout State University, Institute for Vocational Rehabilitation, Materials Development Center, 1968.

Miller, L., & Olson, F. The three faces of client eligibility determination: Implementing federal law in state-federal rehabilitation agencies. *Rehabilitation Research and Practice Review*, 1971, *2*(2), 25–46.

Miller, S. J. Professions, human service. In R. Morris (Ed.), *Encyclopedia of Social Work* (Vol. 2). New York: National Association of Social Workers, 1971.

Mills, C. The development of the Rehabilitation Acts of 1973 and 1974. In W. L. Jenkins, R. M. Anderson, & W. L. Dietrich (Eds.), *Rehabilitation of the severely disabled*. Dubuque, IA: Kendall-Hunt, 1976.

Minneapolis Rehabilitation Center, Inc. *Job seeking skills: Instructing specialists*. Minneapolis: Author, 1971.

Mitra, S. B., Fitzgerald, L., Hilliard, H. S., & Baker, R. N. Effectiveness of paraprofessionals in the rehabilitation process. *Rehabilitation Counseling Bulletin*, 1974, *18*, 112–116.

Molski, J. T. *Work adjustment: Techniques used in reaching its goals*. Unpublished master's thesis, University of Wisconsin-Madison, 1976.

Montan, K. International cooperation in technical aids for the disabled. *International Rehabilitation Review*, 1969, *20*(1), 11, 14.

Mooney, T. D., Cole, T. M., & Chilgren, R. A. *Sexual options for paraplegics and quadriplegics*. Boston: Little, Brown and Company, 1975.

Moor, G., Chervall, E., & West, M. Television as a therapeutic tool. *Archives of General Psychiatry*, 1965, *12*, 217–220.

Moreno, J. L. *Psychodrama*. New York: Beacon House, 1946.

Morgan, C. A. *Some aspects of occupational information and employment for vocational rehabilitation counselors*. Unpublished manuscript, Oklahoma State University, n.d.

Morris, R. *Intercommunity research in community organization*. New York: Columbia University Press, 1961.

Morris, R. Welfare reform 1973: The social services dimension. *Science*, 1973, *181*, 515–522.

Morrow, D. L. Cultural addiction. *Journal of Rehabilitation*, 1972, *38*(3); 30–32, 41.

Moses, H. A., & Patterson, C. H. (Eds.). *Readings in rehabilitation counseling* (2nd ed.). Champaign, IL: Stipes, 1971.

Multi Resource Centers. *Job seeking skills reference manual*. Minneapolis: Author, 1971.

Multi Resource Centers. *Vocational diagnostic interviewing: Reference manual*. Minneapolis: Minneapolis Rehabilitation Center, 1972.

Murphy, W. F. Some clinical aspects of the body, ego, with special reference to phantom limb phenomena. *Psychoanalytic Review*, 1957, *44*, 462–477.

Muthard, J. E. *The role of psychology in the preparation of rehabilitation counselors*. Washington, D.C.: American Psychological Association, Division of Counseling Psychology, December 1963.

Muthard, J. E., & Miller, L. A. *The criteria problem in rehabilitation counseling.* Iowa City: University of Iowa, College of Education, 1966.

Muthard, J. E., & Salomone, P. R. The roles and functions of the rehabilitation counselor. *Rehabilitation Counseling Bulletin*, 1969, *13*(1-SP), 81–168.

Myers, J. S. (Ed.). *An orientation to chronic disease and disability.* New York: Macmillan, 1965.

Myklebust, H. R. *The psychology of deafness: Sensory deprivation, learning, and adjustment.* New York: Grune & Stratton, 1960.

Nadolsky, J. M. Specialization: Its nature and effects. *Vocational Evaluation and Work Adjustment Bulletins*, 1975, *8*(1), 2–7.

Nagi, S. Z. *Disability and rehabilitation: Legal, clinical, and self-concepts and measurement.* Columbus: Ohio State University Press, 1969.

Nagi, S. Z. *Disability concepts and implications to the structure of services.* An address to the American Rehabilitation Counseling Association meeting in Dallas, Texas, March 9, 1977.

National Academy of Sciences. *Prosthetics and Orthotics Research Reference Catalogue.* Washington, D.C.: Author, 1975.

National Association of Manufacturers. *Job opportunities for handicapped workers.* Washington, D.C.: Author, December 1, 1964.

National Association of Sheltered Workshops and Homebound Programs. *A guide to comprehensive rehabilitation services to the homebound disabled* (1st ed.). Washington, D.C.: U.S. Department of Health, Education, and Welfare, Office of Vocational Rehabilitation, April 1961.

National Association of Sheltered Workshops and Homebound Programs. *Sheltered workshops, a handbook* (2nd ed.). Washington, D.C.: Author, 1966.

National Association of Social Workers. *Directory of agencies.* Washington, D.C.: Author, 1975.

National Council on Rehabilitation. *Symposium on the Processes of Rehabilitation.* New York: Author, 1944.

National Industrial Conference Board, Inc. *The company and the physically impaired worker.* New York: Author, 1957.

National Rehabilitation Association. *National Rehabilitation Association.* Washington, D.C.: Author, n.d.

National Rehabilitation Association. *Courage facing handicaps.* N.p.: Author, 1933.

National Rehabilitation Association. Ten years of rehabilitation progress under PL 565 (Special 26-page report). *Journal of Rehabilitation*, 1964, *30*(5), 15–40.

National Rehabilitation Association. NRA views the overriding issue. *NRA Newsletter*, May 1977, pp. 1–2.

National Rehabilitation Counseling Association. RSA Advisory Committee for rehabilitation counselors. *NRCA News*, 1975, *17*(3), 2.

National Rehabilitation Counseling Association-American Rehabilitation Counseling Association. Reorganization threatens rehabilitation in Florida. *NRCA-ARCA News Report*, September 1975.

National Safety Council. *Accident prevention manual for industrial operations.* Chicago: Author, n.d.

National Vocational Guidance Association. Principles and practices of vocational guidance. *Occupations*, 1937, *15*, 772–778.

Nau, L. Why not family rehabilitation? *Journal of Rehabilitation*, 1973, *39*; 14–17, 42.

Neff, W. S. Problems of work evaluation. *Personnel and Guidance Journal*, 1966, *44*, 682–688.

Neff, W. S. (Ed.). *Rehabilitation psychology.* Washington, D.C.: American Psychological Association, 1971.

Neff, W. S. Rehabilitation and work. In W. S. Neff (Ed.), *Rehabilitation psychology* (proceedings of the National Conference on the Psychological Aspects of Disability, held at the Asilomar Conference Center, Monterey, California, October 25–28, 1970). Washington, D.C.: American Psychological Association, 1971a.

Neff, W. S. Assessing vocational potential. In H. Rusalem & D. Malikin (Eds.), *Contemporary vocational rehabilitation.* New York: University Press, 1976.

Nelson, N. *The services of workshops for the disabled in California.* Unpublished manuscript, February 1960.

Nelson, N. *Workshops for the handicapped in the United States: An historical and developmental perspective.* Springfield, IL: Charles C Thomas, 1971.

New York City Central Labor Council AFL-CIO (A final report by G. R. Waters, Sr., J. J. Gehan, & R. A. Barnette). *Job development project: Demonstration of a union-based selective placement program for disabled workers.* New York: Author, June 1970.

New York Life Insurance Company. *Making the most of your job interview.* New York: Author, n.d.

Nicholi, A. M., Jr. (Ed.). *The Harvard guide to modern psychiatry.* Cambridge: Belknap Press, Harvard University Press, 1978.

Nihara, D., Foster, R., Shellhass, M., & Leland, H. *AAMD adaptive behavior scale: Manual* (rev. ed.). Washington, D.C.: American Association on Mental Deficiency, 1974.

Noble, J. H. Actuarial system for weighting case closures. *Rehabilitation Records*, 1973, *9–10*, 34–37.

Noll, V. H. *Introduction to educational measurement* (2nd ed.). Boston: Houghton Mifflin, 1965.

Norris, W., Zeran, F. R., Hatch, R. N., & Engelkes, J. R. *The information service in guidance* (3rd ed.). Chicago: Rand McNally, 1972.

Northen, H. *Social work with groups*. New York: Columbia University Press, 1969.

Northwest Association of Rehabilitation Industries. *Words: Work-oriented rehabilitation dictionary and synonyms* (L. T. Cawood, Ed.). Seattle: Author, 1975.

NRA, *see* National Rehabilitation Association.

Nunnally, J. C., Jr. *Introduction to psychological measurements*. New York: McGraw-Hill, 1970.

Obermann, C. E. The rehabilitation counselor as a professional person. *Journal of Rehabilitation*, 1962, *28*(1), 37–38.

Obermann, C. E. *A history of vocational rehabilitation in America*. Minneapolis: T. S. Denison, 1965.

Oestreich, R. P. NRA wins in Florida! *NRA Newsletter*, May 1978, p. 1.

Ogg, E. *Rehabilitation counselor: Helper of the handicapped* (Public Affairs Pamphlet No. 392). New York: Public Affairs Committee, September 1966.

Ohlsen, M. M. *Group counseling* (2nd ed.). New York: Holt, Rinehart and Winston, 1977.

Olshansky, S. Why do disabled people want to work? *Social and Rehabilitation Record*, 1974, *1*(6), 21–24.

Olshansky, S., & Beach, D. Follow-up of clients placed into regular employment. *Rehabilitation Literature*, 1974, *35*(8), 237–238.

O'Morrow, G. S. *Therapeutic recreation: A helping profession*. Reston, VA.: Reston Publ. Co., 1976.

Ortale, L. *The challenge of placement as a real professional service*. Placement Training Institute. Stillwater: Oklahoma State University, The Clearing House, n.d.

Osipow, S. H. Vocational development problems of the handicapped. In H. Rusalem & D. Malikin (Eds.), *Contemporary vocational rehabilitation*. New York: New York University Press, 1976.

O'Toole, R., O'Toole, A., McMillan, R., & Lefton, M. *The Cleveland rehabilitation complex*. Cleveland: Vocational Guidance and Rehabilitation Services, 1972.

Overby, C. M. Will technology change work-living patterns? *Journal of Rehabilitation*, 1973, *39*(6), 18–19.

Overs, R. P. Scientific observation in work evaluation. In R. E. Hardy & J. G. Cull (Eds.), *Vocational evaluation for rehabilitation services*. Springfield, IL: Charles C Thomas, 1973.

Overs, R. P., O'Connor, E., & DeMarco, B. *Av-ocational activities for the handicapped: A handbook for avocational counseling*. Springfield, IL: Charles C Thomas, 1974.

Oxford English Dictionary. *The compact edition of the Oxford English dictionary*. Oxford: Clarendon Press, 1971.

Page, C. M., Apostal, R. A., & Lipp, L. H. A study of the decision-making process in judging vocational rehabilitation potential. *Rehabilitation Counseling Bulletin*, 1977, *21*(1), 42–46.

Parham, J. A case for consolidating a state human services department. *Social and Rehabilitation Record*, 1977, *4*(2), 24–27.

Parsons, F. *Choosing a vocation*. New York: Houghton Mifflin, 1909.

Parsons, T. Definitions of health and illness in the light of American values and social structure. In E. Jaco (Ed.), *Patients, physicians and illness* (2nd ed.). New York: Free Press, 1972.

Paterson, D. G., & Darley, J. G. *Men, women, and jobs*. Minneapolis: University of Minnesota Press, 1936.

Patterson, C. H. Counselor or coordinator? *Journal of Rehabilitation*, 1957, *23*(5), 13–15.

Patterson, C. H. Is the team concept obsolete? *Journal of Rehabilitation*, 1959, *25*(2); 9–10, 27–28.

Patterson, C. H. (Ed.). *Readings in rehabilitation counseling*. Champaign, IL: Stipes, 1960.

Patterson, C. H. Counseling: Self-clarification and the helping relationship. In H. Borow (Ed.), *Man in a world at work*. Boston: Houghton Mifflin, 1964.

Patterson, C. H. Specialization in rehabilitation counseling. In W. Holbert (Ed.), *Proceedings of a conference on vocational rehabilitation counselor specialization: Cause and effects*. Atlanta, April 29–30, 1965, pp. 11–20.

Patterson, C. H. Specialization in rehabilitation counseling. *Rehabilitation Counseling Bulletin*, 1967, *10*(4), 147–154.

Patterson, C. H. *Theories of counseling and psychotherapy* (2nd ed.). New York: Harper & Row, 1973.

Pattison, H. A. (Ed.). *The handicapped and their rehabilitation*. Springfield, IL: Charles C Thomas, 1957.

Paulson, F. *A system of ethics*. New York: Charles Scribner's Sons, 1899.

Pavlov, I. P. *Conditioned reflexes* (G. V. Anrys, trans.). New York: Liveright, 1927.

Pepper, F. *The value of a pre-admission interview in the selection of students in a graduate program in rehabilitation counseling*. Unpublished doctoral dissertation, University of California-Berkeley, 1976.

Perlman, L. G. *Job placement study*. Washington,

D.C.: National Industries for the Severely Handicapped, 1978.

Perls, F. S. *The gestalt approach and eye witness to therapy*. Palo Alto: Science and Behavior Books, 1973.

Perls, F. S., Goodman, P., & Hefferline, R. F. *Gestalt therapy—Excitement and growth in human personality*. New York: Julian, 1951.

Perls, F. S., Hefferline, R. F., & Goodman, P. *Gestalt therapy*. New York: Dell, 1965.

Pfeiffer, J. W., & Pfeiffer, J. A. A gestalt primer. In J. E. Jones & J. W. Pfeiffer (Eds.), *The 1975 annual handbook for group facilitators*. La Jolla, CA: University Publishers, 1975.

Pflueger, S. S. *Independent living*. Washington, D.C.: Institute for Research Utilization, 1977.

Piccari, J. Vocational evaluation standards. *Vocational Evaluation and Work Adjustment Bulletin*, 1976, *9*(1), 47–51.

Pintner, R., Eisenson, J., & Stanton, M. *The psychology of the physically handicapped*. New York: F. S. Crofts, 1941.

Pomeroy, J. *Recreation for the physically handicapped*. New York: Macmillan, 1964.

Porter, T. L., & Settles, R. B. *Post-entry training programs for rehabilitation counselors*. Preliminary Report of Workshop Proceedings, Atlanta, April 24–26, 1968.

Pratt, J. H. Principles of class treatment and their application to various chronic diseases. *Hospital Social Service*, 1922, *6*, 401.

Pruitt, W. A. Work adjustment: A report on a national opinion study. *Vocational Evaluation and Work Adjustment Bulletin*, 1973, *6*(2), 19–28.

Pruitt, W. A., & Longfellow, R. E. Work evaluation: The medium and the message—guest editorial. *Journal of Rehabilitation*, 1970, *36*(1), 8–9.

Rathbone, J. L., & Lucas, C. *Recreation in total rehabilitation*. Springfield, IL: Charles C Thomas, 1970.

Raush, H. L., & Raush, C. L. *The halfway house movement: A search for sanity*. New York: Meredith Corp., 1968.

Reagles, K. W. *A handbook for follow-up in the human services*. New York: ICD Rehabilitation and Research Center, 1979.

Reagles, K. W., Katz, S., & Wright, G. N. *Rehabilitation in Israel*. Washington, D.C.: B'nai B'rith, 1974.

Reagles, K. W., & Wright, G. N. Economic impact. *Journal of Rehabilitation*, 1972, *38*(1), 25.

Reagles, K. W., Wright, G. N., & Butler, A. J. *A scale of rehabilitation gain for clients of an expanded vocational rehabilitation program*. Madison: University of Wisconsin, Regional Rehabilitation Research Institute, 1970.

Reagles, K. W., Wright, G. N., & Butler, A. J. *Cor-*

relates of client satisfaction in an expanded vocational rehabilitation program. Madison: University of Wisconsin, Regional Rehabilitation Research Institute, 1970a.

Reagles, K. W., Wright, G. N., & Butler, A. J. Toward a new criterion on vocational success. *Rehabilitation Counseling Bulletin*, 1972, *15*(4), 233–241.

Reagles, K. W., Wright, G. N., & Thomas, K. R. Development of a scale of client satisfaction for clients receiving vocational rehabilitation counseling services. *Rehabilitation Research and Practice Review*, Special Spring Issue 1972, *3*(2), 15–22.

Rehabilitation International. *Compendium on the activities of world organizations interested in the handicapped, 1974*. New York: Author, 1974.

Rehabilitation International. *Barrier-free design*. (Report of the United Nations Expert Group Meeting in Barrier-Free Design held June 3–8, 1974 at the United Nations Secretariat, N.Y.) New York: Author, June 1975.

Reid, W. Inter-organizational coordination in social welfare: A theoretical approach to an analysis and intervention. In R. Kramer & H. Sprecht (Eds.), *Readings in community organization practice*. Englewood Cliffs, NJ: Prentice-Hall, 1969.

Rice, B. D. Client participation in evaluation. In S. H. Crow (Ed.), *Positions on the practice of vocational evaluation*. Washington, D.C.: Vocational Evaluation and Work Adjustment Association, 1975.

Richardson, H. D. Preparation for counseling as a profession. *Counselor Education and Supervision*, 1968, *7*(2), 124–131.

Richmond, C. Therapeutic housing. *Rehabilitation Record*, November-December 1972, pp. 8–13.

Riscalla, L. M. Records—A legal responsibility. *Journal of Rehabilitation*, 1974, *40*(1), 12–14.

Ritter, B. Eliminating excessive fears of the environment through contact desensitization. In J. Krumboltz & C. Thoreson (Eds.), *Behavioral Counseling: Cases and techniques*. New York: Holt, Rinehart and Winston, 1969.

Riviere, M. *Rehabilitation of the handicapped: A bibliography 1940–1946*. (Vols. I, II). New York: National Council on Rehabilitation, 1949.

Rizzo, F., & Schworles, T. R. *Mainstreaming the severely disabled student into the community college system: The role of rehabilitation engineering*. Washington, D.C.: U.S. Department of Health, Education, and Welfare, Rehabilitation Services Administration, December 4, 1975.

Robinault, I. P. *Sex, Society, and the Disabled*. Hagerstown, MD: Harper & Row, 1978.

Robinault, I. P. (Ed.). *Functional aids for the mul-*

tiply handicapped. Hagerstown, MD: Harper & Row, 1973.

Robinault, I. P., & Weisinger, M. *Mobilization of community resources: A multi-facet-model for rehabilitation of post-hospitalized mentally ill* (2nd ed.). New York: Research Utilization Laboratory, 1978.

Roe, A. Early determinants of vocational choice. *Journal of Counseling Psychology*, 1957, *4*, 212–217.

Roessler, R., & Bolton, B. *Psychosocial adjustment to disability*. Baltimore: University Park Press, 1978.

Roessler, R., & Mack, G. *Strategies for interagency linkages: A literature review*. Hot Springs: Arkansas Rehabilitation Research and Training Center, 1975.

Roessler, R., & Mack, G. Interagency links: Hang together or hang separately? *American Rehabilitation*, 1977, *2*(3), 30–31.

Rogers, C. R. *Counseling and psychotherapy: Newer concepts in practice*. Boston: Houghton-Mifflin, 1942.

Rogers, C. R. *Client-centered therapy*. Boston: Houghton Mifflin, 1951.

Rogers, C. R. *On becoming a person: A therapist's view of psychotherapy*. Boston: Houghton Mifflin, 1961.

Rose, E. F., & Shay, H. F. The school unit counselor. In J. G. Cull & R. E. Hardy (Eds.), *Vocational rehabilitation: Profession and process*. Springfield, IL: Charles C Thomas, 1972.

Rosenberg, B. The work sample approach to vocational evaluation. In R. E. Hardy & J. G. Cull (Eds.), *Vocational evaluation for rehabilitation services*. Springfield, IL: Charles C Thomas, 1973.

Rosenberg, C. *Assistive devices for the handicapped*. Minneapolis: American Rehabilitation Foundation, 1968.

Rosenstack, F., & Kutner, B. Alienation and family crisis. *Sociological Quarterly*, 1967, Summer, pp. 397–405.

Ross, D. Conceptual model of a professional evaluation. In R. Pacinelli (Ed.), *Research utilization in rehabilitation facilities*. Washington, D.C.: International Association of Rehabilitation Facilities, 1971.

Ross, E. E. *Encyclopedia of job descriptions in manufacturing*. Milwaukee, WI: Sextant Systems, 1969.

Ross, E. M. The coordination of rehabilitation services. *Journal of Applied Rehabilitation Counseling*, 1976, 7(1), 22–26.

Ross, E. M. *Workmen's compensation rehabilitation: A study of the rehabilitation of injured workers in the United States and member jurisdictions of the International Association of Industrial Accident Boards and Commission*. Des Moines, IA: Rehabilitation Committee, September 1976a.

Rosse, A. A., Marra, J. L., & Novis, F. W. The disability adjudicator: Identification of duties and qualifications. *Journal of Rehabilitation*, 1962, *28*(2), 29–30.

Roupe, D. S. Volunteerism: Reawakening to an age-old truth. *Rehabilitation Record*, March-April 1972, pp. 1–6.

Rubin, S. E. A national rehabilitation program evaluation research and training effort: Some results and implications. *Journal of Rehabilitation*, 1977, *43*(2), 28–31.

Rubin, S. E., & Roessler, R. T. *Foundations of the vocational rehabilitation process*. Baltimore: University Park Press, 1978.

Rubin, S. E., & Roessler, R. T. Diagnostic and planning guidelines for the vocational rehabilitation process. *Rehabilitation Literature*, 1979, *40*(2), 34–39.

Rule, W. R. Rehabilitation uses of Adlerian life style counseling. *Rehabilitation Counseling Bulletin*, 1978, *21*(4), 306–316.

Rusalem, H. Penetrating the narrowing circle: A review of the literature concerning the vocational rehabilitation of homebound persons. *Rehabilitation Literature*, 1967, *28*(7), 202–217.

Rusalem, H., & Baxt, R. *Delivering rehabilitation services*. Washington, D.C.: U.S. Department of Health, Education, and Welfare, Social and Rehabilitation Service, 1970.

Rusalem, H., & Cohen, M. The interdependence of public and voluntary rehabilitation agencies in historic perspective. *Journal of Rehabilitation*, 1970, *36*(5), 34–36.

Rusalem, H., & Cohen, M. Alternatives to homebound rehabilitation. In K. Mallik, S. Yuspeh, & J. Mueller (Eds.), *Comprehensive vocational rehabilitation for severely disabled persons*. Washington, D.C.: George Washington University Medical Center, Job Development Laboratory, 1975.

Rusalem, H., & Malikin, D. (Eds.). *Contemporary vocational rehabilitation*. New York: New York University Press, 1976.

Rusk, H. A. *A world to care for*. New York: Random House, 1977.

Rusk, H. A. *Rehabilitation medicine* (4th ed.) (with 35 collaborators, with the editorial assistance of Eugene J. Taylor). St. Louis: Mosby, 1977a.

Rusk, H. A., & Taylor, E. J. *New hope for the handicapped: The rehabilitation of the disabled from bed to job*. New York: Harper, 1949.

Rutherford, T. V. Values of information, referral, and follow-up services: To the client; to agencies; and to the community. *Rehabilitation Literature*, 1968, *29*(12), 363–364.

Safilios-Rothschild, C. *The sociology and social psychology of disability and rehabilitation.* New York: Random House, 1970.

Sales, A. The time has come. *Journal of Rehabilitation,* 1977, *43*(3), 2.

Salhoot, J. T. The use of two group methods with severely disabled persons. In R. E. Hardy & J. G. Cull (Eds.), *Group counseling and therapy techniques in special settings.* Springfield, IL: Charles C Thomas, 1974.

Salomone, P. R., & Rubin, D. C. Job placement: New tactics for securing job leads. *Rehabilitation Counseling Bulletin,* 1979, *22*(4), 338–346.

Samler, J. The counselor in our time. In G. N. Wright (Ed.), *Madison lectures on vocational rehabilitation.* Madison: University of Wisconsin, 1966.

Samuelson, C. O. (Ed.). *The team approach in the placement of the disabled client.* Salt Lake City: University of Utah Medical Center, 1967.

Sands, H., & Radin, J. *The mentally disabled rehabilitant: Post employment services* (2nd ed.). Washington, D.C.: U.S. Department of Health, Education, and Welfare, Office of Human Development, Rehabilitation Services Administration, 1979.

Sankovsky, R. Adjustment services in rehabilitation. *Journal of Rehabilitation,* 1971, *37*(4), 8–10.

Sankovsky, R., & Knight, M. Media workshops in rehabilitation. *Rehabilitation Records,* 1971, *12*(5), 6–8.

Sarason, I. G., & Ganzer, V. J. *Modeling: An approach to the rehabilitation of juvenile offenders.* U.S. Department of Health, Education, and Welfare, Social Rehabilitation Service, June 1971.

Sather, W. S., Wright, G. N., & Butler, A. J. *An instrument for the measurement of counselor orientation.* Madison: University of Wisconsin, Regional Rehabilitation Research Institute, 1968.

Satir, V. *Peoplemaking.* Palo Alto: Science and Behavior Books, 1972.

Sawyer, G. P. Vocational rehabilitation and the industrially injured. In *Proceedings of National Training Institute: The industrially injured.* Washington, D.C.: U.S. Department of Health, Education, and Welfare, Rehabilitation Services Administration, October 1976.

Scherz, F. H. Theory and practice of family therapy. In R. W. Nie and R. H. Nie (Eds.), *Theories of social casework.* Chicago: University of Chicago Press, 1970.

Schneider, E. P. Human sexuality and the handicapped. *Personnel and Guidance Journal,* 1976, *54*(7), 378–380.

Scorzelli, J. F. Situation ethics in rehabilitation counseling. *American Archives of Rehabilitation Therapy,* 1977, *25*(3), 7–8.

Scott, R. B., & Maxwell, L. Contractual counseling sets goals and duties. *Research Review,* 1975, *2*(3), 4–5.

Selby, D. Accountability: Why and how: Challenge and responsibility of sheltered workshops and other rehabilitation facilities today. *Journal of Rehabilitation,* 1977, *43*(2), 25–27.

Seligman, M. (Ed.). *Group counseling and group psychotherapy with rehabilitation clients.* Springfield, IL: Charles C Thomas, 1977.

Shaftel, F. R., & Shaftel, G. *Role-playing for social values: Decision-making in the social studies.* Englewood Cliffs, NJ: Prentice-Hall, 1967.

Sha'ked, A. (Ed.). *Sexuality and disability.* New York: Human Sciences Press, Spring 1978, *1*(1).

Sha'ked, A., Bruyere, S. M., & Wright, G. N. *The assessment of human service needs of persons with epilepsy and cerebral palsy.* Madison: University of Wisconsin, Regional Rehabilitation Research Institute, 1975.

Shartle, C. *Occupational information* (1st ed.). Englewood Cliffs, NJ: Prentice-Hall, 1946.

Shartle, C. *Occupational information: Its development and application* (3rd ed.). Englewood Cliffs, NJ: Prentice-Hall, 1959.

Shaw, K. J. Career development: Client responsibility in rehabilitation planning. *Journal of Rehabilitation,* 1976, *42*(5); 30–33, 39.

Sheets, B. V. *Helping the patient with cerebral palsy to communicate.* New York: United Cerebral Palsy Associations, October 1973.

Shellhase, C. A., & Shellhase, F. E. Role of the family in rehabilitation. *Social Casework,* 1972, *53*, 544–550.

Shoenfeld, E. Deinstitutionalization/Community alternatives. In K. Mallik, S. Yuspeh, & J. Mueller (Eds.), *Comprehensive vocational rehabilitation for severely disabled persons.* Washington, D.C.: George Washington University Medical Center, Job Development Laboratory, 1975.

Shontz, F. C. *The psychological aspects of physical illness and disability.* New York: Macmillan, 1975.

Shworles, T. R. The community college system: Resource for rehabilitation. *American Rehabilitation,* 1976, *1*(3), 8–12.

Shworles, T. R., & Tamagna, I. G. *Development of modern vocational objectives for severely disabled homebound persons: Remote computer programming, microfilm equipment operations, and data entry processes.* Washington, D.C.: George Washington University, Rehabilitation Research and Training Center, 1973.

Sieder, V. M. *The rehabilitation agency and community work: A source book for professional training.* Waltham, MA: Brandeis University, The Florence Heller Graduate School for Advanced Studies in Social Welfare, 1966.

Sieder, V. M. Volunteers. In R. Morris (Ed.), *Encyclopedia of Social Work* (Vol. 1). New York: National Association of Social Workers, 1971.

Siller, J. A., Chipman, A., Ferguson, L., & Vann, D. H. *Studies in reaction to disability. XI: Attitudes of the nondisabled toward the physically disabled.* New York: New York University, School of Education, 1967.

Sindberg, R. M., Roberts, A. F., & Pfeifer, E. J. The usefulness of psychological evaluations to vocational rehabilitation counselors. *Rehabilitation Literature*, 1968, *29*, 290–294.

Sinick, D. *Placement training handbook.* Washington, D.C.: U.S. Department of Health, Education, and Welfare, Office of Vocational Rehabilitation, August 1962.

Sinick, D. *Occupational information and guidance.* Boston: Houghton Mifflin, 1970.

Sinick, D. Rehabilitation counselors on the move. *Personnel and Guidance Journal*, 1973, *52*(3), 167–170.

Sinick, D. Vocational counseling trends in rehabilitation settings. *Journal of Rehabilitation*, 1977, *43*(3); 19–21, 35.

Sinick, D. Can vocational counselors change society? *Vocational Guidance Quarterly*, 1977a, *25*(3); 245–251.

Sink, J. M., & Porter, T. L. Convergence and divergence in rehabilitation counseling and vocational evaluation. *Journal of Applied Rehabilitation Counseling*, 1978, *9*(1), 5–20.

Skinner, B. F. *The behavior of organisms.* New York: Appleton-Century-Crofts, 1938.

Skinner, B. F. *Science and human behavior.* New York: Macmillan, 1953.

Smedley, L. Workmen's compensation—A barrier to rehabilitation? In *Proceedings of National Training Institute: The industrially injured.* Washington, D.C.: U.S. Department of Health, Education, and Welfare, Rehabilitation Services Administration, October 1976.

Smith, B. C. *Instructional materials in independent living.* Menomonie: University of Wisconsin-Stout, Materials Development Center, October 1978.

Smits, S. J. The role and function of the rehabilitation counselor serving the severely disabled. In W. M. Jenkins, R. M. Anderson, & W. L. Dietrich (Eds.), *Rehabilitation of the severely disabled.* Dubuque, IA: Kendall-Hunt, 1976.

Soden, W. H. (Ed.). *Rehabilitation of the handicapped: A survey of means and methods.* New York: Ronald Press, 1949.

Sohoni, N. K. Social barriers and community attitudes concerning the disabled. *International Rehabilitation Review*, January 1977, p. 4.

Spaniol, L. *A model for program evaluation in rehabilitation.* Madison: University of Wisconsin, Regional Rehabilitation Research Institute, 1975.

Springer, D. Remunerative homework for the homebound chronically ill: Observations on the meaning of work. *Personnel and Guidance Journal*, September 1961, pp. 51–57.

State of Iowa, Department of Public Instruction, Rehabilitation Education and Service Branch. *Individual analysis: Individual rehabilitation program.* Des Moines, IA: Author, November 1975.

State of New Jersey Rehabilitation Commission. *The development and administration of an independent living rehabilitation program, 1962–1967.* Washington, D.C.: U.S. Department of Health, Education, and Welfare, Vocational Rehabilitation Administration, 1967.

State of New Mexico Department of Education, Division of Rehabilitation. *Removing architectural barriers.* Santa Fe, NM: Author, 1975.

Steger, J. M. A multidisciplinary model for undergraduate education in rehabilitation. *Rehabilitation Counseling Bulletin*, 1974, *18*, 12–20.

Stein, T. A., & Sessoms, H. D. (Eds.). *Recreation and special populations* (2nd ed.). Boston: Holbrook Press, 1977.

Stolov, W. C., & Clowers, M. R. (Eds.). *Handbook of severe disability.* Washington, D.C.: U.S. Government Printing Office, 1980.

Stone, J. B. The rehabilitation counselor as a client advocate. *Journal of Applied Rehabilitation Counseling*, 1971, *2*(1), 46–54.

Stone, J. B. Counseling and rehabilitation counseling: Differences in emphasis. In B. Bolton & M. E. Jaques (Eds.), *Rehabilitation counseling: Theory and practice.* Baltimore: University Park Press, 1978.

Straus, R. Social change and the rehabilitation concept. In M. B. Sussman (Ed.), *Sociology and rehabilitation.* Washington, D.C.: American Sociological Association, 1965.

Strickland, B. Philosophy-theory-practice continuum: A point of view. *Counselor Education and Supervision*, 1969, *8*(3), 165–175.

Stubbins, J. (Ed.). *Social and psychological aspects of disability.* Baltimore: University Park Press, 1977.

Sullivan, O. M., & Snortum, K. O. *Disabled persons: Their education and rehabilitation.* New York: Century, 1926.

Super, D. E. *The dynamics of vocational adjustment.* New York: Harper, 1942.

Super, D. E. A theory of vocational development. *American Psychologist*, 1953, *8*, 185–190.

Super, D. E., & Crites, J. O. *Appraising vocational fitness by means of psychological tests* (rev. ed.). New York: Harper & Row, 1962.

Sussman, M. B. (Ed.). *Sociology and rehabilitation*. Washington, D.C.: American Sociological Association, 1965.

Sussman, M. B., Haug, M. R., & Krupnick, G. A. *Professional associations and memberships in rehabilitation counseling*. Cleveland: Western Reserve University, Department of Sociology and Anthropology, 1965.

Switzer, M. E. Special education and vocational rehabilitation. In M. E. Frampton & E. D. Gall (Eds.), *Special education for the exceptional* (Vol. 1, *Introduction and problems*). Boston: Porter Sargent, 1955.

Switzer, M. E. Manpower needs in the helping services: The federal government and the helping services. From *Proceedings of the Conference on Education at the Undergraduate Level for the Helping Services*, Durham, NH: New England Board of Higher Education, 1967.

Taylor, F. W. *The principles of scientific management*. New York: Harper & Row, 1911.

Taylor, R. Cooperative and coordinated programming for the vocational education and rehabilitation of the disadvantaged. In R. Taylor & B. Thomason (Eds.), *Vocational education and rehabilitation of the disabled and disadvantaged*. Gainesville: University of Florida, 1970.

Taylor, R. D., Sales, A., & Lavender, H. *Rehabilitation counselor education—A survey of counseling practice*. Gainesville: University of Florida, College of Health Related Professions, Department of Rehabilitation Counseling, 1971.

Terman, L. M. *Genetic studies of genius*. Stanford: Stanford University Press, 1925.

Thomas, G. P., & Ezell, B. The contract as a counseling technique. *Personnel and Guidance Journal*, 1972, *51*(1), 27–31.

Thomas, K. R., Reagles, K. W., Wright, G. N., & Dellario, D. Patterns of rehabilitation service as a function of age and disability. *Industrial Gerontology*, 1974, New Series, *1*(3), 12–23.

Thomason, B. *Counseling the disabled within the total configuration of marital, sexual, and family behavior*. Paper presented before the XIIIth World Congress of Rehabilitation International, Tel Aviv, Israel, June 1976.

Thomason, B., & Barrett, A. M. (Eds.). *Casework performance in vocational rehabilitation* (GTP Bulletin No. 1—Rehabilitation Service Series No. 505). Washington, D.C.: U.S. Department of Health, Education, and Welfare, Office of Vocational Rehabilitation, May 1959.

Thomason, B., & Barrett, A. M. (Eds.). *The placement process in vocational rehabilitation counseling* (compiled from proceedings of Guidance, Training, and Placement workshops). Washington, D.C.: U.S. Department of Health, Educa-tion, and Welfare, Office of Vocational Rehabilitation, 1960.

Thoreson, C., & Hosford, R. Behavioral approaches to counseling. In *Behavior modification in education* (the 72nd yearbook of the National Society for the Study of Education, Part I). Chicago: University of Chicago Press, 1973.

Thorndike, R. L., & Hagen, E. P. *Measurement and evaluation in psychology and education* (4th ed.). New York: John Wiley, 1977.

Thornock, M., Hutchins, T. K., Meyer, S., Kenyon, A., & Williams, M. Attendant care needs of the physically disabled: Institutional perspectives. *Rehabilitation Literature*, 1978, *39*(5), 147–153.

Tiedeman, D. V., & O'Hara, R. P. *Career development: Choice and adjustment*. New York: College Entrance Examination Board, 1963.

Tinsley, H. E. A., & Gaughan, S. M. A cross-sectional analysis of the impact of rehabilitation counseling. *Rehabilitation Counseling Bulletin*, 1975, *18*(3), 147–153.

Tolbert, E. L. *Counseling for career development*. Boston: Houghton Mifflin, 1974.

Towne, A. Homecraft: Source of homebound employment. *Rehabilitation Record*, September-October 1972, pp. 1–5.

Towne, A. Vocational rehabilitation and the work ethic. *Rehabilitation Record*, January-February, 1972a, pp. 7–10.

Trantow, D. J. An introduction to evaluation: Program effectiveness and community needs. *Rehabilitation Literature*, 1970, *31*(1), 2–9.

Tseng, M. S., & Parker, L. E. Toward a placement system empirically established through criterion-group method: Self-employment for the severely handicapped. *Rehabilitation Literature*, 1976, *37*(5), 140–144.

Tyler, L. E. Work and individual differences. In H. Borow (Ed.), *Man in a world at work*. Boston: Houghton Mifflin, 1964.

United Cerebral Palsy Association. *A bill of rights for the handicapped*. New York: Author, May 1973.

United Nations. *Barrier-free design*. New York: Author, 1975.

United Nations, Department of Economic and Social Affairs. *Social barriers to the integration of disabled persons into community life* (report of an expert group meeting, Geneva, June 28–July 5, 1976). New York: Author, 1977.

U.S. Childrens Bureau. *Handbook for recreation*. Detroit: Gale, 1976.

U.S. Civil Service Commission. *A guide for the placement of the physically impaired* (4th ed.). Washington, D.C.: U.S. Government Printing Office, 1947.

U.S. Civil Service Commission. *Employment of handicapped individuals including disabled vet-*

erans in the federal government. Washington, D.C.: Author, 1975.

U.S. Department of Commerce, Bureau of the Census. 1970 census of population: Classified index of industries and occupations. Washington, D.C.: U.S. Government Printing Office, 1971.

U.S. Department of Health, Education, and Welfare, Architectural and Transportation Barriers Compliance Board. Freedom of choice—Report to the President and Congress on Housing Needs of Handicapped Individuals (Vol. 2). Washington, D.C.: Author, October 1975.

U.S. Department of Health, Education, and Welfare, Office of Handicapped Individuals. A summary of selected legislation relating to the handicapped: 1977–1978. Washington, D.C.: U.S. Government Printing Office, May 1979.

U.S. Department of Health, Education, and Welfare, Office of Human Development. Program regulation guide. Washington, D.C.: Author, February 10, 1976.

U.S. Department of Health, Education, and Welfare, Office of the Secretary. Independent living for handicapped individuals: Sources of information. Washington, D.C.: Author, October 1978.

U.S. Department of Health, Education, and Welfare, Office of Vocational Rehabilitation. Small business enterprises for the severely handicapped: A catalog of small business experiences of the homebound and severely handicapped in the state-federal vocational rehabilitation program. Washington, D.C.: Author, 1955.

U.S. Department of Health, Education, and Welfare, Rehabilitation Services Administration. Design for all Americans (a report of the National Commission on Architectural Barriers to Rehabilitation of the Handicapped). Washington, D.C.: Author, 1967.

U.S. Department of Health, Education, and Welfare, Rehabilitation Services Administration. State vocational rehabilitation agency: Program data: Fiscal year 1976. Washington, D.C.: Author, 1976.

U.S. Department of Health, Education, and Welfare, Rehabilitation Services Administration. Program information for rehabilitation training grant program. Washington, D.C.: Author, January 1977.

U.S. Department of Health, Education, and Welfare, Rehabilitation Services Administration. Ready reference guide. Washington, D.C.: U.S. Government Printing Office, 1978.

U.S. Department of Health, Education, and Welfare, Social and Rehabilitation Service. The goal is mobility: Background information on environmental barriers and transportation. Washington, D.C.: Author, 1969.

U.S. Department of Health, Education, and Welfare, Social and Rehabilitation Service, Rehabilitation Services Administration. 50 years of vocational rehabilitation in the U.S.A., 1920–1970. Washington, D.C.: Author, 1970.

U.S. Department of Health, Education, and Welfare, Social Security Administration, Office of Research and Statistics (reported by L. A. Manus). The effects of disability on lifetime earnings. Washington, D.C.: Author, 1978.

U.S. Department of Housing and Urban Development, Office of Policy Development and Research, Study Report by Peoples Housing Inc. Barrier-free communities. Washington, D.C.: U.S. Government Printing Office, 1978.

U.S. Department of Labor. Placing handicapped applicants: An employment service handbook. Washington, D.C.: U.S. Government Printing Office, 1976.

U.S. Department of Labor, Bureau of Labor Statistics. Toward matching personal and job characteristics. Occupational Outlook Quarterly, 1975, 19(1), 2–18.

U.S. Department of Labor, Bureau of Labor Statistics. Employment outlook in counseling occupations. Washington, D.C.: Author, 1976.

U.S. Department of Labor, Bureau of Labor Statistics. Occupational outlook handbook: 1976–77 edition. Washington, D.C.: Author, 1976a.

U.S. Department of Labor, Bureau of Labor Statistics. Occupational outlook handbook: 1980–81 edition. Washington, D.C.: Author, 1980.

U.S. Department of Labor, Employment and Training Administration. Dictionary of occupational titles (4th ed.). Washington, D.C.: Author, 1977.

U.S. Department of Labor, Employment and Training Administration, Office of Information. Program fact sheet. Washington, D.C.: Author, September 1977a.

U.S. Department of Labor, Employment and Training Administration. Guide for occupational exploration. Washington, D.C.: Author, 1979.

U.S. Department of Labor, Employment Standards Administration. Employment of the handicapped: Affirmative action obligations of contractors and sub-contractors. Federal Register, 1974, 39(113), 20566–20571.

U.S. Department of Labor, Employment Standards Administration. Sheltered workshop study: A nationwide report on sheltered workshops and their employment of handicapped individuals. Washington, D.C.: Author, 1977.

U.S. Department of Labor, Manpower Administration. Manual for use of the U.S.E.S.: General aptitude test battery. Washington, D.C.: U.S. Government Printing Office, 1970.

U.S. Department of Labor, Manpower Administration. *A handbook for job restructuring.* Washington, D.C.: Author, 1970a.

U.S. Department of Labor, Manpower Administration. *Handbook for analyzing jobs.* Washington, D.C.: U.S. Government Printing Office, 1972.

U.S. Department of Labor, Manpower Administration. *Task analysis inventories: A method for collecting job information.* Washington, D.C.: U.S. Government Printing Office, 1973.

U.S. DOL, *see* U.S. Department of Labor.

U.S. Executive Office of the President, Office of Management and Budget. *Standard industrial classification manual.* Washington, D.C.: Author, 1972.

U.S. Federal Board for Vocational Education. *Industrial rehabilitation—A statement of policies to be observed in the administration of the Industrial Rehabilitation Act* (Bulletin No. 57, Industrial Rehabilitation Series No. 1). Washington, D.C.: September 1920.

U.S. Federal Board for Vocational Education. Problems of the vocational adjustment and counseling of the disabled soldier and sailor under the Vocational Rehabilitation Act. *The Vocational Summary,* 1920a, *2*(9).

U.S. Federal Board for Vocational Education. *Industrial rehabilitation—General administration and case procedure* (Bulletin No. 64, Industrial Rehabilitation Series No. 2). Washington, D.C.: U.S. Government Printing Office, March 1921.

U.S. Federal Board for Vocational Education. *Bibliography on vocational guidance: A selected list of vocational guidance references for teachers* (Bulletin No. 66, Trade and Industrial Series No. 19). Washington, D.C.: U.S. Government Printing Office, June 1921a.

U.S. Federal Board for Vocational Education. *Industrial rehabilitation: Services of advisement and cooperation* (Bulletin No. 70, Industrial Rehabilitation Series No. 3). Washington, D.C.: U.S. Government Printing Office, October 1921b.

U.S. Federal Board for Vocational Education. *Vocational rehabilitation: Its purposes, scope and methods with illustrative cases.* (Bulletin No. 80, Vocational Rehabilitation Series No. 7). Washington, D.C.: U.S. Government Printing Office, 1923.

U.S. Federal Board for Vocational Education. *A study of rehabilitated persons: A statistical analysis of the rehabilitation of 6391 disabled persons.* (Bulletin No. 132, Civilian Vocational Rehabilitation Series No. 16). Washington, D.C.: U.S. Government Printing Office, 1928.

U.S. Federal Security Agency, Office of Vocational Rehabilitation. *Efficiency of the impaired worker.* Washington, D.C.: U.S. Government Printing Office, 1946.

U.S. GTP, *see* U.S. Rehabilitation Institute Publications.

U.S. HEW, *see* U.S. Department of Health, Education, and Welfare.

U.S. HEW, OVR, *see* U.S. Department of Health, Education, and Welfare, Office of Vocational Rehabilitation.

U.S. HEW, RSA, *see* U.S. Department of Health, Education, and Welfare, Rehabilitation Services Administration.

U.S. HEW, SRS, *see* U.S. Department of Health, Education, and Welfare, Social and Rehabilitation Service.

U.S. HEW, VRA, *see* U.S. Department of Health, Education, and Welfare, Vocational Rehabilitation Administration.

U.S. IRI, *see* U.S. Rehabilitation Institute Publications.

U.S. IRS, *see* U.S. Rehabilitation Institute Publications.

U.S. Rehabilitation Institute Publications

Listed in this section of the References are publications based on institutes and workshops sponsored by the federal rehabilitation agency. These publications are cited in the text as follows: U.S. GTP (Guidance, Training, and Placement Workshop); U.S. IRS (Institute on Rehabilitation Services); U.S. IRI (Institute on Rehabilitation Issues).

General references continue on page 786.

GUIDANCE, TRAINING, AND PLACEMENT WORKSHOP (U.S. GTP) 1947–1962

U.S. GTP, 1947

U.S. Federal Security Agency, Office of Vocational Rehabilitation. *First workshop on training and placement services: Preparation of case work manual, psychological testing and interviewing, standards of case work performance.* Washington, D.C.: Author, 1947.

U.S. GTP, 1949
U.S. Federal Security Agency, Office of Vocational Rehabilitation. *Second workshop on case work standards: Occupational and job information, psychological services, severely disabled.* Washington, D.C.: Author, 1949.

U.S. GTP, 1950
U.S. Federal Security Agency, Office of Vocational Rehabilitation. *Third annual workshop on methods and standards for guidance, training and placement: Developments, case recording, standards, occupational information, psychological services, rehabilitation center, severely disabled, training.* Washington, D.C.: Author, April 1950.

U.S. GTP, 1951
U.S. Federal Security Agency, Office of Vocational Rehabilitation. *Fourth annual workshop on methods and standards for guidance, training and placement: Developments, case work standards, recording, occupational information, psychological services, severely disabled, training.* Washington, D.C.: Author, April 1951.

U.S. GTP, 1951a
U.S. Federal Security Agency, Office of Vocational Rehabilitation. *Fourth annual workshop on methods and standards for guidance, training and placement: Handbook of occupational information materials.* Washington, D.C.: Author, April 1951.

U.S. GTP, 1951b
U.S. Federal Security Agency, Office of Vocational Rehabilitation. *Fourth annual workshop on methods and standards for guidance, training and placement: Employment of severely disabled persons in other than small business enterprises.* Washington, D.C.: Author, 1951.

U.S. GTP, 1951c
U.S. Federal Security Agency, Office of Vocational Rehabilitation. *Fourth annual workshop on guidance, training and placement: Objectives of counseling the disabled for job readiness.* Washington, D.C.: Author, April 1951.

U.S. GTP, 1952
U.S. Federal Security Agency, Office of Vocational Rehabilitation. *Fifth annual workshop on guidance, training and placement—Proceedings, Part I: Total evaluation of the client.* Washington, D.C.: Author, April 1952.

U.S. GTP, 1952a
U.S. Federal Security Agency, Office of Vocational Rehabilitation. *Fifth annual workshop on guidance, training and placement—Proceedings, Part II: Rehabilitation of the mentally retarded and emotionally disturbed.* Washington, D.C.: Author, April 1952.

U.S. GTP, 1952b
U.S. Federal Security Agency, Office of Vocational Rehabilitation. *Fifth annual workshop on guidance, training and placement—Proceedings, Part III: Rehabilitation programs for the homebound.* Washington, D.C.: Author, 1952.

U.S. GTP, 1953
U.S. Department of Health, Education, and Welfare, Office of Vocational Rehabilitation. *Sixth annual workshop on guidance, training and placement—Proceedings, Part I: Diagnostic guides, team approach, sheltered workshops, casework supervision.* Washington, D.C.: Author, June 1953.

U.S. GTP, 1953a
U.S. Department of Health, Education, and Welfare, Office of Vocational Rehabilitation. *Sixth annual workshop on guidance, training and placement—Proceedings, Part II: Community organization, small business enterprises, marketing, rural projects.* Washington, D.C.: Author, June 1953.

U.S. GTP, 1953b
U.S. Department of Health, Education, and Welfare, Office of Vocational Rehabilitation. *Sixth annual workshop on guidance, training and placement—Proceedings, Part III: Rehabilitation of the mentally retarded and the emotionally disturbed.* Washington, D.C.: Author, April 1953.

U.S. GTP, 1954
U.S. Department of Health, Education, and Welfare, Office of Vocational Rehabilitation. *Seventh annual workshop on guidance, training and placement—Proceedings, Part I: Counseling and placement, eligibility.* Washington, D.C.: Author, June 1954.

U.S. GTP, 1954a
U.S. Department of Health, Education, and Welfare, Office of Vocational Rehabilitation. *Seventh annual workshop on guidance, training and placement—Proceedings, Part II: Casework supervision in vocational rehabilitation.* Washington, D.C.: Author, June 1954.

U.S. GTP, 1954b
U.S. Department of Health, Education, and Welfare, Office of Vocational Rehabilitation. *Seventh annual workshop on guidance, training and placement—Proceedings, Part III: Vocational rehabilitation and public assistance: Cooperative programs.* Washington, D.C.: Author, June 1954.

U.S. GTP, 1955
U.S. Department of Health, Education, and Welfare, Office of Vocational Rehabilitation. *Eighth annual workshop on guidance, training and placement—Proceedings, Part I: Rehabilitation counselor training.* Washington, D.C.: Author, June 1955.

U.S. GTP, 1955a
U.S. Department of Health, Education, and Welfare, Office of Vocational Rehabilitation. *Eighth*

annual workshop on guidance, training and placement—*Proceedings, Part I: Manual of rehabilitation case materials useful in the orientation of new counselors.* Washington, D.C.: Author, June 1955.

U.S. GTP, 1955b
U.S. Department of Health, Education, and Welfare, Office of Vocational Rehabilitation. *Eighth annual workshop on guidance, training and placement—Proceedings, Part II: Counseling and placement eligibility.* Washington, D.C.: Author, June 1955.

U.S. GTP, 1956
U.S. Department of Health, Education, and Welfare, Office of Vocational Rehabilitation. *Ninth annual workshop on guidance, training and placement—Proceedings, Part I: Counselor services, eligibility, business enterprises.* Washington, D.C.: Author, June 1956.

U.S. GTP, 1956a
U.S. Department of Health, Education, and Welfare, Office of Vocational Rehabilitation. *Ninth annual workshop on guidance, training and placement—Proceedings, Part II: Community resources, occupational information, placement.* Washington, D.C.: Author, June 1956.

U.S. GTP, 1957
U.S. Department of Health, Education, and Welfare, Office of Vocational Rehabilitation. *Tenth annual workshop on guidance, training and placement—Proceedings, Part I: Utilization of rehabilitation facilities.* Washington, D.C.: Author, April 1957.

U.S. GTP, 1957a
U.S. Department of Health, Education, and Welfare, Office of Vocational Rehabilitation. *Tenth annual workshop on guidance, training and placement—Proceedings, Part II: Handbook on placement, small business enterprises.* Washington, D.C.: Author, April 1957.

U.S. GTP, 1958
U.S. Department of Health, Education, and Welfare, Office of Vocational Rehabilitation. *Eleventh annual workshop on guidance, training and placement—Proceedings, Part I: Supervisory training, counselor training, OASI referrals, business enterprises.* Washington, D.C.: Author, May 1958.

U.S. GTP, 1958a
U.S. Department of Health, Education, and Welfare, Office of Vocational Rehabilitation. *Eleventh annual workshop on guidance, training and placement—Proceedings, Part II: Rehabilitation facility relationships.* Washington, D.C.: Author, May 1958.

U.S. GTP, 1959
U.S. Department of Health, Education, and Welfare, Office of Vocational Rehabilitation. *Twelfth annual workshop on guidance, training and placement—Proceedings, Part I: Supervisory training, non-employed closures.* Washington, D.C.: Author, May 1959.

U.S. GTP, 1959a
U.S. Department of Health, Education, and Welfare, Office of Vocational Rehabilitation. *Twelfth annual workshop on guidance, training and placement—Proceedings, Part II: Rehabilitation of the older client (Evaluation, OASI referrals, business enterprises).* Washington, D.C.: Author, May 1959.

U.S. GTP, 1960
U.S. Department of Health, Education, and Welfare, Office of Vocational Rehabilitation. *Thirteenth annual workshop on guidance, training and placement—Proceedings, Part I: Group leadership, in-service training (supervisors, counselors, secretaries).* Washington, D.C.: Author, May 1960.

U.S. GTP, 1960a
U.S. Department of Health, Education, and Welfare, Office of Vocational Rehabilitation. *Thirteenth annual workshop on guidance, training and placement—Proceedings, Part II: The older client, OASI referrals, small business enterprises.* Washington, D.C.: Author, May 1960.

U.S. GTP, 1961
U.S. Department of Health, Education, and Welfare, Office of Vocational Rehabilitation. *Fourteenth annual workshop on guidance, training and placement—Proceedings, Part I: In-service training, professional publications.* Washington, D.C.: Author, May 1961.

U.S. GTP, 1961a
U.S. Department of Health, Education, and Welfare, Office of Vocational Rehabilitation. *Fourteenth annual workshop on guidance, training and placement—Proceedings, Part II: Operational research, OASI referrals, small business enterprises, Group leadership training.* Washington, D.C.: Author, May 1961.

U.S. GTP, 1962
U.S. Department of Health, Education, and Welfare, Vocational Rehabilitation Administration. *Fifteenth annual workshop on guidance, training and placement—Proceedings: In-service training, independent living, operational research, small business enterprises, group leadership.* Washington, D.C.: Author, May 1962.

INSTITUTE ON REHABILITATION SERVICES
(U.S., IRS) 1963–1973

U.S. IRS, 1963
U.S. Department of Health, Education, and Welfare, Vocational Rehabilitation Administration [1963]. *First institute on rehabilitation services; Training guides in motivation for vocational re-*

habilitation staff. Washington, D.C.: Author, May 1963.

U.S. IRS, 1963a

U.S. Department of Health, Education, and Welfare, Vocational Rehabilitation Administration [1963a]. *First annual institute on rehabilitation services, case recording in rehabilitation.* Washington, D.C.: Author, May 1963.

U.S. IRS, 1963–64

U.S. Department of Health, Education, and Welfare, Vocational Rehabilitation Administration. *First and second institute on rehabilitation services, medical consultation in vocational rehabilitation* (Edited by B. Thomason, University of Florida). Washington, D.C.: Author, May 1963 and 1964.

U.S. IRS, 1964

U.S. Department of Health, Education, and Welfare, Vocational Rehabilitation Administration. *Second institute on rehabilitation services: Training guides in motivation for vocational rehabilitation staff.* Washington, D.C.: Author, May 1964.

U.S. IRS, 1965

U.S. Department of Health, Education, and Welfare, Vocational Rehabilitation Administration. *Third institute on rehabilitation services: Training guides in case load management for vocational rehabilitation staff, final report, committee on case load management* (Edited by J. E. Muthard, University of Iowa). Washington, D.C.: Author, May 1965.

U.S. IRS, 1965a

U.S. Department of Health, Education, and Welfare, Vocational Rehabilitation Administration. *Third institute on rehabilitation services: Training guides in evaluation of vocational potential for vocational rehabilitation staff.* Washington, D.C.: Author, May 1965.

U.S. IRS, 1965b

U.S. Department of Health, Education, and Welfare. Vocational Rehabilitation Administration. *Third institute on rehabilitation services: Development and use of training materials and aids in vocational rehabilitation.* Washington, D.C.: Author, May 1965.

U.S. IRS, 1966

U.S. Department of Health, Education, and Welfare. Vocational Rehabilitation Administration. *Fourth institute on rehabilitation services: Guidelines for organization and operation of vocational evaluation units.* Washington, D.C.: Author, May 1966.

U.S. IRS, 1966a

U.S. Department of Health, Education, and Welfare, Vocational Rehabilitation Administration. *Fourth institute on rehabilitation services: Training methods in vocational rehabilitation.* Washington, D.C.: Author, May 1966.

U.S. IRS, 1967

U.S. Department of Health, Education, and Welfare, Social and Rehabilitation Service, Rehabilitation Services Administration. *Fifth institute on rehabilitation services: Rehabilitation of the public offender.* Washington, D.C.: Author, May 1967.

U.S. IRS, 1967a

U.S. Department of Health, Education, and Welfare, Social and Rehabilitation Service, Rehabilitation Services Administration. *Fifth institute on rehabilitation services: Public information service in rehabilitation.* Washington, D.C.: Author, May 1967.

U.S. IRS, 1968

U.S. Department of Health, Education, and Welfare, Social and Rehabilitation Service, Rehabilitation Services Administration. *Sixth institute on rehabilitation services: Rehabilitation of the alcoholic.* Washington, D.C.: Author, May 1968.

U.S. IRS, 1968a

U.S. Department of Health, Education, and Welfare, Social and Rehabilitation Service, Vocational Rehabilitation Administration. *Sixth institute on rehabilitation services: Use of support personnel in vocational rehabilitation.* Washington, D.C.: Author, May 1968.

U.S. IRS, 1968b

U.S. Department of Health, Education, and Welfare, Social and Rehabilitation Service, Vocational Rehabilitation Administration. *Sixth institute on rehabilitation services: Principles for developing cooperative programs in vocational rehabilitation.* Washington, D.C.: Author, May 1968.

U.S. IRS, 1969

U.S. Department of Health, Education, and Welfare, Social and Rehabilitation Service, Rehabilitation Services Administration. *Seventh institute on rehabilitation services: Recommended standards for closure of cases.* Washington, D.C.: Author, May 1969.

U.S. IRS, 1969a

U.S. Department of Health, Education, and Welfare, Social and Rehabilitation Service, Rehabilitation Services Administration. *Seventh institute on rehabilitation services: A guide to joint vocational rehabilitation and disability determination unit in-service training.* Washington, D.C.: Author, 1969.

U.S. IRS, 1969b

U.S. Department of Health, Education, and Welfare, Social and Rehabilitation Service, Rehabilitation Services Administration. Seventh institute on rehabilitation services: Rehabilitation of individuals with behavioral disorders. Washington, D.C.: Author, May 1969.

U.S. IRS, 1969c

U.S. Department of Health, Education, and Welfare, Social and Rehabilitation Service, Rehabilitation Services Administration. *Seventh institute on rehabilitation services; Expanding the joint use of evaluation facilities by disability determination units and vocational rehabilitation.* Washington, D.C.: Author, 1969.

U.S. IRS, 1970
U.S. Department of Health, Education, and Welfare, Social and Rehabilitation Service, Rehabilitation Services Administration. *Eighth institute on rehabilitation services: Vocational rehabilitation of the disabled disadvantaged in a rural setting.* Washington, D.C.: Author, May 1970.

U.S. IRS, 1970a
U.S. Department of Health, Education, and Welfare, Social and Rehabilitation Service, Rehabilitation Services Administration. *Eighth institute on rehabilitation services: Principles and practices for first-line supervisors in rehabilitation.* Washington, D.C.: Author, May 1970.

U.S. IRS, 1970b
U.S. Department of Health, Education, and Welfare, Social and Rehabilitation Service, Rehabilitation Services Administration. *Eighth institute on rehabilitation services: Guidelines for staff development.* Washington, D.C.: Author, May 1970.

U.S. IRS, 1971
U.S. Department of Health, Education, and Welfare. Social and Rehabilitation Service, Rehabilitation Services Administration. *Ninth institute on rehabilitation services: Placement and follow-up in the vocational rehabilitation process.* Washington, D.C.: Author, May 1971.

U.S. IRS, 1971a
U.S. Department of Health, Education, and Welfare, Social and Rehabilitation Service, Rehabilitation Services Administration. *Ninth institute on rehabilitation services: Selected approaches to expedite the delivery of vocational rehabilitation service.* Washington, D.C.: Author, May 1971.

U.S. IRS, 1971b
U.S. Department of Health, Education, and Welfare, Social and Rehabilitation Service, Rehabilitation Services Administration. *Ninth institute on rehabilitation services: Rehabilitation of the drug abuser.* Washington, D.C.: Author, May 1972.

U.S. IRS, 1972
U.S. Department of Health, Education, and Welfare, Social and Rehabilitation Service, Rehabilitation Services Administration. *Tenth institute on rehabilitation services: Program evaluation: A beginning statement.* Washington, D.C.: Author, 1972.

U.S. IRS, 1972a
U.S. Department of Health, Education, and Welfare, Social and Rehabilitation Service, Rehabilitation Services Administration. *Tenth institute on rehabilitation services: Vocational evaluation and work adjustment services in vocational rehabilitation.* Washington, D.C.: Author, May 1972.

U.S. IRS, 1972b
U.S. Department of Health, Education, and Welfare, Social and Rehabilitation Service, Rehabilitation Services Administration. *Tenth Institute on rehabilitation services: Rehabilitation of disabled public assistance recipients, a training guide, self-training modules for public assistance-vocational rehabilitation teams* (Prepared by D. Brittain). Washington, D.C.: Author, 1972.

U.S. IRS, 1972c
U.S. Department of Health, Education, and Welfare, Social and Rehabilitation Service, Rehabilitation Services Administration. *Tenth institute on rehabilitation services: Rehabilitation of disabled public assistance recipients: A training resource.* Washington, D.C.: Author, 1972.

U.S. IRS, 1973
U.S. Department of Health, Education, and Welfare, Social and Rehabilitation Service, Rehabilitation Services Administration. *Eleventh institute on rehabilitation services: Services to the blind: A community concern.* Washington, D.C.: Author, May 1973.

U.S. IRS, 1973a
University of Arkansas, Rehabilitation Research and Training Center. *Eleventh institute on rehabilitation services: The rehabilitation of the deaf: A training guide.* Hot Springs, AR: Author, 1973.

U.S. IRS, 1973b
West Virginia University, Research and Training Center. *Eleventh institute on rehabilitation services: Rehabilitation of the severely disabled.* Institute, WV: Author, May 1973.

INSTITUTE ON REHABILITATION ISSUES (IRI), 1974–PRESENT

U.S. IRI, 1974
University of Wisconsin-Stout, Research and Training Center. *First institute on rehabilitation issues: Assessment of rehabilitation counselor performance.* Menomonie, WI: Author, April 1974.

U.S. IRI, 1974a
University of Arkansas, Arkansas Research and Training Center. *First institute on rehabilitation issues: Critical issues involved in rehabilitation of the severely handicapped.* Hot Springs, AR: Author, April 1974.

U.S. IRI, 1974b
West Virginia University, Research and Training Center. *First institute on rehabilitation issues: Measurement of outcomes.* Institute, WV: Author, April 1974.

U.S. IRI, 1975
University of Wisconsin-Stout, Research and

Training Center. *Second institute on rehabilitation issues: The delivery of rehabilitation services.* Menomonie, WI: Author, June 1975.

U.S. IRI, 1975a
University of Arkansas Research and Training Center. *Second institute on rehabilitation issues: Consumer involvement: Rehabilitation issues.* Hot Springs, AR: Author, June 1975.

U.S. IRI, 1975b
West Virginia University, Research and Training Center. *Second institute on rehabilitation issues: Placement of the severely handicapped.* Institute, WV: Author, June 1975.

U.S. IRI, 1976
University of Wisconsin-Stout, Research and Training Center. *Third institute on rehabilitation issues: Legal concerns of the rehabilitation counselor.* Menomonie, WI: Author, June 1976.

U.S. IRI, 1976a
University of Arkansas, Arkansas Research and Training Center. *Third institute on rehabilitation issues: Post-employment services in rehabilitation.* Hot Springs, AR: Author, June 1976.

U.S. IRI, 1976b
West Virginia University, Research and Training Center. *Third institute on rehabilitation issues: Affirmative action: Resource manual for vocational rehabilitation.* Institute, WV: Author, June 1976.

U.S. IRI, 1977
University of Wisconsin-Stout, Research and Training Center. *Fourth institute on rehabilitation issues: Rehabilitation facilities: A resource in the vocational rehabilitation of the severely handicapped.* Menomonie, WI: Author, June 1977.

U.S. IRI, 1977a
University of Arkansas, Arkansas Research and Training Center. *Fourth institute on rehabilitation issues: The rehabilitation of the severely handi-capped homebound.* Hot Springs, AR: Author, June 1977.

U.S. IRI, 1977b
West Virginia University, Research and Training Center. *Fourth institute on rehabilitation issues: Utilization of publications of the institute on rehabilitation issues.* Institute, WV: Author, June 1977.

U.S. IRI, 1978
University of Wisconsin-Stout, Research and Training Center. *Fifth institute on rehabilitation issues: Similar benefits.* Menomonie, WI: Author, May 1978.

U.S. IRI, 1978a
University of Arkansas, Arkansas Research and Training Center. *Fifth institute on rehabilitation issues: The role of vocational rehabilitation in independent living.* Hot springs, AR: Author, May 1978.

U.S. IRI, 1978b
West Virginia University, Research and Training Center. *Fifth institute on rehabilitation issues: Vocational rehabilitation of persons with mental disorders.* Dunbar, WV: Author, May 1978.

U.S. IRI, 1979
University of Wisconsin-Stout, Research and Training Center. *Sixth institute on rehabilitation issues: Engineering for rehabilitation—A counselor's guide.* Menomonie, WI: Author, 1979.

U.S. IRI, 1979a
University of Arkansas, Arkansas Research and Training Center. *Sixth institute on rehabilitation issues: Adjustment services for the severely handicapped.* Hot Springs, AR: Author, 1979.

U.S. IRI, 1979b
West Virginia University, Research and Training Center. *Sixth institute on rehabilitation issues: VR and the community or the adventures of Rip Van Rehab: A novel approach.* Dunbar, WV: Author, 1979.

U.S. Veterans Bureau. General Order no. 150-a. Washington, D.C.: Author, November 15, 1924.

U.S. White House Conference on Handicapped Individuals. *Special concerns: State White House Conference workbook.* Washington, D.C.: U.S. Department of Health, Education, and Welfare, Office of Human Development, n.d.

U.S. White House Conference on Handicapped Individuals. *Educational concerns: State White House Conference workbook.* Washington, D.C.: U.S. Department of Health, Education, and Welfare, Office of Human Development, November 1976.

Upham, E. G. Vocational re-education: Selective placement of the handicapped. *The Vocational Summary*, 1919, *2*(2), 35–37.

Urban Institute. *Executive summary of the comprehensive needs study of individuals with the most severe handicaps.* Washington, D.C.: U.S. Department of Health, Education, and Welfare, June 10, 1975.

Urban Institute. *Report of the comprehensive service needs study.* Washington, D.C.: U.S. Department of Health, Education, and Welfare, Office of Human Development, Rehabilitation Services Administration, June 23, 1975a.

Usdane, W. M. The placement process in the rehabilitation of the severely handicapped. *Rehabilitation Literature*, 1976, *37*(6), 162–167.

Vander Kolk, C. J. Counselor stress in relation to disabled and minority clients. *Rehabilitation Counseling Bulletin*, 1977, *20*, 267–274.

Vergason, G. Accountability in special education. *Exceptional Children*, 1973, *39*, 367–373.

VEWAA, *see* Vocational Evaluation and Work Adjustment Association.

Viscardi, H. *A man's stature*. New York: John Day Co., 1952.

Vocational Evaluation and Work Adjustment Association. Vocational Evaluation Project Final Report. Menomonie: University of Wisconsin-Stout, Materials Development Center, 1975. (Reprinted from reports of seven "VEWAA Task Forces" from special issues of *Vocational Evaluation and Work Adjustment Bulletin*, Vol. 8, July, August, and September 1975.)

Vriend, J., & Dyer, W. W. Counseling the reluctant client. *Journal of Psychology*, 1973, *20*(3), 240–246.

Wainwright, C. O., & Couch, R. Work adjustment: Potential and practice. *Journal of Rehabilitation*, 1978, *44*(1), 39–42.

Walker, R. A. *Evaluation*. Minneapolis: Minneapolis Rehabilitation Center, 1966.

Walker, R. A. *Job seeking skills project*. Minneapolis: Minneapolis Rehabilitation Center, 1968.

Walls, R. T., & Moriarty, J. B. The caseload profile: An alternative to weighted closure. *Rehabilitation Literature*, 1977, *38*, 285–291.

Wan, T. H. Correlates and consequences of severe disabilities. *Journal of Occupational Medicine*, 1974, *16*(4), 234–244.

Watson, J. B. *Behaviorism*. New York: Norton, 1930.

Webster's New Collegiate Dictionary. Springfield, MA: G. & C. Merriam, 1976.

Webster's Third New International Dictionary of the English Language (unabridged). Springfield, MA: G. & C. Merriam, 1976.

Wehman, P. Behavioral self-control with the mentally retarded. *Journal of Applied Rehabilitation Counseling*, 1975, *6*(1), 27–34.

Wehman, P. *Helping the mentally retarded acquire play skills*. Springfield, IL: Charles C Thomas, 1977.

Weiner, I. B. (Ed.). *Clinical methods in psychology*. New York: John Wiley, 1976.

Weinstein, E. A., & Kahn, R. L. *The denial of illness*. Springfield, IL: Charles C Thomas, 1955.

Weiss, H. Work adjustment. In R. E. Hardy & J. G. Cull (Eds.), *Services of the rehabilitation facility*. Springfield, IL: Charles C Thomas, 1975.

Westman, W. C. A solid front: Unity, timing, goal oriented counseling break drug addiction cycle. *Journal of Rehabilitation*, 1974, *40*(3), 15–17.

W. E. Upjohn Institute for Employment Research. *Work in America*. Cambridge: M.I.T. Press, 1973.

White, B., Goldston, L., Leeder, B., Soloff, A. *Job placement and job development*. Chicago: Jewish Vocational Service, 1976.

Whitehouse, F. A. Rehabilitation as a dimension of human welfare. Part II. *Journal of Rehabilitation*, September-October, 1961, pp. 19–49.

Whitehouse, F. A. Some professional concepts. In D. Malikin & H. Rusalem (Eds.), *Vocational rehabilitation of the disabled: An overview*. New York: New York University Press, 1969.

Whitehouse, F. A. Some characteristics of comprehensive rehabilitation teamwork. In H. Rusalem & D. Malikin (Eds.), *Contemporary vocational rehabilitation*. New York: New York University Press, 1976.

Whitten, E. B. The voice of dissent: Eligibility and feasibility. *Journal of Rehabilitation*, 1965, *31*(4), 28–29.

Whitten, E. B. Matters for concern. *Journal of Rehabilitation*, 1965a, *31*(2), 2.

Whitten, E. B. The challenge of PL 89-333. *Journal of Rehabilitation*, 1966, *32*(1), 2.

Whitten, E. B. Disadvantaged individuals and rehabilitation. *Journal of Rehabilitation*, 1969, *35*(1), 2.

Whitten, E. B. Handicapped people and the administration. *Journal of Rehabilitation*, 1971, *37*(1), 2.

Whitten, E. B. Disability and physical handicap: Vocational rehabilitation. In R. Morris (Ed.), *Encyclopedia of social work* (Vol. 1). New York: National Association of Social Workers, 1971a.

Whitten, E. B. Rehabilitation in 1973: A reassessment. *Journal of Rehabilitation*, 1973, *39*(3); 2, 43.

Whitten, E. B. A time for decision: Rehabilitation at the crossroads. *Journal of Rehabilitation*, 1973a, *39*(5), 2.

Whitten, E. B. The Rehabilitation Act of 1973 and the severely disabled. *Journal of Rehabilitation*, 1974, *40*(4); 2, 39–40.

Wicas, E. A., & Carluccio, L. Attitudes of counselors toward three handicapped client groups. *Rehabilitation Counseling Bulletin*, 1971, *15*(1), 25–34.

Wilkinson, M. W. Rehabilitation counseling: In critical condition. *Journal of Applied Rehabilitation Counseling*, 1977, *8*(1), 15–21.

Williams, J. C. Some of the most commonly held objections by management to the employment of the handicapped. *Placement institute for vocational rehabilitation counselors and supervisors*. East Lansing: Michigan State University, Kellogg Center, February 1965.

Williams, K. I. Social service exchanges. In R. Morris (Ed.), *Encyclopedia of Social Work* (Vol. 2). New York: National Association of Social Workers, 1971.

Williamson, E. G. *Counseling adolescents*. New York: McGraw-Hill, 1950.

Williamson, E. G. *Vocational counseling: Some historical, philosophical and theoretical perspectives*. New York: McGraw-Hill, 1965.

Williamson, E. G. Vocational counseling: Trait and factor theory. In B. Stefflre & W. H. Grant (Eds.), *Theories of counseling* (2nd ed.). New York: McGraw-Hill, 1973.

Wilson, J., & Litvin, M. *Medicaid: An overview with implications for the developmentally disabled.* Eugene: University of Oregon, Rehabilitation Research and Training Center in Mental Retardation, January 1976.

Wilson, M. *Job analysis for human resource management: A review of selected research and development.* Washington, D.C.: Manpower Management Institute, 1974.

Wolfe, J. Disability is no handicap for DuPont. *The Alliance Review*, Winter 1973–74.

Wolfensberger, W. *Citizen advocacy for the handicapped, impaired and disadvantaged: An overview* (Publication No. (OS) 72–42). Washington, D.C.: U.S. Department of Health, Education, and Welfare, 1972.

Wolpe, J. *Psychotherapy by reciprocal inhibition.* Stanford: Stanford University Press, 1958.

Wolpe, J. *The practice of behavior therapy.* New York: Pergamon Press, 1969.

World Health Organization. *Education and treatment in human sexuality: The training of health professionals* (Technical Report Series No. 572). Geneva: Author, 1975.

World Health Organization. Disability prevention and rehabilitation. *Rehabilitation World*, 1977, *3*(3), 13–22.

Wright, *see* Wright, G.N., unless otherwise indicated.

Wright, B. A. (Ed.). *Psychology and rehabilitation.* Washington, D.C.: American Psychological Association, 1959.

Wright, B. A. *Physical disability—A psychological approach.* New York: Harper & Row, 1960.

Wright, B. A. The question stands: Should a person be realistic? *Rehabilitation Counseling Bulletin*, 1968, *11*(4), 291–296.

Wright, G. N. Wanted—More referrals from high schools. *Journal of Rehabilitation*, 1959, *25*(1), 22–23.

Wright, G. N. *A collection of pamphlets: Horizon special issue.* Chicago: National Epilepsy League, 1960.

Wright, G. N. A report on the epilepsy problems—Article of the month. *Rehabilitation Literature*, 1961, *22*(7), 198–205.

Wright, G. N. Progress report on epilepsy. *Journal of Rehabilitation*, 1965, *31*(6), 17–19.

Wright, G. N. Israel first in counselor training abroad. *Rehabilitation Record*, 1969, *10*(1), 38–40.

Wright, G. N. (Ed.). *Documents pertaining to the proposed Israeli rehabilitation training and research center.* Madison: University of Wisconsin, Regional Rehabilitation Research Institute, 1969a.

Wright, G. N. New needs for professional educa-tion and research in rehabilitation in the world. *Sogo*, 1973, *1*(6), 67–76.

Wright, G. N. (Ed.). *Epilepsy rehabilitation.* Boston: Little, Brown, 1975.

Wright, G. N. (Ed.). *Wisconsin studies in vocational rehabilitation: Series 3, monographs XVII–XXIV.* Madison: University of Wisconsin, Regional Rehabilitation Research Institute, 1976.

Wright, G. N. Epilepsy and the job. *International Journal of Occupational Health and Safety*, 1976a, *45*(1–2), 48–50.

Wright, G. N. *Government support for university education and research in vocational rehabilitation.* A presentation to the Fourth Plenary Session of the Second International Conference on Legislation Concerning the Disabled, Manila, Philippines, January 18, 1978.

Wright, G. N. *Total rehabilitation of severely developmentally disabled adults.* Madison: University of Wisconsin, Rehabilitation Research Institute, 1978a.

Wright, G. N., Berven, N., & Reagles, K. W. Employer ratings of graduates as program evaluation measures. *Rehabilitation Counseling Bulletin*, 1977, *20*(3), 175–184.

Wright, G. N., & Brolin, D. Implementing rehabilitation recommendations for the mentally retarded. *American Journal of Mental Deficiency*, 1971, *75*(5), 586–592.

Wright, G. N., & Butler, A. J. *Rehabilitation counselor functions: Annotated references.* Madison: University of Wisconsin, Regional Rehabilitation Research Institute, 1968.

Wright, G. N., & Butler, A. J. *Wisconsin studies in vocational rehabilitation: Series 1, monographs II-X.* Madison: University of Wisconsin, Regional Rehabilitation Research Institute, 1968a.

Wright, G. N., Butler, A. J., & Aldridge, M. J. *Rehabilitation Information Series.* Madison: University of Wisconsin, Regional Rehabilitation Research Institute, 1968.

Wright, G. N., & Fraser, R. T. *Task analysis for the evaluation, preparation, classification and utilization of rehabilitation counselor-track personnel.* Madison: University of Wisconsin, Regional Rehabilitation Research Institute, 1975.

Wright, G. N., & Fraser, R. T. *Improving manpower utilization: The "rehabilitation task performance scale."* Madison: University of Wisconsin, Rehabilitation Research Institute, 1976.

Wright, G. N., & Fraser, R. T. Improving rehabilitation personnel management: A task performance evaluation scale. *Journal of Rehabilitation*, 1977, *43*(3), 22–24.

Wright, G. N., Gibbs, F. A., & Linde, S. M. (Eds.). *Total rehabilitation of epileptics: Gateway to employment.* Washington, D.C.: U.S. Government Printing Office, 1962.

Wright, G. N., & Katz, S. Rehabilitation counselor psychologists join the rehabilitation team. *Annual of Israel National Society for Rehabilitation of the Disabled*, 1969, 6.

Wright, G. N., & Reagles, K. W. *The economic impact of an expanded program of vocational rehabilitation*. Madison: University of Wisconsin, Regional Rehabilitation Research Institute, 1971.

Wright, G. N., & Reagles, K. W. RCE—Duly accredited? *Journal of Rehabilitation*, 1973, 39(6), 33–35.

Wright, G. N., & Reagles, K. W. (Eds.). *Wisconsin studies in vocational rehabilitation: Series 2, monographs XI–XVI*. Madison: University of Wisconsin, Regional Rehabilitation Research Institute, 1973a.

Wright, G. N., Reagles, K. W., & Butler, A. J. *The Wood County project: An expanded program of vocational rehabilitation*. Madison: University of Wisconsin, Regional Rehabilitation Research Institute, 1969.

Wright, G. N., Reagles, K. W., & Butler, A. J. *An expanded program of vocational rehabilitation: Methodology and description of client population*. Madison: University of Wisconsin, Regional Rehabilitation Research Institute, 1970.

Wright, G. N., Reagles, K. W., & Lewin, I. *A device for systematic planning and evaluation of rehabilitation counselor education*. Madison: University of Wisconsin, Regional Rehabilitation Research Institute, 1970.

Wright, G. N., Reagles, K. W., & Scorzelli, J. F. Measuring the effectiveness and variations of rehabilitation counselor education programs. *Journal of Applied Rehabilitation Counseling*, 1973, 4(2), 76–87.

Wright, G. N., Reagles, K. W., & Thomas, K. R. The Wood County project: An expanded program for the vocationally handicapped. *International Labour Review*, 1971, 104(1–2), 23–25.

Wright, G. N., Reagles, K. W., & Thomas, K. R. Who are the tough rehabilitation cases? *American Archives of Rehabilitation Therapy*, 1973, 21(1), 2–5.

Wright, G. N., & Remmers, H. H. *Handicap problems inventory*. Lafayette, IN: Purdue University Research Foundation, 1960.

Wright, G. N., Smits, S. J., Butler, A. J., & Thoreson, R. W. *A survey of counselor perceptions*. Madison: University of Wisconsin, Regional Rehabilitation Research Institute, 1968.

Wright, G. N., & Trotter, A. B. *Rehabilitation research*. Madison: University of Wisconsin, Regional Rehabilitation Institute, 1968.

Wright, K. C. *Ethics in rehabilitation: Thoughts about values and professional behavior in rehabilitation*. Richmond: Virginia Commonwealth University, 1977.

Wuenschel, R. J., & Brady, J. E. Principles and techniques of placement. *Journal of Rehabilitation*, 1959, 25(2), 16–18.

Yalom, I. D. *The theory and practice of group psychotherapy* (2nd ed.). New York: Basic Books, 1975.

Young, E. B. (Ed.). *Vocational education for handicapped persons: Handbook for program implementation*. Washington, D.C.: U.S. Department of Health, Education, and Welfare, Office of Education, August 1969.

Yuker, H. E., Block, J. R., & Campbell, W. J. *A scale to measure attitudes to disabled persons*. Albertson, NY: Human Resources Foundation, 1960.

Yuker, H. E., Block, J. R., & Young, J. H. *The measurement of attitudes toward disabled persons*. Albertson, NY: Human Resources Center, 1970.

Zaccaria, J. *Theories of occupational choice and vocational development*. Boston: Houghton Mifflin, 1970.

Zadny, J. J., & James, L. F. *Another view on placement: State of the art 1976* (Portland State University Studies in Placement and Job Development for the Handicapped, Studies in Placement Monograph No. 1). Portland, OR: Portland State University, School of Social Work, Regional Rehabilitation Research Institute, 1976.

Zauha, H. Citizen advocacy—Present status and implementation in Nebraska. In C. K. Sigelman (Ed.), *Protective services and citizen advocacy*. Lubbock: Texas Tech University, 1974.

Zimmerman, M. E. Occupational therapy in the ADL program. In H. S. Willard & C. S. Spackman (Eds.), *Occupational therapy* (4th ed.). Philadelphia: Lippincott, 1971.

Index

Index